Textbook of Pharmacognosy and Phytochemistry

Textbook of Pharmacognosy and Phytochemistry

Second Edition

Biren N. Shah
M.Pharm., Ph.D.
Associate Professor
Department of Pharmacognosy and Phytochemistry
Vidyabharti Trust College of Pharmacy
Umrakh, Gujarat

A.K. Seth
M.Pharm., Ph.D.
Principal and Dean
Department of Pharmacy
Sumandeep Vidyapeeth University
Vadodara, Gujarat

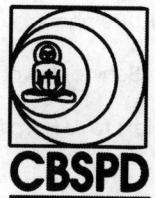

CBSPD

CBS Publishers & Distributors Pvt Ltd

New Delhi • Bengaluru • Chennai • Kochi • Kolkata • Lucknow • Mumbai
Hyderabad • Jharkhand • Nagpur • Patna • Pune • Uttarakhand

Textbook of Pharmacognosy and Phytochemistry
Second Edition

ISBN: 978-93-86217-73-8

Copyright © Authors and Publisher

CBS Edition: 2017
 Reprint: 2018, 2019, 2020, 2022, 2023, 2024, **2025**
First Edition: 2010
Second Edition: 2014

Published by **Satish Kumar Jain** and produced by **Varun Jain** for

CBS Publishers & Distributors Pvt Ltd
4819/XI Prahlad Street, 24 Ansari Road, Daryaganj, New Delhi 110 002, India.
Ph: 011-23266838, 23289259   Website: www.cbspd.com
                                     e-mail: delhi@cbspd.com

Corporate Office: 204 FIE, Industrial Area, Patparganj, Delhi 110 092
Ph: 011-4934 4934   Fax: 011-4934 4935
                                     e-mail: publishing@cbspd.com; publicity@cbspd.com

Branches

• **Bengaluru:** Seema House 2975, 17th Cross, KR Road, Banasankari 2nd Stage, Bengaluru 560 070, Karnataka, India
  Ph: +91-80-26771678/79   Fax: +91-80-26771680   e-mail: bangalore@cbspd.com
• **Chennai:** 18/8B, Subbaraya Street, Shenoy Nagar, Chennai 600 030, Tamil Nadu, India
  Ph: +91-044-42032115, 044-26681266   e-mail: chennai@cbspd.com
• **Kochi:** 42/1325, 1326, Power House Road, Opp KSEB, Power House, Ernakulum Kochi 682 018, Kerala, India
  Ph: +91-484-4059061-65,67   Fax: +91-484-4059065   e-mail: kochi@cbspd.com
• **Kolkata:** 147, Hind Ceramics Compound, 1st Floor, Nilgunj Road, Belghoria, Kolkata-700056, West Bengal, India
  Ph: +033-25633055, 033-25633056   e-mail: kolkata@cbspd.com
• **Lucknow:** Basement, Khushnuma Complex, 7 Meerabai Marg (Behind Jawahar Bhawan), Lucknow-226001, UP, India
  Ph: +0522-4000032   e-mail: tiwari.lucknow@cbspd.com
• **Mumbai:** PWD Shed, Gala no 25/26, Ramchandra Bhatt Marg, Next to JJ Hospital Gate no. 2, Opp. Union Bank of India, Noorbaug, Mumbai-400009, Maharashtra, India
  Ph: 022-66661880/89   e-mail: mumbai@cbspd.com

Representatives

• Gujarat	0-9879558667	• Hyderabad	0-9885175004	• Jharkhand	0-9811541605
• Nagpur	0-8692091830	• Patna	0-9334159340	• Pune	0-9664372571
• Uttarakhand	0-9716462459				

Printed at Chaman Enterprises, Daryaganj, Delhi, India

Preface to the Second Edition

Overwhelming appreciation, whole-hearted acceptance and qualified success of the first edition of *Textbook of Pharmacognosy and Phytochemistry* extended by the students specializing in Pharmacognosy and Phytochemistry, Biotechnology, Pharmaceutical Chemistry, and Chemistry of Natural Products, besides the numerous undergraduate students in bachelor of pharmacy programmes in the reputed pharmacy degree colleges not only in India but also abroad, are very encouraging.

Based on the commendable comments and constructive criticisms received from various academic colleagues across the country, the authors present this meticulously revised and duly expanded second edition. During revision the text has been thoroughly updated, the biosynthetic pathways adequately modified, and chemical structures and tabular contents more explicitly enumerated. Besides, critical definitions, important statements, terminologies and names of chemical constituents have been duly highlighted, facilitating quick location and ease of comprehension to the readers.

It is, however, pertinent to add here that certain extremely preliminary aspects to the related pharmacognostical characteristic features of 'Natural Plant Products', namely morphological structures, adulterants used in herbal products, habitats, method of cultivation, geographical distribution, etc., have been expunged from the text, to which the students invariably obtain sufficient exposure in the early stages of their systematic curriculum follow up.

This is an ultimate textbook in this subject and a boon for students of M.Pharm. (Pharmacognosy) as well as undergraduate students of Pharmacy. Besides the book is of utmost importance for every course comprising a study of plants and their medicinal use.

We are convinced and earnestly believe that this revised and expanded edition of *Textbook of Pharmacognosy and Phytochemistry* shall appropriately fulfill the need of substantial text materials.

—Dr Biren N. Shah
—Dr A.K. Seth

Preface to the First Edition

Textbook of Pharmacognosy and Phytochemistry is the outcome of numerous efforts of authors to assimilate the voluminous knowledge of traditional and modern pharmacognosy, which has long been a requirement of the curricula of various universities across the world.

In times of yore, pharmacognosy was considered as the study of drugs of natural origin. The American Society of Pharmacognosy derived it as the study of physical, chemical, biochemical and biological properties of drug, drug substances or potential drugs or drug substances of natural origin as well as the search for new drugs from natural sources. The world of pharmacognosy has continuously been enriching with multifaceted information considering various aspects of the natural drugs including history, alternative medicinal systems, classification, morphology, identification, cultivation, collection, production and utilization of drugs; trade and utilization of medicinal and aromatic plants and their contribution to national economy; adulteration of drugs of natural origin; evaluation of drugs by their physical, chemical and organoleptic properties; biological screening of herbal drugs; biosynthetic pathways of various phytopharmaceuticals; pharmacognostical study of crude drugs; extraction, isolation and purification of herbal drugs and modern plant biotechnology. Such an enormous information about the natural drug gives rise to a subject that is now recognized as modern pharmacognosy. It is a highly interdisciplinary science, encompassing a broad range of studies involving phytochemical study of medicinal plants and biologically active principles obtained from plants in addition to the traditional pharmacognostical aspects of natural drugs.

Considering all this comprehensive information of the subject, a textbook is premeditated to contribute substantially to the world of pharmacognosist. This modern book of pharmacognosy and phytochemistry emphasizes the biodiversity of plants and encompasses biosynthesis, extraction, isolation of compounds with TLC identification, bioactivity determination and synthesis of plant components of interest in addition to the traditional pharmacognosy comprising cultivation, collection, morphology, microscopy, taxonomy, chemical constituents and uses of drugs of natural origin. A special feature of the book is an additional advantage, that of inclusion of marketed products of the drugs described.

The book is designed to have 35 chapters divided into 10 parts (A to J). Each chapter is written with the aim to give a reasonable background to academician and researchers in the respective topic. A special miscellaneous chapter has been devoted to provide information about ayurvedic, marine medicinal plants, neutraceuticals and cosmeceuticals as well as herbs that have proved to be pesticides or allergens or producing colours, dyes and hallucinogenic effects.

The objective of the authors is fully achieved by systemic assemblage of the well-written chapters with neat and clean well-labelled diagrams wherever necessary.

The authors convey the deep sense of gratitude to their grandparents, parents, spouses and children for motivating them to provide a kind of book badly required collectively for undergraduate, postgraduate and researchers at one place. This is an added advantage the book will give to the readers of any walk of life.

Doubtless, authors are indebted to all who have supported in giving this present shape to the book.

Last but not the least, authors are immensely thankful to our publisher for their support, guidance and cooperation to publish this book.

Suggestions and criticisms will always be solicited by the authors to further improve the quality of the book in real sense.

—Dr Biren N. Shah
—Dr A.K. Seth

List of Reviewers

Dr D. Sathyanarayana
Professor
Department of Pharmacy
Annamalai University, Chidambaram
Tamil Nadu

Dr M.N. Qureshi
Principal
Government Aided AIT Institute of Pharmacy
Malegaon (Nasik), Maharashtra

Dr J. Ravindra Reddy
Professor
Department of Pharmacognosy
Raghavendra Institute of Pharmaceutical
Education and Research (RIPER)
Anantapur, Andhra Pradesh

Dr Gaurav Jain
Asst. Professor
Department of Pharmaceutics
Faculty of Pharmacy
Jamia Hamdard, New Delhi

Rohini Agrawal
Asst. Professor
Department of Pharmacology
United Institute of Pharmacy
Allahabad, Uttar Pradesh

Contents

Chapter 17   Drugs Containing Volatile Oils   298

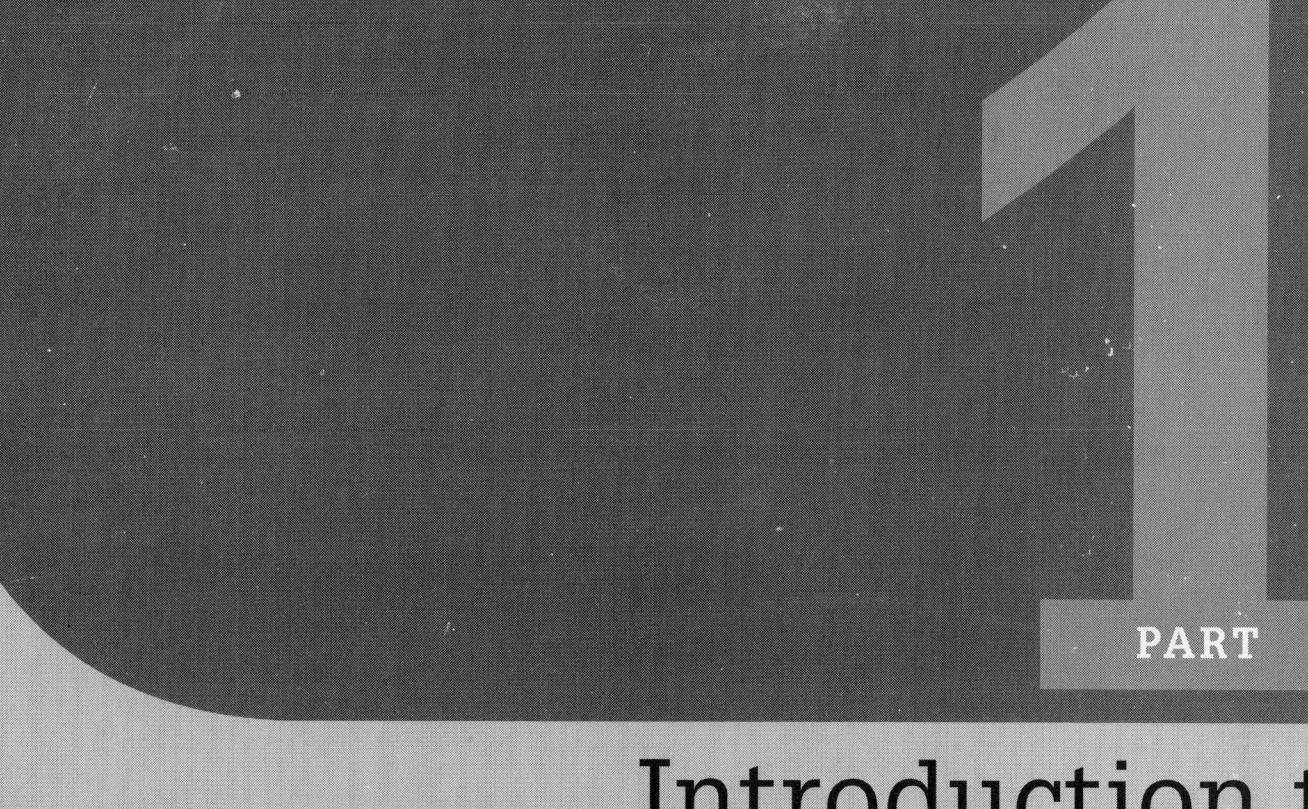

PART 1

Introduction to Pharmacognosy

Section Outline

OVERVIEW

This part provides the information regarding ancient history, evolution and scope of the subject; different traditional system of medicines prevailing in the world; and basic pharmacognostical classification of crude drugs along with the scheme of study for individual drugs.

CHAPTER 1

History, Definition and Scope of Pharmacognosy

CONTENTS

1.1. MEANING OF PHARMACOGNOSY

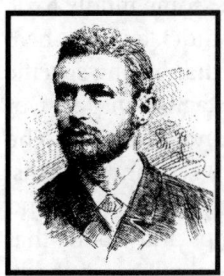

C. A. Seydler

Pharmacognosy, known initially as *materia medica*, may be defined as the study of crude drugs obtained from plants, animals and mineral kingdom and their constituents. There is a historical misinformation about who created the term *pharmacognosy*. According to some sources, it was C. A. Seydler, a medical student at Halle, Germany, in 1815; he wrote his doctoral thesis titled *Analectica Pharmacognostica*. However, recent historical research has found an earlier usage of this term. The physician J. A. Schmidt (Vienna) used that one in his *Lehrbuch der materia medica* in 1811, to describe the study of medicinal plants and their properties. The word *pharmacognosy* is derived from two Latin words *pharmakon*, 'a drug,' and *gignoso*, 'to acquire knowledge of.' It means 'knowledge or science of drugs'.

Crude drugs are plants or animals, or their parts which after collection are subjected only to drying or making them into transverse or longitudinal slices or peeling them in some cases. Most of the crude drugs used in medicine are obtained from plants, and only a small number comes from animal and mineral kingdoms. Drugs obtained from plants consist of entire plants, whereas senna leaves and pods, nux vomica seeds, ginger rhizome and cinchona bark are parts of plants. Though in a few cases, as in lemon and orange peels and in colchicum corm, drugs are used in fresh condition, and most of the drugs are dried after collections. Crude drugs may also be obtained by simple physical processes like drying or extraction with water. Therefore, aloe is the dried juice of leaves of *Aloe* species, opium is the dried latex from poppy capsules and black catechu is the dried aqueous extract from

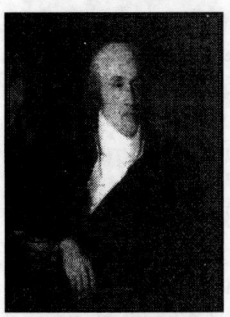

J. A. Schmidt

the wood of *Acacia catechu*. Plant exudates such as gums, resins and balsams, volatile oils and fixed oils are also considered as crude drugs.

Further drugs used by physicians and surgeons or pharmacists, directly or indirectly, like cotton, silk, jute and nylon in surgical dressing or kaolin; diatomite used in filtration of turbid liquid or gums; wax, gelatin, agar used as pharmaceutical auxiliaries of flavouring or sweetening agents or drugs used as vehicles or insecticides are used in pharmacognosy.

Drugs obtained from animals are entire animals, as cantharides; glandular products, like thyroid organ or extracts like liver extracts. Similarly, fish liver oils, musk, bees wax, certain hormones, enzymes and antitoxins are products obtained from animal sources.

Drugs are organized or unorganized. Organized drugs are direct parts of plants and consist of cellular tissues. Unorganized drugs, even though prepared from plants are not the direct parts of plants and are prepared by some intermediary physical processes, such as incision, drying or extraction with water and do not contain cellular tissue. Thus aloe, opium, catechu, gums, resins and other plant exudates are unorganized drugs.

Drugs from mineral sources are kaolin, chalk, diatomite and other bhasmas of Ayurveda.

1.2. ORIGIN OF PHARMACOGNOSY

Views on the beginning of life on planet Earth have forever remained controversial and an unending subject of debate. Nevertheless, we can say with certainty that the vegetable kingdom was already there when man made his appearance on Earth. As man began to acquire closure acquaintance with his environment, he began to know more about plants, as these were the only curative agents he had. As he progressed and evolved, he was not only able to sort on as to which plant served for eating and which did not, but he went beyond and began to associate curative characteristics with certain plants, classifying them as painkillers, febrifuge, antiphlogistics, soporific and so on. This must have involved no doubt, a good deal of trial and error, and possibly some deaths in the beginning also, but as it happened antidotes against poisons were also discovered. As we shall see later, drug substitutes were also forthcoming. All these states of affairs indicate that the origin of pharmacognosy, i.e. the study of natural curative agents points towards the accent of human beings on mother earth, and its historical account makes it clear that pharmacognosy in its totality is not the work of just one or two continental areas but the overall outcome of the steadfast work of many of the bygone civilizations like the Chinese, Egyptian, Indian, Persian, Babylonian, Assyrian and many more. Many of today's wonderful modern drugs find their roots in the medicines developed by the tribal traditions in the various parts of the world.

1.3. HISTORY OF PHARMACOGNOSY

In the early period, primitive man went in search of food and ate at random, plants or their parts like tubers, fruits, leaves, etc. As no harmful effects were observed he considered them as edible materials and used them as food. If he observed other effects by their eating they were considered inedible, and according to the actions he used them in treating symptoms or diseases. If it caused diarrhoea it was used as purgative, if vomiting it was used as memetic and if it was found poisonous and death was caused, he used it as arrow poison. The knowledge was empirical and was obtained by trial and error. He used drugs as such or as their infusions and decoctions. The results were passed on from one generation to the other, and new knowledge was added in the same way.

Ancient China

Chinese pharmacy, according to legend, stems from Shen Nung (about 2700 B.C.), emperor who sought out and investigated the medicinal value of several hundred herbs. He reputed to have tested many of them on himself, and to have written the first *Pen T-Sao*, or *Native Herbal*, recording 365 drugs. These were subdivided as follows: 120 emperor herbs of high, food grade quality which are nontoxic and can be taken in large quantities to maintain health over a long period of time, 120 minister herbs, some mildly toxic and some not, having stronger therapeutic action to heal diseases and finally 125 servant herbs that having specific action to treat disease and eliminate stagnation. Most of those in the last group, being toxic, are not intended to be used daily over a prolonged period of weeks and months. Shen Nung conceivably examined many herbs, barks and roots brought in from the fields, swamps and woods that are still recognized in pharmacy (podophyllum, rhubarb, ginseng, stramonium, cinnamon bark and ephedra).

Inscriptions on oracle bones from the Shang Dynasty (1766–1122 B.C.), discovered in Honan Province, have provided a record of illness, medicines and medical treatment. Furthermore, a number of medical treatises on silk banners and bamboo slips were excavated from the tomb number three at Ma-Huang-Tui in Changsha, Hunan Province. These were copied from books some time between the Chin and Han periods (300 B.C.–A.D. 3) and constitute the earliest medical treatises existing in China.

The most important clinical manual of traditional Chinese medicine is the *Shang Hang Lun* (*Treatise on the Treatment of Acute Diseases Caused by Cold*) written by Chang Chung-Ching (142–220). The fame and reputation of the Shang Han Lun as well as its companion book, *Chin Kuei Yao Lueh* (*Prescriptions from the Golden Chamber*), is the historical origin of the most important classical herbal formulas that have become the basis of Chinese and Japanese-Chinese herbalism (called 'Kampo').

With the interest in alchemy came the development of pharmaceutical science and the creation of a number of books including Tao Hong Jing's (456–536) compilation of the *Pen T'sao Jing Ji Zhu* (*Commentaries on the Herbal Classic*) based on the Shen Nong Pen T'sao Jing, in 492. In that book 730 herbs were described and classified in six categories: (1) stone (minerals), (2) grasses and trees, (3) insects and animals, (4) fruits and vegetables, (5) grains and (6) named but unused. During the Sui dynasty (589–618) the study of herbal medicine blossomed with the creation of specialized books on plants and herbal medicine. Some of these set forth the method for the gathering of herbs in the wild as well as their cultivation. Over 20 herbals were chronicled in the *Sui Shu JingJi Zhi* (*Bibliography of the History of Sui*). These include the books *Zhong Zhi Yue Fa* (*How to Cultivate Herbs*) and the *Ru Lin Cat Yue Fa* (*How to Collect Herbs in the Forest*).

From the Sung Dynasty (960–1276) the establishment of pharmaceutical system has been a standard practice throughout the country. Before the ingredients of Chinese medicine can be used to produce pharmaceuticals, they must undergo a preparation process, e.g. baking, simmering or roasting. The preparation differs according to the needs for the treatment of the disease. Preparation methods, production methods and technology have constantly been improved over time.

In 1552, during the later Ming Dynasty, Li Shi Zhen (1518–1593) began work on the monumental *Pen T'sao Kan Mu* (*Herbal with Commentary*). After 27 years and three revisions, the *Pen T'sao Kan Mu* was completed in 1578. The book lists 1892 drugs, 376 described for the first time with 1160 drawings. It also lists more than 11,000 prescriptions.

Ancient Egypt

The most complete medical documents existing are the *Ebers Papyrus* (1550 B.C.), a collection of 800 prescriptions, mentioning 700 drugs and the *Edwin Smith Papyrus* (1600 B.C.), which contains surgical instructions and formulas for cosmetics. The *Kahun Medical Papyrus* is the oldest—it comes from 1900 B.C. and deals with the health of women, including birthing instructions.

However, it is believed that the *Smith Papyrus* was copied by a scribe from an older document that may have dated back as far as 3000 B.C. Commonly used herbs included: senna, honey, thyme, juniper, cumin, (all for digestion); pomegranate root, henbane (for worms) as well as flax, oakgall, pine-

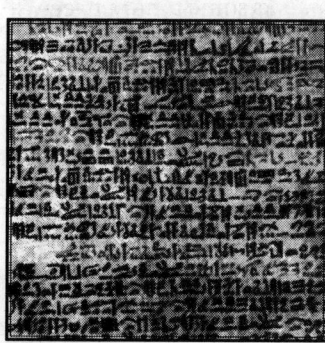

A fragment of Ebers Papyrus

tar, manna, bayberry, ammi, alkanet, aloe, caraway, cedar, coriander, cyperus, elderberry, fennel, garlic, wild lettuce, nasturtium, onion, peppermint, papyrus, poppy-plant, saffron, watermelon, wheat and zizyphus-lotus. Myrrh, turpentine and acacia gum were also used.

Ancient India

In India knowledge of medicinal plants is very old, and medicinal properties of plants are described in *Rigveda* and in *Atharvaveda* (3500–1500 B.C.) from which *Ayurveda* has developed. The basic medicinal texts in this world region— The Ayurvedic writings—can be divided in three main ones (*Charaka Samhita, Susruta Samhita, Astanga Hrdayam Samhita*) and three minor ones (*Sarngadhara Samhita, Bhava Prakasa Samhita, Madhava Nidanam Samhita*). Ayurveda is the term for the traditional medicine of ancient India. Ayur means life and veda means the study of which is the origin of the term. The oldest writing—*Charaka Samhita*—is believed to date back six to seven centuries before Christ. It is assumed to be the most important ancient authoritative writing on Ayurveda. The *Susruta Samhita* is thought to have arisen about the same time period as the *Charaka Samhita*, but slightly after it *Astanga Hrdayam* and the *Astanga Sangraha* have been dated about the same time and are thought to date after the *Charaka* and *Susruta Samhitas*. Most of mentioned medicines origin from plants and animals, e.g. ricinus, pepper, lilly, valerian, etc.

Ancient Greece and Rome

Greek scientists contributed much to the knowledge of natural history. Hippocrates (460–370 B.C.) is referred to as father of medicine and is remembered for his famous oath which is even now administered to doctors. Aristotle (384–322 B.C.), a student of Plato was a philosopher and is known for his writing on animal kingdom which is considered authoritative even in twentieth century. Theophrastus (370–287 B.C.), a student of Aristotle, wrote about plant kingdom. Dioscorides, a physician who lived in the first century A.D., described medicinal plants, some of which like belladonna, ergot, opium, colchicum are used even today. Pliny wrote 37 volumes of natural history and Galen (131–A.D. 200) devised methods of preparations of plant and animal drugs, known as 'galenicals' in his honour.

Pharmacy separated from medicine and materia medica, the science of material medicines, describing collection, preparation and compounding, emerged.

Even up to the beginning of twentieth century, pharmacognosy was more of a descriptive subject akin mainly to botanical science, and it consisted of identification of drugs both in entire and powdered conditions and concerned with their history, commerce, collection, preparation and storage.

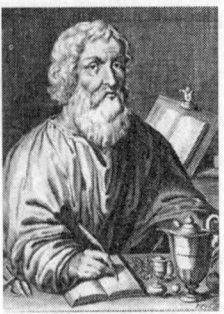
Hippocrates

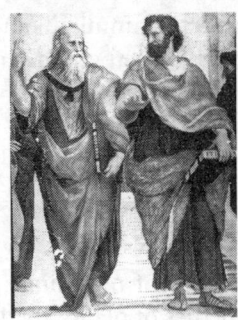
Aristotle And Plato

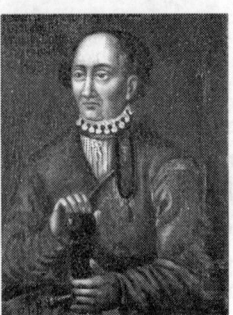
Theophrastus

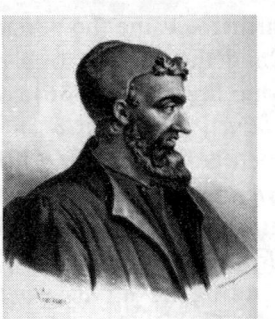
Galen

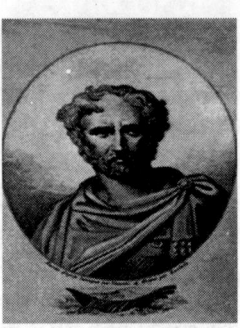
Pliny

The development of modern pharmacognosy took place later during the period 1934–1960 by simultaneous application of disciplines like organic chemistry, biochemistry, biosynthesis, pharmacology and modern methods and techniques of analytic chemistry, including paper, thin layer, and gas chromatography and spectophotometry.

The substances from the plants were isolated, their structures elucidated and pharmacological active constituents studied. The development was mainly due to the following four events:

1. Isolation of penicillin in 1928 by William Fleming and large-scale production in 1941 by Florey and Chain.
2. Isolation of reserpine from rauwolfia roots and confirming its hypotensive and tranquillizing properties.
3. Isolation of vinca alkaloids, especially vincristine and vinblasting. Vincristine was found useful in the treatment of leukaemia. These alkaloids also have anticancer properties.
4. Steroid hormones like progesterone were isolated by partial synthesis from diosgenin and other steroid saponins by Marker's method. Cortisone and hydrocortisone are obtained from progesterone by chemical and microbial reaction.

This period can also be termed antibiotic age, as besides penicillin, active antibiotics like streptomycin, chloramphenicol, tetracycline and several hundred antibiotics have been isolated and studied extensively.

Some of the important aspects of the natural products that led to the modern development of drugs and pharmaceuticals are as follows:

Isolation of phytochemicals

Strong acting substances such as glycosides of digitalis and scilla, alkaloids of hyoscyamus and belladonna, ergot, rauwolfia, morphine and other alkaloids of opium were isolated and their clinical uses studied.

Structure activity relationship

Tubocurarine and toxiferine from curare have muscle relaxant properties because of quaternary ammonium groups. The hypotensive and tranquillizing actions of reserpine are attributed to the trimethoxy benzoic acid moiety which is considered essential. Mescaline and psilocybin have psychoactive properties. Presence of a lactone ring is essential for the action of cardiac glycosides. Likewise anthraquinone glycosides cannot have their action without satisfying the positions at C3, C1, C8, C9 and C10.

Drugs obtained by partial synthesis of natural products

Oxytocic activity of methyl ergometrine is more than that of ergometrine. In ergotamine, by 9:10 hydrogenation, oxytocic activity is suppressed and spasmolytic activity increases. We have already referred to the preparation of steroid hormones from diosgenin by acetolysis and oxidation and further preparation of cortisone by microbial reactions.

Steroid hormones and their semisynthetic analogues represent a multimillion dollar industry in the United States.

Natural products as models for synthesis of new drugs

Morphine is the model of a large group of potent analgesics, cocaine for local anaesthetics, atropine for certain spasmolytics, dicoumarol for anticoagulants and salicin for salicylic acid derivatives. Without model substances from plants a large number of synthetics would have been missed.

Drugs of direct therapeutic uses

Among the natural constituents, which even now cannot be replaced, are important groups of antibiotics, steroids, ergot alkaloids and certain antitumour substances. Further, drugs as digitoxin, strophanthus glycosides, morphine, atropine and several others are known since long and have survived their later day synthetic analogues.

Biosynthetic pathways

Biosynthetic pathways are of primary and secondary metabolites. Some of the important pathways are Calvin's cycle of photosynthesis, shikimic acid pathway of aromatic compounds, acetate hypothesis for anthracene glycosides and isoprenoid hypothesis for terpenes and steroids via acetatemevalonic acid–isopentyl pyrophosphate and squalene.

Progress from 1960 onwards

During this period only a few active constituents mainly antibiotics, hormones and antitumour drugs were isolated or new possibilities for their production were found. From 6-amino penicillanic acid, which has very little antibiotic action of its own, important broad-spectrum semisynthetic penicillins like ampenicillin and amoxicillin were developed.

From ergocryptine, an alkaloid of ergot, bromocryptine has been synthesized. Bromocryptine is a prolactin inhibitor and also has activity in Parkinson's disease and in cancer. By applications of several disciplines, pharmacognosy from a descriptive subject has again developed into an integral and important disciplines of pharmaceutical sciences.

Technical products

Natural products, besides being used as drugs and therapeutic aids, are used in a number of other industries as beverages, condiments, spices, in confectioneries and as technical products.

The coffee beans and tea leaves besides being the source of caffeine are used as popular beverages. Ginger and wintergreen oil are used less pharmaceutically but are more used in preparation of soft drinks. Mustard seed and clove are used in spice and in condiment industry. Cinnamon oil and peppermint oil besides being used as carminatives are used as flavouring agents in candies and chewing gum. Colophony resin, turpentine oil, linseed oil, acacia, pectin and numerous other natural products are used widely in other industries and are called technical products.

Pharmaceuticals aids

Some of the natural products obtained from plants and animals are used as pharmaceutical aids. Thus gums like acacia and tragacanth are used as binding, suspending and emulsifying agents. Guar gum is used as a thickening agent and as a binder and a disintegrating agent in the manufacturing of tablets. Sterculia and tragacanth because of their swelling property are used as bulk laxative drugs. Mucilage-containing drugs like isabgol and linseed are used as demulcents or as soothing agents and as bulk laxatives. Starch is used as a disintegrating agent in the manufacture of tablets and because of its demulcent and absorbent properties it's used in dusting powders. Sodium alginate is used as an establishing, thickening, emulsifying deflocculating, gelling and filming agent. Carbohydrate-containing drugs like glucose, sucrose and honey are used as sweetening agents and as laxative by osmosis.

Agar, in addition to being used as a laxative by osmosis, is also used as an emulsifying agent and in culture media in microbiology. Saponin-containing drugs are used as detergents, emulsifying and frothing agents and as fire extinguishers. Tincture quillaia is used in preparation of coal tar emulsions. Saponins are toxic and their internal use requires great care, and in some countries their internal use as frothing agents is restricted. Glycyrrhiza is used as sweetening agent for masking the taste of bitter and salty preparations.

Fixed oils and fats are used as emollients and as ointment bases and vehicles for other drugs. Volatile oils are used as flavouring agents.

Gelatin is used in coating of pills and tablets and in preparation of suppositories, as culture media in microbiology and in preparation of artificial blood plasma. Animal fats like lard and suet are used as ointment bases. Beeswax is used as ointment base and thickening agent in ointments. Wool fat and wool alcohols are used as absorbable ointment bases.

Thus, from the above description it can be seen that many of the natural products have applications as pharmaceutical aids.

Discovery of new medicines from plants— nutraceutical use versus drug development

Little work was carried out by the pharmaceutical industry during 1950–1980s; however, during the 1980–1990s, massive growth has occurred. This has resulted in new developments in the area of combinatorial chemistry, new advances in the analysis and assaying of plant materials and a heightened awareness of the potential plant materials as drug leads by conservationists. New plant drug development programmes are traditionally undertaken by either random screening or an ethnobotanical approach, a method based on the historical medicinal/food use of the plant. One reason why there has been resurgence in this area is that conservationists especially in the United States have argued that by finding new drug leads from the rainforest, the value of the rainforests to society is proven, and that this would prevent these areas being cut down for unsustainable timber use. However, tropical forests have produced only 47 major pharmaceutical drugs of worldwide importance. It is estimated that a lot more, say about 300 potential drugs of major importance may need to be discovered. These new drugs would be worth $147 billion. It is thought that 125,000 flowering plant species are of pharmacological relevance in the tropical forests. It takes 50,000 to 100,000 screening tests to discover one profitable drug. Even in developed countries there is a huge potential for the development of nutraceuticals and pharmaceuticals from herbal materials. For example the UK herbal materia medica contains around 300 species, whereas the Chinese herbal materia medica contains around 7000 species. One can imagine what lies in store in the flora-rich India.

1.4. SCOPE OF PHARMACOGNOSY

Crude drugs of natural origin that is obtained from plants, animals and mineral sources and their active chemical constituents are the core subject matter of pharmacognosy. These are also used for the treatment of various diseases besides being used in cosmetic, textile and food industries. During the first half of the nineteenth century apothecaries stocked the crude drugs for the preparation of herbal tea mixtures, all kinds of tinctures, extracts and juices which in turn were employed in preparing medicinal drops, syrups, infusions, ointments and liniments.

The second half of the nineteenth century brought with it a number of important discoveries in the newly developing fields of chemistry and witnessed the rapid progress of this science. Medicinal plants became one of its major objects of interest and in time, phytochemists succeeded in isolating the pure active constituents. These active constituents replaced the crude drugs, with the development of semisynthetic and synthetic medicine; they became predominant and gradually pushed the herbal drugs, which had formerly been used, into the background. It was a belief that the medicinal plants are of no importance and can be replaced by man-made synthetic drugs, which in today's scenario is no longer tenable. The drug plants, which were rapidly falling into disuse a century ago, are regaining their rightful place in medicine. Today applied science of pharmacognosy has a far better knowledge of the active constituents and their prominent therapeutic activity on the human beings. Researchers are exploiting not only the classical plants but also related species all over the world that may contain similar types of constituents. Just like terrestrial germplasm, investigators had also diverted their attention to marine flora and fauna, and wonderful marine natural products and their activities have been studied. Genetic engineering and tissue culture biotechnology have already been successful for the production of genetically engineered molecules and biotransformed natural products, respectively.

Lastly, crude drugs and their products are of economical importance and profitable commercial products. When these were collected from wild sources, the amount collected could only be small, and the price commanded was exorbitantly high. All this has now changed. Many of the industrially important species which produced equally large economic profits are cultivated for large-scale crop production. Drug plants, standardized extracts and therapeutically active pure constituents have become a significant market commodity in the international trade. In the light of these glorious facts, scope of pharmacognosy seems to be enormous in the field of medicine, bulk drugs, food supplements, pharmaceutical necessities, pesticides, dyes, tissue culture biotechnology, engineering and so on.

Scope for doctoral graduates in pharmacognosy is going to increase in the coming years. The pharmacognosist would serve in various aspects as follows:

Academics: Teaching in colleges, universities, museums and botanical gardens.

Private industry: Pharmaceutical companies, consumer products testing laboratories and private commercial testing laboratories, the herbal product industries, the cosmetic and perfume industries, etc.

Government: Placement in federal agencies, such as the Drug Enforcement Agency, the Food and Drug Administration, the U.S. Department of Agriculture, Medicinal plant research laboratories, state agencies like forensic laboratories, environmental laboratories, etc.

Undoubtedly, the plant kingdom still holds large number of species with medicinal value which have yet to be discovered. A lot of plants were screened for their pharmacological values like hypoglycaemic, hepatoprotective, hypotensive, anti-inflammatory, antifertility, etc; pharmacognosists with a multidisciplinary background are able to make valuable contributions in the field of phytomedicines.

1.5. FUTURE OF PHARMACOGNOSY

Medicinal plants are of great value in the field of treatment and cure of disease. Over the years, scientific research has expanded our knowledge of the chemical effects and composition of the active constituents, which determine the medicinal properties of the plants. It has now been universally accepted fact that the plant drugs and remedies are far safer than that of synthetic medicines for curing the complex diseases like cancer and AIDS. Enormous number of alkaloids, glycosides and antibiotics have been isolated, identified and used as curative agents. The modern developments in the instrumental techniques of analysis and chromatographical methodologies have added numerous complex and rare natural products to the armoury of phytomedicine. To mention a few, artemisinin as antimalarial, taxol as anticancer, forskolin as antihypertensive, rutin as vitamin P and capillary permeability factor and piperine as bioavailability enhancer are the recent developments. Natural products have also been used as drug substitutes for the semisynthesis of many potent drugs. Ergotamine for dihydroergotamine in the treatment of migraine, podophyllotoxin for etoposide, a potent antineoplastic drug or solasodine and diosgenin that serve for the synthetic steroidal hormones are the first-line examples of the recent days.

In the Western world, as the people are becoming aware of the potency and side effects of synthetic drugs, there is an increasing interest in the plant-based remedies with a basic approach towards the nature. The future developments of pharmacognosy as well as herbal drug industry would be largely dependent upon the reliable methodologies for identification of marker compounds of the extracts and also upon the standardization and quality control of these extracts. Mother earth has given vast resources of medicinal flora and fauna both terrestrial and marine, and it largely depends upon the forthcoming generations of pharmacognosists and phytochemists to explore the wonder drug molecules from this unexploited wealth.

Little more needs to be said about the present-day importance of medicinal plants, for it will be apparent from the foregoing that the plant themselves either in the form of crude drugs or even more important, for the medicinally active materials isolated from them, have been, are and always will be an important aid to the physician in the treatment of disease.

1.6. PHARMACOGNOSTICAL SCHEME

To describe drugs in a systematic manner is known as pharmacognostical scheme, which includes the following headings:

Biological Source

This includes the biological names of plants or animals yielding the drug and family to which it belongs. Botanical name includes genus and species. Often some abbreviations are written after the botanical names, of the biologist responsible for the classification, for example, *Acacia arabica* Willd. Here Willd indicates the botanist responsible for the classification or nomenclature. According to the biennial theory, the botanical name of any plant or animal is always written in italic form, and the first letter of a genus always appears in a capital later.

Biological source also includes the family and the part of the drug used. For example, biological source of senna is, Senna consists of dried leaflets of *Cassia angustifolia*, belonging to family Leguminosae.

Geographical Source

It includes the areas of cultivation, collection and route of transport of a drug.

Cultivation, Collection and Preparation

These are important to mention as these are responsible for quality of a drug.

Morphological Characters

In case of organized drugs, the length, breadth, thickness, surface, colour, odour, taste, shape, etc., are covered under the heading morphological characters, whereas organoleptic properties (colour, odour, taste and surface) should be mentioned, if the drug is unorganized.

Microscopical Characters

This is one of the important aspects of pharmacognosy as it helps in establishing the correct identity of a drug. Under this heading all the detailed microscopical characters of a drug is described.

Chemical Constituents

The most important aspect which determines the intrinsic value of a drug to which it is used is generally described under this heading. It includes the chemical constituents present in the drug. These kinds of drugs are physiologically active.

Uses

It includes the pharmaceutical, pharmacological and biological activity of drugs or the diseases in which it is effective.

Substituents

The drug which is used during nonavailability of original drug is known as substituent. It has the same type of physiological active constituents; however, the percentage quantity of the drug available may be different.

Adulterants

With the knowledge of the diagnostic characters of drugs, the adulterants can be detected. One should have the critical knowledge of substances known to be potential adulterants. Most of the times the adulterants are completely devoid of physiologically active constituents, which leads in the deterioration of the quality. For example, mixing of buffalo milk with goat milk is substitution, whereas mixing of water in the milk is adulteration. In the first case, goat milk is substitute and in the second case water is adulterant.

Chemical Tests

The knowledge of chemical tests becomes more important in case of unorganized drugs whose morphology is not well defined.

Alternative Systems of Medicine

CONTENTS

2.1. INTRODUCTION

Pharmacognosy has been basically evolved as an applied science pertaining to the study of all types of drugs of natural origin. However, its subject matter is directed towards the modern allopathic medicine. During the course of developments, many civilizations have raised and perished but the systems of medicines developed by them in various parts of the world are still practised, and are also popular as the alternative systems of medicine. These are the alternative systems in the sense that modern allopathic system has been globally acclaimed as the principal system of medicine, and so all the other systems prevalent and practised in various parts of the world are supposed to be alternative systems. The philosophy and the basic principles of these so called alternative systems might differ significantly from each other, but the fact cannot be denied that these systems have served the humanity for the treatment and management of diseases and also for maintenance of good health. About 80% of the world population still rely and use the medicines of these traditional systems.

Traditional Chinese medicine in China, *Unani* system in Greece, *Ayurvedic* system in India, *Amachi* in Tibet or more recently *Homoeopathy* in Germany are these systems of medicine which were once practised only in the respective areas or subcontinents of the world, are now popularly practised all over the world. The World Health Organization (WHO) is already taking much interest in indigenous systems of medicine and coming forward to exploit the scientific validity of the medicines used since traditions. The revival of great interest in these age-old systems of health care carries much meaning in the present scenarios. The study of these alternative systems is necessary so as to grasp and receive the best out of it to rescue humanity from the clutches of disease. Modern allopathy has developed many sophisticated and costlier diagnostic methodologies which have made it quite exorbitant and beyond the abilities of common man. Many modern synthetic drugs may harm more than they help in curing the disease by its serious toxic effects. On the contrary, traditional medicines are much more preferred for being safe and without harmful effects and comparatively much cheaper than that of allopathic medicines. However, one fact must be accepted here that the yelling humanity lastly run towards the modern allopathic treatment, which has developed wonderful techniques of diagnosis and highly effective drugs to provide the best and effective treatment than any other system of medicine till date.

2.2. TRADITIONAL CHINESE MEDICINE SYSTEM

The use of herbs as medicine is mentioned in China and Japan. The burial that dates back to 168 B.C. consists of corpus of 11 medical works. The development in the field of medicine had took a drastic change by A.D. 25–220 but people were more confident than the earlier period to understand the nature and they believed that the health and the disease depended on the principles of natural order. The first herbal classic written in China was published in the Qin Dynasty (221–206 B.C.) called the Agriculture Emperors *Materia Medica*. The first plants discovered and used were usually for digestive system disorders (i.e. *Da Huang*), and slowly as more herbs were discovered the herbs became more useful for an increasing number of ailments, and eventually the herbal tonics were created.

Traditional Chinese medicine is based on the principle of *Yin* and *Yang* theory. *Yang* represents the force of light and *Yin* represents the forces of darkness. According to the yellow emperor, *Yin* and *Yang* is the foundation of the entire universe. It underlies everything in creation. It brings about the development of parenthood; it is the root and source of life and death; and it is found with the temples of the gods. In order to treat and cure diseases, one must search for their origins. Heaven was created by the concentration of *Yang* and the Earth by the concentration of Yin. *Yang* stands for peace and serenity; *Yin* stands for confusion and turmoil. *Yang* stands for destruction; *Yin* stands for conservation. *Yang* brings about disintegration; *Yin* gives shape to things. Water is an embodiment of *Yin* and fire is an embodiment of *Yang*. *Yang* creates the air, while *Yin* creates the senses, which belong to the physical body when the physical body dies; the spirit is restored to the air, its natural environment. The spirit receives its nourishment through the air, and the body receives its nourishment through the senses.

Nature has four seasons and five elements. To grant long life, these seasons and elements must store up the power of creation in cold, heat, dryness, moisture and wind. Man has five viscera in which these five climates are transformed into joy, anger, sympathy, grief and fear. The emotions of joy and anger are injurious to the spirit just as cold and heat are injurious to the body. Violent anger depletes *Yin*; violent joy depletes *Yang*. When rebellious emotions rise to Heaven, the pulse expires and leaves the body and when joy and anger are without moderation, then cold and heat exceed all measure, and life is no longer secure. *Yin* and *Yang* should be respected to an equal extent.

When *Yang* is the stronger, the body is hot, the pores are closed, and people begin to pant; they become boisterous and coarse and do not perspire. They become feverish, their mouths are dry and sore, their stomachs feel tight, and they die of constipation. When *Yang* is the stronger, people can endure winter but not summer. When *Yin* is stronger, the body is cold and covered with perspiration. People realize they are ill; they tremble and feel chilly. When they feel chilled, their spirits become rebellious. Their stomachs can no longer digest food and they die. When *Yin* is stronger, people can endure summer but not winter. Thus, *Yin* and *Yang* are alternate. Their ebbs and surges vary, and so does the character of the diseases. The treatment is to harmonize both. When one is filled with vigour and strength, *Yin* and *Yang* are in proper harmony.

Treatment

Every herb has its own properties which include its energy, its flavour, its movement and its related meridians to which it is connected to. The four types of energies are cold, cool, warm and hot. Usually cold or cool herbs will treat fever, thirst, sore throat and general heat diseases. Hot or warm herbs will treat cold sensation in the limbs, cold pain and general cold diseases. The five flavours of herbs are pungent, sour, sweet, salty and bitter. Pungent herbs are generally used to induce perspiration and promote circulation of both blood and *Qi*. Sour herbs exert three functions: constrict, obstruct and solidify. These herbs are good to stop perspiration, diarrhoea, seminal emission and leucorrhoea. Sweet herbs also exert three main functions: nourishing deficiency, harmonizing other herbs or reduce toxicity, relieve pain and slow the progression of acute diseases. Salty herbs soften hardness, lubricate intestines and drain downward. These herbs are used to treat hard stool with constipation or hard swellings as in diseases like goitre. Bitter herbs induce bowel movements; reduce fevers and hot sensations, dry dampness and clear heat. They can also nourish the kidneys and are used to treat damp diseases. After absorption, herbs can move in four different directions: upward towards the head, downward towards the lower extremities, inward towards the digestive organs or outward towards the superficial regions of the body. Upward-moving herbs are used for falling symptoms like prolapsed organs. Downward-moving herbs are used to push down up surging symptoms like coughing and vomiting. Outward-moving herbs are used to induce perspiration and treat superficial symptoms that are moving towards the interior of the body. Inward movements of herbs induce bowel movements and promote digestion. Each herb will have a corresponding meridian or meridians to which it will correspond to. For example, herbs that are active against respiratory tract disorders move to the lungs and can be used for asthma or cough.

2.3. INDIAN SYSTEMS OF MEDICINE

The WHO estimates that about 80% of the populations living in the developing countries rely exclusively on traditional medicine for their primary health care needs. India has an ancient heritage of traditional medicine. Indian traditional medicine is based on different systems including *Ayurveda*, *Siddha* and *Unani*. With the emerging interest in the world to adopt and study the traditional system and to exploit their potentials based on different health care systems, the evaluation of the rich heritage of the traditional medicine is essential.

Almost in all the traditional medicines, the medicinal plants play a crucial role in the traditional medicine. India has a rich heritage of traditional medicine and the traditional health care system have been flourishing for many centuries.

In India, the Ayurvedic system of medicine developed an extensive use of medicines from plants dating from at least 1000 B.C. Western medicine continues to show the influence of ancient practices. For example, cardiac glycosides from *Digitalis purpurea*, morphine from *Papaver somniferum*, reserpine from *Rauwolfia* species, and quinine from *Cinchona* species and artemisinin, an active antimalarial compound from *Artemisia annua*, etc., show the influence of traditional medicine in Western medicine.

Ayurveda—The Indian System of Medicine

Ayurvedic system of medicine is accepted as the oldest written medical system that is also supposed to be more effective in certain cases than modern therapies. The origin of Ayurveda has been lost in prehistoric antiquity, but their concepts were nurtured between 2500 and 500 B.C. in India.

Ayurveda is accepted to be the oldest medical system, which came into existence in about 900 B.C. The word Ayurveda means *Ayur* meaning life and *Veda* meaning science. Thus, Ayurveda literally means science of life. The Indian Hindu mythology states four Veda written by the Aryans: *Rigveda*, *Samveda*, *Yajurveda* and *Atharvaveda*. The Ayurveda is said to be an *Upaveda* (part) of *Atharvaveda*. *Charaka Samhita* (1900 B.C.) is the first recorded book with the concept of practice of Ayurveda. This describes 341 plants and plant products used in medicine. *Sushruta Samhita* (600 B.C.) was the next ayurvedic literature that has special emphasis on surgery. It described 395 medicinal plants, 57 drugs of animal origin, 4 minerals and metals as therapeutic agents.

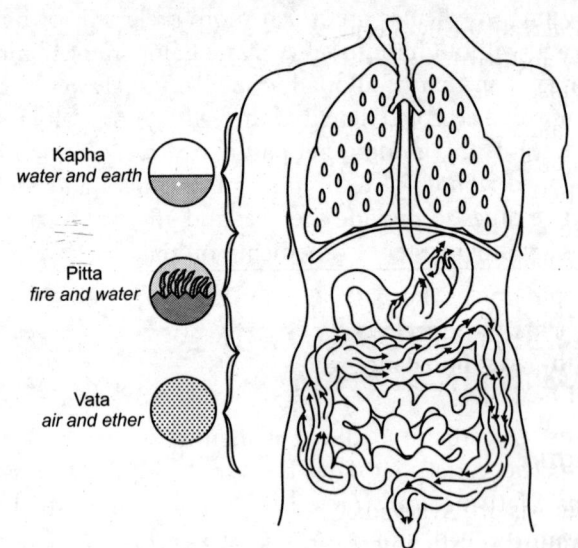

FIG. 2.1 The seats of three doshas: *Vata, Pitta* and *Kapha*

Basic principles of ayurveda

According to ancient Indian philosophy, the universe is composed of five basic elements or *pancha bhutas*: *prithvi* (earth), *jal* (water), *teja* (fire), *vayu* (air) and *akash* (space). Everything in the universe, including food and the bodies were derived from these *bhutas*. A fundamental harmony therefore exists between the macrocosm (the universe) and the microcosm (the individual). The *Pancha Bhuta* theory and the human body: The human body is in a state of continuous flux or dynamic equilibrium. The *pancha bhutas* are represented in the human body as the *doshas, dhatus* and *malas*.

There are three *doshas* in the body. They are *vata, pitta* and *kapha*. There are direct equivalents for these three *doshas*, known as *tridoshas*. However, the factors responsible for movement and sensation in a single cell/whole body are the representatives of *vata*; it explains the entire biological phenomena that are controlled by the functions of central and autonomous nervous system. The factors responsible for digestion, metabolism, tissue building, heat production, blood pigmentation, activities of the endocrine glands and energy are the representatives of *pitta*. The factors responsible for strengthening the stomach and the joints, providing firmness to the limbs, and refreshing the sense organs are the representatives of *kapha*. There are some special areas in the body in which each *dosha* predominates, namely, the chest for *kapha*, digestive organs for *pitta* and the large intestine for *vata*.

The *dhatus* are the body constituents and form the basic structure of the body; each one having its own functions. The *dhatus* are seven in number: *rasa* (food juices), *rakta* (haemoglobin portion of the blood), *mamsa* (muscle tissue), *medas* (fat tissue), *asthi* (bone tissue), *majja* (bone marrow) and *shukra* (semen).

Malas are the by-products of the *dhatus*, partly used by the body and partly excreted as waste matter after the process of digestion is over. These play a supporting role while they are in the body, and when they are eliminated, their supporting role is finished. The useful elements absorbed by the body are retained as *prasad* (useful matter), while those excreted are known as *malas* (waste matter). The chief *malas* are *mutra* (urine), *shakrit* (faeces) and *sweda* (perspiration). The *doshas*, *dhatus* and *malas* should be in a state of perfect equilibrium for the body to remain healthy. Any imbalance among these constituents results in ill health and disease.

Diagnosis

Diagnosis in Ayurveda implies a moment-to-moment monitoring of the interaction between order (health) and disorder (disease). The disease process is a reaction between the bodily *humours* (*doshas*) and tissues (*dhatus*) and is influenced by the environment.

The classical clinical examination in Ayurveda is called *ashta sthana pariksha* (eight-point diagnosis) and includes an assessment of the state of the *doshas* as well as various physical signs. The eight-point diagnoses are *nadi pariksha* (pulse diagnosis), *mutra pariksha* (urine examination), *vata/sparsha* (nervous system assessment), *Pitta/drik* (assessment of digestive fire and metabolic secretions), *kapha/akriti* (mucous and mucoid secretions assessment), *mala pariksha* (stool examination), *jihva pariksha* (tongue examination) and *shabda pariksha* (examination of body sounds).

Treatment

In Ayurveda, before starting the treatment, a person's constitutional type should be determined. Drugs are prescribed based on the patient's body type as well as on what disease or disturbance of the *doshas* they are suffering from. Everything that might affect the patient's health, including their activities, the time of the day, and the season should be taken into consideration. In other words, patients are looked at as individuals as well as in relation to their environment. Ayurvedic treatment attempts to establish a balance among the bodily humours of *vata*, *pitta* and *kapha*, as well as to improve digestion and elimination of *ama* (undigested food).

Ayurvedic therapy often begins with *shodhana* (cleansing) in which toxins, emotional or physical, are eliminated or neutralized. Once *shodhana* is completed, *shamana* (palliative treatment) is used to reduce the intensity of a disease and balance the disordered *doshas*. Finally, *rasayana* (rejuvenation therapy) is used to maintain health and reduce the negative effects of disease.

In Ayurveda, vegetable, animal, mineral substances or metals could be used for their healing effects. The metals mentioned as drugs were gold, silver, copper, lead, tin and iron. Along with these substances elements from the earth, like arsenic, antimony, sand and lime, were also used. Earlier, 600 medicinal plants were recorded in Ayurveda, and it has increased to more than 1200 medicinal plants.

Properties of herbs

Ayurvedic herbs are described and classified according to five major properties: *rasa* (taste), *guna* (physicochemical properties), *veerya* (potency), *vipaka* (postdigestive effect) and *prabhava* (unique effect of the drug). As the digestive process begins, the food or drug is acted upon by the *agnis* (various digestive juices) and enzymes.

Rasa is divided into six major types: *madhura* (sweet), *amla* (sour), *lavana* (salty), *katu* (pungent), *tikta* (bitter) and *kashaya* (astringent) (Table 2.1). Each taste is made up of a combination of two of the five basic elements (earth, water, fire, air and ether). Each taste has their own effects on the three bodily *doshas* (*vata*, *pitta* and *kapha*).

Table 2.1: Different types of Rasa

Rasa	Elements	Action
Madhura (sweet)	Earth + water	Increases *kapha*, decreases *pitta*
Amla (sour)	Earth + fire	Increases *kapha/pitta*, decreases *vata*
Lavana (salty)	Water + fire	Increases *kapha/pitta*, decreases *vata*
Katu (pungent)	Fire + air	Increases *vata/pitta*, decreases *kapha*
Tikta (bitter)	Air + ether	Increases *vata*, decreases *kapha/pitta*
Kashaya (astringent)	Air + earth	Increases *vata*, decreases *kapha/pitta*

Guna represents the physical aspects of a medicinal substance. There are five major classes of *guna*, and each class corresponds to one of the major elements (*mahabhutas*): unctuousness corresponds with water; heaviness with earth; keenness and sharpness with fire; dryness with air; and light with ether. *Gunas* are generally considered in pairs: cold/hot, wet/dry, soft/hard and stable/unstable, etc.

Veerya represents the active principle or potency of a drug. The two divisions are *sita veerya* (indicates *kapha varag*) and *ushna veerya* (indicates *pitta varag*); *vata* remains buffer.

Vipaka is the quality a substance takes on after it has been acted on by the body (after digestion). The three types of *vipaka* are *madhura* (increases *kapha*), sour (increases *pitta*) and *katu* (increases *vata*). The type of food responsible for *madhura*, sour and *katu* are carbohydrates, proteins and fats, respectively.

Prabhava is the activity or influence of a drug in the body. The drugs may have the same *rasa*, *guna*, *veerya* and *vipaka* but the *prabhava* may be different due to the chemical composition.

Branches of ayurveda

Ayurveda maintains that there is a definite relationship between illness and the metaphysical state of an individual. Its approach to medical treatment is to focus on the person rather than the disease.

Ayurveda has eight branches: *Kaya Chikitsa* (Medicine), *Salya Chikitsa* (Surgery), *Salakya Chikitsa* (ENT treatment), *Bala Chikitsa* (Paediatric treatment), *Jara Chikitsa* (treatment related to genetics), *Rasayana Chikitsa* (treatment with chemicals), *Vajikarana Chikitsa* (treatment with rejuvenation and aphrodisiacs), *Graham Chikitsa* (planetary effects) and *Visha Chikitsa* (toxicology).

Tibetan system of medicine which is the main stay of the majority of Tibetan people not only in India, but in neighbouring countries too was developed out of Ayurveda, or was influenced by it. Researches in traditional medicine have confirmed the efficacy of most of the natural substances used by the practitioners of Ayurveda. The principle, treatment and philosophy of Ayurveda are one of the best systems that fulfil the needs of human beings. It has so many good prescriptions without many side effects. Thus, Ayurveda formulates the holistic approach of treatment by subjecting the body as a whole giving least importance to *rogabalam*. This may be the reason for time-consuming treatment in Ayurveda, but the results last long.

2.4. SIDDHA SYSTEM OF MEDICINE

Siddha medicine is practised in Southern India. The origin of the Tamil language is attributed to the sage *Agasthya*, and the origin of *Siddha* medicine is also attributed to him. Before the Aryan occupation of the Sindh region and the Gangetic plain, there existed in the southern India, on the banks of the river Cauvery and Tamirapani, a civilization which was highly organized.

1. This civilization has a system of medicine to deal with problems of sanitation and treatment of diseases. This is the *Siddha* system of medicine. The therapeutics of *Siddha* medicines consists mainly of the use of metals and minerals whereas in the earlier Ayurveda.
2. There is mention of mercury, sulphur, copper, arsenic and gold used as therapeutic agents.

Principle of Siddha system of medicine

The universe consists of two essential entities: matter and energy. The *Siddhas* call them *Siva* (male) and *Shakti* (female, creation). Matter cannot exist without energy inherent in it and vice versa. The two coexist and are inseparable. They are the primordial elements (*bhutas*), and are not to be confused with modern chemistry. Their names are *munn* (solid), *neer* (fluid), *thee* (radiance), *vayu* (gas) and *aakasam* (ether). These five elements (*bhutas*) are present in every

substance, but in different proportions. Earth, water, fire, air and ether are manifestations of five elements.

The human being is made up of these five elements, in different combinations. The physiological function in the body is mediated by three substances (*dravyas*), which are made up of the five elements. They are *vatham*, *pitham* and *karpam*. In each and every cell of the body these three *doshas* coexist and function harmoniously. The tissues are called *dhatus*. *Vatham* is formed by *aakasam* and *vayu*. *Vatham* controls the nervous actions such as movement, sensation, etc. *Pitham* is formed by *thee* and controls the metabolic activity of the body, digestion, assimilation and warmth, etc. *Karpam* is formed by *munn* and *neer* and controls stability. When their equilibrium is upset, disease sets in.

Tridoshas according to Siddha medicine

The *tridoshas* are involved in all functions of the body, physical, mental and emotional.

1. *Vatham:*
   - Characteristic is dryness, lightness, coldness and motility.
   - Formed by *aakasam* and *vayu*, controls the nervous action that constitute movement, activity, sensation, etc. *Vatham* predominates in the bone.
   - *Vatham* predominates in first one-third of life when activities, growth, sharpness of function of sense are greater.

2. *Pitham:*
   - Heat—mover of the nervous force of the body.
   - Formed by *thee*, controls the metabolic activity of the body, digestion, warmth, lustre, intellect, assimilation, etc. *Pitham* predominates in the tissue blood.
   - *Pitham* predominates in the second one third of life.

3. *Karpam:*
   - Smoothness, firmness, viscidity, heaviness.
   - Formed by *munn* and *neer*, controls the stability of the body such as strength, potency, smooth working of joints. *Karpam* predominates in other tissues.
   - *Karpam* predominates in the last one-third of life. Diminishing activity of various organs and limbs.

The seven *dhatus* are as follows:

1. *Rasa* (lymph)
2. *Kurudhi* (blood)
3. *Tasai* (muscle)
4. *Kozhuppu* (adipose tissue)
5. *Elumbu* (bone)
6. *Majjai* (marrow)
7. *Sukkilam* and *artavam* (male and female hormones)

Method of treatment

The treatments for the imbalance of the *Tridoshas* are made up of the five elements. The drugs are made up of the five elements. By substituting a drug of the same constituents (*guna*), the equilibrium is restored. The correction of the imbalance is made by substituting the drug, which is predominately of the opposite nature. An example of *vatham* imbalance is cold, dry; thus the treatment will be oily and warmth. For inactivity of limbs, massage and activity are prescribed. If *pitham dosha* is increased, warmth is produced; to decrease *pitham*, sandalwood is administered, internally or externally because of its cold characteristics.

Five type of *vayu* are as follows:

1. *Prana*: Located in mouth and nostrils (inhaled); aids ingestion.
2. *Apana*: Located at anal extremity (expelled); elimination, expulsion.
3. *Samana*: Equalizer, aids digestion.
4. *Vyana*: Circulation of blood and nutrients.
5. *Udana*: Functions in upper respiratory passages.

Siddha pharmacy

Mercury: Mercury occupies a very high place in *Siddha* medicine. It is used as a catalytic agent in many of its medicines. When mercury is used, it is used in combination with sulphur. The addition of sulphur is to control the fluidity of mercury—this converts to mercuric sulphite which is insoluble in mineral acids.

Siddhas used five forms of mercury:

1. Mercury metal—*rasam*.
2. Red sulphide of mercury—*lingam*.
3. Mercury chloride—*veeram*.
4. Mercury subchloride (mercury chloride)—*pooram*.
5. Red oxide of mercury—*rasa chenduram*. Ordinary *rasa chenduram* (red oxide of mercury) is a poison, but when processed as *poorna chandrodayam* according to *Siddha* practice, it becomes ambrosia.

Classifications of *Siddha* medicine:

1. *Uppu (Lavanam)*: Drugs that dissolve in water and decrepitated when put into fire giving off vapours (water soluble inorganic compounds). There are 25 varieties and are called *kara-charam*, salts and alkalis.
2. *Pashanam*: Drugs that do not dissolve in water but give off vapour when put into fire (water insoluble inorganic compounds).
3. *Uparasam*: Drugs that do not dissolve in water (chemicals similar to *Pashanam* but differing in their actions) such as mica, magnetic iron, antimony, zinc sulphate, iron pyrites, ferrous sulphate.
4. *Loham*: Metals and minerals alloys (water insoluble, melt in fire, solidify on cooling) such as gold, silver copper, iron, tin and lead.
5. *Rasam*: Drugs that are soluble (sublime when put in fire, and changes into small crystals), such as mercury amalgams and compounds of mercury, arsenic.
6. *Gandhakam*: Sulphur insoluble in water, burns off when put into fire.
7. *Ratnas* and *uparatnas*: Thirteen varieties are described, such as coral, *lapis-lazuli*, pearls, diamonds, jade, emerald, ruby, sapphire, opal, *vaikrantham, rajavantham, spatikam harin mani*.

The common preparations of *Siddha* medicines are:

1. *Bhasma* (calcined metals and minerals)
2. *Churna* (powders)
3. *Kashaya* (decoctions)
4. *Lehya* (confections)
5. *Ghrita* (ghee preparations) and *taila* (oil preparations)
6. *Chunna* (metallic preparations which become alkaline)
7. *Mezhugu* (waxy preparations)
8. *Kattu* (preparation that are impervious to water and flames)

Sulphur: Calcined sulphur or red oxide of sulphur can be obtained by solidifying it first by the *Siddha* method of purification. In small doses, it conserves the body, and it is diaphoretic and alterative. Therapeutic ally is used as both external and internal remedy against skin diseases, rheumatic arthritis, asthma, jaundice and blood poisoning.

Arsenic: As per *Siddha kalpa*, purified and consolidated arsenic is effective against all fevers, asthma and anaemia.

Gold: It is alterative, nervine tonic, antidote to poison and a powerful sexual stimulant. Very little is absorbed in the system. Care is taken to see that calcinations of gold is freed from metallic state and lustre to ensure safe absorption in the system.

Thus, these drugs and metallic minerals can be screened for its antiviral, immune stimulant and immuno-modulator activity. As HIV negative people have taken *Kalpha* drugs for rejuvenation and long life, it is believed that if *Kayakalpa* therapy is thoroughly investigated using modern parameters, it might lead one to find whether these drugs could be used in preventative or curative benefits in AIDS or other diseases.

2.5. UNANI SYSTEM OF MEDICINE

Unani system of medicine is originated in Greece by the Greek philosopher, physician Hippocrates (460–377 B.C.), who freed medicine from the realm of superstition and magic, and gave it the status of science. The theoretical framework of *Unani* medicine is based on the teachings of Hippocrates. After him, a number of other Greek scholars followed the system considerably. Among them Galen

(131–212 A.D.) was the one to stabilize its foundation, on which Arab physicians like Raazes (850–925 A.D.) and Avicenna (980–1037 A.D.) constructed an imposing edifice. *Unani* medicine got its importance among the other systems of traditional medicine in Egypt, Syria, Iraq, Persia, India, China and other Middle East and Far East countries. In India, Arabs introduced *Unani* system of medicine, and soon it enriched in India. When Mongols ravaged Persian and central Asian cities, scholars and physicians of *Unani* medicine fled to India. The Delhi Sultans, the Khiljis, the Tughlaqs and the Mughal Emperors provided state patronage to the scholars and even enrolled some as state employees and court physicians. During the 13th and 17th century, *Unani* medicine was firmly rooted in India by Abu Bakr Bin Ali Usman Kasahani, Sadruddin Damashqui, Bahwabin Khwas Khan, Ali Geelani, Akabl Arzani and Mohammad Hoshim Alvi Khan.

Unani considers the human body to be made up of seven components. *Arkan* (elements), *mizaj* (temperaments), *aklath* (humours), *anza* (organs), *arawh* (spirits), *Quo* (faculties) and *afal* (functions), each of which has close relation to the state of health of an individual. A physician takes into account all these factors before diagnosing and prescribing treatment.

Unani medicine is based on the Greece philosophy. According to basic principles of *Unani*, the body is made up of the four basic elements, i.e. Earth, Air, Water and Fire, which have different temperaments, i.e. Cold, Hot, Wet and Dry. After mixing and interaction of four elements, a new compound having new temperament comes into existence, i.e. hot wet, hot dry, cold wet and cold dry. The body has the simple and compound organs, which got their nourishment through four humours, i.e. blood, phlegm, yellow bile and black bile. The humour also assigned temperament as blood is, i.e. hot and wet; phlegm is cold and hot, yellow bile is hot and dry and black bile is cold and dry. Health is a state of body in which there is equilibrium in the humours and functions of the body are normal in accordance to its own temperament and the environment.

When the equilibrium of the humours is disturbed and functions of the body are abnormal, in accordance to its own temperament and environment, that state is called disease. *Unani* medicine believes in promotion of health, prevention of diseases and cure. Health of human is based on the six essentials (*Asbabe Sitta Zaroorya*), if these are followed health is maintained; otherwise, there will be diseases.

Six essentials are atmospheric air, drinks and food, sleep and wakefulness, excretion and retention, physical activity and rest and mental activity and rest.

Diagnosis

Diseases are mainly diagnosed with the help of pulse (*nabz*), physical examination of the urine and stool. Also, patients are examined systematically to make the diagnosis easy as spot diagnosis with the help of simple, modern gadgets.

Treatment

Diseases are treated in the following ways:

1. *Ilajbil Tadbeer* (Regimental Therapy): Some drugless regimens are advised for the treatment of certain ailments, i.e. exercise, massage, hamam (Turkish bath), douches (Cold and Hot) and the regimen for geriatrics.
2. *Ilajbil Ghiza* (Dietotherapy): Different diets are recommended for the patients of different diseases.
3. *Ilajbil Dava* (Pharmacotherapy): The basic concept of treatment is to correct the cause of the disease that may be abnormal temperament due to:

   ■ Environmental factors.
   ■ Abnormal humours either due to internal causes or external causes which may be pathogenic microorganism, through (a) drugs of opposite temperament to the temperament of the disease that is called *Ilaj-bil-zid* or (b) drugs of similar temperament as of the temperament of the disease that is called as *Ilaj-bil-misl*.

4. *Ilajbil Yad* (Surgery).

The drugs used are mostly of the plant origin. Some drugs of animal and mineral origin are also used. Patients are treated either by single drug (crude drugs) or by compound drugs (formulations of single drugs).

There are two types of compound drugs used in the treatment of the diseases, i.e. classical compound drugs which are in use for the hundreds and thousands years and patent/proprietary compound drugs which have been formulated by the individuals or institutions as per their research and experiences. *Unani* system of medicine is one of the oldest systems of medicine in the world; it is still popular and practised in Indian subcontinent and other parts of the world.

2.6. HOMOEOPATHIC SYSTEM OF MEDICINE

Homoeopathy is a specialized system of therapeutics, developed by Dr Samuel Christian Friedrich Hahnemann (1755–1843), a German physician, chemist and a pharmacist, based on natural law of healing: *Similia Similibus Curantur*, which means 'Likes are cured by likes'.

Homois means like (similar) and *pathos* means treatment. Thus, homoeopathy is a system of treating diseases or suffering by the administration of drugs that possess power of producing similar suffering (diseases) in healthy human beings. Dr Hahnemann believed that symptoms are no more than an outward reflection of the body's inner fight to overcome illness: it is not a manifestation of the illness itself. This law of similar for curing diseases has being in use since the time of Hippocrates, father of medicine. But it was Dr Hahnemann who developed it in to a complete system of therapeutics enunciating the law and its application in 1810.

Fundamental Principles of Homoeopathy

Every science has certain basic principles that guide the whole system. Homoeopathy as a science of medical treatment has a philosophy of its own, and its therapeutics is based on certain fundamental principles that are quite distinct and different from those of other school of medical science. These fundamental principles were discussed by Hahnemann in different sections of his medicine and philosophy.

They are as follows:

1. Law of *Similia*
2. Law of simplex
3. Law of minimum
4. Drug proving
5. Drug dynamization or potentization
6. Vital force
7. Acute and chronic diseases
8. Individualization
9. Direction of cure

Law of similia

The therapeutic law on which homoeopathy is based is *Similia Similibus Curentur*, which means 'Let likes be cured by likes'. In this art of healing, the medicine administered to a diseased individual is such that if given to a healthy person it produces same sufferings (diseases) as found in the diseases individual. Thus, the symptoms of the diseased individual are to be matched with the pathogenesis of the medicine, and the medicines which are most similar, viz. *Simillimum* is selected and administered with certainty to cure.

Law of simplex

Simple and single drugs should be prescribed at a time. Thus, medicines are proved on healthy human beings singly and in simple form without admixture of any other substance.

Law of minimum

Drugs are administered in a minimum quantity because of hypersensitivity in disease and the action of drug is always directed towards normal by virtue of altered receptivity of tissue to stimuli in disease. The medicines are just required to arouse a reaction in the body. If they are given in large doses, they cause physiological action producing unwanted side effects and organic damage. The minutest quantity of medicine helps it to reach the disease, which is of very subtle in nature. The curative action of drug can only be expected without any unwanted aggravation by using minimum quantity of medicine.

Drug proving

To apply drugs for therapeutic purposes, their curative power should be known. The curative power of a drug is its ability to produce disease symptoms when employed on a healthy person. The curative power of a drug is known by its pathogenesis and is ascertained by proving the drug singly on healthy human being. This serves the only true record of the curative properties of drug.

Drug dynamization or potentization

Disease is a disturbance or deviation in the normal harmonious flow of life force which is dynamic in nature. Now medicine used to encounter disease should also have dynamic action to act on the dynamic disturbance of life force. Therefore, the drugs are dynamized or potentized liberating their dynamic curative power which lies dormant in them. This dynamization is done by the process of trituration (in case of insoluble substances) or succession (in case of soluble substances).

Preparation of potencies

The potency can be prepared by three different scales, like decimal scale, centesimal scale and millesimal scale.

Decimal scale

This scale was introduced by Dr Constantine Hering. In this scale, the first potency should contain 1/10 part of original drug. The second potency will contain 1/10 part of the first potency, and so on. The potency in this scale is denoted by suffixing the letter 'X' to the number indicating the potency, i.e. the first potency is 1X, the second potency is 2X, and so on.

Centesimal scale

In this scale the first potency should contain 1/100 of original drug and the second potency will contain 1/100 of the first potency, and so on. The potency in this scale is denoted by suffixing the letter 'C' to the number indicating the potency. In practice, it is generally denoted by a simple numerical 1C potency equivalent to 2X potency and 2C potency is equivalent to 4X, and so on.

Millesimal scale

In this scale, the first potency should contain 1/50,000 part of the original drug and second potency will contain 1/50,000 of the first potency, and so on. Potency in this scale is denoted by I, II, V, X, etc., or 0/1, 0/2, 0/5, 0/10, etc. In this scale potency 0/2 is equivalent to 4C = 8X,

0/4 = 8C = 16X and so on. Preparation of potency through trituration is made by either decimal or centesimal, and the preparation of potency though succession is made by decimal, centesimal and millesimal.

Vital force

Disease is nothing but the disharmonious flow of the vital force giving rise to abnormal sensation and functions (symptoms and signs). In order to restore the health, the disordered vital force is to be brought back to normal. Disease and health are two different quantitative states of this vital force of living being, and cure is to be affected here. Vital force has the following characteristics: spiritual, autocratic, automatic, dynamic, unintelligent and instinctive.

Acute and chronic diseases

The diseases are classified into these types depending upon their onset, nature of progress and termination of diseases.

Individualization

No two individuals are alike in the world, so the diseases affecting individuals can never be the same assuming the unique individual picture in each diseased individual. Thus, medicines can never be prescribed on the basis of the name of the disease without individualizing each case of disease.

Direction of cure

Dr. Hering states that cure takes place within outward from above to downward and the symptoms disappears in the reverse of their appearance. If the direction is reverse of that stated then it is not cure but suppression which has occurred.

2.7. AROMATHERAPY

The word aromatherapy means *treatment using scents*. It refers to the use of essential oils in *holistic healing* to improve health and emotional well being, and in restoring balance to the body. Essential oils are aromatic essences extracted from plants, flowers, trees, fruit, bark, grasses and seeds.

There are more than 150 types of oils that can be extracted. These oils have distinctive therapeutic, psychological and physiological properties that improve health and prevent illness. All essential oils have unique healing and valuable antiseptic properties. Some oils are antiviral, anti-inflammatory, pain relieving, antidepressant, stimulating, relaxing, expectorating, support digestion and have diuretic properties too.

Essential oils get absorbed into our body and exert an influence on it. The residue gets dispersed from the body naturally. They can also affect our mind and emotions. They enter the body in three ways: by inhalation, absorption and consumption.

Chemically, essential oils are a mixture of organic compounds like ketones, terpenes, esters, alcohol, aldehyde and hundreds of other molecules which are extremely difficult to classify, as they are small and complex. The essential oils molecules are small. They penetrate human skin easily and enter the bloodstream directly and finally get flushed out through our elementary system.

A concentrate of essential oils is not greasy; it is more like water in texture and evaporates quickly. Some of them are light liquid insoluble in water and evaporate instantly when exposed to air. It would take 100 kg of lavender to get 3 kg of lavender oil; one would need 8 million jasmine flowers to yield barely 1 kg of jasmine oil.

Some of the common essential oils used in aromatherapy for their versatile application are:

1. Clary Sage (*Salvia scared*)
2. Eucalyptus (*Eucalyptus globulus*)
3. Geranium (*Pelargonium graveolens*)
4. Lavender (*Lavandula officinalis*)
5. Lemon (*Citrus limon*)
6. Peppermint (*Mentha piperita*)
7. Rosemary (*Rosmarinus officinalis*)

Origin of Aromatherapy

The title aromatherapy was coined by Gattefosse, a French chemist in the year 1928. He identified the use of aromatic oils accidentally, when he burned his hand while working in his lab, and immediately he pooled his hand inside a bottle containing lavender oil. The burn healed quickly due to lavender oil and left little scarring. The use of aroma oil is known to be as old as 6000 years back, when the God of Medicine and Healing, recommended fragrant oils for bathing and massaging. In 4500 B.C., Egyptians used myrrh and cedar wood oils for embalming their dead and the modern researchers after 6500 years proved the fact that the cedar wood contains natural fixative and strong antibacterial and antiseptic properties that preserved their mummies.

The Greek father of medicine, Hippocrates, recommended regular aromatherapy baths and scented massages. Romans utilized essential oils for pleasure and to cure pain and also for massages. During the great plague in London in 1665, people burnt bundles of lavender, cedar wood and cypress in the streets and carried poises of the same plants as their only defence to combat infectious diseases.

Aromatherapy has received a wider acceptance in the early twentieth century. Dr Jean Volnet, French army surgeon extensively used essential oils in World War II to treat the injured warriors. It was Madame Morquerite Murry (1964), who gave the holistic approach to aroma oils by experimenting with them for individual problems.

Today, researches have proved the multiple uses of aroma oils. Medical research in the recent years has uncovered the fact that the odours we smell have a significant impact on the way we feel. Smells act directly on the brain like a drug. For instance, smelling lavender increases alpha wave frequency in the back of the head, and this state is associated with relaxation.

Mode of Action of Aroma Oils

Dr Alan Huch, a neurologist, psychiatrist and also the director of Smell and Taste Research Centre in Chicago says, 'Smell acts directly on the brain, like a drug'. Our nose has the capacity to distinguish 100,000 different smells, many of which affect us without our knowledge regarding the same.

The aroma enters our nose and connects with cilia, the fine hair inside the nose lining. The receptors in the cilia are linked to the olfactory lobe which is at the end of the smell tract. The end of the tract is in turn connected to the brain itself. Smells are converted by cilia into electrical impulses that are transmitted to the brain through olfactory system. All the impulses reach the limbic system. Limbic system is that part of the brain, which is associated with our moods, emotions, memory and learning. All the smell that reaches the limbic system has a direct chemical effect on our moods.

The molecular sizes of the essential oils are very tiny and they can easily penetrate through the skin and get into the blood stream. It takes anything between a few seconds to two hours for the essential oils to enter the skin, and within four hours, the toxins get out of the body through urine, perspiration and excreta.

Aroma oils work like magic for stress-related problems, psychosomatic disorders, skin infections, hair loss, inflammations and pains arising from muscular or skeletal disorders.

Essential oils are safe to use. The only caution being they should never be used directly because some oils may irritate sensitive skin or cause photosensitivity. They should be blended in adequate proportion with the carrier oils. A patch test is necessary to rule out any reactions.

Application Methods: Essential oils can be utilized in a myriad of ways, such as topically, ingesting or internal and the most common inhalations.

Topical Applications: When using natural products, only your body knows how it is going to respond; therefore, watch for any signs of skin irritation or side effects. Essential oils are soluble with the lipids found in the skin and can penetrate the skin surface and be absorbed into the lymph and circulatory systems. They may be worn as perfumes, ointments, cologne, and can be applied undiluted or diluted using a carrier oil or other base. As a rule, due to the concentrated and potency of pure essential oils, dilution in a carrier is highly recommended for beginners or for those people with sensitive, fair skin, or applications of the face, neck and other sensitive areas and also if you are trying a new oil or blend of oils. Please be careful with children or infants as the dilution's necessary are very minute. When in doubt, always consult.

Baths: Seven to eight drops of essential oil in 30 ml of carrier oil or honey. Add this to running water and mix well before getting in. Be sure to check the safety info for the essential oils that you choose.

Foot baths: Up to six drops in a bowl or footbath of warm water. Soak for approx. 10 minutes. This is great for varicose veins, swollen ankle or tired aching legs.

Compresses: Hot or cold. Five to eight drops of essential oil in a basin filled with either hot or cold water. Agitate the water and place a cotton cloth on top of the water to collect the floating oil. Gently squeeze excess water out and apply directly and immediately to affected area. Wrap another towel over the compress and leave until it reaches body temperature. This can be repeated over and over for relief of pain, headache or to reduce inflammation.

Massage: Add 15–22 drops of essential oil to a 30 ml of carrier oil for a full body massage. Always massage in an upward motion and towards the heart for best effect.

Inhalation Applications: This is one of the simplest and effective methods of dispersing essential oils into the air. Inhalations are a method of introducing essential oils to the lungs via the nose and throat. This can have great benefit for respiratory problems, sinus congestion, flu, coughs, colds, catarrh and sore throats. Use this method once or twice a day.

Facial Steams: Two to three drops of oil into a bowel of boiled water. Drape a towel over your head and lean over the bowl to inhale the steam deeply while keeping eyes shut. Inhale slowly at first, then breathe deeper and deeper. Breathe through your mouth for throat problems, and inhale through your nose for sinus congestion.

Atomizers: Add 12–20 drops of essential oils to distilled water in a spray bottle. Shake well before using and mist on face or into the air.

Vaporizers: 10–12 drops in the top of the vaporizer for a normal size room.

Nebulizers: This electrical unit is designed to disperse the essential oils in a microfine mist. This means that the molecules of oil will hang in the air for much longer due to the minuscule weight of the particles. Research has shown that diffusing in this way may help to reduce bacteria, fungus, mould and unpleasant odours. It not only makes the air fresh, but it also helps you to relax, relieves tension and creates an atmosphere of harmony and peaceful tranquillity.

Direct Inhalation: Put three drops of essential oil into the palm of your hand and rub hands together briefly, and then quickly inhale deeply for greater inhalation. Relieves sinus congestion and is quite invigorating.

Essential oils have being used by the people for thousand years; it has great potential to use in modern days. Appropriate method of cultivation and distillation certainly yield good quality essential oil. The more an essential oil is interfered physically or chemically, the less clinical value it will have. This can be overcome by means of suitable evaluation technique.

2.8. BACH FLOWER REMEDIES

Bach flower remedies were discovered by Dr Bach, renowned physician in London who in 1930 gave up his practice to devote all of his time to the search for a new method of healing. For many years he had sought a natural and pure way to heal people; he had discovered how different people reacted differently to the exact same disease. One could be cheerful and hide his worries while another would be very depressed with no hope for tomorrow. Dr Bach believed that those two patients should be treated differently, not strictly according to the disease, but according to their emotions. It was in 1928 Dr Bach discovered the first 38 essences and started to administer them to his patients, with immediate and successful results. Each of the 38 remedies discovered by Dr Bach is directed at a particular characteristic or emotional state. The cheerful patients would acknowledge their worries, and the depressed patients would regain hope. The essences restored their emotional balance allowing their bodies to heal themselves.

The 38 plants and their indications are as follows:

- Agrimony for people who put a brave face on their troubles
- Aspen for people who are anxious or afraid but don't know why
- Beech for people who are intolerant and critical of others
- Centaury for people who allow others to impose on them
- Cerato for people who doubt their own judgment
- Cherry plum for uncontrolled, irrational thoughts and the fear of doing something awful
- Chestnut bud for people who repeat mistakes and don't learn from experience
- Chicory for over-possessive, selfish people who cling to their loved ones
- Clematis for day dreamers
- Crab apple for those who dislike something about the way they look and as a general cleanser
- Elm for responsible, capable people who in a crisis doubt their ability to cope
- Gentian for people disheartened when something goes wrong
- Gorse for people who have lost hope, often without cause
- Heather for talkative types who are obsessed with their own problems
- Holly for negative feelings of hatred, envy, jealousy and suspicion

- Honeysuckle for people who live in the past
- Hornbeam for mental tiredness at the thought of a coming task
- Impatiens for impatience and irritation at other people's slowness
- Larch for fear of failure and lack of confidence
- Mimulus for people who are afraid of something real that they can name
- Mustard for gloom and depression with no known cause
- Oak for strong, indefatigable people who can over-extend themselves by trying too hard
- Olive for people physically drained by exertion or illness
- Pine for those who blame themselves when things go wrong
- Red chestnut for excessive worry about the welfare of loved ones
- Rock rose for extreme fright and terror
- Rock water for people whose self-discipline and high standards are carried to excess
- Scleranthus for people who find it hard to choose between possible courses of action
- Star of Bethlehem for sudden frights and shock
- Sweet chestnut for utter despair and anguish
- Vervain for enthusiastic people who are always on the go
- Vine for domineering people
- Walnut to help protect against outside influences and the effects of change
- Water violet for private, reserved people who can appear proud and arrogant
- White chestnut for persistent worrying thoughts
- Wild oat for people unable to find a direction for their lives
- Wild rose for people who resign themselves without complaint or effort to everything life throws at them
- Willow for people who are full of self-pity, resentment and bitterness

Dr Bach's remedies are still made today at the Bach Centre, Mount Vernon, in England. Since 1991, practitioner courses have been running at the Centre and are now running in the United States, Canada, Spain, Holland and Ireland as well. As a result more than 350 trained practitioners are now registered with the Centre.

2.9. TIBETAN SYSTEM OF MEDICINE

Tibetan medicine is an ancient synthesis of the art of healing, drawing on the knowledge of medical systems existing in a wide region of Southeast and Central Asia. The history of Tibetan medical system dates back to some 3800 years to the time of the non-Buddhist culture of Tibet's native religion. It has continued to evolve since then to the time of the strong emergence of Buddhist culture in India. The Tibetans made use of their countries abundant natural resources of flora and fauna to fight against diseases. The seventh and eighth century observed the real development in the field of Tibetan medicine. Ayurveda has contributed a great deal in enriching Tibetan medicine. The *Gyudshi* or the Four Great *Tantras* is the most authoritative classic of Tibetan medicine, and bears ample proof of its loyal allegiance to Ayurvedic classics like *Charaka, Susruta* and *Astanga* hydra of *Vaghbhata*. One of the unique features of Tibetan medical system is its ideological structure of medical theory and practice in the image of a tree known as Allegorical Tree.

Like the phenomena of conditioned existence, diseases are also the product of causes and conditions. There are two main causes of the disease: a long-term cause and short-term cause. Ignorance or unawareness is the ultimate cause of all diseases. Because of ignorance or delusion, one cannot see the reality of the phenomena and thereby clings to personal self or ego which in turn gives rise to the three mental poisons: desire, hatred and stupidity. So ignorance and three mental poisons constitute the long-term cause of disease. Secondly, the short-term causes of disease are the three humours: wind energy (*Tib. rlung*), bile energy (*Tib. mkhris pa*) and phlegm (*Tib. bad kan*). They are produced by the three mental poisons: desire gives rise to wind, hatred to bile and stupidity to phlegm. These three humours constitute the basic energy system in the body. They are interrelated to all vital functions of the body, organs, seven constituents and three excretions. Seven constituents of the body are: food (nutrition), blood, flesh, fat, bone, marrow and semen. The three excrements are sweat, urine and faeces.

When the three humours, seven body constituents and the three excrements are balanced, one is healthy; when they are unbalanced one becomes sick. There are four factors responsible for the imbalance; they are improper climate, influence of demons, improper diet and improper behaviour. Since everything is interrelated, imbalance in one organ or one of the humours affects the rest of the organism. Because of the interdependence of humours and body constituents, etc., their imbalance can be diagnosed by the methods specially used by Tibetan doctors. The methods are:

Interrogation

Considering the patient's history.

Visual Examination

Visual examination consists of examining the patient's physical structure, eyes, tongue, urine, etc.

Tactile Examination

This method of diagnosis is concerned with things such as temperature, inflammations, etc. Most important here is diagnosis by pulse.

Treatments

There are four methods of treatment. They are diet, behaviour modification, medicine and physical therapy. The most important therapeutic technique is to restore the balance of the three 'NYES-PA' (humours) and to ensure that the seven constituents of the body are always in a healthy state. These seven constituents are: essential nutrient (*dangsma*), blood (*khark*), fat (*tsil*), muscle tissues (*sha*), bone (*rus*), marrow (*kang*) and regenerative fluid (*khuwa*).

Diet

The first treatment involves the prescribing of a proper diet. For example, if the patient is suffering from a bile disorder, he should not take alcohol and should drink cool boiled water.

Behaviour Modification

For example, a patient with a bile disorder should not do heavy physical activities. He should rest in the shade, and not sleep during the day. If these two factors fail to bring about a positive result, further treatment should be carried out.

Medicine

Prescription of natural drugs. Here again the physician starts with less-potent concoctions and turns to stronger forms, if necessary. The drugs can be classified in 10 forms: decoction, pills, powder, granules, medicinal butter, medicinal calxes, concentrated extractions, medicinal wine, gem medicine and herbal medicine.

Physical Therapy

Apart from natural drugs, the physician may also have to depend on other therapeutic techniques, like massage, hot and cold compresses, mineral spring bath therapy and medicinal bath are the gentle techniques. Blood, letting, cauterization, moxibustion, cupping and golden needle therapy are considered as rough techniques. There is also some minor surgery such as the draining of abscesses.

Tibetan medical philosophy is a holistic philosophy involving the harmonious operation and balance of all the energies that constitute the human psychophysical being. Theses energies are the psychologically originating three 'NYES-PA' or humours, which correspond to the three mental poisons and the five cosmophysical energies that are at the basis of all phenomena. If all the factors that influence these energies (seasonal factors; diet and nutrition, life style and mental attitudes) are positively disposed, then these energies remain in balanced operation, and health is experienced. It is the objective of Tibetan medicine that the balance in these energies should be maintained.

CHAPTER 3

Classification of Drugs of Natural Origin

CONTENTS

- Introduction
  - ▶ Organized Drugs
  - ▶ Unorganized Drugs
- Classification of Crude Drugs

- ▶ Alphabetical Classification
- ▶ Taxonomical Classification
- ▶ Morphological Classification
- ▶ Pharmacological Classification

- ▶ Chemical Classification
- ▶ Chemotaxonomical Classification
- ▶ Serotaxonomical Classification

3.1. INTRODUCTION

The flora and fauna of mother earth has a great diversity. The number of plant species divided in about 300 families and 10,500 genera are supposed to be about 2–2.5 lacs. At least 100–150 species of medicinal plants are currently cultivated and about 30–40 of them are the large-scale field corps. Drugs of the animal and mineral origin have also been used since the beginning and even today many such crude drugs are important, commercial products. All these drugs of natural origin have been used as the curative agents and even in this age of scientific discoveries and invention, natural drug have been the primary choice as a source of drug. Human inquisitiveness has gone beyond the terrestrial regions and exploited the seas and oceans which contain about 5 lacs species of marine organisms. Therapeutically active constituents found in these organisms open yet another great natural source of drugs of unending search.

Crude drugs can be regarded as the substances either used directly or indirectly as a drug which have not been changed or modified in its chemical composition.

The crude drugs of natural origin can be divided into two main categories as organized crude drugs and unorganized crude drugs.

Organized Drugs

Organized drugs consist of the cellular organization in the form of anatomical features. These are mostly the crude drugs from plant sources. Almost all of the morphological plant parts or the entire plant itself can be called as an organized drugs. A long list can be made of such crude drugs. To mention few of them, like, Cinchona bark, Sandalwood, Quassia wood, Senna, Digitalis leaves, Nux vomica seeds, Rauwolfia roots and many other examples of above-mentioned groups or crude drugs exemplified by some other morphological organs can be quoted as the example of organized crude drugs.

Microscopical and anatomical studies are preeminent for such crude drugs. These can be used directly in medicine or can be used by modifying or by extracting the active ingredient from it. The simple medicines prepared from these drugs are herbal teas, extracts, tinctures, etc., and it may be extensively processed for the isolation and purification of pure therapeutically active constituent which is ultimately responsible for the action of the drug.

Unorganized Drugs

The unorganized drugs do not have the morphological or anatomical organization as such. These are the products which come directly in the market but their ultimate source remains the plants, animals or minerals. Microscopical studies are not required for such crude drugs. These includes products like plant exudates as gums, oleogums, oleogumresins, plant lattices like that of opium, aloetic juices like aloes or dried extracts of black and pale catechu, agar, alginic acid, etc., are products coming under this group. Other products like essential oils, fixed oils, fats and waxes obtained from vegetable or animal sources, although hydro-distilled or extracted from plant, become the direct commodity for use. Unorganized crude drugs may be miscellaneous mineral products like *shilajit*. These products may be solid, semisolid or liquid and the physical, chemical and analytical standards may be applied for testing their quality and purity.

3.2. CLASSIFICATION OF CRUDE DRUGS

The most important natural sources of drugs are higher plant, microbes and animals and marine organisms. Some useful products are obtained from minerals that are both organic and inorganic in nature. In order to pursue (or to follow) the study of the individual drugs, one must adopt some particular sequence of arrangement, and this is referred to a system of classification of drugs. A method of classification should be:

(a) simple,
(b) easy to use and
(c) free from confusion and ambiguities.

Because of their wide distribution, each arrangement of classification has its own merits and demerits, but for the purpose of study the drugs are classified in the following different ways:

1. Alphabetical classification
2. Taxonomical classification
3. Morphological classification
4. Pharmacological classification
5. Chemical classification
6. Chemotaxonomical classification
7. Serotaxonomical classification

Alphabetical Classification

Alphabetical classification is the simplest way of classification of any disconnected items. Crude drugs are arranged in alphabetical order of their Latin and English names (common names) or sometimes local language names (vernacular names). Some of the pharmacopoeias, dictionaries and reference books which classify crude drugs according to this system are as follows:

1. Indian Pharmacopoeia
2. British Pharmacopoeia
3. British Herbal Pharmacopoeia
4. United States Pharmacopoeia and National Formulary
5. British Pharmaceutical Codex
6. European Pharmacopoeia

In European Pharmacopoeia these are arranged according to their names in Latin where in United States Pharmacopoeia (U.S.P.) and British Pharmaceutical Codex (B.P.C.), these are arranged in English.

Merits

- It is easy and quick to use.
- There is no repetition of entries and is devoid of confusion.
- In this system location, tracing and addition of drug entries is easy.

Demerits

There is no relationship between previous and successive drug entries.

Examples: Acacia, Benzoin, Cinchona, Dill, Ergot, Fennel, Gentian, Hyoscyamus, Ipecacuanha, Jalap, Kurchi, Liquorice, Mints, Nux vomica, Opium, Podophyllum, Quassia, Rauwolfia, Senna, Vasaka, Wool fat, Yellow bees wax, Zeodary.

Taxonomical Classification

All the plants possess different characters of morphological, microscopical, chemical, embryological, serological and genetics. In this classification the crude drugs are classified according to kingdom, subkingdom, division, class, order, family, genus and species as follows.

Class: Angiospermae (Angiosperms) are plants that produce flowers and Gymnospermae (Gymnosperms) which don't produce flowers.

Subclass: Dicotyledonae (Dicotyledons, Dicots) are plants with two seed leaves; Monocotyledonae (Monocotyledons, Monocots) with one seed leaf.

Superorder: A group of related plant families, classified in the order in which they are thought to have developed their differences from a common ancestor. There are six superorders in the Dicotyledonae (*Magnoliidae, Hamamelidae, Caryophyllidae, Dilleniidae, Rosidae, Asteridae*), and four superorders in the Monocotyledonae (*Alismatidae, Commelinidae, Arecidae* and *Liliidae*). The names of the superorders end in –idae.

Order: Each superorder is further divided into several orders. The names of the orders end in –ales.

Family: Each order is divided into families. These are plants with many botanical features in common, and are the highest classification normally used. At this level, the similarity between plants is often easily recognizable by the layman. Modern botanical classification assigns a type plant to each family, which has the particular characteristics that separate this group of plants from others, and names the family after this plant.

The number of plant families varies according to the botanist whose classification you follow. Some botanists recognize only 150 or so families, preferring to classify other similar plants as subfamilies, while others recognize nearly 500 plant families. A widely accepted system is that devised by Cronquist in 1968, which is only slightly revised today. The names of the families end in –*aceae*.

Subfamily: The family may be further divided into a number of subfamilies, which group together plants within the family that have some significant botanical differences. The names of the subfamilies end in –*oideae*.

Tribe: A further division of plants within a family, based on smaller botanical differences, bin still usually comprising many different plants. The names of the tribes end in –*eae*.

Subtribe: A further division based on even smaller botanical differences, often only recognizable to botanists. The names of the subtribes end in –*inae*.

Genus: This is the part of the plant name that is most familiar; the normal name that you give a plant—Papaver (Poppy), Aquilegia (Columbine) and so on. The plants in a genus are often easily recognizable as belonging to the same group.

Species: This is the level that defines an individual plant. Often, the name will describe some aspect of the plant—the colour of the flowers, size or shape of the leaves, or it may be named after the place where it was found. Together, the genus and species name refer to only one plant, and they are used to identify that particular plant. Sometimes, the species is further divided into subspecies that contain plants not quite so distinct that they are classified as varieties. The name, of the species should be written after the genus name, in small letters, with no capital letter.

Variety: A variety is a plant that is only slightly different from the species plant, but the differences are not so insignificant as the differences in a form. The Latin is *varietas*, which is usually abbreviated to var. The name follows the genus and species name, with var. before the individual variety name.

Form: A form is a plant within a species that has minor botanical differences, such as the colour of flower or shape of the leaves. The name follows the genus and species name, with form (or f.) before the individual variety name.

Cultivar: A cultivar is a cultivated variety—a particular plant that has arisen either naturally or through deliberate hybridization, and can be reproduced (vegetatively or by seed) to produce more of the same plant.

The name follows the genus and species name. It is written in the language of the person who described it, and should not be translated. It is either written in single quotation marks or has cv. written in front of the name.

Kingdom	Plants
Subkingdom	Tracheobionta—Vascular plants
Superdivision	Spermatophyta—Seed plants
Division	Magnoliophyta—Flowering plants
Class	Magnoliopsida—Dicotyledons
Subclass	Asteridae
Order	Asterales
Family	Asteraceae—Aster family
Genus	*Tridax* L.—Tridax

Merits

Taxonomical classification is helpful for studying evolutionary developments.

Demerits

This system also does not correlate in between the chemical constituents and biological activity of the drugs.

Morphological Classification

In this system, the drugs are arranged according to the morphological or external characters of the plant parts or animal parts, i.e. which part of the plant is used as a drug, e.g. leaves, roots, stem, etc. The drugs obtained from the direct parts of the plants and containing cellular tissues are called as *organized* drugs, e.g. rhizomes, barks, leaves, fruits, entire plants, hairs and fibres. The drugs which are prepared from plants by some intermediate physical processes such as incision, drying or extraction with a solvent and not containing any cellular plant tissues are called *unorganized* drugs. Aloe juice, opium latex, agar, gambir, gelatin, tragacanth, benzoin, honey, beeswax, lemon grass oil, etc., are examples of unorganized drugs.

Organized drugs

Woods: Quassia, Sandalwood and Red Sandalwood.

Leaves: Digitalis, Eucalyptus, Gymnema, Mint, Senna, Spearmint, Squill, Tulsi, Vasaka, Coca, Buchu, Hamamelis, Hyoscyamus, Belladonna, Tea.

Barks: Arjuna, Ashoka, Cascara, Cassia, Cinchona, Cinnamon, Kurchi, Quillia, Wild cherry.

Flowering parts: Clove, Pyrethrum, Saffron, Santonica, Chamomile.

Fruits: Amla, Anise, Bael, Bahera, Bitter Orange peel, Capsicum, Caraway, Cardamom, Colocynth, Coriander, Cumin, Dill, Fennel, Gokhru, Hirda, Lemon peel, Senna pod, Star anise, Tamarind, Vidang.

Seeds: Bitter almond, Black Mustard, Cardamom, Colchicum, Ispaghula, Kaladana, Linseed, Nutmeg, Nux vomica, Physostigma, Psyllium, Strophanthus, White mustard.

Roots and rhizomes: Aconite, Ashwagandha, Calamus, Calumba, Colchicum corm, Dioscorea, Galanga, Garlic, Gention, Ginger, Ginseng, Glycyrrhiza, Podophyllum, Ipecac, Ipomoea, Jalap, Jatamansi, Rauwolfia, Rhubarb, Saussurea, Senega, Shatavari, Turmeric, Valerian, Squill.

Plants and herbs: Ergot, Ephedra, Bacopa, Andrographis, Kalmegh, Yeast, Vinca, Datura, Centella.

Hair and fibres: Cotton, Hemp, Jute, Silk, Flax.

Unorganized drugs

Dried latex: Opium, Papain.

Dried juice: Aloe, Kino.

Dried extracts: Agar, Alginate, Black catechu, Pale catechu, Pectin.

Waxes: Beeswax, Spermaceti, Carnauba wax.

Gums: Acacia, Guar Gum, Indian Gum, Sterculia, Tragacanth.

Resins: Asafoetida, Benzoin, Colophony, copaiba Guaiacum, Guggul, Mastic, Coal tar, Tar, Tolu balsam, Storax, Sandarac.

Volatile oil: Turpentine, Anise, Coriander, Peppermint, Rosemary, Sandalwood, Cinnamon, Lemon, Caraway, Dill, Clove, Eucalyptus, Nutmeg, Camphor.

Fixed oils and fats: Arachis, Castor, Chalmoogra, Coconut, Cotton seed, Linseed, Olive, Sesame, Almond, Theobroma, Cod-liver, Halibut liver, Kokum butter.

Animal products: Bees wax, Cantharides, Cod-liver oil, Gelatin, Halibut liver oil, Honey, Shark liver oil, shellac, Spermaceti wax, wool fat, musk, Lactose.

Fossil organism and minerals: Bentonite, Kaolin, Kieselguhr, Talc.

Merits

Morphological classification is more helpful to identify and detect adulteration. This system of classification is more convenient for practical study especially when the chemical nature of the drug is not clearly understood.

Demerits

- The main drawback of morphological classification is that there is no correlation of chemical constituents with the therapeutic actions.
- Repetition of drugs or plants occurs.

Pharmacological Classification

Grouping of drug according to their pharmacological action or of most important constituent or their therapeutic use is termed as pharmacological or therapeutic classification of drug. This classification is more relevant and is mostly a followed method. Drugs like digitalis, squill and strophanthus having cardiotonic action are grouped irrespective of their parts used or phylogenetic relationship or the nature of phytoconstituents they contain.

S. no.	Pharmacological category	Example
1.	Drug acting on G.I.T.	
	Bitter	Cinchona, Quassia, Gentian
	Carminative	Fennel, Cardamom, Mentha
	Emetic	Ipecac
	Antiamoebic	Kurchi, Ipecac
	Laxative	Agar, Isabgol, Banana
	Purgative	Senna, Castor oil
	Cathartic	Senna
2.	Drug acting on Respiratory system	
	Expectorant	Vasaka, Liquorice, Ipecac
	Antitussive	Opium (codeine)
	Bronchodilators	Ephedra, Tea
3.	Drug acting on Cardiovascular system	
	Cardio tonic	Digitalis, Strophanthus, Squill
	Cardiac depressant	Cinchona, Veratrum
	Vasoconstrictor	Ergot
	Antihypertensive	Rauwolfia
4.	Drug acting on Autonomic nervous system	
	Adrenergic	Ephedra
	Cholinergic	Physostigma, Pilocarpus
	Anticholinergic	Datura, Belladonna
5.	Drug acting on Central nervous system	
	Central analgesic	Opium (morphine)
	CNS depressant	Belladonna, Opium, Hyoscyamus
	CNS stimulant	Tea, Coffee
	Analeptic	Nuxvomica, Camphor, Lobelia
6.	Antispasmodic	Datura, Hyoscyamus, Opium, Curare
7.	Anticancer	Vinca, Podophyllum, Taxus
8.	Antirheumatic	Aconite, Colchicum, Guggul
9.	Anthelmintic	Quassia, Vidang
10.	Astringent	Catechu, Myrobalans
11.	Antimalarial	Cinchona, Artemisia
12.	Immunomodulatory	Ginseng, Ashwagandha, Tulsi
13.	Immunizing agent	Vaccines, Sera, Anti toxin
14.	Drug acting on skin membrane	Beeswax, Wool fat, Balsam of Tolu, Balsam of Peru
15.	Chemotherapeutic	Antibiotics
16.	Local Anaesthetic	Coca

Merits

This system of classification can be used for suggesting substitutes of drugs, if they are not available at a particular place or point of time.

Demerits

Drugs having different action on the body get classified separately in more than one group that causes ambiguity and confusion. Cinchona is antimalarial drug because of presence of quinine but can be put under the group of drug affecting heart because of antiarrhythmic action of quinidine.

Chemical Classification

Depending upon the active constituents, the crude drugs are classified. The plants contain various constituents in them like alkaloids, glycosides, tannins, carbohydrates, saponins, etc. Irrespective of the morphological or taxonomical characters, the drugs with similar chemical constituents are grouped into the same group. The examples are shown in this table.

S. no.	Chemical constituent group	Examples
1.	Alkaloids	Cinchona, Datura, Vinca, Ipecac Nux vomica
2.	Glycosides	Senna, Aloe, Ginseng, Glycyrrhiza, Digitalis
3.	Carbohydrates and its derived products	Acacia, Tragacanth, Starch, Isabgol
4.	Volatile oil	Clove, Coriander, Fennel, Cinnamon, Cumin
5.	Resin and Resin combination	Benzoin, Tolu Balsam, Balsam of peru
6.	Tannins	Catechu, Tea
7.	Enzymes	Papain, Caesin, Trypsin
8.	Lipids	Beeswax, Kokum butter, Lanolin

Merits

It is a popular approach for phytochemical studies.

Demerits

Ambiguities arise when particular drugs possess a number of compounds belonging to different groups of compounds.

Chemotaxonomical Classification

This system of classification relies on the chemical similarity of a taxon, i.e. it is based on the existence of relationship between constituents in various plants. There are certain types of chemical constituents that characterize certain classes of plants. This gives birth to entirely a new concept of chemotaxonomy that utilizes chemical facts/characters for understanding the taxonomical status, relationships and the evolution of the plants.

For example, tropane alkaloids generally occur among the members of Solanaceae, thereby, serving as a chemotaxonomic marker. Similarly, other secondary plant metabolites can serve as the basis of classification of crude drugs. The berberine alkaloid in Berberis and Argemone, Rutin in Rutaceae members, Ranunculaceae alkaloids among its members, etc., are other examples.

It is the latest system of classification that gives more scope for understanding the relationship between chemical constituents, their biosynthesis and their possible action.

Serotaxonomical Classification

The serotaxonomy can be explained as the study about the application or the utility of serology in solving the taxonomical problems. Serology can be defined as the study of the antigen–antibody reaction. Antigens are those substances which can stimulate the formation of the antibody. Antibodies are highly specific protein molecule produced by plasma cells in the immune system. Protein are carriers of the taxonomical information and commonly used as antigen in serotaxonomy.

It expresses the similarities and the dissimilarities among different taxa, and these data are helpful in taxonomy. It determines the degree of similarity between species, genera, family, etc., by comparing the reaction with antigens from various plant taxa with antibodies present against a given taxon.

Serology helps in comparing nonmorphological characteristics, which helps in the taxonomical data. This technique also helps in the comparison of single proteins from different plant taxa.

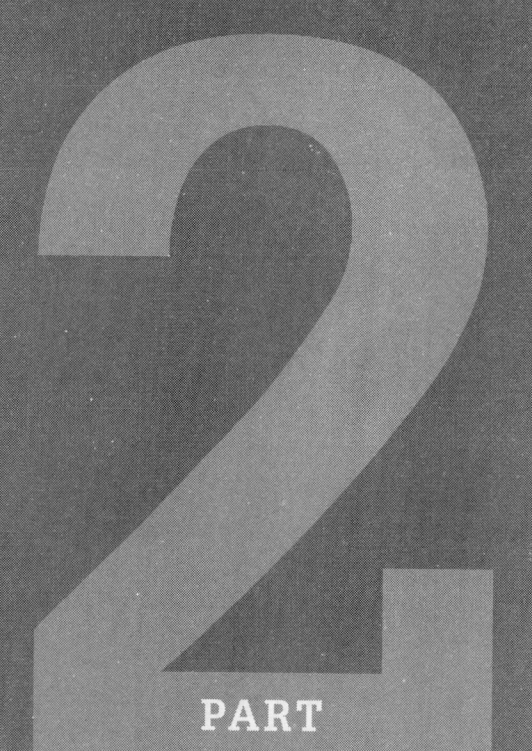

PART

Pharmaceutical Botany

Section Outline

OVERVIEW

This part provides the information regarding detail knowledge of pharmaceutical botany. It includes the detail morphological characteristics of different parts of the plants along with the study of their respective families by floral formula and floral diagrams.

Morphology of Different Plant Parts

CONTENTS

4.1. INTRODUCTION

Arrangements of plants into groups and subgroups are commonly spoken as classification. Various systems of classifying plants have gradually developed during past few centuries which have emerged as a discipline of botanical science known as taxonomy or systematic botany. The Taxonomy word is derived from two Greek words 'Taxis' meaning an arrangement and 'nomos' meaning laws. Therefore, the systemization of our knowledge about plants in an orderly manner becomes subject matter of systematic botany.

The aim and objective of taxonomy is to discover the similarities and differences in the plants, indicating their closure relationship with their descents from common ancestry. It is a scientific way of naming, describing and arranging the plants in an orderly manner.

The classification of plants may be based upon variety of characters possessed by them. Features like specific morphological characters, environmental conditions, geographical distribution, colours of flowers and types of adaptations or reproductive characteristics can be used as a base for taxonomical character.

KEY TERMS

4.2. HISTORY

Many attempts were made in the earlier days to name and distinguish the plants as well as animals. Earliest mentions of classifications are credited to the Greek scientist Aristotle (384–322 B.C.) who is also called as the father of natural history. Aristotle attempted a simple artificial system for classifying number of plants and animals on the basis of their morphological and anatomical resemblances. It worked with great success for more than two thousand years.

Theophrastus (370–285 B.C.), the first taxonomist who wrote a systematic classification in a logical form was a student of Aristotle. He attempted to extend the botanical knowledge beyond the scope of medicinal plants. Theophrastus classified the plants in about 480 taxa, using primarily the most obvious morphological characteristics, i.e. trees, shrubs, undershrubs, herbs, annuals, biennials and perennials. He recognized differences based upon superior and inferior ovary, fused and separate petals and so on. He is called father of botany. Several of the names mentioned by him in his treatise, 'De Historia Plantarum' was later taken up by Linnaeus in his system of classification.

A. P. de Tournfort (1658–1708) carried further the promotional work on genus. He had a clear idea of genera and many of the names used by him in his *Institutions Rei Herbariae* (1700) were adopted by Linnaeus. Tournfort's system classified about 9000 species into 698 genera and 22 classes. This system although artificial in nature was extremely practical in its approach.

Most of the taxonomists after Tournfort used the relative taxonomic characterization as a basis for classification. This natural base helped to ascertain the nomenclature and also showed its relative affinities with one another. All the modern systems of classification are thus natural systems.

John Ray (1682), an English Botanist used a natural system based on the embryo characteristics. Most important of his works were *Methodus Plantarum Nova* (1682), *Historia Plantarum* (1686) and *Synopsis Methodica Stirpium Britanicarum* (1698). He classified the plants into two main groups: *Herbae*, with herbaceous stem and *Arborae*, with woody stem.

The main groups of flowerless and flowering plants were subdivided distinctly into 33 smaller groups. He divided flowering plants in monocotyledonae and dicotyledonae, which later worked as a great foundation for the further developments of systematic botany

Carrolus Linnaeus (1707–1778), a Swedish botanist, introduced the system of binomial nomenclature. His artificial system was based on particular names of a substantive and objective nature. It is best known as *binomial system of nomenclature* in which the first general name indicates the genus and the second specific name denotes the species. Linnaeus characterized and listed about 4378 different species of plants and animals in his works *Species Plantarum* and *Genera Plantarum* (1753). He classified plants on the basis of reproductive organs, i.e. stamens and carpels—and hence this system is also known as the sexual system of classification. According to this system, plants are divided into 24 classes having 23 phanerogams and one cryptogam. Phanerogams were classified on the basis of unisexual and bisexual flowers. Further classification is based on the number and types of stamens and carpels.

A French Botanist A. P. de Candolle (1819) extensively worked and improved the natural system of classification. Along with the recognition of cotyledons, corolla and stamen characteristics, Candolle introduced the arrangement of fibrovascular bundles as a major character. He also provided a classification system for lower plants; Candolle mainly divided plants into vascular and cellular groups, i.e. plants with cotyledons and without cotyledons. There groups were further divided and subdivided on the basis of cotyledons and floral characteristics.

Bentham and Hooker's System

George Bentham (1830–1884) and Joseph Hooker (1817–1911) two British Botanists, adopted a very comprehensive, natural system of classification in their published work *Genera Plantarum* (1862–1883), which dominated the botanical science for many years. It is an extension of Candolle's work.

According to this system, the plant kingdom comprises about 97,205 species of seed plants which are distributed in 202 orders and were further divided in families. Dicotyledons have been divided in three divisions on the basis of floral characteristics namely: polypetalae, gamopetalae and monochlamydeae—all the three divisions consisting of total 163 families. Polypetalae have both calyx and corolla with free petals and indefinite number of stamens along with carpels. Gamopetalae have both calyx and corolla, but the latter is always gamopetalous or fused. Stamens are definite and epipetalous along with carpels. In monochlamydeae flowers are incomplete because of the absence of either calyx or corolla, or both the whorls. It generally includes the families which do not come under the above two subclasses.

Following the above scheme of classification Indian senna, *Cassia angustifolia* and Ginger, *Zingiber officinalis* may be referred to its systematic position as mentioned in Table 4.1.

Table 4.1: Scheme of systematic classification of drugs

Division	Phanerogam	Phanerogam
Subdivision	Angiosperm	Angiosperm
Class	Dicotyledonae	Monocotyledonae
Subclass	Polypetalae	–
Series	Calyciflorae	Epigynae
Order	Resales	Scitamineae
Family	Leguminosae	Zingiberaceae
Subfamily	Caesalpinieae	–
Genus	*Cassia*	*Zingiber*
Species	*angustifolia*	*officinalis*

Bentham and Hookers system of classification was accepted throughout the British Empire and in the United States, and was adapted to lesser extent by Continental botanists. It was regarded as the most convenient and suitable for practical utility.

Adolf Engler (1844–1930), a German Botanist published his system of classification in *Die Naturlichen Pflanzenfamilien* in 23 volumes, covering the whole plant kingdom. The increasing complexity of the flowers is considered for classification. Engler believed that woody plants with unisexual and apetalous flowers are most primitive in origin. This is a natural system which is based on the relationships and is compatible with evolutionary principles.

Hutchinson's System of Classification

A British systematic Botanist J. Hutchinson published his work, *The Families of Flowering Plants* in 1926 on Dicotyledons and in 1934 on monocotyledons. Hutchinson made it clear that the plants with sepals and petals are more primitive than the plants without petals and sepals on the assumption that free parts are more primitive than fused ones. He also believed that spiral arrangement of floral parts, numerous free stamens and hermaphrodite flowers are more primitive than unisexual flowers with fused stamens. He considered monochlamydous plants as more advanced than dicotyledons. Hutchinson's system indicates the concept of phylogenetic classification and seems to be an advanced step over the Bentham and Hooker system of classification. Hutchinson accepted the older view of woody and herbaceous plants and fundamentally called them as Lignosae and Herbaceae. He revised the scheme of classification in 1959. Hutchinson placed the gymnosperms first, then the dicotyledons and lastly the monocotyledons.

H. H. Rusby (1931) worked on phylogenic classification. His work is the scathing criticism on the phylogenic system attempted by M. C. Nair, 'Angiosperm Phylogeny on a Chemical basis.' While criticizing M. C. Nair, he indicated that the taxonomists need to study and use all the criteria including chemical nature while working on phylogenic system. He stubbornly criticized a publication on Cinchona that when the whole genus has been thoroughly investigated for its morphology; chemistry, reproduction, embryology, horticulture, ecology and geography, all the information is ignored in the chemotaxonomical study which is a great misfortune to Cinchona literature.

M. P. Morris (1954) worked on chemotaxonomy of toxic cyanogenetic glycosides of *Indigofera endecaphylla* and pointed out that *p*-nitropropionic acid, a hydrolysis product of Hiptagenic acid, occurs in a free state in the plants. His work provided the direction to chemotaxonomy of cyanogenetic principles.

4.3. STUDY OF DIFFERENT TISSUE SYSTEMS

The flowering plants have highly evolved organizations which indicate the structural and functional specialization. Externally these organizations may be regarded as the morphological parts, but internally it can be categorized in cells, tissues and tissue systems. The morphologically

most easily and clearly recognizable units of the plant body are the cells. The united masses of cells are distinct from one another structurally as well as functionally. Such groupings of cells may be referred to as tissues which further may develop into a simpler or complex cellular organization.

The arrangement of various tissues or tissue systems in the plant indicates its specialized nature. For example, vascular tissues are mainly concerned with the conduction of food and water, and for the efficient functioning; a complex network is developed with the places of water intake, sites of food synthesis and with areas of growth, development and storage. In the same way nonvascular tissues are also continually arranged which indicates the specific interrelationship of vascular tissues, storage tissues and supportive tissues. Plant tissues are generally categorized into two categories (as shown in Fig. 4.1).

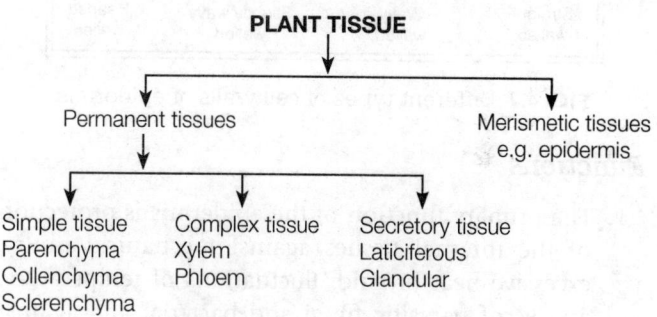

FIG. 4.1. Types of plant tissue

Table 4.2: Difference between merismetic and permanent tissues		
S. no.	**Merismetic Tissue**	**Permanent Tissue**
1.	Comprises of young cells which have the power to redivide and multiply.	These cells are living or dead having attained their definite form and size.
2.	These cells are present at growing points, i.e. tips of roots, shoots and epidermis.	Usually present in the ground tissue and make the fundamental tissue system.
3.	These cells are closely packed without intracellular spaces.	Intracellular spaces are present.

In the plant body, the following three tissue systems can be distinguished.

(A) **Dermal tissue system:** It represents the outer most part of the plant which forms a protective covering line. It includes epidermis, periderm, etc.

(B) **Vascular tissue system:** It is concerned with transmission of material in the plant and represents stellar structures like xylem and phloem.

(C) **Ground tissue system:** It consists of simple cells which may be strengthened by addition of thickened cells. It represents ground tissue made up of parenchyma, collenchyma and sclerenchyma.

Dermal Tissue System

Epidermis

The epidermal tissue system is derived from the dermatogen of the apical meristem and forms the epidermis (*epi - upon, derma - skin*) or outermost skin layer, which extends over the entire surface of the plant body. Epidermis is the outermost layer of the plant consisting normally of a single layer of flattened cells. The walls may be straight, wavy or beaded and often covered with a layer of cuticle made up of cutin (Fig. 4.2).

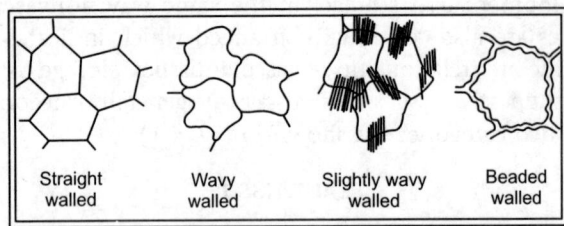

Straight walled | Wavy walled | Slightly wavy walled | Beaded walled

FIG. 4.2 Different types of cell walls of epidermis

Functions

1. The primary function of the epidermis is protection of the internal tissues against mechanical injury, excessive heat or cold, fluctuations of temperature, attacks of parasitic fungi and bacteria, and against the leaching effect of rain. This is possible due to the presence of cuticle, hairs, tannin, gum, etc.
2. Prevention of excessive evaporation of water from the internal tissues by the development of thick cuticles, wax and other deposition, cutinized hairs, scales, multiple epidermis, etc., is another important function of the epidermis.
3. Strong cuticles and cutinized hairs, particularly a dense coating of hairs, protect the plant against intense illumination (i.e. strong sunlight) and excessive radiation of heat.
4. The epidermis also acts as a storehouse of water, as in desert plants.
5. The epidermis sometimes has some minor functions like photosynthesis, secretion, etc.

Stomata (Fig. 4.3)

Stomata are minute openings usually found in the epidermis of the leaves as in Digitalis, Senna, etc., or in young green stems as in Ephedra, in flower as in clove and in fruit as in fennel, orange peel. These openings are surrounded with a pair of kidney-shaped cells called guard cells. The term 'stoma' is often applied to the stomatal arrangement, which consists of slit like opening along with the guard cells. The epidermal cells surrounding the guard cells are called neighbouring cells or subsidiary cells. These, in many cases, as in Digitalis resemble the other epidermal cells, but in large number of plants they differ in size, arrangement and shape from the other epidermal cells.

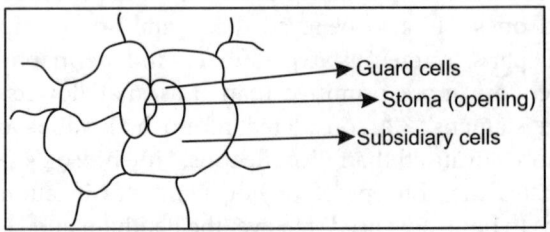

Guard cells
Stoma (opening)
Subsidiary cells

FIG. 4.3 Stomata

Types of stomatal arrangement: According to the arrangement of the epidermal cells surrounding the stomata, they have been grouped as follows (Fig. 4.4):

1. **Diacytic or caryophyllaceous (cross celled):** The stoma is accompanied by two subsidiary cells, the long axis of which is at right angles to that of the stoma. This type of stoma is also, called the Labiatae type as it is found in many plants of the family Labiatae such as vasaka, tulsi, spearmint and peppermint.
2. **Anisocytic or cruciferous (unequal celled):** The stoma is surrounded by usually three subsidiary cells of which one is markedly smaller than the others. This type of stoma is also called the Solanaceous type as it is found in many plants of the family Solanaceae, such as Belladonna, Datura, Hyoscyamus, Stramonium, Tobacco; it is also found in many plants of the family Compositae.

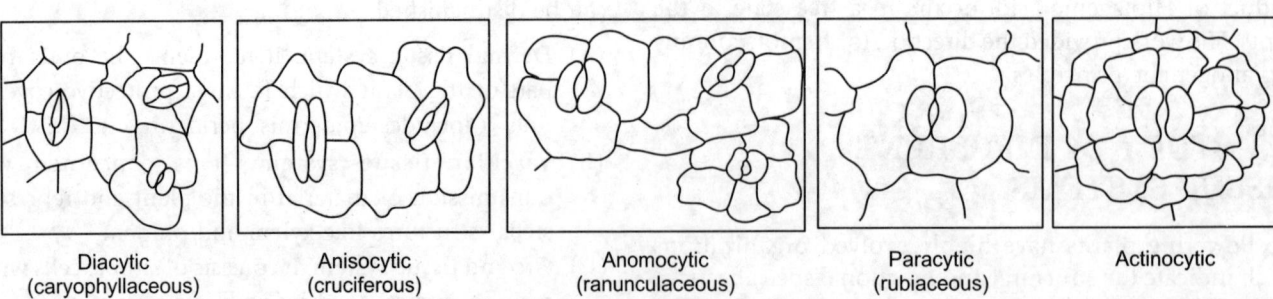

Diacytic (caryophyllaceous) | Anisocytic (cruciferous) | Anomocytic (ranunculaceous) | Paracytic (rubiaceous) | Actinocytic

FIG. 4.4 Different types of stomata

3. **Anomocytic or ranunculaceous (irregular celled):** The stoma is surrounded by a varying number of cells in no way differing from those of the epidermal cells as in Digitalis, eucalyptus, henna, lobelia, neem, etc.

4. **Paracytic or rubiaceous (parallel celled):** The stoma is surrounded usually by two subsidiary cells, the long axis of which are parallel to that of stoma as in Senna and many Rubiaceous plants.

5. **Actinocytic (radiate celled):** The stoma is surrounded by circle of radiating cells, as in *Uva ursi*.

Functions and distributions of stomata: Stomata perform the function of gaseous exchange and transpiration in the plant body. They are most abundant in the lower epidermis of a dorsiventral leaf and less abundant on the upper epidermis. In isobilateral leaves, stomata remain confined to the upper epidermis alone; in submerged leaves no stoma is present. In Buchu and Neem, stomata are present only on lower surface, while in case of Belladonna, Datura, Senna, etc., stomata are present on the both surfaces. The distribution of stoma shows great variation between upper and lower epidermis. In desert plants and in those showing xerophytic adaptations, e.g. Ephedra, Agave, Oleander, etc., stomata are situated in grooves or pits in the stem or leaf. This is a special adaptation to reduce excessive evaporation, as the stomata sunken in pits are protected from gusts of wind.

Trichomes

Trichomes are more elongated outgrowths of one or more epidermal cells, and consist of two carts, a foot or root embedded in the epidermis and a free projecting portion termed as body. Trichomes usually occur in leaves but are also found to be present on some other parts of the plant as in Kurchi, Nux vomica and Strophanthus seeds, Andrographis and Belladonna stem, Cummin, and Lady's finger fruits, etc. Trichomes are rarely present on the leaves of Bearberry, Buchu, Henna, etc., and are absent in glabrous leaves like Coca, Hemlock, Savin, etc.

Functions of trichomes: Trichomes or hairs are adapted to many different purposes. A dense covering of trichomes prevents the damage by insects and the clogging of stomata due to accumulation of dust. Trichomes also aid the dispersion of seeds of Milkweed (Asclepias) and Madar (Calotropis), which are readily scattered by wind. In Peppermint, Rosemary, Tulsi, etc., trichomes perform the function of secreting volatile oil.

Types of trichomes: Broadly, the trichomes are classified as:

1. Covering trichomes or clothing hairs or nonglandular trichomes and
2. Glandular trichomes

Depending upon the structure, shape and number of cells, they are further classified as follows:

[A] *Covering trichomes* (Fig. 4.5)

(a) Unicellular trichomes

1. Linear, strongly waved, thick walled trichomes—*Yerba santa*
2. Linear, thick walled and warty trichomes—*Damiana*
3. Short. conical trichomes—*Tea*
4. Short, conical, warty trichomes—*Senna*
5. Large, conical, longitudinally striated trichomes—*Lobelia*
6. Long, tubular, flattened and twisted trichomes—*Cotton*
7. Lignified trichomes—*Nux vomica, strophanthus*
8. Short, sharp, pointed, curved, conical trichomes—*Cannabis*
9. Unicellular, stellate trichomes—*Deutzia scabra*

(b) Multicellular unbranched trichomes

1. Uniseriate, bicellular, conical—*Datura*
2. Biseriate—*Calendula officinalis*
3. Multiseriate—*Male fern*

(c) Multicellular branched trichomes

1. Stellate (star shaped)—*Hamamelis, Kamala*

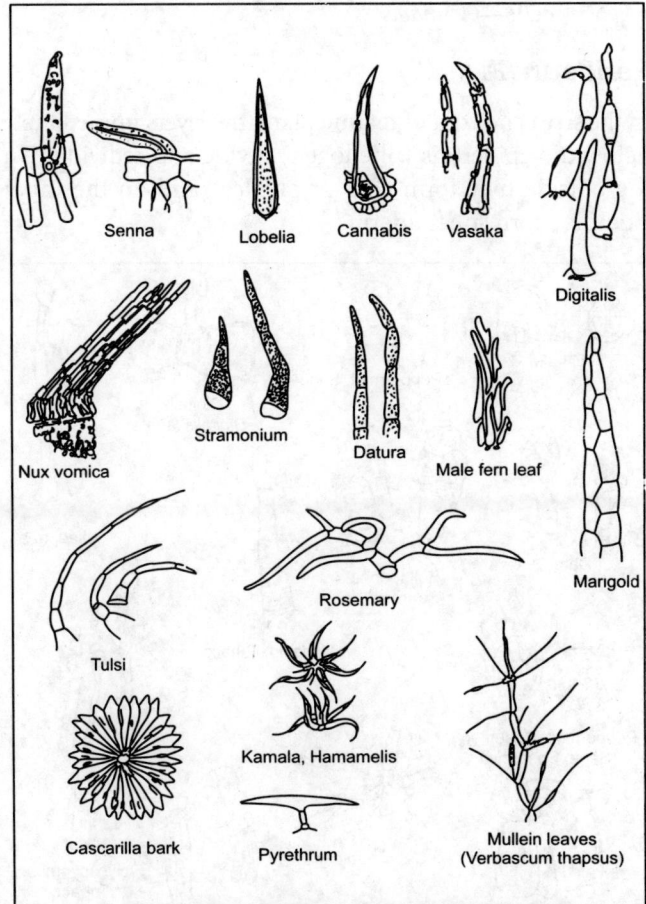

FIG. 4.5 Covering trichomes

2. Peltate (shield-like structure)—*cascarilla*
3. Candelabra (branched)—*Rosemary, Verbascum thapsus*
4. T-shaped trichomes—*Pyrethrum*

[B] Glandular trichomes (Fig. 4.6)

(a) Unicellular glandular trichomes

1. Sessile trichomes—Without stalk - *Piper betel, Vasaka*

(b) Multicellular glandular trichomes

1. Unicellular stalk with single spherical secreting cell at the apex—*Digitalis purpurea*
2. Uniseriate, multicellular stalk with single spherical cell at the apex—*Digitalis thapsi*
3. Uniseriate stalk and bicellular head—*Digitalis purpurea*
4. Multicellular, uniseriate stalk and multicellular head—*Hyoscyamus*
5. Biseriate stalk and biseriate secreting head—*Santonica*
6. Short, unicellular stalk and head formed by a rosette of two to eight club-shaped cells—*Mentha*
7. Multiseriate, multicellular cylindrical stalk and a secreting head of about eight radiating club-shaped cells—*Cannabis*

Periderm (Fig. 4.7)

In the stem and root of mature plant, the layers immediately below the epidermis (phellogen) divide and redivide. On the outside they form cork or phellem and on the inner side they form phelloderm.

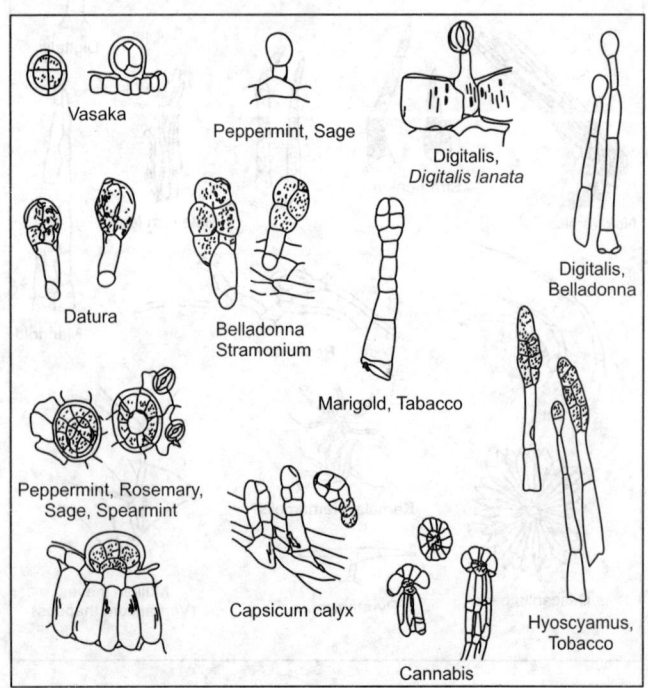

FIG. 4.6 Glandular trichomes

Phellem + Phellogen + Phelloderm = Periderm

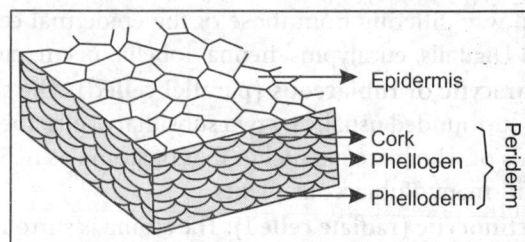

FIG. 4.7 Periderm

The cork cells are rectangular brick shaped or polygonal; phelloderm cells are mostly parenchymatous in nature. Lenticels are present in the periderm, especially in the bark of old plants which are similar in function to stomata. These are open pores with absence of guard cells. The cork cells are impregnated with a layer of suberin. The various types of cork cells are shown in Figure 4.8.

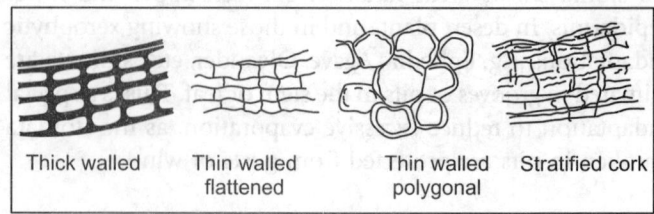

Thick walled | Thin walled flattened | Thin walled polygonal | Stratified cork

FIG. 4.8 Various types of cork cells

Vascular Tissue System

This system consists of a number of vascular bundles which are distributed in the stele. The stele is the central cylinder of the stem and the root surrounded by the endodermis. It consists of vascular bundles, pericycle, pith and medullary rays. Each bundle is made up of xylem and phloem, with a cambium in dicotyledonous stems, or without a cambium in monocotyledonous stems, or only one kind of tissue xylem or phloem, as in roots.

Function

The function of this system is to conduct water and raw food material from the roots to the leaves, and prepared food material from leaves to the storage organs and the growing regions.

The vascular bundle of a dicotyledonous stem, when fully formed, consists of three well-defined tissues:

1. Xylem or wood
2. Phloem or bast
3. Cambium

[1] Xylem

Xylem or wood is a conducting tissue and is composed of elements of different kinds, viz. (a) tracheids, (b) vessels or tracheae, (c) wood fibres and (d) wood parenchyma. Xylem, as a whole, is meant to conduct water and mineral salts upwards from the root to the leaf to give mechanical strength to the plant body.

(a) Tracheids: These are elongated, tube-like cells with hard, thick and lignified walls and large cell cavities. Their ends are tapering, either rounded or chisel-like and less frequently, pointed. They are dead, empty cells and their walls are provided with one or more rows of bordered pits (Fig. 4.9a). Tracheids may also be annular, spiral, scalariform or pitted (with simple pits) (Fig. 4.9b). In transverse section, they are angular—either polygonal or rectangular. Tracheids (and not vessels) occur alone in the wood of ferns and gymnosperms, whereas in the wood of angiosperms, they are associated with the vessels. Their walls being lignified and hard, their function is conduction of water from the root to the leaf.

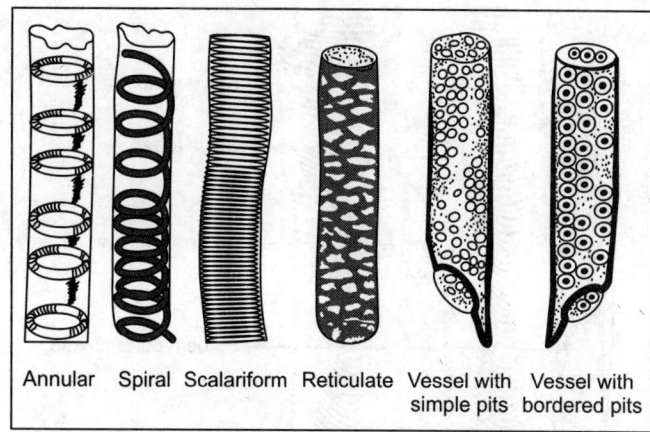

FIG. 4.10 Different kinds of vessels

walled. The wood parenchyma assists, directly or indirectly, in the conduction of water, upwards, through the vessels and the tracheids. It also serves to store food.

[2] Phloem

The phloem or bast is another conducting tissue, and is composed of the following elements: (a) sieve tubes, (b) companion cells, (c) phloem parenchyma and (d) bast fibres (rarely). Phloem, as a whole, is meant to conduct prepared food materials from the leaf to the storage organs and growing regions.

(a) Sieve tubes: Sieve tubes are slender, tube-like structures, composed of elongated cells which are placed end to end. Their walls are thin and made of cellulose. The transverse partition walls are, however, perforated by a number of pores. The transverse wall then looks very much like a sieve, and is called the sieve plate. The sieve plate may sometimes be formed in the side (longitudinal) wall (Fig. 4.11). In some cases, the sieve plate is not transverse (horizontal), but inclined obliquely, and then different areas of it become perforated. A sieve plate of this nature is called a compound plate. At the close of the growing season, the sieve plate is covered by a deposit of colourless, shining substance in the form of a pad, called the callus or callus pad. This consists of carbohydrate, called callose. In winter, the callus completely clogs the pores, but in spring, when the active season begins, it gets dissolved. In old sieve tubes, the callus forms a permanent deposit. The sieve tube contains no nucleus, but has a lining layer of cytoplasm, which is continuous through the pores. Sieve tubes are used for the longitudinal transmission of prepared food materials—proteins and carbohydrates—downward from the leaves to the storage organs, and later upward from the storage organs to the growing regions. A heavy deposit of food material is found on either side of the sieve plate with a narrow median portion.

(b) Companion cells: Associated with each sieve lube and connected with it by pores is a thin-walled, elongated cell

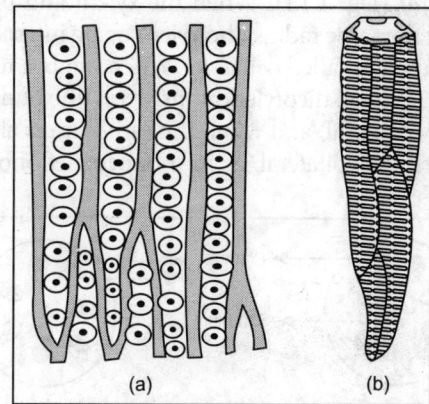

FIG. 4.9 (a) Tracheids with bordered pits; (b) scalariform tracheid

(b) Vessels or tracheae: Vessels are cylindrical, tube-like structures. They are formed from a row of cells placed end to end, from which the transverse partition walls break down. A vessel or trachea is, thus, a tube-like series of cells, very much like a series of water pipes forming a pipeline. Their walls are thickened in various ways, and vessels can be annular, spiral, scalariform, reticulate, or pitted, according to the mode of thickening (Fig. 4.10). Associated with the vessels are often some tracheids. Vessels and tracheids form the main elements of the wood or xylem of the vascular bundle. They serve to conduct water and mineral salts from the roots to the leaves. They are dead, thick-walled and lignified, and as such, they also serve the mechanical function of strengthening the plant body.

(c) Xylem (wood) fibres: Sclerenchymatous cells associated with wood or xylem are known as wood fibres. They occur abundantly in woody dicotyledons and add to the mechanical strength of the xylem and of the plant body as a whole.

(d) Xylem (wood) parenchyma: Parenchymatous cells are of frequent occurrence in the xylem, and are known as wood parenchyma. The cells are alive and generally thin

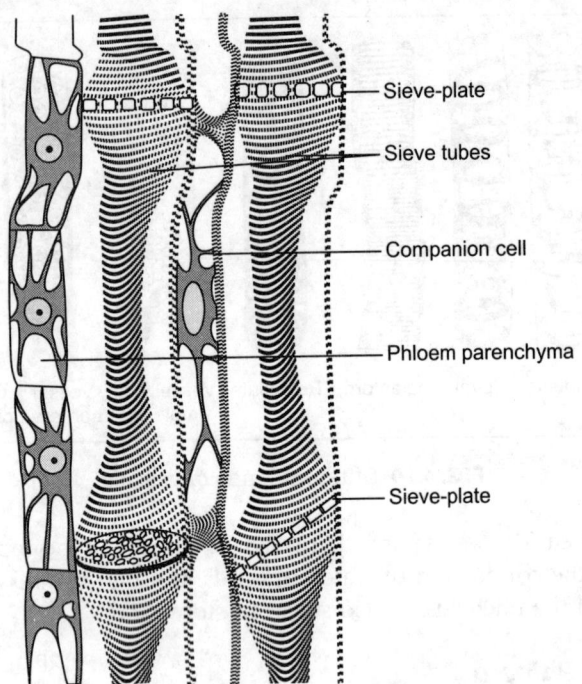

FIG. 4.11 A sieve tube in longitudinal section

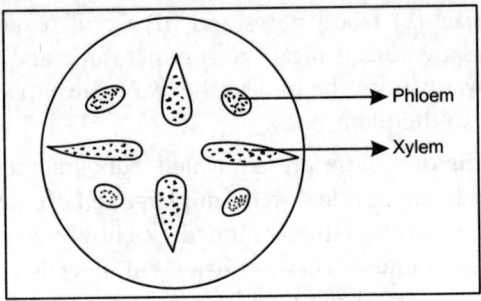

FIG. 4.12 Radial vascular bundle

known as the companion cell. It is living and contains protoplasm and an elongated nucleus. The companion cell is present only in angiosperms (both dicotyledons and monocotyledons). It assists the sieve tube in the conduction of food.

(c) Phloem parenchyma: There are always some parenchymatous cells forming a part of the phloem in all dicotyledons, gymnosperms and ferns. The cells are living, and often cylindrical. They store up food material and help to conduct it. Phloem parenchyma is, however, absent in most monocotyledons.

(d) Bast fibres: Sclerenchymatous cells occurring in the phloem or bast are known as bast fibres. These are generally absent in the primary but occur frequently in the secondary phloem.

[3] Cambium

This is a thin strip of primary meristem lying between the xylem and phloem. It consists of one or a few layers of thin-walled and roughly rectangular cells. Although cambial cells look rectangular in transverse section, they are very elongated, often with oblique ends. They become flattened tangentially, i.e. at right angles to the radius of the stem.

Types of Vascular Bundles

According to the arrangement of xylem and phloem, the vascular bundles are of the following types:

(A) Radial vascular bundle (Fig. 4.12): When the xylem and phloem form separate bundles which lie on different radii,

alternating with each other, as in roots. The radial vascular bundle is the most primitive type of vascular bundles.

(B) Conjoint vascular bundle: When the xylem and phloem combine into one bundle, it is called as conjoint vascular bundle. There are different types of conjoint vascular bundles.

(1) Collateral (Fig. 4.13): When the xylem and phloem lie together on the same radius, the xylem being internal and the phloem external is called collateral. When cambium is present in collateral as in all dicotyledonous stems, the bundle is said to be open collateral, and when the cambium is absent, it is said to be closed collateral, as in monocotyledonous stems.

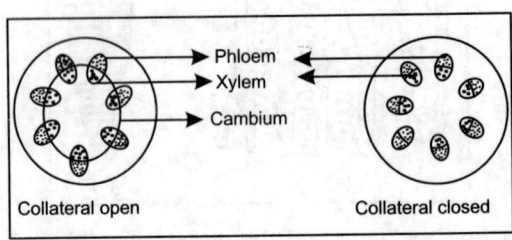

FIG. 4.13 Collateral vascular bundle

(2) Bicollateral (Fig. 4.14):

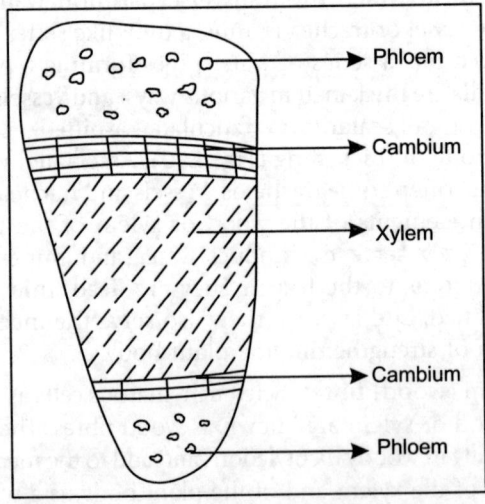

FIG. 4.14 Bicollateral vascular bundle

When the both phloem and cambium occur twice in a collateral bundle—once on the outer side of the xylem and again on the inner side of it, is called as bicollateral. The sequence is outer phloem, outer cambium, xylem, inner cambium and inner phloem. Bicollateral bundles are characteristics of Cucurbitaceae. They are also often found in Solanaceae, Apocynaceae, Convolvulaceae, Myrtaceae, etc. A bicollateral bundle is always open.

(C) Concentric vascular bundle (Fig. 4.15): When one kind of vascular tissue (xylem or phloem) is surrounded by the other is called as concentric vascular bundle. Evidently, there are two types, according to whether one is central or the other one is so. When the phloem lies in the centre and is surrounded by xylem, as in some monocotyledonous, the concentric bundle is said to be amphivasal (leptocentric). When, on the other hand, the xylem lies in the centre and is surrounded by phloem, the concentric bundle is said to be amphicribral (Hadrocentric). A concentric bundle is always closed.

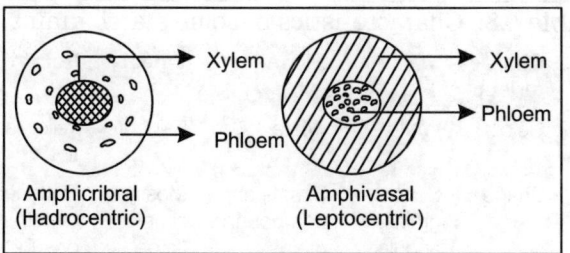

FIG. 4.15 Concentric vascular bundle

Ground Tissue System

Ground tissue system is represented by the cortex, hypodermis, pith, mesophyll and portion of midrib of leaves and comprises of the following tissues.

(a) Parenchyma

The parenchyma consists of a collection of cells which are more or less isodiametric, that is, equally expanded on all sides (Fig. 4.16a). Typical parenchymatous cells are oval, spherical or polygonal. Their walls are thin and made of cellulose. They are usually living. Parenchymatous tissue is of universal occurrence in all the soft parts of plants. Its main function is storage of food material. When parenchymatous tissue contains chloroplasts, it is called chlorenchyma (Fig. 4.16b). Its function is to manufacture food material. A special type of parenchyma develops in many aquatic plants and in the petiole of banana. The wall of each such cell grows out in several places, like rays radiating from a star and is, therefore, stellate or star-like in general appearance. These cells leave a lot of air cavities between them, where air is stored up. Such a tissue is often called aerenchyma (Fig. 4.16c).

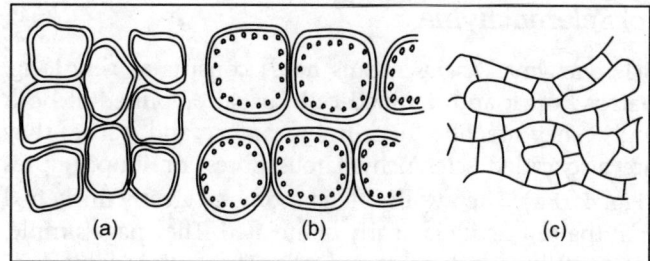

FIG. 4.16 (a) Parenchyma, (b) Chlorenchyma and (c) Aerenchyma

(b) Collenchyma (Fig. 4.17a and b)

This tissue consists of somewhat elongated, parenchymatous cells with oblique, slightly rounded or tapering ends. The cells are much thickened at the corners against the intercellular spaces. They look circular, oval or polygonal in a transverse section of the stem. The thickening is due to a deposit of cellulose, hemicellulose and protopectin. Although thickened, the cells are never lignified. Simple pits can be found here and there in their walls. Their thickened walls have a high refractive index and, therefore, this tissue in section is very conspicuous under the microscope. Collenchyma is found under the skin (epidermis) of herbaceous dicotyledons, e.g. sunflower, gourd, etc., occurring there in a few layers with special development at the ridges, as in gourd stem. It is absent from the root and the monocotyledon, except in special cases. The cells are living and often contain a few chloroplasts. Being flexible in nature, collenchyma gives tensile strength to the growing organs, and being extensible, it readily adapts itself to rapid elongation of the stem. Since it contains chloroplasts, it also manufactures sugar and starch. Its function is, therefore, both mechanical and vital.

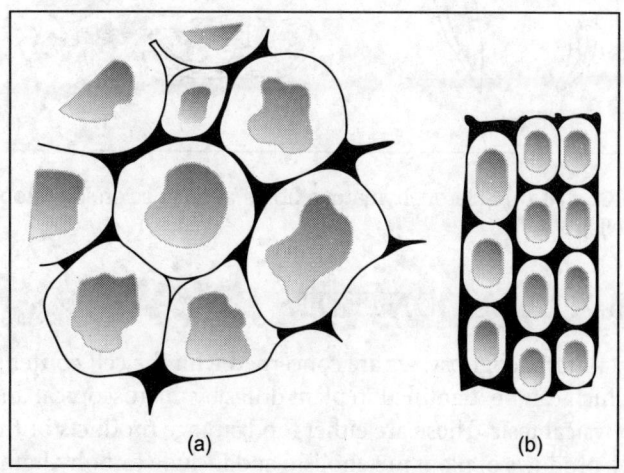

FIG. 4.17 (a) Collenchyma in transaction and (b) Collenchyma in longitudinal section

(c) Sclerenchyma

Sclerenchyma (*scleros* means hard) consists of very long, narrow, thick and lignified cells, usually pointed at both ends. They are fibre-like in appearance and hence, they are also called sclerenchymatous fibres, or simply fibres (Fig. 4.18a). Their walls often become so greatly thickened that the cell cavity is nearly obliterated. They have simple, often oblique, pits in their walls. The middle lamella is conspicuous in sclerenchyma. They are dead cells and serve a purely mechanical function, i.e. they give the requisite strength, rigidity, flexibility and elasticity to the plant body and thus enable it to withstand various strains.

Sclereids: Sometimes, special types of sclerenchyma develop in various parts of the plant body to meet local mechanical needs. They are known as sclereids or stone cells (Fig. 4.18b). They may occur in the cortex, pith, phloem, hard seeds, nuts, stony fruits, and in the leaves and stems of many dicotyledons and also gymnosperms. The cells, though very thick-walled, hard and strongly lignified (sometimes cutinized or suberized), are not long and pointed like sclerenchyma, but are mostly isodiametric, polyhedral, short-cylindrical, slightly elongated or irregular in shape. Usually, they have no definite shape. They are dead cells, and have very narrow cell cavities, which may be almost obliterated, owing to excessive thickness of the cell wall. They may be somewhat loosely arranged or closely packed. They may also occur singly. They contribute to the firmness and hardness of the part concerned.

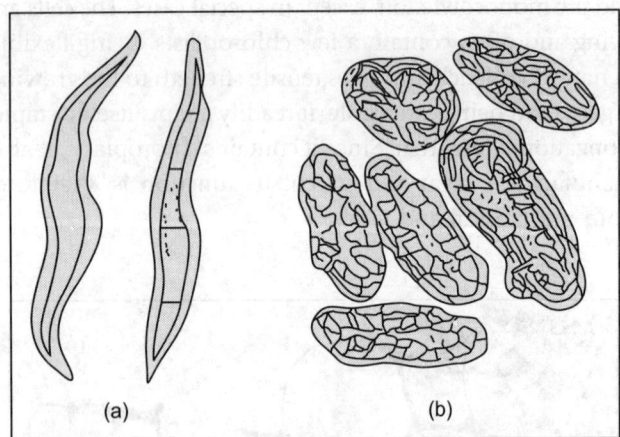

(a)   (b)

FIG. 4.18 (a) Sclerenchymatous fibres and (b) sclereids (stone cells)

4.4. CELL CONTENTS

In pharmacognosy, we are concerned with the cell contents which can be identified in plant drugs by microscopical and physical tests. These are either food storage products or the by-products of plant metabolism and include carbohydrates, proteins, lipids, calcium oxalate, calcium carbonate, tannins, resins, etc. Some of these cell contents of diagnostic importance can be briefly described as follows.

Starch

Starch is present in different parts of the plant in the form of granules of varying size. Starch is found abundantly in fruit, seed, root, rhizome and as smaller grains in chlorophyll containing tissue of the plant such as leaf. Starches of different origins can be identified by studying their size, shape and structure, as well as, position of the hilum and striations. Chemically, starches are polysaccharides containing amylopectin and β-amylose. Starch turns blue to violet when treated with iodine solution.

Starches of pharmaceutical interest are obtained from maize, rice, wheat and potato (Fig. 4.19). These starches can be differentiated from each other by microscopical examination. A comparative account of their macroscopical, microscopical and physical characteristics is given in the Table 4.3. For purpose of microscopical studies, the powder should be mounted in Smiths starch reagent containing equal parts of glycerin, water and 50% acetic acid.

Table 4.3: Characteristics of some starch grains

S. no.	Characteristic	Maize	Rice	Wheat	Potato
1.	Colour	White	White	Faint grey	Yellowish tint
2.	Shape	Simple grains, angular, hilum central, rarely compound grains	Simple or compound grains (2–150 components), polyhedral with sharp angles	Mostly simple (large and small) grains, faint striations, Hilum appears as line	Flattened ovoid or sub-spherical, well-marked striations, hilum eccentric.
3.	Size in µm	5–30	2–10	Small 2–9 Large 10–45	10–100
4.	pH	Neutral	Alkaline	Acidic	Acidic
5.	Moisture content (%v/w)	13	13	13	20
6.	Ash content (%w/w)	0.3	0.6	0.3	0.3

A systematic description of starch grains should include:

1. *Shape*—Ovoid, spherical, subspherical, ellipsoidal, polyhedral, etc.
2. *Size*—Dimensions in µm.
3. *Position of hilum*—Central, eccentric, pointed, radiate, linear, etc.
4. *Aggregation*—Simple, compound; number of components present in a compound grain.

5. Appearance between crossed polaroids.
6. *Location*—Loose, present in type of cell and tissue.
7. *Frequency*—Occasional, frequent, abundant.

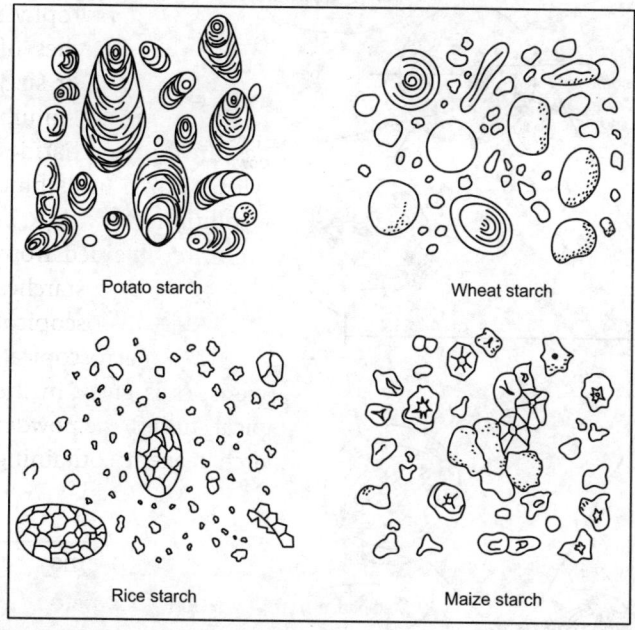

Potato starch   Wheat starch

Rice starch   Maize starch

FIG. 4.19 Starch grains obtained from the different sources

Aleurone Grain

Protein is stored in the form of aleurone grain by plants. Aleurone grain consists of a mass of protein surrounded by a thin membrane, and is found abundantly in the endosperm of the seed. The ground mass of protein, however, often encloses an angular body (crystalloid) arid one or more rounded bodies (globoids).

Defat thin sections containing aleurone grains and treat with the following reagents.

1. *Alcoholic picric acid*—Ground tissue and crystalloid are stained yellow.
2. *Millon's reagent*—Protein is stained red on warming.
3. *Iodine solution*—Only crystalloid and ground substance are stained yellowish brown.

Calcium Oxalate Crystals

Calcium oxalate crystals are considered as excretory products of plant metabolism. They occur in different forms and provide valuable information for identification of crude drugs in entire and powdered forms.

1. *Microsphenoidal or sandy crystals*—Belladonna.
2. *Single acicular crystals*—Cinnamon, gentian,
3. *Prismatic crystals*—Quassia, hyoscyamus, senna, rauwolfia, cascara.
4. *Rosettes crystals*—Stramonium, senna, cascara, rhubarb.
5. *Bundles of acicular crystals*—Squill, ipecacuanha.

The sections to be examined for calcium oxalate should be cleared with caustic alkali or chloral hydrate. These reagents very slowly dissolve the crystals, so the observation should be made immediately after clearing the section. The polarizing microscope is useful in the detection of small crystals.

Mount the cleared section or powder in the following reagents and observe the crystals.

1. *Acetic acid*—Insoluble.
2. *Caustic alkali*—Insoluble.
3. *Hydrochloric acid*—Soluble.
4. *Sulphuric acid* (60% w/w)—Soluble, on standing replaced by needles of calcium sulphate.

Calcium Carbonate

Aggregates of crystals of calcium carbonate are called 'cystoliths', which appear like small bunches of grapes in the tissue. Calcium carbonate dissolves with effervescence in acetic, hydrochloric or sulphuric acid. When treated with 60% w/w sulphuric acid, needled shaped crystals of calcium sulphate slowly separate out.

Fixed Oils and Fats

Fixed oils and fats are widely distributed in both vegetative and reproductive parts of the plant. They are more concentrated in the seeds as reserved lipids. Fixed oils occur as small refractive oil globules, usually present in association with aleurone grains. Fixed oil and fat show certain common characteristics and respond to the following tests:

1. They are generally soluble in ether and alcohol with few exceptions.
2. 1% solution of osmic acid colours them brown or black.
3. Dilute tincture of alkanna stains them red on standing for about 30 minutes.
4. A mixture of equal parts of strong solution of ammonia and saturated solution of potash slowly saponifies fixed oil and fat.

Mucilage

Mucilages are polysaccharide complexes of sugar and uronic acids, usually formed from the cell wall. They are insoluble in alcohol but swell or dissolve in water. The following tests are useful for the detection of mucilage in cells.

1. Solution of ruthenium red stains the mucilage pink. Lead acetate solution is added to prevent undue swelling or solution of the substance being tested.
2. Solution of corallin soda and 25% sodium bicarbonate solution (alkaline solution of corallin) stain the mucilage pink.

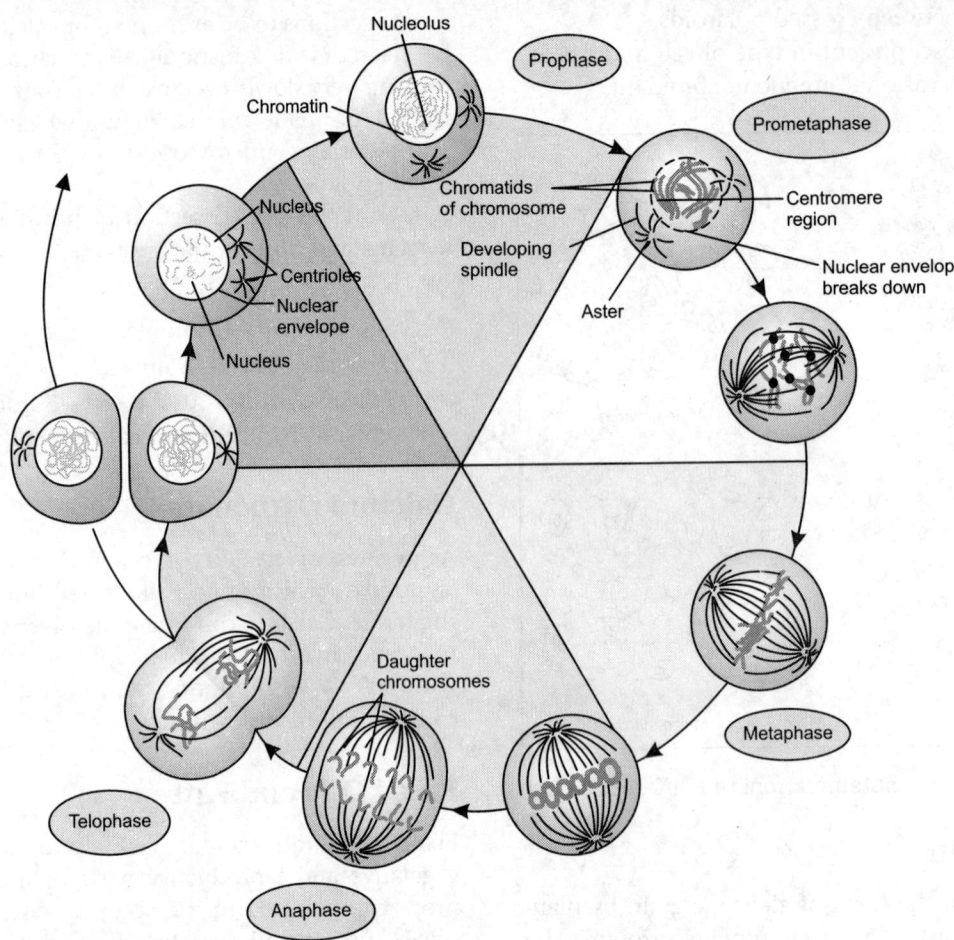

FIG. 4.20 Phases of mitotic cell division

4.5. CELL DIVISION

From the smaller plants like algae to the large trees like eucalyptus, all starts their growth from a single cell called as egg cell. It is brought about by the development of new cells. Two important processes are continued which ultimately helps in the vegetative growth and also in the preservation of hereditary characteristics. It includes the division of nucleus termed as mitosis and the division of cell cytoplasm, referred to as cytokinesis.

Mitosis

Mitosis is a somatic cell division which is responsible for the development of vegetative body of the plants. A German Botanist Stransburger (1875) first studied it in detail. The process of mitotic cell division consists of four important stages, viz. prophase, metaphase, anaphase and telophase (Figure 4.20).

Prophase

This phase of chromosome fixation is the longest one in the mitotic cell division. Firstly, the indistinct chromosomes appear as the recognizable thread. Chromosomes are closely occurring double threads of which each longitudinal half becomes chromatid. Gradually chromosomes are thickened. Chromatid starts dividing longitudinally into two halves along with chromosomal substance matrix around it. Some gap start appearing in the chromosomes which is called as centromeres. At the end of prophase, nucleoli become smaller, matrix becomes clearer and the nucleus enters into metaphase.

Metaphase

During this phase nuclear membrane vanishes and the spindle formation takes place; Bipolar spindle is made up of delicate fibres. Later the nuclear membrane is removed; spindle appears into the nuclear region. Movement of chromosomes to the equatorial plane of spindle separates them from one another. Centromeres are along the equators while the arms of the chromosomes are directed towards the cytoplasm where they are most clearly revealed.

Protometaphase

Nuclear envelope fragments. Microtubes of spindle invade nuclear area and are able to interact with chromosomes. Chromosomes are more condensed. The two chromatids have kinetochore-protein structure. Microtubes attach to kinetochore and move the chromosomes back and forth. The kinetochore that do not attach interact with others from the opposite pole.

Anaphase

In anaphase, chromatid halves move away equatorially at two opposite poles with the tractile fibres. The chromatid separates completely from each other. The spindle undergoes maximum elongation to facilitate separation of diploid chromatids. It is a shortest phase of mitosis.

Telophase

In telophase, chromatids forms the close groups. The polar caps of the spindle disappear and the formation of nuclear membrane takes place around the groups of chromosomes. The matrix and spindle body disappears completely. Appearance of nucleoli and nuclear sap makes them recognizable as two distinct nuclei.

Once again nucleus formed grows in size and starts working as metabolic nuclei to enter again in the cycle of mitotic cell division. It mainly depends upon types of plants, plant part and temperature.

Cytokinesis

Cytokinesis is the partition of cytoplasmic material. It takes place either by formation of new cell walls or by cytoplasmic breakdown. New cells are formed by deposition of cellulosic material in the equatorial zones, which forms the membrane and divide cytoplasm into newly formed cells.

Meiosis

Meiosis is a process of nuclear division in which the numbers of chromosomes are reduced to half (n) from the basic nucleus of 2n chromosomes. A German botanist Stransburger (1888) was the first researcher of this complex genetic process. Chromosomes are called as the carriers of hereditary characters, so the meiosis is the process of transmission of these genetic characteristics. All sexually reproducing plants and animals are gametes with haploid number of chromosomes. Fusion of the male and female gametes results into zygote whereby doubling of chromosomes to 2n takes place to develop offspring.

Meiosis involves two successive divisions: the first process of division I is reduction division, while the second process of division II is similar to that of mitosis, (Figure 4.21).

Division I

In this process of meiosis mother nucleus undergoes complicated changes which can be subdivided into various phases as given below.

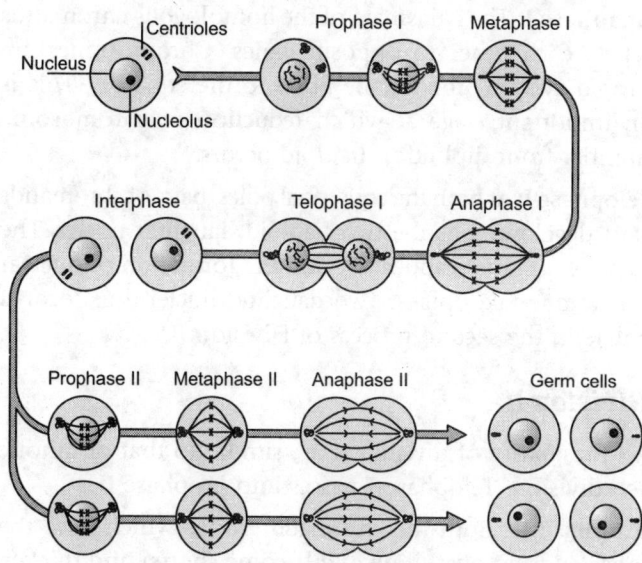

FIG. 4.21 Phases of meiosis

Prophase I: In this phase chromosomes are systematically arranged. This phase is again divided into five different stages:

- *Leptotene:* This is an early prophase in which diploid chromosomes are found as long, single threads of identical pairs. Coiling of these threads of chromosomes occurs.
- *Zygotene:* Identical chromosomes gets attracted towards each other and the pairs are developed throughout their length. This pairing is termed as synapsis. The chromosomes thus paired are homologous in nature.
- *Pachytene:* The pairs of chromosomes go shorter and thicker due to coiling. Longitudinal splitting in it gives rise to four chromatids from each chromosome. This is a longer phase of prophase I.
- *Diplotene:* This is a stage where separation of chromatids takes place. Their point of attachment remains at a single point known as chiasmata. At this stage the exchange of the genetic material occurs due to crossing over, a prominent feature of meiosis. With further thickening and shortening of chromosomes, diplotene ends into diakinesis.
- *Diakinesis:* In this last stage of prophase I, two halves of the chromosome starts moving equatorially. Chiasmata remain as a point of attachment. Nucleolus disappears and nuclear membrane gets dissolved to release the chromosomes in cytoplasm. Nuclear spindle formation begins at the end of diakinesis.

Metaphase I: In this phase both the chromatids starts moving to two opposite poles of the spindle. In mitotic metaphase chromosomes are lined up at the opposite poles while in meiosis chiasmata remains attached to spindle fibres at the opposite poles.

Anaphase I: The chiasmata of the homologous chromatids repels each other to opposite poles. Chromosomes are carried away by the tractile fibres to the equators. This is an important stage at which reduction of chromosome number from diploid to haploid occurs.

Telophase I: At both the equatorial poles, pairs of chromatids start developing as the two haploid daughter nuclei. The nucleolus starts reappearing and the formation of nuclear membrane takes place. Two daughter nuclei thus formed enters in the second process of Division II.

Division II

All the phases of division II are similar to that of mitotic cell division. Telophase I passes into prophase II.

Prophase II: Both the chromatid groups which have the loose ends go on coiling and become shorter and thicker. Nucleolus and nuclear membrane vanishes and spindle fibres show its appearance.

Metaphase II: In Metaphase II, chromatids once again starts separating equatorially at two opposite poles. Pairs of chromatids separate completely with its own centromere and ends in Anaphase II.

Anaphase II: At the stage of Anaphase II, two sister chromatids of each pair of chromosome move to opposite poles of the spindle as directed by the centromeres.

Telophase II: In Telophase II, both the polar groups of chromosomes are converted to the nuclei by formation of nuclear membrane.

Lastly via cytokinesis four daughter cells are formed each having the haploid or 'n' number of chromosomes.

4.6. MORPHOLOGICAL STUDY

The abundance of plants and their size from bacteria to huge trees make it difficult to study their morphological characters. Classification of plants has solved the problem to a greater extent. Still it is impossible to define precisely the plant body as made up of certain parts only. Plants exhibit vividness in several respects.

The details of morphological characters of these plant organs are as under.

Morphology of Bark

The bark (in commerce) consists of external tissues lying outside the cambium, in stem or root of dicotyledonous plants. Following are the tissues present in bark:

Cork (phellem), phellogen and phelloderm (collectively known as periderm), cortex, pericycle, primary phloem and secondary phloem.

In Botany, the bark consists of periderm phytissues lying outside it, i.e. cork, phellogen and phelloderm.

Methods of collection of barks

Bark is generally collected in spring or early summer because the cambium is very active and thin walled and gets detached easily. Following are the methods of collection of barks.

1. Felling method: The fully grown tree is cut down near the ground level by an axe. The bark is removed by making suitable longitudinal and transverse cuts on the stem and branches. The disadvantages of this method are (a) the plant is fully destroyed and (b) the root bark is not utilized.

2. Uprooting method: In this method, the stem of definite age and diameter are cut down, the root is dug up and bark is collected from roots, stems and branches. In Java, cinchona bark is collected by this method.

3. Coppicing method: The plant is allowed to grow up to certain age and diameter. The stems are cut at a certain distance from ground level. Bark is collected from stem and branches. The stumps remaining in the ground are allowed to grow up to certain level; again the shoots are cut to collect the bark in the same manner. Cascara bark and Ceylon cinnamon bark are collected by this method.

The following features may be used to describe the morphology of bark (Fig. 4.22).

1. Shape: The shape of the bark depends upon the mode of cuts made and the extent and shrinkage occurred during drying.

(a) Flat: When the large piece of the bark is collected from old trunk and dried under pressure, the bark is flat, e.g. Quillaia and Arjuna bark.

(b) Curved: Here, both the sides of the bark are curved inside, e.g. Wild cherry, Cassia and Cascara barks.

(c) Recurved: Both sides of bark are curved outside, e.g. Kurchi bark.

(d) Channelled: When the sides of bark are curved towards inner side to form channel, e.g. Cascara, Cassia and Cinnamon barks.

(e) Quill: If one edge of bark covers the other edge, it is called quill, e.g. Ceylon, Cinnamon and Cascara barks.

(f) Double quill: Here, both the edges curve inward to form double quill, e.g. Cinnamon and Cassia barks.

(g) Compound quill: When the quills of smaller diameter are packed into bigger quills, it is called compound quills. Compound quills are formed to save the space in packing and transportation, e.g. Cinnamon bark.

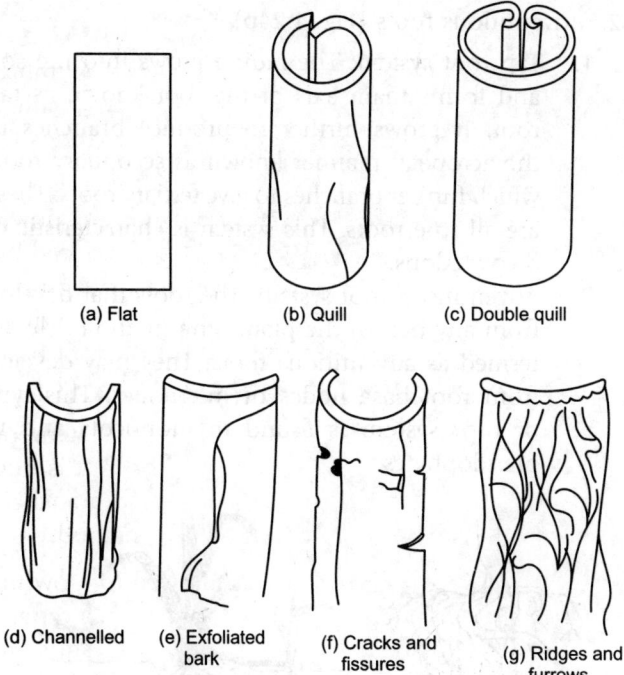

(a) Flat   (b) Quill   (c) Double quill

(d) Channelled   (e) Exfoliated bark   (f) Cracks and fissures   (g) Ridges and furrows

FIG. 4.22 Morphological characters of bark

2. Outer surface:

(a) Smooth: When development of cork is even, e.g. Arjuna bark.

(b) Lenticels: They are transversely elongated holes formed on outer surface because of lateral pressure, e.g. Wild Cherry and Cascara barks.

(c) Cracks and fissures: They are formed due to increase in diameter, e.g. Cinchona bark.

(d) Longitudinal wrinkles: They are formed because of shrinkage of soft tissues, e.g. Cascara bark.

(e) Furrows: If troughs between wrinkles are wide, it is called furrows, e.g. Cinchona calisaya bark.

(f) Exfoliation: Sometimes the cork of bark flakes off exposing cortex, e.g. in Wild cherry bark.

(g) Rhytidoma: It is composite dead tissue consisting of alternate layers of cork, cortex and/or phloem, e.g. Quillaia and Tomentosa barks. Sometimes it is removed during peeling.

(h) Corky warts: They are the small circular patches, found sometimes in old barks, e.g. in *Cinchona succirubra* and Ashoka bark.

(i) Epiphytes: Such as moss, lichen and liverworts are sometimes seen in bark, e.g. Cascara bark.

3. Inner surface: The colour and condition of inner surface is of diagnostic value.

(a) Striations: When parallel longitudinal ridges are formed during drying, it is called striations; it may be fine or coarse, e.g. Cascara bark.

(b) Corrugations: They are the parallel transverse wrinkles formed due to longitudinal shrinkage, e.g. Cascara bark.

4. Fracture: The appearance of exposed surface of transversely broken bark is called fracture. Different types of fracture, their descriptions and examples are given in Table 4.4.

TABLE 4.4: Various types of fracture of bark

S. no.	Type	Description	Examples of barks
1.	Short	Smooth	Cassia, Cinnamon, Cascara
2.	Granular	Shows grain-like minute prominences	Wild cherry
3.	Splintery	Shows uneven projecting points	Quillaia
4.	Fibrous	Shows thread-like fibres	Cascara
5.	Laminated	Shows tangentially elongated layers	Quillaia

Histology of barks

The bark shows following microscopical character:

(i) Tabular, radially arranged cork cells, may be suberized or lignified (e.g. in Cassia bark).

(ii) Thin-walled cellulosic parenchymatous phellogen and phelloderm.

(iii) Collenchymatous and/or parenchymatous cortex.

(iv) Parenchymatous or sclerenchymatous pericycle; may contain band of stone cells and fibres.

(v) Primary phloem which is generally crushed, e.g. in Cascara and Arjuna.

(vi) Secondary phloem consisting of sieve tubes, companion cells, phloem parenchyma, phloem fibres and stone cells. Phloem fibres are thick walled, lignified, e.g. in Cinchona and Cascara; stone cells are thick, lignified with narrow lumen, e.g. Kurchi and Cinnamon barks; sometimes branched stone cells are seen in Wild cherry bark.

(vii) Thin walled, living radially elongated medullary ray cells which are uni-, bi- or multiseriate and straight or wavy.

(viii) Starch, calcium oxalate, oil cells, mucilage, etc., are often present in cortex.

Morphology of Roots

Root is a downward growth of the plant into the soil. It is positively geotropic and hydrotropic. Radicle from the germinating seed grows further into the soil to form the root. It produces similar organs. Root does not have nodes or internodes. Branching of the root arises from the pericyclic tissues. Roots are covered by root caps or root heads.

[A] Functions of roots

1. Roots fix the plant to the soil and give mechanical support to the plant body.
2. Roots absorb water and the minerals dissolved in it from the soil and transport them to the aerial parts where they are needed.
3. At times, the root undergoes modification and performs special functions like storage, respiration, reproduction, etc.

[B] Various parts of a root

A typical underground root exhibits the following parts (Fig. 4.23):

1. Root cap: The tip of the root is very delicate and is covered by root cap. Root cap protects the growing cells and as and when it is worn out it is replaced by the underlying tissues immediately.
2. Region of cell division: The next layer of tissue lying immediately after the root cap towards the stem is the meristematic tissue producing new cells, known as region of cell division or growing region.
3. Region of elongation: The newly formed cells in the growing region grow further by elongation in this region resulting in the increase in the length of the root.
4. Region of root hairs: Above the region of elongation is the region of root hairs wherein the root hairs, the unicellular, tubular outgrowths formed by the epiblema are formed. They are responsible for strengthening the hold of root into the soil and also for the absorption of water.
5. Region of maturation: It is located above the region of root hairs. It does not absorb anything, but is mainly responsible for the absorbed material by roots. The root branches or the lateral roots are produced in this region.

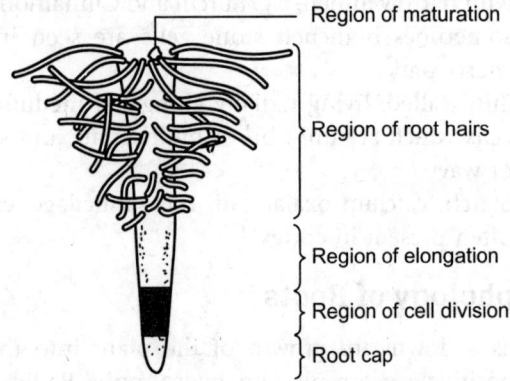

FIG. 4.23 Apex of root showing different regions

[C] Types of roots

There are two types of root systems:

1. Tap root system or primary roots (Fig. 4.24a)

2. Adventitious roots (Fig. 4.24b)

1. Tap root system: The radicle grows into the soil and forms main axis of the root known as tap root. It grows further to produce branches in the acropetal manner known as secondary roots which further branches to give tertiary roots. These are all true roots. This system is characteristic of dicotyledons.
2. Adventitious root system: The roots that develop from any part of the plant other than radicle are termed as adventitious roots. They may develop from root base nodes or internodes. This type of root system is found in monocots and in pteridophytes.

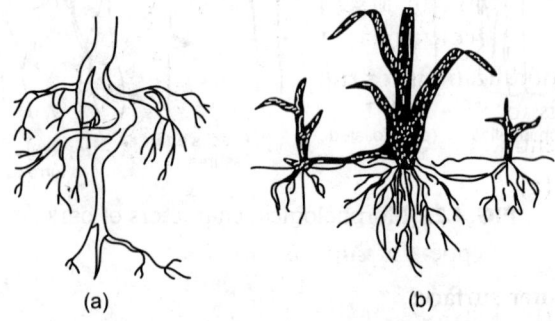

(a)   (b)

FIG. 4.24 (a) Tap root system and (b) adventitious root system

I. Modification for storage of food: This type of modification is shown by both the types of roots, i.e. tap roots and adventitious roots. They store carbohydrates and are used during early growth of successive season.

(i) Tap roots show the following three types of modifications:

(a) Conical (Fig. 4.25a): These are cone-like, broader at the base and tape-ring at the tip, e.g. carrot.
(b) Fusiform (Fig. 4.25b): These roots are more or less spindle shaped, i.e. tapering at both the ends, e.g. radish.
(c) Napiform (Fig. 4.25c): These are spherical shaped and very sharply tapering at lower part, e.g. beat and turnip.

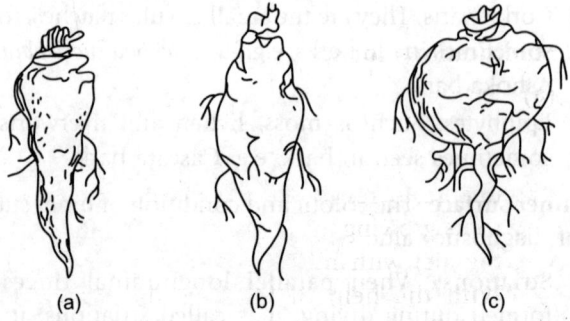

(a)   (b)   (c)

FIG. 4.25 (a) Conical root, (b) fusiform root and (c) napiform root

(ii) Adventitious root show the following types of modifications. They store carbohydrates but do not assume any special shape.

(a) Tuberous roots: These get swollen and form single or isolated tuberous roots which are fusiform in shape, e.g. sweet potato, jalap, aconite.

(b) Fasciculated tuberous roots: When several tuberous roots occur in a group or cluster at the base of a stem they are termed as fasciculated tuberous roots as in dahlia, asparagus.

(c) Palmated tuberous roots: When they are exhibited like palm with fingers as in common ground orchid.

(d) Annulated roots: The swollen portion is in the form of a series of rings called annules as in ipecacuanha.

II. Modifications for support: Plant develops special aerial roots to offer additional support to the plant by way of adventitious roots.

(a) Clinging or climbing roots (Fig. 4.26a): These types of roots are developed by plants like black pepper for support or for climbing purposes at nodes.

(b) Stilt roots (Fig. 4.26b): This type of root is observed in maize and screw-pine, which grow vertically or obliquely downwards and penetrate into soil and give additional support to the main plant.

(c) Columnar roots (Fig. 4.26c): In certain plants like banyan, the additional support is given by specially developed pillars or columnar roots. They even perform the function of regular roots.

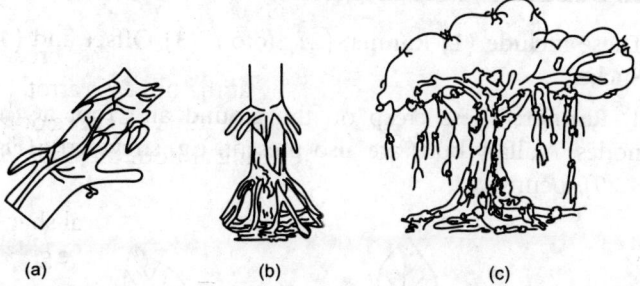

(a)   (b)   (c)

FIG. 4.26 (a) Climbing root, (b) stilt root and (c) columnar root

III. Modifications for special functions:

(a) Respiratory roots or pneumatophores (Fig. 4.27): The roots of the plant growing in marshy places on seashores due to continuous water logging are unable to respire properly. They develop some roots growing against the gravitational force (in the air) with minute openings called lenticels. With the help of lenticels they carry on the exchange of gases. They look like conical spikes around the stems. This type of root is observed in case of plants called mangroves found in creeks, i.e. avicennia.

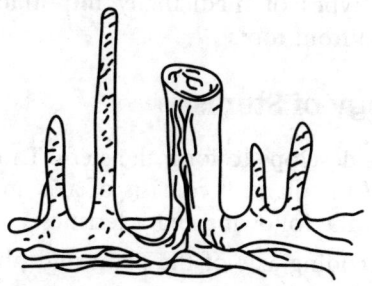

FIG. 4.27 Respiratory roots

(b) Sucking roots or haustoria: The plants, which are total parasites on the host, develop special type of roots for the purpose of absorption of food material from, the host. These roots neither possess root caps nor root hairs, and are known as sucking roots, e.g. cuscuta, striga and viscum.

(c) Photosynthetic roots: Aerial roots in some cases, specially in leafless epiphytes become green in colour on exposure to sunlight and perform photosynthesis and are known as photosynthetic roots as in case of *Tinospora cordifolia*.

(d) Epiphytic or assimilatory roots: The plants which grow on the branches or stems of the plants without taking any food from them are called epiphytic and the roots developed by them are the epiphytic roots. They consist of the following:

(i) Clinging roots with which they get fixed with the host and

(ii) Aerial roots which hang freely in the air, which are normally long greenish white in colour and absorb moisture from the atmosphere with the help of porous tissue. These roots are devoid of root caps and root hairs. They carry on photosynthesis. These are developed in the plants growing in humid atmosphere. Bulbophyllum, uanda are the examples of this type.

(e) Nodulated roots or root tubercles: The plants belonging to leguminosae family develop nodules or tubercles. These are formed by nitrogen fixing bacteria and getting carbohydrates from the plants. Roots and bacteria are symbiotic to each other. These swellings developed by roots are nodulated roots.

Uses of roots

1. Source of food and vegetables: Most of vegetables constitute roots only, i.e. radish, turnip, beet, carrot, etc. They are rich sources of vitamins or their precursors.

Some of them like sweet potato and tapioca are rich in starch, and hence are consumed as food.

2. Various types of medicinally important drugs are obtained from roots.

Morphology of Stems

The plumule develops to form the stem. Thus stem is an aerial part of the plant. It consists of axis and the leaves. Stem has got the following characteristics:

1. It is ascending axis of the plant and phototropic in nature.
2. It consists of nodes, internodes and buds.
3. It gives rise to branches, leaves and flowers.
4. Stems may be aerial, subaerial and underground.

Depending upon the presence of mechanical tissues, the stems may be weak, herbaceous or woody.

[A] Weak stems: When the stems are thin and long, they are unable to stand erect, and hence may be one of the following types:

1. Creepers or prostate stem: When they grow flat on the ground with or without roots, e.g. grasses, gokhru, etc.
2. Climbers: These are too weak to stand alone. They climb on the support with the help of tendrils, hooks, prickles or roots, e.g. *Piper betel, Piper longum.*
3. Twinners: These coil the support and grow further. They are thin and wiry, i.e. ipomoea.

[B] Herbaceous and woody stems: These are the normal stems and may be soft or hard and woody, i.e. sunflower, sugarcane, mango, etc.

1. Produce leaves and exposes them properly to sunlight for carrying out photosynthesis.
2. Conducts water and minerals from roots to leaves and buds.
3. Foods produced by leaves are transported to nongreen parts of the plant.
4. Produce flowers and fruits for pollination and seal dispersal.
5. Depending upon the environment it gets suitably modified to perform special functions like storage of foods, means of propagation, etc.

I. Underground modifications of stems

Underground modifications of stems are of the following types:

1. Rhizome
2. Tuber
3. Bulb
4. Corm

1. **Rhizomes:** Grow horizontal under the soil. They are thick and are characterized by the presence of nodes, internodes and scale leaves. They also possess bud in the axil of the scale leaves, e.g. ginger, turmeric, rhubarb, male fern, etc.

2. **Tubers:** Tubers are characterized by the presence of 'eyes' from the vegetative buds which grow further and develop into a new plant. Tubers are the swollen underground structure of the plant, e.g. potato, jalap, aconite, etc.

3. **Bulb:** In this case, the food material is stored in fleshy scales that overlap the stem. They are present in the axils of the scales, and few of them develop into new plant in the spring season at the expense of stored food material in the bulb. Adventitious roots are present at the base of the bulb. The reserve food material formed by the leaves is stored at their bases, and the new bulbs are produced next year, e.g. squill, garlic (Fig. 4.28a) and onion (Fig. 4.28b).

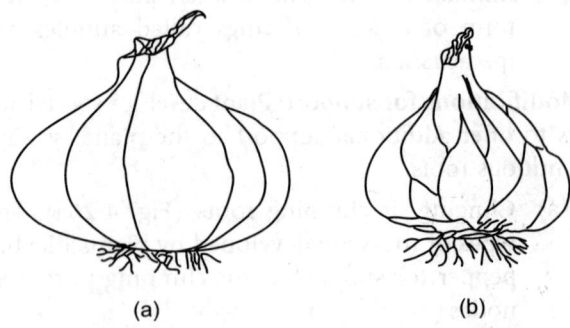

(a)   (b)

FIG. 4.28 Bulbs: (a) onion and (b) garlic

4. **Corm:** Corms are generally stout, and grow in vertical direction. They bear bud in the axil of the scaly leaves, and these buds then develop further to form the new plant. Adventitious roots are present at the base of the corm, e.g. saffron, colchicum, dioscorea, etc.

II. Subaerial modifications of stems

These include (1) Runner, (2) Stolon, (3) Offset and (4) Sucker.

1. **Runner:** These creep on the ground and root at the nodes. Axillary buds are also present, e.g. strawberry (Fig. 4.29), pennywort.

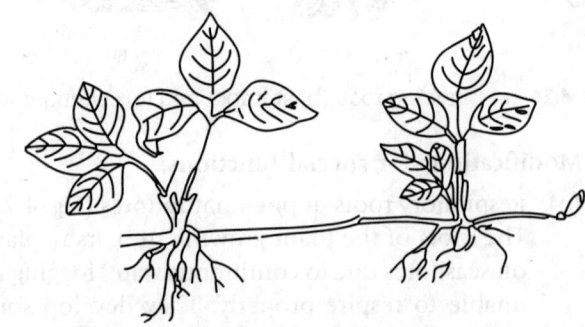

FIG. 4.29 Strawberry runner

2. **Stolon:** These are lateral branches arising from the base of the stems which grow horizontally. They are characterized by the presence of nodes and internodes. Few branches

growing above the ground develop into a new plant, e.g. glycyrrhiza, arrowroot, jasmine, etc.

3. **Offsets:** These originate from the axil of the leaf as short, thick horizontal branches and also characterized by the presence of rosette type leaves and a cluster of roots at their bottom, e.g. aloe, valerian.

4. **Sucker** (Fig. 4.30): These are lateral branches developed from underground stems. Suckers grow obliquely upwards, give rise to a shoot which develop further into a new plant, e.g. mentha species, chrysanthemum, pineapple, banana, etc.

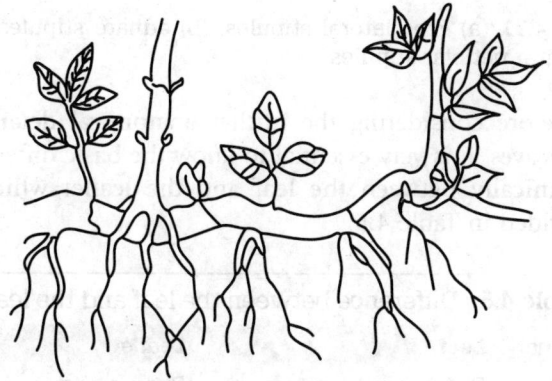

FIG. 4.30 Sucker of mentha

III. Aerial modification of stems

As the name indicates they grow into the air above the soil to a certain height, as follows:

1. **Phylloclades:** At times, the stem becomes green and performs the function of leaves. Normally this is found in the plants growing in the desert (xerophytes). Phylloclades are characterized by the presence of small leaves or pointed spines, e.g. opuntia, ruscus, euphorbia, etc.

Cladode is a type of phylloclade with one internode, i.e. *asparagus.*

2. **Thorns and prickles:** This is another type of aerial modification meant for protection. Thorns are hard, pointed, straight structures, such as duranta (Fig. 4.31a), lemon, etc. Prickles and thorns are identical in function. Prickles get originated from outer tissues of the stem. Thus, they are superficial outgrowths. Prickles are sharp, pointed and curved structures. They are scattered all over the stem. Rose (Fig. 4.31b), smilax can be quoted as examples of the same.

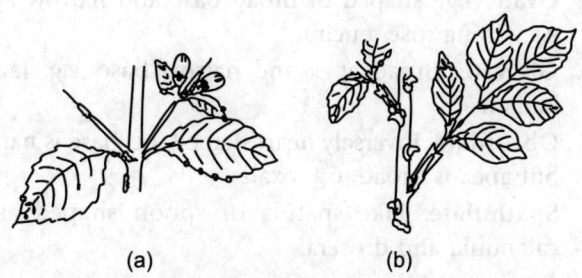

(a)   (b)

FIG. 4.31 (a) Thorns of duranta and (b) rose prickles

3. **Stem tendrils:** In certain plants, the buds develop into tendrils for the purpose of support. Terminal buds in case of vitis, axillary bud in case of passiflora are suitable examples.

4. **Bulbils:** These are modifications of floral buds meant for vegetative propagation, such as *Dioscorea* (Fig. 4.32) and *Agave.*

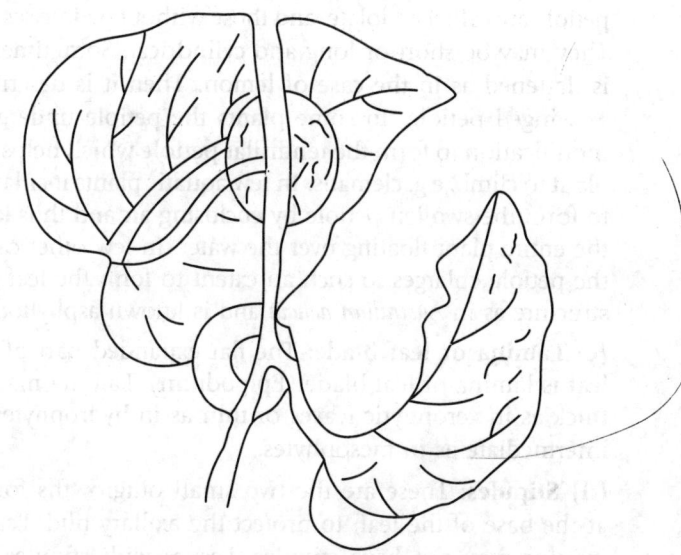

FIG. 4.32 Bulbil of *Dioscorea*

Uses of stems

Depending upon the structural and chemical contents, stems are used for various purposes.

1. Underground stems in their various forms are either used as food spices or for culinary purposes like, potato, amorphophallus, colocasia, garlic, ginger and onion.
2. Jowar, rice and other stems are used as fodder.
3. Stems of jute, hemp and flax as sources of industrial fibres used for various purposes.
4. Sugarcane stems are used as source of sucrose while latex from stems of *Hevea brasiliensis* is used as rubber.
5. Woods from stems of several plants are used as drugs like quassia, guaicum, sandalwood, etc.
6. The stems of several plants are injured to produce gums for their multiple industrial uses like gum-acacia, gum-tragacanth, gum-sterculia, etc.

Morphology of Leaves

Leaves are flat, thin green, appendages to the stem, containing supporting and conducting strands in their structure. They develop in such a way that older leaves are placed at the base while the younger ones at the apex.

[A] A typical angiospermic leaf consists of the following parts:

(a) Leaf base or hypopodium: By means of which it is attached to the stem.

(b) Petiole: It is the stalk of leaf with which leaf blade is attached to the stem. It is also known as mesopodium. It may be present in leaf or may be absent in leaf. Leaves with petiole are called petiolate, and those without petiole sessile. They may be short or long and cylindrical. Sometimes, it is flattened as in the case of lemon. Then it is described as winged petiole. In some plants the petiole undergoes modification to form the tendrillar petiole which helps the plant to climb, e.g. clematis. In few aquatic plants it enlarges to form the swollen petiole by enclosing air and thus keep the entire plant floating over the water. In few other cases, the petiole enlarges to such an extent to form the leaf like structure as in *Australian acacia* and is known asphyllode.

(c) Lamina or leaf blade: The flat expanded part of the leaf is lamina or leaf blade (Epipodium). Lamina may be thick as in xerophytic leaves or thin as in hydrophytes or intermediate as in mesophytes.

(d) Stipules: These are the two small outgrowths found at the base of the leaf, to protect the axillary bud. Leaves may or may not have stipules. Leaves with stipules are described as stipulate, while those without stipules are described as ex-stipulate.

Some stipules perform special functions and hence are put into following types:

1. *Tendrillar stipules:* The stipules get modified into coiled, tendrils helping the plant to climb, i.e. Indian sarsaparilla (Smilax microphylla).

2. *Foliaceous stipules:* In case of plants with compound leaves some of the leaflets get converted into tendril and the stipules expand to form the flat surface and carry on photosynthesis, i.e. *Lathyrus or Pisum.*

3. *Bud stipules:* Scaly stipules of the *Ficus sp.* are characteristic, which protect the terminal vegetative bud. With the development and unfolding of the leaf the bud stipule falls off.

4. *Spiny stipules:* In some plants, the stipules get converted into spines and help against browsing animals as in the case of *Acacia* and *Zizyphus.*

There are five types of stipules which are as under:

1. *Free lateral* (Fig. 4.33a): These are free and located on either side of the leaf as in China rose.

2. *Adnate* (Fig. 4.33b): When the stipules unite with the petioles forming wing like structure are known as adnate stipules, i.e. Groundnut, rose, etc.

3. *Inter-petiolar* (Fig. 4.33c): When stipules are located in between the two petioles of two leaves as in ixora.

4. *Axillary:* When two stipules unite becoming axillary to the leaves.

5. *Ochreate stipules:* These form a hollow tube around the stem as in *Polygonum.*

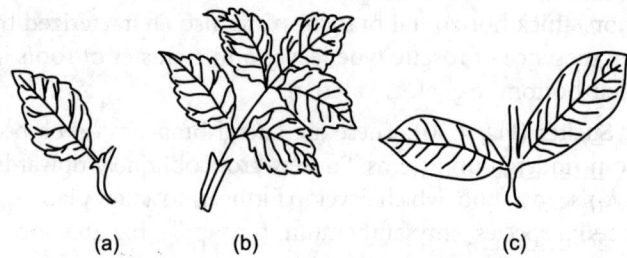

FIG. 4.33 (a) Free lateral stipules, (b) adnate stipules and (c) inter petiolar stipules

Before considering the further anatomical details of the leaves, it is very essential to know the basic difference botanically between the leaf and the leaflet which is provided in Table 4.5.

Table 4.5: Difference between the leaf and the leaflet

S. no.	Leaf	Leaflet
1.	Bud or branch is present in the axil	Bud is absent
2.	Leaves are solitary and are arranged spirally	These are arranged in pairs
3.	These lie in different planes	Leaflets lie in the same plane
4.	Symmetrical at the bases, i.e. *belladonna, vasaka, eucalyptus,* etc.	Asymmetrical at bases, i.e. *rose, senna, acacia, etc.*

[B] Shape of the lamina of leaves (Fig. 4.34)

Various shapes of the leaves are due to various types or shapes of lamina. It may be one of the following:

1. **Acicular:** Needlelike, i.e. *pinus.*
2. **Subulate:** With acute apex and recurved point, i.e. Ephedra sinica.
3. **Linear:** When it is long, narrow and flat, i.e. grasses.
4. **Oblong:** Broad leaves with two parallel margins and abruptly tapering apex, i.e. banana.
5. **Lanceolate:** Which look like lance or spear shaped, e.g. nerium, senna.
6. **Ovate:** Egg shaped or broad base and narrow apex, e.g. China rose, buchu.
7. **Obovate:** Broad apex and narrow base, e.g. Jangli-badam.
8. **Obcordate:** Inversely heart shaped, i.e. base is narrow but apex is broad, e.g. oxalis.
9. **Spathulate:** Like spatula or spoon shaped as in calendula and drosera.
10. **Cuneate:** Wedge shaped as in pista.
11. **Cordate:** Heart shaped, i.e. betel.

12. **Sagittate:** Arrow shaped such as in arum.
13. **Hastate:** When the two lobes of sagittate leaf are directed outwards as in ipomoea.
14. **Reniform:** Kidney shaped, i.e. Indian pennywort.
15. **Auriculate:** When the leaf has got ear like projections at the base.
16. **Lyrate:** When it is lyre shaped or the blade is divided into lobes with large marginal lobe, i.e. radish mustard.
17. **Runcinate:** With the lobes convex before and straight behind, pointing backward like the teeth of the double saw, i.e. dandelion leaf.
18. **Rotund (Orbicular):** When the blade is circular or round, e.g. lotus.
19. **Elliptical or oval:** When the leaves are narrow at the base and apex but broad in the middle such as guava, vinca, etc.
20. **Peltate:** When the lamina is shield shaped and fixed to the stalk by the centre.

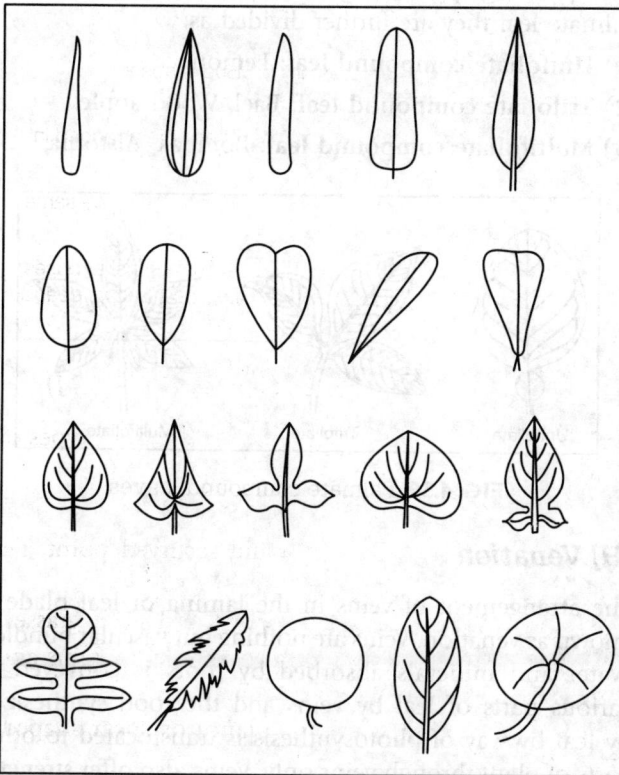

FIG. 4.34 Shape of the lamina of leaves

[C] Leaf margins (Fig. 4.35)

Leaf margin may be of the following types:
1. **Entire:** When it is even and smooths, i.e. senna, eucalyptus.
2. **Sinuate or wavy:** With slight undulations like Ashoka.
3. **Crenate:** When the teeth are round as in digitalis.

4. **Dentate:** Toothed margin, teeth directing outwards such as margosa, melon.
5. **Serrate:** When it is like the teeth of the saw such as rose, China rose, etc.
6. **Ciliated:** It is fringed with hairs.
7. **Biserrate:** Lobed serrate margin.
8. **Bicrenate:** Lobed crenate margin.

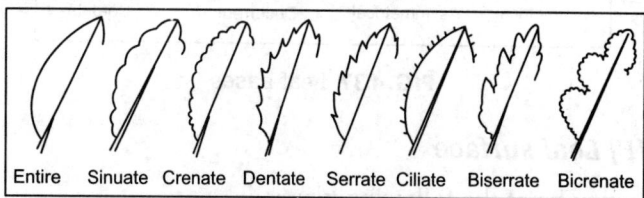

FIG. 4.35 Margins of leaves

[D] Leaf apices (Fig. 4.36)

The apex of the leaf may be one of the following kinds:
1. **Obtuse:** Rounded tip, i.e. banyan.
2. **Acute:** When it is pointed to form acute angle, but not stiff, i.e. hibiscus.
3. **Acuminate:** Pointed tip with much elongation, peepal.
4. **Recurved:** When the apex is curved backward.
5. **Cuspidate:** With spiny tip like date palm.
6. **Mucronate:** Rounded apex ending abruptly in a short point, i.e vinca, ixora.
7. **Retuse:** Broad tip with slight notch, i.e. pistia.
8. **Emarginate:** When tip is deeply notched as in bambinia.
9. **Tendrillar:** Tip forming a tendril such as Gloriosa superba.

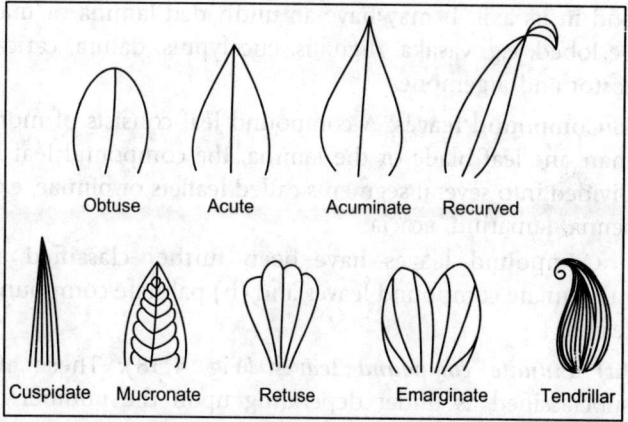

FIG. 4.36 Leaf apices

[E] Leaf bases (Fig. 4.37)

The lower extremity of the lamina of the leaf may exhibit one of the following shapes:
1. **Symmetrical:** Equal as in vasaka.
2. **Asymmetrical:** Unequal as in senna or datura.

3. **Decurrent**: As in digitalis.
4. **Cordate**: As in betel.

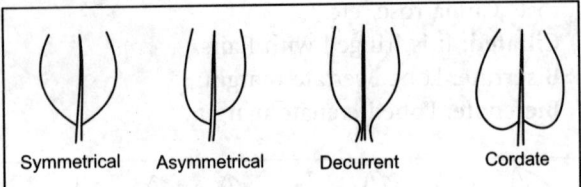

FIG. 4.37 Leaf bases

[F] Leaf surface

It may be of the following types:

1. **Glabrous**: When surface is smooth and free of hair or any outgrowth, i.e. vasaka, datura.
2. **Rough**: When harsh to touch, digitalis.
3. **Hairy**: When covered with hairs.
4. **Glutinous**: When covered with sticky substance, tobacco.
5. **Glaucous**: When covered with waxy coating, castor.
6. **Pubescent**: Covered with straight, short hair, i.e. senna.

[G] Types of leaves

Taking into consideration the nature of the lamina of the leaves, they are classified into two main groups:

1. Simple leaves and
2. Compound leaves.

1. **Simple leaves**: A leaf which has only one leaf blade or lamina is called a simple leaf. It may be stipulate or exstipulate, petiolate or sessile, but always possess axillary bud in its axil. It may have an undivided lamina or may be lobed, e.g. vasaka, digitalis, eucalyptus, datura, carica, castor and argemone.

2. **Compound leaves**: A compound leaf consists of more than one leaf blade or the lamina, the compound leaf is divided into several segments called leaflets or pinnae, e.g. senna, tamarind, acacia.

Compound leaves have been further classified as (a) pinnate compound leaves and (b) palmate compound leaves.

(a) Pinnate compound leaves (Fig. 4.38): These are subclassified as under depending upon the number of rachis (an axis bearing the leaflets in pinnate compound leaf is known as rachis):

1. **Unipinnate compound leaves**: Wherein only one rachis bearing the leaflets is present. When an even number of leaflet is present, it is known as paripinnate, e.g. Tamarind, Gulmohar; if the number of leaflet is odd, it is described as imparipinnate, e.g. rose, margosa, etc.

2. **Bipinnate compound leaves**: It consists of primary rachis and secondary rachis. The secondary rachis only bears the leaflets, e.g. acacia.

3. **Tripinnate compound leaves**: These contain primary, secondary and even tertiary rachis. Tertiary rachii only bear the leaflets as in moringa, oroxylon.

4. **Decompound leaf**: Wherein compound leaf is much divided irregularly as in coriander, carrot, anise, etc.

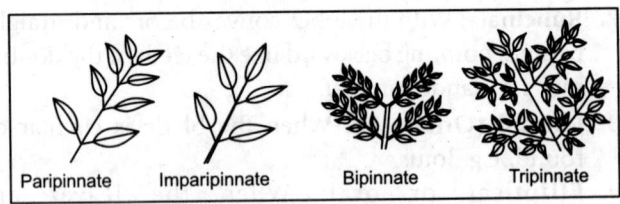

FIG. 4.38 Pinnate compound leaves

(b) Palmate compound leaves (Fig. 4.39): In this type the leaflets are born by the petiole of the leaf.

Depending upon the number of leaflets in a compound palmate leaf they are further divided as:

(1) **Unifoliate compound leaf**: Lemon.

(2) **Trifoliate compound leaf**: Bael, Wood apple.

(3) **Multifoliate compound leaf**: Bombax, Alstonia.

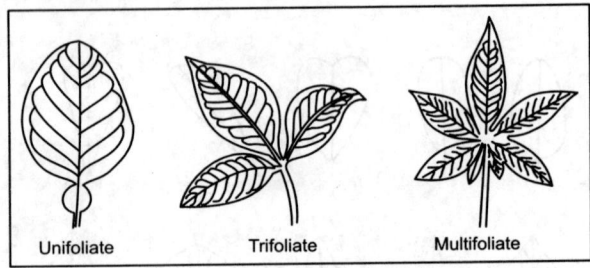

FIG. 4.39 Palmate compound leaves

[H] Venation

The arrangement of veins in the lamina or leaf blade is known as venation. Veins are nothing but vascular bundles. Water and minerals absorbed by roots is conveyed to various parts of leaf by veins and the food synthesized by leaf by way of photosynthesis is translocated to other parts of plant through veins only. Veins also offer strength, support and shape to the lamina of the leaf. The prominent vein in the centre of the leaf is known as midrib. In the flowering plants two types of venations exist: (1) reticulate and (2) parallel.

1. **Reticulate venation** (Fig. 4.40): This type of venation is characterized by the fact that many veins and veinlets in the lamina of the leaf are arranged in the form of network or reticulars. This type of venation is characteristic to dicotyledonous leaves. It is further subclassified as:

(a) Unicostate-reticulate venation: Where the leaf contains only one midrib and several veins are given out on both the sides to form the network such as henna, eucalyptus, peepal, etc.

(b) Multicostate-reticulate venation: In this type many veins of equal strength arise from the end of the petiole. Each vein further branches to give rise to veinlets that form the network. The veins may be convergent (meeting at the apex) or divergent (diverge towards the margin) as in castor, carica and cucurbita.

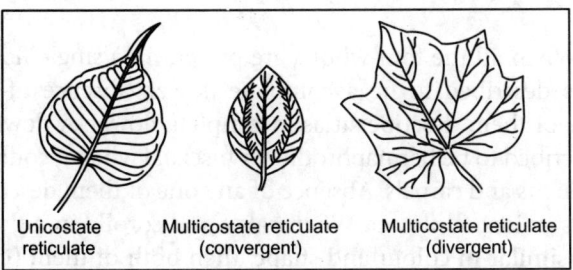

FIG. 4.40 Reticulate venation

2. **Parallel venation** (Fig. 4.41): In this type the vein and veinlets in leaf blade are arranged parallel to one another. It is characteristic to monocotyledonous plants with few exceptions like dioscorea and sarsaparilla.

Like reticulate venation, it may also be unicostate parallel venation or multicostate parallel venation as under:

(a) Unicostate parallel venation: Wherein the leaf consists of only one midrib running from apex to the petiole of the leaf. The veinlets and veins arise parallel to one another on each side as in banana and canna.

(b) Multicostate parallel venation: In case of multicostate parallel venation many number of main veins of equal strength arise from the tip or the petiole and run parallel to each other. It may be convergent as in case of several grasses and bamboo or divergent as in case of fan palm.

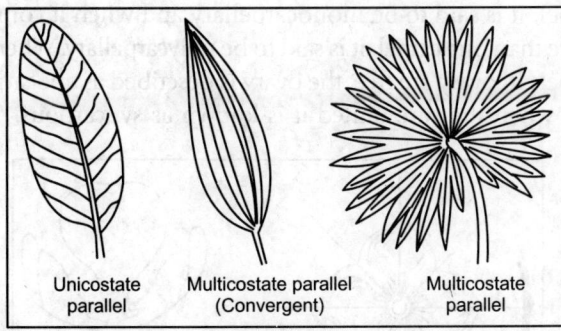

FIG. 4.4I Parallel venation

[I] Phyllotaxy

It is the mode of arrangement of leaves on the stem. Since the leaves are the chief organs of photosynthesis they must be exposed to sunlight favourably. This is done by arranging the leaves in systematic manner. Following are the various types of phyllotaxy (Fig. 4.42):

1. **Alternate or spiral:** This phyllotaxy is characterized by the presence of one leaf at each node and all leaves together make a spiral path on the axis, i.e. tobacco, mustard and sunflower.

2. **Opposite:** When two leaves are placed at the same node and are opposite to one another. This is farther divided into two:

   (a) **Opposite decussate:** In this type a pair of leaves of one node is at right angles to the pair of leaves at the next node such as madar, sacred basil, vinca.

   (b) **Opposite superposed:** When one pair of leaves is placed above the other exactly in the same plane, i.e. Rangoon creeper, ixora.

3. **Whorled:** When more than two leaves are present in a single node and are arranged in a circle as in nerium, alstonia.

4. **Leaf mosaic:** In this type, the leaves are so arranged that there will not be any overshading and all the leaves are exposed properly. The older leaves have longer petiole while younger leaves have short petiole and are placed in the space left by the older leaves. It recalls the arrangement of glass bits in a mosaic and hence the name, e.g. *Oxalis* and *acalypha*.

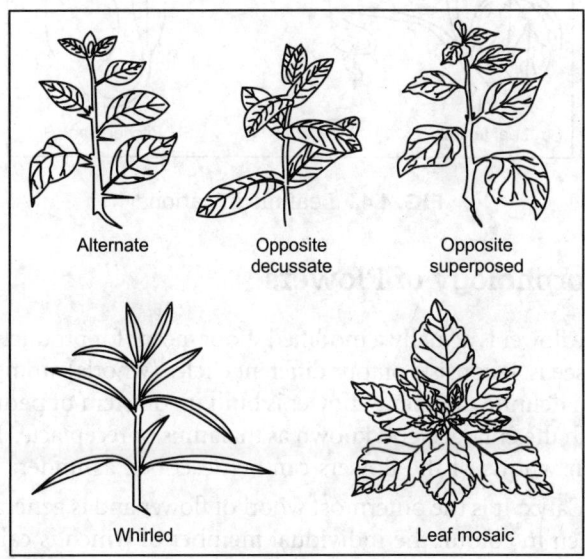

FIG. 4.42 Types of phyllotaxy

[J] Modifications of Leaves

Under the functions of leaves, it is stated that leaves have to perform two types of functions, i.e. primary functions and secondary functions. Under the primary function, leaves are known to perform three main functions like photosynthesis, gaseous exchange and transpiration. The secondary functions which the leaf has to perform are support, protection, storage of food material, etc.

To perform these secondary functions the leaf undergoes structural and physiological changes called modifications. There are at least five types of leaf modifications known (Fig. 4.43).

1. **Leaf tendrils:** Leaves get modified into slender, coiled and wiry structures as seen in *Lathyrus* peas and *gloriosa* for support to the plant.

2. **Leaf spines:** For the sake of protection certain leaves get converted into spines as seen in *Aloe, argemone, acacia,* etc.

3. **Phyllode:** Petiole gets modified to flat leaf-like phyllode to reduce the transpiration, e.g. *Australian acacia.*

4. **Scale leaves:** In *ginger* and *potato* they protect the terminal buds, while in *onion* and *garlic* they store food material.

5. **Pitcher and bladder:** These are specially developed modifications of leaves to capture and digest insects in case of carnivorous plants, e.g. Utricularis Bladder wort and *Nepenthes.*

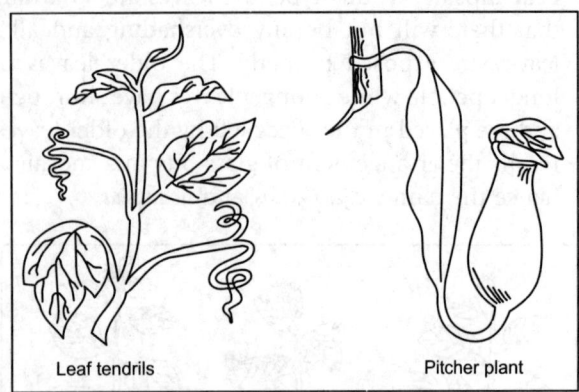

Leaf tendrils   Pitcher plant

FIG. 4.43 Leaf modifications

Morphology of Flowers

The flower is actually a modified shoot meant for production of seeds. It consists of four different circles (whorls) arranged in a definite manner. A flower is built up on stem or pedicel with the enlarged end known as thalamus or receptacle. The four whorls of the flowers can be described as under:

1. **Calyx:** It is the outermost whorl of flower and is generally green in colour, the individual member of which is called sepal.

2. **Corolla:** It is the second whorl of flower and is either white or bright coloured, each member of which is known as petal.

3. **Androecium:** It is the third circle of flower and constitutes the male part. The individual component is called stamen and each stamen consists of filament, anther and connective.

4. **Gynoecium:** This is the fourth circle of the flower and constitutes the female part. Each component is known as carpel or pistil and is made of stigma, style and ovary.

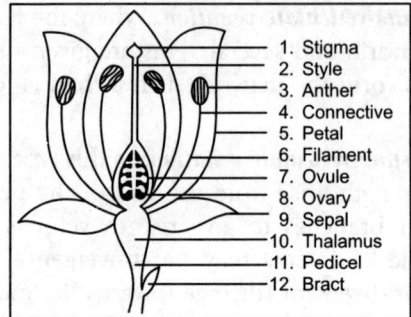

1. Stigma
2. Style
3. Anther
4. Connective
5. Petal
6. Filament
7. Ovule
8. Ovary
9. Sepal
10. Thalamus
11. Pedicel
12. Bract

FIG. 4.44 Typical parts of flower

When all the four whorls are present in a single flower, it is described to be a complete flower, absence of any one of them describes it as incomplete flower. A flower is described to be hermaphrodite or bisexual when it contains stamens and carpels. Absence of any one of them describes it as unisexual flower. When calyx and corolla in a flower are similar in colour and shape, then both of them (calyx and corolla) together are called perianth, i.e. garlic, onion, asparagus.

When a flower is divided into two equal parts by any vertical section passing through the centre, then it is described as regular or symmetrical or actinomorphic flower (Fig. 4.45a) as in ipomoea, rose, datura and shoe flower. But when it cannot be divided equally into two parts by one vertical section, then it is described as irregular or asymmetrical or zygomorphic flower (Fig. 4.45b).

When the stamens arise from petals instead of thalamus, the petals are called epipetalous. When the stamens get united with gynaecium the structure is known as gynostemium. The union of stamens among themselves is known as cohesion. When the filaments of stamen get united to form a single bundle, it is known as monoadelphous. When it forms two bundles, it is known as diadelphous. When anthers get united to form a column (but filaments are free), the stamens are known as syngenesious. When ovary consists of only one carpel, it is said to be monocarpellary and when it contains more than one carpel, it is said to be polycarpellary. When the carpels in ovary are free, the ovary is described as apocarpous and when they are united it is known as syncarpous.

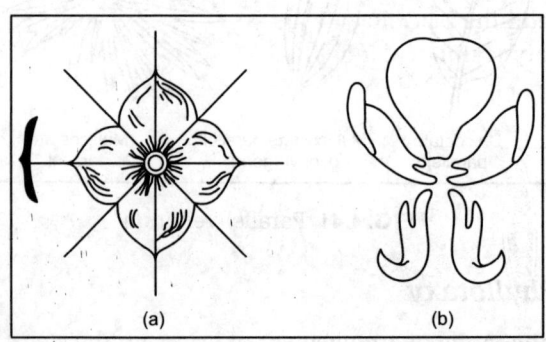

(a)   (b)

FIG. 4.45 (a) Actinomorphic flower and (b) zygomorphic flower

Arrangement of Floral Parts on Thalamus

Depending upon the arrangement of floral parts on thalamus, the flowers may be of three types.

(i) **Hypogynous flower (Superior ovary)** (Fig. 4.46a): Herein the thalamus is conical, flat, convex and stamens, sepals and petals are arranged at base and ovary at the apex, e.g. *brinjal, china rose, mustard*, etc.

(ii) **Perigynous flowers (Half-superior Ovary)** (Fig. 4.46b): Thalamus is flat, sepals and stamens grow around the ovary. The flowers are said to be perigynous as in *rose, strawberry peach*.

(iii) **Epigynous flower (Inferior ovary)** (Fig. 4.46c): The thalamus is fused with ovary wall, calyx, corolla, stamen appear at the top and the gynaecium at the bottom as in *sunflower, cucumber, apple*, etc.

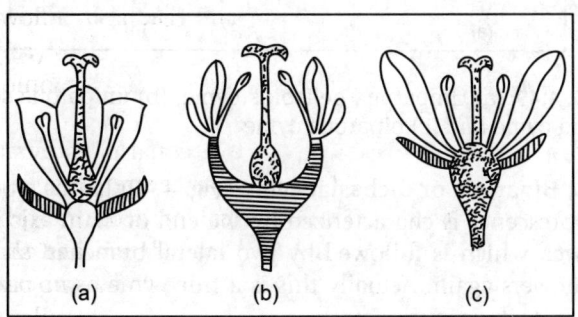

FIG. 4.46 (a) Superior ovary, (b) half-superior ovary and (c) inferior ovary

Placentation

The type of distribution of placentae in the ovary is called placentation. They are of the following types (Fig. 4.47).

1. **Marginal:** It is characteristic to monocarpellary ovary and placentae arise on ventral suture, e.g. bean and pea.

2. **Axile:** It is characteristic to polycarpellary syncarpous, bilocular or multilocular ovary. Ventral sutures of each carpel meet at the centre and each of them have marginal placentation, e.g. onion, china rose, ipomoea.

3. **Parietal:** It is characteristic to polycarpellary syncarpous ovary and the placentae develop on the ventral suture but the ovary is unilocular as in papaya and cucurbita.

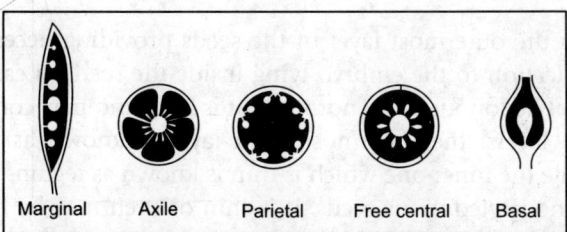

| Marginal | Axile | Parietal | Free central | Basal |

FIG. 4.47 Types of placentation

4. **Free central:** It is characteristic to polycarpellary syncarpous ovary, which is unilocular. Ovules arise on the central axis, but it is not connected with the peripheral wall, e.g. dianthus, saponaria, portulaca.

5. **Basal:** It is characteristic to polycarpellary and unilocular ovary. Only one ovule is present and it arises from its base as in sunflower.

Pollination

Pollination is the process of transference of pollen grains from the anther of a flower to the stigma of the same flower or another flower of the same or allied species. Pollen grains are produced by bursting the anther and are carried by various agencies to the stigma.

The agencies may be insects of various types, wind or even water. There are two types of pollination, i.e. (a) self-pollination or autogamy and (b) cross pollination or allogamy.

(a) Self-pollination: There are two types of self-pollination, i.e.

- **Homogamy:** In this case the anthers and stigmas of a flower mature at the same time.
- **Cleistogamy:** It is found in flowers which never open or in the underground flowers of *Commelina benghalensis*.

(b) Cross-pollination: Pollination through the agency of insects, animals (such as snails, bats, squirrels, birds and even human being) wind and water is cross-pollination

Pollination by insects is known as entomophily. To attract various insects, plants adapt different means such as colour, nectar and scent. Entomophilous pollination is very common in plants.

Morphology of Inflorescence

Plant bear flowers either solitary or in groups. The flowers which are large and showy are normally borne solitary, but which are not so prominent and are small, occur in group or bunches.

The form of natural bunch of flowers in which they occur is called inflorescence. Depending upon the type of branching various forms of inflorescences are known. The axis on which the flowers are arranged is known as peduncle while the stalks of flowers are known as pedicels.

Types of inflorescences

Following are the types of inflorescences (Fig. 4.48):

(A) Racemose or indefinite inflorescence:

1. **Raceme:** In this type of inflorescence the peduncle is long. Flowers are stalked and born in acropetal succession and peduncle has indefinite growth and goes

on producing flowers as in mustard, radish, dwarf gold mohur, etc. When the main axis is branched and the lateral branches bear the flowers, it is said to be compound raceme or panicle or branched raceme as in Gulmohar, Peltophorum, Yuchr, etc.

2. Spike: This is similar to raceme, with sessile flowers as in Rangoon creeper, vasaka. A branched spike of polyanthus and terminalia species is known.

3. Spadix: In this inflorescence the peduncle is short with numerous small unisexual flowers, which are sessile and covered with boat shaped bract known as Spathe, i.e. banana, arum, palms and coconut are the example of compound spadix.

4. Catkin: A spike with unisexual sessile flowers on long peduncle as in mulberry and oak.

5. Umbel: Axis is shortened and bears flowers at its top which are having equal stalk and arranged in centripetal succession. A whorl of bracts is present at the base of inflorescence as in coriander, caraway, cumin, fennel, etc.

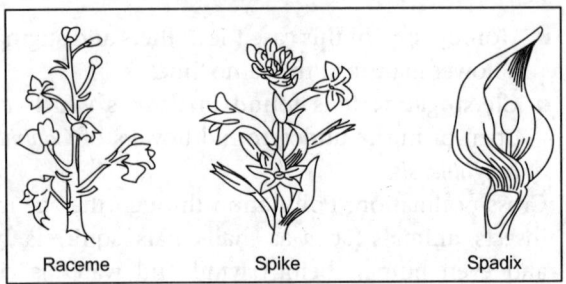

FIG. 4.48 Types of inflorescence

6. Spikelet: It is present in family *Gramineae* characterized by small and branched spikes. Spikelets are provided with two bracts at the base known as glumes, and bracteole called palea.

7. Corymb: Peduncle is short, flowers bracteate, bisexual oldest flower is lower most and youngest at apex. Lowermost has longest stack and youngest has shortest, lying at same level.

8. Capitulum or head: In this type flattened and expanded peduncle is present, called as receptacle. Base of receptacle is covered with bracts. The flowers are small and sessile (florets). Flowers towards the periphery are older, while at the centre, they are younger and open later. Two types of flowers are present, i.e. ray florets (strap shaped) and disc florets (tubular shaped), e.g. zinnia, cosmos, sunflower.

9. Capitate: Inflorescence similar to umbel type, except the flowers are sessile, i.e. acacia.

(B) Cymose inflorescence: In this type the growth of the main axis or peduncle is stopped by producing the flower. The order of opening is centrifugal. Its types are as under:

(i) Solitary cyme: In this type the inflorescence ends in a single flower as in datura, capsicum, China rose, etc.

(ii) Uniparous or monochasial cyme: In this type, axis ends in a flower only; one branch arises just behind and ends in a flower. Uniparous depending upon the type of branching is again subdivided into (a) *Hellicoid uniparous* (Fig. 4.49a) and (b) *Scorpioid uniparous* (Fig. 4.49b).

Hellicoid uniparous is characterized by branching on one side only, while scorpioid uniparous cyme by branching on alternate side.

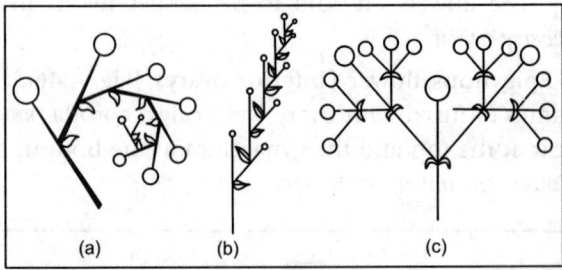

FIG. 4.49 (a) Uniparous helicoids cyme, (b) uniparous scorpioid cyme and (c) biparous cyme

(iii) Biparous or dichasial cyme (Fig. 4.49c): This type of inflorescence is characterized by the end of main axis in a flower, which is followed by two lateral branches ending in flowers again. Actually this is a true cyme as in case of ixora, teak, jasmine, etc.

(iv) Multiparous or polychasial: The main axis ends in a flower and numbers of flowers are produced laterally in the same manner, i.e. in nerium, calotropis, etc.

(v) Special type: In this type hypanthodium (like peepal and fig), verticillasters (sacred basil, mentha, coleus blumei) cymose-umbel (onion) are included. Each of them has its special characters not covered in any type described above.

Morphology of Seeds

The seed is a fertilized ovule and is a characteristic of Phanerogams. Parenchymatous body of the ovule known as nucellus contains embryo-sac in which fertilization of pollen cells takes place giving rise to embryo. The seeds are characterized by the presence of three parts known as embryo, endosperm and seed coat.

Seed coat

It is the outermost layer of the seeds providing necessary protection to the embryo lying inside the seed. In case of dicotyledonous seeds normally, it is hard and may contain two layers; the outermost thick layer is known as testa while the inner one which is thin is known as tegumen. In monocotyledonous seeds, it is thin or even may be fused with the wall of the fruit.

Embryo

It is the main part of the seed. It consists of an axis having apical meristem for plumule, radicle the origin or root and adhered to it are one or two cotyledons, differentiating the plants as monocot or dicot.

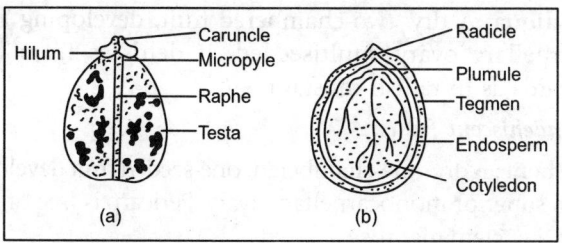

FIG. 4.50 (a) Castor seed (b) L.S. of Castor seed

Endosperm

It is the nutritive tissue nourishing the embryo. It may be present or may not be present in the seed. Depending upon the presence or absence the seeds are classified as under:

1. Endospermic or albuminous seeds.
2. Nonendospermic or exalbuminous seeds.
3. Perispermic seeds.

1. Endospermic or albuminous seeds: In this seed, the part of the endosperm remains even up to the germination of seed and is partly absorbed by embryo. Therefore, seeds are known as endospermic seeds as in colchicum, isabgol, linseed, nux vomica, strophanthus, wheat and rice.

2. Nonendospermic or exalbuminous seeds: During the development of these seeds, the endosperm is fully absorbed by embryo and endosperm, and is not represented in the seeds; hence, they are known as nonendospermic, e.g. sunflower, tamarind, cotton and soya bean.

3. Perispermic seeds: Herein the nucleus develops to such an extent that it forms a big storage tissue and seeds are found to contain embryo, endosperm, perisperm and seed coat; e.g. pepper, cardamom, nutmeg, guinea grains.

Seeds are characterized by the following descriptive terms:

(a) **Hilum:** This is the point of attachment of seed to its stalk.
(b) **Micropyle:** It is the minute opening of the tubular structure, wherefrom water is provided for the germination of seeds.
(c) **Raphe:** Raphe is described as longitudinal marking of adherent stalk of anatropous ovule.
(d) **Funicle:** It is the stalk of the ovule attaching it to the placenta.
(e) **Chalaza:** This is the basal portion of ovule where stalk is attached.

Special features of seeds (Fig. 4.51)

Sometimes, apart from the regular growth of seeds, additional growth is visible in the form of appendages which attribute to their special features. They are described as:

(i) **Aril:** Succulent growth from hilum covering the entire seeds as in nutmeg (mace) and yew seeds.
(ii) **Arillode:** Outgrowth originating from micropyle and covering the seeds as in cardamom.
(iii) **Arista (awn):** Stiff bristle-like appendage with many flowering glumes of grasses and found in strophanthus.
(iv) **Caruncle:** A warty outgrowth from micropyle, i.e. castor, croton, viola moringa.
(v) **Hairs:** Gossypium and calotropis are examples of this type of outgrowth.

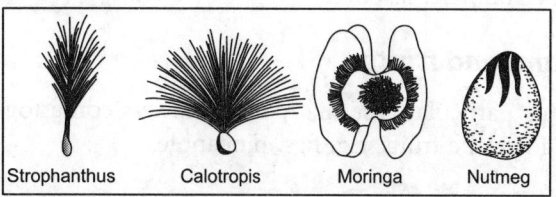

FIG. 4.51 Special features of seeds

Functions of Seeds

Seed performs the following functions:

1. Reproduction, i.e. it germinates into new plant.
2. Spread of the species.
3. Species and varieties do not come to an end by successive formation of seeds by plant. Thus seeds are 'means of perennation'.

Morphology of Fruits

Phanerogams are said to be matured when they reach the flowering stage. The ovules of the flowers after fertilization get converted into seeds, whereas the ovary wall develops further to form the protective covering over the seed, which is known as fruit. In botany, this particular coating is also called pericarp.

Pericarp consists of three different layers, one after the other as:

1. **Epicarp:** The outermost coating of the pericarp and may be thin or thick.
2. **Mesocarp:** A layer in between epicarp and endocarp, and may be pulpy or made up of spongy parenchymatous tissue.
3. **Endocarp:** The innermost layer of the pericarp, may be thin or thick or even woody.

It is not necessary that the fruits should have seeds. If the ovules do not fertilize, the seedless fruits are formed. Depending upon the number of carpels present in the flowers, and other structures, the fruits fall into (1) simple fruits, (2) aggregate fruits and (3) compound fruits (Fig. 4.52).

Simple fruits

Formed from the single carpel or from syncarpous gynoecium. Once again depending upon the mesocarp, whether it is dry or fleshy, they are classified as dry fruits and fleshy fruits. Dry fruits are further subclassified into dehiscent and indehiscent fruits.

Aggregate fruits

These fruits get formed from many carpels or apocarpous gynoecium, e.g. raspberry.

Compound fruits

In this particular case many more flowers come together and form the fruits, e.g. figs, pineapple.

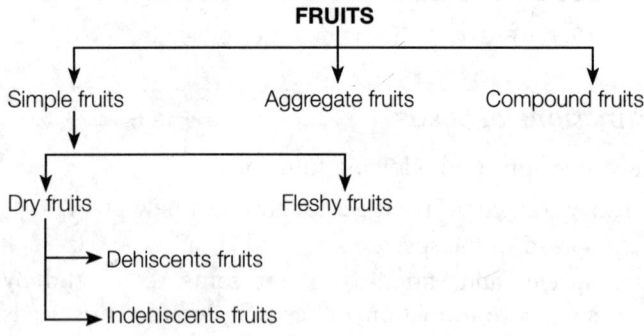

FIG. 4.52 Types of fruits

False fruits

Sometimes it so happens that apart from the ovary and the other floral parts like thalamus, receptacle or calyx grow and form the part of the fruit, known as false fruit or pseudocarp. Following are the few examples of pseudocarp in which other parts of the flower forming important part of the fruits are shown in the bracket. Strawberry (thalamus), cashew nut (peduncle and thalamus), apple (thalamus), marking nut (peduncle) and rose (thalamus).

I. Dehiscent capsular fruits:

1. **Legume or pod:** It is a dry monocarpellary fruit developing from superior ovary, dehiscing by both the margins, i.e. senna, tamarind, pea.

2. **Capsule:** It is a dry one to many-chambered fruit, developing from superior or poly carpellary ovary dehiscing in various forms, i.e. cardamon, cotton, datura, lobelia, colchicum, digitalis, poppy.

3. **Follicle:** Similar to legumes and dehisces at one margin only, i.e. rauwolfia, anise, calotropis.

4. **Siliqua:** A dry, two-chambered fruit, developing from bicarpellary ovary, multiseeded. It dehisces from base upwards as in radish mustard, etc.

II. Indehiscent fruits:

1. **Achene:** A dry, one-chambered, one-seeded fruit developed from superior monocarpellary ovary. Pericarp is free of seed coat, i.e. clematis, rose.

2. **Caryopsis or grain:** Small, dry, one-seeded fruits, developing from simple pistil, pericarp fused with seed coat as in maize, rice, bamboo.

3. **Nut:** Dry, one-seeded fruits developing from superior ovary, pericarp hard and woody, i.e. areca nut, marking nut, cashew nut.

4. **Samara:** Dry, one- or two-seeded, winged fruit from superior bi- or tricarpellary ovary, i.e. dioscorea, shorea, etc.

5. **Schizocarp:** These are further divided into two sub-classes.

   (i) **Lomentum:** In this type of pod of legume is partitioned into one-seeded compartments as observed in acacia, ground nut, cassia fistula.

   (ii) **Cremocarp:** Dry, two-chambered fruit, developing from an inferior bicarpellary ovary. Splitting into two, indehiscent one-seeded pieces are called mericarps, i.e. coriander, cumin, fennel, dill, etc.

Fleshy fruits (Fig. 4.53):

1. **Drupe (stone fruit):** A fleshy one or more seeded fruit, with pericarp well differentiated into epicarp, fleshy mesocarp and hard endocarp as in mango, olive, coconut, etc.

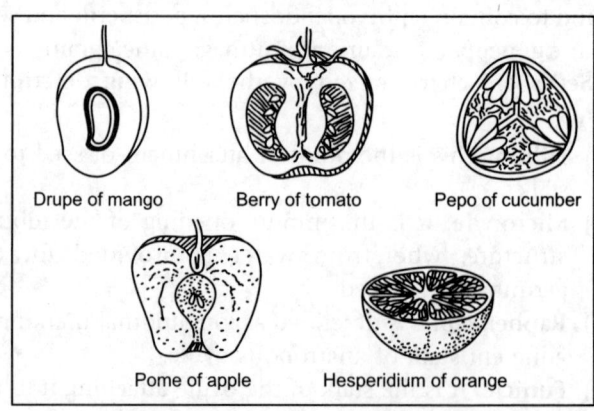

FIG. 4.53 Types of flashy fruits

2. **Berry**: A fleshy, many-seeded fruit developed from superior, single carpel, i.e. tomato, guava, grapes, banana.

3. **Pepo**: Pulpy, many-seeded fruit developing from one- or three celled inferior ovary, i.e. cucumber gourd, colocynth, water melon.

4. **Pome**: Fleshy, one- or more-celled syncarpous fruit. Fleshy, part is thalamus, while actual fruit lies inside, e.g. apple, pear.

5. **Hesperidium**: A superior, many-seeded fleshy fruit endocarp forming chambers; epicarp and mesocarp fused to form skin, e.g. orange, lemon.

Uses of fruits

1. Apart from the main source of food grains, i.e. wheat, jowar, fruits are also used for their high sugar value, minerals and vitamins.
2. Fleshy fruits like, papaya, mango and apple are used commercially as source of pectin.
3. Bayberry wax and olive oil are obtained industrially from fruits only.
4. Several fruits like chilli, black pepper, caraway and cumin are used on large scale for the preparation of spices.

Study of Different Families

CONTENTS

5.1. INTRODUCTION

A British systematic botanist J. Hutchinson published his work, *The Families of Flowering Plants* in 1926 on dicotyledons and in 1934 on monocotyledons. Hutchinson made it clear that the plants with sepals and petals are more primitive than the plants without petals and sepals on the assumption that free parts are more primitive than fused ones. He also believed that spiral arrangement of floral parts, numerous free stamens and hermaphrodite flowers are more primitive than unisexual flowers with fused stamens. He considered monochlamydous plants as more advanced than dicotyledons. Hutchinson's system indicates the concept of phylogenetic classification and seems to be an advanced step over the Bentham and Hooker system of classification. Hutchinson accepted the older view of woody and herbaceous plants, and fundamentally called them as Lignosae and Herbaceae. He revised the scheme of classification in 1959. He has divided the flowering plants into two phyla: phylum I—Gymnospermae (not elaborated by him) and phylum II—Angiospermae. The latter are divided into two subphyla: subphylum I—Dicotyledons and subphylum II—Monocotyledons.

The division of angiosperms into these two large classes is based on the following factors:

(1) In dicotyledons, the embryo bears two cotyledons, and in monocotyledons, it bears only one.

(2) In dicotyledons, the primary root persists and gives rise to the tap root, while in monocotyledons, the primary root soon perishes and is replaced by a cluster of adventitious (fibrous) roots.

(3) As a rule, venation is reticulate in dicotyledons and parallel in monocotyledons. Among monocotyledons, aroids, sarsaparilla (*Smilax*) and yams (*Dioscorea*), however, show reticulate venation, and among dicotyledons, Alexandrian laurel (*Calophyllum*) shows parallel venation. Further, in dicotyledons, the veinlets end freely in the mesophyll of the leaf, whereas in monocotyledons, veins or veinlets do not end freely.

(4) The dicotyledonous flower usually has a pentamerous symmetry, sometimes tetramerous (as in Cruciferae and Rubiaceae), while the monocotyledonous flower has a trimerous symmetry.

(5) In the dicotyledonous stem, the vascular bundles are arranged in a ring and are collateral and open, i.e. they contain a strip of cambium which gives rise to secondary growth. In the monocotyledonous stem, however, the bundles are scattered in the ground tissue and are collateral and closed. Hence, there is no secondary growth (with but few exceptions). Also the bundles are more numerous in monocotyledons than in dicotyledons. Further, they are more or less oval in monocotyledons and wedge shaped in dicotyledons.

(6) In the dicotyledonous root, the number of xylem bundles varies from 2 to 6, seldom more, but in the monocotyledonous root there are many, seldom a limited number (5–8). It may also be noted that the cambium soon makes its appearance in the dicotyledonous root as a secondary meristem and gives rise to secondary growth, but in the monocotyledonous root, the presence of cambium is rare. Hence, there is no secondary growth.

Floral Diagram

The number of parts of a flower, their general structure, arrangement and the relation they bear to one another (aestivation), adhesion, cohesion and position with respect to the mother axis may be represented by a diagram known as the floral diagram. The floral diagram is the ground plan of a flower. In the diagram, the calyx lies outermost, the corolla internal to the calyx, the androecium in the middle and the gynoecium in the centre. Adhesion and cohesion of members of different whorls may also be shown clearly by connecting the respective parts with lines. The black dot on the top represents the position of the mother axis (not the pedicel), which bears the flower. The axis lies behind the flower and, therefore, the side of the flower nearest to the axis is called the posterior side, and the other side away from the axis the anterior side. The floral characteristics of species may be well represented by a floral diagram, whereas more than one diagram may be necessary to represent a genus or family.

Floral Formula

The different whorls of a flower, their number, cohesion and adhesion may be represented by a formula known as the floral formula. In the floral formula, K stands for calyx, C for corolla, P for perianth, A for androecium and G for gynoecium The figures following the letters K, C, P, A and G indicate the number of parts of those whorls. Cohesion of a whorl is shown by enclosing the figure within brackets, and adhesion is shown by a line drawn on top of the two whorls concerned. In the case of the gynoecium, the position of the ovary is shown by a line drawn above or below G on the figure. If the ovary is superior, the line should be below it; and if inferior, the line should be on top. Thus, all the parts of a flower are represented in a general way by a floral formula.

Besides, some symbols are used to represent certain features of flowers. Thus ♂ represents male, ♀ female, H hermaphrodite, ♂♀ dioecious, ♂-♀ monoecious, ♂ ♀ H polygamous, ⊕ actinomorphic, ·↿· zygomorphic, ∞ indefinite number of parts, etc.

Features used in descriptions of angiospermic plants:

- **Habitat:** Natural abode of the plant.
- **Habit:** Herb (erect, prostrate, decumbent, diffuse, trailing, twining or climbing), shrub (erect, straggling, twining or climbing), tree or any other peculiarity in the habit.
- **Root:** Nature of the foot; any special form.
- **Stem:** Kind of stem—herbaceous or woody; cylindrical or angular; hairy or smooth; jointed or not; hollow or solid; erect, prostrate, twining or climbing; nature of modification, if any.
- **Leaf:** Arrangement—whether alternate, opposite (super-posed or decussate) or whorled; stipulate or exstipulate; nature of the stipules, if present, simple or compound; nature of the compound leaf and the number of leaflets; shape and size; hairy or smooth; deciduous or persistent: venation; margin; apex; and petiole.
- **Inflorescence:** Type of inflorescence.
- **Flower:** Sessile or stalked; complete or incomplete; unisexual or bisexual; regular, zygomorphic or irregular; hypogynous, epigynous or perigynous; bracteate or ebracteate; nature of bracts and bracteoles, if present; shape, colour and size of the flower.
- **Calyx:** Polysepalous or gamosepalous; number of sepals or lobes; superior or inferior; aestivation; shape, size and colour.
- **Corolla:** Polypetalous or gamopetalous; number of petals or lobes; superior or inferior; aestivation; shape, size colour and scent; corona or any special feature. (When there is not much difference between the calyx and the corolla, the term perianth should be used. It may be sepaloid or petaloid, polyphyllous or gamophyllous, or free or epiphyllous).
- **Androecium:** Number of stamens—definite (10 or less) or indefinite (more than 10); free or united; nature of cohesion—monadelphous, diadelphous, polyadelphous, syngenesious or synandrous; nature of adhesion—epipetalous or gynandrous, or any special feature; whether alternating with the petals (or corolla lobes) or opposite them. Length of stamens—general length; inserted or exerted; didynamous or tetradynamous; position of stamens—hypogynous, perigynous or epigynous; attachment of the anther and its dehiscence; anther lobes or appendages, if any.

- Gynoecium or pistil: Number of carpels; syncarpous or apocarpous; nature of style—long or short; stigmas— simple, lobed or branched; their number and nature—smooth or papillose; ovary—superior or inferior; number of lobes; number of chambers (loculi); nature of placentation; number and form of ovules in each loculus of the ovary.
- Fruit: Kind of fruit.
- Seeds: Number of seeds in the fruit; shape and size; albuminous or exalbuminous; nature of endosperm, if present.

5.2. APOCYNACEAE (Fig. 5.1)

- Habit: These are mostly twining or erect shrubs and lianes, a few herbs and trees with latex. Bicollateral bundles or internal phloem often present.
- Leaves: The leaves are simple, opposite or whorled, rarely alternate.
- Flowers: The flowers are regular, bisexual and hypogynous, in cymes. They are usually salver or funnel shaped, often with corona.
- Calyx: The sepals are five in number, and rarely four, gamosepalous and often united only at the base.
- Corolla: There are five petals, rarely four. They are gamopetalous and twisted.
- Androecium: There are five stamens, rarely four. They are epipetalous, alternating with the petals, included within the corolla tube. The anthers usually connate around the stigma and apparently adnate to it. The disc is ring like or glandular.
- Gynoecium: The carpels are two or (2), apocarpous or syncarpous, superior. When apocarpous, each ovary is one-celled with marginal placentation, and when syncarpous the ovary may be one celled with parietal placentation, or two celled with axile placentation. There are 2-∞ ovules in each.
- Fruit: There is a pair of follicles, barriers or drupes.
- Seeds: The seeds often have a crown of long, silky hairs and they mostly have endosperm.

Floral formula: $\oplus$ or $\cdot | \cdot H\ K_5\ C_5\ A_5\ \bar{G}_{(2)}$

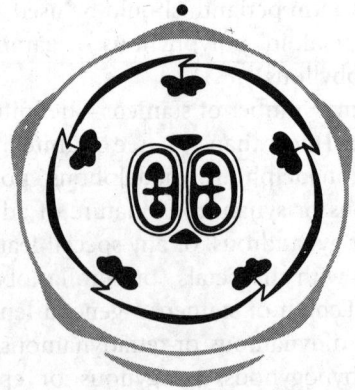

FIG. 5.1 Floral diagram of Apocynaceae

Examples: Rauwolfia, kurchi, devil tree, etc.

5.3. COMPOSITAE (Fig. 5.2)

- Habit: These are herbs and shrubs, rarely twiners, e.g. *Mikania scandens*, or trees, e.g. *Vernonia arborea*. They sometimes have internal phloem. Some genera have latex, e.g. *Sonchus, Crvpis, Lactuca, Picris*, etc.
- Leaves: The leaves are simple, alternate or opposite, rarely compound.
- Inflorescence: The inflorescence is a head (or capitulum), with an involucre of bracts.
- Flowers (florets): The flowers are of two kinds—the central ones (called disc florets) are tubular, and the marginal ones (called ray florets) are ligulate. Sometimes all florets are of one kind, either tubular or ligulate. The disc flowers are regular, tubular, bisexual and epigynous, each usually in the axil of a bracteole.
- Calyx: The calyx is often modified into a cluster of hairs called pappus, as in *Tridax* and *Ageratum*, or into scales, as in sunflower and *Eclipta*, or absent, as in water cress (*Enhydra*).
- Corolla: There are (5) petals. It is gamopetalous and tubular.
- Androecium: The five stamens are epipetalous. The filaments are free but the anthers united (syngenesious).
- Gynoecium: The carpels are (2), syncarpous. The ovary inferior, one-celled with one basal, anatropous ovule. There is one style and the stigma is bifid.
- Fruit: The fruit is a cypsela.

Floral formula: $\oplus\ H\ Kpappus$ or $C_{(5)}\ \overline{A_{(5)}}\ \bar{G}_{(2)}$

- The ray florets are zygomorphic, ligulate, unisexual (female), or sometimes neuter, as in sunflower, and epigynous, each usually in the axil of a bracteole. The calyx is usually modified into pappus. Sometimes it is scaly or absent. The corolla has (5) petals, is gamopetalous and ligulate (strap shaped). The gynoecium has disc florets shape.

Floral formula: $\cdot | \cdot\ ♀\ Kpappus$ or $o\ C_{(5)}\ \bar{G}_{(2)}$

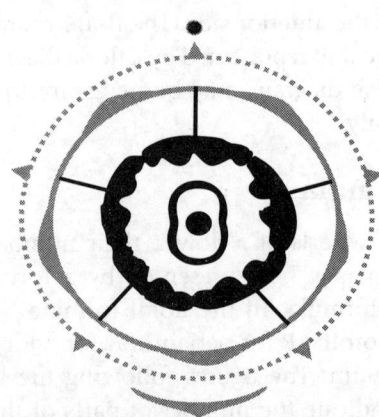

FIG. 5.2 Floral diagram of Compositae (disc floret)

Examples: Sunflower, pyrethrum, artemisia, etc.

5.4. CONVOLVULACEAE (Fig. 5.3)

- Habit: These are mostly twiners, often with latex and bicollateral vascular bundles or internal phloem.
- Leaves: The leaves are simple, alternate and exstipulate.
- Inflorescence: The inflorescence is cymose. The flowers are regular, bisexual, hypogynous, often large and showy.
- Calyx: There are five sepals, usually free. The odd one is posterior, imbricate and persistent.
- Corolla: There are (5) petals, is gamopetalous, funnel shaped, twisted in bud and sometimes imbricate.
- Androecium: The five stamens are epipetalous, alternating with the petals.
- Gynoecium: There are (2) carpels, rarely more, connate. The ovary is superior, with a disc at the base. It is two celled, with two ovules in each cell, or sometimes four-celled with one ovule in each cell. The placentation is axile.
- Fruit: The fruit is a berry or a capsule.

Floral formula: $\oplus$ H K_5 $C(_5)$ A_5 $\underline{G}(_2)$

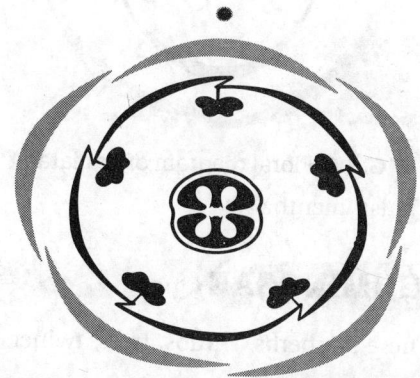

FIG. 5.3 Floral diagram of Convolvulaceae

Examples: Sweet potato (*Ipomoea batatas*), jalap (*Ipomoea purga*), etc.

5.5. CRUCIFERAE (Fig. 5.4)

- Habit: These are annual herbs.
- Leaves: The leaves are radical and cauline, simple, alternate, often lobed, or rarely pinnately compound.
- Inflorescence: A raceme (corymbose towards the top).
- Flowers: The flowers are regular and cruciform, bisexual and complete hypogynous.
- Calyx: They are sepals, 2 + 2, which are free, and in two whorls.
- Corolla: There are four petals, free, in one whorl. They alternate with the sepals. They are cruciform. Each petal has distinct limb and claw.
- Androecium: There are six stamens in two whorls, two short, outer ones and four long, inner ones (tetradynamous).
- Gynoecium: There are two syncarpous carpels. The ovary is superior, at first one-celled, but later two-celled owing

to the development of a false septum. There are often many ovules in each cell, sometimes only two. They are anatropous or campylotropous. The placentation is parietal.
- Fruit: The fruit is a long, narrow siliqua or a short, broad silicula.
- Seeds: These are exalbuminous. The embryo is curved. The seeds remain attached to a wiry framework, called the replum, which surrounds the fruit.

Floral formula: $\oplus$ H K_{2+2} C_4 A_{2+4} $\underline{G}_{(2)}$

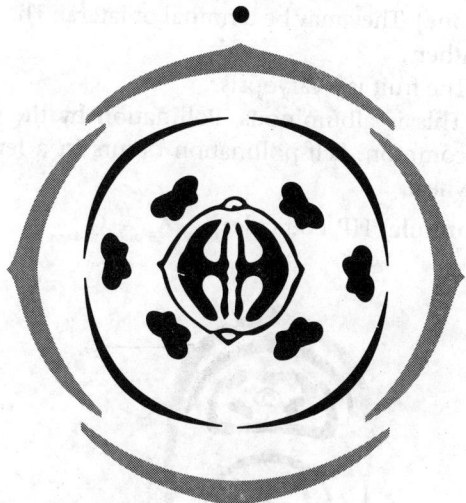

FIG. 5.4 Floral diagram of Cruciferae

Examples: Black mustard (*Brassica nigra*).

5.6. GRAMINEAE (Fig. 5.5)

- Habit: These are herbs, rarely woody, as bamboos. They are very widely distributed all over the earth.
- Stem: This is cylindrical and has distinct nodes and internodes (sometimes hollow), called culm.
- Leaves: These are simple, alternate and distichous. They have a sheathing leaf base that is split open on the side opposite the leaf blade. There is a hairy structure, called the ligule, at the base of the leaf blade.
- Inflorescence: This is usually a spike or a panicle of spikelets. Each spikelet consists of one or few flowers (not exceeding five), and its base-bears two empty bracts or glumes (G_I, G_{II}), one placed a little above and opposite the other. A third glume, called the lemma or flowering glume, stands opposite the second glume. The lemma encloses a flower in its axil. It may have a bristle-like appendage, long or short, known as the awn. Opposite the flowering glume or lemma, there is a somewhat smaller, two-nerved glume called the palea. The spikelet may be sessile or stalked.
- Flowers: These are usually bisexual, sometimes unisexual and monoecious.

- Perianth: This is represented by 2- or 3-minute scales, called the lodicules, at the base of the flower. These are considered to form the rudimentary perianth.
- Androecium: There are three stamens, or sometimes six, as in rice and bamboo. The anthers are versatile and pendulous.
- Gynoecium: The carpels are generally considered to number (three), reduced to one by their fusion or by the suppression of two. The ovary is superior and one-celled, with one ovule. The styles usually number two (three in bamboos, and two fused into one in maize, rarely one). They may be terminal or lateral. The stigmas are feathery.
- Fruit: The fruit is a caryopsis.
- Seed: This is albuminous. Pollination by the wind is most common. Self-pollination occurs in a few cases, as in wheat.

Floral Formula: HP Lodicules$_{2 \text{ or } 3}$ A$_{3 \text{ or } 6}$ $\underline{G}_{(3) \text{ or } 1}$

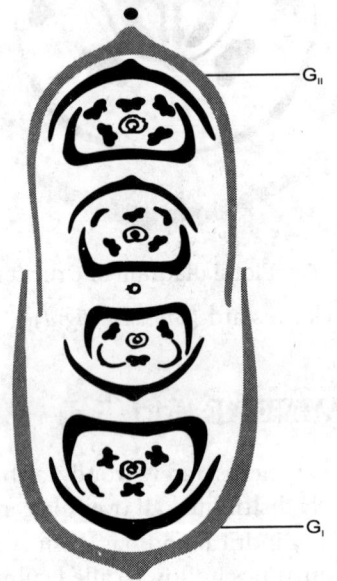

FIG. 5.5 Floral diagram of Gramineae

Examples: Rice, maize, bamboo, etc.

5.7. LABIATAE (Fig. 5.6)

- Habit: These are herbs and undershrubs with square stems.
- Leaves: These are simple, opposite or whorled, exstipulate and have oil glands.
- Flowers: This is a zygomorphic, bilabiate, hypogynous and bisexual.
- Inflorescence: This is a verticillaster. It is often reduced to a true cyme, as in tulsi.
- Calyx: The petals are (five in number), gamopetalous and bilabiate, i.e. two lipped. The aestivation is imbricate.

- Androecium: The stamens are four and didynamous. Sometimes there are only two, as in *sage*. They are epipetalous.
- Gynoecium: The carpels are (2) and syncarpous. The disc is prominent. The ovary is four-lobed and four-celled, with one ovule in each cell, ascending from the base of ovary. The style is gynobasic, i.e. it develops from the depressed centre of the lobed ovary. The stigma is bifid.
- Fruit: This is a group of four nutlets, each with one seed. The seed has only scanty endosperm, or even none.

Floral formula: $\cdot \vert \cdot$ H K$_{(5)}$ $\overline{C_{(5)}}$ $\overline{A}_4$ $\underline{G}_{(2)}$

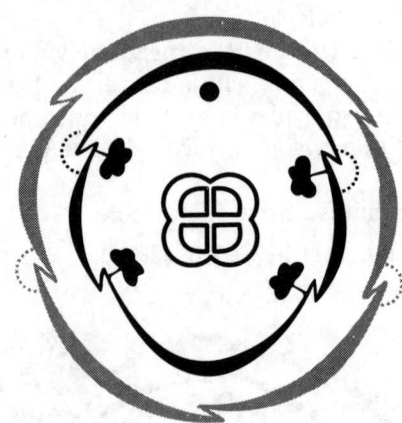

FIG. 5.6 Floral diagram of Labiatae

Examples: Tulsi, mentha, etc.

5.8. LEGUMINOSAE

- Habit: These are herbs, shrubs, trees, twiners or climbers.
- Roots: The roots of many species, particularly of Papilionaceae, have tubercles.
- Leaves: These are alternate, pinnately compound, and rarely simple, as in rattlewort (*Crotalaria sericea*), camel's foot tree (Bauhinia) and some species of desmodium, e.g. *D. gangeticum*, with a swollen leaf-base known as the pulvinus. There are two, usually free, stipules.
- Flowers: These are bisexual and complete, regular or zygomorphic or irregular, and hypogynous or slightly perigynous.
- Calyx: There are usually 5 or (5) sepals, with the odd one anterior (away from the axis). Sometimes there are four sepals. They may be united or free.
- Corolla: There are usually five petals, with the odd one posterior (towards the axis). Sometimes there are four petals, free or united.
- Androecium: There are usually 10 or more stamens (often less than 10 by reduction) free or united.
- Gynoecium: There is one carpel. The ovary is one-celled, with one to many ovules. It is superior and the placentation is marginal. The ovary often borne on a long or short stalk is called the stipe or gynophore.

- Fruit: This is mostly a legume or pod (dehiscent), or sometimes a lomentum (indehiscent).

This is the second biggest family among the dicotyledons, and has varying characteristics. As such, it has been divided into the following subfamilies: Papilionaceae, Caesalpinieae and Mimoseae.. The division is primarily based on the characteristics of the corolla and the stamens.

Papilionaceae (Fig. 5.7)

- Habit: Herbs, shrubs, trees and climbers.
- Leaves: Unipinnate, sometimes trifoliate, rarely simple; stipels often present.
- Inflorescence: Usually a raceme.
- Flowers: Zygomorphic, polypetalous and papilionaceous.
- Calyx: Usually has five sepals, gamosepalous, often imbricate, sometimes valvate.
- Corolla: Usually has five petals, free, of very unequal sizes, the posterior and largest one being the vexillum or standard, the two lateral ones being the wings or alae, and the two innermost ones (apparently united) forming the keel or carina; aestivation vexillary.
- Androecium: Stamens 10, diadelphous (9) + 1, rarely 10, free, as in coral tree (erythrina), or (10), connate, as in rattlewort (crotalaria).

Floral formula: $\cdot | \cdot \, H \, K_{(5)} \, C_5 \, A_{(9)+1} \, \underline{G}_1$

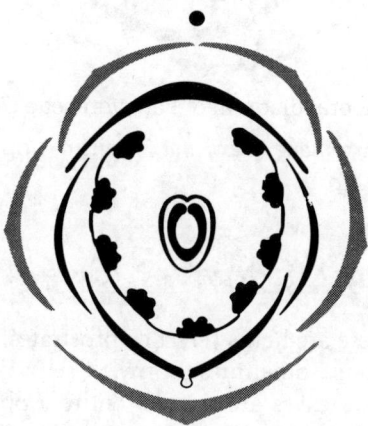

FIG. 5.7 Floral diagram of Papilionaceae

Examples: Methi, indigo, bengal gram, etc.

Caesalpinieae (Fig. 5.8)

- Habit: Shrubs trees, rarely climbers or herbs.
- Leaves: Unipinnate or bipinnate, rarely simple, as in camel's foot tree (Bauhinia); stipels absent.
- Inflorescence: Mostly a raceme.
- Flowers: Zygomorphic or irregular and polypetalous.
- Calyx: Sepals usually have five, polysepalous (sometimes gamosepalous), imbricate.
- Corolla: Usually have five petals, free, subequal or unequal, the odd or posterior one (sometimes very small) always innermost; aestivation imbricate.

- Androecium: There are 10 stamens, or less by reduction; free.

Floral formula: $\cdot | \cdot \, H \, K_5 \, C_5 \, A_{10} \, \underline{G}_1$

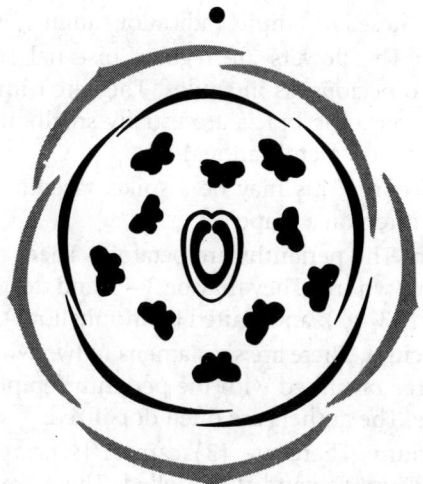

FIG. 5.8 Floral diagram of Caesalpinieae

Examples: Indian Senna, *Saraca indica*, etc.

Mimoseae (Fig. 5.9)

- Habit: Shrubs and trees, sometimes herbs or woody climbers.
- Leaves: Bipinnate; stipels present or absent.
- Inflorescence: A head or a spike.
- Flowers: Regular, often small and aggregated in spherical heads.
- Calyx: (5) or (4) sepals, generally gamosepalous, valvate.
- Corolla: (5) or (4) petals, mostly gamopetalous; aestivation valvate.
- Androecium: Usually ∞ stamens, sometimes 10 (as in *Entada, Neptunia, Prosopis* and *Parkia*), free, often united at the base; pollen often united in small masses.

Floral formula: $\oplus \, H \, K_{(5 \, or \, 4)} \, C_{(5 \, or \, 4)} \, A_{\infty \, or \, 10} \, G_1$

Examples: Catechu and other species of acacia, *Mimosa pudica*, etc.

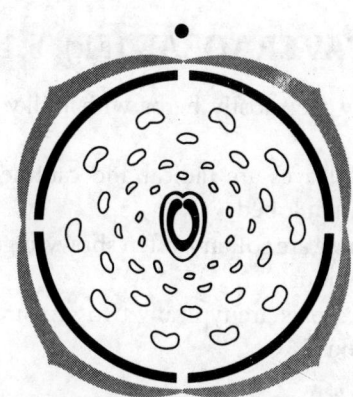

FIG. 5.9 Floral diagram of Mimoseae

5.9. LILIACEAE (Fig. 5.10)

- Habit: These are herbs and climbers, and rarely shrubs or trees with a bulb or rhizome, or with fibrous roots.
- Leaves: These are simple, radical or cauline, or both.
- Flowers: The flowers are regular, bisexual (rarely unisexual) dioecious, as in smilex. They are trimerous and hypogynous. The bracts are usually small and scarious (thin, dry and membranous).
- Inflorescence: This may be a spike, raceme, panicle or umbel, often on a scape.
- Perianth: The perianths are petaloid. There are usually six in two whorls. They may be 3 + 3 and free (polyphyllous), or (3 + 3), and united (gamophyllous).
- Androecium: There are six stamens in two whorls, 3 + 3, rarely free or united with the perianth (epiphyllous) at the base. The anthers are often dorsifixed.
- Gynoecium: There are (3) carpels (syncarpous). The ovary is superior and three celled. There are usually ∞ ovules in two rows in each loculus. The placentation is axile. There are (3) or 3 styles.
- Fruit: This may be a berry or capsule.
- Seeds: The seeds are albuminous.

Floral formula: $\oplus \text{ H } P_{3+3 \text{ or } (3+3)} A_{3+3} \underline{G}_{(3)}$

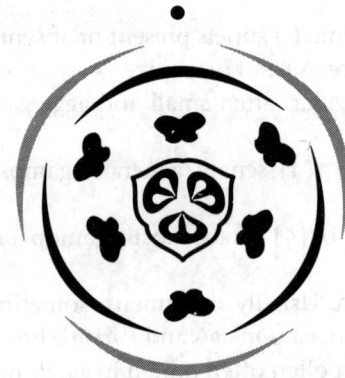

FIG. 5.10 Floral diagram of Liliaceae

Examples: Onion, garlic, aloe, colchicum, etc.

5.10. PAPAVERACEAE (Fig. 5.11)

- Habit: They are mostly herbs with milky or yellowish latex.
- Leaves: The leaves are radical and cauline, simple and alternate, often lobed.
- Flowers: These are solitary, often showy, regular, bisexual and hypogynous.
- Calyx: The sepals are typically two or sometimes three, free, caducous.

- Corolla: There are petals 2 + 2 or 3 + 3, arranged rarely more, in two whorls (rarely three), large, free, rolled or crumpled in the bud, caducous and imbricate.
- Androecium: Stamens α, sometimes two or four. They are free.
- Gynoecium: The carpels (2–∞), (4–6) in argemone. It is syncarpous. The ovary is superior, 1-chambered, or spuriously 2- to 4-chambered, with 2–∞ parietal placentae which may project inwards, as in poppy (Papaver). The stigmas are distinct or sessile and rayed over the ovary, as in poppy. The ovules are numerous.
- Fruit: This is a septicidal capsule dehiscing by or opening by pores. There are many seeds, with oily endosperm.

Floral formula: $\oplus \text{ H K}_{2 \text{ or } 3} C_{2+2 \text{ or } 3+3} A_{\infty} \underline{G}_{(2-\infty)}$

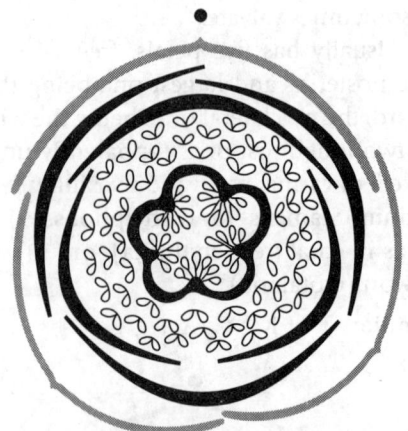

FIG. 5.11 Floral diagram of Papaveraceae (Argemone)

Examples: *Argemone mexicana*, Opium poppy (*Papavera somniferum*), etc.

5.11. RUBIACEAE (Fig. 5.12)

- Habit: These are herbs (erect or prostrate), shrubs, trees and climbers, sometimes thorny.
- Leaves: The leaves are simple, entire, opposite (decussate) or whorled, with interpetiolar (sometimes intrapetiolar) stipules.
- Flowers: The flowers are regular, bisexual, epigynous, sometimes dimorphic, as in some species of randia and oldenlandia.
- Inflorescence: The inflorescence is typically cymose, frequently dichasial and branched, sometimes in globose heads.
- Calyx: There are usually four sepals, sometimes five. It is gamosepalous. The calyx tube adnates to the ovary.
- Corolla: There are usually four sometimes five. It is gamopetalous, generally rotate. The aestivation is valvate, imbricate or twisted.

- Androecium: The stamens are as epipetalous, inserted within or at the mouth of the corolla tube, alternating with the corolla lobes.
- Gynoecium: The carpels are two, syncarpous. The ovary is inferior, commonly two-locular, with 1–∞ ovules in each. The disc is usually annular, at the base of the style.
- Fruit: The fruit is a berry, drupe or capsule.
- Seeds: The seed has fleshy or horny endosperm.

Floral formula: $\oplus \, H \, K_{(4 \, or \, 5)} \, \overline{C_{(4 \, or \, 5)}} \, A_{4 \, or \, 5} \, \overline{G}_2$

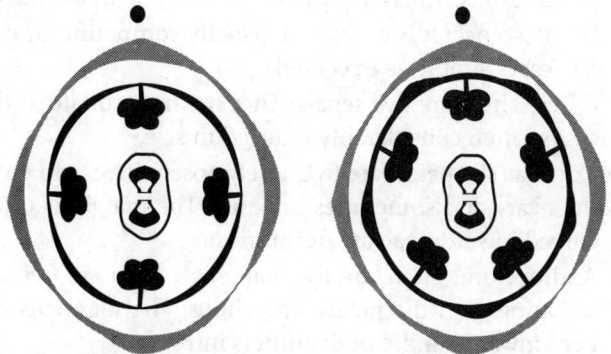

FIG. 5.12 Floral diagram of Rubiaceae

Examples: *Cinchona, Ipecac,* etc.

5.12. RUTACEAE (Fig. 5.13)

- Habit: These are shrubs and trees (rarely herbs).
- Leaves: The leaves are simple or compound, alternate or rarely opposite and gland dotted.
- Flowers: These are regular, bisexual and hypogynous. The disc below the ovary is prominent and ring or cap like.
- Calyx: There are four or five sepals free or connate below and imbricate.
- Corolla: Petals four or five, free, imbricate.
- Androecium: The number of stamens varies, they can be as many, or more often twice, as many, as the petals (obdiplostemonous), or numerous, as in citrus and aegle. They are free or united in irregular bundles (polyadelphous), and inserted on the disc.
- Gynoecium: There are generally (4) or (5) carpels, or ∞, as in citrus. They are syncarpous or free at the base and united above, and either sessile or seated on the disc. The ovary is generally four- or five-locular, or multilocular as in citrus, with axile placentation (parietal in limonia only). There are usually 2–∞ (rarely 1) ovules in each loculus, arranged in two rows.
- Fruit: This is a berry, capsule or hesperidium.
- Seeds: The seeds may or may not have an endosperm. Polyembryony is frequent in *Citrus*, e.g. lemon and orange (but not pummelo and citron).

Floral formula: $\oplus \, H \, K_{4 \, or \, 5} \, C_{4 \, or \, 5} \, A_{8, \, 10 \, or \, \infty} \, \underline{G}_{(4, \, 5 \, or \, \infty)}$

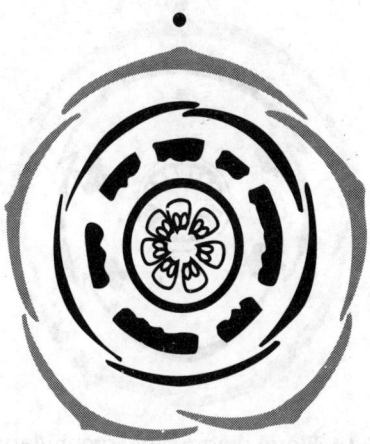

FIG. 5.13 Floral diagram of Rutaceae

Examples: *Citrus limon, Citrus aurantium, Aegle marmelos* (wood apple).

5.13. SCROPHULARIACEAE (Fig. 5.14)

- Habit: These are mostly herbs and under-shrubs.
- Leaves: These are simple, alternate, opposite or whorled, exstipulate, and sometimes exhibit heterophylly.
- Inflorescence: This is usually racemose (raceme or spike), and sometimes cymose (dichasium). It can be axillary or terminal. The flowers are solitary in some species.
- Flowers: These are zygomorphic, two-lipped and sometimes personate. They often have a great diversity of form. They are bisexual and hypogynous. Bracts and bracteoles are generally present.
- Calyx: The sepals are (5), gamosepalous, five-lobed and often imbricate.
- Corolla: The petals are (5), gamopetalous, often two-lipped and sometimes spurred or saccate. They are medianly zygomorphic, very rarely regular (as in *Scoparia*), and imbricate.
- Androecium: The stamens are four, didynamous, sometimes two, arching over in pairs. The posterior stamen is absent or a staminode. The anthers are divaricate.
- Gynoecium: The carpels are (2) and syncarpous. The ovary is superior, bilocular and antero-posterior (and not oblique as in solanaceae). The placentation is axile. The stigma is simple or bilobed. There are usually many ovules, though sometimes only a few. The disc is ring-like around the base of the ovary, sometimes unilateral.
- Fruit: This is mostly a capsule and sometimes a berry.
- Seeds: These are usually numerous, minute and endospermic.

Floral formula: $\cdot | \cdot$ H $K_{(5)}$ $\overline{C_{(5)} A_{4 \text{ or } 2}}$ $\underline{G}_{(2)}$

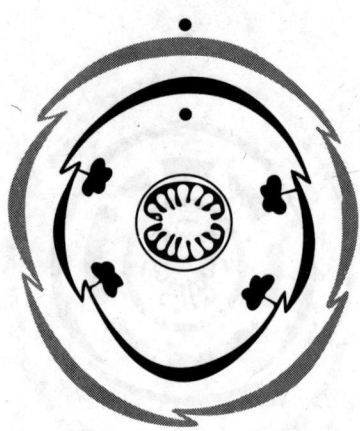

FIG. 5.14 Floral diagram of Scrophulariaceae

Examples: *Digitalis purpurea*, brahmi *(Bacopa monnieri)*, etc.

5.14. SOLANACEAE (Fig. 5.15)

- **Habit:** These are herbs and shrubs; bicollateral bundles or internal phloem are often present.
- **Leaves:** These are simple, sometimes pinnate, as in tomato, and alternate.
- **Flowers:** These are regular, seldom zygomorphic, as in *Brunfelsia*, bisexual and hypogynous.
- **Calyx:** The sepals are (5), united and persistent.
- **Corolla:** The petals are (5) and united. It is usually funnel or cup shaped, five lobed. The lobes are valvate or twisted in the bud.
- **Androecium:** The stamens are five, epipetalous and alternate with the corolla lobes. The anthers are apparently connate and often open by means of pores.
- **Gynoecium:** The carpels are (2) and syncarpous. The ovary is superior and obliquely placed. It is two celled or sometimes four celled, owing to the development of a false septum, as in *tomato* and thorn apple. There are many ovules in each chamber. The placentation is axile.
- **Fruit:** The fruit is a berry or capsule with many seeds.

Floral formula: $\oplus$ H $K_{(5)}$ $\overline{C_{(5)} A_5}$ $\bar{G}_{(2)}$

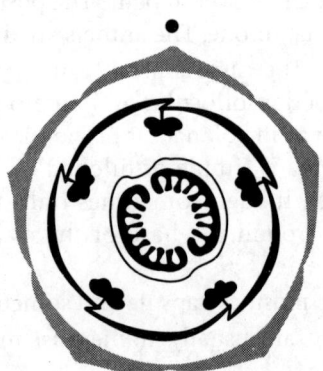

FIG. 5.15 Floral diagram of Solanaceae

Examples: *Atropa belladona*, tomato, capsicum, datura, etc.

5.15. UMBELLIFERAE (Fig. 5.16)

- **Habit:** These are herbs (rarely shrubs). The stem is usually fistular.
- **Leaves:** The leaves are alternate, simple, often much divided, sometimes decompound; petiole usually sheathing at the base.
- **Flowers:** The flowers are regular (actinomorphic) or sometimes zygomorphic, epigynous, bisexual or polygamous. The outer flowers are sometimes rayed; mostly protandrous. The bracts are in the form of an involucre.
- **Inflorescence:** It is an umbel, usually compound or in a few cases simple as in centella.
- **Calyx:** There are five sepals. They are free, adnate to the ovary, often considerably reduced in size.
- **Corolla:** The petals are five, rarely absent, free, adnate to the ovary and sometimes unequal. The margin is often curved inwards, valvate or imbricate.
- **Androecium:** There are five stamens, which are free, alternating with the petals, epigynous. The filaments are bent inwards in the bud; anthers introrse.
- **Gynoecium:** The carpels are two, syncarpous. The ovary is inferior, two-celled, antero-posterior, crowned by a two-lobed, epigynous disc (stylopodium), with two free styles arising from it. The stigmas capitate. There are two ovules, solitary in each cell and pendulous.
- **Fruit:** The fruit is a cremocarp consisting of two indehiscent carpels laterally or dorsally compressed, breaking up into two parts, called mericarps, which are attached to a slender, often forked axis *(carpophore)*. Each mericarp usually shows five longitudinal ridges and oil canals *(vittae)* in the furrows.
- **Seeds:** There are two seeds, one in each mericarp; albuminous.

Floral formula: $\oplus$ or $\cdot | \cdot$ H K_5 C_5 A_{10} $\underline{G}_{(2)}$

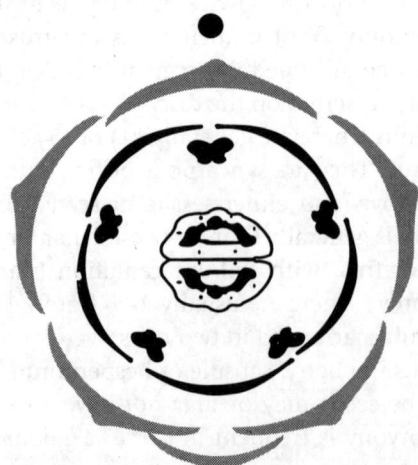

FIG. 5.16 Floral diagram of Umbelliferae

Examples: Fennel, coriander, caraway, dill, etc.

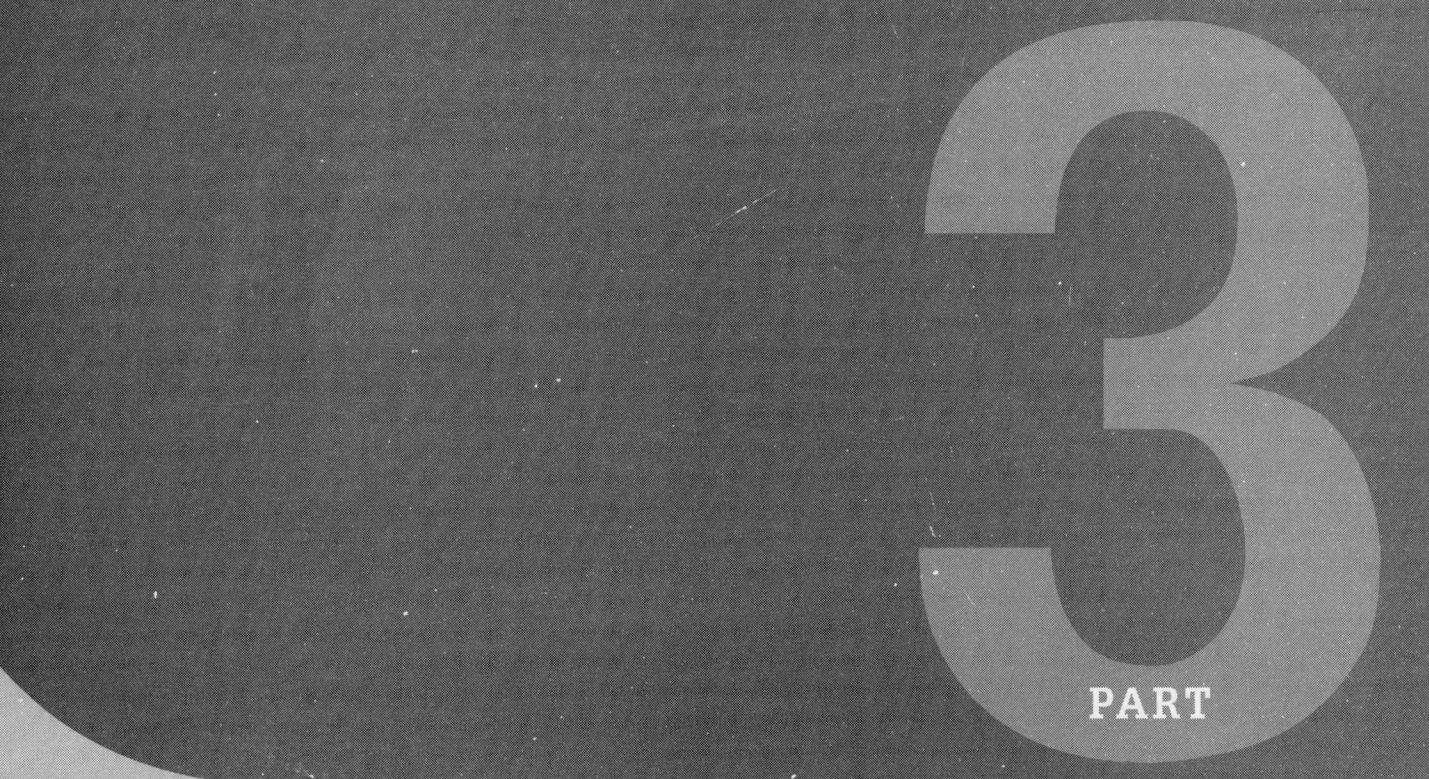

PART 3

PART

Cultivation, Collection, Production and Utilization of Herbal Drugs

Section Outline

OVERVIEW

The crude drugs that reach the market and pharmaceutical industries will have passed through different stages that have some effect on the nature and amount of active constituents responsible for therapeutic activity. Those stages are to be concerned more in order to make a drug useful to the mankind by all means. This part concerns regarding those parameters that have some effect over plants. This part also deals with the current trade of medicinal plant, worldwide growth of herbal industries and role of herbal industries in national economy.

CHAPTER 6

Cultivation, Collection and Processing of Herbal Drugs

CONTENTS

6.1. INTRODUCTION

The crude drugs which reach the market and pharmaceutical industries will have passed through different stages that have some effect in the nature and amount of active constituents responsible for therapeutic activity. Those stages are to be concerned more in order to make a drug useful to the mankind by all means. This chapter concerns regarding such parameters which has some effect over plants.

Cultivation produces improved quality of plants. It helps in selecting the species, varieties or hybrids that have the desired phytoconstituents due to the controlled environmental growth better plant product is obtained and makes the collection and processing steps easier when compared to wild sources. Cultivation results in obtaining plants with maximum secondary metabolites. It leads to industrialization in the country by the regular supply of plants. Serves as a useful tool for research purposes.

The advantages of cultivation may be briefly summarized as follows:

1. It ensures quality and purity of medicinal plants. Crude drugs derive their utility from chemical contents in them. If uniformity is maintained in all operations during the process of cultivation, drugs of highest quality can be obtained. Cultivation of rhizomes demands an adequate quantity of fertilizers and proper irrigation. Systematic cultivation results in raising a crop with maximum content of volatile oil and other constituents. The examples of ginger, turmeric and liquorice can be cited to illustrate this point. If the cultivated plants are kept free of weeds, the contamination of crude drugs can be conveniently avoided.

KEY TERMS

2. Collection of crude drugs from cultivated plants gives a better yield and therapeutic quality. However, it is a skilled operation and requires some professional excellence, if the collection of crude drugs for market is done from cultivated plants by skilled and well-experienced personnel, the high yield and therapeutic quality of drugs can be maintained. For example, collection of latex from poppy capsules and oleo-resins from Pinus species, if done by experienced persons, can result in better yield of crude drugs. Preservation of green colour of senna leaves and minimizing the deterioration of cardiac glycosides in freshly collected leaves of digitalis can be achieved only by highly skilled labour.

3. Cultivation ensures regular supply of a crude drug. In other words, cultivation is a method of crop-planning. Planning a crop cultivation regularizes its supply and as a result the industries depending upon crude drugs do not face problem of shortage of raw material.

4. The cultivation of medicinal and aromatic plants also leads to industrialization to a greater extent. The cultivation of coffee and cocoa in Kerala has given rise to several cottage and small-scale industries. The cultivation of cinchona in West Bengal has led to the establishment of the cinchona-alkaloid factory near Darjeeling. The government owned opium factory at Ghaziabad is an eloquent testimony to the significance of well planned cultivation of poppy.

5. Cultivation permits application of modern technological aspects such as mutation, polyploidy and hybridization.

6.2. SOILS, SEEDS AND PROPAGATION MATERIAL

The physical, chemical and microbiological properties of the soil play a crucial role in the growth of plants. Water holding capacity of different sizes of soil too affects the plants. The calcium present in the soil would be very much useful for some plants where as the others does not require calcium. The seed to be used for cultivation should be identified botanically, showing the details of its species, chemotype and origin. The seeds should be 100% traceable. The parent material should meet standard requirements regarding the purity and germination. It should be free from pests and diseases in order to guarantee healthy plant growth. Preference should be given to the resistant or tolerant species. Plant materials or seeds derived from genetically modified organisms have to comply with national and European Union regulations. Season when the seeds should be sown and at what stage a seed should be sown should be predetermined. Few seeds such as cinnamon losses its viability if stored for long period and the percentage of germination would be less for the seeds which were long stored.

Methods of Plant Propagation

Medicinal plants can be propagated by two usual methods as applicable to nonmedicinal plants or crops. These methods are referred as sexual method and asexual method. Each of these methods has certain advantages, and also, disadvantages.

1. Sexual method (seed propagation)

In case of sexual method, the plants are raised from seeds and such plants are known as seedlings. The sexual method of propagation enjoys following advantages:

1. Seedlings are long-lived (in case of perennial drugs) and bear more heavily (in case of fruits). Plants are more sturdier.
2. Seedlings are comparatively cheaper and easy to raise.
3. Propagation from seed has been responsible for production of some chance-seedlings of highly superior merits which may be of great importance to specific products, such as orange, papaya, etc.
4. In case of plants where other vegetative methods cannot be utilized, propagation from seeds is the only method of choice.

Sexual method suffers from following limitations:

1. Generally, seedling trees are not uniform in their growth and yielding capacity, as compared to grafted trees.
2. They require more time to bear, as compared to grafted plants.
3. The cost of harvesting, spraying of pesticides, etc., is more as compared to grafted trees.
4. It is not possible to avail of modifying influence of root stocks on scion, as in case of vegetatively propagated trees.

For propagation purpose, the seeds must be of good quality. They should be capable of a high germination rate, free from diseases and insects and also free from other seeds, used seeds and extraneous material. The germination capacity of seeds is tested by rolled towel test, excised embryo test, etc. The seeds are preconditioned with the help of scarification to make them permeable to water and gases, if the seeds are not to be germinated in near future, they should be stored in cool and dry place to maintain their germinating power. Long storage of seeds should be avoided.

Before germination, sometimes a chemical treatment is given with stimulants like gibberellins, cytokinins, ethylene, thiourea, potassium nitrate or sodium hypochlorite. Gibberellic acid (GA_3) promotes germination of some type of dormant seeds and stimulates the seedling growth. Many freshly harvested dormant seeds germinate better after soaking in potassium nitrate solution. Thiourea is used for those seeds which do not germinate in dark or at high temperatures.

Methods of sowing the seeds

Numerous methods of sowing the seeds of the medicinal plants are in practice. Few of them using seeds for cultivation are described:

Broadcasting: If the seeds are extremely small the sowing is done by broadcasting method. In this method the seeds are scattered freely in well prepared soil for cultivation. The seeds only need raking. If they are deeply sown or covered by soil, they may not get germinated. Necessary thinning of the seedlings is done by keeping a specific distance, e.g. Isabgol, Linseed, Sesame, etc.

Dibbling: When the seeds of average size and weight are available, they are sown by placing in holes. Number of seeds to be put in holes vary from three to five, depending upon the vitality, sex of the plants needed for the purpose and the size of the plant coming out of the seeds.

For example, in case of fennel four to five fruits are put in a single hole keeping suitable distance in between two holes. In case of castor, only two to three seeds are put. In case of papaya, the plants are unisexual and only female plants are desired for medicinal purposes. Hence, five to six seeds are put together and after the sex of the plants is confirmed, healthy female plant is allowed to grow while male plants and others are removed.

Miscellaneous: Many a time the seeds are sown in nursery beds. The seedlings thus produced are transplanted to farms for further growth, such as cinchona, cardamom, clove, digitalis, capsicum, etc.

Special treatment to seeds: To enhance germination, special treatments to seeds may be given, such as soaking the seeds in water for a day, e.g. castor seeds and other slow-germinating seeds. Sometimes, seeds are soaked in sulphuric acid, e.g. henbane seeds. Alternatively, testa is partially removed by grindstone or by pounding seeds with coarse sand, e.g. Indian senna. Several plant hormones like gibberellins, auxins are also used.

2. Asexual method

In case of asexual method of vegetative propagation, the vegetative part of a plant, such as stem or root, is placed in such an environment that it develops into a new plant.

Asexual propagation enjoys following advantages:

1. There is no variation between the plant grown and plant from which it is grown. As such, the plants are uniform in growth and yielding capacity. In case of fruit trees, uniformity in fruit quality makes harvesting and marketing easy.
2. Seedless varieties of fruits can only be propagated vegetatively, e.g. grapes, pomegranates and lemon.
3. Plants start bearing earlier as compared to seedling trees.

4. Budding or grafting encourages disease-resistant varieties of plants.
5. Modifying influence of root-stocks on scion can be availed of.
6. Inferior or unsuitable varieties can be over-looked.

It suffers from following disadvantages:

1. In comparison to seedling trees, these are not vigorous in growth and are not long-lived.
2. No new varieties can be evolved by this method.

Asexual method of vegetative propagation consists of three types:

(a) Natural methods of vegetative propagation.
(b) Artificial methods of vegetative propagation.
(c) Aseptic method of micropropagation (tissue culture).

(a) Natural methods of vegetative propagation: It is done by sowing various parts of the plants in well prepared soil. The following are the examples of vegetative propagation.

Bulbs	Squill, garlic
Corms	Colchicum, saffron
Tubers	Jalap, aconite, potato
Rhizomes	Ginger, turmeric
Runners	Peppermint
Suckers	Mint, pineapple, chrysanthemum, banana
Offsets	Aloe, valerian
Stolons	Arrow-root, Liquorice

(b) Artificial methods of vegetative propagations: The method by which plantlets or seedlings are produced from vegetative part of the plant by using some technique or process is known as artificial method of vegetative propagation. These methods are classified as under:

1. Cuttings
(i) Stem cuttings
   (a) Soft wood cuttings: Berberry
   (b) Semi-hardwood cuttings: Citrus, camellia
   (c) Hardwood cuttings: Orange, rose and bougainvillea
(ii) Root cuttings: Brahmi
(iii) Leaf cuttings: Bryophyllum
(iv) Leaf bud cuttings

2. Layering
(i) Simple layering: Guava, lemon
(ii) Serpentine layering: Jasmine, clematis
(iii) Air layering (Gootee): Ficus, mango, bougainvillea, cashew nut
(iv) Mount layering

(v) Trench layering

(vi) Tip layering

3. Grafting

(i) Whip grafting: Apple and rose

(ii) Tongue grafting

(iii) Side grafting: Sapota and cashew nut

(iv) Approach grafting: Guava and sapota

(v) Stone grafting: Mango

(c) Aseptic method of micropropagation (tissue culture): It is a novel method for propagation of medicinal plants. In micropropagation, the plants are developed in an artificial medium under aseptic conditions from fine pieces of plants like single cells, callus, seeds, embryos, root tips, shoot tips, pollen grains, etc. They are also provided with nutritional and hormonal requirements.

Preparation and Types of Nursery Beds

For various genuine reasons, seeds cannot be sown directly into soil, i.e. very small size (isabgol, tulsi) high cost, poor germination rate and long germination time (cardamom, coriander). Under such circumstances, seeds are grown into the nursery bed which not only is economical, but one can look after the diseases (if any) during germination period. Small size of beds can be irrigated conveniently along with fertilizers, as and when necessary. There are four types of nursery beds.

1. Flat bed method
2. Raised bed method
3. Ridges and furrow method
4. Ring and basin method

Taking into consideration the amount of water and type of soil required for a particular seed one should select the type.

Methods of Irrigation

Water is essential for any type of cultivation. After studying the availably and requirement of water for a specific crop, one has to design his own irrigation system at the reasonable cost.

Following methods of irrigation are known traditionally in India. The cultivation has an option after giving due consideration to the merits and demerits of each.

1. *Hand watering:* Economical and easy to operate.
2. *Flood watering:* Easy to operate, results in wastage of water.
3. *Boom watering:* Easy to operate, but restricted utility.
4. *Drip irrigation:* Scientific, systematic and easy to operate; costly.
5. *Sprinkler irrigation:* Costly, gives good results.

6.3. GOOD AGRICULTURAL PRACTICES

Depending on the method of cultivation different standard operating procedures for cultivation should be followed by the cultivators. A suitable area for the cultivation and the standard operation procedures for the cultivation should be developed depending upon the needs of the plants. Medicinal and aromatic plants should not be grown in soils which are contaminated by sludge and not contaminated by heavy metals, residues of plant protection products and any other unnatural chemicals, so the chemical products (pesticide and herbicide) used should be with as minimum negative effect as possible, human faeces should be avoided. Depending upon the soil fertility and the nutritional requirement of medicinal plants the type of the fertilizer and the amount of the fertilizer to be used is determined. Products for chemical plant protection have to conform to the European Union's maximum residue limits. Proper irrigation and drainage should be earned out according to the climatic condition and soil moisture. The soil used for cultivation should be well aerated. The use of pesticides and herbicides has to be documented. Irrigation should be minimized as much as possible and only be applied according to the needs of the plant. Water used for irrigation should be free from all possible forms of contaminants and should comply with national and European Union quality standards. The area for cultivation should be strictly prohibited from the contaminations like house garbage, industrial waste, hospital refuse and faeces. Field management should be strengthened and proper measures like pruning, shading, etc., should be provided for increasing the yield of the active constituent and maintain the consistency of the yield. The pests used should give high efficacy, hypotoxicity and low residue at the minimum effective input so that the residue of pesticides are also reduced and protected from ecological environment.

Application and storage of plant protection products have to be in conformity with the regulations of manufacturers and the respective national authorities. The application should only be earned out by qualified staff using approved equipment. The nutrient supply and chemical plant protection, should secure the marketability of the product. The buyer of the batch should be informed about the brand, quantity and date of pesticide use in written.

Though several countries in the world have a rich heritage of herbal drugs, very few have their claim for their procurement of crude drugs only from cultivated species. Our reliance on wild sources of crude drugs and the lack of information on the sound cultivation and maintaining technology of crude drugs have resulted in gradual depletion of raw material from wild sources. Though the cultivation of medicinal plants offers wide range of advantages over the wild sources, it can be an uneconomical process for some crude drugs which occur abundantly in nature, e.g.

nux vomica, acacia, etc. On the other hand, crude drugs like cardamom, clove, poppy, tea, cinchona, ginger, linseed, isabgol, saffron, peppermint, fennel, etc., are obtained majorly from cultivated plants. The cultivation of crude drugs involves keen knowledge of various factors from agricultural and pharmaceutical sphere, such as soil, climate, rainfall, irrigation, altitude, temperature, use of fertilizers and pesticides, genetic manipulation and biochemical aspects of natural drugs. When all such factors are precisely applied, the new approach to scientific cultivation technology emerges out.

6.4. FACTORS AFFECTING CULTIVATION

Cultivation of medicinal plants offers wide range of advantages over the plants obtained from wild sources. There are few factors to concern which have a real effect on plant growth and development, nature and quantity of secondary metabolites. The factors affecting cultivation are altitude, temperature, rainfall, length of day, day light, soil and soil fertility, fertilizers and pests. The effects of these factors have been studied by growing particular plants in different environmental conditions and observing variations. For example, a plant which is subjected to a particular environment may develop as a small plant which, when analysed shows high proportion of metabolite than the plants attained the required growth. Nutrients have the ability to enhance the production of secondary metabolites, at the same time they may reduce the metabolites as well.

Altitude

Altitude is a very important factor in cultivation of medicinal plants. Tea, cinchona and eucalyptus are cultivated favourably at an altitude of 1000–2000 metres. Cinnamon and cardamom are grown at a height of 500–1000 metres, while senna can be cultivated at sea level. The following are the examples of medicinal and aromatic plants indicating the altitude for their successful cultivation (Table 6.1).

Table 6.1: Altitude for Drug cultivation

Plant	Altitude (metres)
Tea	1000–1500
Cinchona	1000–2000
Camphor	1500–2000
Cinnamon	250–1000
Coffee	1000–2000
Clove	Up to 900
Saffron	Up to 1250
Cardamom	600–1600

Temperature

Temperature is a crucial factor controlling the growth, metabolism and there by the yield of secondary metabolites of plants. Even though each species has become adapted to its own natural environment, they are able to exist in a considerable range of temperature. Many plants will grow better in temperate regions during summer, but they lack in resistance to withstand frost in winter.

Table 6.2: Optimum temperature for drug cultivation

Plant	Optimum temperature (°F)
Cinchona	60–75
Coffee	55–70
Tea	70–90
Cardamom	50–100

Rainfall

For the proper development of plant, rainfall is required in proper measurements. Xerophytic plants like aloes do not require irrigation or rainfall. The effects of rainfall on plants must be considered in relation to the annual rainfall throughout the year with the water holding properties of the soil. Variable results have been reported for the production of constituents under different conditions of rainfall. Excessive rainfall could cause a reduction in the secondary metabolites due to leaching of water soluble substances from the plants.

Day Length and Day Light

It has been proved that even the length of the day has an effect over the metabolites production. The plants that are kept in long day conditions may contain more or less amount of constituents when compared to the plants kept in short day. For example peppermint has produced menthone, menthol and traces of menthofuran in long day conditions and only menthofuran in short day condition.

The developments of plants vary much in both the amount and intensity of the light they require. The wild grown plants would meet the required conditions and so they grow but during cultivation we have to fulfil the requirements of plants. The day light was found to increase the amount of alkaloids in belladonna, stramonium, cinchona, etc. Even the type of radiation too has an effect over the development and metabolites of plants.

Soil

Each and every plant species have its own soil and nutritive requirements. The three important basic characteristics of soils are their physical, chemical and microbiological properties. Soil provides mechanical support, water and essential foods for the development of plants. Soil consists of air, water, mineral matters and organic matters. Variations in particle size result in different soils ranging from clay, sand and gravel. Particle size influences the water holding capacity of soil. The type and amount of minerals plays a vital role in plant cultivation. Calcium favours the growth of certain plants whereas with some plants it does not produce any effects. The plants are able to determine their own soil pH range for their growth; microbes should be taken in to consideration which grows well in certain pH. Nitrogen containing soil has a great momentum in raising the production of alkaloids in some plants.

Depending upon the size of the mineral matter, the following names are given to the soil (Table 6.3).

Table 6.3: Type of soil on the basis of particle size

Particle size (diameter)	Type of soil
Less than 0.002 mm	Fine clay
0.002–0.02 mm	Coarse clay or silt
0.02–0.2 mm	Fine sand
0.2–2.0 mm	Coarse sand

Depending upon the percentage covered by clay, soils are classified as under (Table 6.4).

Table 6.4: Type of soil on the basis of percentage covered by clay

Type of soil	Percentage covered by clay
Clay	More than 50% of clay
Loamy	30–50% of clay
Silt loam	20–30% of clay
Sandy loam	10–20% of clay
Sandy soil	More than 70% sand
Calcarious soil	More than 20% of lime

Soil Fertility

It is the capacity of soil to provide nutrients in adequate amounts and in balanced proportion to plants. If cropping is done without fortification of soil with plant nutrients, soil fertility gets lost. It is also diminished through leaching and erosion. Soil fertility can be maintained by addition of animal manures, nitrogen-fixing bacteria or by application of chemical fertilizers. The latter is time saving and surest of all above techniques.

Fertilizers and Manures

Plant also needs food for their growth and development. What plants need basically for their growth are the carbon dioxide, sun-rays, water and mineral matter from the soil.

Thus, it is seen that with limited number of chemical elements, plants build up fruits, grains, fibres, etc., and synthesize fixed and volatile oils, glycosides, alkaloids, sugar and many more chemicals.

(a) Chemical fertilizers

Animals are in need of vitamins, plants are in need of sixteen nutrient elements for synthesizing various compounds. Some of them are known as primary nutrients like nitrogen, phosphorus and potassium. Magnesium, calcium and sulphur are required in small quantities and hence, they are known as secondary nutrients. Trace elements like copper, manganese, iron, boron, molybdenum, zinc are also necessary for plant growths are known as micronutrients. Carbon, hydrogen, oxygen and chlorine are provided from water and air. Every element has to perform some specific function in growth and development of plants. Its deficiency is also characterized by certain symptoms.

(b) Manures

Farm yard manure (FYM/compost), castor seed cake, poultry manures, neem and karanj seed cakes vermin compost, etc., are manures. Oil-cake and compost normally consists of 3–6% of nitrogen, 2% phosphates and 1–1.5% potash. They are made easily available to plants. Bone meal, fish meal, biogas slurry, blood meal and press mud are the other forms of organic fertilizers.

(c) Biofertilizers

Inadequate supply, high costs and undesirable effects if used successively are the demerits of fertilizers or manures and hence the cultivator has to opt for some other type of fertilizer. Biofertilizers are the most suitable forms that can be tried. These consist of different types of microorganisms or lower organisms which fix the atmospheric nitrogen in soil and plant can use them for their day to day use. Thus they are symbiotic. Rhizobium, Azotobacter, Azospirillum, Bijericcia, Blue-green algae, Azolla, etc., are the examples of biofertilizers.

Pests and Pests Control

Pests are undesired plant or animal species that causes a great damage to the plants. There are different types of pests; they are microbes, insects, non insect pests and weeds.

Microbes

They include fungi, bacteria and viruses. Armillaria Root Rot (Oak Root Fungus) is a disease caused by fungi *Armillaria mellea* (Marasmiaceae) and in this the infected plant become nonproductive and very frequently dies within two to four years. Plants develop weak, shorter shoots as they are infected by the pathogen. Dark, root-like structures (rhizomorphs), grow into the soil after symptoms develop on plants. The fungus is favoured by soil that is continually damp. Powdery mildew is another disease caused by fungus *Uncinula necato* on leaves, where chlorotic spots appear on the upper surface of leaf. On fruit the pathogen appears as white, powdery masses that may colonize the entire berry surface. Summer Bunch Rot is a disease in which masses of black, brown or green spores develop on the surface of infected berries caused by a variety microbes like *Aspergillus niger, Alternaria tennis, Botrytis cinerea, Cladosporium herbarum, Rhizopus arrhizus,* Penicillium sp. and others.

Fomitopsis pinicola (Sw.) P. Karst. Belonging to family Fomitopsidaceae causes a diseases known as red-belted fungus. Several other fungi attacks the medicinal plants, like *Pythium aphanidermatum* causes pythium rhizome rot, *Septoria digitalis* causing leaf spot, little leaf disease by *Phytophthora cinnamomi* Rands (Pythiaceae), etc.

Crown gall disease caused by *Agrobacterium tumefaciens* (Rhizobiaceae). Galls may be produced on canes, trunks, roots and cordons and may grow to several inches in diameter. Internally galls are soft and have the appearance of disorganized tissue. The pathogen can be transmitted by any agent that contacts the contaminated material. Galls commonly develop where plants have been injured during cultivation or pruning. *Xylella fastidiosa* is a bacterium causes Pierce's Disease, in this leaves become slightly yellow or red along margins and eventually leaf margins dry or die.

Many viruses are also reported to cause necrosis of leaves, petioles and stems, they are tobacco mosaic virus, mosaic virus, cucumber mosaic virus, tobacco ring spot virus, yellow vein mosaic, etc.

Controlling techniques: Chemical fumigation of the soil, fungicide, bactericide, pruning, proper water and fertilizer management, good sanitation, heat treatment of planting stock, cut and remove the infected parts, genetically manipulating the plants for producing plants to resist fungi and bacteria are practices that are used to prevent or minimize the effects produced by microbes.

Insects

Ants, they are of different varieties—Argentine ant: *Linepithema humile,* Grey ants: *Formica aerata* and *Formica perpilosa,* Pavement ant: *Tetramorium caespitum,* Southern fire ant: *Solenopsis xyloni,* Thief ant: *Solenopsis molesta.* They spoil the soil by making nest and they feed honey dew secreted in plants.

Branch and Twig Borer *(Melalgus confertus)* burrow into the canes through the base of the bud or into the crotch formed by the shoot and spur. Feeding is often deep enough to completely conceal the adult in the hole. When shoots reach a length of 10–12 inches, a strong wind can cause the infected parts to twist and break. The click beetle *(Limonius canus)* can feed on buds. Cutworms *(Peridroma saucia, Amathes c-nigrum,*

Orthndes rufula) injures the buds and so the buds may not develop. Leafhoppers *(Erythroneura elegantula, Erythroneura variabilis)* remove the contents of leaf cells, leaving behind empty cells that appear as pale yellow spots.

Oak twig pruners *(Anelaphiis* spp. Linsley) are known as shoot, twig and root insects that affects the above mentioned parts.

Controlling techniques: Tilling the soil will also affect the nesting sites of ants and help to reduce their populations, collection and destruction of eggs, larvae, pupae and adults of insects, trapping the insects, insecticides, creating a situation to compete among males for mating with females, cutworms can be prevented by natural enemies like predaceous or parasitic insects, mammals, parasitic nematodes, pathogens, birds and reptiles.

Non insect pests

They are divided into vertebrates and invertebrates. Vertebrates that disrupt the plants are monkeys, rats, birds, squirrels, etc. Non vertebrates are Webspinning Spider Mites *(Tetranychus pacificus, Eotetranychus willamettei, Tetranychus urticae),* which causes discoloration in leaves and yellow spots. Nematode *(Meloidogyne incognita, Xiphinema americanutri, Criconemella xenoplax)* produces giant cell formation, disturbs the uptake of nutrients and water, and interferes with plant growth. Crabs, snails are the other few invertebrates that causes trouble to the plant.

Controlling techniques: Construction of concrete ware houses, traps, biological methods, rodenticides, etc.

Weeds

Weeds reduce growth and yields of plants by competing for water, nutrients and sunlight. Weed control enhances the establishment of new plants and improves the growth and yield of established plants. The skilled persons have many weed management tools available to achieve these objectives; however, the methods of using these tools vary from year to year and from place to place.

Soil characteristics are important to weed management. Soil texture and organic matter influence the weed species that are present, the number and timing of cultivations required, and the activity of herbicides. Annual species, such as puncturevine, crabgrass, horseweed and Panicum spp., or perennials like Johnson grass, nutsedge and bermudagrass are more prevalent on light-textured soil while perennials such as curly dock, field bindweed, and dallisgrass are more common on heavier-textured soils. Less pre-emergent herbicide is required for weed control on sandy, light soils, but residual control may be shorter than on clay or clay loam soils. Use low rates of herbicide on sandy soils or those low in organic matter. Clay soils are slower to dry for effective cultivation than sandy loam soils; thus, more frequent cultivation is practiced on lighter soils than heavy soils.

Few common weeds are:

Bermudagrass: It is a vigorous spring- and summer-growing perennial. It grows from seed but its extensive system of rhizomes and stolons can also be spread during cultivation.

Dallisgrass: It is a common perennial weed that can be highly competitive in newly planted plants; in established plants area it competes for soil moisture and nutrients. Dallisgrass seedlings germinate in spring and summer, and form new plants on short rhizomes that developed from the original root system. The other weeds are pigweeds Amaranthus spp. pineapple-weed *Chamomilla suaveolens*, nightshades Solanum spp., etc.

Apart from these, parasitic and epiphytic plants like dodder (Cuscuta spp. L.), mistletoe (Phoradendron spp. Nutt.), American squawroot (*Conopholis americana*), etc., too affect the growth of plants.

Controlling techniques: Use of low rates of herbicides: Herbicides are traditionally discussed as two groups: those that are active against germinating weed seeds (pre-emergent herbicides) and those that are active on growing plants (postemergent herbicides). Some herbicides have both pre- and postemergent activity. Herbicides vary in their ability to control different weed species.

Pre-emergent herbicides are active in the soil against germinating weed seedlings. These herbicides are applied to bare soil and are leached into the soil with rain or irrigation where they affect germinating weed seeds. If herbicides remain on the soil surface without incorporation, some will degrade rapidly from sunlight. Weeds that emerge while the herbicide is on the surface, before it is activated by rain or irrigation, will not be controlled. Postemergent herbicides are applied to control weeds already growing in the vineyard. They can be combined with pre-emergent herbicides or applied as spot treatments during the growing season. In newly planted plants, selective postemergent herbicides are available for the control of most annual and perennial grasses, but not broadleaf weeds.

Frequent wetting of the soil promotes more rapid herbicide degradation in the soil. Herbicide degradation is generally faster in moist, warm soils than in dry, cold soils.

Table 6.5: General methods of pest controls

Controlling techniques	Methods involved
Cultural	Changing the time of sowing and harvesting, maintenance of storage, special cultivation methods, proper cleaning, using trap crops and resistant varieties
Physical	Mechanical control, utilization of physical factors (temperature, less oxygen concentration, humidity, passing CO_2)
Biological	Using predators, parasites, pathogens, sterilization, genetic manipulation, pheromones
Chemical	Use of pesticides, herbicides, antifeedants

Other Factors that Affect the Cultivated Plants

Air Pollution

Chemical discharges into the atmosphere have increased dramatically during this century, but the total effect on plants is virtually unknown. It has been demonstrated that air pollutants can cause mortality and losses in growth of plants. Nearly all species of deciduous and coniferous trees are sensitive to some pollutants. There are many chemicals released into the atmosphere singly and as compounds. In addition, other compounds are synthesized in the atmosphere. Some chemicals can be identified through leaf tissue analysis and by analysing the air. Generally, pollution injury first appears as leaf injury. Spots between the veins, leaf margin discoloration and tip burns are common. These symptoms can also be influenced by host sensitivity, which is effected by genetic characteristics and environmental factors.

Herbicide

Herbicides should be handled very carefully; misapplication of herbicides can often damage nontarget plants. The total extent of such damage remains unclear, but localized, severe damage occurs. Symptoms of herbicide injury are variable due to chemical mode of action, dosage, duration of exposure, plant species and environmental conditions. Some herbicides cause growth abnormalities such as cupping or twisting of foliage while others cause foliage yellowing or browning, defoliation, or death.

6.5. PLANT HORMONES AND GROWTH REGULATORS

Plant hormones (phytohormones) are physiological intercellular messengers that control the complete plant lifecycle, including germination, rooting, growth, flowering, fruit ripening, foliage and death. In addition, plant hormones are secreted in response to environmental factors such as excess of nutrients, drought conditions, light, temperature and chemical or physical stress. So, levels of hormones will change over the lifespan of a plant and are dependent upon season and environment.

The term *plant growth factor* is usually employed for plant hormones or substances of similar effect that are administered to plants. Growth factors are widely used in industrialized agriculture to improve productivity. The application of growth factors allows synchronization of plant development to occur. For instance, ripening fruits can be controlled by setting desired atmospheric ethylene levels. Using this method, fruits that are separated from their parent plant will still respond to growth factors; allowing commercial plants to be ripened in storage during and after transportation. This way the process of harvesting can be run much more efficiently and effectively. Other applications include rooting of seedlings or the suppression of rooting with the simultaneous promotion of cell division as required by plant cell cultures. Just like with animal hormones, plant growth factors come in a wide variety, producing different and often antagonistic effects. In short, the right combination of hormones is vital to achieve the desired behavioural characteristics of cells and the productive development of plants as a whole. The plant growth regulators are classified into synthetic and native. The synthetic regulators are also known as exogenous regulators and the native are called endogenous.

Five major classes of plant hormones are mentioned: auxins, cytokinins, gibberellins, abscisic acid and ethylene. However as research progresses, more active molecules are being found and new families of regulators are emerging; one example being polyamines (putrescine or spermidine). Plant growth regulators have made the way for plant tissue culture techniques, which were a real boon for mankind in obtaining therapeutically valuable secondary metabolites.

Auxins

The term *auxin* is derived from the Greek word *auxein* which means 'to grow'. Generally compounds are considered as auxins if they are able to induce cell elongation in stems and otherwise resemble indoleacetic acid (the first auxin isolated) in physiological activity. Auxins usually affect other processes in addition to cell elongation of stem cells but this characteristic is considered critical of all auxins and thus *helps* define the hormone.

Auxins were the first plant hormones discovered. Charles Darwin was among the first scientists to pool in plant hormone research. He described the effects of light on movement of canary grass coleoptiles in his book 'The Power of Movement in Plants' presented in 1880. The coleoptile is a specialized leaf originating from the first node which sheaths the epicotyl in the plants seedling stage protecting it until it emerges from the ground. When unidirectional light shines on the coleoptile, it bends in the direction of the light. If the tip of the coleoptile was covered with aluminium foil, bending would not occur towards the unidirectional light. However if the tip of the coleoptile was left uncovered but the portion just below the tip was covered, exposure to unidirectional light resulted in curvature towards the light. Darwin's experiment suggested that the tip of the coleoptile was the tissue responsible for

perceiving the light and producing some signal which was transported to the lower part of the coleoptile where the physiological response of bending occurred. When he cut off the tip of the coleoptile and exposed the rest of the coleoptile to unidirectional light curvature did not occur confirming the results of his experiment.

Salkowski (1885) discovered indole-3-acetic acid (IAA) in fermentation media. The isolation of the same product from plant tissues would not be found in plant tissues for almost 50 years. IAA is the major auxin involved in many of the physiological processes in plants. Fitting in 1907 put his efforts in studying signal transaction by making incisions on the light or dark side of the plant. He failed because the signal was capable of crossing or going around the incision. In 1913, modification was made in Fitting's experiment by Boysen-Jensen, in that they inserted pieces of mica to block the transport of the signal and showed that transport of auxin towards the base occurs on the dark side of the plant as opposed to the side exposed to the unidirectional light. In 1918, Paal confirmed Boysen-Jensen's results by cutting off coleoptile tips in the dark, exposing only the tips to the light, replacing the coleoptile tips on the plant but off centered to one side or the other. Results showed that whichever side was exposed to the coleoptile, curvature occurred towards the other side. Soding (1925) followed Paal's idea and showed that if tips were cut off there was a reduction in growth but if they were cut off and then replaced growth continued to occur.

In 1926, Fritz Went reported a plant growth substance, isolated by placing agar blocks under coleoptile tips for a period of time then removing them and placing them on decapitated Avena stems. After placement over the agar, the stems resumed growth. In 1928, again Went developed a method of quantifying this plant growth substance. His results suggested that the curvatures of stems were proportional to the amount of growth substance in the agar. This test was called the avena curvature test. Much of our current knowledge of auxin was obtained from its applications. It was Went's work, which had a great influence in stimulating plant growth substance research. He is often credited with dubbing the term auxin but it was actually Kogl and Haagen-Smit who purified the compound auxentriolic acid (auxin A) from human urine in 1931. Later Kogl isolated other compounds from urine which were similar in structure and function to auxin A. One of which was indole-3 acetic acid (IAA) initially discovered by Salkowski in 1885. In 1954 a committee of plant physiologists was set up to characterize the group auxins.

Indole acetic acid (IAA) is the principle natural auxin and other natural auxins are indole-3-acetonitrile (IAN), phenyl acetic acid and 4-chloroindole-3-acetic acid. The exogenous or synthetic auxins are indole-3-butyric acid (IBA), α-naphthyl acetic acid (NAA), 2-naphthyloxyacetic acid

IAA, IBA, NOA, NAA, NAD, 2,4-D

(NOA), 1-naphthyl acetamide (NAD), 5-carboxymethyl-N, N-dimethyl dithiocarbamate, 2,4-dichlorophenoxy acetic acid (2,4-D), etc.

Production and occurrence

Produced in shoot and root meristematic tissue, in young leaves, mature root cells and small amounts in mature leaves. Transported throughout the plant parts and the production of IAA will be more in day time. It is released by all cells when they are experiencing conditions which would normally cause a shoot meristematic cell to produce auxin. Ethylene has direct or indirect action over to enhance the synthesis auxin.

IAA is chemically similar to the amino acid tryptophan which is generally accepted to be the molecule from which IAA is derived. Three mechanisms have been suggested to explain this conversion:

- Tryptophan is converted to indolepyruvic acid through a transamination reaction. Indolepyruvic acid is then converted to indoleacetaldehyde by a decarboxylation reaction. The final step involves oxidation of indoleacetaldehyde resulting in indoleacetic acid.
- Tryptophan undergoes decarboxylation resulting in tryptamine. Tryptamine is then oxidized and deaminated to produce indoleacetaldehyde. This molecule is further oxidized to produce indoleacetic acid.
- IAA can be produced via a tryptophan-independent mechanism. This mechanism is poorly understood, but has been proven using tip (-) mutants. Other experiments have shown that, in some plants, this mechanism is actually the preferred mechanism of IAA biosynthesis.

The enzymes responsible for the biosynthesis of IAA are most active in young tissues such as shoot apical meristems and growing leaves and fruits. These are the same tissues where the highest concentrations of IAA are found. One way plants can control the amount of IAA present in tissues at a particular time is by controlling the biosynthesis of the hormone. Another control mechanism involves the production of conjugates which are, in simple terms, molecules which resemble the hormone but are inactive. The formation of conjugates may be a mechanism of storing and transporting the active hormone. Conjugates can be formed from IAA via hydrolase enzymes. Conjugates can be rapidly activated by environmental stimuli signalling a quick hormonal response. Degradation of auxin is the final method of controlling auxin levels. This process also has two proposed mechanisms outlined below.

The oxidation of IAA by oxygen resulting in the loss of the carboxyl group and 3-methyleneoxindole as the major breakdown product. IAA oxidase is the enzyme which catalyses this activity. Conjugates of IAA and synthetic auxins such as 2,4-D can not be destroyed by this activity.

C-2 of the heterocyclic ring may be oxidized resulting in oxindole-3-acetic acid. C-3 may be oxidized in addition to C-2 resulting in dioxindole-3-acetic acid. The mechanisms by which biosynthesis and degradation of auxin molecules occur are important to future agricultural applications. Information regarding auxin metabolism will most likely lead to genetic and chemical manipulation of endogenous hormone levels resulting in desirable growth and differentiation of important plant species.

Functions of auxin

- Stimulates cell elongation.
- The auxin supply from the apical bud suppresses growth of lateral buds. Apical dominance is the inhibiting influence of the shoot apex on the growth of axillary buds. Removal of the apical bud results in growth of the axillary buds. Replacing the apical bud with a lanolin paste containing IAA restores the apical dominance. The mechanism involves another hormone, ethylene. Auxin (IAA) causes lateral buds to make ethylene, which inhibits growth of the lateral buds.
- Differentiation of vascular tissue (xylem and phloem) is stimulated by IAA.

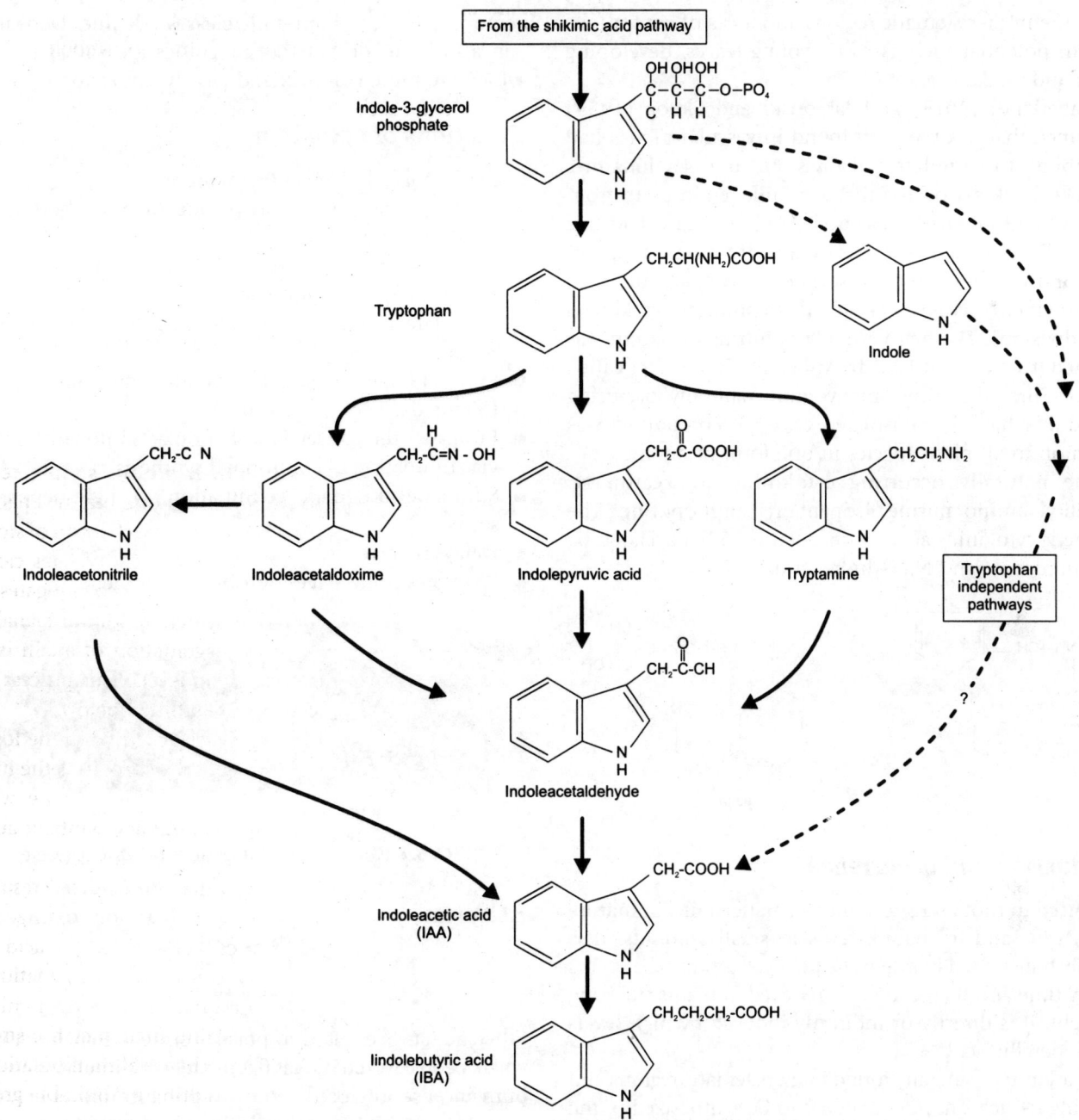

FIG. 6.1 Pathways of IAA biosynthesis

- Auxin stimulates root initiation on stem cuttings and lateral root development in tissue culture (adventitious rooting).
- Auxin mediates the tropistic response of bending in response to gravity and light (this is how auxin was first discovered).
- Auxin has various effects on leaf and fruit abscission, fruit set, development, and ripening, and flowering, depending on the circumstances.

Cytokinins

Cytokinins are compounds with a structure resembling adenine which promote cell division and have other similar functions to kinetin. They also regulate the pattern and frequency of organ production as well as position and shape. They have an inhibitory effect on senescence. Kinetin was the first cytokinin identified and so named because of the compounds ability to promote cytokinesis (cell division). Though it is a natural compound, it is not made in plants, and is therefore usually considered a 'synthetic' cytokinin. The common naturally occurring cytokinin in plants today is called zeatin which was isolated from corn.

Cytokinin have been found in almost all higher plants as well as mosses, fungi, bacteria, and also in many prokaryotes and eukaryotes. There are more than 200 natural and synthetic cytokinins identified. Cytokinin concentrations are more in meristematic regions and areas of continuous growth potential such as roots, young leaves, developing fruits and seeds.

Haberlandt (1913) and Jablonski and Skoog (1954) identified that a compound found in vascular tissues had the ability to stimulate cell division. In 1941, Johannes van Overbeek discovered that the milky endosperm from coconut and other various species of plants also had this ability. The first cytokinin was isolated from herring sperm in 1955 by Miller and his associates. This compound was named kinetin because of its ability to promote cytokinesis (cell division). The first naturally occurring cytokinin was isolated from corn in 1961 by Miller and it was later called zeatin. Since that time, many more naturally occurring cytokinins have been isolated and the compound was common to all plant species in one form or another.

The naturally occurring cytokinins are zeatin, N^6 dimethyl amino purine, isopentanyl aminopurine. The synthetic cytokinins are kinetin, adenine, 6-benzyl adenine benzimidazole and N,N'-diphenyl urea.

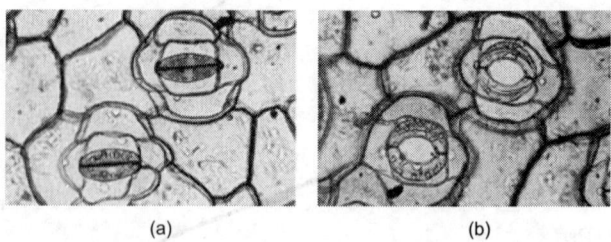

Kinetin   Zeatin

Production and occurrence

Produced in root and shoot meristematic tissue, in mature shoot cells and in mature roots in small amounts. If is rapidly transported in xylem stream. Peak production occurs in day time and their activity is reduced in plants suffering drought. It is directly or indirectly induced by high levels of Gibberellic acid.

Cytokinin is generally found in meristematic regions and growing tissues. They are believed to be synthesized in the roots and translocated via the xylem to shoots. Cytokinin biosynthesis happens through the biochemical modification of adenine. They are synthesized by following pathway.

A product of the mevalonate pathway called isopentyl pyrophosphate is isomerized. This isomer can then react with adenosine monophosphate with the aid of an enzyme called isopentenyl AMP synthase. The result is isopentenyl adenosine-5'-phosphate (isopentenyl AMP). This product can then be converted to isopentenyl adenosine by removal of the phosphate by a phosphatase and further converted to isopentenyl adenine by removal of the ribose group. Isopentenyl adenine can be converted to the three major forms of naturally occurring cytokinins.

Other pathways or slight alterations of this one probably lead to the other forms. Degradation of cytokinins occurs largely due to the enzyme cytokinin oxidase. This enzyme removes the side chain and releases adenine. Derivatives can also be made but the difficulties are with pathways, which are more complex and poorly understood.

Functions of cytokinin

- Stimulate cell division (cytokinesis).
- Stimulate morphogenesis (shoot initiation/bud formation) in tissue culture.
- Stimulate the growth of lateral (or adventitious) buds-release of apical dominance.
- Stimulate leaf expansion resulting from cell enlargement.
- May enhance stomatal opening in some species (Figure 6.2).
- Promotes the conversion of etioplasts into chloroplasts via stimulation of chlorophyll synthesis.
- Stimulate the dark germination of light-dependent seeds.
- Delays senescence.
- Promotes some stages of root development.

(a)   (b)

FIG. 6.2 Effect of cytokinin on stomatal opening

Ethylene

Ethylene

Ethylene has been used in practice since the ancient times, where people would use gas figs in order to stimulate ripening, burn incense in closed rooms to enhance the ripening of pears. It was in 1864, that leaks of gas from street lights showed stunting of growth, twisting of plants, and abnormal thickening of stems. In 1901, a Russian scientist named Dimitry Neljubow showed that the active component was ethylene. Doubt 1917, discovered that ethylene stimulated abscission. In 1932 it was demonstrated that the ethylene evolved from stored apple inhibited the growth of potato shoots enclosed with them. In 1934 Gane reported that plants synthesize ethylene. In 1935, Crocker proposed that ethylene was the plant hormone responsible for fruit ripening as well as inhibition of vegetative tissues. Ethylene is now known to have many other functions as well.

Production and occurrence

Production is directly induced by high levels of Auxin, root flooding and drought. It is found in germinating seeds and produced in nodes of stems, tissues of ripening fruits, response to shoot environmental, pest, or disease stress and in senescent leaves and flowers. Light minimizes the production of ethylene. It is released by all cells when they are experiencing conditions which would normally cause a mature shoot cell to produce ethylene.

Ethylene is produced in all higher plants and is produced from methionine in essentially all tissues. Production of ethylene varies with the type of tissue, the plant species and also the stage of development. The mechanism by which ethylene is produced from methionine is a three step process. ATP is an essential component in the synthesis of ethylene from methionine. ATP and water are added to methionine resulting in loss of the three phosphates and S-adenosyl methionine (SAM). 1-amino-cyclopropane-l-carboxylic acid synthase (ACC-synthase) facilitates the production of ACC from SAM. Oxygen is then needed in order to oxidize ACC and produce ethylene. This reaction is catalysed by an oxidative enzyme called ethylene forming enzyme. The control of ethylene production has received considerable study. Study of ethylene has focused around the synthesis promoting effects of auxin, wounding and drought as well as aspects of fruit-ripening. ACC synthase is the rate limiting step for ethylene production and it is this enzyme that is manipulated in biotechnology to delay fruit ripening in the 'flavour saver' tomatoes.

Functions of ethylene

- Production stimulated during ripening, flooding, stress, senescence, mechanical damage, infection.
- Regulator of cell death programs in plants (apoptosis).
- Stimulates the release of dormancy.
- Stimulates shoot and root growth and differentiation (triple response).
- Regulates ripening of climacteric fruits.
- May have a role in adventitious root formation.
- Stimulates leaf and fruit abscission.
- Flowering in most plants is inhibited by ethylene. Mangoes, pineapples and some ornamentals are stimulated by ethylene.
- Induction of femaleness in dioecious flowers.
- Stimulates flower opening.
- Stimulates flower and leaf senescence.

Gibberellins

Gibberellic acid

Unlike the classification of auxins which are classified on the basis of function, gibberellins are classified on the basis of structure as well as function. All gibberellins are derived from the ent-gibberellane skeleton. The gibberellins are named GA_1. GA_n in order of discovery. Gibberellic acid was the first gibberellin to be structurally characterized as GA_3. There are currently 136 GAs identified from plants, fungi and bacteria.

They are a group of diterpenoid acids that functions as plant growth regulators influencing a range of developmental processes in higher plants including stem elongation, germination, dormancy, flowering, sex expression, enzyme induction and leaf and fruit senescence. The origin of research into gibberellins can be traced to Japanese plant pathologists who were investigating the causes of the 'bakanae' (foolish seedling) disease which seriously lowered the yield of rice crops in Japan, Taiwan and throughout the Asian countries. Symptoms of the disease are pale yellow, elongated seedlings with slender leaves and stunted roots. Severely diseased plants die whereas plants with slight symptoms survive but produce poorly developed grain, or none at all.

Bakanae is now easily prevented by treatment of seeds with fungicides prior to sowing. In 1898 Shotaro Hori demonstrated that the symptoms were induced by infection with a fungus belonging to the genus Fusarium, probably *Fusarium heterosporum* Necs.

In 1912, Sawada suggested that the elongation in rice-seedlings infected with bakanae fungus might be due to a stimulus derived from fungal hyphae.

Subsequently, Eiichi Kurosawa (1926) found that culture filtrates from dried rice seedlings caused marked elongation in rice and other subtropical grasses. He concluded that bakanae fungus secretes a chemical that stimulates shoot elongation, inhibits chlorophyll formation and suppresses root growth.

Although there has been controversy among plant pathologists over the nomenclature of bakanae fungus, in the 1930s, the imperfect stage of the fungus was named *Fusarium moniliforme* (Sheldon) and the perfect stage, was named as *Gibberella fujikuroi* (Saw.) Wr. by H. W. Wollenweber. The terms 'Fujikuroi' and 'Saw' in *Gibberella fujikuroi* (Saw.) Wr. were derived from the names of two distinguished Japanese plant pathologists, Yosaburo Fujikuro and Kenkichi Sawada.

In 1934, Yabuta isolated a crystalline compound from the fungal culture filtrate that inhibited growth of rice seedlings at all concentrations tested. The structure of the inhibitor was found to be 5-*n*-butylpicolinic acid or fusaric acid. The formation of fusaric acid in culture filtrates was suppressed by changing the composition of the culture medium. As a result, a noncrystalline solid was obtained from the culture filtrate that stimulated the growth of rice seedlings. This compound was named gibberellin by Yabuta.

In 1938, Yabuta and his associate Yusuke Sumiki finally succeeded in crystallizing a pale yellow solid to yield gibberellin A and gibberellin B. (The names were subsequently interchanged in 1941 and the original gibberellin A was found to be inactive.) Determination of the structure of the active gibberellin was hampered by a shortage of pure crystalline sample. In the United States, the first research on gibberellins began after the Second World War. In 1950, John E. Mitchell reported optimal fermentation procedures for the fungus, as well as the effects of fungal extracts on the growth of bean *(Vicia faba)* seedlings. In Northern USDA Regional Research Laboratories in Peoria, large-scale fermentations were carried out with the purpose of producing pure gibberellin A for agricultural uses but initial fermentations were found to be inactive. Further researches were carried out by Sumiki in 1951, Stodola et al., 1955, and Curtis and Cross, 1954 regarding gibberellins and finally the gibberellic acid was determined by its chemical and physical properties.

In 1955, members of Sumuki group, succeeded in separating the methyl ester of gibberellin A into three components, from which corresponding free acids were obtained and named gibberellins A1, A2 and A3. Gibberellin A3 was found to be identical to gibberellic acid. In 1957, Takahashi et al. isolated a new gibberellin named gibberellin A4 as a minor component from the culture filtrate.

In the mid 1950s, evidence that gibberellins were naturally occurring substances in higher plants began to appear in the literature. Margaret Radley in the UK demonstrated the presence of gibberellin-like substances in higher plants. In the United States, Bernard Phinney et al were the first to report gibberellin-like substance in maize. This was followed by the isolation of crystalline gibberellin A1, A5, A6 and A8 from runner bean *(Phaseolus multiflorus)*. After 10 years the number of gibberellins reported in the literature isolated from fungal and plant origins rapidly increased. In 1968, J. MacMillan and N. Takahashi concluded that all gibberellins should be assigned numbers as gibberellin A1-x, irrespective of their origin. Over the past 20 years using modern analytical techniques many more gibberellins have been identified. At the present time the number of gibberellins identified is 126.

Production and occurrence

Produced in the roots, embryo and germinating seeds. The level of gibberellins goes up in the dark when sugar cannot be manufactured and will be reduced in the light. It is released in mature cells (particularly root) when they do not have enough sugar and oxygen to support both themselves and released by all cells when they are experiencing conditions which would normally cause a mature root cell to produce GA.

Gibberellins are diterpenes synthesized from acetyl CoA via the mevalonic acid pathway. They all have either 19 or 20 carbon units grouped into either four or five ring systems. The fifth ring is a lactone ring as shown in the structures above attached to ring A. Gibberellins are believed to be synthesized in young tissues of the shoot and also the developing seed. It is not clear whether young root tissues also produce gibberellins. There is also some evidence that leaves may also contain them. The gibberellins are formed through the pathway, three acetyl CoA molecules are oxidized by two NADPH molecules to produce three CoA molecules as a side product and mevalonic acid. Mevalonic acid is then phosphorylated by ATP and decarboxylated to form isopentyl pyrophosphate. Four of these molecules form geranylgeranyl pyrophosphate which serves as the donor for all GA carbon atoms.

This compound is then converted to copalylpyrophosphate which has 2 ring systems. Copalylpyrophosphate is then converted to kaurene which has 4 ring systems. Subsequent oxidations reveal kaurenol (alcohol form), kaurenal (aldehyde form) and kaurenoic acid, respectively.

Kaurenoic acid is converted to the aldehyde form of GA12 by decarboxylation. GA12 is the first true gibberellane ring system with 20 carbons. From the aldehyde form of GA12 arise both 20 and 19 carbon gibberellins but there are many mechanisms by which these other compounds arise. During active growth, the plant will metabolize most gibberellins by hydroxylation to inactive conjugates quickly with, the exception of GA3. GA3 is degraded much slower which helps to explain why the symptoms initially associated with the hormone in the disease bakanae are present. Inactive conjugates might be stored or translocated via the phloem and xylem before their release (activation) at the proper time and in the proper tissue.

Functions of gibberellins

- Stimulates stem elongation by stimulating cell division and elongation. GA controls internode elongation in the mature regions of plants. Dwarf plants do not make enough active forms of GA.
- Flowering in biennial plants is controlled by GA. Biennials grow one year as a rosette and after the winter, they bolt (rapid expansion of internodes and formation of flowers).
- Breaks seed dormancy in some plants that require stratification or light to induce germination.
- Stimulates α-amylase production in germinating cereal grains for mobilization of seed reserves.
- Juvenility refers to the different stages that plants may exist in. GA may help determine whether a particular plant part is juvenile or adult.
- Stimulates germination of pollen and growth of pollen tubes.
- Induces maleness in dioecious flowers (sex expression).

- Can cause parthenocarpic (seedless) fruit development or increase the size of seedless fruit (grapes).
- Can delay senescence in leaves and citrus fruits.
- May be involved in phytochrome responses.

Abscisic Acid

Natural growth inhibiting substances are present in plants and affect the normal physiological process of them. One such compound is abscisic acid, a single compound unlike the auxins, gibberellins, and cytokinins. It was called 'abscisin II' originally because it was thought to play a major role in abscission of fruits. At about the same time another group was calling it 'dormin' because they thought it had a major role in bud dormancy. Though abscisic acid generally is thought to play mostly inhibitory roles, it has many promoting functions as well.

Abscisic acid (Abscisin II)

In 1963, when Frederick Addicott and his associates were the one to identify abscisic acid. Two compounds were isolated and named as abscisin I and abscisin II. Abscisin II is presently called abscisic acid (ABA). At the same time Philip Wareing, who was studying bud dormancy in woody plants and Van Steveninck, who was studying abscission of flowers and fruits discovered the same compound.

Production and occurrence

ABA is a naturally occurring sesquiterpenoid (15-carbon) compound in plants, which is partially produced via the mevalonic pathway in chloroplasts and other plastids. Because it is synthesized partially in the chloroplasts, it makes sense that biosynthesis primarily occurs in the leaves. The production of ABA is by stresses such as water loss and freezing temperatures. The biosynthesis occurs indirectly through the production of carotenoids. Breakdown of these carotenoids occurs by the following mechanism: Violaxanthin (forty carbons) is isomerized and then splitted via an isomerase reaction followed by an oxidation reaction. One molecule of xanthonin is produced from one molecule of violaxanthonin and it is not clear what happens to the remaining byproducts. The one molecule of xanthonin produced is unstable and spontaneously changed to ABA aldehyde. Further oxidation results in ABA. Activation of the molecule can occur by two methods. In the first method, an ABA-glucose ester can form by attachment of glucose to ABA. In the second method, oxidation of ABA can occur to

form phaseic acid and dihyhrophaseic acid. Both xylem and phloem tissues carries ABA. It can also be translocated through parenchyma cells. Unlike auxins, ABA is capable of moving both up and down the stem.

Functions of abscisic acid

- The abscisic acid stimulates the closure of stomata (water stress brings about an increase in ABA synthesis) (Figure 6.3).
- Involved in abscission of buds, leaves, petals, flowers and fruits in many, if not all, instances, as well as in dehiscence of fruits.
- Production is accentuated by stresses such as water loss and freezing temperatures.
- Involved in bud dormancy.
- Prolongs seed dormancy and delays germination (vivipary).
- Inhibits elongation.
- ABA is implicated in the control of elongation, lateral root development and geotropism, as well as in water uptake and ion transport by roots.
- ABA coming from the plastids promotes the metabolism of ripening.
- Promotes senescence.
- Can reverse the effects of growth stimulating hormones.

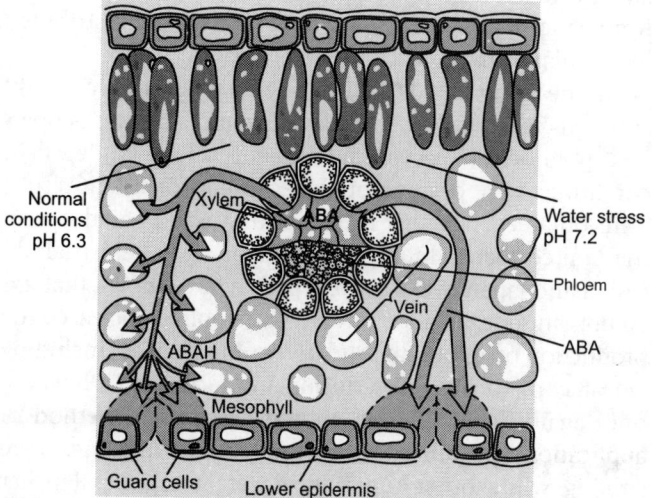

FIG. 6.3 Closure of stomata and water stress brings about an increase in ABA synthesis

Polyamines

Polyamines are unique as they are effective in relatively high concentrations. Typical concentrations range from 5 to 500 mg/L. Polyamines influence flowering and promote plant regeneration. Few examples are spermine, spermidine and putrescine. They play a major role in basic genetic processes such as DNA synthesis and gene expression. Spermine and spermidine bind to the phosphate backbone of nucleic acids. The interaction is mostly based on electrostatic interactions between negatively charged phosphates of the nucleic acids and the positively charged ammonium groups of the polyamines.

Polyamines are responsible for cell migration, proliferation and differentiation in plants. They represent a group of plant growth hormones, but they also have an effect on skin, hair growth, female fertility, fat depots, pancreatic integrity and regenerative growth in mammals. In addition, spermine is an important reagent widely used to precipitate DNA in molecular biology protocols. Spermidine is a standard reagent in PCR applications.

Spermine and spermidine are derivatives of putrescine (1,4-diaminobutane) which is produced from L-ornithine by action of ODC (ornithine decarboxylase). L-Ornithine is the product of L-arginine degradation by arginase. Spermidine is a triamine structure that is produced by spermidine synthase (SpdS) which catalyses monoalkylation of putrescine (1,4-diaminobutane) with decarboxylated S-adenosylmethionine (dcAdoMet) 3-aminopropyl donor. The formal alkylation of both amino groups of putrescine with the 3-aminopropyl donor yields the symmetrical tetraamine spermine.

Brassinosteroids

There are approximately 60 naturally occurring polyhydroxy steroids known as brassinosteroids (BRs). They are named after the first one identified, brassinolide, which was isolated from rape in 1979. They appear to be widely distributed in the plant kingdom.

In the early 1980s USDA scientists showed that BR could increase yields of radishes, lettuce, beans, peppers and potatoes. However, subsequent results under field conditions were disappointing because inconsistent results were obtained. For this reason testing was phased out in the United States. More recently large-scale field trials in China and Japan over a six-year period have shown that 24-epibrassinolide, an alternative to brassinolide, increased the production of agronomic and horticultural crops (including wheat, corn, tobacco, watermelon and cucumber). However, once again depending on cultural conditions, method of application and other factors, the results sometimes were striking while other times they were marginal. Further improvements in the formulation, application method, timing, effects of environmental conditions and other factors need to be investigated further in order to identify the reason for these variable results.

Brassinosteroids may be a new class of plant growth substances. They are widely distributed within the plant kingdom, they have an effect at extremely low concentrations, both in bioassays and whole plants, and they have a range of effects that are different from the other classes of plant substances. Finally, they can be applied to one part of the plant and transported to another location where, in very low amounts, they elicit a biological response.

Functions of brassinosteroids

- Promote shoot elongation at low concentrations.
- Strongly inhibit root growth and development.
- Promote ethylene biosynthesis and epinasty.
- Interfere with ecdysteroids (moulting hormones) in insects.
- Have had contradictory effects in tissue culture. 24-epibrassinolide has been shown to mimic culture conditioning factors and to be synergistic with these factors in promoting carrot cell growth. However, in transformed tobacco cells brassinosteroids in low concentrations significantly inhibited cell growth.
- Enhance xylem differentiation.
- Decrease fruit abortion and drop.
- Enhance resistance to chilling, disease, herbicide and salt stress.
- Promotion of germination.
- Promote changes in plasmalemma energization and transport, assimilate uptake.
- Increase RNA and DNA polymerase activities and synthesis of RNA, DNA and protein.

Salicylic Acid

Salicylic acid has been known to be present in some plant tissues for quite some time, but has only recently been recognized as a potential PGR. Salicylic acid is synthesized from the amino acid phenylalanine. SA is thought by some to be a new class of plant growth regulator. It is a chemically characterized compound, ubiquitously found in the plant kingdom and has an effect on many physiological processes in plants at low concentrations. Further molecular studies on SA signal transduction should yield insights into the mechanism of action of this important regulatory compound.

Functions of salicylic acid

- Promotes flowering.
- Stimulates thermogenesis in *Arum* flowers.
- Stimulates plant pathogenesis protein production (systemic acquired resistance).
- May enhance longevity of flowers.
- May inhibit ethylene biosynthesis.
- May inhibit seed germination.
- Blocks the wound response.
- Reverses the effects of ABA.

Jasmonates

Jasmonates are represented by jasmonic acid (JA) and its methyl ester. They were first isolated from the jasmine plant in which the methyl ester is an important product in the perfume industry. JA is synthesized from linolenic acid, which is an important fatty acid. JA is considered by some to be a new class of plant growth regulator. It is a chemically characterized compound and has been identified in many plant species. It has physiological effects at very low concentrations and indirect evidence suggests that it is transported throughout the plant.

Biosynthesis of jasmonates

In the early 1980s, the pathway for jasmonic acid biosynthesis was elucidated by Vick and Zimmerman (Fig. 6.4). Jasmonic acid was shown to be synthesized from linolenic acid, which is first oxygenated by lipoxygenase (LOX), to yield 13(S)-hydroperoxy linolenic acid (13-HPOT). Zimmerman and Feng observed that this fatty acid hydroperoxide can be cyclized to 12-oxophytodienoic acid (OPDA) and the apparent hydroperoxide cyclase activity was found to be present in many plant species. We know now that the cyclization is achieved by the consecutive action of two enzymes, namely, allene oxide synthase (AOS) and allene oxide cyclase (AOC). Vick and Zimmerman continued to

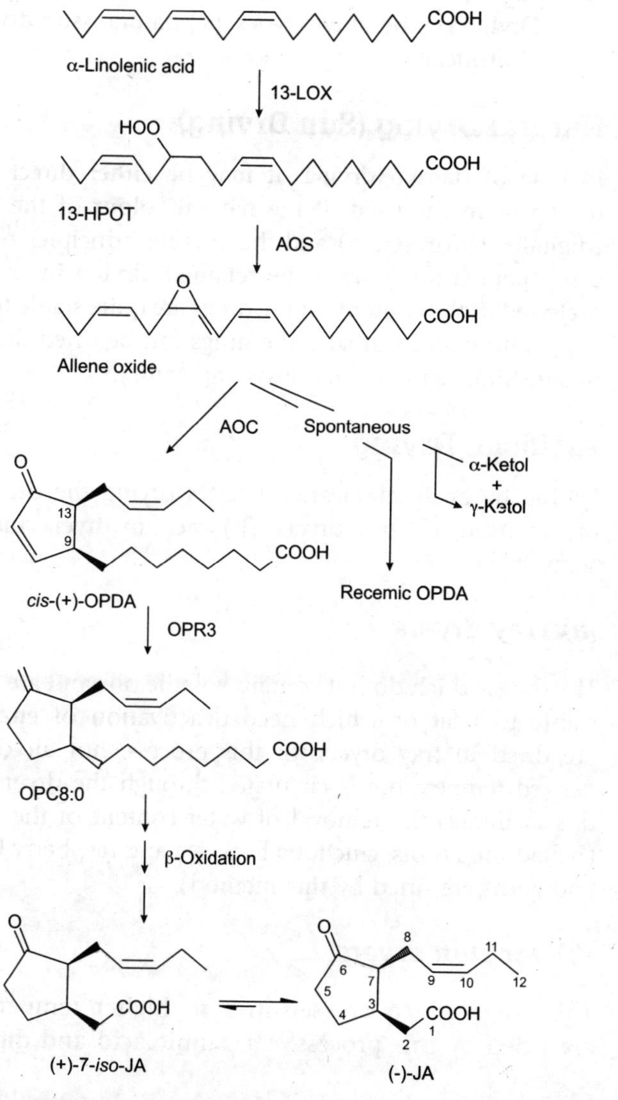

show that OPDA is further metabolized to jasmonic acid. This includes the reduction of the cyclopentenone ring of OPDA to yield the respective cyclopentanone (OPC 8:0) followed by three cycles of beta-oxidation resulting in the shortening of the octanoic acid side chain and the formation of jasmonic acid.

Functions of jasmonates

- Inhibition of many processes such as seedling longitudinal growth, root length growth, mycorrhizial fungi growth, tissue culture growth, embryogenesis, seed germination, pollen germination, flower bud formation, carotenoid biosynthesis, chlorophyll formation, rubisco biosynthesis and photosynthetic activities.
- Promotion of senescence, abscission, tuber formation, fruit ripening, pigment formation, tendril coiling, differentiation in plant tissue culture, adventitious root formation, breaking of seed dormancy, pollen germination, stomatal closure, microtubule disruption, chlorophyll degradation, respiration, ethylene biosynthesis and protein synthesis.
- They play an important role in plant defense by inducing proteinase synthesis.

6.6. COLLECTION OF CRUDE DRUGS

Collection is the most important step which comes after cultivation. Drugs are collected from wild or cultivated plants and the tasks for collection depends upon the collector, whether he is a skilled or unskilled labour. Drugs should be collected when they contain maximum amount of constituents in a highly scientific manner. The season at which each drug is collected is so important, as the amount, and sometimes the nature, of the active constituents could be changed throughout the year. For example, Rhubarb is collected only in summer seasons because no anthraquinone derivatives would be present in winter season but anthranols are converted to anthraquinones during summer. Not only the season but also the age of the plant should be taken into great consideration since it governs not only the total amount of active constituents produced in the plants but also the proportions of the constituents of the active mixture. High proportion of pulegone in young plants of peppermint will be replaced by menthone and menthol and reduction in the percentage of alkaloids in datura as the plant ages are examples of the effect of aging in plants. Moreover the composition of a number of secondary plant metabolites varies throughout the day and night, and it is believed that some interconversion would happen during day and night.

Generally the leaves are collected just before the flowering season, e.g. vasaka, digitalis, etc., at this time it is assumed that the whole plant has come to a healthy state and contain an optimum amount of metabolites, flowers are

FIG. 6.4 The Vick and Zimmerman pathway for jasmonic acid biosynthesis collected before they expand fully, e.g. clove, saffron, etc., and underground organs as the aerial parts of plant cells die, e.g. liquorice, rauwolfia, etc. Since it is very difficult to collect the exact medicinally valuable parts, the official pharmacopoeia has fixed certain amount of foreign matter that is permissible with drug. Some fruits are collected after their full maturity while the others are collected after the fruits are ripe. Barks are usually collected in spring season, as they are easy to separate from the wood during this season. The barks are collected using three techniques, felling (bark is peeled off after cutting the tree at base), uprooting (the underground roots are dug out and barks are collected from branches and roots) and coppicing (plant is cut one metre above the ground level and barks are removed).

Underground parts should be collected and shaken, dusted in order to remove the adhered soil; water washing could be done if the adhered particles are too sticky with plant parts. The unorganized drugs should be collected from plants as soon as they oozes out, e.g. resins, latex, gums, etc. Discoloured drugs or drugs which were affected by insects should be rejected.

6.7. HARVESTING OF CRUDE DRUGS

Harvesting is an important operation in cultivation technology, as it reflects upon economic aspects of the crude drugs. An important point which needs attention over here is the type of drug to be harvested and the pharmacopoeial standards which it needs to achieve. Harvesting can be done efficiently in every respect by the skilled workers. Selectivity is of advantage in that the drugs other than genuine, but similar in appearance can be rejected at the site of collection. It is, however, a laborious job and may not be economical. In certain cases, it cannot be replaced by any mechanical means, e.g. digitalis, tea, vinca and senna leaves. The underground drugs like roots, rhizomes, tubers, etc., are harvested by mechanical devices, such as diggers or lifters. The tubers or roots are thoroughly washed in water to get rid of earthy matter. Drugs which constitute all aerial parts are harvested by binders for economic reasons. Many a times, flowers, seeds and small fruits are harvested by a special device known as seed stripper. The technique of beating plant with bamboos is used in case of cloves. The cochineal insects are collected from branches of cacti by brushing. The seaweeds producing agar are harvested by long handled forks. Peppermint and spearmint are harvested by normal method with mowers, whereas fennel, coriander and caraway plants are uprooted and dried. After drying, either they are thrashed or beaten and the fruits are separated by winnowing. Sometimes, reaping machines are also used for their harvesting.

6.8. DRYING OF CRUDE DRUGS

Before marketing a crude drug, it is necessary to process it properly, so as to preserve it for a longer time and also to acquire better pharmaceutical elegance. This processing includes several operations or treatments, depending upon the source of the crude drug (animal or plant) and its chemical nature. Drying consists of removal of sufficient moisture content of crude drug, so as to improve its quality and make it resistant to the growth of microorganisms. Drying inhibits partially enzymatic reactions. Drying also facilitates pulverizing or grinding of a crude drug. In certain drugs, some special methods are required to be followed to attain specific standards, e.g. fermentation in case of *Cinnamomum zeylanicum* bark and gentian roots. The slicing and cutting into smaller pieces is done to enhance drying, as in case of glycyrrhiza, squill and calumba. The flowers are dried in shade so as to retain their colour and volatile oil content. Depending upon the type of chemical constituents, a method of drying can be used for a crude drug. Drying can be of two types: (1) natural (sun drying) and (2) artificial.

Natural Drying (Sun Drying)

In case of natural drying, it may be either direct sun-drying or in the shed. If the natural colour of the drug (digitalis, clove, senna) and the volatile principles of the drug (peppermint) are to be retained, drying in shed is preferred. If the contents of the drugs are quite stable to the temperature and sunlight, the drugs can be dried directly in sunshine (gum acacia, seeds and fruits).

Artificial Drying

Drying by artificial means includes drying the drugs in (a) an oven, i.e. tray dryers, (b) vacuum dryers and (c) spray dryers.

(a) Tray dryers

The drugs which do not contain volatile oils and are quite stable to heat or which need deactivation of enzymes are dried in tray dryers. In this process, hot air of the desired temperature is circulated through the dryers and this facilitates the removal of water content of the drugs (belladonna roots, cinchona bark, tea and raspberry leaves and gums are dried by this method).

(b) Vacuum dryers

The drugs which are sensitive to higher temperature are dried by this process, e.g. tannic acid and digitalis leaves.

(c) Spray dryers

Few drugs which are highly sensitive to atmospheric conditions and also to temperature of vacuum drying are dried by spray-drying method. The technique is followed for quick drying of economically important plant or animal constituents, rather than the crude drugs. Examples of spray drying are papaya latex, pectin, tannins, etc.

6.9. GARBLING (DRESSING)

The next step in preparation of crude drug for market after drying is garbling. This process is desired when sand, dirt and foreign organic parts of the same plant, not constituting drug are required to be removed. This foreign organic matter (extraneous matter) is removed by several ways and means available and practicable at the site of the preparation of the drugs. If the extraneous matter is permitted in crude drugs, the quality of drug surfers and at times, it dose not pass pharmacopoeial limits. Excessive stems in case of lobelia and stramonium need to be removed, while the stalks, in case of cloves are to be deleted. Drugs constituting rhizomes need to be separated carefully from roots and rootlets and also stem bases. Pieces of iron must be removed with the magnet in case of castor seeds before crushing and by shifting in case of vinca and senna leaves. Pieces of bark should be removed by peeling as in gum acacia.

6.10. PACKING OF CRUDE DRUGS

The morphological and chemical nature of drug, its ultimate use and effects of climatic conditions during transportation and storage should be taken into consideration while packing the drugs. Aloe is packed in goat skin. Colophony and balsam of tolu are packed in kerosene tins, while asafoetida is stored in well closed containers to prevent loss of volatile oil. Cod liver oil, being sensitive to sunlight, should be stored in such containers, which will not have effect of sunlight, whereas, the leaf drugs like senna, vinca and others are pressed and baled. The drugs which are very sensitive to moisture and also costly at the same time need special attention, e.g. digitalis, ergot and squill. Squill becomes flexible; ergot becomes susceptible to the microbial growth, while digitalis looses its potency due to decomposition of glycosides, if brought in contact with excess of moisture during storage. Hence, the chemicals which absorb excessive moisture (desiccating agents) from the drug are incorporated in the containers. Colophony needs to be packed in big masses to control autoxidation. Cinnamon bark, which is available in the form of quills, is packed one inside the other quill, so as to facilitate transport and to prevent volatilization of oil from the drug. The crude drugs like roots, seeds and others do not need special attention and are packed in gunny bags, while in some cases bags are coated with polythene internally. The weight of certain drugs in lots is also kept constant, e.g. Indian opium.

6.11. STORAGE OF CRUDE DRUGS

Preservation of crude drugs needs sound knowledge of their physical and chemical properties. A good quality of the drugs can be maintained, if they are preserved properly. All the drugs should be preserved in well closed and, possibly, in the filled containers. They should be stored in the premises which are water proof, fire proof and rodent proof. A number of drugs absorb moisture during their storage and become susceptible to the microbial growth. Some drugs absorb moisture to the extent of 25% of their weight. The moisture not only increases the bulk of the drug, but also causes impairment in the quality of crude drug. The excessive moisture facilitates enzymatic reactions resulting in decomposition of active constituents, e.g. digitalis leaves and wild cherry bark. Gentian and ergot receive mould infestation due to excessive moisture. Radiation due to direct sunlight also causes destruction of active chemical constituents, e.g. ergot, cod liver oil and digitalis. Form or shape of the drug also plays very important role in preserving the crude drugs. Colophony in the entire form (big masses) is preserved nicely, but if stored in powdered form, it gets oxidized or looses solubility in petroleum ether. Squill, when stored in powdered form becomes hygroscopic and forms rubbery mass on prolonged exposure to air. The fixed oil in the powdered ergot becomes rancid on storage. In order to maintain a good quality of ergot, it is required that the drug should be defatted with lipid solvent prior to storage. Lard, the purified internal fat of the abdomen of the hog, is to be preserved against rancidity by adding siam benzoin. Atmospheric oxygen is also destructive to several drugs, and hence they are filled completely in well closed containers, or the air in the container is replaced by an inert gas like nitrogen; e.g. shark liver oil, papain, etc.

Apart from protection against adverse physical and chemical changes, the preservation against insect or mould attacks is also important. Different types of insects, nematodes, worms, moulds and mites infest the crude drugs during storage. Some of the more important pests found in drugs are Coleoptera (*Stegobium paniceum* and *Calandrum granarium*), Lepidoptera (*Ephestia kuehniella* and *Tinea pellionella*) and Archnida or mites (*Tyroglyphus farinae* and *Glycyphagus domesticus*). They can be prevented by drying the drug thoroughly before storage and also by giving treatment of fumigants. The common fumigants used for storage of crude drugs are methyl bromide, carbon disulphide and hydrocyanic acid. At times, drugs are given special treatment, such as liming of the ginger and coating of nutmeg. Temperature is also very important factor in preservation of the drugs, as it accelerates several chemical reactions leading to decomposition of the constituents. Hence, most of the drugs need to be preserved at a very low temperature. The costly phytopharmaceuticals are required to be preserved at refrigerated temperature in well closed containers. Small quantities of crude drugs could be readily stored in airtight, moisture proof and light proof containers such as tin, cans, covered metal tins or amber glass containers. Wooden boxes and paper bags should not be used for storage of crude drugs.

6.12. QUALITY MANAGEMENT

The herbal drug manufacturers should establish a quality management department which is responsible for supervision and quality control for the entire production process, and should have adequate staff, premises, instruments and equipment to meet the standard requirements of the scale of production and species identification. The quality management department should monitor the environment and hygienic management, test production materials, packaging materials and the crude drugs, and issue testing reports, develop training plans and supervise their implementation; and also they should manage the original records of production, packaging, testing, etc. Prior to packaging, the quality control department should test each batch of the crude drugs in accordance with the national or approved standards for crude drugs. The testing procedures should include macroscopic characters and identification, impurities, moisture, ash and acid insoluble ash, extracts and assay for marker or active constituents. Pesticide residue, heavy metals and microbiological limits should comply with the national standards and the relevant requirements. The testing reports should be signed by the operator and the responsible person of the quality control department, and then filed. As far as the personnel and facilities are concerned, they should possess qualifications of college education or above in pharmacy, knowledge in alternative systems of medicines, agronomy, animal husbandry or the relevant specialties, trained on production techniques, safety, and hygiene and have experience in the production of crude drugs, quality management of crude drugs. Staff engaged in the field work should be familiar with cultivation techniques, especially the use of pesticides and safety protection; those engaged in rearing should be familiar with rearing techniques.

The personnel engaged in processing, packaging or testing should undergo health examinations regularly and those suffering from infectious diseases, dermatitis or open wounds shall not be allowed to do work which is in direct contact with crude drugs. The producer should designate a person to be responsible for checking sanitation and hygiene. The applicable range and precision of instruments, metres, measures, weighers and balances, etc., used in production and testing, should conform to the relevant requirements, their performance status should be clearly indicated and calibration should be conducted regularly.

6.13. DOCUMENTATION

The producer should maintain its standard operating procedures for production and quality management. Detailed records for the entire production process of each crude drug should be documented, and if necessary, photos or images might be attached, which should include, origin of seeds, strains and propagation materials, production techniques and process, sowing time, quantity and area of medicinal plants, seedling, transplantation, and the type, application schedule, quantity arid usage of fertilizer, quantity, application schedule and usage of pesticide, microbicide or herbicide, collection time and yield, fresh weight and processing, drying and drying loss, transport and storage of medicinal parts. Quality evaluations of crude drugs: description of macroscopic characters of crude drugs and records of test results. All these records, production plans and their details, contracts or agreements, etc., should be filed and kept properly by a designated person.

CHAPTER 7

Indian Trade in Medicinal and Aromatic Plants

CONTENTS

7.1. INTRODUCTION

Recently there has been a shift in universal trend from synthetic to herbal medicine, which we can say 'Return to Nature'. Medicinal plants have been known for millennia and are highly esteemed all over the world as a rich source of therapeutic agents for the prevention of diseases and ailments. Nature has bestowed our country with an enormous wealth of medicinal plants; therefore, India has often been referred to as the medicinal garden of the world. Countries with ancient civilizations, such as China, India, South America, Egypt, etc., are still using several plant remedies for various conditions. In this regard, India has a unique position in the world, where a number of recognized indigenous systems of medicine, viz. Ayurveda, Siddha, Unani, Homoeopathy, Yoga and Naturopathy are being utilized for the health care of people. No doubts that the herbal drugs are popular among rural and urban community of India. The one reason for the popularity and acceptability is the belief that all natural products are safe. The demand for plant-based medicines, health products, pharmaceuticals, food supplement, cosmetics, etc., are increasing in both developing and developed countries due to the growing recognition that the natural products are nontoxic, have less side effects and easily available at affordable prices. Nowadays, there is a revival of interest with herbal-based medicine due to the increasing realization of the health hazards associated with the indiscriminate use of modern medicine, and the herbal drug industries is now very fast growing sector in the international market. But unfortunately, India has not done well in this international trade of herbal industry due to lack of scientific input in herbal drugs. So, it would be appropriate to highlight the market potential of herbal products that would open floodgate for development of market potential in India. With these objects, we reviewed here the market potential of herbal medicine in India.

The export of medicinal plants and herbs from India has been quite substantial for the last few years. India has a large endemic flora. There are more than 80,000 medicinal plants known, and nearly 180 plant-derived chemical compounds have been developed as modern pharmaceuticals, which are included in the Pharmacopoeia of India. The

KEY TERMS

domestic ayurvedic market is estimated to be US$ 1 billion, and is growing at the rate of 15–20% annually. India has been the major supplier of medicinal plants in the world market until 1977, when it was kept to second position by South Korea with export worth only Rs 16 crore during 1978–79. The quantum of export had dropped to almost half of what it was in 1976–77 when India exported medicinal plants worth around Rs 29.8 crore. The items of export value were opium, psyllium husks and seeds, *Vinca rosea*, kuth roots and senna leaves and pods. At present the annual trade of Indian medicinal plants is estimated to be 37,200 tonnes valued around US$ 93,540,272.00, which is expected to be increased to US$ 629,194,624.00 by 2005. During 1980s, India was the largest supplier of medicinal plants to the world market with the supply of 10.555 metric tonnes of medicinal plant material and about 14 metric tonnes of plant-derived products and their derivatives. The annual turn over was around US$ 300 million. In 1995, psyllium husk, seeds and senna were the main export items from India. During 1998–99, India exported psyllium husk worth US$ 19.6 million and senna leaves worth US$ 22.4. India also exported finished ayurvedic and unani medicine during the year 2000–01. It exported medicine worth around US$ 128 million to various countries including United States, Germany, Russia, UK, Hong Kong and Malaysia.

The global herbal industry is estimated to be US$ 50 billion annually and growing at the rate of 5.5–6.5% annually. The Indian contribution to the global industry is around 10% only. One of the important items of export, covering approximately 80% of the world requirement, is a proteolytic enzyme, papain mainly manufactured in Maharashtra from raw papaya fruits. The commercial production of pectin from thalamus of sunflower is also carried out at Jalgaon in Maharashtra.

India is one of the few countries in the world where essential oils industry was developed at a very early stage. The essential oils, perfumes and flavours have been associated with Indian civilization for several thousand years. Because of its vast area and a variety of soil and climate, essential oils containing plants of all types can be grown in one or the other parts of the country. India produces essential oils from wild and commercially grown plants in appreciable quantities such as palmarosa, citronella, calamus, cardamom, celery seed, cedarwood, dill, ginger, lemon grass, vetiver and rose oil. The annual production of coriander is about 243,000 tonnes, which constitute approximately 80% of the world demand. About 30% of global demand in cardamom and 15% in saffron are met by India. The annual production of saffron is approximately 150 tonnes.

The most significant export is of the sandalwood oil, for which our country is the major producer, exporting approximately 50–60 tonnes to the world market. India is a leader in the production of menthol as mentha oil steadily expanded in the last decade during the year 2000–01. India exported about 3,870 tonnes of mint oil worth about Rs 1.26 billion. India is also a leader in the production and export of high value perfumes (attars) for the world market.

The domestic market of Indian traditional system of medicine comprising of ayurveda, unani, siddha and homoeopathy has been reported to the tune of approximately Rs 5000 crore only, and India is at present exporting herbal medicines and materials to the value of about Rs 550 crore only. In the domestic market, the ayurvedic medicines account for a major portion, about 85% as compared to unani, siddha and homoeopathy system. The total patent and proprietary medicines of these systems are manufactured by over 9500 licensed pharmacies/herbal manufacturing units spread all over India.

With the development of phytochemical industry in India, domestic requirement for various medicinal plants grew considerably. Consequently, the Govt of India has adopted restrictive export policy in respect of those crude drugs, which were indiscriminately exploited in the forest, such as rauwolfia, podophyllum, Indian rhubarb, dioscorea, kuth, jatamansi, *Atropa acuminata*, *Artemisia brevifolia*, berberis, colchicum, *Ephedra gerardiana*, *Gentiana kurroa*, *Picrorhiza kurroa*, *Swertia chirata*, *Valerian wallichii*, etc. However, with due permission from the Chief Conservator of Forest or officer authorized by him; the material of plantation or of nursery origin certificate can be exported.

These medicines are mainly consumed within the country and some of these are also exported to the Middle East. Major destination countries are the United States, Nepal, Japan, Sri Lanka, Russia, Germany, Italy, Nigeria and UAE, and according to the survey reports, Sri Lanka, Egypt, Bangladesh and Mauritius are the countries having maximum export potential.

The major pharmaceuticals exported from India in the recent years were isabgol, vinca extract, senna derivatives, castor oil in dehydrated form, beta ionone, papain, berberine hydrochloride and opium alkaloids.

India's export of essential oils during last few years has shown the erratic trends. The sandalwood oil share is more than 50% in the total export; the United States accounted for major share of exports of this item followed by the erstwhile USSR. The mentha oil has the same export trend as the cheaper quality is being exported by China. India is also exporting volatile oils to France, Japan, Sudan, Germany and Switzerland. The other important items of export value are cardamom oil, lemon grass oil, palmarosa oil, pudina oil, peppermint oil, clove oil, geranium oil, vetiver oil and lavender oil.

7.2. INDIAN HERBAL TRADE IN WORLD SCENARIO

The utilization of herbal drugs is on the flow, and the market is growing step by step. The annual turnover of the Indian herbal medicinal industry is about Rs 2300 crore as against the pharmaceutical industry's turnover of Rs 14,500 crore, with a growth rate of 15%. The export of medicinal plants and herbs from India has been quite substantial in the last few years. India is the second largest producer of castor seeds in the world, producing about 125,000 tonnes per annum. The major pharmaceuticals exported from India in the recent years are isabgol, opium alkaloids, senna derivatives, vinca extract, cinchona alkaloids, ipecac root alkaloids, solasodine, diosgenine/16DPA, menthol, gudmar herb, mehndi leaves, papian, rauwolfia, guar gum, jasmine oil, sandalwood oil, etc. The turnover of herbal medicines in India as over-the-counter products, ethical and classical formulations and home remedies of traditional systems of medicine is about US$ 1 billion and export of herbal crude extract is about US$ 80 million. The herbal drug market in India is about US$1 billion. Some of the medicinal plants, whose market potential is very high, have been identified and summarized in Table 7.1.

Table 7.2: Manufacturer of herbal formulation

S. no.	Name of the company
1.	Ansar Drug Laboratories, Surat
2.	Acis Laboratories, Kanpur
3.	Aimil Pharmaceutical, New Delhi
4.	Allen Laboratories, Kolkata
5.	Bharti Rasanagar, Kolkata
6.	Dabur India Ltd., Ghaziabad
7.	Dattatraya Krishan Sandu Bros., Mumbai
8.	Herbals Pvt. Ltd., Patna
9.	Herbo-med (P) Ltd., Kolkata
10.	The Himalaya Drug Co., Bangalore
11.	Indian Herb and Research Supply Co., Saharanpur
12.	J & J Dechane Laboratories Pvt. Ltd., Hyderabad
13.	Madona Pharmaceutical Research Pvt. Ltd., Kolkata
14.	Kruzer Herbals, New Delhi
15.	Shilpachem, Indore
16.	Hamdard (Wakf) Laboratories, Delhi
17.	Zandu Pharmaceutical Works Ltd., Mumbai
18.	Baidyanath Ayurveda Bhavan, Jhansi
19.	Charak Pharmaceuticals, Mumbai

Table 7.1: List of high-market-potential medicinal plants

Aconitum ferox (Ranunculaceae)	Garcinia camboga (Guttiferae)
Aconitum heterophyllum (Ranunculaceae)	Gymnema sylvestre (Asclepiadaceae)
Allium sativum (Liliaceae)	Holarrhena antidysenterica (Apocynaceae)
Azadirachta indica (Meliaceae)	Ocimum teniflorum (Labiatae)
Andrographis paniculata (Acanthaceae)	Picrorhiza kurroa (Scrophulariaceae)
Asparagus recemosus (Liliaceae)	Plantago ovata (Plantaginaceae)
Berberis aristata (Berberidaceae)	Saraca indica (Leguminosae)
Commiphora wightii (Burseraceae)	Saussurea costus (Asteraceae)
Crocus sativus (Iridaceae)	Solanum nigrum (Solanaceae)
Nardostachys jatamansi (Valerianaceae)	Tinospora cordifolia (Menispermaceae)
Embelica officinalis (Euphorbiaceae)	Withania somnifera (Solanaceae)

7.3. MEDICINAL PLANT-BASED INDUSTRIES IN INDIGENOUS SYSTEM OF MEDICINE

In India, it is estimated that there are about 25,000 licensed pharmacy of Indian system of medicine. Presently, about 1000 single drugs and about 3000 compound formulations are registered. Herbal industry in India uses about 8,000 medicinal plants. Table 7.2 contains some important manufacturer of herbal formulation. However, none of the pharma has standardized herbal medicines using active compounds as markers linked with confirmation of bioactivity of herbal drugs in experimental animal models. From about 8000 drug manufactures in India, there are however not more than 25 manufactures that can be classified as large-scale manufactures. The annual turnover of Indian herbal industry was estimated around US$ 300 million in ayurvedic, and unani medicine was about US$ 27.7 million. In 1998–99, it again went up to US$ 31.7 million and in 1999–2000 of the total turnover was US$ 48.9 million of ayurvedic and herbal products. Export of herbal drugs in India is around US$ 80 million. Some of the highly consumed medicinal plants are presented in Table 7.3 with reference to their turnover. Figure 7.1(a–d) are the graphical representation of some highly consumed Indian medicinal plants vs. estimated consumption per annum (in tonnes).

Table 7.3: Important plants with reference to trade

S. no.	Plant name	Common name	Plant part	Estimated consumption (tonnes)
1.	Aconitum heterophyllum	Atis	Root	20
2.	Acorus calamus	Vacha	Rhizome	150
3.	Aloe vera	Aloes	Leaf	200
4.	Anacyclus pyrethrum	Akarkara	Fruit	50
5.	Andrographis paniculata	Kalmegh	Aerial part	250
6.	Asparagus recemosus	Shatavari	Root	500
7.	Berberis aristata	Daru haldi	Root	500
8.	Cedrus deodara	Deodar	Heart Wood	200
9.	Chlorophytum borivil-ianum	Safed musli	Root	25
10.	Cinnamomum zeylanicum	Dalchini	Bark	200–300
11.	Commiphora wightii	Guggul	Gum resin	500
12.	Crocus sativus	Kesar	Stigma	5
13.	Cyprus rotundus	Nagar motha	Rhizome	150
14.	Eclipta alba	Bhringraj	Aerial part	500
15.	Elettaria cardamomum	Elaichi	Seed	60
16.	Embelia ribes burm	Vidanga	Fruit	200
17.	Glycyrrhiza glabra	Mulethi	Root	5000
18.	Hedychium spicatum	Kapur kachri	Rhizome	400
19.	Hemidesmus indicus	Anantmool	Root	200
20.	Holarrhena pubescens	Kurchi	Bark	150
21.	Justicia adhatoda	Vasaka	Leaf	500
22.	Mucuna pruriens	Kaunch beej	Seed	200
23.	Myristica fragrans	Jaiphal	Fruit	500
24.	Nardostachys grandiflora	Jatamansi	Root	200
25.	Embelica officinalis	Amla	Fruit	10,000
26.	Picrorhiza kurroa	Kutki	Root	200
27.	Piper cubeba	Cubeb	Fruit	150
28.	Piper longum	Pipramul	Fruit	200
29.	Piper nigrum	Black pepper	Fruit	150
30.	Plumbago zeylanica	Chitrak	Root	500
31.	Pueraria tuberosa	Vidari kanda	Root	200
32.	Saraca indica	Ashoka	Bark	1200
33.	Senna alexandrina	Senna	Leaf and pod	1000
34.	Strychnos nux vomica	Nux vomica seed	Seed	1000
35.	Swertia chirata	Chirayita	Whole plant	300
36.	Syzygium aromaticum syn Eugenia aromaticum	Laung	Flower bud	150
37.	Syzygium cumini	Jaman beej	Seed	300
38.	Trachyspermum ammi	Ajwain	Fruit	200
39.	Terminalia bellirica	Bahera	Fruit	500
40.	Terminalia chebula	Harar	Fruit	500
41.	Tinospora cordifolia	Guduchi	Stem	1000
42.	Valeriana jatamansi	Tagar	Root and Rhizome	150

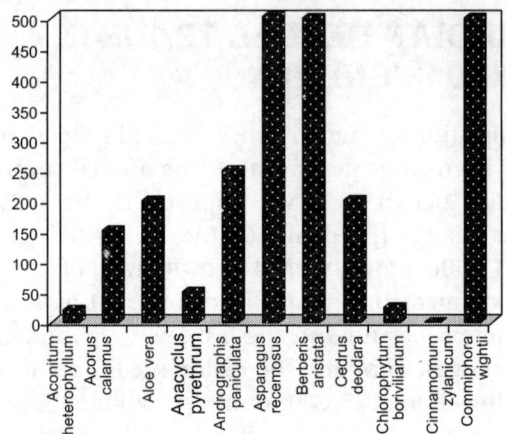

FIG. 7.1(A) Important Indian medicinal plants vs. estimated consumption per annum (in tonnes)

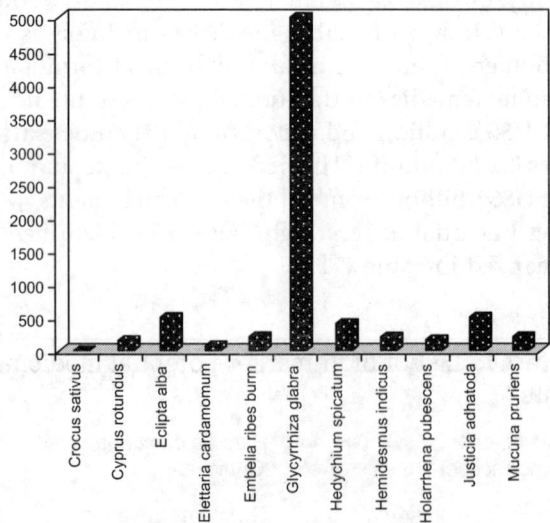

FIG. 7.1(B) Important Indian medicinal plants vs. estimated consumption per annum (in tonnes)

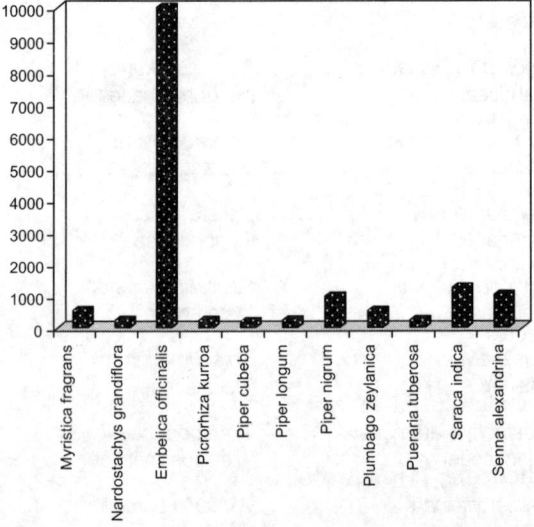

FIG. 7.1(C) Important Indian medicinal plants vs. estimated consumption per annum (in tonnes)

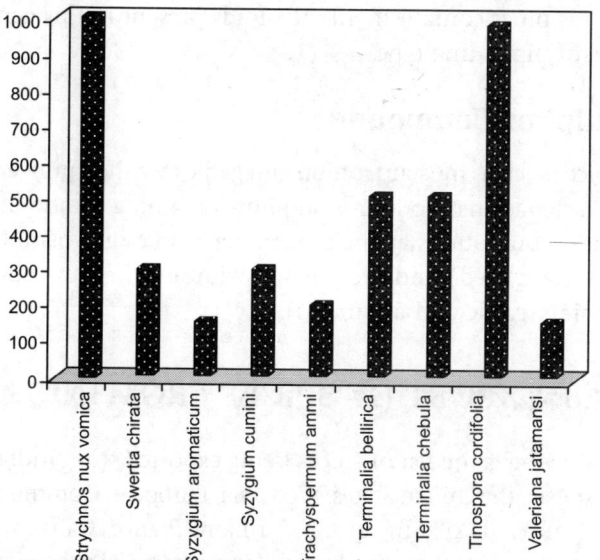

FIG. 7.1(D) Important Indian medicinal plants vs. estimated consumption per annum (in tonnes)

7.4. EXPORT POTENTIAL OF INDIAN PHYTOPHARMACEUTICAL PRODUCTS

Indian phytopharmaceutical products, which are in demand in the international market for their quality and potency, are:

■ **Artemisinin:** This is sesquiterpene lactone obtained from herb *Artemisia annua*, family Asteraceae, effective in treating malaria including cerebral malaria.

■ **Berberine hydrochloride and berberine sulphate:** This is benzyl isoquinoline alkaloidal salt obtained from Berberis spp. viz. *B. aristata*, *B. vulgaris*. It is used as tonic astringent, febrifuge, hepatic dysfunction, diabetes and in gastroenteritis.

■ **Colchicine:** This is a yellowish benzyl tetra-hydroisoquinoline type alkaloid, obtained from many species of Colchicum (e.g. *C. luteum.*, *C. speciosum*) and also from genera Androcymbium, Gloriosa, Iphigenia, Littonia and Sandersonia. It is used to relieve gout and rheumatic problems.

■ **Diosgenin, Hecogenin and Solasodine:** These are natural steroidal sapogenins, obtained from Dioscorea species (e.g. *D. deltoidea*, *D. maxicana*, *D. compositae* and *D. floribunda*); Agave spp. and Solanum spp. respectively used in various hormonal preparations including birth control pills.

■ **Ephedrine:** It is a protoalkaloid obtained from various spp. of Ephedra (Ma-huang) and may also be prepared by synthesis. It is used for the relief of asthma and hay fever.

■ **Hyoscine and Hyoscyamine:** These are tropane alkaloids obtained from *D. stramonium*, *Hyoscyamus niger* and *H. muticus*. It is used as sedative in preoperative medication before the induction of anaesthesia and in ophthalmic practice to dilate the pupil of the eye.

■ **Morphine, Codeine and Papaverine:** These are the opium alkaloids obtained from the latex of *Papaver somniferum*. It is used as a pain killer (morphine) and antitussive (codeine).

■ **Psoralen:** This is furanocoumarin obtained from *Psoralea corylifolia*. It is used in leucoderma and skin problems.

■ **Quinine and Quinidine:** These are quinoline alkaloids obtained from various spp. of Cinchona bark used as antimalarials.

■ **Reserpine and Ajmalicine:** These are the indole alkaloids obtained from *Rauwolfia serpentine*, used to treat hypertension and as a vasodilator.

■ **Rutin:** This is yellow coloured crystalline flavonol glycoside obtained from buckwheat, i.e. *Fagopyrum esculentum* (Polygonaceae). It is included in dietary supplements and claimed to be benefit in treating conditions characterized by capillary bleeding.

■ **Sennosid   es A and B:** This is anthraquinone glycoside obtained from *Cassia senna* and is used to treat habitual constipation.

■ **Taxol (Paclitaxel):** This is diterpene ester obtained from Taxus species (e.g. *T. brevifolia* and *T. wallichiana*; Taxaceae), used as anticancer agent.

■ **Xanthotoxin:** This is furanocoumarin obtained from *Ammi majus* and *Heracleum candicans*, used in leucoderma and other skin problems.

7.5. INDIAN MEDICINAL PLANTS USED IN COSMETIC AND AROMATHERAPY

Following is the list of few Indian medicinal plants, which are in demand in the domestic as well as international market being useful in herbal cosmetic and in aromatherapy.

Aloe vera (Kumari)	Rosa damascena (Rose)
Pelargonium graveolens (Geranium)	Matricaria chamomilla
Ocimum basilicum and O. sanctum	Lawsonia inermis (Mehndi)
Hibiscus rosa-sinensis (Japa)	Mentha piperita (Peppermint oil)
Mentha arvensis (Mint oil)	Eucalyptus globulus (Eucalyptus oil)

7.6. INDIAN MEDICINAL PLANTS IN CRUDE FORM

The following list of Indian medicinal plants having export potential in the crude form as well as their phytopharmaceutical products:

Aconitum spp. (Vatsanabha)	Acorus calamus (Vacha)
Adhatoda vasica (Vasa)	Herberts aristata (Daruhaldi)
Cassia senna (Senna)	Colchicum luteum (Colchicum)
Hedychium spicatum (Kapur kachri)	Heracleum candicans (Kaindal)
Inula racemosa (Pushkarmool)	Juglans regia (Akhrot)
Juniperus spp. (Aarar)	Plantago ovata (Isabgol)
Picrorhiza kurroa (Kutki)	Podophyllum hexandrum (Bankakri)
Punica granatum (Anar)	Rauwolfia serpentina (Sarpagandha)
Rheum australe (Revandchini)	Swertia chirata (Chirata)
Valeriana wallichii (Tagar)	Zingiber officinale (Adrak)

7.7. SPICES

Spices form an important ingredient of culinary preparations in the tropics. They are added to the food in minor quantities to alter the taste and flavour of the preparation. Though they do not contribute to the energy content of the diet, they help to increase the digestion of the diet by enhancing the secretion of the digestive enzyme in the alimentary tract and by increasing the perspiration. There are four major groups of active constituents present in the spices, responsible for all these properties:

1. Volatile oils
2. Phenolics
3. Alkaloids
4. Sulphur-containing compounds

Volatile Oils

Volatile oils are sweet-smelling liquids, and they emit fragrance to the food and are also slight bitter in taste. Thus, they help to enhance the secretion of digestive enzyme in the alimentary tract. All spices belonging to the apiaceae (umbelliferous fruits and their leaves) and the lamiaceae (leafy spices) are rich in volatile oils. Since the oils are lost on cooking, these spices are mostly added as condiments.

Phenolics

Phenolics component contribute to the taste, colour and flavour of a number of spices. The phenols present in spices are simple in structure mostly containing single aromatic ring, e.g. gingerols (ginger), phenolic amines are the pungent principles (capsaicins) in red pepper and phenylpropenes are present in cloves (eugenol) and fennel (anethole).

Alkaloids

Alkaloids are the largest group of nitrogenous natural organic compounds but only a few spices belonging to the genus piper contain them. Alkaloids present in this genus are of piperidine type.

Sulphur Compounds

Spices such as mustard, onion and garlic owe their pungency and characteristic odour to sulphur-containing compounds. These compounds are present in the form of glucosinolate (mustard seed) and are volatile with an offensive odour (onion, garlic and asparagus).

7.8. EXPORT OF SPICES FROM INDIA

Following is the list of spices being exported from India to East Asia, the United States, West Asia, European Community and Africa, UAE, Singapore, Germany, France, Canada, Sri Lanka, Japan, Malaysia, Russia, Bangladesh, Pakistan, Saudi Arabia and Netherlands.

Although other countries like China, Brazil, Thailand, etc., have also started export of spice, but even then the demand for Indian spices is not being affected.

Spices exports have registered substantial growth during the last decade, registering an annual average growth rate of 11.1% in value terms. During the year 2007–08, the export earnings from spices have surpassed US$ 1 billion mark for the first time and registered an all time high both in terms of quantity and value in spice exports. In 2007–08, the export of spices from India has been 444,250 tonnes valued US$ 1101.80 million registering an increase of 39% in value over 2006–07. India commands a formidable position in the World Spice Trade with 48% share in volume and 44% in value (Table 7.4 and Figure 7.2).

The history of Indian spice is very old, as there are evidences of India having trade of vegetable drugs and spices with Greece even before Alexander's invasion in 327 B.C. India's glory for the land of spice and perfumery attracted foreigners (French, British, Arab, Portuguese and Dutch). Portuguese invaded India and controlled over the spice trade of the country. They were taken over by Dutch, who exploited spices of India for many years. Later the British Empire took over and shared most of the world spice trade with Holland. Arabs had taken the spice products from southern India and established it even after independence. Spices have continued to be the main attraction of international trade in India. The Government of India had established separate board as 'Spice Board of India', for promoting the spice trade which control their production and quality. Besides, the Spice Board, the Indian Institute of Spices Research (HSR) was established at Calicut in 1986, which is responsible for providing latest biotechnology for more production of spices.

Southern states of India remained the main centre of region of spice production. Even today, Southern states of the country produce most of the spices.

Table 7.4: Item wise export of spices from India

Item	2005–06 Quantity (MT)	2005–06 Value (Rs lakh)	2005–06 Value (MLS US $)	2006–07 Quantity (MT)	2006–07 Value (Rs lakh)	2006–07 Value (MLS US $)	2007–08 Quantity (MT)	2007–08 Value (Rs lakh)	2007–08 Value (MLS US $)
Pepper	17,363	15,095	34.06	28,750	30,620	67.90	35,000	51,950	129.05
Cardamom (S)	863	2682	6.05	650	2236	4.96	500	2475	6.15
Cardamom (L)	1046	1155	2.61	1500	1695	3.76	1325	1500	3.73
Chilli	113,174	40,301	90.93	148,500	80,775	179.13	209,000	109,750	272.62
Ginger	9411	4296	9.69	7500	3975	8.81	6700	2800	6.96
Turmeric	46,405	15,286	34.49	51,500	16,480	36.55	49,250	15,700	39.00
Coriander	23,756	6771	15.28	20,500	7462	16.55	26,000	11,025	27.39
Cumin	12,879	9819	22.16	26,000	20,150	44.68	28,000	29,150	72.41
Celery	4165	1501	3.39	3550	1321	2.93	2900	1325	3.29
Fennel	5725	2782	6.28	3575	2380	5.28	5250	2850	7.08
Fenugreek	15,525	3403	7.68	8500	2699	5.98	11,100	3300	8.20
Other seeds (1)	12,670	3322	7.50	8000	2240	4.97	8850	3125	7.76
Garlic	34,688	4798	10.83	11,500	2128	4.72	675	400	0.99
Tamarind	14,101	3078	6.95	10,200	3000	6.65	11,250	3100	7.70
Nutmeg and Mace	1530	3117	7.03	2100	4274	9.48	1300	2875	7.14
Vanilla	72	1227	2.77	125	1996	4.43	200	1775	4.41
Other spices (2)	7033	4415	9.96	9300	4280	9.49	7750	5000	12.42
Curry powder	9340	7838	17.69	9500	8693	19.28	11,500	11,100	27.57
Mint products (3)	14,544	81,321	183.49	16,250	110,095	244.15	21,100	128,050	318.08
Oils and Oleoresins	6074	50557	114.08	6250	51,079	113.27	6600	56,300	139.85
TOTAL	**350,363**	**262,762**	**592.89**	**373,750**	**357,575**	**792.95**	**444,250**	**443,550**	**1,101.80**

(1) Includes bishops weed (Ajwain seed), dill seed, poppy seed, aniseed, mustard, etc.
(2) Includes asafoetida, cinnamon, cassia, cambodge, saffron, spices (NES), etc.
(3) Includes menthol, menthol crystals and mint oils.

* *Source:* DGCI&S., Calcutta/Shipping Bills/Exporters' Returns.

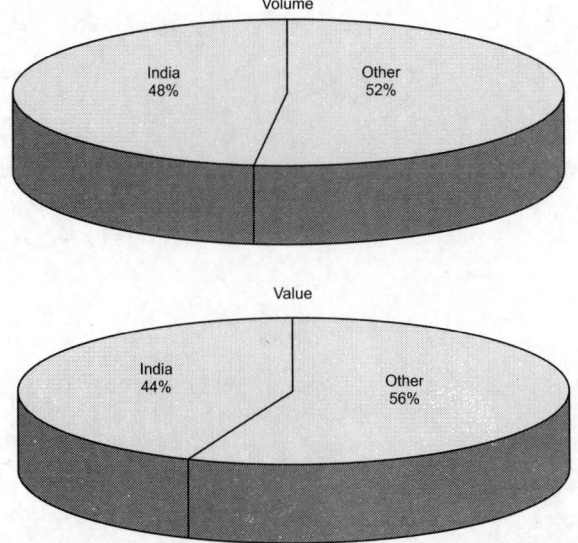

FIG. 7.2 India's share in world trade of spices (2007–08)

At present Kerala tops in the production of black pepper, cardamom and ginger, while producing substantial quantities of long pepper and turmeric; Andhra Pradesh has monopoly in the production of turmeric and chillies. More than half of the country's chillies and turmeric production is produced by the state of Andhra Pradesh alone. Currently about 50 million tonnes of chillies were produced by the Andhra Pradesh.

The spices export during April–December 2008 is estimated as 334,150 tonnes valued Rs 3810.95 crore (US$ 860.40 million) as against 325,320 tonnes valued Rs 3,320.00 crore (US$ 821.45 million) in the corresponding period of the last financial year. Compared to last year, the export has shown an increase of 15% in rupee value and a 3% in quantity. In dollar terms, the increase is 5%, according to data released by Spices Board.

Spice oils and oleoresins including mint products contributed 42% of the total export earnings. Chilli contributed 21% followed by pepper 8%, cumin 8% and turmeric 5%.

During April–December 2008, export of most of the major spices have shown an increasing trend both in terms of quantity and value as compared to the same period of last year. However, exports of pepper and chilli have declined both in terms of quantity and value as compared to last year. During the period, export of ginger and mint products has declined in quantity only.

During April–December 2008, the export of pepper from India has been 19,100 tonnes valued at Rs 317.77 crore as against 27,580 tonnes valued Rs 400.20 crore of last year. The average export price of pepper has gone up from Rs 145.11 per kg in 2007 to Rs 166.37 per kg in 2008. The low inventory in the major international markets due to the economic recession is reported to be the major reason for the decline in exports.

During the period, India has exported 141,000 tonnes of chilli and chilli products valued Rs 793.18 crore as against 149,755 tonnes valued Rs 807.03 crore of last year. The traditional buyers of Indian chilli, viz. Malaysia, Indonesia and Sri Lanka continued their buying this year also. It is expected that the export will pick up in the coming months as the new crop comes to market.

The export of seed spices has shown an increasing trend both in the quantity and value as compared to last year. The export of coriander seed during April–December 2008 has been 19,600 tonnes valued at Rs 137.23 crore as against 19,150 tonnes valued at Rs 77.69 crore of last year, registering an increase of 77% in value. The unit value of export has gone up from Rs 40.57/kg in 2007 to Rs 70.01/kg in 2008.

The export of cumin seed during April–December 2008 has increased considerably and the export has been 28,500 tonnes valued at Rs 296.13 crore as against 18,885 tonnes valued at Rs 199.09 crore. The export of cumin up to December 2008 is an all-time record both in terms of quantity and value. The export of cumin has shown an increase of 51% in quantity and 49% in value terms as compared to last year. The reported crop failure in other major producing countries, viz. Syria, Turkey and Iran has helped India to achieve this substantial increase in the export of cumin.

The export of value-added products like curry powder and spice oils and oleoresins have also shown substantial increase both in terms of quantity and value as compared to last year. During April–December 2008, a total quantity of 10,500 tonnes of curry powder and *masalas* valued Rs 124.45 crore has been exported as against 8375 tonnes valued at Rs 81.10 crore of last year. During April–December 2008, the export of spice oils and oleoresins has been 5550 tonnes valued at Rs 574.23 crore as against 4815 tonnes valued at Rs 404.04 crore of last years, registering an increase of 42% in value and 15% in volume.

Against the export target of 425,000 tonnes valued Rs 4350.00 crore (US$ 1,025.00) for the year, the achievement of 334,150 tonnes valued Rs 3810.95 crore (US$ 860.40 million) up to December 2008 is 79% in quantity, 88% in rupee value and 84% in dollar terms of value. The export of spices like cumin, fenugreek, nutmeg and mace, vanilla and other seeds have already achieved the respective targets fixed for the year 2008–09.

CHAPTER 8

Utilization of Aromatic Plants and Derived Products

CONTENTS

8.1. INTRODUCTION

Aromatic plants are plants that possess aromatic compounds, most of which are essential oils which are volatile in room temperature. These compounds are synthesized and stored in a special structure called gland, which is located in different parts of plant such as leaves, flowers, fruits, seeds, barks and roots. These essential oils can be extracted by various physical and chemical processes, such as steam distillation, maceration, expression, enfleurage and solvent extraction. They are mainly used as flavours and fragrances. However, from ancient times, these plants have been used as raw materials for cosmetics, pharmaceuticals, botanical pesticides, etc.

Importance of Aromatic Plants

Aromatic plants can be divided into four groups based on how they are utilized, viz.

- ■ *As raw materials for essential oils extraction:* This is the major use of aromatic plants and is the one dealt with in this aromatic plant.
- ■ *As spices:* These are plants in which their nonleafy parts are used as a flavouring or seasoning.
- ■ *As herbs:* These are plants in which their leafy or soft flowering parts are used as a flavouring or seasoning.
- ■ *Miscellaneous group:* These are aromatic plants used in some ways other than the ones mentioned above, e.g. as medicines, cosmetics, dyes, air fresheners, disinfectants, botanical pesticides, herbal drinks/teas, potpourri, insect repellents, etc.

People have made extensive use of aromatic plants from time immemorial. The Egyptian, the Persian and the Babylonian were known to grow and use aromatic plants in making perfumes and other scented waters from a distillation of rose petals and orange blossoms. Oriental people were also fond of aromatic plants. These aromatic plants were grown in the palace compounds and used as raw materials to make perfumes, scented water and a dozen of other aromatic products.

8.2. IMPACT OF INDUSTRIALIZATION

The techniques of essential oils extraction from aromatic plants have been known for thousands of year. These essential oils have been used in home-made perfumes, scented water, traditional medicine, etc. These plants were normally grown in the backyard and collected for use whenever there was a need. With the advance of industrialization through large-scale production and modern facilities for processing and utilization, aromatic plants and their products have become very popular. However, as production costs become more and more expensive, it is necessary to come up with practical solution, i.e. the invention of synthetic compounds that are almost the same as natural materials. This has considerably reduced the use of natural flavour and fragrant materials.

Volatile Oil

A substance of oily consistency and feel, derived from a plant and containing the principle to which the odour and taste of the plant are due (essential oils), in contrast to a fatty oil, a volatile oil evaporates when exposed to the air and thus is capable of distillation It may also be obtained by expression or extraction as many volatile oils identical to or closely resembling the natural oils can be made synthetically. This is also known as ethereal oil.

The essential oils industry was traditionally a cottage industry in India. Since 1974, a number of industrial companies have been established for large-scale production of essential oils, oleo resins and perfume. The essential oils from plants being produced in India include ajwain oil, cedar wood oil, celery oil, citronella oil, davana oil, eucalyptus oil, geranium oil, lavender oil, lemon grass oil, mentha oil, palmarosa oil, patchouli rose oil, sandalwood oil, turpentine oil and vetiver oil. The manufacture of turpentine oil and resin from pine is a sizable and well-established industry in India having 10,000–25,000 tonnes annual production of the oil—α-pinine and δ-3-carene being two vital components produced from the oil. α-Ionone from lemon grass oil for perfumery and β-ionone for vitamin A synthesis are produced in India. Before 1960, menthol was not produced in India but the introduction of Japanese mint, *Mentha arvensis* and subsequent improvements therefore enabled India to produces over 500 tonnes of menthol, and now tops the world market in export of natural menthol. Although the production of major oils is highly organized as a number of developing countries have volatile oil rich flora not fully utilized or cultivated.

Essential Oils

The chemical components of essential oils can be divided into two main categories: the hydrocarbon monoterpenes, diterpenes and sesquiterpenes, as well as some oxides, phenolics and sulphur- and nitrogen-containing material. Common terpenes include limonene, which occurs in most citrus oils and the antiseptic pine, found in pine and terpene oils. Important sesquiterpenes include chamazulene and farnesene, which occur in chamomile oil and which have been widely studied for anti-inflammatory and bactericidal properties.

The extensive occurrence of ester in essential oils includes linalyl acetate, which is a component of bergamot and lavender, and geranyl acetate that is found in sweet marjoram. Other common esters are the bornyl, eugenyl and lavandulyl acetate. The characteristic fruity aromas of esters are claimed to have sedative and fungicidal properties.

Aldehydes are also clamed to have sedative properties, the most common being citronellal and neral found in lemon scanted oils; citral also has antiseptic properties. Equally pungent to the aldehydes in many instances are the ketones, such as jasmone and funchone found in jasmine and fennel oil, respectively. Ketones, such as camphor, carnone, methone and pine comphone, found in many proprietary preparations are effective in upper respiratory tract complaints. However, some ketones are also among the more toxic components of essential oils, and are found in pennyroyal and buchu.

The alcohol within essential oils is generally nontoxic. Commonly occurring terpene alcohols include citronellal found in rose, lemon and eucalyptus, also geramnial, borneol, farnesol, menthol, nerol and linalool occurring in rose wood and lavender. Alcohol has antiseptic and antiviral properties, and in aromatherapy, they are claimed to have an uplifting quality.

A wide range of oxides occur in essential oils including ascaridole, bisabolol and bisabolene oxides and linalool oxide from hyssop. The most important oxide, however, is cineole. Also known as eucalyptus oil, it occurs extensively in other oils such as bay laurel, rosemary and cajuput. It is used medicinally for its expectorant properties. Utilization of essential oils in different industries has been summarized in Figure 8.1.

Indian scenario

India is one of the few countries in the world having varied agroclimatic zones suitable for the cultivation of a host of essential oils bearing plants. Due to increased awareness of health hazards associated with synthetic chemicals coupled with the increase coast of petroleum products, the use of essential oils has been gradually increasing. The consumers are showing increasing preference for natural material over the synthetic. During the last few years with the spurt in the production of essential oils, it is emerging as a potential agro-based industry in India. At present in India about 30% of the fine chemical used annually in perfumes and flavours come from essential oils. The total consumption of perfumery and flavouring

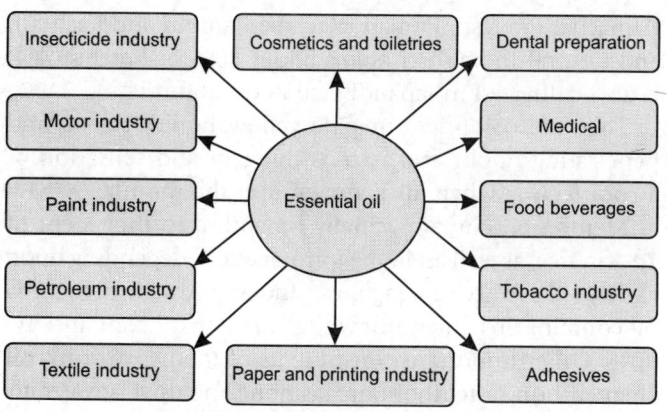

FIG. 8.1 Utilization of essential oils

material in India is abut 3800 MT/annum valued at Rs 100 crore. Food, dental, pharmaceutical flavours share is around 700 MT, and the rest represents perfumery. The estimated production of perfumery raw material is around 500 tonnes/annum valued at Rs 400 crore. According to Trade Development Authority of India, the total production of fragrance excluding formulation for captive consumption by the user industry is about Rs 120 crore/annum. A number of essential oils form palmarosa, citronella, ginger grass, basil, mint, lemon grass, eucalyptus, cedar wood, lavender oil, davana oil, celery seed oil, fennel and other oils have been widely used in a variety of products in India. Out of these the essential oils currently being produced in India are oil of citronella, lemon grass, basil, mint, sandalwood, palmarosa, eucalyptus, cedar wood, vetiver and geranium. Rose oil, lavender, davana oil, oil of khus and ginger grass are produced in small quantities. During last forty year, the importance of developing essential oils bearing plants is being increasingly realized. With the introduction of Japanese mint and subsequent improvement there upon, India produces 5000 tonnes of menthol valued at Rs 100 crore and is one of the leading menthol-producing country. Presently, the areas under mint cultivation are estimated to be around 40,000 hectares, mainly in Uttar Pradesh, Punjab, Haryana and to some extent in Bihar and Madhya Pradesh. The export of essential oils during the year 1991–92 has been Rs 53.6 crore as against Rs 40 crore during the year 1990–91, thereby registering an increases of 37% over the last year. An amount of Rs 61 crore has been saved in foreign exchange annually by means of production of certain oils of mint, aromatic grass, linalool, geranium, lavender and rose oil during 1991–92. With the increase in production of above essential oils, it would be possible for the country to save more valuable foreign exchange in the coming years.

The magic items of export are ginger oil, sandalwood oil, lemon grass oil, jasmine oil and other essential oils. During the year 1991–92, export of sandalwood oil has registered a recorded figure of Rs 13 crore compared to Rs 6.2 crore during 1990–91. The major buyers of Indian essential oils being Russia, United States, France, UK, Netherlands, UAE, Saudi Arabia, Spain, Morocco, Germany, Australia, Pakistan, Korea, Taiwan, etc. Similarly, citronella oil production has reached 500 tons when it was totally imported 55 years ago. Also jasmine and tuberose concentrate from South India have created a marks in world marked. Thus, an interesting scenario in the development of natural essential oils in India has enraged.

World scenario

India ranks 26th in import and 14th in respect of export in world in the trade of essential oils. United States, France and Germany are the top three countries in the world in the trade of essential oils. India holds around 7% of import and 1.1% of export. The values of export from India during 1991–92 to three major countries like United States, France and Germany have been to the tune of Rs 21.2 crore with major share going to the United States (Rs 8.2 crore) and France (Rs 7.39 crore).

The world trade in essential oils and its product is vast, and the oils of major importance are aniseed, citronella, clove, geranium, lemon grass, peppermint oil, patchouli, sandalwood, vetiver, mint oil, lemon grass, palmarosa, etc.

Future demand

Approximately 90% of the present requirement of essential oils in the country is met by the indigenous production and 10% from import. In 1950, the production was hardly 7580 tonnes, which has since been rising to 8000 tonnes. This has been both vertical and horizontal growth in the production of essential oils. Peppermint, spearmint and other mint oil constitute 68% of total volume of production of essential oils in the country. Other important varieties which constitute 28% of the total production are basil oil, citronella oil, eucalypts oil, lemon grass, palmarosa, and sandalwood and vetiver oil. The annual growth rate of pharmaceutical industry in terms of volume and value is expected to be between 11% and 13% in the next five years. The other important sector showing rapid expansion is the processed food industry particularly ice cream and confectionery items. Fragrance finds use in toiletries and personal care products. Volume wise toiletries constitute 90% of all these products. The annual production of toiletries has been estimated by Toilet Makers Association from 3.5 lakh tonnes in 1991 to 4.8 lakh tonnes in 1995, at an annual growth rate of 8%. The requirement of essential oils by consumer industries under fragrances, flavour and aroma chemicals are 60%, 20% and 20%, respectively.

The association of essential oils manufactures estimated growth in export value from Rs 50 corer in 1991–92 to Rs 125 corer in 1995–96. India ranks 14th in the world export trade, and its share being at an average 0.6–0.8% of the total. These are an ample room for penetration into the foreign market especially to the newly developing countries of the middle and for east.

Export of major essential oils from India

Mentha arvensis and mint oil, cedar wood oil, clove oil, eucalyptus oil, tuberose concentrate, palmarosa oil, patchouli oil, sandalwood oil, lemon grass oil, davana oil, coriander oil, dill oil, spearmint oil, rose oil, *Mentha piperita*, jasmine concentrate, Jasmine oil.

8.3. TOXICITY OF ESSENTIAL OILS

With the latest therapeutic trend towards aromatherapy and excessive use of essential oils under the labels of natural products, the knowledge of toxicity of essential oils has become important to avoid their abusive use.

As a general rule, the acute toxicity of essential oils by the oral route is low or very low; e.g. many of the oils used have an LD_{50} between 2 and 5 g/kg body weight (e.g. anise, eucalyptus and clove) and for most of them greater than 5 g/kg body weight (e.g. chamomile, citronella, lavender, marjoram and vetiver). Other oils have further low LD_{50} between 1 and 2 g/kg for sweet basil, tarragon, hyssop (1.5 g/kg), savoury (1.37 g/kg), sassafras (1.9 g/kg), winter green (0.9–3.25 g/kg), chenopodium (0.25 g/kg), thuja (0.83 g/kg), pennyroyl (0.4 g/kg) and mustard oil (0.34 g/kg).

A review of the available literature shows that serious accident involves the young children, due to the ingestion of oils such as clove (eugenol) eucalyptus, pennyroyl (pulegone), winter green (methyl salicylate deadly) and parsley (apiol) in large quantity.

The chronic toxicity of essential oils is also not well known at least for uses, such as aromatherapy as well as for any other route of administration as the doses in which they are used are too low for chronic toxicity.

At present in India about 30% of the fine chemicals used annually in perfumes and flavour are obtained from essential oils. The total consumption of perfumery and flavouring materials in India is about 4800 metric tonne/annum. The food technology, oral hygiene and pharmaceutical flavour share around 900 metric tonnes and rest represents perfumery.

8.4. UTILIZATION OF AROMATIC PLANTS

Mentha Oil

The oil is obtained by stream distillation of the fresh flowering tops of the plants known as *Mentha piperita* Linn; *Mentha arvensis var. piperascens* (Japanese Mint; Family: Labiatae). Mentha oil is commercially cultivated in Uttar Pradesh,

Himachal Pradesh, Punjab, Haryana, Jammu and Kashmir, and Central India. It contains about 80% of *l*-menthol. It is also cultivated in Japan, Brazil and California.

They are colourless or pale yellow liquid; strong and penetrating odour and taste is pungent and sensation of a cool feeling when air is drawn into the mouth.

Mentha oil contains chiefly *l*-menthol to the extent of 70% in free, as well as, in the form of esters, depending upon variety (like American, Japanese, Indian). American mentha oil contains 80% menthol while Japanese oil contains 70–90%. Other important constituents of the peppermint oil are menthone, menthofuran, jasmone, menthyl isovalerate, menthyl acetate and several other terpenes derivatives. The other terpene includes 1-limonene, isopulegone, cineole, pinene, camphene, etc. Jasmone and esters are responsible for pleasant flavour, while menthofuran causes resinification and develops dirty smell.

Utilization of mentha oil and derived products

1. Carminative.
2. Spasmolytic.
3. Mild antidiarrhoeic.
4. Aromatic stimulant.
5. Cholagogue.
6. In tooth paste preparations as a taste corrector.
7. The oil is used for flavouring in pharmaceuticals, dental preparation, mouth washes, cough drops, soaps, chewing gum.
8. It is widely used in flatulence, nausea and gastralgia.
9. The oil has mild antiseptic and local anaesthetic properties.
10. It is used externally in rheumatism, neuralgia, congestive, headache and toothache.
11. The menthol is antipruritic and used on the skin or mucous membrane as counter-irritant, antiseptic and stimulant. Internally, it has a depressant effect on the heart.
12. The menthol is used in food industries such as liquor, soda, syrup, confectionary (candy, chewing gum and chocolate).
13. The menthol is used in cosmetic preparation like shaving cream, tooth paste, lotion, deodorant and aftershave lotion, etc.

Eucalyptus Oil

It is a volatile oil obtained by steam distillation from fresh leave *Eucalyptus globules* and other species of eucalyptus (Family: Myrtaceae). It should contain not less than 65% of cineole.

It is indigenous to Australia and Tasmania. It is cultivated in the United States (California), Spain, Portugal and in India. *E. citriodora*, known as citron scented or lemon scented gum, is grown on large scale basis in Kerala, Tamil Nadu and other states.

The odour of oil is aromatic and camphoraceous. It is colourless or pale yellow liquid, having pungent and camphorous taste followed by the sensation of cold. It is soluble in 90% alcohol, fixed oils, fats and in paraffin.

Eucalyptus oil chiefly contains cineole, also known as eucalyptol. It also contains pinene, camphene and traces of phellandrene, citronellal, gallotannins, methyl ester of *p*-coumaric acid, and cinnamic acid in combined form.

Citriodorol (from *E. citriodora*): It also contains small quantity of butyric, valerenic and caproic aldehyde.

Cineole   Camphene

Phellandrene

Utilization of eucalyptus oil

1. Eucalyptus oil is used as a counter-irritant, an antiseptic and expectorant.
2. Antibacterial and antituberculosis (citriodorol).
3. Diaphoretic.
4. It is used to relieve cough and in chronic bronchitis in the form of inhalation.
5. Solution of eucalyptus oil is used as nasal drops.
6. It is used in infections of the upper respiratory tract, malaria and certain skin diseases, in ointment for burns and as mosquito repellent.
7. If mixed with an equal amount of olive oil, it is useful as a rubefacient for rheumatism.

Geranium Oil

Geranium oil is obtained by steam distillation of the tender parts of the plants of various species like *Pelargonium* (Geraniaceae) (*P. graveolens, P. capitatum and P. odoratissium Linn*).

It is indigenous to South Africa and cultivated in Algeria, Morocco, Spain, France and Italy. Indian geranium oil is obtained from other species and is known as palmarosa oil.

All varieties of geranium generally contain 0.08–0.4% of fragrant volatile oil. Geranium oil contains two types of constituents, i.e. alcohol and esters. The alcohols are β-citranellol and geraniol about 60–70% of the oil. While esters namely geranyl geranyl-tiglate, citronellyl formate and citranellyl acetate contribute about 20–30% oil. Several sesquiterpenes alcohols are also reported in the oil, and are responsible for pleasant fragrance.

Beta-citranellol   Geraniol

Utilization of geranium oil

1. As a flavouring agent for creams, lotions, soap, perfumes and other products. It is also used in alcoholic, nonalcoholic beverages, candy and other dairy products at 0.001%.
2. The oil is used in the treatment of inflammation, with its mild soothing effect.
3. It is a stimulant of the adrenal cortex and can be used to balance the production of androgens which occurs during the menopause.
4. The oil is good insecticide.

Vetiver Oil (Khus Oil)

It is obtained by steam distillation from roots of the plant of *Vetiveria zizanioides* Stapf (Family: Gramineae).

The plant is found growing in India, Myanmar, Sri Lanka and East and West Africa. It is cultivated in Indonesia, Caribbean Islands, Malaysia and the United States. In India, it is found abundant in Punjab, Rajasthan, Kerala, Karnataka and Tamil Nadu.

Cultivation of vetiver grass is done by sowing the seeds or from slips. A well-drained sandy loam is most suitable for cultivation. The temperature ranging from 25–38°C and rainfall of 100–200 cm are desired. It thrives best in marshy places and humid climate. Planting of slips is done just before the outbreak of monsoon. The distance between two plants and between two rows is approximately 2.5 cm. Proper arrangements for irrigation must be made after rainy season is over. Fertilizers and manures are provided to produce sturdy grass and roots. The grass attains the height of 1–1.5 metre above the guard. When the plant is about 15–18 months of age, the roots are collected by uprooting in dry months of the year. If necessary, digging is done for collection of roots. The drug is slashed, cut into small pieces and used for extraction of oil.

Colour of oil is light brown to deep brown or green and odour is characteristics. It is soluble in fixed oil and alcohol.

The vetiver oil mainly contains alcohol (45–60%), i.e. vetivenol, vetiverol, and 8–35% ketone namely 3-vetivones. Indian vetiver oil contains khusal, khusitol and khusinol.

Utilization of vetiver oil

1. It is used as stimulant, refrigerant, flavouring agent, aromatic, stomachic and in the treatment of prickly heat or itches.
2. It is used as antiseptic, antispasmodic and rubefacient.
3. It is also used in burns, sores and as diaphoretic.
4. It is also used in preparation of sherbet, soap, perfumery and toilet preparations and as a fixative of volatile oils.

Sandalwood Oil

Sandalwood oil is obtained by distillation of dried heart wood from the plant *Santalum album* Linn (Family: Santalaceae).

The sandal tree is available in India and Malaya. In India, the trees are available in Tamil Nadu, Mysore, Maharashtra, Uttar Pradesh, Madhya Pradesh, Assam, Bihar, Rajasthan and Gujarat.

Sandalwood oil is yellowish and pale reddish viscous liquid. It has strong fragrance, taste is slightly bitter.

Sandalwood oil contains mixture of two isomers α- and β-santolol (90%), α and β-santalene, santalone, santanone, isovaleraldehyde, α- and β-santalic acids, etc.

Utilization of sandalwood oil

1. Oil is used as perfuming agent in various cosmetic preparations and incense sticks.
2. It is used for wound and blisters caused by small pox vaccination, gonorrhoea, cough and dysuria.
3. Sandalwood oil along with neem oil is used as a contraceptive.
4. Sandalwood oil along with double quantity of mustard oil used for treatment for pimples on the nose.
5. Sandalwood oil and sandalwood are considered as cooling, diuretic, diaphoretics and expectorant drugs.
6. It is very gentle antiseptic and diuretic and is useful in urinary problem like cystitis.

Utilization of sandalwood

1. Sandalwood is used for preparing several articles such as small boxes, cabinet panels, combs, book mark, walking stick, pen-holder, card cases, paper cutter, picture frames, etc.
2. Sawdust from heartwood is mostly used as incense for scenting cloths and cupboards, and for stuff in pincushions.
3. Fine powder of sandalwood is used as a cosmetic.

Lemon Grass Oil

Lemon grass oil is the oil distilled from *Cymbopogon flexuosus* Stapf or from *C. citrates* Staf (Family: Gramineae).

Lemon grass oil is a reddish yellow or brown. It has odour resembling that of lemon oil. It is almost entirely soluble in 70% alcohol; the solubility gradually decreases on storage.

Lemon grass oil mainly contains citral and citronellal (75–85%). The other terpene is geraniol, nerol, linalool, methyl heptenol, limonene, etc.; beta-ionone is derived from citral.

Utilization of lemon grass oil

1. It is used as flavouring and perfuming agent.
2. It is also used as a mosquito repellent.
3. It is used as a source of citral for the preparation of beta-ionone.
4. The β-ionone is used as precursor of vitamin A.
5. The oil is used in perfumery, soaps and cosmetics.

CHAPTER 9

Role of Medicinal Plants in National Economy

CONTENTS

- Introduction
- Economic Growth Potential in Natural Health and Cosmetic Products
- Future Economic Growth
- Development of Herbal Medicinal Industry
- Contribution to Economy of the People

9.1. INTRODUCTION

Since ancient times, mankind all over the world mainly depended upon plant kingdom to meet all their needs of medicines: for alleviating ailments, search for eternal health, longevity and to seek remedy to relieve pain and discomfort, fragrance, favours and foods. It had prompted the early man to explore his immediate natural surrounding and try many plant, animal products, mineral and develop a variety of therapeutic agents.

Medicinal plants still play an important role in emerging and developing countries of Asia, both in preventive and curative treatments, despite advances in modern Western medicine. They also generate income to the people of many Asian countries, who earn their livelihood from selling collected materials from the forest or by cultivating on their farms. Thus, the medicinal plants constitute a very important national resource. People in India and China are known to have used plants in organized health care regime for over 5,000 years. European herbal medicines blossomed in the Greco-Roman era and remained in mainstream until six decades ago. The ancient civilization of India, China, Greece, Arab and other countries of the world developed their own systems of medicine independent of each other, but all of them were predominantly plant based. But the theoretical foundation and the in sights or in depth understanding on the practice of medicine was much superior in ayurveda among organized system of medicine. It is perhaps the oldest (6000 B.C.) among the organized traditional medicine. People from other countries of the world as China, Cambodia, Indonesia and Baghdad used to come to the ancient universities of India, like Takshila (700 B.C.) and Nalanda (500 B.C.) to learn health sciences of India particularly ayurveda. From history, we learn that since ancient times, plants remained major natural resource in the world.

One of the oldest repositories of human knowledge, the *Rigveda* (4500–4600 B.C.) mentioned the use of medicinal plants for the treatment of one or other disease. In the long struggle to overcome the powerful forces of nature, the human beings have always turned to plants. There are reports available about the local communities in the Asian, African and Latin American countries having a long history of dependence on traditional remedies, largely based on plants, for immediate access to relatively safe, cost-effective, efficacious and culturally acceptable solutions to primary health care.

The World Health Organization (WHO) estimated that 80% of the population of developing countries relies on traditional medicines, mostly plant drugs for their primary health care needs. Even the modern pharmacopoeia still contains at least 25% drugs derived from plants and many others, which are semisynthetic, built on prototype compounds isolated from plants. Medicinal plants are the major components of all indigenous or alternative systems of medicine. For example, they are common elements in ayurveda, homoeopathy, naturopathy, Oriental and Native American Indian medicine. Demand for herbal drugs is increasing throughout the world due to growing recognition of natural plant-based products, being nontoxic, having no side effects, easily available at affordable prices and sometimes the only source of health care available to the poor. Hence, medicinal plant sector has traditionally occupied an important position in the sociocultural, spiritual, economic values of rural and tribal lives of both developing and developed countries. Millions of rural households are using medicinal plants in self-help mode.

About 90% of medicinal plants used by the industries are collected from the wild source. While over 800 species are used by industries, not more than 20 species of plant are under the commercial cultivation. Hence, more than 70% plant collection involved destructive harvesting because of the use of parts like root, bark, stem, wood and whole plant (in the case of herbs). This process is a definite threat to the genetic stock and diversity of medicinal plant resources, and ultimately to the economy of the country if the biodiversity is not sustainably used.

The other main source of medicinal plants is from cultivation. The cultivated material is definitely more appropriate for use in the production of drugs. Indeed, standardization, whether for pure products, extracts or crude drugs, is critical and becomes easier. Hence, higher cost for cultivated material and cultivation are often done under contract. More recently growers have set up cooperative or collaborative ventures in an attempt to improve their negotiating power and achieve higher prices, and thus medicinal plants in a wider context generate income to the people of many Asian countries who earn their livelihood from selling collected materials from the wild forest, or by cultivating on their farms.

International trade in medicinal plants both within South Asian countries and East Asia, Europe and North America is growing in economic importance, e.g. Nepal is earning an estimated US$ 8.6 million annually from the export of medicinal plants; thus, the medicinal plants and other forest products influence local, national and international economics.

There is widespread belief that 'green' drugs are healthier than synthetic product. Recent reports have witnessed an upsurge in the popularity of herbal medicines. In most industrialized countries, use of medicinal plants has increased dramatically in the last decade; there has been a rising trend in *Ayurvedic* (herbal) products—an area where India's expertise dates back centuries. But it is not only in the last decade that the country has truly seen the commercialization on the herbal concept. Herbal has now become full-fledged wave composing of both in beauty care and health care products. As well as herbal over-the-counter (OTC) drugs have gained substantial ground. Currently, according to industry estimate, total pharmaceutical market is around Rs 5000 crore; the total herbal market share is Rs 1200 crore, of which the OTC market constitutes around Rs 400 crore.

The importance and value of traditional and indigenous herbal medicine was the subject of campaign of the WHO. Its effort, in the 1970s, led an appeal to all member countries to do their utmost to preserve their national heritage in the form of ethnomedicine and ethnopharmacology and to bring back the use of known and tested medicinal plants and derivatives into primary health care in rural areas as alternatives when modern medicines are not available.

In India, plants have been traditionally used for human and veterinary health care and also, in the food and textile industry. Ninety percent of the local food resources known to indigenous people were undocumented to nutritional literature, trade, cosmetics and perfumes; but India has a special position in area of herbal medicines, since it is one of the few countries which are capable of cultivating most of the important plants used both in modern and traditional systems of medicine. This is because India has vast area with wide variation in climate, soil, altitude/latitude and rich flora.

The herbal drug market itself is growing at a rate of between 20% and 30% annually, with individual company registering different growth rates. The healthy growth rate of this market can also be attributed to the government policy of encouraging the manufacturers of purely herbal products. This coupled with absence of any pricing guidelines. Unlike Drug Price Control Order (DPCO), pricing guidelines for ethical drugs has resulted in this segment being perceived as a highly lucrative alternative source of revenue. The new patent policy under 'GATT', which came into effective by the year 2005, has encouraged the herbal market.

While the domestic market (about US$ 1 billion of Ayurvedic medicine) is opening up to the herbal phenomenon; the export market is also showing promise. Many pharmaceutical companies are targeting export as the prime source in the coming years. World trade in plant medicines is of billions of dollar. In 1994, China exported US$ 5 billion of plant drugs; Germany imported about US$ 105 millions of plant drugs. The number of medicinal plants trade too is astonishing. Now Germany export market is about Rs 600 crore, and is expected to expand to Rs 20,000 crore in the next decade. The present export volume of crude drugs from India stands at 36,200 tonnes valued around US$ 24 millions. China and India are two great producers of medicinal plants having more than 40% of global diversity.

In developing countries, plants are the main source of alternative medicine. According to the WHO, as many as 80% of the world's people rely on traditional medicines for their primary health care, most types of which use remedies from plants. The use of traditional medicine in developing countries is increasing because population is increasing. Government wants to encourage indigenous forms of medicine rather than to rely on imported drugs, and there are strong moves to revive traditional cultures; being easy access and cost effectiveness ultimately affect the national economy.

For example, traditional medicine is an important part of African culture. It varies with cultural group and region. The Western pharmaceuticals are inaccessible especially to rural-based population. Therefore, more than 80% of Africans rely on plant-based medicine. About 70–90% of the population in South Africa, Zambia, Nigeria, Mozambique, Ethiopia and Democratic Republic of Congo, among others, relies on traditional medicine for their health care. In South Africa, at national level, 20,000 tonnes of medicinal plant materials are traded, corresponding to a value of about US$ 60 millions. In Zambia, trade in traditional medicine is worth over US$ 43 millions per annum. Traditional systems of medicine are also predominant medical systems in practice in Malawian rural areas.

Medicinal plants based medicine also has significant role in most Latin American countries. About 70–80% of the Latin American population relies on traditional medicines for their health care needs. For example, about 80% of Ecuadorians rely on medicinal plants or products derived from plants. There is lack of access to modern drugs in a significant part of Latin America. In India, annual turnover of herbal industry was estimated around US$ 250 million in 1995. According to Chemexcil report, export value of Ayurvedic and Unani medicine was about US$ 41.6 million during 1999–2000; the major OTC products contribute around US$ 30.5 million.

9.2. ECONOMIC GROWTH POTENTIAL IN NATURAL HEALTH AND COSMETIC PRODUCTS

Medicinal plants also play a great role in food supplements for health care as well as in personal care of the mankind alongside the therapeutically active substances, thus medicinal plant based nutraceuticals and cosmeceuticals industry is a promising sector with enormous economic growth potential. The United States leads the market, followed by countries of Western Europe and Japan. In

1999, the global health food products market was US$ 6.8 billion, almost thrice the value in 1987. The global demand for herbal extract in food products grew to US$ 3 billion in 1999 from US$ 0.76 million in 1997, almost 4.5 fold rise in demand (Table 9.1). There are reports that Asia and Pacific Latin America, Africa and Middle East are set to provide the fastest growth for food-based (nutraceuticals) industry. The United States, Japan and major European countries are the largest global producers and consumers of neutraceuticals, owing to higher level of consumer income.

Globally, the market for plant-based cosmeceuticals has been estimated to US$ 22 billions, and the fastest growing sector in this market is antiaging products. The developed countries like the United States, Japan, Australia and Europe are the most dominant market for cosmeceuticals, and China, Malaysia, Russia and Latin America have a strong potential for long-term growth. In the United States, the market for cosmeceuticals was estimated at US$ 2.5 billion, where the market for medicinal plant ingredients used in cosmetics and toiletries stood at US$ 345 million in 1998, forecasted to increase 7.9% annually to reach US$ 503 million by 2005 and 760 million by 2008.

Table 9.1 Medicinal plant extracts demand in cosmetics from 1989 to 1998

Item	Demand value (million US$)		
	1989	1993	1998
Aloe extract	38	46	63
Botanical extract	180	230	345
Others	22	34	67
Plant acids/enzymes	19	37	65
Essential oils	101	113	150
Other natural products	85	115	180
Total	**445**	**575**	**870**

9.3. FUTURE ECONOMIC GROWTH

Throughout the world, about 35,000–70,000 species of plants have been used at one time or another for medicinal, neutraceuticals and cosmeceuticals purposes. In India, about 1000 plant species, in Nepal about 700 species, about 700 species in Peninsular Malaysia and its neighbouring Islands and in Chinese medicine about 9905 plant materials are used but only a relatively very small number of them are used in any significant volume. According to the International Trade Centre (ITC) report, there is generally upward trend except for 1990, when it dipped slightly before rising again to US$ 1.08 billion in 1991. The world trade in medicinal plants and raw material from plants parts averaged US$ 1.28 billion during 1995–1999. Thus, there is lot of scope in future for new plant-based drugs that are still to be introduced, and the economic significance of these plant-based pharmaceuticals is considerable which is based on the following two aspects:

1. The value of the current plant-based pharmaceuticals.
2. The value of potential plant-based pharmaceuticals, which are yet to be introduced.

The values of these drugs are described both in terms of their market value and their economic value.

Market value is a subset of economic value, which includes all benefits to society. Market value of the drugs is attributable to the plants raw materials, development and manufacturing costs as well as the incorporation of research cost for the failed efforts and above all the existence of consumer's surplus.

Economic value represents all the social benefits of particular type of product including market value. Economic value can be viewed as an expression of the total benefit of a product.

The relationship between the economic value of a medicinal plant species and market price of the drugs derived from it, is not a direct one. However, it is true that the market prices are minimum valuations assuming that:

- the demand for the drug is inelastic,
- that it is appropriate to value an essential input as its own cost plants, and
- the economic rent obtained from it plus the associated consumer's surplus.

For example, the market value of a stand of forest could be measured by translating the wood volume there in into an equivalent quantity of paper and then taking the market value of the paper. In contrast, economic value to society includes not only the value of the paper (or whatever the other commodity is selected), but also what may be referred to as the *in situ* benefit of trees as forest that is the contribution as:

- the forest checks the soil erosion, stabilizing the water table, converting carbon dioxide into oxygen (environmental effects);
- providing protection to wild life and;
- providing recreational opportunities; hence, the economic value is much larger in magnitude but also much more difficult to quantify.

For example, an economic value for medicinal plant species would be examining the current cost to society of a disease whose impact might be diminished in the future by drug derived from plants, e.g. in the case of cancer disease which is the major cause of about 5 lakh deaths per year in the United States and cost about US$ 14 billion annually in treatment, whereas the value of each life estimated to be about US$ 8 million, then the total value will be about US$ 4 trillion annually. Anticancer drugs save about 75,000 lives annually in the United States (an estimated 15% of 500,000 lives), and plant-based drugs comprise about 40% of total group of anticancer drugs. Combining those estimates, approximately 30,000 lives are saved annually in the United States as result of the use of plant-based drugs. Multiplying the lives saved by the value per life, the annual economic value of plant-based drugs in the United States alone is estimated to be about US$ 250 billion. Since this estimate reflect only a part of the total economic value of all plant-based pharmaceuticals; moreover, these values include none of the nonpharmaceuticals benefits provided by the plants responsible for these drugs. The above mentioned data is on the basis of information by Violette and Chestnut 1986, in EPA-230-06-86016 Feb. 1986, and information available from the economic value of biological diversity among medicinal plants. These values would be tripled to US$ 750 billion annually to account for anticancer application in all Organization for Economic Cooperation and Development (OECD) countries.

This reflects that medicinal plants and their products have taken an increasing medical and economical importance with respect to product categories like health food, cosmetics and personal care products containing natural ingredients—the demand for medicinal plants is growing exponentially. The fastest growing world market in herbal products is opening up new opportunities for the developing countries to benefit from the rising green consumerism, trend to develop their export potential. However, this requires a grand strategic plan, which takes a holistic view of the entire situation to boost the export.

9.4. DEVELOPMENT OF HERBAL MEDICINAL INDUSTRY

To cope up with the increasing demand for quality herbal medicines in the domestic as well as export markets, the successful development of herbal medicines industry will contribute to positive impact for the development of the national health care systems, improvement of people welfare, creation of competitive pharmaceutical products and encouragement of new drug discovery in the pharmaceutical industry, which will ultimately contribute to the economy of the people.

9.5. CONTRIBUTION TO ECONOMY OF THE PEOPLE

A partnership scheme among institutions involved, i.e. the farmers, general public, research and higher education, government health care services providers and the industry, taking into consideration the interest of each constituent, is to be directed to an integrated National Herbal Medicine Industry.

The industry is expected to have better access to the market and the customers of the commodities for further processing to produce added value. The industry and its technology will play its role in creating and enhancing the competitiveness of the products, and the results in the form of revenue will be distributed to the farmers through the procurement of farmer's products in an agreed reasonable price. Research and higher education institution with the support from government will provide the knowledge and technical assistance required by the farmers. The farmers will then have all the requirements to participate and contribute to activities that will ultimately and positively impact the economy of the farmer. The scheme will result multiplier effects through creation of new jobs.

Herbal medicines will be the leading products in pharmaceutical business in the future. The abundant sources of many varieties and uniqueness of medicinal plants for herbal medicines open opportunity for the development of competitive pharmaceutical products to supply the domestic and export market.

Analytical Pharmacognosy

OVERVIEW

This part provides the information regarding various analytical techniques to determine the quality, purity and efficacy of herbal drugs, which is considered as the major factor for acceptance of herbal formulations in world market. Various basic to advance methods for evaluation of crude drugs and methods for their biological screenings are described in this part.

CHAPTER 10

Drug Adulteration

CONTENTS

- Introduction
- Adulteration
- ▶ Types of Adulterants
- ▶ Unintentional Adulteration
- ▶ Intentional Adulteration

10.1. INTRODUCTION

Medicinal plants constitute an effective source of traditional (e.g. ayurvedic, chinese, homoeopathy and unani) and modern medicine. Herbal medicine has been shown to have genuine utility. Germany and France, together represent 39% of the $14 billion global retail market. In India, about 80% of the rural population depends on medicinal herbs and/or indigenous systems of medicine. In fact today, approximately 70% of 'synthetic' medicines are derived from plants. Popularity among the common people increased the usage of medicinal plants/herbal drugs. Herbal adulteration is one of the common malpractices in herbal raw-material trade. Adulteration is described as intentional substitution with another plant species or intentional addition of a foreign substance to increase the weight or potency of the product or to decrease its cost. In general, adulteration is considered as an intentional practice. However, unintentional adulterations also exist in herbal raw-material trade due to various reasons, and many of them are unknown even to the scientific community. The present chapter deals with different intentional and unintentional adulterations, reasons behind them and methods for easy identification of the spurious plant and authentication of the authentic plant.

10.2. ADULTERATION

A treatise published two centuries ago (in 1820) on adulterations in food and culinary materials is a proof for this practice as an age-old one. Due to adulteration, faith in herbal drugs has declined. Adulteration in market samples is one of the greatest drawbacks in promotion of herbal products. Many researchers have contributed in checking adulterations and authenticating them. It is invariably found that the adverse event reports are not due to the intended herb, but rather due to the presence of an unintended herb. Medicinal plant dealers have discovered the 'scientific' methods in creating adulteration of such a high quality that without microscopic and chemical analysis, it is very difficult to trace these adulterations.

Definition: The term adulteration is defined as substituting original crude drug partially or wholly with other similar-looking substances. The substance, which is mixed, is free from or inferior in chemical and therapeutic property.

Types of Adulterants

Adulteration in simple terms is debasement of an article. The motives for intentional adulteration are normally commercial and are originated mainly with the intension of enhancement of profits. Some of the reasons that can be cited here are scarcity of drug and its high price prevailing in market. The adulteration is done deliberately, but it may occur accidentally in some cases. Adulteration involves different conditions such as deterioration, admixture, sophistication, substitution, inferiority and spoilage. Deterioration is impairment in the quality of drug, whereas admixture is addition of one article to another due to ignorance or carelessness or by accident. Sophistication is the intentional or deliberate type of adulteration. Substitution occurs when a totally different substance is added in place of original drug. Inferiority refers to any substandard drug, and spoilage is due to the attack of microorganisms.

Unintentional Adulteration

Unintentional adulteration may be due to the following reasons:

1. confusion in vernacular names between indigenous systems of medicine and local dialects,
2. lack of knowledge about the authentic plant,
3. nonavailability of the authentic plant,
4. similarity in morphology and or aroma,
5. careless collection and
6. other unknown reasons.

Name confusion

In ayurveda, 'Parpatta' refers to *Fumaria parviflora*. In siddha, 'Parpadagam' refers to *Mollugo pentaphylla*. Owing to the similarity in the names in traditional systems of medicine, these two herbs are often interchanged or adulterated or substituted. Because of the popularity of siddha medicine in some parts of south India, traders in these regions supply *M. pentaphylla* as Parpatta/Parpadagam and the north Indian suppliers supply *F. parviflora*. These two can be easily identified by the presence of pale yellow to mild brown-coloured, thin wiry stems and small simple leaves of *M. pentaphylla* and black to dark brown-coloured, digitate leaves with narrow segments of *F. parviflora*. *Casuarina equisetifolia* for *Tamarix indica* and *Aerva lanata* for *Bergenia ciliata* are some other examples of adulterations due to confusion in names.

Lack of knowledge about authentic source

'Nagakesar' is one of the important drugs in ayurveda. The authentic source is *Mesua ferrea*. However, market samples are adulterated with flowers of *Calophyllum inophyllum*. Though the authentic plant is available in plenty throughout the Western Ghats and parts of the Himalayas, suppliers are unaware of it. There may also be some restrictions in forest collection. Due to these reasons, *C. inophyllum* (which is in the plains) is sold as Nagakesar. Authentic flowers can be easily identified by the presence of two-celled ovary, whereas in case of spurious flowers they are single celled.

Similarity in morphology

Mucuna pruriens is the best example for unknown authentic plant and similarity in morphology. It is adulterated with other similar papilionaceae seeds. *M. utilis* (sold as white variety) and *M. deeringiana* (sold as bigger variety) are popular adulterants. Apart from this, *M. cochinchinensis*, *Canavalia virosa* and *C. ensiformis* are also sold in Indian markets. Authentic seeds are up to 1 cm in length with shining mosaic pattern of black and brown colour on their surface. *M. deeringiana* and *M. utilis* are bigger (1.5–2 cm) in size. *M. deeringiana* is dull black, whereas *M. utilis* is white or buff coloured.

Lack of authentic plant

Hypericum perforatum is cultivated and sold in European markets. In India, availability of this species is very limited. However, the abundant Indo-Nepal species *H. patulum* is sold in the name of *H. perforatum*. Market sample is a whole plant with flowers, and it is easy to identify them taxonomically. Anatomically, stem transverse section of *H. perforatum* has compressed thin phloem, hollow pith and absence of calcium oxalate crystals. On the other hand, *H. patulum* has broader phloem, partially hollow pith and presence of calcium oxalate crystals.

Similarity in colour

It is well known that in course of time, drug materials get changed to or substituted with other plant species. 'Ratanjot' is a recent-day example. On discussion with suppliers and nontimer forest product (NTFP) contractors, it came to be known that in the past, roots of *Ventilago madraspatana* were collected from Western Ghats, as the only source of 'Ratanjot'. However, that is not the practice now. It is clearly known that *Arnebia euchroma var euchroma* is the present source. Similarity in yielding a red dye, *A. euchroma* substitutes *V. madraspatana*. The description to identify these two is unnecessary because of the absence of *V. madraspatana* in market. Whatever is available in the market, in the name of Ratanjot, was originated from *A. euchroma*.

Careless collections

Some of the herbal adulterations are due to the carelessness of herbal collectors and suppliers. *Parmelia perlata* is used in ayurveda, unani and siddha. It is also used as grocery. Market samples showed it to be admixed with other species (*P. perforata* and *P. cirrhata*). Sometimes, *Usnea* sp. is also mixed with them. Authentic plants can be identified by their thallus nature.

Unknown reasons

'Vidari' is another example of unknown authentic plant. It is an important ayurvedic plant used extensively. Its authentic source is *Pueraria tuberosa*, and its substitute is *Ipomoea digitata*. However, market samples are not derived from these two. It is interesting to know that an endangered gymnosperm *Cycas circinalis* is sold in plenty as Vidari. The adulterated materials originated from Kerala, India. Although both the authentic plant and its substitute are available in plenty throughout India, how *C. circinalis* became a major source for this drug is unknown. *P. tuberosa* can be easily identified by the presence of papery flake-like tubers, *I. digitata* by the presence of its concentric rings of vascular bundles and their adulterant *C. circinalis* by its leaf scars and absence of vessel elements.

Intentional Adulteration

Intentional adulteration may be due to the following reasons:

1. adulteration using manufactured substances,
2. substitution using inferior commercial varieties,
3. substitution using exhausted drugs,
4. substitution of superficially similar inferior natural substances,
5. adulteration using the vegetative part of the same plant,
6. addition of toxic materials,
7. adulteration of powders and
8. addition of synthetic principles.

Adulteration using manufactured substances

In this type of adulteration the original substances are adulterated by the materials that are artificially manufactured. The materials are prepared in a way that their general form and appearance resemble with various drugs. Few examples are cargo of ergot from Portugal was adulterated with small masses of flour dough moulded to the correct size and shape and coloured, first using red ink, and then into writing ink. Bass-wood is cut exactly the required shape of nutmegs and used to adulterate nutmegs. Compressed chicory is used in place of coffee berries. Paraffin wax is coloured yellow and is been substituted for beeswax, and artificial invert sugar is used in place of honey.

Substitution using inferior commercial varieties

In this type, the original drugs are substituted using inferior quality drugs that may be similar in morphological characters, chemical constituents or therapeutic activity. For example hog gum or hog tragacanth for tragacanth gum, mangosteen fruits for bael fruits, Arabian senna, obovate senna and Provence senna are used to adulterate senna, ginger being adulterated with Cochin, African and Japanese ginger. *Capsicum annuum* fruits and Japanese chillies are used for fruits of *C. minimum*.

Substitution using exhausted drugs

In this type of substitution the active medicaments of the main drugs are extracted out and are used again. This could be done for the commodities that would retain its shape and appearance even after extraction, or the appearance and taste could be made to the required state by adding colouring or flavouring agents. This technique is frequently adopted for the drugs containing volatile oils, such as clove, fennel, etc. After extraction, saffron and red rose petals are recoloured by artificial dyes. Another example is balsam of Tolu that does not contain cinnamic acid. The bitterness of exhausted gentian is restored by adding aloes.

Substitution of superficially similar inferior natural substances

The substituents used may be morphologically similar but will not be having any relation to the genuine article in their constituents or therapeutic activity. Ailanthus leaves are substituted for belladona, senna, etc., saffron admixed with saff flower; peach kernels and apricot kernels for almonds; clove stalks and mother cloves with cloves; peach kernel oil used for olive oil; chestnut leaves for hamamelis leaves and Japan wax for beeswax are few examples for this type of adulteration.

Adulteration using the vegetative part of the same plant

The presence of vegetative parts of the same plant with the drug in excessive amount is also an adulteration. For example, epiphytes, such as mosses, liverworts and lichens that grow over the barks also may occur in unusual amounts with the drugs, e.g. cascara or cinchona. Excessive amount of stems in drugs like lobelia, stramonium, hamamelis leaves, etc., are few example for this type of adulteration.

Addition of toxic materials

In this type of adulteration the materials used for adulteration would be toxic in nature. A big mass of stone was found in the centre of a bale of liquorice root. Limestone pieces with asafetida, lead shot in opium, amber-coloured glass pieces in colophony, barium sulphate to silvergrain cochineal and manganese dioxide to blackgrain cochineal, are few examples in this adulteration.

Adulteration of powders

Powdered drugs are found to be adulterated very frequently. Adulterants used are generally powdered waste products of a suitable colour and density. Powdered olive stones for powdered gentian, liquorice or pepper; brick powder for barks; red sanders wood to chillies; dextrin for powdered ipecacuanha, are few adulterants.

Addition of synthetic principles

Synthetic pharmaceutical principles are used for market and therapeutic value. Citral is added to lemon oil, whereas benzyl benzoate is added to balsam of Peru. Apart from these, the herbal products labelled to improve sexual performance in men, when analysed, contained sildenafil. Brand names included Actra-Rx, Yilishen, Hua Fo, Vinarol and Vasx, Sleeping Buddha containing estazolam, Diabetes Angel containing glyburide and phenformin are few examples under this category.

Evaluation of Crude Drugs

CONTENTS

11.1. INTRODUCTION

Evaluation of a drug ensures the identity of a drug and determines the quality and purity of drugs. The main reasons behind the need for evaluation of crude drugs are biochemical variation in the drug, effect of treatment and storage of drugs, and the adulterations and substitutions.

Improvements in analytical methods have definitely led to improvements in harvesting schedules, cultivation techniques, storage, activity, stability of active compounds and product purity. All of these gains have resulted in tremendous improvements in the quality of herbal preparations now available.

Methods currently employed in evaluating herbs are organoleptic, microscopic, physical, chemical and biological parameters.

11.2. ORGANOLEPTIC EVALUATION

Organoleptic evaluation means the study of drugs using organs of senses. It refers to the methods of analysis like colour, odour, taste, size, shape and special features, such as touch, texture, etc. Obviously, the initial sight of the plant or extract is so specific that it tends to identify itself. If this is not enough, perhaps the plant or extract has a characteristic odour or taste. Organoleptic analysis represents the simplest, yet the most human form of analysis.

Talka gum, which is used as a substitute for acacia gum could be identified by its colour and form. Talka gum is usually broken and also some tears are brown in colour and other colourless, whereas acacia is white to yellow in colour. Mangosteen fruits are a substitute for bael fruits and can be identified by darker rind and the wedge-shaped radiate stigmas. Cuprea Bark (*Remijia pedunculata*) differs in its morphological character with cinchona. Blood Root used as an adulterant for hydrastis is dark reddish-brown in colour, whereas hydrastis is yellow in colour. *Rheum rhaponticum* are much smaller than those of the Chinese rhubarb and are easily distinguished.

KEY TERMS

Ginger and capsicum have pungent taste, whereas gentian and chirata have bitter taste. Morphological differentiation of leaves and pods of Indian senna and Alexandrian senna, sweet taste of liquorice, odours of umbelliferous fruits, disc-shaped structure of nux vomica, conical shape of aconite, quills of cinnamon, etc., are few examples of this organoleptic evaluation.

11.3. MICROSCOPICAL EVALUATION

Microscopic evaluation is indispensable in the initial identification of herbs, as well as in identifying small fragments of crude or powdered herbs, and in the detection of adulterants (e.g. insects, animal faeces, mould, fungi, etc.) as well as identifying the plant by characteristic tissue features. Every plant possesses a characteristic tissue structure, which can be demonstrated through study of tissue arrangement, cell walls and configuration when properly mounted in stains, reagents and media. Lignin stains red or pink with a drop of phloroglucinol and concentrated hydrochloric acid. Mucilage is stained pink with ruthenium red, and N/50 iodine solution stains starch and hemicellulose blue.

The characteristic features of cell walls, cell contents, starch grains, calcium oxalate crystals, trichomes, fibres, vessels, etc., have been studied in details. Surinam quassia is recognized by the absence of calcium oxalate and presence of uniseriate medullary rays, crystal fibres, and wavy medullary rays of cascara bark, lignified trichomes and plasmodesma in nux vomica. Stone cells are absent in the frangula bark, whereas they are present in cascara. Presence of pith in rhizomes and absence in roots, warty trichomes of senna, and presence or absence of crystals of aloin indicates different varieties of aloes, glandular trichomes of mint, etc. The powder of clove stalks contains sclereids and calcium oxalate crystals, but cloves do not contain these two. *Rauwolfia micrantha*, *R. densiflora* and *R. perokensis* are found to serve as an adulterant for *R. serpentine*. The roots of these species can be differentiated from *R. serpentine* by the presence of sclerenchyma in the above species which is absent in *R. serpentine*.

The techniques like microscopic linear measurements, determination of leaf constants and quantitative microscopy are also used in this evaluation.

Linear measurements include size of starch grains, length and width of fibres, trichomes, etc. The diameter of starch grains present in ipecacuanha assists in distinguishing its varieties. The diameter of starch grains in cassia bark distinguishes from cinnamon and detects senna stalk in powdered senna leaf. The size of the stomata in leaves of *Barosma betulina* distinguishes it from other species of Barosma. The diameter of phloem fibres aids the detection of cassia in cinnamon, and the width of the vessel helps to detect clove stalks in powdered cloves. Measurements

of diameter for the identification of commercial starches and for the detection in them of foreign starch are few examples of linear measurements.

Determination of leaf constants include stomatal number, stomatal index, vein islet, veinlet termination number and palisade ratios. Stomatal number is average number of stomata per sq. mm of epidermis of the leaf.

Stomatal index: It is the percentage which the numbers of stomata form to the total number of epidermal cells, each stoma being counted as one cell. Stomatal index can be calculated by using the following formula:

$$\text{Stomatal index (S.I.)} = \frac{S}{E + S} \times 100$$

where,

S = number of stomata per unit area and

E = number of epidermal cells in the same unit area.

Timmerman (1927) and Rowson (1943) were amongst the first few to investigate leaf drugs for stomatal number and stomatal index.

Vein-islet number: It is defined as the number of vein islets per sq. mm of the leaf surface midway between the midrib and the margin. It is a constant for a given species of the plant and is used as a characteristic for the identification of the allied species. Levin in 1929 determined vein-islet numbers of several dicot leaves.

Veinlet termination number: It is defined as the number of veinlet termination per sq. mm of the leaf surface midway between midrib and margin. A vein termination is the ultimate free termination of veinlet. Hall and Melville in 1951 determined veinlet termination number of distinguishing between Indian and Alexandrian Senna.

Palisade ratio: It is defined as the average number of palisade cells beneath each epidermal cell. Unlike vein-islet number for the determination of which an unbroken portion of the leaf is required, palisade ratio can be determined with the powdered drug. The technique of palisade ratio determination was introduced by Zorning and Weiss (1925) in their studies on Compositae.

One example is vein-islet number of Alexandrian senna is 25–29.5, whereas Indian senna is 19.5–22.5. Stomatal index of Alexandrian senna is 10–15, whereas that of Indian Senna is 14–20.

Quantitative Microscopy (Lycopodium Spore Method)

This is an important technique employed in identification of crude drug when chemical and physical methods are inapplicable. Using this, one can determine the proportions of the substances present by means of the microscope, using the Lycopodium spore method.

The powdered drugs with well-defined particles which may be counted—for example, starch grains or single-layered cells or tissues—the area of which may be traced under suitable magnification or the objects of uniform thickness, and the length of which, can be measured under suitable magnification and actual area calculated are usually evaluated using this method.

Adulterated starchy drugs can be determined by counting the number of starch grains per mg and calculating the amount from the known number of starch grains per mg of the pure starch or starchy material.

Thus, if spent ginger is the adulterant, one knows that ginger contains 286,000 starch grains per mg, and the amount used as an adulterant can be calculated by using this figure. The percentage purity of an authentic powdered ginger is calculated using the following equation:

$$\frac{N \times W \times 94,000 \times 100}{S \times M \times P} = \% \text{ purity of drugs}$$

where,

N = number of characteristic structures (e.g. starch grains) in 25 fields;

W = weight in mg of lycopodium taken;

S = number of lycopodium spores in the same 25 fields;

M = weight in mg of the sample, calculated on basis of sample dried at 105°C and

P = 286,000 in case of ginger starch grains powder.

If the material is one for which a constant is not available, it is necessary to determine one by a preliminary experiment.

11.4. CHEMICAL EVALUATION

The chemical evaluation includes qualitative chemical tests, quantitative chemical tests, chemical assays and instrumental analysis. The isolation, purification and identification of active constituents are chemical methods of evaluation. Qualitative chemical tests include identification tests for various phytoconstituents like alkaloids, glycosides, tannins, etc. The procedures for the identification tests of various phytoconstituents are given under their respective chapters in the text, where it could be referred. Examples of identification of constituents are: copper acetate used in the detection of colophony present as an adulterant for resins, balsams and waxes; Holphen's test for cottonseed oil and Baudouin's test for sesame oil in olive oil; the test with acetic and nitric acids for Gurjun balsam in copaiba; Van Urk's reagent for ergot; Vitali's morins reaction for tropane alkaloids; iodine for starch; murexide test for purine bases, etc., are examples of this evaluation.

Quantitative chemical tests such as acid value (resins, balsams), saponification value (balsams), ester value (balsams, volatile oils), acetyl value (volatile oils), etc., are also useful in evaluation of a drug by means of chemical treatment.

Chemical assays include assays for alkaloid, resin, volatile oil, glycoside, vitamins or other constituent. Few examples are the assay of total alkaloid in belladonna herb, the total alkaloid and nonphenolic alkaloid in ipecacuanha, the alkaloid strychnine in nux vomica, the resin in jalap, and the vitamins in cod-liver oil. The results obtained can conclude the presence of inferior or exhausted drug and, by proving absence of the assayed constituent, it will suggest complete substitution of a worthless article.

Instrumental analyses are used to analyse the chemical groups of phytoconstituents using chromatographic and spectroscopic methods. Chromatographic methods include paper chromatography, thin-layer chromatography, gas chromatography, high-performance liquid chromatography and high-performance thin-layer chromatography. Spectroscopic methods include ultraviolet and visible spectroscopy, infrared spectroscopy, mass spectroscopy, and nuclear magnetic spectroscopy.

11.5. PHYSICAL EVALUATION

In crude plant evaluation, physical methods are often used to determine the solubility, specific gravity, optical rotation, viscosity, refractive index, melting point, water content, degree of fibre elasticity and other physical characteristics of the herb material.

Solubility

Drug specific behaviour towards solvents are taken into consideration. This is useful for the examination of many oils, oleoresins, etc. Few examples are the solubility of colophony in light petroleum, the solubility of balsam of Peru in solution of chloral hydrate, the solubility of castor oil in half its volume of light petroleum and the turbidity produced with two volumes of the solvent; the solubility of balsam of Peru in an equal volume of alcohol, 90%, and the production of a turbidity with a larger volume; castor oil is soluble only in three volumes of 90% alcohol, while the adulterated form it shows good solubility in alcohol. Alkaloidal bases are soluble in organic solvents and alkaloidal salts are soluble in polar solvents.

Optical Rotation

Anisotropic crystalline solids and samples containing an excess of one enantiomer of a chiral molecule can rotate the orientation of plane-polarized light. Such substances are said to be optically active, and this property is known as optical rotation. The enantiomer that rotates light to the right, or clockwise when viewing in the direction of light propagation, is called the dextrorotatory (d) or (+) enantiomer, and the enantiomer that rotates light to the left, or counterclockwise, is called the levorotatory (l) or (-) enantiomer. Few examples of drugs with this property are eucalyptus oil (0° to +10°), honey (+3° to -15°), Chenopodium oil (-30° to -80°), etc.

Refractive Index

Refractive index is defined as the property of a material that changes the speed of light, computed as the ratio of the speed of light in a vacuum to the speed of light through the material. When light travels at an angle between two different materials, their refractive indices determine the angle of transmission refraction of the light beam. In general, the refractive index varies based on the frequency of the light as well; thus, different colours of light travel at different speeds. High intensities can also change the refractive index. This could be used as a parameter in evaluating the herbal drugs; for example castor oil 1.4758–1.527, clove oil 1.527–1.535, etc.

Specific Gravity

It is also known as relative density. The ratio of the mass of a solid or liquid to the mass of an equal volume of distilled water at 4°C (39°F) or of a gas to an equal volume of air or hydrogen under prescribed conditions of temperature and pressure. Some examples of specific gravity of drugs are cottonseed oil 0.88–0.93, coconut oil 0.925, castor oil 0.95, etc.

Viscosity

Viscosity is the resistance of a fluid to flow. This resistance acts against the motion of any solid object through the fluid and also against motion of the fluid itself past stationary obstacles. Viscosity of a liquid is constant at a given temperature and is an index of its composition. Viscosity also acts internally on the fluid between slower- and faster-moving adjacent layers. Since it is constant at a given temperature, it is used as an evaluation parameter; for example, pyroxylin kinematic viscosity, 1100–2450 centistokes.

Melting Point

The melting point of a solid is the temperature at which it changes state from solid to liquid. Plant constituents have very sharp and constant melting points. As far as crude drugs are concerned, melting point range has been fixed due to mixed chemicals. The following drugs could be evaluated using this parameter; for example, beeswax 62–65°C, wool fat 34–44°C, agar melts at 85°C, etc.

Moisture Content

The moisture content of a drug will be responsible for decomposition of crude drugs either producing chemical change or microbial growth. So the moisture content of a drug should be determined and controlled. The moisture content is determined by heating a drug at 105°C in an oven to a constant weight. Following are the examples of two crude drugs with their moisture content limit: the moisture content of digitalis and ergot should not be more than 5% w/w and 8% w/w, respectively.

Ultraviolet Light

Certain drugs fluoresce when the cut surface or the powder is exposed to ultraviolet radiation, and it is useful in the identification of those drugs. Some pieces of rhapontic, Indian and Chinese rhubarb are very difficult to distinguish, and it is very difficult in powdered form, but examination in ultraviolet light gives such marked differences in fluorescence that the varieties can be easily distinguished from each other.

Ash Values

The determination of ash is useful for detecting low-grade products, exhausted drugs, and excess of sandy or earthy matter. Different types of ash values are used in detection of crude drugs like, total ash, acid-insoluble ash, water-soluble ash and sulphated ash.

Total ash is useful in detecting the crude drugs that are mixed with various mineral substances like sand, soil, calcium oxalate, chalk powder or other drugs with different inorganic contents to improve their appearance, as is done with nutmegs and ginger. The maximum temperature used for total ash should be not more than 450°C because alkali chlorides that may be volatile in higher temperatures would be lost.

Acid-insoluble ash means the ash insoluble in dilute hydrochloric acid. It is often of more value than the total ash. The majority of crude drugs contain calcium oxalate, and the quantity of calcium oxalate varies very frequently. So total ash of a crude drug vary within wide limits for specimens of genuine drug, for example, rhubarb, total ash range from 8 to 40%. In this case, the total ash is useless to detect earthy matter adherent to such a drug. So acid-insoluble ash would be preferable for rhubarb. The calcium oxide or carbonate, yielded by the incinerated oxalate, will be soluble in hydrochloric acid when the ash is treated with hydrochloric acid; the remaining ash is weighed, which is known as the acid-insoluble ash. By this we can detect the presence of excessive earthy matter, which is likely to occur with roots and rhizomes and with leaves which are densely pubescent, like those of foxglove, clothed with abundant trichomes secreting resin, as in henbane, and tend to retain earth matter splashed on to them during heavy rainstorms.

The water-soluble ash is used to detect the presence of material exhausted by water. Sulphated ash is done by addition of sulphuric acid in order to get sulphate salts, and the percentage ash is calculated with reference to the air-dried drug. The temperature used for this is above 600°C. The total ash and acid-insoluble ash values of Guduchi are not more than 16 and 3%, respectively. The total ash value and water-soluble ash values of ginger are 6 and 1.7%, respectively.

Extractive Values (Table 11.1)

The extracts obtained by exhausting crude drugs with different solvents are approximate measures of their chemical constituents. Various solvents are used according to the type of the constituents to be analysed. Water-soluble extractive is used for crude drugs containing water-soluble constituents like glycosides, tannins, mucilage, etc.; alcohol-soluble extractive is used for crude drugs containing tannins, glycosides, resins, etc.; and ether-soluble extractives are used for drugs containing volatile constituents and fats.

Table 11.1: Extractive values of some crude drugs

Water-soluble extractive (% w/w)		Alcohol-soluble extractive (% w/w)		Ether-soluble extractive (% w/w)	
Aloe	Not less than 25.0	Aloe	Not less than 10.0	Linseed	Not less than 25.0
Glycyrrhiza	Not less than 20.0	Asafoetida	Not less than 50.0	Capsicum	Not less than 12.0

Foreign Organic Matters

The parts of the organ or organs other than those parts of drugs mentioned in the definition and description of the drug are known as foreign organic matters. They may be insect, moulds, earthy material, animal excreta, etc. Each and every vegetable drug has their own limits. Few examples of such limits are garlic should not contain more than 2%, saffron should not contain more than 2%, shatavari should not contain more than 1%, etc.

11.6. BIOLOGICAL EVALUATION

The plant or extract can then be evaluated by various biological methods to determine pharmacological activity, potency and toxicity. The biological evaluation would serve better than the physical and chemical evaluation for drugs that could not be satisfactorily assayed by these last two methods. Moreover, this is an important method, the crude drugs are considered important only because of their biological effects and this evaluation would conclude the effect. These methods are considered to be less precise, more time-consuming and more expensive. Bioassays should be as simple as possible, and attempts should be made to have access to a large number of different tests so that many biological properties can be screened. The bioassay methods are of three types: they are toxic, symptomatic and tissue or organ methods. Different animals are used in toxic and symptomatic method and isolated organ or tissue is used in the third method.

These assays are conducted by determining the amount of drug of known potency required to produce a definite effect on suitable test animals or organs under standard conditions. Reference standard are used in certain bioassay procedures to minimize errors.

Toxicity studies are performed in suitable animal models to decide the lethal dose and effective dose of crude drags. Mice are used to test the effects of various vaccines.

Oxytocic activity of vasopressin injection is tested on guinea pigs, and oxytocic injection is assayed on young domestic chickens by injecting into an exposed crural or brachial vein and noticing the changes in blood pressure. Pigeons are used to assay digitalis glycosides by transfusing the drug through the alar vein to the blood stream and observing the lethal effects. Depressor activities and mydriatic effects of certain drugs are tested in cats and cat's eye, respectively. Anthelmintic drugs are evaluated on worms.

The drugs that have an effect in eyes are assayed on rabbit's eyes. Dogs are used to assay the drugs that exhibit cardiac and gastrointestinal activities. Effects of ergot are carried out on cock's comb or rabbit's intestine or its uterus. Next to the animals, the studies are carried out in human beings also. In some instances, the effects that are observed from animal studies would be different when tested in humans. The tested biological activities include hepatoprotective activity, hypoglycaemic activity, anti-inflammatory activity, antiulcer activity, immunomodulatory activity, etc.

Microbiological assays are carried out to determine the effects of drug in various microorganisms, and this is employed in the identification of antimicrobial drugs. The methods used in this type of assays are agar well-diffusion method, disc-diffusion method and turbidimetric method. In other microbiological methods, the living bacteria yeast moulds are used for assaying vitamins.

CHAPTER 12

Biological Screening of Herbal Drugs

CONTENTS

- Introduction
- Need for Phytopharmacological Evaluation
- New Strategies for Evaluating Natural Products
- Errors in Screening Procedures
- Screening Methods for Analgesic Agents
- Screening Methods for Antidiabetic Agents
- Evaluation of Antidiarrhoeal Agents
- Screening Methods for Antifertility Agents
- Screening Methods for Anti-inflammatory Agents
- Screening Methods for Antipyretic Agents
- Screening Methods for Antiulcer Agents
- Screening Methods for Diuretic Agents
- Screening Methods for Hepatoprotective Agents
- Screening Methods for Wound-Healing Agents

12.1. INTRODUCTION

It is well-known that drugs when administered to the body never produce 'new' effects but get by modifying existing physiological systems. Observation of visible effects of plant extracts on intact animals can give information of their pharmacological activity and possible use as therapeutic agents. The species commonly used for this purpose are mouse and rat. Availability of suitable worksheets is essential to enable systematic observation of valuable symptoms. Elaborate procedures, using mice and cats, have been described by Irwin (1964). Reinhard (1982) has published a simplified scheme for mice. His article also contains descriptions of a number of tests for specific activities, which can be performed in mice. Malone (1977) has devised screening protocols for rats, which are suitable for working with natural products, partly purified fractions or pure compounds. Rats are injected intraperitoneally with the samples and observed at defined time intervals for one day. Observations are then performed once a day for one week, after which the animals are killed and examined. The test protocol contains observation of 58 parameters and has been named by Hippocrates, the 'father of medicine'. Sandberg (1967) made minor modifications to the original protocol (55 parameters). Malone (1977) has published a modified worksheet with 63 parameters and has also discussed computerization of the procedure, allowing comparison of the pharmacological profile of an unknown sample with similar profiles of known drugs.

Modern chemical methods have led to a dramatic increase in the number of natural or synthetic molecules available for pharmacological research. At the same time, recent developments in cellular and molecular pharmacology provide an increasing number of selective tests able to identify the activity and the mechanisms of action of biologically active molecules. Paradoxically, however, the availability of numerous sophisticated techniques do not necessarily make pharmacological research much easier. Molecular graphics have not yet proven very serviceable in the investigation of novel molecules. On the other hand, the probability of assessing the biological activity of new drugs by stochastic screening with modern reliable methods remains limited, unless viable working hypotheses can first be made as to their overall effect.

This difficulty could be partly overcome by intermediate screening methods, on the basis of global or functional tests. Such methods have been developed in various domains of biology, such as cardiovascular research or in the identification of antimitotic or immunosuppressive drugs. However, only very few methods are available as yet for application to the cases of neurotropic substances. Most global tests for screening neurotropic drugs are outdated; adequate behavioural tests are only capable of detecting a few transmitters like activities, and such a situation represents three limiting factor in an area characterized by particularly rapid developments. The number of identified transmitter substances has increased from less than 10 to over 50 in a few years. In addition, several are neuropeptides, an important, but still relatively unexplored class of biologically active molecules. Peptides of marine origin represent an important source of natural substances still awaiting systematic screening.

12.2. NEED FOR PHYTO-PHARMACOLOGICAL EVALUATION

To demonstrate a pharmacological effect, nothing can replace observation of animal models; but as they are expensive and often difficult to interpret, simpler tests are used. These tests require less effort and also make possible a better understanding of the mechanisms of action of substances being tested. Nonanimal models are becoming smaller and smaller while still remaining representative of a living organism.

By means of finely adjusted multidisciplinary efforts and of a choice of tests that accurately represent future therapeutic applications, research centres, such as the National Cancer Institute in the United States, have been able to select active substances with some success. Thus, the combination of several selective, sensitive and specific tests (such as the model of P-338 leukaemia in vivo versus astrocytoma in vitro) has made it possible to detect directly up to 90% of clinically active antitumour compounds. These methods have also helped to eliminate substances that give false positive results, such as cardenolides, saponosides, flavonoids and terpenic lactones. At the cost of a huge effort applied to more than 100,000 plant extracts, only about 10 particularly promising antileukaemic substances were selected. Among these were indicine N-oxide, maytansine, homoharringtonine, taxol and its derivatives, and 4-beta-hydroxywithanolide E (whose 17-alpha side chain removes all its cardioactivity).

Of course, most pharmacochemical researches are performed with more limited means, but the scientific literature flows with interesting results. These may be categorized into two groups according to the possible methods of approach. One approach is to demonstrate new pharmacological activities, or even future clinical applications, from raw materials or natural substances already known. For example, hypericin inhibits monoamine oxidases A and B from rat brain, which may explain its antidepressive properties; 5–6 g of pectin ingested daily significantly decrease cholesterol levels by inhibiting the reabsorption of bile; trigonelline, from fenugreek, displays a hypoglycaemic effect in animals with experimental alloxan-induced diabetes; sulphur compounds from garlic and onions, and phenylpropane derivatives from the essential oil of nutmeg, have displayed good properties against platelet aggregation; gossypol, obtained from raw cottonseed oil, is well known as a male contraceptive agent, acting after 4–5 weeks of treatment, without affecting the testosterone level—its molecular mechanism of action towards lipid membranes has been elucidated.

The second type of approach is the discovery of new natural substances displaying pharmacological or even new therapeutic effects. This is the royal road par excellence that most often leads to patents being taken out. Publications in this field are numerous, which can be further explained by the following examples.

(1) Withanolide F has an anti-inflammatory action, demonstrated by the classical plantar oedema test in rats, which is five times that of phenylbutazone and comparable to that of hydrocortisone (a substance with no effect on the central nervous system).

(2) Certain tetracylic sesquiterpenes isolated from sponges of the genus phyllospongia have comparable anti-inflammatory effects in vivo.

(3) New triterpenic saponosides, such as dianosides A and B isolated from *Dianthus superbus* L. var *longicalycinus* (Carycphyilaceae) have analgesic properties at subcutaneous doses of 10–30 mg/kg as measured by the acetic acid test in mice.

These few results, taken as examples, demonstrate—if such a demonstration is necessary—that this approach to research leads along an extremely interesting trail. It is a technique permitting innovation of the type currently much sought. The accumulation of scientific knowledge also leads to the development of a rigorous pharmacological vigilance, particularly with regard to natural substances that are considered a priority to be of secondary therapeutic value. Examples that come to mind are glycyrrhizin, whose not inconsiderable mineralocorticoid activity induces iatrogenic hypertension with hypokalaemic and metabolic alkalosis; the pyrrolizidine alkaloids present in the Boraginaceae and Astgeraceae (particularly the genera *Senecic* and *Eupatorium*), which induce fatty degeneration of liver cells and eventually necrosis and fibrosis, caused by certain bifunctional alkylating pyrrole metabolites that bind to DNA; diterpene esters of the phorbol and ingenol types, present in the Euphorbiaceae and Thymeliaceae, which are in fact cocarcinogenic substances.

The terpenes, as with the flavonoids, certain molecules in the environment, though considered inactive in their normal state, may nevertheless show some activity when combined with an appropriate vector. Such is the case of epoxylathyrol, a diterpene present in the latex and seeds of *Euphorbia lathysis L.* This plant contains natural esters that have no activity on cultures of hepatic tumour cells. However, Schroeder et al. (1979) have synthesized a series of aliphatic esters with chain lengths ranging from 2 to 20 carbon atoms and have performed tests in vitro. The cytotoxicity curves demonstrate that the dibutyrate ester represents the optimal chain length, revealing an activity that the nonesterified epoxylathyrol does not possess. All this shows how greatly the interaction between the human body and molecules in our environment may be modifiable, and how research on substances thought to be devoid of interest may lead to surprises.

12.3. NEW STRATEGIES FOR EVALUATING NATURAL PRODUCTS

The fundamental problem for chemists working on natural products used to be that of choosing which pharmacological principles and methods to use to understand the possible biological use of any given substance.

The RICB (Reseau d'interaction chimie—Bioiogique or Chemical Biological Interaction Network) has come up with lots of objectives for helping the chemists as described below.

The RICB helps chemists by providing assistance from biologists, who use their knowledge and sophisticated methods of observation for the pharmacological activity of any given substance. Rather than the current classical procedure of observing an overall pharmacological effect (e.g. measurement of femoral artery blood flow in dogs), it is now possible to observe the effect of the substance on any one of the underlying components of the overall peripheral pharmacological effect (e.g. binding to α- or β-adrenergic receptors, or to angiotensin or vasopressin receptors, or the effect of posterior pituitary vasopressin). The RICB aids biologists by providing new tools for examining receptors, neuromediators, ion channels and membrane-coupling mechanisms. It can thus be said that, thanks to derivatives of yohimbine (indole alkaloids from the Rubiaceae and Apocynaceae), the alpha-1 and alpha-2 subtypes of adrenergic receptors were distinguished. Likewise, forskolin, a labdane diterpene, enabled progress to be made in understanding the adenylate cyclase system. Morphine, ouabain and tetrodotoxin are other examples

of biological agents derived from the chemistry of natural materials. Biologists can also make use of the chemists' extra skills in resolving certain problems at the frontiers of biology, such as extraction, labelling and molecular modelling.

In general, the RICB has also provided a discussion forum for a collaboration between two disciplines that are relatively unfamiliar with each other and for developing new strategies in the evaluation of natural or synthetic substances. By using different animal models, the phyto-pharmacological potentials of different plant species, including *Nelumbo nucifera* and *Leucas lavandulaefolia* have been reported.

12.4. ERRORS IN SCREENING PROCEDURES

Any screening procedure has a characteristic error rate. This is inevitable because in high-throughput screening it is necessary to compromise with some accuracy or precision to achieve the requisite speed. Thus when a large number of compounds are carried through a particular screen, some of the compounds are classified incorrectly. A screen may be used in an absolute sense, so that compounds that pass a certain criterion are termed positives, whereas those that fail to meet the criterion are termed negatives. Compounds that pass, but should have failed, are false positives. In general, false positives are tolerable, if they are not too numerous, because they will be rectified later. Compounds that fail, but should have passed, are false negatives. False negatives are lost forever if the failure eliminates them from further testing.

All screening procedures are based on assumptions of analogy. They have different degrees of relevance or predictability. Studies in phase II clinical trials predict the results with high probability in large clinical trails. But even here there is the possibility of false-positive or false-negative results. The relevance of a test is much less in early pharmacological tests, such as used in high-throughput screening. Generally, the relevance is inversely proportional to the simplicity of the test.

In any case, one is confronted with the problem of false-positive results (type I errors) and false-negative results (type II errors).

In each step, two sources of error for false-positive results have to be taken in to account:

1. a = error of the first type due to the model
2. α = error of the first type due to statistics

In the error of the first type, a compound is considered to be active, but is actually ineffective. This type of error is clarified during further development, after negative clinical trials at the latest.

However, there are two sources of error for false-negative results:

1. b = error of the second type due to the model
2. β = error of the second type due to statistics

In the error of the second type, a compound is considered to be ineffective, but is actually effective.

This type of error will never be clarified; an effective drug has just been missed. Perhaps another investigator will test this compound under different aspects.

The statistical errors derive from the fact that a pharmacological test is performed only several times or in a limited number of animals. One can specify the probability that a decision made is incorrect, that is, a drug candidate is erroneously identified as effective when it is actually ineffective. Usually this risk is set to 5% ($P < 0.05$) and is called the statistical error of the first type or type I error. The error of the second type or type II error is connected to the type I error by statistical rules.

Usually, screening is performed sequentially. Tests in high-throughput screening are followed by tests in isolated organs, then in small animals, and special tests in higher animals, until the compound is recommended for further development and for studies in human beings. From each step, not only errors of type I, but also from type II, arise. As a consequence, many effective compounds are lost.

There are two ways to circumvent this obstacle: (1) to increase the number of compounds entering the screening procedure dramatically, hope for a reasonable number of true positives, and accept a high rate of false-negative results (White 2000) as followed in the ultra high-throughput screening; or (2) to perform tests with high relevance, meaning tests with high predictive value in whole animals at an early stage (Vogel and Vanderbeeke 1990).

The literature on high-throughput screening includes some publications dealing with false-negative results (Jones and King 2003; Colland and Daviet 2004; Heller-Uszynska and Kilian 2004).

Zhang et al. (1999, 2000) studied the role of false-negative results in high-throughput screening procedures. They presented a statistical model system that predicts the reliability of hits from a primary test as affected by the error in the assay and the choice of the hit threshold. The hit confirmation rate, as well as false-positive (representing substances that initially fall above the hit limit but whose true activity is below the hit limit) and false-negative (representing substances that initially fall below the hit limit but whose true activity is in fact greater than the hit limit) rates have been analysed by computational simulation. The Z-factor and the Zi-factor were introduced to characterize the reliability of high-throughput assays.

The problem of type II errors, that is, false-negative results, also exists in many other physiological and pharmacological studies (Martorana et al. 1982; Bar- ros et al. 1991; Sandkühler et al. 1991; Waldeck 1996; Williams et al. 1997). For example, Pollard and Howard (1986) reinvestigated the staircase test, a well-accepted primary screening method for anxiolytics, and found several false-negative results for clinically active anxiolytics.

12.5. SCREENING METHODS FOR ANALGESIC AGENTS

Centrally Acting Analgesics

Hot plate method

The paws of mice and rats are very sensitive to heat even at temperatures which do not damage the skin. They respond by jumping, withdrawal of paws and licking of paws. The time until these responses occur can be prolonged after administration of centrally acting analgesics, whereas peripheral analgesics of the acetyl salicylic acid or phenyl acetic acid type do not generally affect these responses.

The hot plate consists of an electrically heated surface. The temperature is controlled for 55–56°C. Adult albino rats are used for the test. The animals are placed on the hot plate, and the time until either licking or jumping occurs is recorded by a stopwatch. The delay in response is recorded after administration of the standard or the test compound.

Haffner's tail clip method

In this method, the raised tail phenomena in mice are observed. Six mice per group are used. A clip is applied to the base of the tail of mice, and the reaction time is noted. The test compounds are administered orally to fasted animals. The animal quickly responds to the stimuli by biting the clip or the tail near the location of the clip. The time between stimulation onset and response is measured by a stopwatch.

Tail immersion test

This method is based on the observation that morphine-like drugs are selectively capable of prolonging the reaction time of the typical tail-withdrawal reflex in rats induced by immersing the end of the tail in warm water of 55°C. Adult albino rats are used for the test. They are placed in individual cages leaving the tail hanging out freely. The animals are allowed to adapt to the cages for 30 min before testing. The lower 5 cm portion of the tail is marked. This part of the tail is immersed in a cup of freshly filled water of exactly 55°C. Within a few seconds, the rat reacts by withdrawing the tail. A stopwatch records the reaction time. The reaction time is determined before and periodically after either oral or subcutaneous administration of the test substance. A withdrawal time of more than 6 s is regarded as a positive response.

Radiant heat method

This test is useful for quantitative measurements of pain threshold against thermal radiation in man and for evaluation of analgesic activity. It is very useful for discriminating between centrally acting morphine-like analgesics and nonopiate analgesics.

The animal is put into a small cage with an opening for the tail at the rear wall. The investigator holds the tail gently. By the opening of a shutter, a light beam exerting radiant heat is directed at the end of the tail. For about 6 s, the reaction of the animal is observed. The mouse tries to pull the tail away and turns the head. The shutter is closed with a switch as soon as the investigator notices this reaction. Mice with a reaction time of more than 6 s are not used in the test. The escape reaction is the end point of this test. Before administration of the test compound or the standard, the normal reaction time is determined. The test compounds and the standard are administered either orally or subcutaneously. The analgesiometer can also be used to measure analgesic activities.

Formalin test in rats

Rats weighing 180–300 g are administered 0.05 ml of 10% formalin into the lower surface of the front paw. The test drug is administered simultaneously either subcutaneously or orally. Each individual rat is placed in a clear plastic cage for observation. Readings are taken and scored according to a pain scale. Pain responses are indicated by elevation of the paw or excessive licking and biting of the paw. Analgesic response or protection is indicated if both paws are resting on the floor with no elevation of the injected paw.

Tooth pulp stimulation

This test is based on the fact that stimulation of the tooth pulp induces characteristic reactions, such as licking, biting, chewing and head flick which can be observed easily.

Adult healthy rabbits are used for the test. Rabbits are anaesthetized and their pulp chambers exposed with a high-speed dental drill. On the day of the experiment, clamping electrodes are placed into the drilled holes. After an accommodation period of 30 min, stimulation is started to determine the threshold value. The stimulus is applied with a frequency of 50 Hz and duration of 1 s. The electrical current is started at 0.2 mA and increased until the phenomenon of licking occurs. The test substance is either injected intravenously or given orally. The animals serve as their own controls.

Grid shock test

This test measures the analgesic properties by the 'flinch-jump' procedure in rats. The floor of the box used is wired with stainless steel wire, spaced about 1 mm apart. The stimulus is given in the form of an electric current, 30 cycles per second with duration of 2 ms per pulse. With increasing shock intensities, the mice flinch exhibit a startling reaction, increase locomotion or attempt to jump. The behaviour is accurately reflected on the oscilloscope by marked fluctuations of the pulse and defined as the pain threshold response. The current as measured in milliamperes is recorded for each animal before and after administration of the drug.

Electrical stimulation of the tail

This method is based on the fact that since the tail of mice is known to be sensitive to any stimulus, the stimulus can be varied either by the duration of the electric shock or by an increase in the electric current to check the efficacy of the analgesic agent.

Male mice weighing 20 g are placed in special cages. A pair of clips is attached to the tail, and the positive electrode is placed at the end of the tail. Electric current at an intensity of 40–50 V is applied. The frequency of the stimulation is 1 shock/second, and the pulse duration is 2.5 ms. The normal response time range of the stimuli is 3–4 sec. Following administration of the drug, the response time is registered at 15 min intervals until the reaction time returns to control levels.

Peripherally Acting Analgesics

Pain in inflamed tissue (Randall–Selitto test)

This method is based on the principle that inflammation increases the peripheral analgesic sensitivity to pain. Inflammation decreases the pain reaction threshold, but the threshold is readily elevated by nonnarcotic analgesics of the salicylate-amidopyrine type as well as by the narcotic analgesics.

Groups of healthy albino rats (130–175 g) are used. The animals are starved 18 to 24 h before administration. To induce inflammation, 0.1 ml of a 20% suspension of Brewer's yeast in distilled water is injected subcutaneously into the plantar surface of the left hind paw of the rat. After three hours, pressure is applied through a tip to the plantar surface of the rat's foot at a constant rate to the point when the animal struggles, squeals or attempts to bite. Each animal is tested for its control pain threshold. Any animal with a control pain threshold greater than 80 g is eliminated and replaced. The mean applied force is determined for each time interval.

Writhing test

Pain is induced by injection of irritants into the peritoneal cavity of mice. The animals react with a characteristic stretching behaviour which is called writhing. The test is suitable to detect analgesic activity. An irritating agent such as phenyl quinone or acetic acid is injected intraperitoneally to mice, and the stretching reaction is evaluated.

Mice of either sex of weight 20–25 g are used. Phenyl quinone in a concentration of 0.02% is suspended in a 1% suspension of carboxy methyl cellulose. About 0.25 ml of this suspension is injected intraperitoneally. The mice are placed individually into glass beakers and are observed for a period often one minute. The number of writhes is recorded for each animal. A writhe is indicated by a stretching of the abdomen with simultaneous stretching of at least one hind limb.

12.6. SCREENING METHODS FOR ANTIDIABETIC AGENTS

Diabetes mellitus is a metabolic disorder characterized by increased blood glucose level associated with discharge of glucose in urine. There are two major types of diabetes mellitus, that is, insulin-dependent diabetes mellitus (IDDM) and noninsulin-dependent diabetes mellitus (NIDDM). Insulin-dependent diabetes mellitus, also called type 1 diabetes, occurs due to complete loss of pancreatic β-islet cells and hence there is insulin deficiency. Noninsulin-dependent diabetes mellitus, also called as type 2 diabetes, is due to insulin resistance. Insulin resistance is developed due to defects at the receptor level or insulin signalling at the postreceptor level. This defect may be in the effector cells such as the skeletal muscle, the adipose tissue, etc., or in the β-islet cells. A large number of drugs including herbs and minerals with suspected antidiabetic activity have been successfully tested in the laboratory. The various animal models to screen antidiabetic activity are listed in this section.

Models for Insulin-Dependent Diabetes Mellitus

Alloxan-induced diabetes

Alloxan is a cyclic urea compound which induces permanent diabetes. It is a highly reactive molecule which produces free radical damage to β-islet cells and causes cell death. Alloxan at a dose level of 100 mg/kg in rats produces diabetes. In rabbits, a dose level of 150 mg/kg infused through a marginal ear vein produces diabetes in 70% of the animals.

Albino rats of either sex weighing 150–200 g are injected with a single dose of alloxan monohydrate (100 mg/kg body weight) dissolved in normal saline (0.9%) by intraperitoneal route. The animals are kept for 48 h during which food and water is allowed ad libitum. The blood glucose level shows the triphasic response with hyperglycaemia for 1 h followed by hypoglycaemia that lasts for 6 h and stable hyperglycaemia after 48 h. The animals showing fasting blood glucose level above 140 mg/dl after 48 h of alloxan administration are considered diabetic. Drug samples to be screened are administered orally for a period of six weeks. After six weeks of treatment, blood samples are collected from 8 h fasting animals through a caudal vein. Serum is separated by cooling centrifuge (2–4°C) at 3000 r.p.m. for 10 min. The serum glucose level is estimated by glucose oxidase-peroxidase method (GOD-POD kit) using an autoanalyser.

Streptozotocin-induced diabetes

Streptozotocin is a broad-spectrum antibiotic which causes β-islet cells damage by free radical generation. Streptozotocin induces diabetes in almost all species of animals excluding rabbits and guinea pigs. The diabetogenic dose of Streptozotocin varies with species. In mice, the dose level is 200 mg/kg through i.p. and in beagle dogs 15 mg/kg through i.v. for three days. Adult albino rats of either sex weighing 150–200 g are injected with Streptozotocin (60 mg/kg body weight) prepared in citrated buffer (pH 4.5) solution by i.p. route. The citrated buffer is prepared by mixing 53.9 parts of 0.1 M citric acid and 46.1 parts of 0.2 M disodium hydrogen orthophosphate and finally adjusted to a pH of 4.5. The blood glucose level shows the same triphasic response as seen in alloxan-treated animals. Animals showing fasting blood glucose level above 140 mg/dl after 48 h of Streptozotocin administration are considered diabetic. Drug samples to be screened are administered orally for a period of six weeks. After six weeks of treatment, blood samples are collected from 8 h fasted animals through a caudal vein. Serum is separated by cooling centrifuge (2–4°C) at 3000 r.p.m. for 10 min. The serum glucose level is estimated by glucose oxidase-peroxidase method (GOD-POD kit) using an autoanalyser.

Virus-induced diabetes

Viruses are one of the etiological agents for IDDM. They produce diabetes mellitus by infecting and destroying β-islet cells of pancreas. Various human viruses used for inducing diabetes include: RNA picornavirus, coxsackie B4 (CB-4) and encephalomyocarditis (EMC-D).

Six- to eight-week-old mice are inoculated by 0.1 ml of 1:50 dilution of D-variant encephalomyocarditis (EMC) through i.p. route. The 0.1 ml of the above dilution contains 50 PFU (plaque-forming units) of EMC virus. Mortality due to this concentration of virus is approximately 10–20%. A less-infecting variant produces a comparable damage by eliciting autoimmune reactivity to the β-islet cells. Infected animals are considered hyperglycaemic if their nonfasting levels exceed by 250 mg/dl the levels of uninfected animals of the same strain. Drug samples to be screened are administered orally for a period of six weeks. After six weeks of drug treatment, blood glucose estimation is done to determine the antidiabetic activity.

Insulin antibodies-induced diabetes

A transient diabetic syndrome can be induced by injecting guinea pigs with anti-insulin serum. It neutralizes the endogenous insulin with insulin antibodies. Diabetes persists as long as the antibodies are capable of reacting with the insulin remaining in circulation.

Preparation of Antibody: Bovine insulin, dissolved in acidified water (pH 3.0) at a dose of 1 mg is injected to guinea pigs weighing 300–400 g. Anti-insulin sera is collected after two weeks of antigenic challenge.

Adult albino rats are injected with 0.25–1.0 ml of guinea pig anti-insulin serum. Insulin antibodies induce a dose-dependent increase of blood glucose level up to 300 mg/dl. Slow rate intravenous infusion or an intra-peritoneal injection prolongs the effect for more than a few hours. However, large doses and prolonged administration are accompanied by ketonaemia. The drug sample to be screened is administered by a suitable route, and blood glucose level is analysed to determine the activity.

Hormone-induced diabetes

Dexamethasone: Dexamethasone is a steroid possessing immunosupression action which causes an autoimmune reaction in the islets and produces type 1 diabetes.

Adult rats weighing 150–200 g are injected with dexamethasone at a dose level of 25 mg/kg body weight by i.p. twice a day. The repeated injection of the same dose level is carried out for a period of 20–30 days resulting in IDDM. The sample to be screened is administered through a suitable route, and blood glucose level is analysed to determine the activity.

Genetic Models

Nonobese diabetic mouse

Nonobese diabetic mouse (NOD) is a model of IDDM. Hypoinsulinaemia is developed which is caused by autoimmune destruction of pancreatic β-islet cells in association with autoantibody production.

Mice are breed at the laboratory by sib-mating over 20 generations. After 20 generations of sib-mating, spontaneous development of IDDM in mice is obtained. Diabetes develops abruptly between 100 and 200 days of age. Weight loss, polyurea and severe glucosuria are common. The animals are treated with the drug sample to be screened. Blood sample is analysed for glucose level to determine activity.

Bio-breeding rat

Diabetes is inherited as an autosomal recessive trait and develops with equal frequency and severity among males and females. Insulin deficiency and insulitis are due to autoimmune destruction of pancreatic β-islet cells.

Spontaneous diabetes is diagnosed in a noninbreed but closed out-breed colony of rats at bio-breeding laboratories.

Rats are breed at the laboratory by sib-mating over 20 generations. After 20 generations of sib-mating, spontaneous development of IDDM in rats is obtained. The onset of clinical diabetes is sudden and occurs at about 60–20 days of age. The clinical presentation of diabetes in the bio-breeding (BB) rat is simiiar to that of its human counterpart. Marked hyperglycaemia, glycosuria and weight loss occur within a day of onset and are associated with decreased plasma insulin, that if untreated will result in ketoacidosis. The animals are treated with the drug sample to be screened for a required period of time. The blood sample is analysed for glucose level to determine activity.

Models for NIDDM

Streptozotocin-induced neonatal model for NIDDM

Streptozotocin causes severe pancreatic β-cells destruction, accompanied by a decrease in pancreatic insulin stores and a rise in plasma glucose level. In contrast to adult rats, the treated neonates partially regenerate and become normoglycaemic by three weeks of age. In the next few weeks, the β-cell number increase, mainly from the proliferation of cells derived from ducts, leads to hyperinsulinaemia, and shows symptoms similar to insulin resistance.

Neonatal rats are treated with Streptozotocin (90 mg/kg body weight) prepared in citrated buffer (pH 4.5) by i.p. at birth or within the first 5 days following birth. After six weeks, the rats develop symptoms similar to NIDDM. Rats showing fasting blood glucose level above 140 mg/dl are considered diabetic. Further steps are similar to that of the alloxan-induced model. The drug sample to be screened is administered by a suitable route, and blood glucose level is analysed to determine the activity.

Other Chemically Induced NIDDM Models

Adrenaline-induced acute hyperglycaemia

Adrenaline is a counter-regulatory hormone to insulin. It increases the rate of glycogenolysis and glucose level in blood causing acute hyperglycaemia.

Adult albino rats are injected at a dose level of 0.1 mg/kg through s.c. route. The dose produces peak hyperglycaemic effect at 1 h and lasts up to 4 h. The drug sample to be analysed is administered through a suitable route, and blood glucose level is determined. Oral hypoglycaemic agents can be screened by this method.

Chelating Agents

Dithizone-induced diabetes

Organic agents react with zinc in the islets of Langerhans causing the destruction of β-islet cells, producing diabetes.

Severe necrosis and disintegration of β-cells (insulin-producing cells) were observed, while α-cells (cells which produce glucoagon which maintains the glucose level in the blood) remain unaltered. Compounds such as dithizone, EDTA, 8-hydroxy quinoline are used to induce spontaneous type 2 diabetes in experimental animals. Dithizone at a dose level of 40–100 mg/kg (i.v.) produces type 2 diabetes in mice, cats, rabbits and golden hamsters.

Adult rabbits weighing 1.8–2 kg are divided into two groups of six animals each. An exactly weighed amount of dithizone is dissolved in dilute ammoniacal solution (0.2 to 0.5%). The solution is warmed to 60 -70°C for 10 min to aid solubility of dithizone. Dithizone injection at a dose level of 50–200 mg/kg produces triphasic glycaemic reaction. Initial hyperglycaemia is observed after 2 h and normoglycaemia after 8 h, which persists for up to 24 h. Permanent hyperglycaemia is observed after 24–72 h. The drug sample to be analysed is administered through a suitable route, and the blood glucose level is determined.

Models for Insulin Sensitivity and Insulin-like Activity

Euglycaemic clamp technique

This method has proved to be a useful technique of quantifying in vivo insulin sensitivity. A variable glucose infusion is delivered to maintain euglycaemia during insulin infusion. The net glucose uptake is quantified, and the sensitivity of the body tissue to insulin is determined.

Adult albino rats weighing 150–200 g are fasted overnight and anaesthetized with pentobarbital (40 mg/kg i.p.). Catheters are inserted into a jugular vein and a femoral vein for blood collection and insulin and glucose infusion, respectively. To evaluate the insulin action under physiological hyperinsulinaemia (steady-state plasma insulin concentration during the clamp test is around 100 μU/dl) and maximal hyperinsulinaemia, two insulin infusion rates, that is, 6 and 30 mU/kg/min are used. The blood glucose concentrations are determined from samples collected at 5 min intervals during the 90-min clamp test. The glucose infusion rate is adjusted so as to maintain basal level. The glucose metabolic clearance rate is calculated by dividing the glucose infusion rate by the steady-state blood glucose concentration. The drug sample to be analysed is administered through a suitable route, and the blood glucose level is determined.

Assay for insulin and insulin-like activity

This assay involves comparing two standard solutions of insulin with the test drug for its insulin-like activity.

Four groups of six rabbits weighing at least 1.8 kg are used. Two standard solutions of insulin containing one unit and two units respectively and two dilutions of sample whose potency is being examined are prepared. As diluent, a solution of 0.1 to 0.25% w/v of either m-cresol or phenol and 1.4 to 1.8 w/v of glycerol acidified with hydrochloric acid to a pH between 2.5 and 3.5 is used. Each of the prepared solution (0.5 ml) is injected subcutaneously. After 1 h and 2.5 h of each injection, a suitable blood sample is taken from the ear vein of each rabbit, and the blood sugar level is determined preferably by glucose oxidase method.

12.7. EVALUATION OF ANTIDIARRHOEAL AGENTS

Castor Oil-Induced Diarrhoea in Rats

The method followed here is the method of Awouters et al. (1978) with modification. The original method included only male wistar rats (220–250 g), where they were starved overnight before treatment with the selected drug in the next morning. In the present study, rats of either sex (180–200 g) are fasted for 18 hours. Animals are housed in six in each. Varying doses of the test drugs are administered orally by gavage as suspension to different groups of animals. The next group received dipehnoxylate (5 mg/kg) orally as suspension as standard drug for comparison. Other group that served as control is treated with the control vehicle only.

One hour after treatment, each animal receives 1 ml of castor oil orally by gavage and then observed for defecation. Up to 4th hour after the castor oil challenge, the presence of characteristic diarrhoeal droppings are noted in the transparent plastic dishes placed beneath the individual rat cages.

The effects of the test drug like the standard antidiarrhoeal agent, diphenoxylate, are calculated based on the frequency of defecation when compared to untreated rats. Both substances also should reduce greatly the wetness of faecal droppings.

Gastrointestinal Motility Tests

Rats are fasted for 18 h and placed in different cages containing six in each. Each animal is administered orally with 1 ml of charcoal meal (3% deactivated charcoal in 10% aqueous tragacanth). Immediately after that the first few groups of animals are administered orally with the test drug at varying doses. Next group receives atropine (0.1 mg/kg, i.p.), the standard drug for comparison. The last group is treated with aqueous tragacanth solution as control. Thirty minutes later, each animal is killed and the intestinal distance moved by the charcoal meal from the pylorus is cut and measured and expressed as a percentage of the distance, the charcoal meal has moved from the pylorus to the caecum.

The antidiarrhoeal test drugs decrease propulsion of the charcoal meal through the gastrointestinal tract when compared with the control group by this model which is comparable to that of atropine (standard drug) which reduces the motility of the intestine significantly.

PGE$_2$-Induced Enteropooling

In this method, rats of the same stock as above are deprived of food and water for 18 h and are placed in six perforated cages with six animals per cage. The first few groups of rats are treated with varying doses of the test drug. The last two groups are treated with 1 ml of 5% v/v ethanol in normal saline (i.p.). The last group of this is then treated with the control vehicle, which served as control. Immediately afterwards, PGE$_2$ is administered orally to each rat (100 μg/kg) in 5% v/v ethanol in normal saline. After 30 minutes, each rat is killed and the whole length of the intestine from the pylorus to the caecum dissected out and its contents are collected in a test tube and the volume is measured.

PGE$_2$ induces significant increase in the fluid volume of rat intestine when compared with control animals receiving only ethanol in normal saline and control vehicle. The antidiarrhoeal test drugs inhibit this PGE$_2$-induced enteropooling. Statistical analysis is performed by student's 't' test, and in all the cases results are expressed as mean ± SE.

12.8. SCREENING METHODS FOR ANTIFERTILITY AGENTS

Antifertility agents are substances which prevent reproduction by interfering with various normal reproductive mechanisms in both males and females. An ideal contraceptive agent is one which possess 100% efficacy, reversibility of action, which is free from side effects and is easy to use.

Ancient literature has mentioned the use of a number of plants/preparations for regulation of fertility in the form of emmenagogues, ecbolics, abortifacients and local contraceptives. For centuries, virtually every indigenous culture has been using plants and/or their various parts in one or the other form to restrict its population. Women have used herbs since time immemorial to control their fertility. The information was passed on from mother to daughter; midwives and wise women all possessed this knowledge, but most of these plant's activities and their mechanism of action were not scientifically studied.

There are approximately 250,000 species growing on earth. It stands to reason that not all of them can be used to regulate fertility; therefore some criteria have to be laid down for selecting plants to evaluate their antifertility potential. Three options are available:

1. Investigation of plants that have folkloric/traditional reputation as contraceptives;
2. Evaluation of plants that are known to contain constituents which theoretically affect the female cycle and thus produce antifertility effects, for example, oestrogenic sterols, isoflavones and coumestans or those which have a potential to contract the uterus; and
3. Random collection of plants for mass screening.

During the last six decades, sporadic attempts have been made by Indian investigators to evaluate antifertility plants. But there is variation in the reports given by various investigators on the same plant part (from inactivity to 100% activity). This appears to be due to inadequate attention given to proper botanical identification, authentication and testing procedure. In spite of the detailed description of plants found in ancient ayurvedic and unani literature, documented experimental or clinical data on them are lacking. Furthermore the efficacies of these plants have not yet been confirmed through repeated investigations.

Screening Methods for Antifertility Activity in Females

Antifertility action of drugs acting in females may be due to:

1. Inhibition of ovulation
2. Prevention of fertilization
3. Interference with transport of ova from oviduct to endometrium of the uterus
4. Implantation of fertilized ovum
5. Distraction of early implanted embryo

Screening Methods for Antiovulatory Activity

Cupric acetate-induced ovulation in rabbits

Rabbits are reflex ovulators. They ovulate within a few hours after mating or after mechanical stimulation of vagina or sometimes even the mere presence of a male or administration of certain chemicals like cupric acetate.

In this screening method, cupric acetate is used for the induction of ovulation. The rabbit ovulates within a few hours after an i.v. injection of cupric acetate (0.3 mg/kg using 1% cupric acetate in 0.9% saline). Injection of antiovulatory drugs, 24 h before the induction procedure prevents ovulation.

Sexually mature female albino rabbits, weighing 3–4 kg, are used for the study. Animals are kept in isolation for at least 21 days to ensure that they are not pregnant and to prevent the induction of ovulation by mating. They are then treated with the test drug, and 24 h later an i.v. injection of cupric acetate is given. The rabbits are sacrificed and the ovaries are examined 18–24 h later.

The total number of ovulation points on both the ovaries is recorded for each animal. Then the ovaries and uterus are excised and preserved in 10% buffered formalin and subjected to histopathological evaluation.

HCG-induced ovulation in rats

Immature female albino rats do not ovulate spontaneously and do not show cyclic changes of the vaginal epithelium. Priming with human chorionic gonadotropin (HCG) induces follicular maturation, followed by spontaneous ovulation two days later. Injection of an antiovulatory drug before the induction procedure will prevent ovulation. This principle is used for screening potential antiovulatory agents.

Immature female albino rats (24–26 days old) are used for the experiment. The animals are treated with various test drugs in different dose levels. After the administration of the test drug, exogenous HCG is given to induce ovulation. After two days, the animals are sacrificed. Their ovaries are preserved in a 10% buffered formalin and subjected to histopathological evaluation. The results are compared with the control group.

Screening Methods for Oestrogenic Compounds: In Vivo Methods

A primary therapeutic use of oestrogen (both in vivo and in vitro) is in contraception. The rationale for these preparations is that excess exogenous oestrogen inhibits FSH and LH and thus prevents ovulation.

Assay for water uptake

The principle of the assay is based on the observation that the uterus responds to oestrogens by increased uptake and retention of water. A peak in the uptake is observed six hours after administration.

Ovariectomized adult animals may be used for this experiment. It is simpler to use immature 18-day-old mice or 22-day-old rats obtained two days before the beginning of the experiment. The animals are randomly grouped. The control group is given 0.1 ml of cottonseed oil (vehicle for estradiol) subcutaneously. The oestrogen control group is given doses ranging from 0.01 to 0.1 µg to establish a dose-response curve. In the initial test, the test compound is given to groups at a high and low dose. In subsequent tests, it is given over a range of doses to provide the dose-response curve. All doses are given in 0.1 ml of cottonseed oil.

Five hours after treatment, the animals are killed by cervical fracture and the uteri are quickly excised. The operation is begun by a longitudinal slit through the skin of the abdomen and through the body wall. The uterus is picked up with the forceps and severed from the vagina. The uterine horns are separated from the connective tissues and are then cut at their constriction point near the ovary. The uteri are kept moist by placing them on dump (not wet) filter paper and by covering them with damp filter paper. They are then rapidly weighed in a sensitive balance. The uteri are dried in an oven at 60°C, for 24 h and are reweighed. The percentage increase in water over control can be calculated and compared with the values of other groups.

Procedure for ovariectomy: The animals are anaesthetized with ether. A single transverse incision is made in the skin of the back. This incision can be shifted readily from one side to the other, so as to lie over each ovary in turn. A small puncture is then made over the site of the ovary, which can be seen through the abdominal wall, embedded in a pad of fat. The top of a pair of fine forceps is introduced, and the fat around the ovary is grasped, care being taken not to rupture the capsule around the ovary itself. The tip of the uterine horn is then crushed with a pair of artery forceps and the ovary together with the fallopian tube removed with a single cut using a pair of fine scissors. Usually no bleeding is observed. The muscular wound is closed by absorbable sutures, and the outer skin wound is closed by nylon suture.

Four-day uterine weight assay

This assay is based on the observation that oestrogens cause an increase in protein synthesis and thus bring about an increase in uterine weight. A peak is observed after about 40 h.

Immature or Ovariectomized albino mice or rats can be given the test drug intramuscularly in cottonseed oil for three consecutive days. On the fourth day, animals are killed by cervical fracture, the uteri rapidly excised and the uterine contents gently squeezed out (results are unreliable if the uterine contents are not removed). The uteri are weighed immediately in the wet state. They are then dehydrated in an oven at 100°C for 24 h and reweighed to obtain the dry weight increase. The log dose is plotted against the wet weight to produce a sigoid curve, and the ED_{50} can be determined for comparison of the test compound with estradiol.

Vaginal opening

This assay is based on the principle that vaginal opening occurs in immature female albino mice and rats when treated with oestrogenic compounds. Complete vaginal opening is considered a sign of oestrogenic activity.

Immature female animals (18-day-old mice, 21-day-old rats) are used for the study. The test and standard drugs are administered to the animals intramuscularly in cottonseed oil. The vaginal opening is observed to determine oestrogenic activity.

Vaginal cornification

This assay is based on the fact that rats and mice exhibit a cyclical ovulation with associated changes in the secretion of hormones. This leads to changes in the vaginal epithelial cells. The estrus cycle is classified into the proestrus, estrus, metestrus and diestrus stage. Drugs with oestrogenic activity change the animals from whatever stage they were into the estrus stage.

Adult female albino rats having a regular estrus cycle are used for the study. Animals are treated with various test and standard drugs. Change in the vagina can be observed by taking vaginal smears and examining these for cornified cells, leucocytes, and epithelial cells in the normal animals and treated animals twice daily over a period of four days. Any drug which changes the animals into the estrus stage skipping other stages is considered to have oestrogenic activity.

The experimental procedure for taking vaginal smears

Holding the animal on the ventral side up, a drop of normal saline is inserted into the vagina with a Pasteur pipette. Care must be taken to avoid damage or injury to the vagina so as to prevent pseudopregnancy. The drop of normal saline should be aspirated and replaced several times. It is then transferred to a microscope slide and allowed to dry. The smears are fixed by placing the slide in absolute alcohol for 5 sec, allowing it to dry, and staining it with a 5% aqueous methylene blue solution for 10 min. The excess stain is washed off with tap water, and the slide is dried and observed using a low power microscope.

Chick oviduct method

The weight of the oviduct of young chicken increases depending on the dose of natural and synthetic oestrogen. This principle is used for the screening of oestrogenic compounds.

Seven-day-old pullet chicks are injected subcutaneously twice daily with solutions of the test compound in various doses for six days. Doses (0.02–0.5 µg) of 17β-estradiol per animal serve as standard. Six to ten chicks are used for each dosage group. On the day after the last injection, the animals are sacrificed and the weight of the body and oviduct is determined.

Screening Methods for Oestrogenic Compounds: *In Vitro* Methods

Potency assay

This assay determines the affinity of the test compound for oestrogen receptor sites in the uterus.

The uptake of titrated estradiol by immature uteri must be established. The inhibition of this uptake by pretreatment with a test compound will then indicate the oestrogenic potency of the compound.

Four immature female mice (20 days old) are killed. The uteri are quickly excised and are placed in a Krebs–Ringer phosphate buffer. Pieces of diaphragm are taken from each animal to serve as control tissue for nonspecific uptake of estradiol. The uteri are divided at the cervix into two horns; this helps as one horn can be used as the control and the other for testing the compound. The tissues are placed in vials containing 5.0 ml of Krebs–Ringer phosphate buffer, incubated and shaken at 37°C with 95% oxygen; 5% carbon dioxide is bubbled through. The radiochemical purify of the ^{3}H-estradiol can be checked chromatographically. Buffer solution of radioactive estradiol is made up so that each 5 ml of buffer contains 0.0016 µg of radioactive estradiol (0.25 µci). A stock solution can be made and kept refrigerated for up to 6 weeks.

The excised tissues are treated as follows:

Control: Four pieces of diaphragm are incubated and shaken with 5 ml of buffer solution for 15 min at 37°C and are then shaken for 1 h with 5 ml of buffer containing the radioactive estradiol and 2% w/v bovine albumin.

Experimental: Four uterine horns are incubated and are shaken in 5 ml of buffer at 37°C for 15 min. They are then incubated and shaken with 5 ml of buffer containing 2% of albumin and radioactive estradiol at 37°C for 1 h. Both control and experimental tissue are removed and washed with buffer at 37°C for 5 min, kept in damped filter paper, and weighed. The tissues are then prepared for counting. Samples of 100 µl of the incubation solution are also taken for counting.

Treatment of tissues for counting: The tissues are dried to determine constant weight and the dry weight recorded. Each piece of tissue is placed in a glass counting vial and incubated at 60°C in a shaking water bath with 0.5 ml of hyamine hydrochloride 10× until the tissue has completely dissolved. If the solution is discoloured, 50 µl of 20% hydrogen peroxide may be added. A total of 50 µl of concentrated HCl and 15 ml of phosphor solution are added to each vial. The vials are allowed to equilibrate in the packed liquid scintillation counter, and counts are taken. Counting efficiency is determined by the addition of an internal standard. The results are expressed as disintegrations per minutes per unit of wet weight (dpm/mg). Test compounds can be incubated with the labelled oestrogen. This helps in assaying their effectiveness in competing for the receptors in the uterus.

Oestrogen receptor-binding assay

Oestrogen receptor-binding assay uses the principle of competitive binding of labelled and unlabelled oestrogen on the oestrogenic receptors. Oestrogenic compounds displace the labelled oestrogen in a concentration-dependent manner from the oestrogen receptor.

Cytosol preparation: Uteri from 18-day-old female albino mice are removed and homogenized at 0°C in 1:50 (w/v) of Tris-sucrose buffer in a conical homogenizer. Human endometrium from menopausal women frozen within 2 h of hysterectomy and stored in liquid nitrogen can also used. The frozen endometrium is pulverized and homogenized in l:5 (w/v) of Tris-sucrose buffer. Homogenates are centrifuged for 1 h at 105,000 r.p.m.

Screening Methods for Antioestrogens: *In Vivo* Methods

Antagonism of physiological effects of oestrogens

Antioestrogenic compounds inhibit some or all of the physiological effect of oestrogen, such as water uptake of uterus, uterotrophy and vaginal cornification. This principle is used for the screening of antioestrogenic activity.

The assay techniques used for antioestrogens are modifications of the oestrogenic assays. The dose of oestrogen used is that which is required to produce 50% of the maximum possible response. The test compound can be injected simultaneously or at varying times before or after the oestrogen. The procedure for assays of water uptake, uterotrophy and vaginal cornification are followed as described earlier except that the test compounds are given with the oestrogen.

Screening Methods for Antioestrogens: *In Vitro* methods

Aromatase inhibition

This assay is based on the principle that some compounds which inhibit aromatase (oestrogen synthase) can produce antioestrogenic activity. Antioestrogenic activity of compounds can be evaluated indirectly by evaluating aromatase-inhibiting ability.

Ovarian tissue from adult golden hamsters is used. The estrus cycle is monitored for at least three consecutive four-day estrus cycles before the experiment. The experiments for evaluating inhibitor effects are performed with ovaries obtained from animals sacrificed on day 4 (proestrus) of the cycle. The ovaries are excised free from adhering fat tissue and quartered. The quarters are transferred into plastic incubation flasks with 2 ml of Krebs–Ringer bicarbonate salt (KBR) solution (pH 7.6) containing 8.4 mM glucose. The flasks are gassed with O_2:CO_2 (95%:5%), tightly closed and placed in a shaker/water bath (37°C) for incubation of the fragments. The incubation media are replaced with fresh KBR after preincubation for 1 h. The ovaries are further incubated for 4 h in the presence or absence of inhibitors. 4-OH androstenedione is used as standard in concentrations between 0.33 and 330 µM/l. At the end of the experiment, the incubation media are removed and centrifuged. In the supernatant oestrogen, progesterone and testosterone are determined by radioimmunoassays. The data of control and test group are compared with suitable statistical analysis.

Screening Methods for Progestins: *In Vivo* Methods

Proliferation of uterine endometrium in oestrogen-primed rabbits: Clauberg–McPhail test

Female rabbits weighing 800–1000 g are primed with estradiol. They are then administered with progestational compounds leading to the proliferation of endometrium and converted into the secretary phase. This principle is used for the screening of progestational compounds.

Female rabbits weighing 800–1000 g are primed with a daily injection of oestradiol 0.5 µg/ml in aqueous solution. On day 7, the drug treatment is begun. The total dose is given in five equally divided fractions daily over five days. Twenty-four hours after the last injection, the animals are killed. The uteri are dissected out, and frozen sections of the middle portion of one horn is prepared and examined for histological interpretation. For interpretation of progestational proliferation of endometrium, the beginning of glandular development may be graded 1 and endometrium consisting only of glandular tissue may be graded 4.

Pregnancy maintenance test

Progesterone is responsible for the maintenance of pregnancy. This principle is used for the screening of progestational compound.

Ovariectomy is done on day 5/10/15 day of pregnancy in different groups of pregnant rats. The animals are treated with different test and standard drugs. Pregnant rats are killed 5/10/15 days later. An average of living foetuses at the end of the experiment is compared with the standard and the control group (without ovariectomy). The ED_{50} of progesterone is 5 mg/day in rat and less than 0.5 mg/day in mouse.

Carbonic anhydrase activity in rabbit's endometrium

There is a linear dose-response relationship between dose of progestogens and carbonic anhydrase activity in rabbit endometrium. This principle is used for the screening of progestational compounds.

Immature female albino rabbits are used in this study. The animals are primed with estradiol and administered test and standard drugs. After the drug treatment, the animals are sacrificed and their uterus removed. The endometrial extract of the uterus is evaluated for the carbonic anhydrase activity calorimetrically.

Prevention of abortion in oxytocin-treated pregnant rabbits

Administration of oxytocin by i.v. route to pregnant rabbits on the 30th day of pregnancy causes abortion. Prior administration of progestational compounds prevents the abortion. This principle is used for the detection and screening of progestational compounds.

Ten units of oxytocin are administered to pregnant rabbits on day 30 of pregnancy. Test and standard drugs in oil are injected 24 hours before. The control animal not receiving any drugs aborts within 2–30 min after administration of oxytocin. Drugs which have progestational activity prevent abortion.

Deciduoma reaction in rats

This study is based on the phenomenon of maternal/placental tumour formation due to progestational drugs in traumatized uterus of ovariectomized rats. This phenomenon is used for the screening of progestational compounds.

Ovariectomized adult female albino rats weighing between 150 and 200 g are used for the study. The rats are primed with four injections of 1 μg oestrone. This is followed by nine days of drug therapy. On day five, one uterine horn is exposed and 1 mg of histamine dihydrochloride injected into the lumen. Twenty-four hours after the last dose of drug, the animals are killed, the uterine horn cut off, weighed and histologically examined.

Screening Methods for Progestins: *In Vitro* Methods

Progesterone receptor-binding assay

Progesterone receptor-binding assay uses the principle of competitive binding of labelled and unlabelled progesterone on progesterone receptors. Progestational compounds displace the labelled progesterone in a concentration-dependent manner from the progesterone receptor.

Human uteri obtained after hysterectomy is frozen in liquid nitrogen and stored at 80°C until use. For cytosol preparation, uterine tissues are minced and homogenized with a homogenizer at 0–4°C in ice-cold PENG buffer composed of 10 mM KH_2PO_4, 10 mM K_2HPO_4, 1.5 mM EDTA, 3 mM NaN_3, 10% glycerol, pH 7.5. The homogenates are then centrifuged at 10,5000 g at 4°C for 30 min. The supernatant is taken as cytosol.

The cytosol preparations are incubated with ^{3}H-R5020 as radio-ligand at a concentration of 8 nmol/l and increased concentrations (1×10^{-10} to 1×10^{-5} mol/l) of the competitor steroid overnight at 4°C. Then unbound steroids are adsorbed by incubating with 0.5 ml of DCC (0.5% carbon (Norit A), 0.05% dextran T400 in PENG buffer) for 10 min at 4°C. After centrifugation (10 min at 1,500 g at 4°C), 0.5 ml of the supernatant is withdrawn

and counted for radioactivity. To calculate the relative binding affinity, the percentage of radio-ligand bound in the presence of the competitor compared to that bound in its absence is plotted against the concentration of unlabelled competing steroid.

Screening Method for Antiprogestational Activity

Antagonism of physiological effect of progesterone

The antiprogestational compound inhibits some or all the physiological effect of progesterones. This principle is used to screen the antiprogestational activity of drugs.

The procedures for assay of the Clauberg–McPhail test and deciduoma formation are as described for progestational activity except that the test compounds are given along with the progesterone.

Screening Method for Anti-implantation Activity

Female albino rats of established fertility in the proestrus or estrous stage are mated with mature male rats of established fertility (in the female to male ratio of 3:1). Each female is examined for the presence of spermatozoa in the early morning vaginal smear. The day on which this sign of mating is seen is taken as day 1 of pregnancy. The female is then separated and caged singly. The test drug is administered orally to the animals once daily on specific days of pregnancy at different concentrations. On day 10th of pregnancy, the animals are laparotomized, and the number of implants present in both the uterine horns as well as the number of corpora lutea (CL) on each ovary is counted. The animals are allowed to complete the gestation period (usually 21–23 days) and the number of litters delivered, if any are counted. Preimplantation loss and postimplantation loss are calculated using the following formula.

Preimplantation loss = No. of CL on 10th day—No. of implants on 10th day

Post implantation loss = No. of implants on 10th day—No. of litters delivered

$$\% \text{ preimplantation loss} = \frac{\text{No. of CL - No of implants}}{\text{No. of CL}} \times 100$$

$$\% \text{ preimplantation loss} = \frac{\text{No. of implants - No of litters}}{\text{No. of implants}} \times 100$$

The animal is anaesthetized with ether and the limbs tied to a rat board (waxed) with the ventral side up. The hairs on the area around the midline abdominal region are clipped with a curved scissor and the region cleaned with 70% alcohol. An incision of 2 cm length is made along the midline to expose the viscera. The superficially tying coils of ileum are lifted to expose the two uterine horns. The horns are examined for implantation sites. Implants are visible as clear swellings on the uterine horns giving the uterine tube a beaded appearance. Embryos with a bright red dish aspect and a clear margin are considered to be healthy. Those of a dull blue colour with no clear margin and orientation with some exudates are considered resorbing. The number of implants and resorption sites per horn are counted. The ovaries, which lie on the upper end of the uterine horns, show corpora lutea as yellow spots over the surface. The number of corpora lutea present on each ovary is also noted.

After counting, the organs are replaced back. A small quantity of neosporin powder is sprinkled over the organs to prevent any infection. The incision through the muscular layer is closed with a continuous suture using absorbable catguts. The skin layer is closed with continuous sutures using silk thread. An antiseptic, povidone iodine solution, is applied on the sutured area after wiping with 70% alcohol. The animal is maintained on light ether anaesthesia throughout the experiment. After laparotomy, the rats are transferred to a warm place till they recover from the anaesthesia.

Screening Methods for Abortifacient Activity

Adult female albino rabbits are used for the study. The pregnancy date is counted from the date of observed mating. The existence of pregnancy may be confirmed by palpation after the 12th day of pregnancy. Intra-amniotic and intra-placental injections are administered to the rabbits under ether anaesthesia on the 20th day of pregnancy. The uterus is exposed through a midline incision, its various parts are identified by transillumination from a strong source of light and a particular site chosen for injection. Then the material is injected in 0.1 ml of solvent into the amniotic fluid or in 0.05 ml of solvent into the placenta.

Alternatively, the drugs can be given through any route and duration from the 20th day of pregnancy. The effect of the drug is determined by looking for vaginal bleeding, changes in weight, abdominal palpation and by postmortem examination.

Screening Methods for Antifertility Activity in Males

Developing male antifertility agent involves interference with spermatogenesis without loss of libido and varying sexual characteristics.

The general approaches include:

1. Emergent spermatozoa made nonfunctional
2. Production of oligospermia/aspermia

In vivo methods

Fertility test: Fertility test is based on the evaluation of the average litter size. Antifertility agents negatively affect the average litter size.

Groups of 5–10 male rats of proven fertility are treated with the drug and are paired with fertile females in the ratio of 1:3. Daily vaginal smears are examined for the presence of sperms; normally within one week all females which have passed through one estrus cycle would have mated. The mated animals are kept separately till the gestational period. The litters are counted and using the following formula; the average litter size is calculated.

$$\text{Average litter size} = \frac{\text{Total litter}}{\text{No. of females mated}}$$

If vaginal smear shows leucocytes in 10–14 days, pseudopregnancy is confirmed. If insemination is not detected then inhibition of libido or aspemic copulation might be the cause. Fertility patterns can be obtained from changes in average litter size.

Cohabitation test: This test determines the time interval for litter production after placing treated males with two females each. The date of mating is calculated from the date of parturition. This method is suitable for drugs known to cause sterility for several weeks.

Adult female and male albino rats of proven fertility are used for the study. They are kept for mating in the ratio of 2:1 till both females deliver litters. The date of mating is calculated from the date of parturition. The time interval for litter production after placing treated males with the two females is calculated.

Subsidiary test: This test determines the changes in spermatozoa count with time. The antifertility drugs affect the spermatozoa count negatively.

Adult male albino rats weighing between 150 and 250 g are used for the study. They are kept in a cage containing artificial or animal vagina. The vagina is artificially stimulated by a cylindrical plastic jacket with a rubber liner filled with water at 5°C. About 0.5 ml of ejaculate is diluted with saline containing traces of formalin. The resulting suspension is counted on a haemocytometer.

In vitro methods

Spermicidal activity: Spermicidal drugs are diluted with normal saline and serial dilutions are made. About 0.2 ml of human seminal fluid is mixed with 1 ml of spermicidal solution. Then the mixture is incubated at 37°C for 30 min. A drop of the mixture is placed immediately on a slide, and at least five fields are microscopically observed under high power (×400) for assessment of sperm morphological changes and motility. Effective agents can immobilize and kill the sperms.

Immobilization assay: The cauda portion of the epididymes of a ram is isolated and minced in 0.9% saline solution (pH 7.5). It is filtered through a piece of cheese cloth to get a sperm suspension. For human samples, ejaculates (n = 10) from normal subjects after 72–96 h of sexual abstinence are subjected to routine semen analysis following liquefaction at 37°C. Sperm count above 100 million/ml and viability above 60% with normal morphology and rapid and progressive motility is employed for the test.

Ram epididymal sperm suspension (100–200 million/ml) or human ejaculate (100–150 million/ml) are mixed thoroughly in a 1:1 ratio with different concentration of drugs. A drop of the mixture is placed immediately on a slide and at least five fields are microscopically observed under high power (×400) for assessment of sperm motility. The mixture is then incubated at 37°C for 30 min, and the above process is repeated.

Nonspecific aggregation estimation: Different concentrations of drugs are treated with ram sperm suspension in a 1:1 ratio and kept at 37°C for 1 h. One drop of the sedimented sperm is then taken from the bottom of the micro centrifuge tube, placed on a slide, and the percent aggregation examined microscopically under 400× magnifications. Since the nonaggregated spermatozoa remain in the supernatant, the latter is collected and the turbidity determined spectrophotometrically at 545 nm. The aggregation is indirectly proportional to the sperm viability.

Sperm revival test: This assay determines the extent of spermicidal and immobilization capability of drugs by evaluating the revival of sperm motility.

To study the revival of sperm motility, after completion of the immobilization assay, the spermatozoa are washed twice in physiological saline. They are then incubated once again in the same medium free of drug at 37°C for 30 min to observe the reversal of sperm motility.

Assessment of plasma membrane integrity: To assess the sperm plasma membrane, integrity ram sperm suspension (100–200 million/ml) or human ejaculated sperm (100–150 million/ml) are mixed with the drug at the minimum effective concentration, at a ratio of 1:1 and incubated for 30 min at 37°C. Sperm samples mixed with saline in a similar manner serve as controls. For viability assessment, one drop each of 1% aqueous solution of eosin Y and of 10% aqueous solution of nigrosin was placed in a micro centrifuge tube. A drop of well-mixed sperm sample is added to it and mixed thoroughly. The mixture is dropped onto a glass slide and observed under 400× magnification.

For the hypoosmotic swelling test (HOS), 0.1 ml of aliquot is taken from each of the treated and control sample, mixed thoroughly with 1 ml of HOS medium (1.47% fructose and 2.7% sodium citrate at a 1:1 ratio) and incubated for 30 min at 37°C. The curling tails are examined under phase contrast microscope using 100× magnification.

5-Nucleotidase is released possibly due to destabilization of plasma membrane. This can be estimated to determine the effect of the drug on the plasma membrane integrity of the sperm. The activity of 5'-nucleotidase can be determined by measuring the rate of release of inorganic phosphate from adenosine 5'-monophosphate. After incubating the sperm suspension with the drug, the sperm pellet is collected by centrifugation at 3000 g at 37°C. It is then washed twice in 0.9% saline and suspended in 0.1 mol/l Tris-HCl buffer (pH 8.5) with each reaction system containing (100–200) million spermatozoa. An aliquot of 0.1 ml suspension of sperm is added to 0.9 ml of buffered substrate containing 3 mmol/l adenosine 5'-monophosphate and 50 mmol/l $MgCl_2$ dissolved in 0.1 mol/l Tris-HCl buffer. The tubes are incubated at 37°C for 30 min, and 0.5 ml 20% TCA (0–4°C) is added to the mixture to stop the reaction. The mixture is then centrifuged at 10,000 g at 4°C. The pellet is discarded and the supernatant kept for phosphate estimation. The activity of 5'-nucleotidase is expressed in terms of μg of phosphate released. The activity of 5'-nucleotidase is indirectly proportional to the plasma membrane integrity.

Evaluation of acrosomal status: This method evaluates the acrosomal status of sperm. The acrosome is the cap-like structure on the head of the spermatozoa. It breaks down just before fertilization, releasing a number of enzymes that assist penetration between the follicle cells that surround the ovum. The most widely studied acrosomal enzyme is the acrosin that has been shown to be associated with acrosoraes of all mammalian spermatozoa. The highest substrate specificity was obtained with BAEE (N-benzoyl-L-argine ethyl ester).

Different concentrations of drugs are mixed with ram sperm suspension in a 1:1 ratio and kept at 37°C for 1 h. The suspension is centrifuged and the pellets collected. The pellets are extracted with 3 μmol/l HCl at pH 3 and the enzyme activity is measured, following the hydrolysis of 0.5 μmol/l BAEE dissolved in 0.05 mol/l Tris-HCl buffer containing 0.05 mol/l $CaCl_2$ at pH 8. The activity of acrosin is expressed in terms of mIU. One mIU activity means the amount of enzyme, which causes the hydrolysis of one nano mole of BAEE in 1 min at 25°C. The activity of acrosin is directly proportional to the fertilizing capability of sperms.

Androgenic and antiandrogenic activities: Androgenic compounds increase the weight of the testes and seminal vesicles of immature male mice. Antiandrogenic compounds suppress the increase in weight responses of testosterone. This principle is used for the screening of androgenic and antiandrogenic activity.

Immature male mice weighing around 20 g are used for the study. The drugs are administered for seven days alone and along with testosterone. Twenty-four hours after the last dose, the animals are weighed and sacrificed with an over dose of ether. The testes and seminal vesicles are removed and weighed rapidly in a sensitive balance. The weights are compared with the control group.

12.9. SCREENING METHODS FOR ANTI-INFLAMMATORY AGENTS

WHO has identified 2000–2010 as the decade for musculoskeletal disorders. Herbal drugs like holy basil (tulsi; *Ocimum sanctum*), turmeric *(Curcuma longa)*, Indian olibanum tree *(Boswellia serrata)*, ginger *(Zingiber officnale)*, etc., are widely used for the treatment of various inflammatory disorders. They are not only found to be safer and have fewer side effects, but they also cover a large domain of mechanisms involved in inflammation thus proving to be more beneficial than synthetic drugs. Inflammation expresses the response to damage of cells and vascular tissues. The five basic symptoms of inflammation—redness, swelling, heat, pain and deranged function—have been known since the ancient Greek and Roman era.

The major events occurring during this response are an increased blood supply to the affected tissue by vasodilation, increased capillary permeability caused by retraction of the endothelial cells which allows the soluble mediators of immunity to reach the site of inflammation and leukocytes migration out of the capillaries into the surrounding tissues. Neutrophils, monocytes and lymphocytes also migrate towards the site of infection. The development of inflammatory reactions is controlled by the following systems: cytokines, complement, kinin and fibrinocytic pathways; by lipid mediators (prostaglandins and leukotrienes) released from different cells; and by vasoactive mediators released from mast cells, basophils and platelets.

The response is accompanied by the clinical signs of erythema, oedema, hyperalgesia and pain. Inflammatory responses occur in three distinct phases, each apparently mediated by different mechanisms:

Acute transient phase: Characterized by local vasodilatation and increased capillary permeability.

Subacute phase: Characterized by infiltration of leukocytes and phagocytic cells.

Chronic proliferative phase: Tissue degeneration and fibrosis occur.

Drugs preventing acute and subacute inflammation can be tested using the following models: paw oedema in rats, croton oil ear oedema, pleurisy tests, UV-erythema in guinea pigs, oxazolone-induced ear oedema in mice, granuloma pouch technique and vascular permeability. The effectiveness of drugs which work at the proliferative phase can be measured by methods for testing granuloma formation, such as the cotton pellet granuloma, adjuvant-induced arthritis, glass rod granuloma and PVC sponge granuloma.

Testing of Drugs Preventing Acute and Subacute Inflammation

Paw oedema

This technique is based upon the ability of anti-inflammatory agents to inhibit the oedema produced in the hind paw of the rat after injection of a phlogistic agent (irritant). Rats with a body weight between 100 and 150 g are required. Many irritants have been used, such as brewer's yeast, formaldehyde, dextran, egg albumin, kaolin, Aerosil® and sulphated polysaccharides like carrageenan. The animals are fasted overnight. The control rats receive distilled water while the test animals receive drug suspension orally. Thirty minutes later, the rats are subcutaneously injected with 0.1 ml of 1% solution of carrageenan in the foot pad of the left hind paw. The paw is marked with ink and immersed in the water cell of a plethysmometer up to this mark. The paw volume is measured plethysmographically immediately after injection, 3 and 6 h after injection, and eventually 24 h after injection. The paw volumes for the control group are then compared with those of the test group.

Croton oil ear oedema in rats and mice

This method mainly evaluates the antiphlogistic activity of topically applied steroids.

For this method, mice (22 g) or rats (70 g) are required. For tests in mice, the irritant is composed of (v/v): 1 part croton oil, 10 parts ethanol, 20 parts pyridine and 69 parts ethyl ether; for rats the irritant is composed of (v/v): 4 parts croton oil, 10 parts ethanol, 20 parts pyridine and 66 parts ethyl ether. The standard and the test compound are dissolved in this solution. Irritants are applied on both sides of the right ear (0.01 ml in mice or 0.02 ml in rats under ether anaesthesia). Controls receive only the irritant solvent. The left ear remains untreated. Four hours after application, the animals are sacrificed under anaesthesia. Both ears are removed and discs of 8 mm diameter are cut. The discs are weighed immediately and the weight difference between the treated and untreated ear is recorded indicating the degree of inflammatory oedema.

Pleurisy test

Pleurisy is the phenomenon of exudative inflammation in man. In experimental animals, pleurisy can be induced by several irritants, such as carrageenan, histamine, bradykinin prostaglandins, mast cell degranulators and dextran. Leukocyte migration and various biochemical parameters involved in the inflammatory response can be measured easily in the exudate.

Male rats weighing 220–260 g are required. The animal is lightly anaesthetized with ether and placed on its back. The hair from the skin over the ribs on the right side is removed and the region cleaned with alcohol. A small incision is made into the skin under the right arm. The wound is opened and 0.1 ml of 2% carrageenan solution is injected into the pleural cavity through this incision. The wound is closed with a clip. One hour before this injection and 24 and 48 h thereafter, rats are treated (subcutaneously or orally) with the standard or the test compound. A control group receives only the vehicle. The animals are sacrificed 72 h after carrageenan injection and pinned on a dissection board with the forelimbs fully extended. About 1 ml of heparinized Hank's solution is injected into the pleural cavity through an incision. The cavity is gently massaged to mix its contents. The fluid is aspirated out of the cavity using a pipette. The aspirated exudates are collected in a graduated plastic tube. About 1 ml (the added Hank's solution) is subtracted from the measured volume. The values of each experimental group are averaged and compared with the control group. The white blood cell number in the exudate is measured using a Coulter counter or a haematocytometer.

Ultraviolet erythema in guinea pigs

Anti-inflammatory agents delay the development of ultraviolet erythema on albino guinea pigs. They are shaved on the back 18 h before testing. The test compound is suspended in the vehicle and half the dose of the test compound is administered orally 30 min before ultraviolet exposure. Control animals are treated with the vehicle alone. The guinea pigs are placed in a leather cuff with a hole of 1.5–2.5 cm size punched in it, allowing the ultraviolet radiation to reach only this area. An ultraviolet burner is warmed up for about 30 min before use and placed at a constant distance (20 cm) above the animal. Following a 2 min ultraviolet exposure, the remaining half of the test compound is administered. The erythema is scored 2 h and 4 h after exposure.

Oxazolone-induced ear oedema in mice

The oxazolone-induced ear oedema in mice is a model of delayed contact hypersensitivity that permits the quantitative evaluation of the topical and systemic anti-inflammatory activity of a compound following topical administration.

Mice of either sex (25 g) are required. A fresh 2% solution of oxazolone in acetone is prepared. This solution (0.01 ml) is injected on the inside of both ears under anaesthesia. The mice are injected 8 days later, again under anaesthesia, with 0.01 ml of 2% oxazolone solution (control) or 0.01 ml of oxazolone solution in which the test compound or the standard is dissolved, on the inside of the right ear. The

left ear remains untreated. The maximum of inflammation occurs 24 h later. At this time the animals are sacrificed under anaesthesia and a disc of 8 mm diameter is punched from both ears. The discs are immediately balance. The weight difference is an indicator of the inflammatory oedema.

Granuloma pouch technique

Irritants such as croton oil or carrageenan produce aseptic inflammation resulting in large volumes of exudate, which resembles the subacute type of inflammation. Rats (150–200 g) are selected for the study; the back of the animals is shaved and disinfected. With a very thin needle, an air pouch is made by injection of 20 ml of air under ether anaesthesia. Into the resulting air pouch 0.5 ml of a 1% solution of croton oil in sesame oil is injected. After 48 h, the air is withdrawn from the pouch and 72 h later any resulting adhesions are broken. Instead of croton oil, 1 ml of a 20% suspension of carrageenan in sesame oil can be used as irritant. Starting with the formation of the pouch, the animals are treated every day either orally or subcutaneously with the test compound or the standard. On the fifth day, the animals are sacrificed under anaesthesia. The pouch is opened and the exudate collected in glass cylinders. The average value of the exudate of the controls and the test groups is calculated.

Vascular permeability

This test is used to evaluate the inhibitory activity of drugs against increased vascular permeability, which is induced by a phlogistic substance. Mediators of inflammation, such as histamine, prostaglandins and leucotrienes are released following stimulation of mast cells. This leads to a dilation of arterioles and venules and to an increased vascular permeability. As a consequence, fluid and plasma proteins are released and edemas are formed. Vascular permeability is increased by subcutaneous injection of the mast cell-degranulating compound 48/80. The increase of permeability can be recognized by the infiltration of the injected sites of the skin with the dye Evan's blue.

Male rats (160 and 200 g) are used. About 5 ml/kg of 1% solution of Evan's blue is injected intravenously. One hour later, the animals are dosed with the test compound orally or intraperitoneally. After 30 min, the animals are lightly anaesthetized with ether and 0.05 ml of 0.01% solution of compound 48/80 is injected subcutaneously at three sites. About 90 min after the injection of compound 48/80, the animals are sacrificed by ether anaesthesia. The abdominal skin is removed and the dye-infiltrated areas of the skin measured. The percent inhibition in the treated animals as compared to the control group is calculated.

Testing of Drugs Preventing the Proliferative Phase (Granuloma Formation) of Inflammation

Cotton pellet granuloma

Foreign body granulomas are induced in rats by the subcutaneous implantation of pellets of compressed cotton. After several days, histologically giant cells and undifferentiated connective tissue can be observed besides fluid infiltration. The amount of newly formed connective tissue can be measured by weighing the dried pellets after removal. More intensive granuloma formation has been observed if the cotton pellets are impregnated with carrageenan.

Male and female rats with an average weight of 200 g are used. The back skin is shaved and disinfected with 70% ethanol. An incision is made in the lumbar or neck region. Subcutaneous tunnels are formed and a sterilized cotton pellet is placed with the help of a blunted forceps. The animals are treated for seven days subcutaneously or orally. They are then sacrificed, the pellets taken out and dried. The net dry weight, that is, after subtracting the weight of the cotton pellet is determined. The average weight of the pellets of the control group as well as that of the test group is calculated. The percent change of granuloma weight relative to the vehicle control group is determined.

Adjuvant arthritis in rats

Adjuvant-induced arthritis in rats exhibit many similarities to human rheumatoid arthritis. An injection of complete Freund's adjuvant into the rat's paw induces inflammation as a primary lesion with a maximum inflammation after three to five days. Secondary lesions occur after a delay of approximately 11–12 days and are characterized by inflammation of noninjected sites (hind legs, forepaws, ears, nose and tail), a decrease in weight and immune responses.

Male rats with an initial body weight of 130–200 g are used. On day 1, rats are injected in the subplantar region of the left hind paw with 0.1 ml of complete Freund's adjuvant. The adjuvant consists of 6 mg mycobacterium butyricum thoroughly ground with a mortar and pestle and suspended in heavy paraffin oil (Merck) to give a concentration of 6 mg/ml. Dosing with the test compounds or the standard is started on the same day and continued for 12 days. Both paw volumes and body weight are recorded on the day of injection. The paw volume is measured plethysmographically with equipment as described in the paw oedema tests. On day 5, the volume of the injected paw is measured again, indicating the primary lesion and the influence of therapeutic agents on this phase. The severity of the induced adjuvant disease is determined by measuring the noninjected paw (secondary lesions) with a plethysmometer. The animals are not dosed with the test compound or the standard from day 12 to 21. On day 21, the body weight is determined again and the severity of the secondary lesions evaluated visually and graded according to the following scheme:

Ears	Aabsence of nodules and redness	0
	Presence of nodules and redness	1
Nose	No swelling of connective tissue	0
	Intensive swelling of connective tissue	1
Tail	Absence of nodules	0
	Presence of nodules	1
Forepaws	Absence of inflammation	0
	Inflammation of at least 1 joint	1
Hind paws	Absence of inflammation	0
	Slight inflammation	1
	Moderate inflammation	2
	Marked inflammation	3

Sponge implantation technique

Foreign body granulomas are induced in rats by subcutaneous implantation of a sponge. Sponges used for implantation are prepared from polyvinyl foam sheets (thickness: 5 mm). Discs are punched out to a standard size and weight (10.0 ± 0.02 mg). The sponges are then soaked in 70% v/v ethanol for 30 min, rinsed four times with distilled water and healed at 80°C for 2 h. Before implantation in the animal, the sponges are soaked in sterile 0.9% saline in which either drugs, antigens or irritants have been suspended. Typical examples include 1% carrageenan, 1% yeast, 1% zymosan A, 6% dextran, heat-killed Bordetella pertussis or 0.5% heat-killed Mycobacterium tuberculosis.

Sponges are implanted in rats weighing 150–200 g under ether anaesthesia. An incision is made and separate cavities are formed into which sponges are inserted. Up to 8 sponges may be implanted per rat. The incision is closed with Michel clips and the animals maintained at a constant temperature of 24°C. For short-term experiments, the animals are treated with the test drug or standard once before implantation orally or subcutaneously. For long-term experiments, the rats are treated daily up to 3 weeks.

Glass rod granuloma

Glass rod-induced granulomas reflect the chronic proliferate phase of inflammation. Of the newly formed connective tissue, not only can the wet and dry weight be measured, but also the chemical composition and mechanical properties. Glass rods with a diameter of 6 mm are cut to a length of 40 mm and the ends rounded off. They are sterilized before implantation. Rats are anaesthetized with ether, the back skin shaved and disinfected. From an incision in the back region, a subcutaneous tunnel is formed with a blunted forceps. A glass rod is introduced into this tunnel. The incision wound is closed by sutures. The animals are kept in separate cages. The rods remain in situ for 20 or 40 days. Animals are treated orally. At the end of 20 days the animals are sacrificed. The glass rods are removed together with the surrounding connective tissue, which forms a tube around the glass rod. By incision at one end, the glass rod is extracted and the granuloma sac inverted forming a plain piece of pure connective tissue. Wet weight of the granuloma tissue is recorded. The specimens are kept in a humid chamber until further analysis. Biochemical analyses, such as determination of collagen and glycosaminoglycans, can also be performed.

12.10. SCREENING METHODS FOR ANTIPYRETIC AGENTS

Treatment with antipyretics has been very important in the preantibiotic era. Nevertheless, for treatment of acute viral diseases and for treatment of protozoal infections like malaria, reduction of elevated body temperature by antipyretics is still necessary. For anti-inflammatory compounds, an antipyretic activity is regarded as a positive side effect. To evaluate these properties, fever is induced in rabbits or rats by injection of lipopolysaccharides or Brewer's yeast.

Antipyretic Testing in Rats

The subcutaneous injection of Brewer's yeast suspension is known to produce fever in rats. A decrease in temperature can be achieved by administration of compounds with antipyretic activity.

Procedure

A 15% suspension of Brewer's yeast in 0.9% saline is prepared. Groups of six male or female wistar rats with a body weight of 150 g are used. By insertion of a thermocouple to a depth of 2 cm into the rectum the initial rectal temperatures are recorded. The animals are fevered by injection of 10 ml/kg of Brewer's yeast suspension subcutaneously in the back below the nape of the neck. The site of injection is massaged in order to spread the suspension beneath the skin. The room temperature is kept at 22–24°C. Immediately after yeast administration, food is withdrawn. 18 h post challenge, the rise in rectal temperature is recorded. The measurement is repeated after 30 min. Only animals with a body temperature of at least 38°C are taken into the test. The animals receive the test compound or the standard drug by oral administration. Rectal temperatures are recorded again 30, 60, 120 and 180 min postdosing.

Evaluation

The differences between the actual values and the starting values are registered for each time interval. The maximum reduction in rectal temperature in comparison to the control group is calculated. The results are compared with the effect of standard drugs, for example, aminophenazone 100 mg/kg p.o. or phenacetin 100 mg/kg p.o.

Modifications of the method

Stitt and Shimada (1991) and Shimada et al. (1994) induced fever in rats by microinjecting 20 ng PGE_1 directly into one of the brain's circumventricular organs of the rat known as the organum vasculosum laminae terminalis.

Luheshi et al. (1996) induced fever by intraperitoneal injection of 100 µg/kg lipopolysaccharide into rats and measured the inhibition of fever by interleukin-1 receptor antagonist.

Telemetry has been used to record body temperature in animals (Riley et al. 1978; Gallaher et al. 1985; Clement et al. 1989; Guillet et al. 1990; Kluger et al. 1990; Bejanian 1991; Watkinson et al. 1996; Miller et al. 1997).

Antipyretic Testing in Rabbits

Lipopolysaccharides from Gram-negative bacteria, for example, E. coli, induce fever in rabbits after intravenous injection. Only lipopolysaccharide fractions are suitable, which cause an increase of body temperature of 1°C or more at a dose between 0.1 and 0.2 µg/kg after 60 min. In the rabbit, two maxima of temperature increases are observed. The first maximum occurs after 70 min and the second after 3 h.

Procedure

Rabbits of both sexes and of various strains with a body weight between 3 and 5 kg can be used. The animals are placed into suitable cages and thermocouples connected with an automatic recorder are introduced into the rectum. The animals are allowed to adapt to the cages for 60 min. Then 0.2 ml/kg containing 0.2 µg lipopolysaccharide are injected intravenously into the rabbit ear. After 60 min, the test compound is administered either subcutaneously or orally. Body temperature is monitored for at least 3 h.

Evaluation

A decrease of body temperature for at least 0.5°C for more than 30 min as compared with the temperature value before administration of the test compound is regarded as positive effect. This result has been found after 45 mg/kg phenylbutazone s.c. or 2.5 mg/kg indomethacin s.c.

Modifications of the method

Cashin and Heading (1968) described a simple and reliable assay for antipyretic drugs in mice, using intracerebral injection of pyrogens. Davidson et al. (1991) tested the effect of human recombinant lipocortin on the pyrogenic action of the synthetic polyribonucleotide polyinosini:polycytidylic acid in rabbits. Yeast-induced pyrexia in rats has been used for antipyretic efficacy testing by Loux et al. (1982) and Cashin et al. (1977). van Miert et al. (1977) studied the effects of antipyretic agents on fever and ruminal stasis induced by endotoxins in conscious goats. Petrova et al. (1978) used turpentine-induced fever in rabbits to study antipyretic effects of dipyrone and acetylsalicylic acid. Lee et al. (1985) studied the antipyretic effect of dipyrone on endotoxin fever of macaque monkeys. Loza Garcia et al. (1993) studied the potentiation of chlorpromazine-induced hypothermia by the antipyretic drug dipyrone in anaesthetized rats. Shimada et al. (1994) studied the mechanism of action of the mild analgesic dipyrone preventing fever induced by injection of prostaglandin E1 or interleukin-1β into the organum vasculosum terminalis of rat brain.

12.11. SCREENING METHODS FOR ANTIULCER AGENTS

An ulcer is a local defect, or excavation of the surface of an organ, or tissue, which is produced by the sloughing of inflammatory necrotic tissue. The term 'peptic ulcer' refers to a group of ulcerative disorders of the upper GIT, which appears to have in common, the participation of acid pepsin in their pathogenesis. A peptic ulcer probably results due to an imbalance between aggressive (acid, pepsin and *H. pylori*) and defensive (gastric mucous, bicarbonate secretion, prostaglandins, innate resistance of the mucosal cells) factors. In gastric ulcers, acid secretion is normal or low.

Pylorus Ligation in Rats

This principle is based on ulceration induced by accumulation of acidic gastric juice in the stomach (Shay et al. 1945).

The requirements include stereo microscope, adult albino rats (150–170 g), anaesthetic ether, plastic cylinder and 0.1 N sodium hydroxide.

Adult albino rats weighing 150–170 g are starved for 48 h although they have access to drinking water. Normally ten animals are used per dose and as control. After they are ether anaesthetized, a midline abdominal incision is made and the pylorus ligated. The abdominal wall is closed by sutures and test compounds are given either orally by gavage or injected subcutaneously. The animals are placed for 19 h in plastic cylinders with an inner diameter of 45 mm being closed on both ends by a wire mesh. The animals are then sacrificed using carbon dioxide

anaesthesia. The abdomen is opened, and a ligature is placed around the oesophagus close to the diaphragm. The stomach is removed and the contents drained into a centrifuge rube. Along the greater curvature, the stomach is opened and pinned onto a cork plate. The mucosa is then examined with a stereo microscope.

The evaluation is done by counting the numbers of ulcers and the severity graded according to the following scores:

0 = no ulcers; 1 = superficial ulcers; 2 = deep ulcers; 3 = perforations

The volume of gastric content is measured after centrifugation. Acidity is determined by titration with 0.1 N NaOH. Ulcer index U is calculated using the following formula:

$$U_1 = U_n + U_s + U_p \times 10^{-1}$$

where U_n = the average number of ulcers per animal, U_s = average of severity score and U_p = percentage of animals with ulcers.

Ulcers Through Immobilization Stress

The principle behind this method involves psychogenic factors, such as stress, which play a major role in the pathogenesis of gastric ulcers in man.

The requirements include adult albino rats, anaesthetic ether, CO_2 anaesthesia and a stereo microscope.

A group of 10 adult albino rats (150–170 g) per dose of the test drug and for controls are used. Food and water are withdrawn 24 h before the experiment. After oral and subcutaneous administration of the test compound or a placebo solution, the animals are slightly anaesthetized with ether. Both the upper and lower extremities are fixed together and the animals wrapped in wire gauge. They are horizontally suspended in the dark at 20°C for 24 h and finally sacrificed using carbon dioxide anaesthesia. The stomach is removed, fixed on a cork plate, and the number and severity of the ulcers registered with a stereo microscope.

Stress Ulcer by Cold Water Immersions

The principle behind this assay is that cooling the rats in water when they are restrained according to the previous model accelerates the occurrence of gastric ulcers and shortens the time of necessary immobilization. In this model, the gastric ulcer formation is mainly due to gastric hypermotility, which could lead to mucosal over-friction.

The requirements include wistar rats, cages, Evans blue dye, 2% formol saline, CO_2 anaesthesia and a magnifier.

Groups of 8–10 wistar rats weighing 150–200 g are used. After oral administration of the test compounds, the rats are placed vertically in individual restraint cages in water at 22°C for 1 h. They are then removed, dried, and injected intravenously through a tail vein with 30 mg/kg Evans blue. After 10 min, they are sacrificed using CO_2 anaesthesia and their stomachs removed. Formol saline (2% v/v) is then injected into the totally ligated stomachs for storage overnight. The next day, the stomachs are opened along the greatest curvature, washed in warm water and examined under a threefold magnifier.

The evaluation is done by measuring the lengths of the longest diameter of the lesions. This is summated to give a total lesion score (in mm) for each animal; the mean count in control rats should be about 25 (range 20–28). Inhibition of the lesion production is expressed as a percentage value.

Indomethacin-Induced Ulcers in Rats

This assay is based on the fact that use of nonsteroidal anti-inflammatory agents like indomethacin and acetyl salicylic acid induces gastric lesions in man and in experimental animals by inhibition of gastric cyclooxygenase.

The requirements include wistar rats, 0.1% Tween 80, 2% formol saline and CO_2 anaesthesia.

Groups of 8–10 wistar rats weighing 150–200 g are used. The test drugs are administered orally in 0.1% Tween 80 solutions 10 min before an oral administration of indomethacin (20 mg/kg). After 6 h, the rats are sacrificed in CO_2 anaesthesia and their stomachs removed. Formol saline (2% v/v) is then injected into the totally ligated stomachs for storage overnight. The next day, the stomachs are opened along the greatest curvature, washed in warm water and examined.

The mean score is calculated in control rats. It should be about 25 (range 20–28). Inhibition of the lesion production is expressed as a percentage value.

12.12. SCREENING METHODS FOR DIURETIC AGENTS

Drugs that induce diuresis (enhances urine outflow) are known as diuretics. Many herbal plants like cantaloupe (*Cucitmis melo*), *Dolichos biflorus* (virus), radish (*Raphanus sativus*), kanguni (*Satania italica*), Oriental sweet gum (*Liquidamber orientalis*) and kapok tree (*Ceibia pentandra*) possess diuretic activity. Extracts from these drugs are used in various diseases like hypertension, congestive heart failure, oedema, nephrolithiasis and urolithiasis. The diuretic activity of these drugs can be evaluated by the following methods.

Diuretic Activity in Rats (Lipschitz Test)

This test is based on the principle that water and sodium excretion in test animals is different as compared to rats treated with a high dose of urea. The 'Lipschitz value' is the quotient between excretion by test animals and excretion by the urea control.

Adult albino rats weighing 100–200 g are used for the study. Six animals per group are placed in metabolic cages individually provided with a wire mesh bottom and a funnel to collect the urine. Stainless steel sieves are placed in the funnel to retain faeces and allow the urine to pass. The rats are fed with standard diet and water ad libitum. Food and water are withdrawn 17–24 h before the experiment. The test compound is administered orally. The other group is treated with urea (1 g/kg) orally. Additionally 5 ml of 0.9% NaCl solution per 100 g of body weight are given by gavage. Urine excretion is recorded after 5 and 24 h. The sodium content of the urine is determined by flame photometer.

Urine volume excreted per 100 g body weight is calculated for each animal, in the group. Results are expressed as the 'Lipschitz value', that is, the ratio T/U in which T is the response of the test compound and U that of urea treatment. The value of 1.0 and more are regarded as a positive effect. Potent diuretics having a Lipschitz value of 2.0 and more have been found.

Chronic Renal Failure in Rats

Chronic renal failure is a frequent pathological condition in man. The following assay is used for special pharmacological studies as well as evaluation of renal toxicity of new chemicals.

Albino rats weighing between 150 and 200 g are used for the study. Rats are anaesthetized by i.m. injection of ketamine (40 mg/kg) and droperidol (0.25 mg/kg). An incision is made in the abdominal wall, and the small bowel and caecum are lifted and placed on saline-soaked sponges. The right kidney is exposed and dissected from the retroperitoneal area, the vascular and ureteric pedicles are ligated with silk sutures, and the kidney removed. The renal artery of the left kidney is dissected into the hilum to expose the three main segmental renal arteries. The kidney is not dissected out of the peritoneum. The anterior caudal branch of the artery is then temporarily ligated to establish the volume of renal tissue supplied. The area of ischemia becomes demarcated within 10–15 s. If this approximates ¼ to ⅓ of the kidney, a permanent ligature is placed. The viscera are then carefully replaced in the abdomen and peritoneum and linea alba is closed with a continuous suture. The skin is closed with stainless steel clips.

Blood for serum creatinine is collected by retro orbital puncture under anaesthesia at various time intervals up to 12 months. In association with this, urine is collected every 24 h for the measurement of creatinine, protein and specific gravity.

Compounds which posses diuretic activity will increase the volume, accompanied by decrease in urine specific gravity which indicates the decrease in concentrating ability of the kidney. Proteinuria is also significantly increased. Terminal uremia occurs after 14–15 months.

Diuretic and Saluretic Activity in Dogs/Cat

Renal physiology of the dog is claimed to be closer to man than that of rats. So dogs have been extensively used to study renal physiology and the action of diuretics. Using catheters, periodic collection of urine can be made with more reliability than in rats.

Dogs or cats are anaesthetized using sodium pentobarbitone 35–50 mg/kg. The lower abdomen is opened. The femoral vein is exposed and cannulated with a suitable venous cannula. The venous cannula is used for the administration of test drugs and saline. The control group receives only water. The standard group receives 1 g/kg urea or 5 mg/kg furosamide per day. The test groups receive different test drugs. The urinary bladder is catheterized through the urethra and connected to a measuring cylinder. The urine is collected, the volume measured and analysed for Na^+/K^- ions using flame photometry. Chloride ions are estimated using argentometry. The urine volume and electrolyte concentration of test compounds are compared with the control group to determine the diuretic activity.

12.13. SCREENING METHODS FOR HEPATOPROTECTIVE AGENTS

A toxic or repeated dose of a known hepatotoxin is administered to induce liver damage in experimental animals. The test substance is administered before or after the toxin treatment. If the hepatotoxicity is prevented or reduced, the test substance is effective. There are various models of inducing hepatotoxicity in rodents (rats and mice).

Hepatitis in Long-Evans Cinnamon Rats

The Long-Evans Cinnamon strain of rats has been recommended as a useful model to study genetically transmitted hepatitis and chronic liver disease. It has been speculated that this strain of rats is prone to liver diseases due to excessive copper accumulation in the liver.

Long-Evans Cinnamon rats are housed in temperature and humidity controlled rooms at a 12:12 light/dark cycle. Groups of 6–10 rats are given different diets based on a 15% purified egg protein diet and supplemented with vitamins or drugs. Drugs are applied via mini-pumps intraperitoneally implanted under ether anaesthesia. The occurrence of jaundice is easily observable as the time when the ears and tail turn yellow and the urine becomes bright orange, staining the fur in the lower abdominal region. Usually, the jaundice progressively worsens, ending in death of the animal within about a week. Incidence of jaundice and mortality versus time are used as parameters to measure the extent of hepatoprotective activity.

Allyl Alcohol-Induced Liver Necrosis in Rats

In this method allyl alcohol is used as a liver necrosis-inducing agent in rats.

Albino rats weighing 120–150 g are used. On the first day, food but not water is withdrawn. After 6 h, the compounds to be tested for protective activity are administered i.p. or orally. After 1 h, the animals are dosed orally with 0.4 ml/kg of a 1.25% solution of allyl alcohol in water. Next morning, the treatment with the potentially protective drugs is repeated. Food but not water is withheld until the third day. Next morning, the animals are sacrificed and the liver is removed. The parietal sides of the liver are checked using a stereomicroscope with 25 times magnification. Focal necrosis is observed as white-green or yellowish hemorrhagic areas clearly separated from unaffected tissue. The diameter of the necrotic areas is determined using an ocularmicrometer. These values are added for each animal to obtain an index for necrosis.

Carbon Tetrachloride-Induced Liver Fibrosis in Rats

Chronic administration of carbon tetrachloride to rats induces severe disturbances of hepatic function together with histologically observable liver fibrosis. This model is used for the screening of hepatoprotective agents.

Albino rats are treated orally twice a week with 1 mg/kg carbon tetrachloride, dissolved in olive oil 1:1, over a period of 8 weeks. The animals are kept under standard conditions (day/night rhythm: 8:00 a.m. to 8:00 p.m.; 22°C room temperature; standard diet; water ad libitum). Twenty animals serve as controls receiving only olive oil; 40–60 animals receive only the carbon tetrachloride. Groups of 20 rats receive in addition to carbon tetrachloride, the compound under investigation in various doses by gavage twice daily (with the exception of the weekends, when only one dose is given) on the basis of the actual body weight. The animals are weighed weekly. At the end of the experiment (8 weeks), the animals are anaesthetized and exsanguinated through the caval vein.

The serum is analysed for parameters like total bilirubin, total bile acids, 7 S fragment of type IV collagen, procollagen III N-peptide. The liver, kidney, aortic wall and tail tendons are prepared for determination of hydroxyproline. They are weighed and completely hydrolysed in 6 N HCl. Hydroxyproline is measured by HPLC and expressed as mg/mg wet weight of the organs.

For histological analysis, three to five pieces of the liver weighing about 1 g are fixed in formalin and Carnoy solution. Three to five sections of each liver are embedded, cut, and stained with azocarmine aniline blue (AZAN) and evaluated for the development of fibrosis using a score of 0–IV.

Grade 0	Normal liver histology.
Grade I	Tiny and short septa of connective tissue without influence on the structure of the hepatic lobules.
Grade II	Large septa of connective tissue, flowing together and penetrating into the parenchyma; tendency to develop nodules.
Grade III	Nodular transformation of the liver architecture with loss of the structure of the hepatic lobules.
Grade IV	Excessive formation and deposition of connective tissue with subdivision of the regenerating lobules and development of scars.

The values of all the parameters of the test group are compared with the control group using suitable statistical methods.

Bile Duct Ligation-Induced Liver Fibrosis in Rats

Ligation of the bile duct in rats induces liver fibrosis, which can be evaluated histologically and by determination of serum collagen parameters. This model is used for the screening of hepatoprotective agents.

Albino rats are anaesthetized and laparotomy is performed under aseptic conditions. A midline incision in the abdomen is made from the xiphosternum to the pubis, exposing the muscle layers and the linea alba, which is then incised over a length corresponding to the skin incision. The edge of the liver is then raised and the duodenum pulled down to expose the common bile duct, which pursues an almost straight course of about 3 cm from the hilum of the liver to its opening into the duodenum. There is no gall bladder, and the duct is embedded for the greater part of its length in the pancreas, which opens into it by numerous small ducts. A blunt aneurysm needle is passed under the part of the duct selected, the pancreas is stripped away with care, and the duct is double ligatured with cotton thread.

The peritoneum and the muscle layers as well as the skin wound are closed with cotton stitches. The animals receive normal diet and water ad libitum throughout the experiment. Groups of 5–10 animals receive the test compound in various doses or the vehicle twice daily for 6 weeks. They are then sacrificed and the blood harvested for determination of bile acids. 7 S fragment of type IV collagen, and procollagen III N-peptide. The liver is used for histological studies and for hydroxyproline determinations. Control animals show excessive bile duct proliferation as well as formation of fibrous septa. This is consistent with complete biliary cirrhosis. The value of the test is compared with the control using suitable statistical analysis.

Galactosamine-Induced Liver Necrosis

A single dose or a few repeated doses of D-galactosamine causes acute hepatic necrosis in rats. Prolonged administration leads to cirrhosis. This model is used for the screening of hepatoprotective agents.

Adult albino rats weighing 110–180 g are injected intraperitoneally three times weekly with 500 mg/kg D-galactosamine over a period of one to three months. The test substances are administered orally with food or by gavage. The control group receives only vehicle or food without drugs. The rats are sacrificed at various time intervals and the livers excised and evaluated by light microscopy and immunohistology using antibodies against macrophages, lymphocytes and the extracellular matrix component.

Countrymade Liquor Model

Countrymade liquor (CML, containing 28.5% alcohol) is used to produce hepatotoxicity in this model. CML is administered orally at a dose of 3 ml/100 g/day for 30 days, which results in severe fatty changes in liver.

Rats are divided into groups of eight each. The control group receives 1% gum acacia as vehicle, corn oil (1 ml/100 g/day) and glucose isocaloric to the amount of alcohol. The positive control group receives CML (3 ml/100 mg/day) in two divided doses and corn oil (1 ml/100 g/day) in a single dose. Other test groups receive drugs in respective doses along with CML (3 ml/100 g/day) and corn oil.

After 21 days, the blood is withdrawn for analysis of SGOT, SGPT, alkaline phosphatase, serum cholesterol, albumin, total proteins, bilirubin, glucose and creatinine. The rats are sacrificed and the livers dissected out for histopathological analysis. The value of the test is compared with the control using suitable statistical analysis.

Paracetamol Model

This model is used to produce experimental liver damage only in mice, since rats are resistant to paracetamol-induced hepatotoxicity. Paracetamol administered orally as a single dose of 500 mg/kg in mice produces hepatotoxicity.

Adult albino mice are used for the study. Paracetamol is administered as a single dose of 500 mg/kg. After 48 h, they are treated with the test drugs for 5 days. At the end of the experiment, blood is withdrawn for biochemical analysis of SGOT, SGPT, alkaline phosphatase, serum cholesterol, albumin, total proteins, bilirubin, glucose and creatinine. The liver is subjected to histopathological studies. The value of the test is compared with the control using suitable statistical analysis.

Partial Hepatectomy Model

In this method, partial hepatectomy (removal of 70% of liver mass) is done and the action of drugs on the regeneration of liver cells studied. Hepatoprotective agents improve the regeneration capability of liver.

Rats are used for this study as they can withstand surgical infections better than mice. They are anaesthetized using light ether anaesthesia. A median line incision reaching 3–4 mm posteriorly from the xiphoid process of the sternum is done and the large median lobe of the liver with the left lateral lobe taken out. These lobes are ligated by coarse linen and excised. Around 68 ± 2% of the total hepatic parenchyma is also removed. The peritoneum is closed using absorbable suture and the integument closed using nonabsorbable surgical suture. Various hepatoprotective drugs can be screened for their activity using these hepatectomized rats.

At the end of the screening experiments, the blood is collected for analysis of the serum. The following parameters are determined: SGOT, SGPT, alkaline phosphatase, serum cholesterol, albumin, total proteins, bilirubin, glucose and creatinine. The animals are sacrificed. The liver is excised out, weighed and subjected to histopathological evaluation. The value of the test is compared with the control using suitable statistical analysis.

12.14. SCREENING METHODS FOR WOUND-HEALING AGENTS

The extracts obtained from plants are usually made into different formulations, either as ointment or as lotion and applied to the skin wound. Sometimes it is used internally or even injected if required depending on the nature of the constituents. The models usually used for the evaluation of the wound-healing activity can be described as follows.

Excision Wound Model

Four groups of animals containing ten in each group are to be anaesthetized by open mask method with anaesthetic ether. The rats are depilated on the back. One excision, wound is inflicted by cutting away 500 mm² full thickness of skin of a predetermined area. Rats are left undressed to the open environment. Then the drug, that is, the reference standard (0.2% w/w nitrofurazone ointment), simple ointment BP (control) and test drug ointment or different other forms are administered till the wound is completely healed. This model is used to monitor wound contraction and epithelialization time. Epithelialization time is noted as the number of days after wounding required for the scar to fall off leaving no raw wound behind. Wound contraction is calculated as percent reduction in wound area. The progressive changes in wound area are monitored planimetrically by tracing the wound margin on a graph paper every alternate day. To determine the changes in healing of wound measurement of wound, area on graph paper is expressed as unit (mm²). For histopathological examination, tissues are collected from the completely healed wound when the scar is removed. A transverse section of tissue is prepared from each group of rat and stained with haematoxylin and eosin to reveal the tissue section clearly. Then the tissues are observed under microscope to study different histopathological phenomenon.

Incision Wound Model

Four groups of animals containing ten in each group are anaesthetized, and two paravertebral long incisions of 6 cm length are made through the skin and cutaneous muscles at a distance of about 1.5 cm from midline on each side of the depilated back of rat. Full aseptic measures are not taken and no local or systemic antimicrobials are used throughout the experiment. All the groups are treated in the same manner as mentioned in case of excision wound model. No ligature is to be used for stitching. After the incision is made, the parted skin is kept together and stitched with black silk by 0.5 cm apart. Surgical thread (No. 000) and curved needle (No. 11) are used for stitching. The continuous threads on both wound edges are tightened for good adoption of wound. The wound was left undressed. The ointment of extract, standard drug (nitrofurazone ointment) and simple ointment BP is applied to the wound twice daily or feeded daily until complete recovery, to the respective groups of animals.

Tensiometer

It consists of a 6 × 12-inch wooden board with one arm of 4-inch long, fixed on each side of the possible longest distance of the board. The board is placed at the edge of a table. A pulley with bearing is mounted on the top of one arm. An alligator clamp with 1-cm width is tied on the tip of another arm by a fishing line (20-lb test monofilament) in such a way that the clamp could reach the middle of the board. Another alligator clamp is tied on a longer fishing line with 1 litre polyethylene bottle on the other end.

Tensile strength of wound represents the promotion of wound healing. Usually wound-healing agents promote the gaining of tensile strength. Tensile strength (the force required to open the healing skin) was used to measure the amount of healing. The instrument used for this purpose is called as tensiometer, which is explained as above. This was designated on the same principle as the thread tested in textile industry. One day before performing the experiment (measurement of tensile strength) the sutures are removed from the stitched wounds of rats after recovery and tensile strength is measured as follows.

Determination of Tensile Strength

The sutures are removed on ninth day of wounding and the tensile strength is measured on 10th day. Extract ointments along with simple ointment (control) and nitrofurazone ointment (standard) are administered through out the period, twice daily for 9 days. On 10th day again the rats are anaesthetized, and each rat is placed on a stack of paper towels on the middle of the board. The amount of the towels could be adjusted in such a way so that the wound is on the same level of the tips of the arms. The clamps are then carefully clamped on the skin of the opposite sides of the wound at a distance of 0.5 cm away from the wound. The longer pieces of the fishing line are placed on the pulley and finally to polyethylene bottle, and the position of the board is adjusted so that the bottle receive a rapid and constant rate of water from a large reservoir, until the wound began to open. The amount of water in the polyethylene bag is weighed and considered as tensile strength of the wound. The mean determinations are made on both sides of the animals and are taken as the measures of the tensile strength of the wound. The tensile strengths of the extract and nitrofurazone ointment treated wounds are compared with control. Tensile strength increment indicates better wound-healing promotions of the applied drug.

Dead Space Wound

Three groups of animals containing ten in each group are anaesthetized by open mask method with anaesthetic ether. Dead space wounds are created by subcutaneous implantation of sterilized polypropylene tubes (2.5 × 5 cm). The test drug is administered at different doses based on the design of the experiment for a period of ten days. The granuloma tissues formed on the tubes are harvested on the 10th postwounding day. The buffer extract of the wet granuloma tissue is used for the determination of lysyl oxidase activity, protein content and tensile strength. Part of granuloma tissue is dried, and the acid hydrolysate is used for the determination of hydroxyproline, hexosamine and hexuronic acid.

The progresses of wound healing in excision and incision wound method have to be studied. The measurement of the tensile strength, that is, the effect of the extract and standard drug on the wound-healing process by incision wound method have to be studied. Results are expressed as mean ± SE and compared with the corresponding control (simple ointment) values; p-values are calculated by student's t-test by comparing with control. Percentages of wound contractions are calculated with respect to the corresponding 0 day's wound area (mm^2).

The contractions of wound with all the drugs comparing with simple ointment (control) are measured. The epithelialization period of the wound area of the extract treated group are compared with standard drug treated group. Tensile strength of wounds of rats treated with standard drug (nitrofurazone ointment), in case of incision wound model is measured increment in tensile strength indicates better wound healing.

The histopathological examination of the tissues of the wound area treated with extract, standard drug is performed. In these studies, test drugs (herbals) with good activity showed rapid increase in tissue regeneration in skin wounds, more relative fibrosis. The skin adrenal structures like pilosebaceous glands, sweat glands, etc., are better presented in wounds treated with extract compared to standard drug treated animal wounds.

The changes in the biochemical parameters affecting wound healing in dead space wound model like, granuloma weight, lysyl oxidase activity, as well as protein content are to be measured which is usually increased with effective test drugs. The hydroxyproline, hexuronic acid, hexosamine level are measured which are increased considerably. The observed increase in tensile strength could be attributed to the increase in lysyl oxidase activity which is responsible for cross-linking and maturation of collagen. The reduction in granuloma weight is also due to better maturation of collagen, which invariably leads to shrinkage of granulation tissue. However in this case, the observed increase in tensile strength is not only due to increased cross linking via lysyl oxidase but also due possibly to interactions (noncovalent, electrostatic) with the ground substance as evidenced by a highly significant increase in the hexosamine content.

Wound healing involves different phases such as contraction, epithelialization, granulation, collagenation, etc. The glycosidal mixture of extract of *Centella asiatica* has been reported to be responsible to enhance incised wounds healing (Rosen et al., 1967) and in stimulating collagen in human skin fibroblast cell (Vogel and DeSouza, 1980).

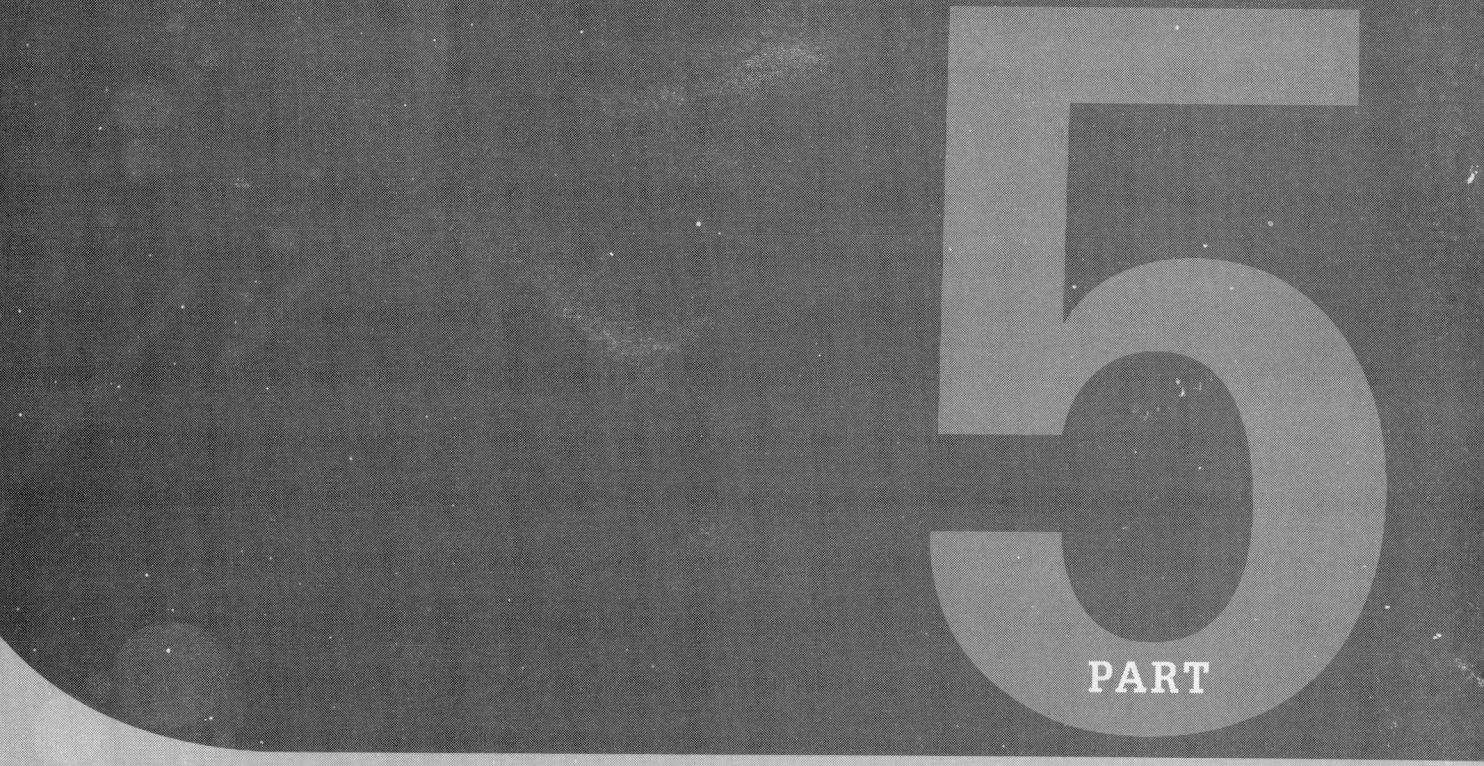

Biogenesis of Phytopharmaceuticals

Section Outline

OVERVIEW

All organisms need to transform and interconvert a vast number of organic compounds to enable them to live, grow and reproduce. They need to provide themselves with energy in the form of ATP, and a supply of building blocks to construct their own tissues. An integrated network of enzyme-mediated and carefully regulated chemical reactions is used for this purpose, collectively referred to as *intermediary metabolism*, and the pathways involved are termed *metabolic pathways*. Some of the crucially important pathways are discussed in this part.

CHAPTER 13

General Biosynthetic Pathways of Secondary Metabolites

CONTENTS

13.1. INTRODUCTION

All organisms need to transform and interconvert a vast number of organic compounds to enable them to live, grow and reproduce. They need to provide themselves with energy in the form of ATP, and a supply of building blocks to construct their own tissues. An integrated network of enzyme-mediated and carefully regulated chemical reactions is used for this purpose, collectively referred to as 'intermediary metabolism', and the pathways involved are termed 'metabolic pathways'. Some of the crucially important molecules of life are carbohydrates, proteins, fats and nucleic acids.

Despite the extremely varied characteristics of living organisms, the pathways for generally modifying and synthesizing carbohydrates, proteins, fats and nucleic acids are found to be essentially the same in all organisms, apart from minor variations. These processes demonstrate the fundamental unity of all living matter, and are collectively described as 'primary metabolism', with the compounds involved in the pathways being termed 'primary metabolites'. Thus degradation of carbohydrates and sugars generally proceeds via the well-characterized pathways known as glycolysis and the Krebs/citric acid/tricarboxylic acid cycle, which release energy from the organic compounds by oxidative reactions. Oxidation of fatty acids from fats by the sequence called β-oxidation also provides energy.

In contrast to these primary metabolic pathways, which synthesize, degrade and generally interconvert compounds commonly encountered in all organisms, there also exists an area of metabolism concerned with compounds which have a much more limited distribution in nature. Such compounds, called 'secondary metabolites', are found in only specific organisms, or groups of organisms, and are an expression of the individuality of species. Secondary metabolites are not necessarily produced under all conditions, and in the vast majority of cases the function of these compounds and their benefit to the organism is not yet known. Some are undoubtedly produced for easily appreciated reasons, for example, as toxic materials providing defence against predators, as volatile attractants towards the same or other species, or as colouring agents to attract or warn other species, but it is logical to assume that all do play some vital role for the well-being of the producer. It is this area of 'secondary metabolism' that provides most of the pharmacologically active

KEY TERMS

natural products. It is thus fairly obvious that the human diet could be both unpalatable and remarkably dangerous if all plants, animals and fungi produced the same range of compounds.

13.2. THE BUILDING BLOCKS

The building blocks for secondary metabolites are derived from primary metabolism as indicated in Figure 13.1. This scheme outlines how metabolites from the fundamental processes of photosynthesis, glycolysis and the Krebs cycle are tapped off from energy-generating processes to provide biosynthetic intermediates. The number of building

blocks needed is surprisingly few, and as with any child's construction set a vast array of objects can be built up from a limited number of basic building blocks. By far the most important building blocks employed in the biosynthesis of secondary metabolites are derived from the intermediates acetyl coenzyme A (acetyl-CoA), shikimic acid, mevalonic acid and 1-deoxyxylulose 5-phosphate. These are utilized respectively in the acetate, shikimate, mevalonate and deoxyxylulose phosphate pathways.

In addition to acetyl-CoA, shikimic acid, mevalonic acid and deoxyxylulose phosphate, other building blocks based on amino acids are frequently employed in natural product synthesis.

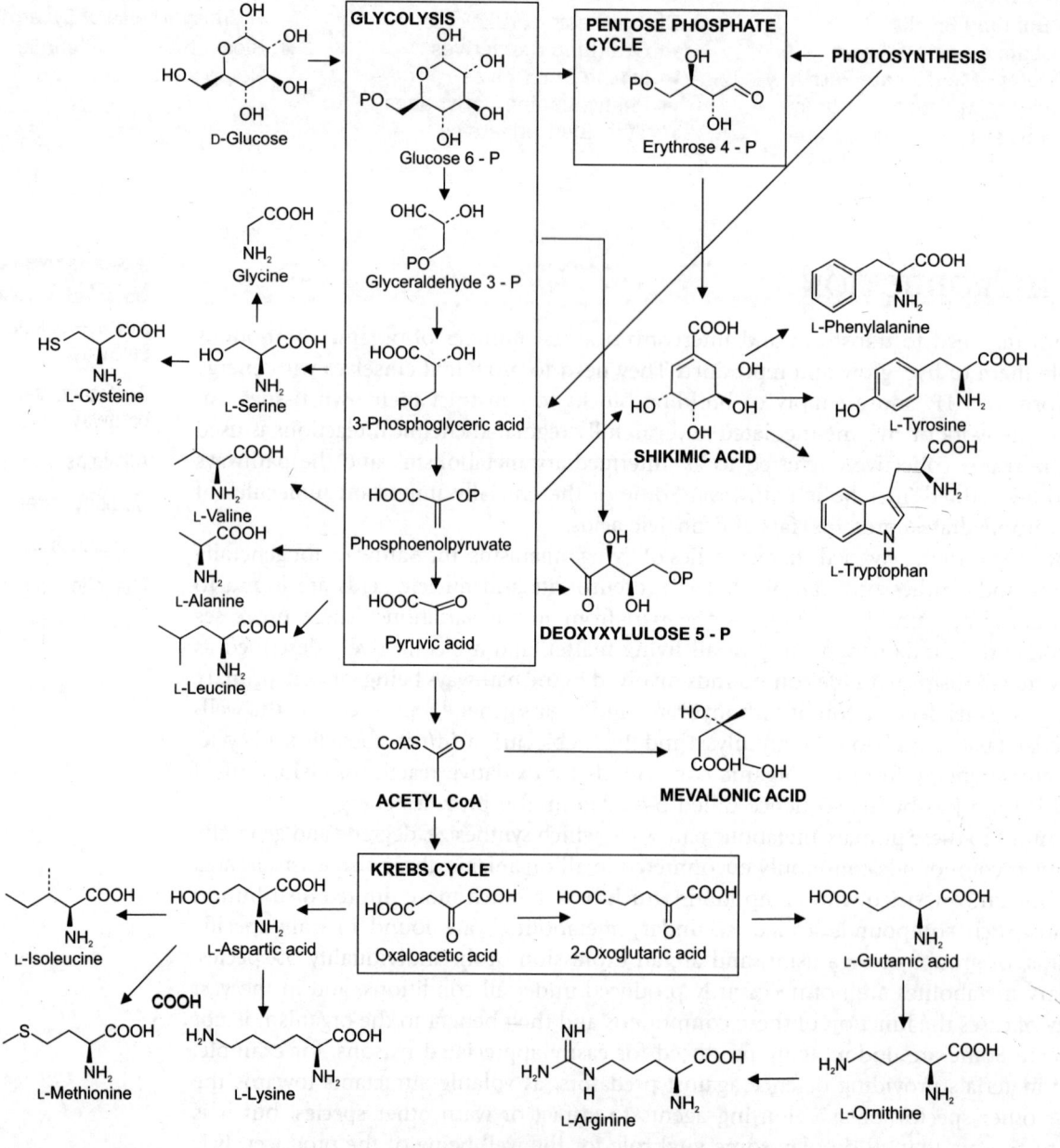

FIG. 13.1 Primary metabolismic pathways

Peptides, proteins, alkaloids and many antibiotics are derived from amino acids, and the origins of the most important amino acid components of these are briefly indicated in Figure 13.1. Intermediates from the glycolytic pathway and the Krebs cycle are used in constructing many of them, but the aromatic amino acids phenylalanine, tyrosine and tryptophan are themselves products from the shikimate pathway. Ornithine, a nonprotein amino acid,

and its homologue lysine, are important alkaloid precursors having their origins in Krebs cycle intermediates.

Relatively few building blocks are routinely employed, and the following list, though not comprehensive, includes those most frequently encountered in producing the carbon and nitrogen skeleton of a natural product.

The structural features of these building blocks are shown in Figure 13.2.

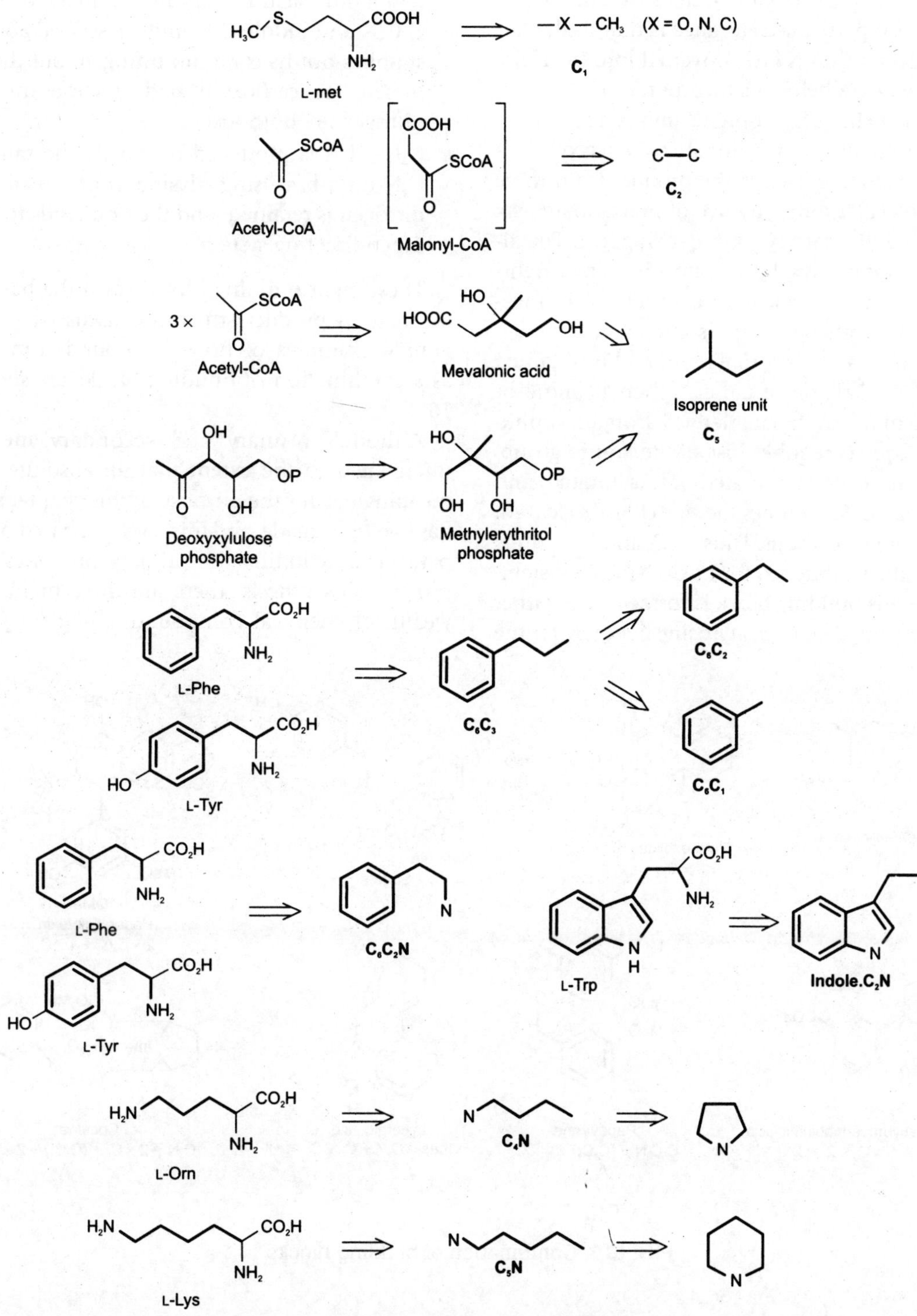

FIG. 13.2 The building blocks

- C_1: The simplest of the building blocks is composed of a single carbon atom, usually in the form of a methyl group, and most frequently it is attached to oxygen or nitrogen, but occasionally to carbon. It is derived from the S-methyl of L-methionine. The methylenedioxy group (OCH_2O) is also an example of a C_1 unit.

- C_2: A two-carbon unit may be supplied by acetyl-CoA. This could be a simple acetyl group, as in an ester, but more frequently it forms part of a long alkyl chain (as in a fatty acid) or may be part of an aromatic system (e.g. phenols). Of particular relevance is that in the latter examples, acetyl-CoA is first converted into the more reactive malonyl-CoA before its incorporation.

- C_5: The branched-chain C_5 'isoprene' unit is a feature of compounds formed from mevalonate or deoxyxylulose phosphate. Mevalonate itself is the product from three acetyl-CoA molecules, but only five of mevalonate's six carbons are used, the carboxyl group being lost. The alternative precursor deoxyxylulose phosphate, a straight-chain sugar derivative, undergoes a skeletal rearrangement to form the branched chain isoprene unit.

- C_6C_3: This refers to a phenylpropyl unit and is obtained from the carbon skeleton of either L-phenylalanine or L-tyrosine, two of the shikimate-derived aromatic amino acids. This, of course, requires loss of the amino group. The C_3 side chain may be saturated or unsaturated, and may be oxygenated. Sometimes the side chain is cleaved, removing one or two carbons. Thus, C_6C_2 and C_6C_1 units represent modified shortened forms of the C_6C_3 system.

- C_6C_2N: Again, this building block is formed from either L-phenylalanine or L-tyrosine, L-tyrosine being by far the more common. In the elaboration of this unit, the carboxyl carbon of the amino acid is removed.

- Indole.C_2N: The third of the aromatic amino acids is L-tryptophan. This indole-containing system can undergo decarboxylation in a similar way to L-phenylalanine and L-tyrosine so providing the remainder of the skeleton as an indole.C_2N unit.

- C_4N: The C_4N unit is usually found as a heterocyclic pyrrolidine system and is produced from the nonprotein amino acid L-ornithine. In marked contrast to the C_6C_2N and indole.C_2N units described above, ornithine supplies not its α-amino nitrogen, but the δ-amino nitrogen. The carboxylic acid function and the α-amino nitrogen are both lost.

- C_5N: This is produced in exactly the same way as the C_4N unit, but using L-lysine as precursor. The ε-amino nitrogen is retained, and the unit tends to be found as a piperidine ring system.

These eight building blocks form the basis of many of the natural product structures discussed in this chapter. Simple examples of how compounds can be visualized as a combination of building blocks are shown in Figure 13.3.

Although primary and secondary metabolism are interrelated to the extent that an absolute distinction is meaningless, for the purpose of this chapter some division has had to be made, and this has been based on biosynthetic pathways. Excluding the primary processes of sugar and protein biosynthesis, there are three main routes to the wealth of chemical compounds found in plants, that is,

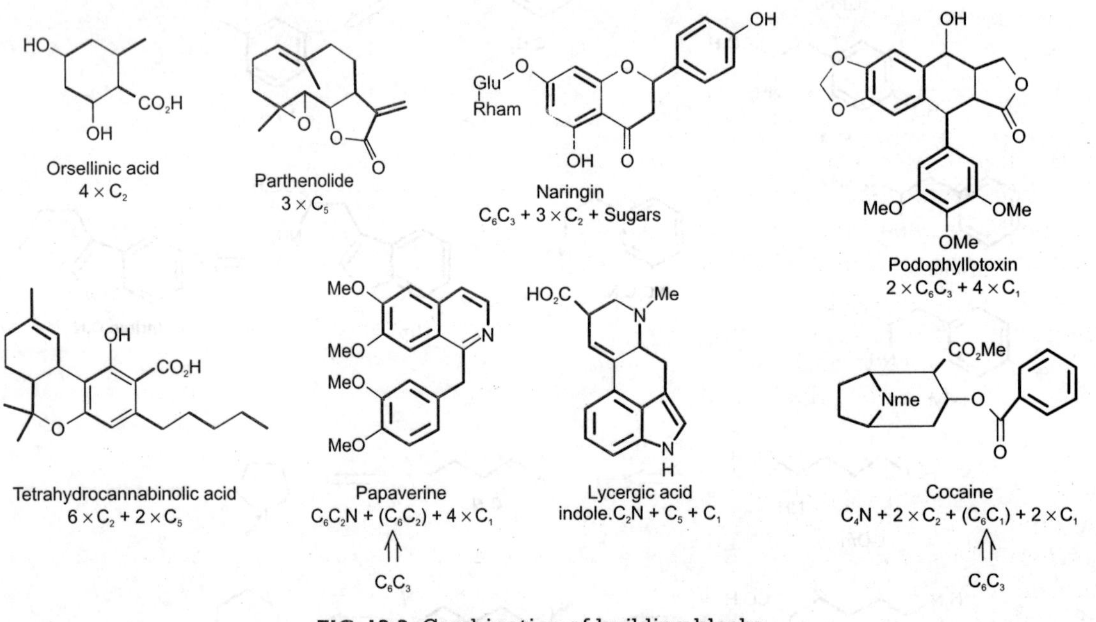

Orsellinic acid
$4 \times C_2$

Parthenolide
$3 \times C_5$

Naringin
$C_6C_3 + 3 \times C_2$ + Sugars

Podophyllotoxin
$2 \times C_6C_3 + 4 \times C_1$

Tetrahydrocannabinolic acid
$6 \times C_2 + 2 \times C_5$

Papaverine
$C_6C_2N + (C_6C_2) + 4 \times C_1$
⇑
C_6C_3

Lysergic acid
indole.$C_2N + C_5 + C_1$

Cocaine
$C_4N + 2 \times C_2 + (C_6C_1) + 2 \times C_1$
⇑
C_6C_3

FIG. 13.3 Combination of building blocks

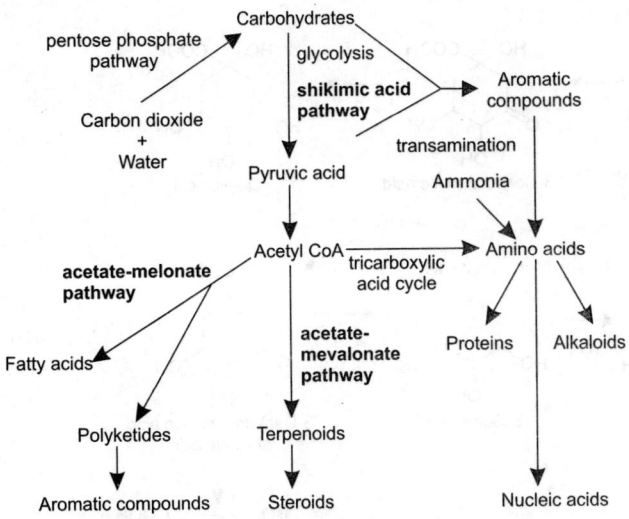

FIG. 13.4 Biosynthetic pathways in plants

shikimic acid pathways, acetate-malonate and acetate-mevalonate pathways, which are interrelated as shown in Figure 13.4.

Shikimic Acid Pathway

The shikimate pathway provides an alternative route to aromatic compounds, particularly the aromatic amino acids L-phenylalanine, L-tyrosine and L-tryptophan. This pathway is employed by microorganisms and plants, but not by animals, and accordingly the aromatic amino acids feature among those essential amino acids for men whom have to be obtained in the diet. A central intermediate in the pathway is shikimic acid, a compound which had been isolated from plants of *Illicium* species (Japanese 'shikimi') many years before its role in metabolism had been discovered. Most of the intermediates in the pathway were identified by a careful study of a series of *Escherichia coli* mutants prepared by UV irradiation. Their nutritional requirements for growth, and any by-products formed, were then characterized. A mutant strain capable of growth usually differs from its parent in only a single gene, and the usual effect is the impaired synthesis of a single enzyme. Typically, a mutant blocked in the transformation of compound A into compound B will require B for growth whilst accumulating A in its culture medium. In this way, the pathway from phosphoenolpyruvate (from glycolysis) and D-erythrose 4-phosphate (from the pentose phosphate cycle) to the aromatic amino acids was broadly outlined. Phenylalanine and tyrosine form the basis of C_6C_3 phenylpropane units found in many natural products, for example, cinnamic acids, coumarins, lignans and flavonoids, and along with tryptophan are precursors of a

wide range of alkaloid structures. In addition, it is found that many simple benzoic acid derivatives, for example, gallic acid and p-aminobenzoic acid (4-aminobenzoic acid) are produced via branch points in the shikimate pathway (Figure 13.5).

The precursors, that is, D-erythrose 4-phosphate and phosphoenolpyruvate combine to form 3-deoxy-D-arabino-heptulosonic acid-7-phosphate (DAHP), a reaction catalysed by phospho-2-oxo-3-deoxyheptonate aldolase. The enzyme, 3-dehydroquinate synthase, catalysing the cyclization of DAHP to 3-dehydroquinic acid, requires cobalt (II) and nicotinamide adenine dinucleotide (NAD) as cofactors.

The shikimic acid pathway contains several branch points, the first of these, dehydroquinic acid, can be converted either to 3-dehydroshikimic acid, which continues the pathway, or to quinic acid. The enzymes catalysing the dehydration of dehydroquinic acid are of two kinds. Form 1, associated with shikimate dehydrogenase, is independent of shikimate concentration, while form 2 is specifically activated by shikimate.

It has been suggested that the two forms provide a control in the utilization of dehydroquinic acid producing either shikimic acid or protocatechuic acid.

After phosphorylation, catalysed by shikimate kinase, shikimic acid adds on enol pyruvate to form 3-enolpyruvylshikimic acid-5-phosphate. This reaction is catalysed by enolpyruvylshikimate phosphate synthase, whereas conversion to chorismic acid is catalysed by chorismate synthase.

The formation of chorismic acid is an important branch point in the shikimic acid pathway as this compound can undergo three different types of conversion. The name 'chorismic' is derived from a Greek word for separate, indicating the multiple role of this compound. In the presence of glutamine, chorismic acid is converted to anthranilic acid, whereas chorismate mutase catalyses the formation of prephenic acid. Chorismic acid is also converted into p-aminobenzoic acid.

Then after anthranilic acid is converted first to phosphoribosylanthranilic acid and then to carboxyphenylaminodeoxyribulose-5-phosphate, these reactions being catalysed by anthranilate phosphoribosyl transferase and phosphoribosylanthranilate isomerase, respectively. Ring closure to form indolyl-3-glycerol phosphate is catalysed by indolylglycerol phosphate synthase. The enzyme catalysing the final reaction, that is, tryptophan synthase consists of two components; component A catalyses the dissociation of indolylglycerol phosphate to indole and glyceraldehydes-3-phosphate, whereas component B catalyses the direct condensation of indole with serine to form tryptophan.

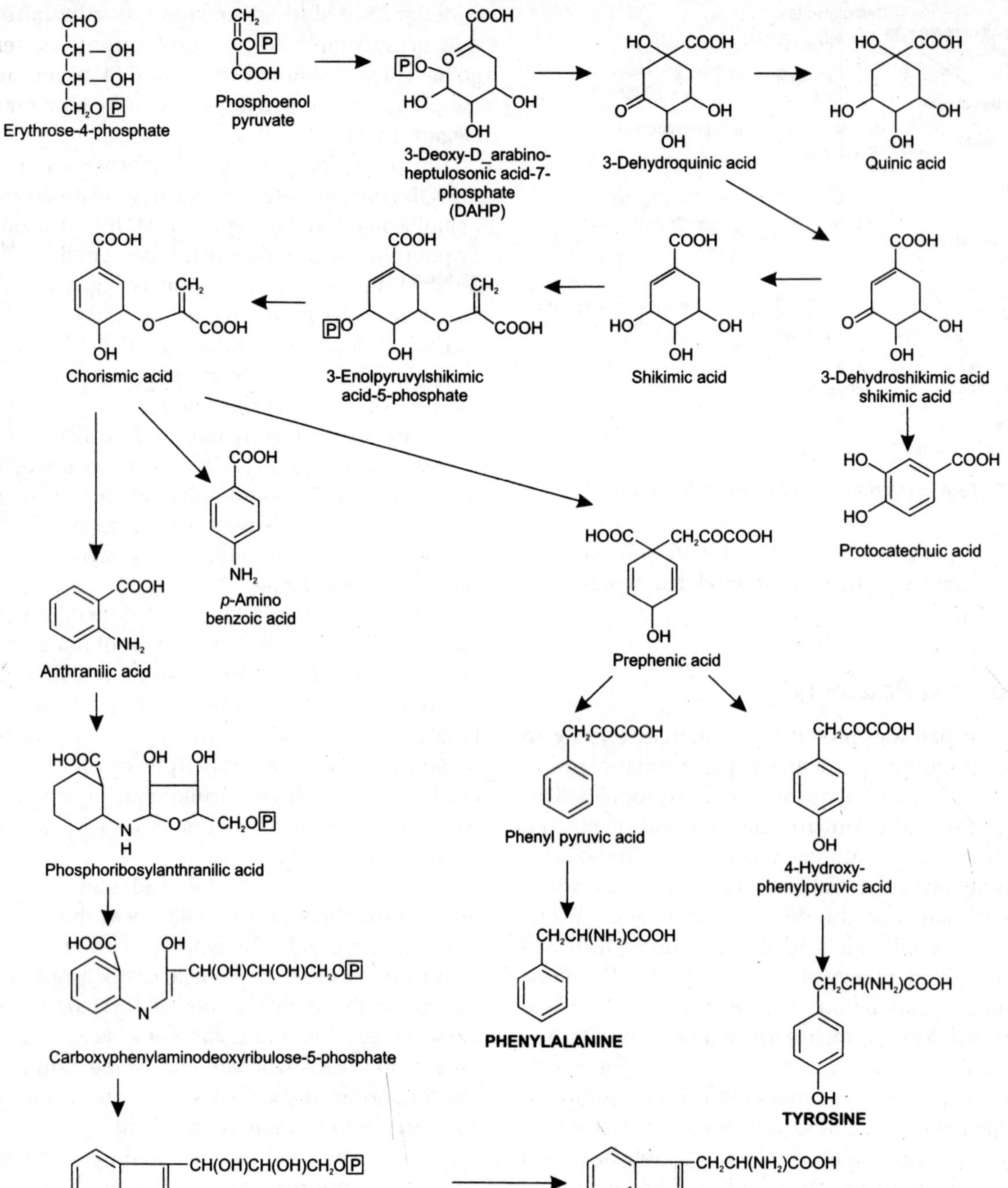

FIG. 13.5 Shikimic acid pathway

Tyrosine and phenylalanine are both biosynthesized from prephanic acid, but by independent pathways.

In the formation of tyrosine, prephanic acid is first aromatized to 4-hydroxyphenylpyruvic acid, a reaction catalysed by prephenate dehydrogenase. Transamination, catalysed by tyrosine aminotransferase, then gives tyrosine.

The biosynthesis of phenylalanine involves first the aromatization of prephanic acid to phenylpyruvic acid,

a reaction catalysed by prephenate dehydratase, and then transamination catalysed by phenylalanine aminotransferase, which gives phenylalanine.

Acetate-Mevalonate Pathway

Since a long time biochemists were aware of the involvement of acetic acid in the synthesis of cholesterol, squalene and rubber-like compounds. The discovery of acetyl coenzyme A called as 'active acetate' in 1950, further supported the role of acetic acid in biogenetic pathways. Later, mevalonic acid was found to be associated with the acetate. Mevalonic acid further produced isopentenyl pyrophosphate (IPP) and its isomer dimethylallyl pyrophosphate (DMAPP). These two main intermediates IPP and DMAPP set the 'active isoprene' unit as a basic building block of isoprenoid compounds. Both of these units yield geranyl pyrophosphate (C_{10}-monoterpenes) which further association with IPP produces farnesyl pyrophosphate (C_{15}-sesquiterpenes).

Farnesyl pyrophosphate with one more unit of IPP develops into geranyl—eranyl pyrophosphate (C_{20}-diterpenes). The farnesyl pyrophosphate multiplies with its own unit to produce squalene, and its subsequent cyclization gives rise to cyclopentanoperhydrophenantherene skeleton containing steroidal compounds like cholesterols and other groups like triterpenoids. The acetate-mevalonate pathway thus works through IPP and DMAPP via squalene to produce two different skeleton containing compounds,

that is, steroids and triterpenoids. It also produces vast array of monoterpenoids, sesquiterpenoids, diterpenoids, carotenoids, polyprenols, and also the compounds like glycosides and alkaloids in association with other pathways (Figure 13.6).

Acetate-Malonate Pathway

Acetate pathway operates functionally with the involvement of acyl carrier protein (ACP) to yield fatty acyl thioesters of ACP. These acyl thioesters forms the important intermediates in fatty acid synthesis. These C_2 acetyl CoA units at the later stage produces even number of fatty acids from n-tetranoic (butyric) to n-eicosanoic (arachidic acid). The synthesis of fatty acids is thus explained by the reactions given in Figure 13.7. Unsaturated fatty acids are produced by subsequent direct dehydrogenation of saturated fatty acids. Enzymes play important role in governing the position of newly introduced double bonds in the fatty acids.

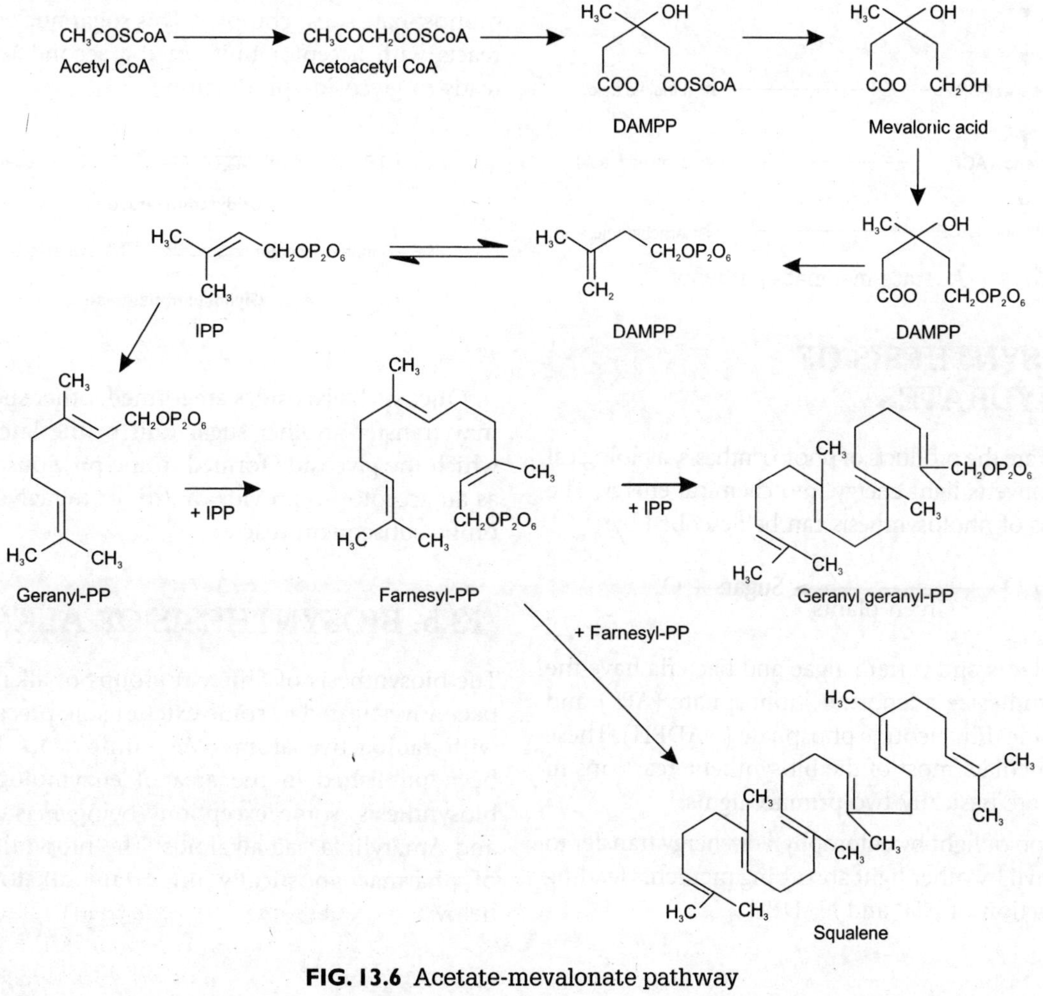

FIG. 13.6 Acetate-mevalonate pathway

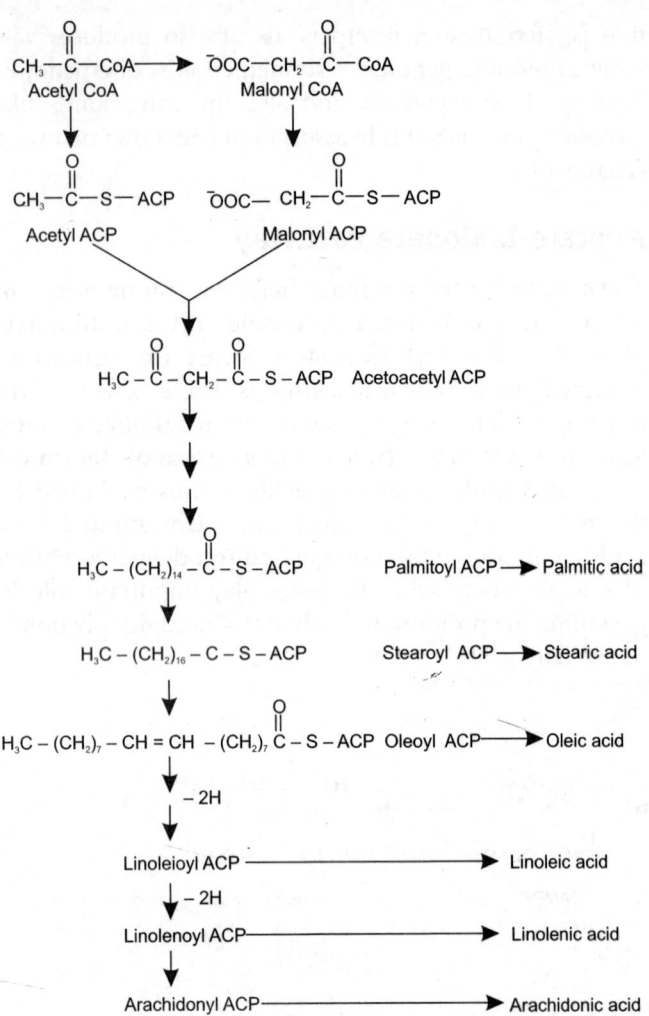

FIG. 13.7 Acetate-malonate pathway

13.3. BIOSYNTHESIS OF CARBOHYDRATES

Carbohydrates are the products of photosynthesis, a biological process that converts light energy into chemical energy. The general process of photosynthesis can be described by:

$$CO_2 + H_2O \xrightarrow[\text{Green plants}]{} \text{Sugars} + O_2$$

All green plants and certain algae and bacteria have the capacity to synthesize adenosine triphosphate (ATP) and nicotine adenine dinucleotide phosphate (NADPH). These compounds mediate most of the biosynthetic reactions in plants. There are basically two primary lights:

1. Absorption of light by chlorophyll or energy transfer to chlorophyll by other light absorbing pigments leading to production of ATP and NADPH.

2. Photolysis of water to produce oxygen and electrons which are transferred via carrier species and produces ATP and NADPH, two reactive molecules which work as activating and reducing agents.

Blackmann Reaction: In the subsequent 'dark reaction', carbon dioxide is reduced to produce four, five, six and seven carbon sugars. The reactions were firstly given by Blackmann and hence called as Blackmann reaction. It is estimated that about 4000×10^9 tons of CO_2 is fixed annually through the photosynthetic process. The path of carbon in photosynthesis was first given by Calvin is termed as Calvin cycle.

$$CO_2 + 2\ NADPH_2 + 2\ ATP \longrightarrow (CH_2O)_n + H_2O + 2\ ADP + 2\ NADPH$$
$$\text{(Carbohydrate)}$$

13.4. BIOSYNTHESIS OF GLYCOSIDES

The glycosides are the condensation products of sugar and the acceptor unit called as aglycone. The reaction occurs in two parts as given below. Firstly sugar phosphates bind with uridine triphosphate (UTP) to produce sugar—uridine diphosphate sugar complex. This sugar nucleotide complex reacts with acceptor units in the second reaction which leads to glycoside production.

UTP + Sugar 1-P $\rightleftharpoons$ UDP - Sugar + Ppi
(1)
Uridyl transferase

UDP - Sugar + Acceptor $\rightleftharpoons$ Acceptor - Sugar + UDP
(2)
Glycosyl transferase

Once such glycosides are formed, other specific enzymes may transfer another sugar unit in the later reactions in which the glycoside formed in the previous reaction work as an acceptor to provide di-, tri- or tetraglycosides and so on by subsequent reactions.

13.5. BIOSYNTHESIS OF ALKALOIDS

The biosynthesis of different groups of alkaloids has now been investigated to some extent using precursors labelled with radioactive atoms. Very little work has, however, been published in the area of enzymology of alkaloid biosynthesis, some exceptions being in studies of ergot and Amaryllidaceae alkaloids. The biosynthetic pathways of pharmacognostically important alkaloids are given below.

Ornithine Derivatives

L-Ornithine is a nonprotein amino acid forming part of the urea cycle in animals, where it is produced from L-arginine in a reaction catalysed by the enzyme arginase. In plants it is formed mainly from L-glutamate. Ornithine contains both δ- and α-amino groups, and it is the nitrogen from the former group which is incorporated into alkaloid structures along with the carbon chain, except for the carboxyl group. Thus ornithine supplies a C_4N building block to the alkaloid, principally as a pyrrolidine ring system, but also as part of the tropane alkaloids (Figure 13.8).

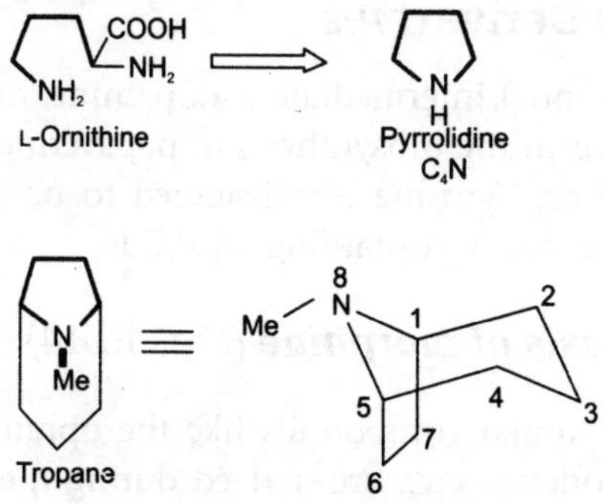

FIG. 13.8 C_4N building block

Ornithine is a precursor of the cyclic pyrrolidines that occur in the alkaloids of tobacco (nicotine, nornicotine) and in solanaceae family. Most of the tobacco alkaloids have nicotine as the starting compound. Few of the intermediates produced during the biosynthesis of tropane are also the starting compounds for hyosycamine and cocaine.

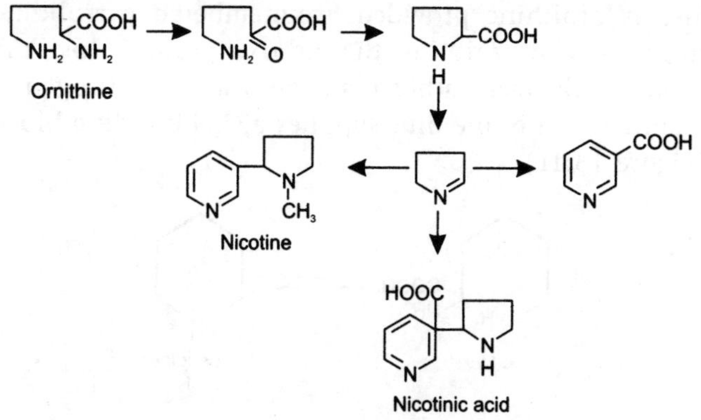

FIG. 13.9 Biosynthesis of nicotine

Biosynthesis of tropane

The starting compound of this synthesis is ornithine and methylornithine is the first intermediate.

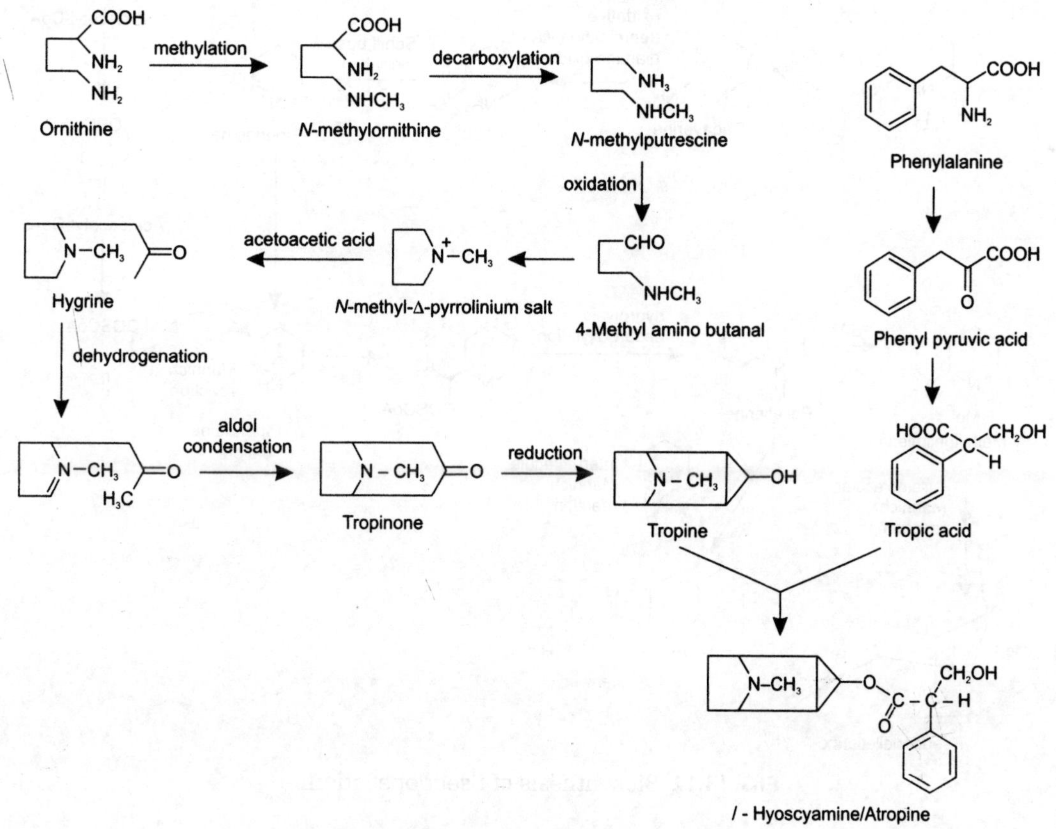

FIG. 13.10 Biosynthesis of atropine

Lysine Derivatives

L-Lysine is the homologue of L-ornithine, and it too functions as an alkaloid precursor, using pathways analogous to those noted for ornithine. The extra methylene group in lysine means this amino acid participates in forming six-membered piperidine rings, just as ornithine provided five-membered pyrrolidine rings. As with ornithine, the carboxyl group is lost, the ε-amino nitrogen rather than the α-amino nitrogen is retained, and lysine thus supplies a C_5N building block (Figure 13.11).

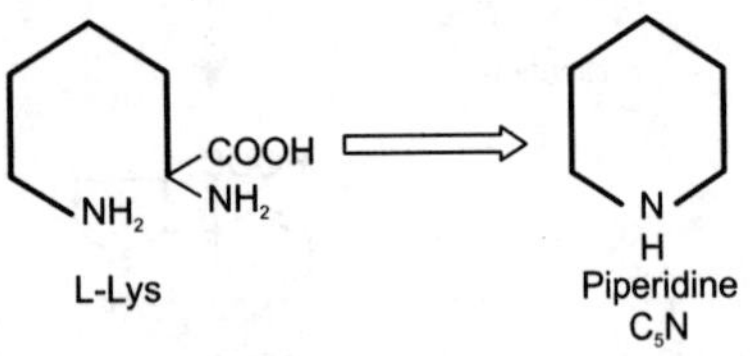

FIG. 13.11 C_5N building block

Lysine is a precursor for piperidine. Piperidine forms the basic skeleton for numerous alkaloids. Lysine and its derivatives are responsible for the biogenesis of some of the bitter principles of the lupine, lupinine, lupanine, anabasine, pelletierine and some other alkaloidal compounds.

Lycopodium, a substance obtained from Lycopodium spp., also belongs to this group.

Phenylalanine Derivatives

Whilst the aromatic amino acid L-tyrosine is a common and extremely important precursor of alkaloids, L-phenylalanine is less frequently utilized, and usually it contributes only carbon atoms, for example, C_6C_3, C_6C_2, or C_6C_1 units, without providing a nitrogen atom from its amino group. Ephedrine (Figure 13.13.), the main alkaloid in species of *Ephedra* (Ephedraceae) and a valuable nasal decongestant and bronchial dilator, is a prime example.

Tyrosine Derivatives

The first essential intermediate is dopamine; dopamine is the precursor in the biosynthesis of papaverine, berberine and morphine. Tyrosine is considered to be a precursor for the huge family containing alkaloids.

Biosynthesis of morphine (Fig. 13.14)

A range of similar compounds like the opium alkaloids, thebaine, codeine, etc., are derived during the formation of morphine.

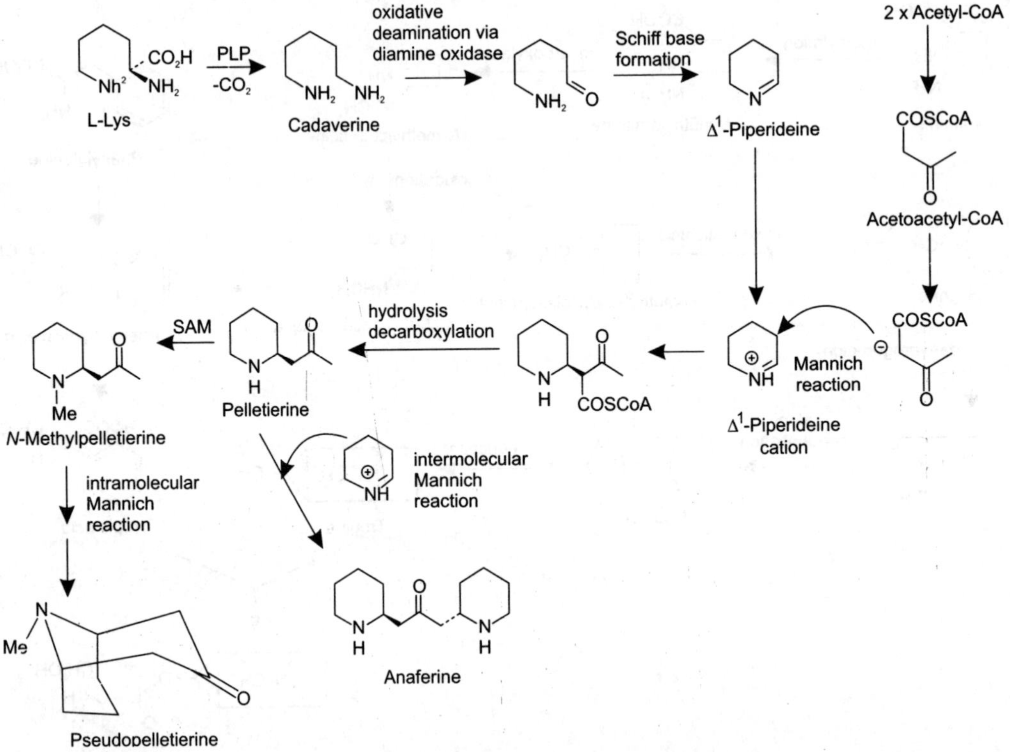

FIG. 13.12 Biosynthesis of pseudopelletierine

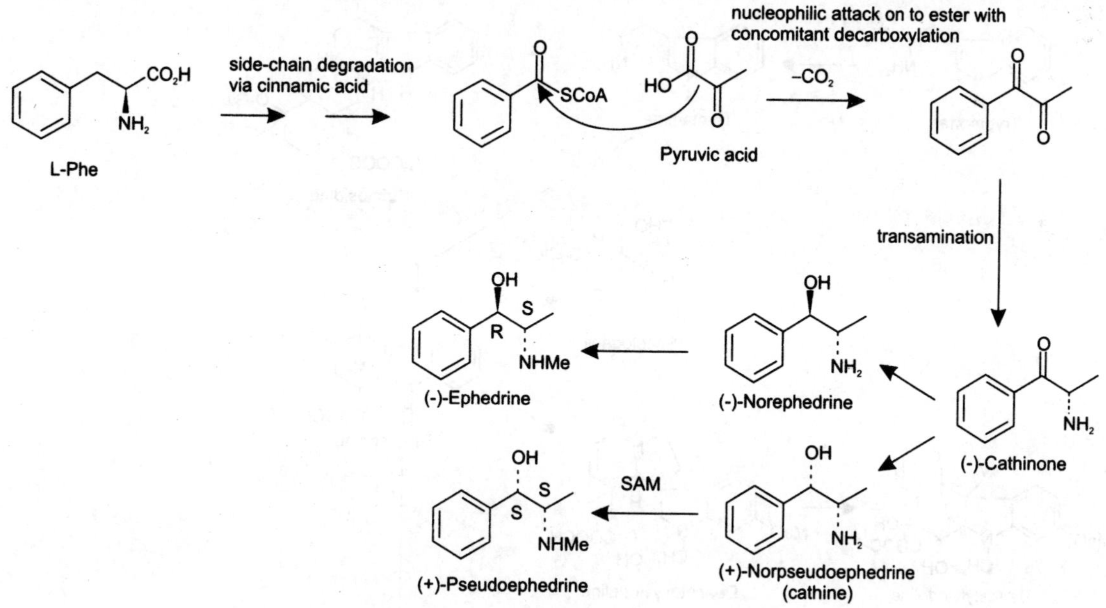

FIG. 13.13 Biosynthesis of ephedrine

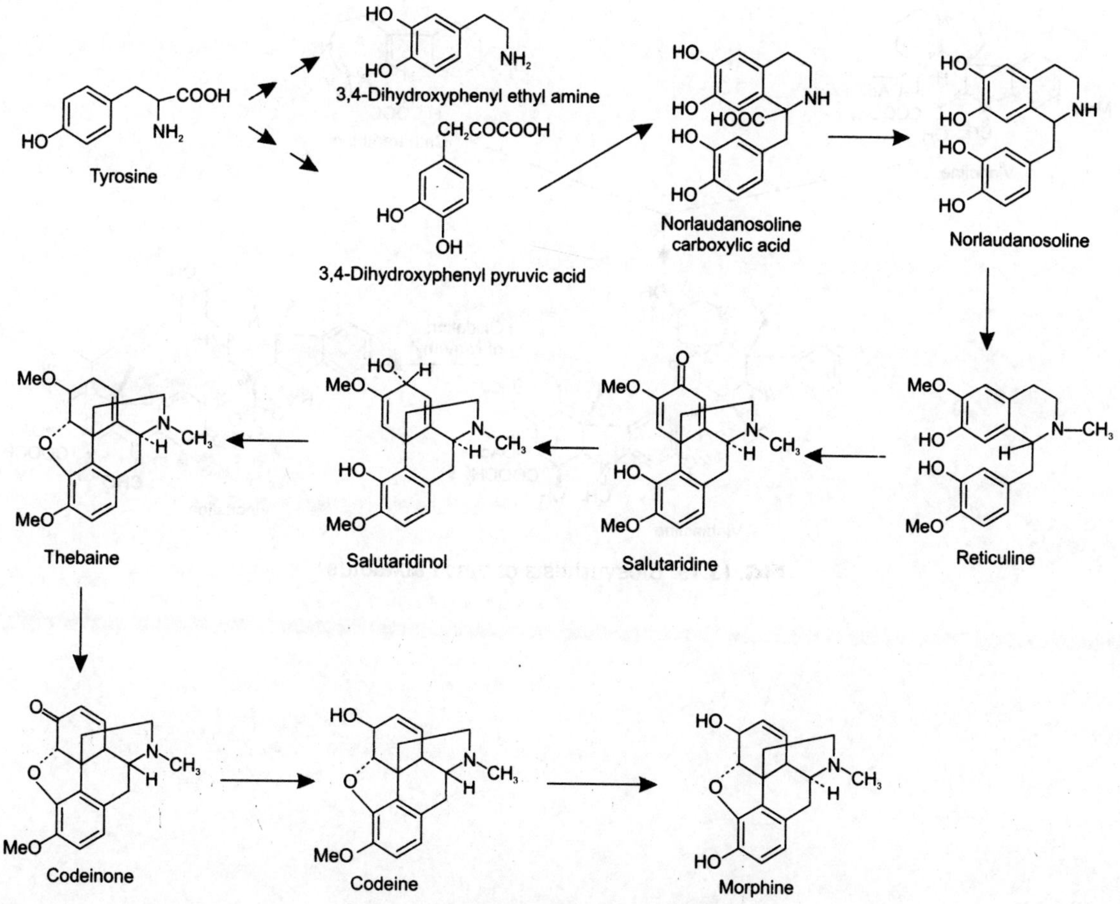

FIG. 13.14 Biosynthesis of morphine

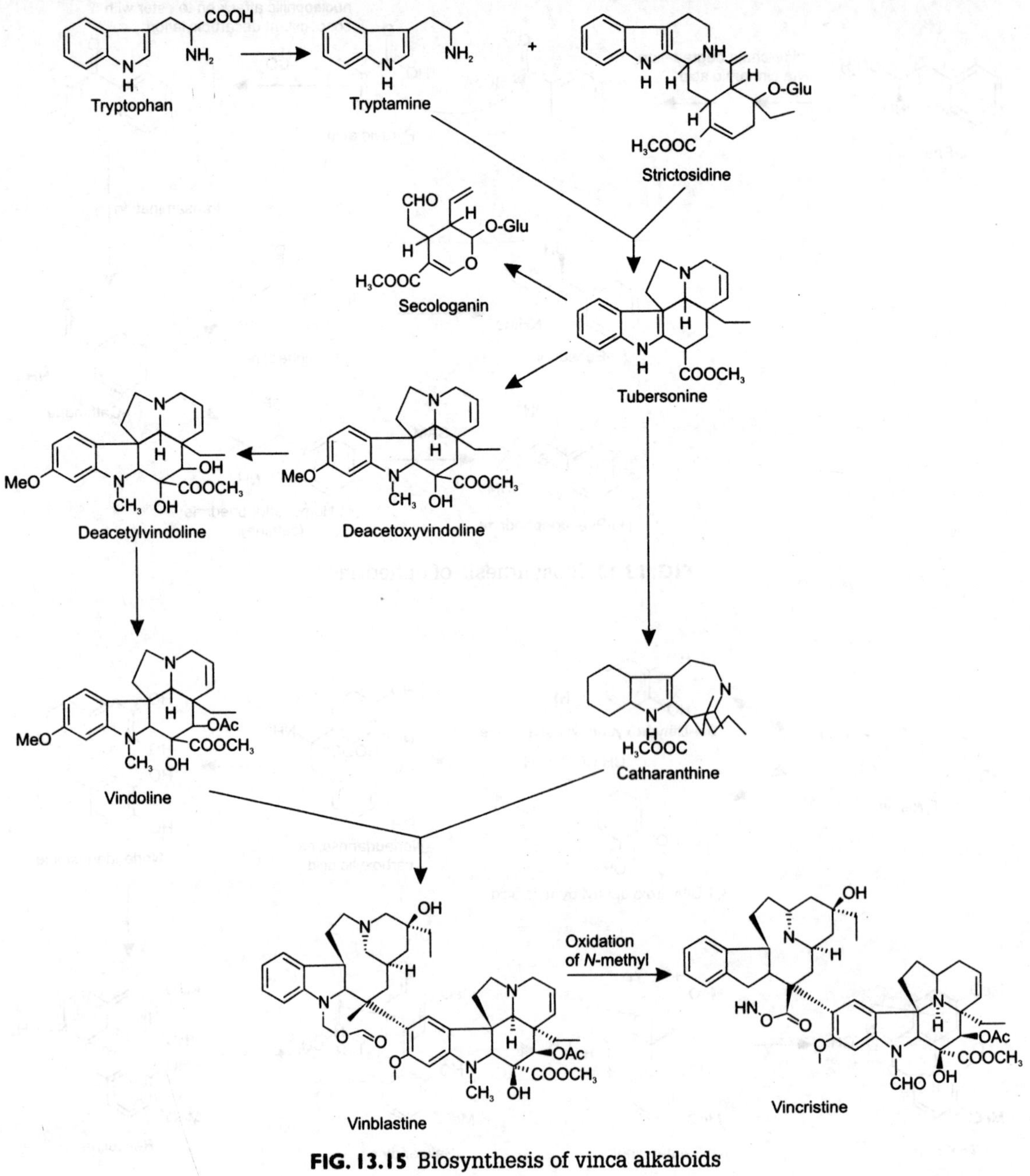

FIG. 13.15 Biosynthesis of vinca alkaloids

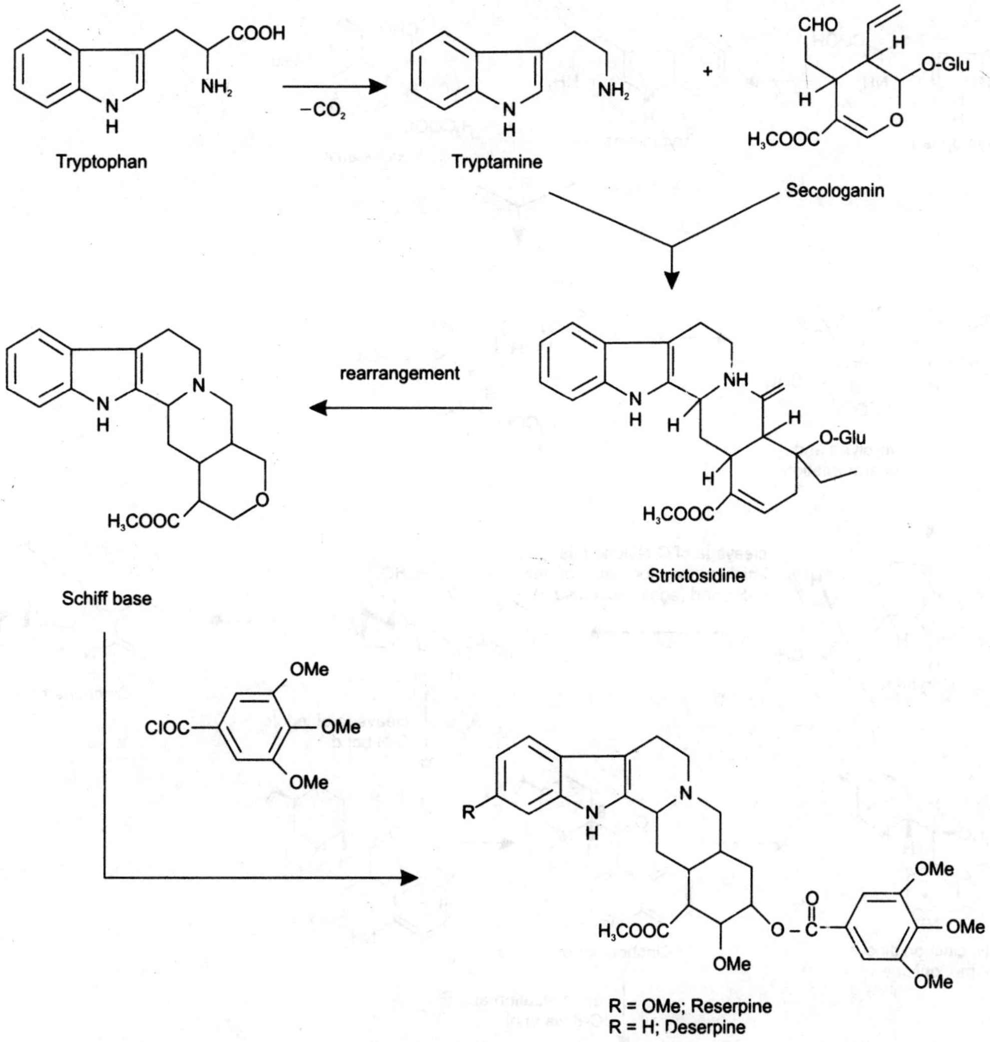

FIG. 13.16 Biosynthesis of reserpine

Tryptophan Derivatives

About 1200 dissimilar compounds, the entire of which are tryptophan derivatives have been isolated till today. The tryptophan derivatives correspond to 25% of all known alkaloids and many of them are medicinally valuable. Tryptophan and its decarboxylated product (tryptamine) are precursors for the biosynthesis of broad range of indole alkaloids of which the vinca and rauwolfia alkaloids are examples; and also in the alkaloids belonging to families like Apocynaceae, Loganiaceae and Rubiaceae. D-Tubocurarine, the active components of curare, is also a tryptophan derivative. Tryptamine on condensation with secologanin produces vincoside a nitrogenous glucoside. Some of the indole alkaloids in vinca are formed from vincoside.

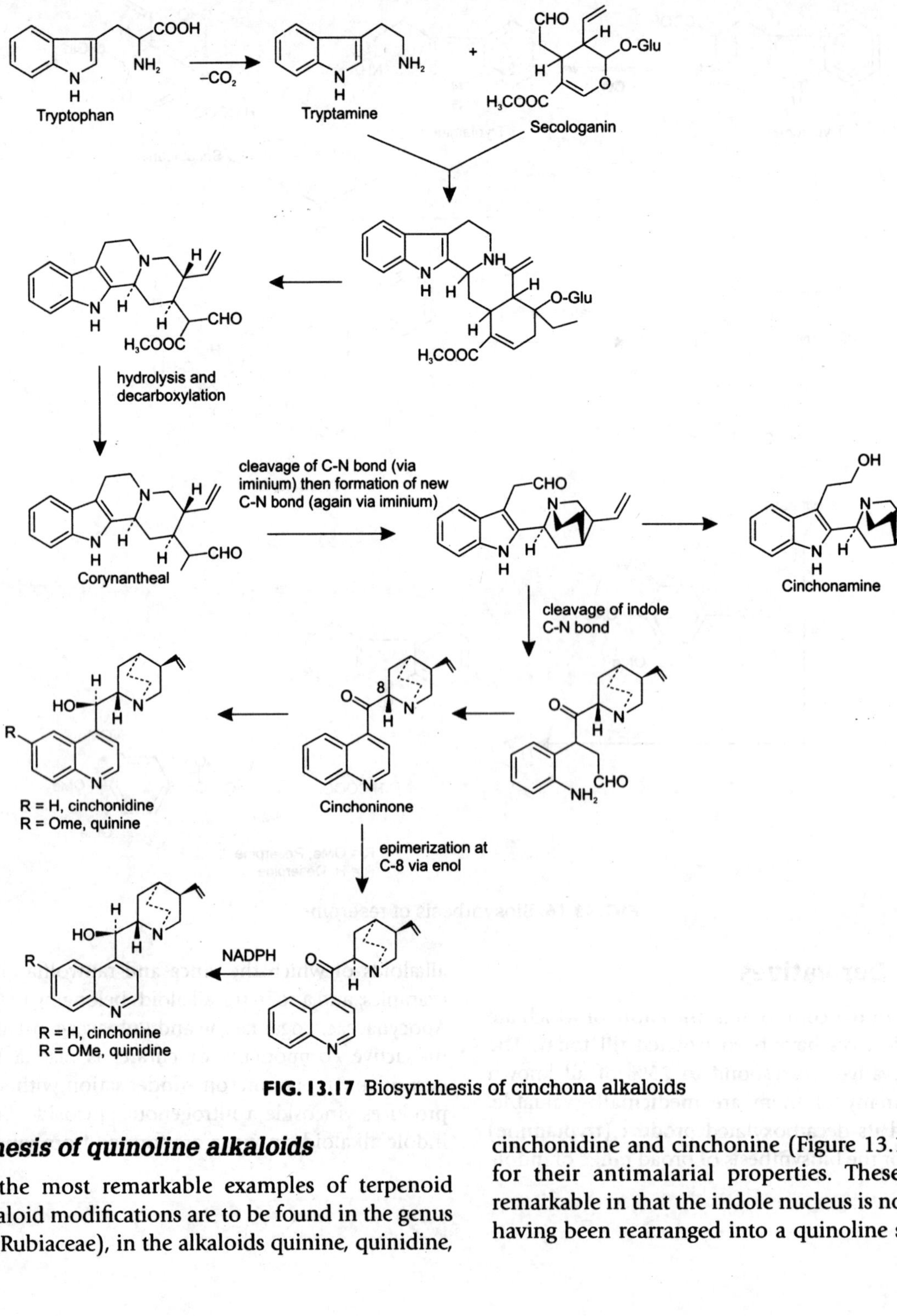

FIG. 13.17 Biosynthesis of cinchona alkaloids

Biosynthesis of quinoline alkaloids

Some of the most remarkable examples of terpenoid indole alkaloid modifications are to be found in the genus *Cinchona* (Rubiaceae), in the alkaloids quinine, quinidine, cinchonidine and cinchonine (Figure 13.17), long prized for their antimalarial properties. These structures are remarkable in that the indole nucleus is no longer present, having been rearranged into a quinoline system.

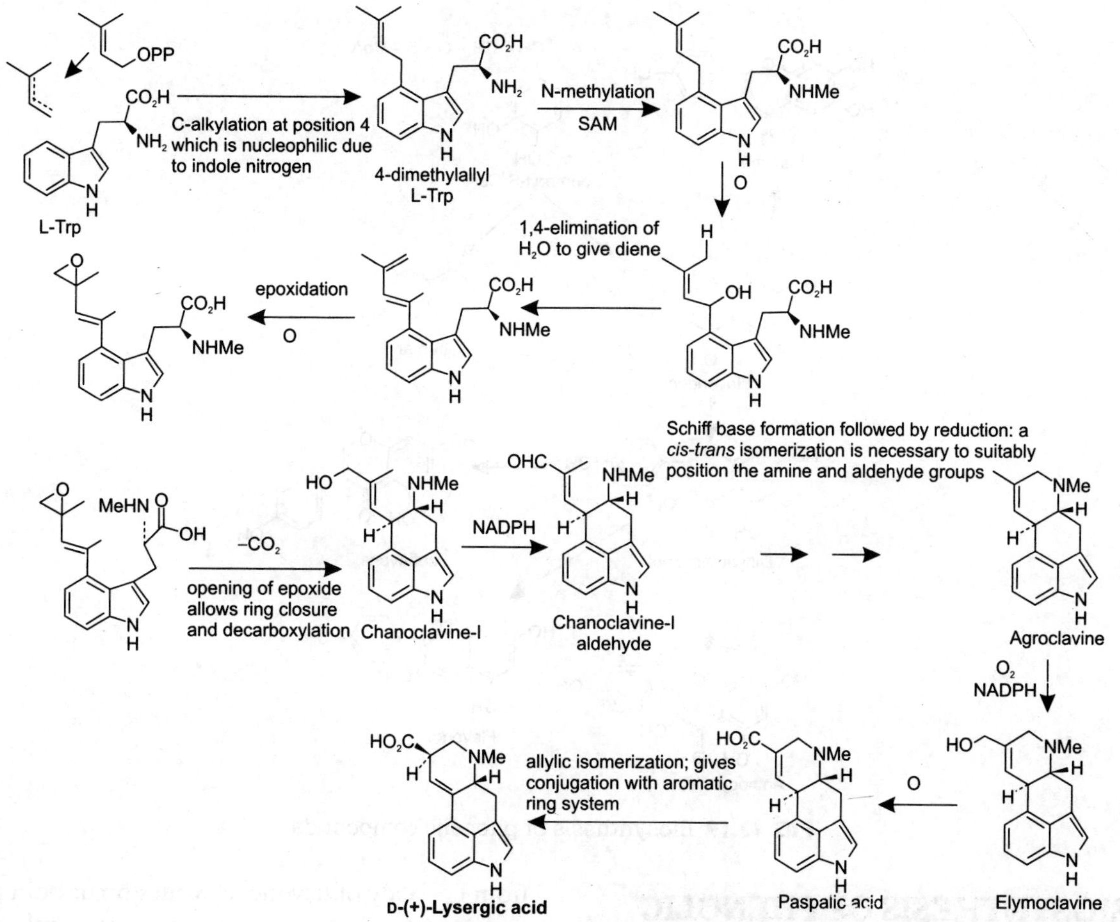

FIG. 13.18 Biosynthesis of lysergic acid

Biosynthesis of Lysergic Acid

The building blocks for lysergic acid are tryptophan (less the carboxyl group) and an isoprene unit (Figure 13.18). Alkylation of tryptophan with dimethylallyl diphosphate gives 4-dimethylallyl-L-tryptophan, which then undergoes N-methylation. Formation of the tetracyclic ring system of lysergic acid is known to proceed through chanoclavine-I and agroclavine, though the mechanistic details are far from clear. Labelling studies have established that the double bond in the dimethylallyl substituent must become a single bond on two separate occasions, allowing rotation to occur as new rings are established. This gives the appearance of *cis–trans* isomerizations as 4-dimethylallyl-L-tryptophan is transformed into chanoclavine-I, and as chanoclavine-I aldehyde cyclizes to agroclavine. A suggested sequence to account for the first of these is shown. In the later stages, agroclavine is hydroxylated to elymoclavine, further oxidation of the primary alcohol occurs giving paspalic acid, and lysergic acid then results from a spontaneous allylic isomerization.

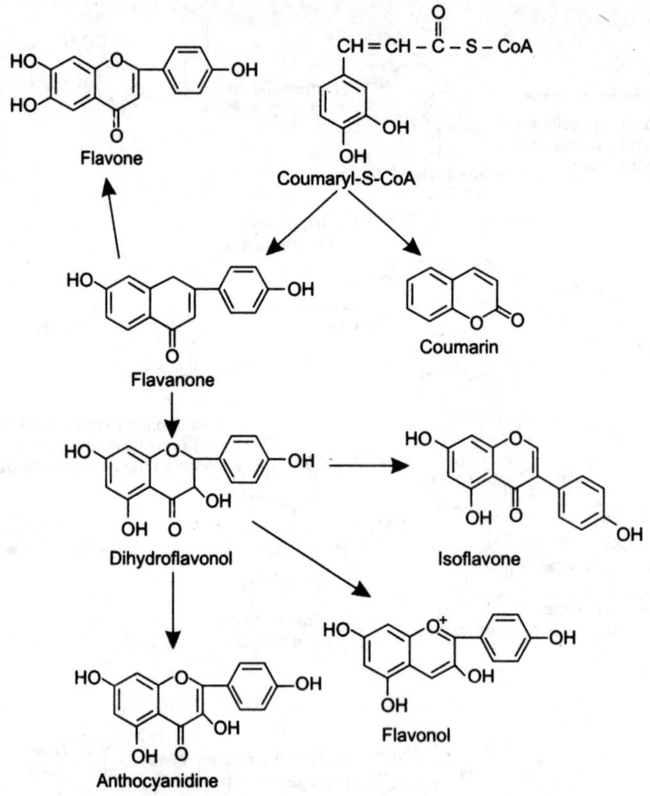

FIG. 13.19 Biosynthesis of phenolic compounds

13.6. BIOSYNTHESIS OF PHENOLIC COMPOUNDS (FIG. 13.19)

Most of the phenolic compounds belong to the category of flavonoids, with acidic nature due to the presence of –OH group in it. The flavonoids have their basic structure from C_{15} body of flavone. Flavones occur both as coloured and in colourless nature, for example, anthocyanins are normally red or yellow. They also form chelate complexes with metals and get easily oxidized to form a polymer. Some of the common phenolic compounds are coumarin, flavone, flavonol, anthrocyanidines, etc.

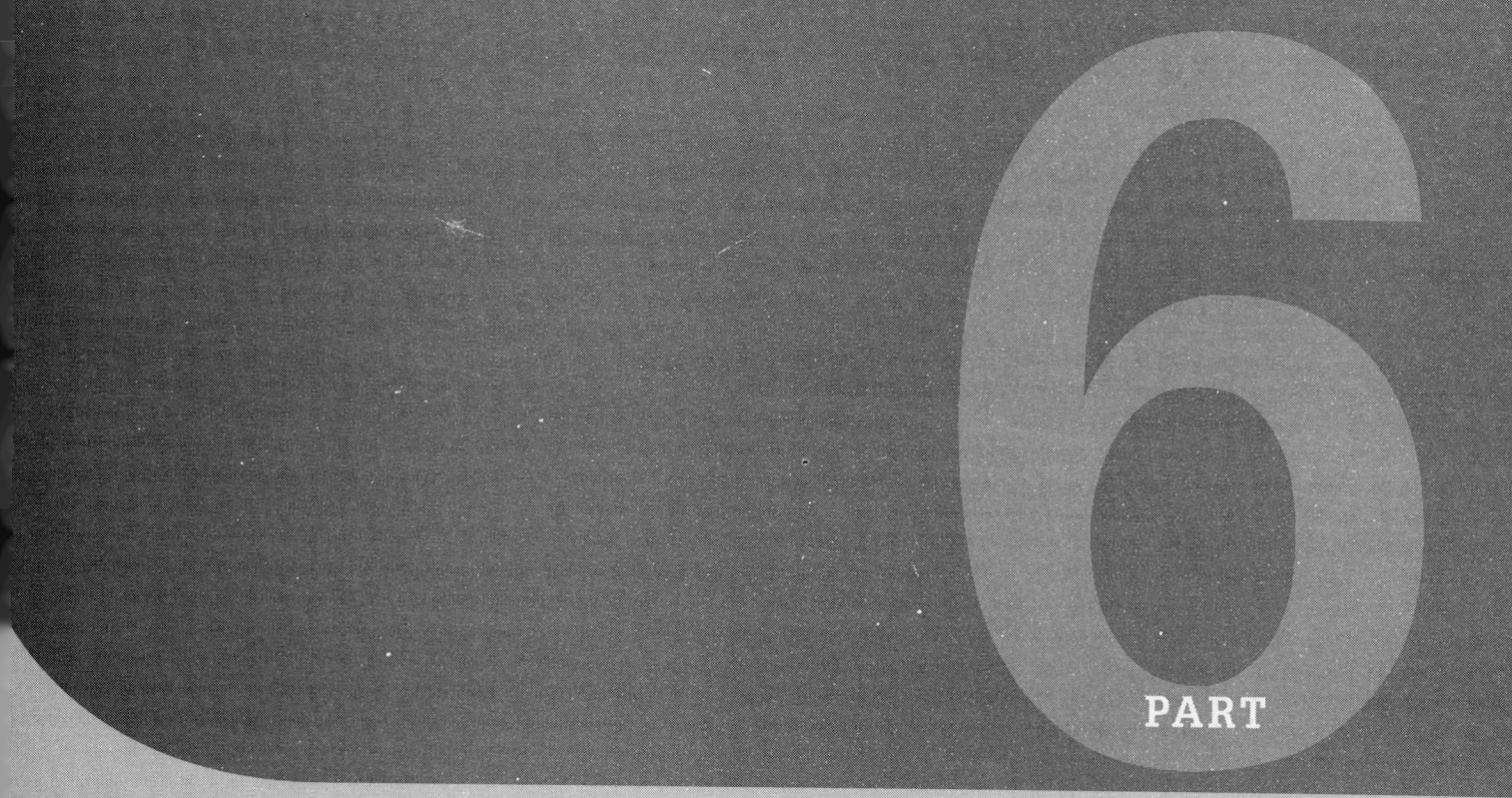

Pharmacognostical Study of Crude Drugs

Section Outline

OVERVIEW

This part provides the basic and detail information regarding the pharmacognostical study of various crude drugs coming under the category of carbohydrates, glycosides, alkaloids, resins, tannins, volatile oils, minerals and fixed oils. This part also makes students aware about the various herbal formulations of particular drugs available in the market.

CHAPTER 14

Drugs Containing Carbohydrates and Derived Products

CONTENTS

- Introduction
- Classification
- Tests for Carbohydrates
- Biosynthesis of Carbohydrates
- Acacia Gum
- Guar Gum
- Honey
- Tragacanth

- Sodium Alginate
- Pectin
- Karaya Gum
- Bael
- Agar
- Manna
- Xanthan Gum
- Ghatti Gum

- Ispaghula
- Tamarind
- Chitin
- Carrageenan
- Locust Bean Gum
- Starch

14.1. INTRODUCTION

Carbohydrates, as the name suggest, were defined as a group of compounds composed of carbon, hydrogen and oxygen in which the latter two elements are in the same proportion as in water and were expressed by a formula $(CH_2O)_n$, that is, hydrates of carbon.

The term *carbohydrates* arose from the mistaken belief that substances of this kind were hydrates of carbon, because the molecular formula of many substances could be expressed in the form $C_x(H_2O)_y$, for example, glucose ($C_6H_{12}O_6$), sucrose ($C_{12}H_{22}O_{11}$), etc. In these examples, the hydrogen and oxygen are present in the same ratio as in water. But this definition has certain drawbacks as given below:

- It should be kept in mind that all organic compounds containing hydrogen and oxygen in the proportion found in water are not carbohydrates. For example, formaldehyde HCHO for the present purpose written as $C(H_2O)$; acetic acid CH_3COOH written as $C_3(H_2O)_2$; and lactic acid $CH_3CHOHCOOH$ written as $C_3(H_2O)_3$ are not carbohydrates.

- Also, a large number of carbohydrates such as rhamnose ($C_6H_{12}O_5$), cymarose ($C_7H_{14}O_4$), digitoxose ($C_6H_{12}O_4$), etc., are known which do not contain the usual proportions of hydrogen to oxygen.

- Finally, certain carbohydrates are also known which contain nitrogen or sulphur in addition to carbon, hydrogen and oxygen.

From the above discussion, it can be concluded that the definitions described above are not correct; however, carbohydrates are now defined chemically as polyhydroxy aldehyde or polyhydroxy ketones or compound that on hydrolyses produce either of the above.

Carbohydrates are among the first products to arise as a result of photosynthesis. They constitute a large proportion of the plant biomass and are responsible, as cellulose, for the rigid cellular framework and, as starch, for providing an important food reserve. Of special pharmacognostical importance is the fact that sugars unites with a wide variety of other

KEY TERMS

compounds to form glycosides and secondary metabolites. Mucilage, as found in marshmallow root and psyllium seeds, act as water-retaining vehicles, where as gums and mucilage, which are similar in composition and properties, are formed in the plant by injury or stress and usually appear as solidified exudates; both are typically composed of uronic acid and sugar units. The cell walls of the brown seaweeds and the middle lamellae of higher plant tissues contain polysaccharides consisting almost entirely of uronic acid components.

Low molecular weight carbohydrates are crystalline, soluble in water and sweet in taste, for example, glucose, fructose, sucrose, etc. The high molecular weight carbohydrates (polymers) are amorphous, tasteless and relatively less soluble in water, for example, starch, cellulose, inulin, etc.

14.2. CLASSIFICATION

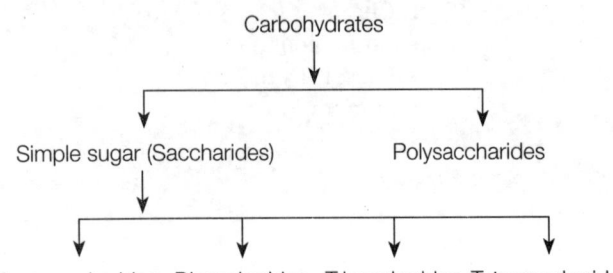

Monosaccharides

The term *monosaccharides* is employed for such sugars that on hydrolysis yield no further, lower sugars. The general formula of monosaccharides is $C_nH_{2n}O_n$. The monosaccharides are subdivided as bioses, trioses, tetroses, pentoses, hexoses, heptoses, depending upon the number of carbon atoms they possess.

Bioses

They contain two carbon atoms. They do not occur free in nature.

Trioses

They contain three carbon atoms, but in the form of phosphoric esters, for example, glyceraldehydes.

Tetroses

They contain four carbon atoms, for example, erythrose, threose, etc.

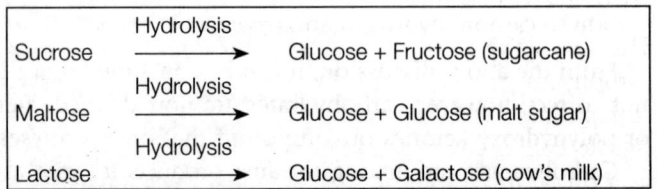

Pentoses

They are very common in plants and are the products of hydrolysis of polysaccharides like hemicelluloses, mucilages and gums, for example, ribose, arabinose and xylose.

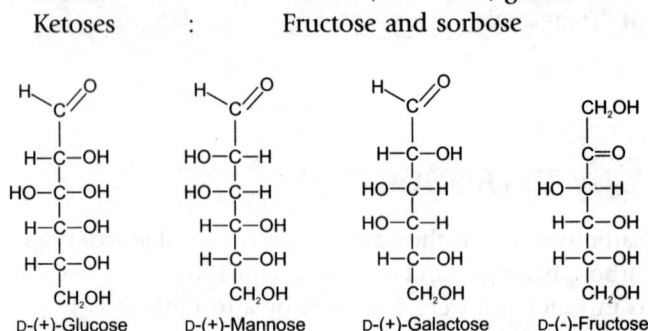

Hexoses

They are monosaccharides containing six carbon atoms and are abundantly available carbohydrates of plant kingdom. They are further divided into two types: aldoses and ketoses. They may be obtained by hydrolysis of polysaccharides like starch, insulin, etc.

Aldoses	:	Glucose, mannose, galactose
Ketoses	:	Fructose and sorbose

Heptoses

They contain seven carbon atoms, vitally important in the photosynthesis of plant and glucose metabolism of animals and are rarely found accumulated in plants, for example, glucoheptose and manoheptose.

Disaccharides

Carbohydrates, which upon hydrolysis yield two molecules of monosaccharides, are called as disaccharides.

Sucrose	Hydrolysis →	Glucose + Fructose (sugarcane)
Maltose	Hydrolysis →	Glucose + Glucose (malt sugar)
Lactose	Hydrolysis →	Glucose + Galactose (cow's milk)

Trisaccharides

As the name indicates, these liberate three molecules of monosaccharides on hydrolysis.

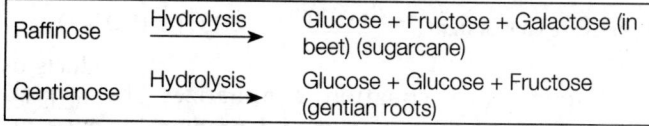

| Raffinose | Hydrolysis → | Glucose + Fructose + Galactose (in beet) (sugarcane) |
| Gentianose | Hydrolysis → | Glucose + Glucose + Fructose (gentian roots) |

Tetrasaccharides

Stachyose, a tetrasaccharide, yields on hydrolysis, four molecules of monosaccharide, found in manna.

Polysaccharides

On hydrolysis they give an indefinite number of monosaccharides. By condensation, with the elimination of water, polysaccharides are produced from monosaccharides. Depending upon the type of product of hydrolysis these are further classified as Pentosans and Hexosans. Xylan is pentosan, whereas starch, insulin and cellulose are the examples of hexosans.

Cellulose is composed of glucose units joined by β-1, 4 linkages, whereas starch contains glucose units connected with α-1, 4 and α-1, 6 units. Polyuronides, gums and mucilages are the other pharmaceutically important polysaccharide derivatives.

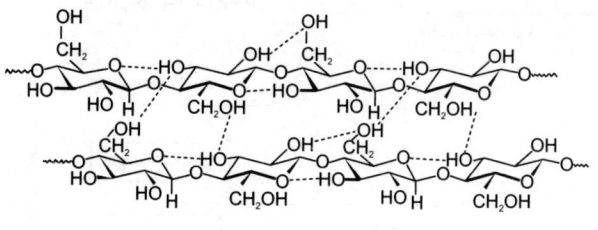

Cellulose β-1, 4 linkages

14.3. TESTS FOR CARBOHYDRATES

The following are some of the more useful tests for sugars and other carbohydrates.

Reduction of Fehling's Solution

To the solution of carbohydrate, equal quantity of Fehling's solutions A and B is added. After heating, brick red precipitate is obtained.

Molisch Test

The test is positive with soluble as well as insoluble carbohydrates. It consists of treating the compounds with α-naphthol and concentrated sulphuric acid which gives purple colour. With a soluble carbohydrate this appears as a ring if the sulphuric acid is gently poured in to form a layer below the aqueous solution. With an insoluble, carbohydrate such as cotton wool (cellulose), the colour will not appear until the acid layer is shaken to bring it in contact with the material.

Osazone Formation

Osazones are sugar derivatives formed by heating a sugar solution with phenylhydrazine hydrochloride, sodium acetate and acetic acid. If the yellow crystals which form are examined under the microscope they are sufficiently characteristic for certain sugars to be identified. It should be noted that glucose and fructose form the same osazone (glucosazone, m.p. 205°C). Before melting points are taken, osazones should be purified by recrystallization from alcohol. Sucrose does not form an osazone, but under the conditions of the above test sufficient hydrolysis takes place for the production of glucosazone.

Resorcinol Test for Ketones (Selivanoff's Test)

A crystal of resorcinol is added to the solution and warmed on a water bath with an equal volume of concentrated hydrochloric acid. A rose colour is produced if a ketone is present (e.g. fructose, honey or hydrolysed inulin).

Test for Pentoses

Heat a solution of the substance in a test tube with an equal volume of hydrochloric acid containing a little phloroglucinol. Formation of a red colour indicates pentoses.

Keller-Kiliani Test for Deoxysugars

A deoxysugar (found in cardiac glycosides) is dissolved in acetic acid containing a trace of ferric chloride and transferred to the surface of concentrated sulphuric acid. At the junction of the liquids a reddish-brown colour is produced which gradually becomes blue.

Furfural Test

A carbohydrate sample is heated in a test tube with a drop of syrupy phosphoric acid to convert it into furfural. A disk of filter paper moistened with a drop of 10% solution of aniline in 10% acetic acid is placed over the mouth of the test tube. The bottom of the test tube is heated for 30–60 s. A pink or red stain appears on the reagent paper.

Benedict's Test

Reducing sugars are usually detected with *Benedict's reagent*, which contains Cu^{2+} ions in alkaline solution with sodium citrate added to keep the cupric ions in solution. The alkaline conditions of this test causes isomeric transformation of ketoses to aldoses, resulting in all monosaccharides and most disaccharides reducing the blue Cu^{2+} ion to cuprous oxide (Cu_2O), a brick red-orange precipitate.

One millilitre of a sample solution is placed in a test tube, 2 ml of Benedict's reagent (a solution of sodium citrate and sodium carbonate mixed with a solution of copper sulphate) is added to it. The solution is then heated in a boiling water bath for 3 minutes. The formation of a reddish precipitate within 3 minutes indicates the presence of carbohydrates.

Barfoed's Test

Barfoed's solution contains cupric ions in an acidic medium. The milder condition allows oxidation of monosaccharides but does not oxidize disaccharides. If the time of heating is carefully controlled, disaccharides do not react while reducing monosaccharides give the positive result (red Cu_2O precipitate). Ketoses do not isomerize with this reagent.

One millilitre of a sample solution is placed in a test tube. Three millilitre of Barfoed's reagent (a solution of cupric acetate and acetic acid) is added to it. The solution is then heated in a boiling water bath for 3 minutes. The formation of a reddish precipitate within 3 minutes indicates the presence of carbohydrates.

Bial's Test

Bial's reagent contains orcinol (5-methylresorcinol) in concentrated HCl with a small amount of $FeCl_3$ catalyst. Pentoses are converted to furfural by this reagent, which forms a blue-green colour with orcinol. This test is used to distinguish pentoses from hexoses.

Two millilitre of a sample solution is placed in a test tube and 2 ml of Bial's reagent (a solution of orcinol, HCl and ferric chloride) is added. The solution is then heated gently on a Bunsen burner or in hot water bath. If the colour is not obvious, more water can be added to the tube. The formation of a bluish product indicates the presence of pentoses. All other colours indicate a negative result for pentoses. Note that hexoses generally react to form green, red or brown products.

14.4. BIOSYNTHESIS OF CARBOHYDRATES

Production of Monosaccharides by Photosynthesis

Carbohydrates are products of photosynthesis, a biologic process that converts electromagnetic energy into chemical energy. In the green plant, photosynthesis consists of two classes of reactions. One class comprises the so-called light reactions that actually convert electromagnetic energy into chemical potential. The other class consists of the enzymatic reactions that utilize the energy from the light reactions to fix carbon dioxide into sugar. These are referred to as the dark reactions. The results of both of these types of reactions are most simply summarized in the following equation:

$$2H_2O + CO_2 + light \xrightarrow{\text{chlorophyll}} (CH_2O) + H_2O + O_2$$

Although this equation summarizes the overall relationships of the reactants and products, it gives no clue as to the nature of the chemical intermediates involved in the process. The elucidation of the reactions by which carbon dioxide is accepted into an organic compound and ultimately into sugars with regeneration of the carbon dioxide acceptor was a major achievement in biosynthetic research. The pathway of carbon in photosynthesis, as worked out primarily by Calvin and coworkers, is presented in Figure 14.1.

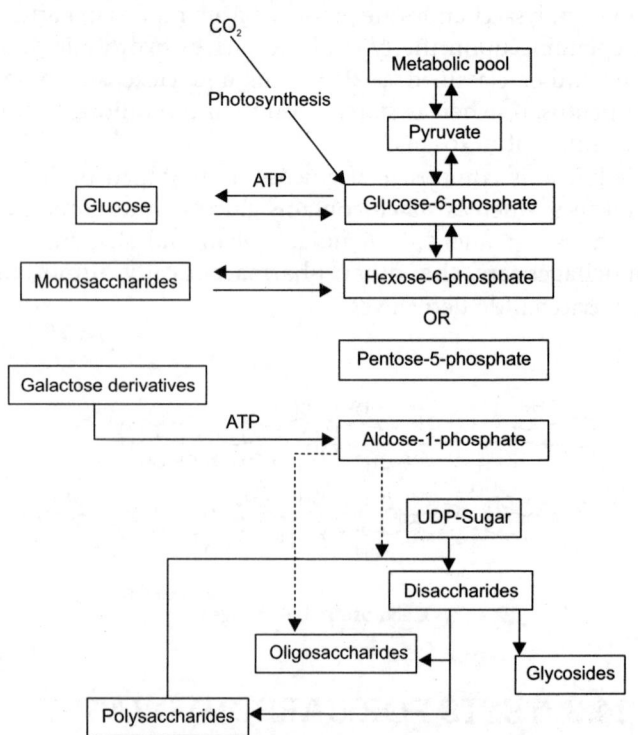

FIG. 14.1 Carbohydrate biosynthesis

Production of sucrose

Sucrose is of considerable metabolic importance in higher plants. Studies have shown that sucrose is not only the first sugar formed in photosynthesis but also the main transport material. Newly formed sucrose is, therefore, probably the usual precursor for polysaccharide synthesis. Although an alternative pathway consisting of a reaction between glucose 1-phosphate and fructose is responsible for sucrose production in certain microorganisms, the biosynthesis of this important metabolite in higher plants apparently occurs as shown in Figure 14.2.

Fructose 6-phosphate, derived from the photosynthetic cycle, is converted to glucose 1-phosphate, which, in turn, reacts with UTP to form UDP-glucose. UDP-glucose either reacts with fructose 6-phosphate to form first sucrose phosphate and ultimately sucrose, or with fructose to form sucrose directly. Once formed, the free sucrose may either remain *in situ* or may be translocated via the sieve tubes to various parts of the plants. A number of reactions, for example, hydrolysis by invertase or reversal of the synthetic sequence, convert sucrose to monosaccharides from which other oligosaccharides or polysaccharides may be derived.

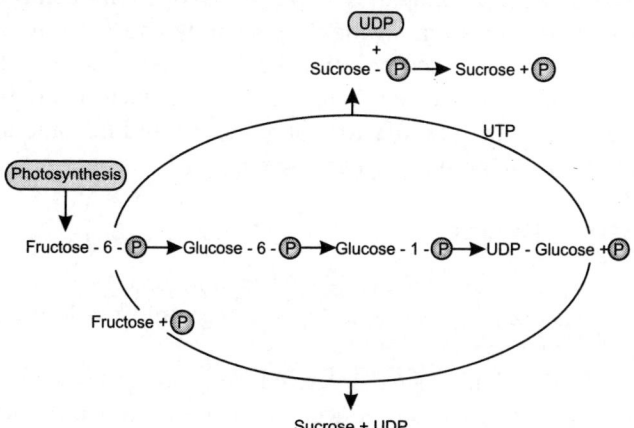

FIG. 14.2 Pathways of sucrose biosynthesis

ACACIA GUM

Synonyms

Acacia gum, Acacia vera, Egyptian thorn, Gummi africanum, Gum Senegal, Gummae mimosae, Kher, Sudan gum arabic, Somali gum, Yellow thorn, Indian Gum and Gum Arabic.

Biological Source

According to the USP, acacia is the dried gummy exudation obtained from the stems and branches of *Acacia senegal* (L.) Willd or other African species of Acacia. In India, it is found as dried gummy exudation obtained from the stems and branches of *Acacia arabica* Willd, belonging to family Leguminosae

Geographical Source

Acacia senegal (Fig. 14.3) is the characteristic species in the drier parts of Anglo-Egyptian Sudan and the northern Sahara, and is to be found throughout the vast area from Senegal to the Red Sea and to eastern India. It extends southwards to northern Nigeria, Uganda, Kenya, Tanzania and southern Africa. The plant is extensively found in Arabia, Kordofan (North-East Africa), Sri Lanka and Morocco. In India it is found chiefly in Punjab, Rajasthan and Western Ghats. Sudan is the major producer of this gum and caters for about 85% of the world supply.

Cultivation and Collection

Acacia is a thorny tree up to 6 m in height. In Sudan, gum is tapped from specially cultivated trees while in Senegambia,

because of extremes of climate; cracks are produced on the tree and the gum exudes and is collected from the wild plants. Acacia trees can be cultivated by sowing the seeds in the poor, exhausted soil containing no minerals. The trees also grow as such by seed-dispersal.

Gum is collected by natives from 6 to 8 years old trees, twice a year in dry weather in November or in February—March. Natives cut the lower thorny branches to facilitate the working and by means of an axe make 2–3 ft long and 2–3 inches broad incision on the stem and branches, loosen the bark by axe and remove it, taking care not to injure the cambium and xylem. Usually they leave a thin layer of bark on xylem. If xylem is exposed, white ant enters the plant and gum is not produced. After injury in winter gum exudes after 6–8 weeks while in summer after 3–4 weeks. It is believed that bacteria finding their way through the incision are more active in summer and gum is produced quickly. The exuded gum is scraped off, collected in leather bags and then is cleaned by separating debris of bark and wood and separating sand, etc., by sieving.

Gum is dried in the sun by keeping it in trays in thin layers for about 3 weeks when bleaching takes place and it becomes whiter. This result in uneven contraction and cracks and fissures are formed on its outer surface and as a result original transparent gum becomes opaque. This process is called ripening of the gum.

Morphology

Colour	Tears are usually white, pale-yellow and sometimes creamish-brown to red in colour. The powder has off-white, pale-yellow or light-brown in appearance.
Odour	Odourless
Taste	Bland and mucilaginous
Shape and size	Tears are mostly spheroidal or ovoid in shape and having a diameter of about 2.5–3.0 cm
Appearance	Tears are invariably opaque either due to the presence of cracks or fissures produced on the outer surface during the process or ripening. The fracture is usually very brittle in nature and the exposed surface appears to be glossy.

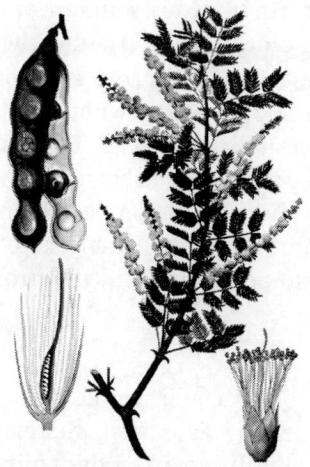

FIG. 14.3 *Acacia senegal*

History

Gum was brought from the Gulf of Aden to Egypt in the 17th B.C., and in the works of Theophrastus it is spoken of as a product of Upper Egypt. The West African product was imported by the Portuguese in the fifteenth century. Until quite recently, commerce in the Sudan was in the hands of a number of local merchants, but it is now entirely controlled by the Gum Arabic Company Ltd., a concessional company set up by the Sudanese Government. This Company alone produces about 40,000 tonnes per annum.

Chemical constituents

Acacia consists principally of arabin, which is a complex mixture of calcium, magnesium and potassium salts of arabic acid. Arabic acid is a branched polysaccharide that yields L-arabinose, D-galactose, D-glucuronic acid and L-rhamnose on hydrolysis. 1,3-Linked D-galactopyranose units form the backbone chain of the molecule and the terminal residues of the 1,6-linked side chains are primarily uronic acids. Acacia contains 12–15% of water and several occluded enzymes such as oxidases, peroxidases and pectinases. The total ash content should be in the range of 2.7–4.0%.

Chemical Tests

1. **Lead acetate test:** An aqueous solution of acacia when treated with lead acetate solution yields a heavy white precipitate.
2. **Reducing sugars test:** Hydrolysis of an aqueous solution of acacia with dilute HCl yields reducing sugars whose presence are ascertained by boiling with Fehling's solution to give a brick-red precipitate of cuprous oxide.
3. **Blue colouration due to enzyme:** When the aqueous solution of acacia is treated with benzidine in alcohol together with a few drops of hydrogen peroxide (H_2O_2), it gives rise to a distinct blue colour due to the presence of oxidases enzyme.
4. **Borax test:** An aqueous solution of acacia affords a stiff translucent mass on treatment with borax.
5. **Specific test:** A 10% aqueous solution of acacia fails to produce any precipitate with dilute solution of lead acetate (a clear distinction from Agar and Tragacanth); it does not give any colour change with Iodine solution (a marked distinction from starch and dextrin); and it never produces a bluish-black colour with $FeCl_3$ solution (an apparent distinction from tannins).

Uses

The mucilage of acacia is employed as a demulcent. It is used extensively as a vital pharmaceutical aid for emulsification and to serve as a thickening agent. It finds its enormous application as a binding agent for tablets, for example, cough lozenges. It is used in the process of 'granulation' for the manufacturing of tablets. It is considered to be the gum of choice by virtue of the fact that it is quite compatible with other plant hydrocolloids as well as starches, carbohydrates and proteins. It is used in combination with gelatin to form conservates for micro-encapsulation of drugs. It is employed as colloidal stabilizer. It is used extensively in making of candy and other food products. Gum acacia solution has consistency similar to blood and is administered intravenously in haemodialysis. It is used in the manufacture of adhesives and ink, and as a binding medium for marbling colours.

Allied Drugs

Talka gum is usually much broken and of very variable composition, some of the tears being almost colourless and others brown.

Ghatti or *Indian gum* is derived from *Anogeissus latifolia* (Combretaceae). It is produced in much the same localities as sterculia gum, and is harvested and prepared in a similar manner. It resembles talka in possessing tears of various colours. Some of the tears are vermiform in shape and their surface shows fewer cracks than even the natural acacia. Aqueous dispersions of the gum have a viscosity intermediate between those of acacia and sterculia gums.

West African Gum Combretum, obtained from *Combretum nigricans,* is not permitted as a food additive but is exploited as an adulterant of gum arabic. Unlike the latter in which the rhamnose and uronic acid units are chain terminal, in gum combretum these moieties are located within the polysaccharides chain.

Many other gums of the acacia type are occasionally met with in commerce, and many gum exudates of the large genus *Acacia* have been given chemotaxonomic consideration.

Toxicology

Acacia is essentially nontoxic when ingested. Allergic reactions to the gum and powdered forms of acacia have been reported and include respiratory problems and skin lesions.

Acacia contains a peroxidase enzyme, which is typically destroyed by brief exposure to heat. If not inactivated, this enzyme forms coloured complexes with certain amines and phenols and enhances the destruction of many pharmaceutical products including alkaloids and readily oxidizable compounds, such as some vitamins. Acacia gum reduces the antibacterial effectiveness of the preservative methyl-*p*-hydroxybenzoate against *Pseudomonas aeruginosa* presumably by offering physical barrier protection to the microbial cells from the action of the preservative. A trypsin inhibitor also has been identified, but the clinical significance of the presence of this enzyme is not known.

Marketed Product

Dental cream and Evecare syrup and capsule manufactured by Himalaya Drug Company.

GUAR GUM

Synonyms

Guar gum, Jaguar gum, Guar flour and Decorpa.

Biological Source

Guar gum is a seed gum produced from the powdered endosperm of the seeds of *Cyamopsis tetragonolobus* Linn. belonging to family Leguminosae (Fig. 14.4).

Geographical Source

Guar or cluster bean is a drought-tolerant annual legume that was introduced into the United States from India in 1903. Commercial production of guar in the United States began in the early 1950s and has been concentrated in northern Texas and south-western Oklahoma. The major world suppliers are India, Pakistan and the United States, Australia and Africa. Rajasthan in western India is the major guar-producing state, accounting for 70% of the production. Guar is also grown in Gujarat, Haryana, Punjab and in some parts of Uttar Pradesh and Madhya Pradesh. India grows over 850,000 tons, or 80% of the total guar produced all over the world. 75% of the guar gum or derivatives produced in India are exported, mainly to the United States and to European countries.

Cultivation, Collection and Preparation

The plant of gaur gum is draught resistance and quite hardy in its constitutions. It is generally shown in May–June and harvested in September–October. At the stage of full maturity, the plant yields 600–800 lb of seeds per acre under un-irrigated conditions but the production nearly doubles under irrigated conditions.

First of all the fully developed white seeds of guar gum are collected and freed from any foreign substances. The sorted seeds are fed to a mechanical 'splitter' to obtain the bifurcated guar seeds which are then separated into husk and the respective cotyledons having the 'embryo'. The gum is found into the endosperm. Generally, the guar seeds comprise the endosperm 35–40%, germ (or embryo) 45–50% and husk 14–17%.

The cotyledons, having a distinct bitter taste are separated from the endosperm by the process called 'winnowing'. The crude guar gum, that is, the endosperms is subsequently pulverized by means a 'micro-pulverizer' followed by grinding. The relatively softer cotyledons sticking to the endosperms are separated by mechanical 'sifting' process.

Thus, the crude guar gum is converted to a purified form (i.e. devoid of cotyledons), which is then repeatedly pulverized and shifted for several hours till a final white powder or granular product is obtained.

Morphology

Colour	It is colourless or pale yellowish-white coloured powder
Odour	Characteristic
Taste	Gummy

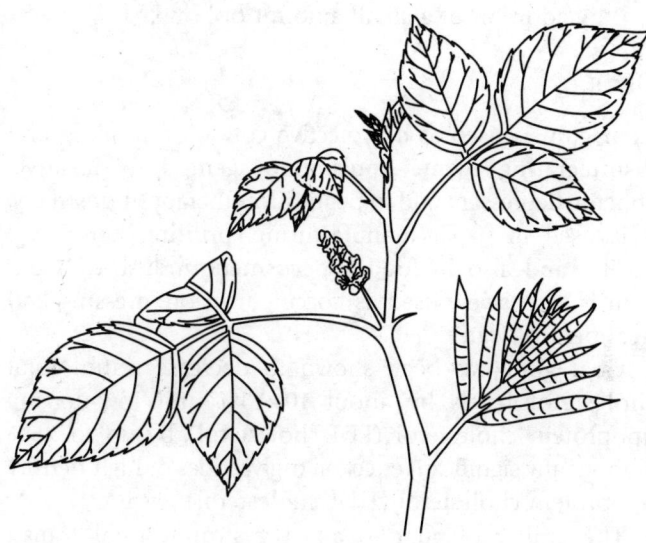

FIG. 14.4 *Cyamopsis tetragonolobus*

History

Guar gum is a dietary fibre obtained from the endosperm of the Indian cluster bean. The endosperm can account for more than 40% of the seed weight and is separated and ground to form commercial guar gum.

Guar gum has been used for centuries as a thickening agent for foods and pharmaceuticals. It continues to find extensive use for these applications and also is used by the paper, textile and oil-drilling industries.

Chemical Constituents

The water-soluble part of guar gum contains mainly of a high molecular weight hydrocolloidal polysaccharide, that is, galactomannan, which is commonly known as guaran. Guaran consists of linear chains of $(1{\rightarrow}4)$—β—D—mannopyranosyl units with α—D—galactopyranosyl units attached by $(1{\rightarrow}6)$ linkages. However, the ratio of D—galactose to D—mannose is 1: 2. The gum also contains about 5–7% of proteins.

Chemical Tests

1. On being treated with iodine solution (0.1 N), it fails to give olive-green colouration.

2. It does not produce pink colour when treated with ruthenium red solution (distinction from sterculia gum and agar).
3. A 2% solution of lead acetate gives an instant white precipitate with guar gum (distinction from sterculia gum and acacia).
4. A solution of guar gum (0.25 g in 10 ml of water) when mixed with 0.5 ml of benzidine (1% in ethanol) and 0.5 ml of hydrogen peroxide produces no blue colouration (distinction from gum acacia).
5. Aqueous solution of guar gum is converted to a gel by addition of a small amount of borax.

Uses

Guar gum is used as a protective colloid, a binding and disintegrating agent, emulsifying agent, bulk laxative, appetite depressant and in peptic ulcer therapy. Industrially, it is used in paper manufacturing, printing, polishing, textiles and also in food and cosmetic industries. Guar gum is extensively used as flocculent in ore-dressing and treatment of water.

Guar gum has been shown to decrease serum total cholesterol levels by about 10–15% and low-density lipoprotein cholesterol (LDL-cholesterol) by up to 25% without any significant effect on triglycerides or high-density lipoprotein cholesterol (HDL-cholesterol) levels.

The ability of guar to affect gastrointestinal transit may contribute to its hypoglycemic activity. Guar reduces postprandial glucose and insulin levels in both healthy and diabetic subjects and may be a useful adjunct in the treatment of noninsulin-dependent diabetes.

Guar gum remains important ingredient in over-the-counter weight loss preparations. Even in the absence of weight loss, guar supplementation for 2 weeks reduced blood pressure by 9% in moderately overweight men.

Toxicology

In the colon, guar gum is fermented to short-chain fatty acids. Both guar and its resultant by-products do not appear to be absorbed by the gut. The most common adverse effects, therefore, are gastrointestinal, including gastrointestinal pain, nausea, diarrhoea and flatulence. Approximately half of those taking guar experience flatulence; this usually occurs early in treatment and resolves with continued use. Starting with doses of about 3 g three times a day, not to exceed 15 g per day, can minimize gastrointestinal effects.

Guar gum may affect the absorption of concomitantly administered drugs. Bezafibrate, acetaminophen (e.g. Tylenol), digoxin (e.g. Lanoxin), glipizide (e.g. Glucotrol) or glyburide (e.g. DiaBeta, Micronase) are generally unaffected by concomitant administration. The ingestion of more than 30 g of guar per day by diabetic patients did not adversely affect mineral balances after six months. Guar gum in a weight-loss product has been implicated in oesophageal obstruction in a patient who exceeded the recommended dosage. In a recent review, 18 cases of oesophageal obstruction, seven cases of small bowel obstruction, and possibly one death were associated with the use of Cal-Ban 3000, a guar gum containing diet pill. The water-retaining capacity of the gum permits it to swell to 10- to 20-fold and may lead to luminal obstruction, particularly when an anatomic predisposition exists. Guar always should be taken with large amounts of liquid. Occupational asthma has been observed among those working with guar gum. Because of its potential to affect glycemic control, guar gum should be used cautiously by diabetic patients.

Marketed Product

Ascenta *Omega Smooth* Orange Sensation by Ascenta Health Ltd.

HONEY

Synonyms

Madhu, Madh, Mel, Purified Honey.

Biological Source

Honey is a viscid and sweet secretion stored in the honey comb by various species of bees, such as *Apis mellifera, Apis dorsata, Apis florea, Apis indica* and other species of *Apis*, belonging to family Apideae (Order: Hymenoptera).

Geographical Source

Honey is available in abundance in Africa, India, Jamaica, Australia, California, Chile, Great Britain and New Zealand.

Collection and Preparation

The nectar of the flowers is a watery solution containing 25% sucrose and 75% water. The worker bee sucks this nectar through its hollow tube of mouth (proboscis) and deposits in honey-sac located in abdomen. The enzyme invertase present in saliva of the bee converts nectar into invert sugar, which is partially utilized by the bee and the remaining is deposited into honey comb. Honey comb is smoked to remove the bees and honey is obtained by applying the pressure to it or allowing it to drain naturally. The honey of commerce is heated to 80°C and allowed to stand. The impurities which float over the surface are skimmed off and the liquid is diluted with water to produce honey of 1.35 density. Natural honey has the density of 1.47. Many-a-time, honey is extracted from the comb by centrifugation. It must be free from foreign substances. Honey is liable to fermentation, unless it is suitably processed. Honey is heated to 80°C before it is sent to the market, so as to avoid fermentation. It should be cooled rapidly or else it darkens in colour on keeping. If necessary (and if not prepared by centrifugation method), honey is required to be filtered through wet cloth or funnel.

Morphology

Colour	Pale yellow to reddish brown viscid fluid
Odour	Pleasant and characteristic
Taste	Sweet, slightly acrid
Extra features	However, the taste and odour of honey solely depends upon the availability of surrounding flowers from which nectar is collected. On prolonged storage it usually turns opaque and granular due to crystallization of dextrose and is termed as 'Granulated honey'

History

The honey used for flavouring medicinal was first known historically as a flavoured sweetening agent and was once the official honey of the National Formulary. Its use dates back to ancient times, with Egyptian medical texts (between 2600 and 2200 B.C.) mentioning honey in at least 900 remedies. Almost all early cultures universally hailed honey for its sweetening and nutritional qualities, as well as its topical healing properties for sores, wounds and skin ulcers. During war time it was used on wounds as an antiseptic by the ancient Egyptians, Greeks, Romans, Chinese and even by the Germans as late as World War I.

The 1811 edition of *The Edinburgh New Dispensatory* states, 'From the earliest ages, honey has been employed as a medicine, it forms an excellent gargle and facilitates the expectoration of viscid phlegm; and is sometimes employed as an emollient application to abscesses, and as a detergent to ulcers'. It has consistently appeared in modern use for the same purposes by the laity and medical profession. Today, bees are commonly kept in Europe, the Americas, Africa and Asia; at least 300,000 tons of honey is produced annually.

Chemical Constituents

The average composition of honey is as follows: Moisture 14–24%, Dextrose 23–36%, Levulose (Fructose) 30–47%, Sucrose 0.4–6%, Dextrin and Gums 0–7% and Ash 0.1–0.8%. Besides, it is found to contain small amounts of essential oil, beeswax, pollen grains, formic acid, acetic acid, succinic acid, maltose, dextrin, colouring pigments, vitamins and an admixture of enzymes, for example diastase, invertase and inulase. Interestingly, the sugar contents in honey varies widely from one country to another as it is exclusively governed by the source of the nectar (availability of fragment flowers in the region) and also the enzymatic activity solely controlling the conversion into honey.

Chemical Tests

Adulteration in honey is determined by the following tests:

1. **Fiehe's Test for Artificial Invert Sugar:** Honey (10 ml) is shaken with petroleum or solvent ether (5 ml) for 5–10 min. The upper ethereal layer is separated and evaporated in a china dish. On addition of 1% solution of resorcinol in hydrochloric acid (1 ml) a transient red colour is formed in natural honey while in artificial honey the colour persists for sometime.

2. **Reduction of Fehling's Solution:** To an aqueous solution of honey (2 ml) Fehling's solutions A and B are added and the reaction mixture is heated on a steam bath for 5–10 min. A brick red colour is produced due to the presence of reducing sugars.

3. **Limit Tests:** The limit tests of chloride, sulphate and ash (0.5%) are compared with the pharmacopoeial specifications.

Uses

Honey shows mild laxative, bactericidal, sedative, antiseptic and alkaline characters. It is used for cold, cough, fever, sore eye and throat, tongue and duodenal ulcers, liver disorders, constipation, diarrhoea, kidney and other urinary disorders, pulmonary tuberculosis, marasmus, rickets, scurvy and insomnia. It is applied as a remedy on open wounds after surgery. It prevents infection and promotes healing. Honey works quicker than many antibiotics because it is easily absorbed into the blood stream. It is also useful in healing of carbuncles, chaps, scalds, whitlows and skin inflammation; as vermicide; locally as an excipient, in the treatment of aphthae and other infection of the oral mucous membrane. It is recommended in the treatment of preoperative cancer. Honey, mixed with onion juice, is a good remedy for arteriosclerosis in brain. Diet rich in honey is recommended for infants, convalescents, diabetic patients and invalids.

Honey is an important ingredient of certain lotions, cosmetics, soaps, creams, balms, toilet waters and inhalations. It is used as a medium in preservation of cornea.

Today, as in earlier times, honey is used as an ingredient in various cough preparations. It is also used to induce sleep, cure diarrhoea and treat asthma. A review of literature found at least 25 scientific articles verifying honey's wound and topical ulcer healing powers.

Interestingly, potent antibacterial peptides (apidaecins and abaecin) have been isolated and characterized in the honeybee (*Apis mellifera*) itself and a new potent antibacterial protein named royalisin has been found in the royal jelly of the honeybee.

Adulterant and Substitutes

Due to the relatively high price of pure honey, it is invariably adulterated ether with artificial invert sugar or simply with cane-sugar syrup. These adulterants or cheaper substituents not only alter the optical property of honey but also its natural aroma and fragrance.

Toxicology

Generally, honey is considered safe as a sweet food product, a gargle and cough-soothing agent, and a topical product for minor sores and wounds. However, medical reports indicate that honey can be harmful when fed to infants because some batches contain spores of *Clostridium botulinum*, which can multiply in the intestines and result in botulism poisoning. Infant botulism is seen most commonly in 2- to 3-month-old infants after ingestion of botulinal spores that colonize in the GIT as well as toxin production *in vivo*. Infant botulism is not produced by ingestion of preformed toxin, as is the case in food borne botulism. Clinical symptoms include constipation fallowed by neuromuscular paralysis (starting with the cranial nerves and then proceeding to the peripheral and respiratory musculature). Cases are frequently related to ingestion of honey, house dust and soil contaminated with *Clostridium botulinum*. Intense management under hospital emergency conditions and trivalent antitoxin are recommended, although use of the latter in infant botulism has not been adequately investigated.

Marketed Product

OLBAS Cough Syrup manufactured by Olbas Herbal Remedies, Philadelphia is mainly used for the treatment of cough and sore throat.

TRAGACANTH

Synonyms

Goat's thorn, gum dragon, gum tragacanth, hog gum.

Biological Source

It is the air dried gummy exudates, flowing naturally or obtained by incision, from the stems and branches of *Astragalus gummifer* Labill and certain other species of *Astragalus*, belonging to family Leguminosae (Fig. 14.5).

Geographical Source

Various species of *Astragalus* which yield gum are abundantly found in the mountainous region of Turkey, Syria, Iran, Iraq and the former USSR at an altitude of about 1000–3000 m. Two important varieties of tragacanth, that is, Persian tragacanth and Smyrna or Anatolian tragacanth come from Iran and turkey respectively. In India it is found wild in Kumaon and Garhwal region.

The approximate distribution of a number of gum-producing species found in the areas where tragacanth is collected is shown in Table 14.1.

Table-14.1: Distribution of gum producing *Astragalus* species.

Species	Geographical distribution
A. gummifer	Anatolia and Syria
A. kurdics	Northern Iraq, Turkey and Syria
A. brachycalyx	Western and South western Iran
A. eriostylus	Southern west Iran
A. verus	Western Iran
A. leioclados	Western and central Iran
A. echidnaeformis	Isfahan region of Iran
A. gossypinus	Isfahan region of Iran
A. microephalus	Shiraz and Kerman regions of Iran, Turkey
A. adscendens	South western and southern Iran
A. strobiliferus	Eastern Iran
A. heratensis	Khorasan to Afghanistan

Cultivation, Collection and Preparation

Most of the plants from which tragacanth is collected grow at an altitude of 1000–3000 m. The shrubs are very thorny; each of their compound leaves has a stout, sharply pointed rachis which persists after the fall of the leaflets. The mode of collection varies somewhat in different districts, but the following details of collection in the province of Far are typical.

Gums can be obtained from the plants in their first year but is then said to be of poor quality and unfit for commercial use. The plants are therefore tapped in the second year. The earth is taken away from the base to depth of 5 cm, and the exposed part is incised with a sharp knife having a thin cutting edge. A wedge-shaped piece of wood is used by the collector to force open the incision so that the gum exudes more freely. The wedge is generally left in the cut for some 12–24 h before being withdrawn. The gum exudes and is collected 2 days after the incision. Some of the plants are burned at the top after having had the incision made. The plant then sickens and gives off a greater quantity of gum. However, this practice is not universal, as many plants can not recover their strength and are killed by the burning. The gum obtained after burning is of lower quality than that obtained by incision only, and is reddish and dirty looking. The crop becomes available in August–September.

After collection, the gum is graded as ribbons and flakes which are further categorized into various subgrades on the basis of shape, size and colour (Table 14.2). The best grades form the official drug, while the lower grades are used in the food, textile and other industries.

Table 14.2: Grades of tragacanth

Grade		Description
Ribbon	No. 1	Fine flat druggists' ribbon
	No. 2	White flat druggists' ribbon
	No. 3	Light-cream curly ribbon
	No. 4	Mid-cream flat ribbon
	No. 5	Pinkish mixed ribbon
Flake	No. 26	Mid-cream thin flake
	No. 27	Amber thick flake
	No. 28	Amber-brown thick flake
	No. 55	Reddish-brown mixed hoggy flake

Morphology

Colour	The flakes are white or pale yellowish-white
Odour	Odourless
Taste	Mucilaginous
Shape and size	Tragacanth occurs in the form of ribbon or flakes. Flakes are approximately 25 × 12 × 2 mm in size
Appearance	The gum is horny, translucent with transverse and longitudinal ridges. Fracture is short

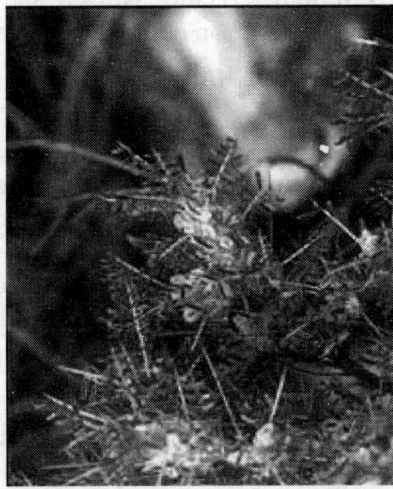

FIG. 14.5. *Astragalus gummifer*

Chemical Constituents

Interestingly, tragacanth comprises two vital fractions: first, being water soluble and is termed as *tragacanthin* and the second, being water insoluble and is known as *bassorin*. Both are not soluble in alcohol. The said two components may be separated by carrying out the simple filtration of very dilute mucilage of tragacanth and are found to be present in concentrations ranging from 60% to 70% for bassorin and 30–40% for tragacanthin. Bassorin actually gets swelled up

in water to form a gel, whereas tragacanthin forms an instant colloidal solution. It has been established that no methoxyl groups are present in the tragacanthin fraction, whereas the bassorin fraction comprised approximately 5.38% methoxyl moieties. Rowson (1937) suggested that the gums having higher methoxyl content, that is, possessing higher bassorin contents yielded the most viscous mucilage.

Tragacanth gum is composed mainly of sugars and uronic acid units and can be divided into three types of constituents. The acidic constituents tragacanthic acid on hydrolysis yields galactose, xylose and galacturonic acid. A neutral polysaccharide affords galactose and arabinose after its hydrolysis while a third type is believed to be steroidal glycoside.

Chemical Tests

1. An aqueous solution of tragacanth on boiling with conc. HCl does not develop a red colour.
2. It does not produce red colour with ruthenium red solution.
3. When a solution of tragacanth is boiled with few drops of $FeCl_3$ [aqueous 10% (w/v)], it produces a deep-yellow precipitate.
4. It gives a heavy precipitate with lead acetate.
5. When tragacanth and precipitated copper oxide are made to dissolve in conc. NH_4OH, it yields a meager precipitate.

Uses

It is used as a demulcent in cough and cold preparations and to manage diarrhoea. It is used as an emollient in cosmetics. Tragacanth is used as a thickening, suspending and as an emulsifying agent. It is used along with acacia as a suspending agent. Mucilage of tragacanth is used as a binding agent in the tablets and also as an excipient in the pills. Tragacanth powder is used as an adhesive. It is also used in lotions for external use and also in spermicidal jellies. It is also used as a stabilizer for ice cream in 0.2–0.3% concentration and also in sauces. Tragacanth has been reported to inhibit the growth of cancer cells in vitro and in vivo.

Adulterant and Substitutes

Tragacanth gum of lower grades known as hog tragacanth is used in textile industry and in the manufacture of pickles. The gum varies from yellowish brown to almost black. Citral gum obtained from *A. strobiliferus* is also used as an adulterant.

Karaya gum which is sometimes known as sterculia gum or Indian tragacanth is invariably used as a substitute for gum tragacanth.

Toxicology

Tragacanth is generally recognized as safe (GRAS) in the United States for food use. There is no indication that dietary supplementation for up to 21 days has any significant adverse effects in man. Tragacanth is highly susceptible to bacterial degradation and preparations contaminated with enterobacteria have been reported to have caused fetal deaths when administered intraperitoneally (i.p.) to pregnant mice. A cross sensitivity to the asthma-induced effects of quillaja bark has been observed for gum tragacanth.

SODIUM ALGINATE

Synonyms

Algin, Alginic acid sodium salt, Sodium polymannuronate, Kelgin, Minus, Protanal.

Biological Source

Sodium alginate is the sodium salt of alginic acid. Alginic acid is a polyuronic acid composed of reduced mannuronic and glucuronic acids, which are obtained from the algal growth of the species of family Phaeophyceae. The common species are *Macrocystis pyrifera*, *Laminaria hyperborea*, *Laminaria digitata*, *Ascophyllum nodosum* and *Durvillaea lessonia*. It is a purified carbohydrate extracted from brown seaweed (algae) by treatment of dilute alkali.

Geographical Source

Sea-weeds are found in Atlantic and Pacific oceans, particularly in coastal lines of Japan, United States, Canada, Australia and Scotland. In India, it is found near the coast of Saurashtra. The largest production of algin is in the United States and UK.

Collection and Preparation

The brown coloured algae are used for extraction of alginic acid. The colour is due to carotenoid pigment present in it. *M. pyrifera*, the principal source for global supply, is a perennial plant that lives from 8 to 12 years, and grows, as much as, 30 cm per day. This giant kelp is found mainly in Pacific Ocean. It grows on stands from 15 m to 1.5 km in width and several km in length. The mechanical harvesting is done about four times a year.

Alginic acid is present in the cell wall. The seaweeds are harvested, dried, milled and extracted with dilute sodium carbonate solution which results in a pasty mass. It is then diluted to separate insoluble matter. Soft water is only used for extraction purposes, so as to avoid incompatibilities. It is treated with calcium chloride or sulphuric acid for conversion into either calcium alginate or insoluble alginic acid, which is collected and purified by thorough washing. If calcium is used, it is treated with hydrochloric acid. Alginic acid so collected is treated with sodium carbonate for neutralization and converted into sodium salt. The alginic acid content on dry solid basis varies from 22% to 35% in all the varieties of brown algae.

Morphology

Colour	White to buff coloured powder
Odour	Odourless
Taste	Tasteless
Appearance	It is available either as a coarse or fine powder. It is readily soluble in water forming viscous colloidal solution and insoluble in alcohol, ether, chloroform and strong acids. 1% solution of gum at 20°C may have a viscosity in the range of 20–400 centipoises.

History

Alginic acid, a hard, horny polysaccharide, was first isolated by the English chemist Stanford in 1883 and in Britain was first marketed in 1910. The commercial production of algin first began in 1929 in United States Since then it is produced in the UK, France, Norway and Japan. The present total algin production is estimated to be more than 15,000 tones per annum.

Identification Tests

1. Precipitate formation with calcium chloride: To a 0.5% solution of the sample in sodium hydroxide, add one-fifth of its volume of a 2.5% solution of calcium chloride. A voluminous, gelatinous precipitate is formed. This test distinguishes sodium alginate from gum arabic, sodium carboxymethyl cellulose, carrageenan, gelatin, gum ghatti, karaya gum and tragacanth gum.

2. Precipitate formation with ammonium sulphate: To a 0.5% solution of the sample in sodium hydroxide, add one-half of its volume of a saturated solution of ammonium sulphate. No precipitate is formed. This test distinguishes sodium alginate from agar, sodium carboxymethyl cellulose, carrageenan, methyl cellulose and starch.

3. Test for alginate: Moisten 1–5 mg of the sample with water and add 1 ml of acid ferric sulphate. Within 5 min, a cherry-red colour develops that finally becomes deep purple.

4. 1% solution in water forms heavy gelatinous precipitate with dilute sulphuric acid.

Chemical Constituents

Algin consists chiefly of the sodium salt of alginic acid, a linear polymer of L-guluronic acid and D-mannuronic acid; the chain length is long and varies (mol. wt. from 35,000 to 1.5×10^6) with the method of isolation and the source of the algae. Mannuronic acid is the major component. The alginic acid molecule appears to be a copolymer of 1, 4-linked mannopyranosyluronic acid units, of 1,4-linked gulopyranosyluronic acid units, and of segments where these uronic acids alternate with 1,4-linkages.

Uses

High and medium viscosity grades of sodium alginate are used in the preparation of paste, creams and for thickening and stabilizing emulsions. It is a good suspending and thickening agent, but a poor emulsifying agent. It is used as binding and disintegrating agent in tablets and lozenges. In food industry, it is used for the preparation of jellies, ice cream, etc. It is also used in textile industry. For pharmaceutical purposes, when desired, it is sterilized by heating in an autoclave. The solution of sodium alginate should not be stored in metal containers. It is preserved by the addition of 0.1% of chloroxylenol, chlorocresol, benzoic acid or parabenes. Potassium, aluminium and calcium alginates are also used medicinally.

Capsules containing sodium alginate and calcium carbonate are used to protect inflamed areas near the entrance to the stomach. The acidity of the stomach causes formation of insoluble alginic acid and carbon dioxide; the alginic acid rises to the top of the stomach contents and forms a protective layer.

Marketed Product

Each 100 ml of Lamina G solution manufactured by Taejoon Pharm Co. Ltd, Seoul contains 5.0 g of sodium alginate. It is mainly used for the treatment of gastric and duodenal ulcer, erosive gastritis, reflux oesophagitis (usual dosage is 20–60 ml orally three to four times daily before meal) and haemostasis in gastric biopsy (usual dosage is 10–30 ml by endoscope, followed by 30 ml orally).

PECTIN

Pectin, in general, is a group of polysaccharides found in nature in the primary cell walls of all seed bearing plants and are invariably located in the middle lamella. It has been observed that these specific polysaccharides actually function in combination with both cellulose and hemicellulose as an intercellular cementing substance. One of the richest sources of pectin is lemon or orange rind which contains about 30% of this polysaccharide. Evaluation and standardization of pectin is based on its 'Gelly-grade' that is, its setting capacity by the addition of sugar. Usually, pectin having 'gelly-grade' of 100, 150 and 200 are recommended for medicinal and food usages.

Biological Source

Pectin is a purified polysaccharide substance obtained from the various plant sources such as inner peel of citrus fruits, apple, raw papaya, etc. Numbers of plants sources of pectin are mentioned below:

Common Name	Botanical Name	Family
Lemon	Citrus lemon	Rutaceae
Orange	Citrus aurantium	Rutaceae
Apple	Pyrus malus	Rosaceae
Papaya	Carica papaya	Caricaceae
Sunflower heads	Helianthus tuberosus	Asteraceae
Guava	Psidium guyava	Myrtaceae
Beets	Beta vulgaris	Chenopodiaceae
Carrot	Daucus carota	Apiaceae
Mangoes	Mangifera indica	Anacardiaceae

Geographical Source

Lemon and oranges are mostly grown in India, Africa and other tropical countries. Apple is grown in the Himalayas, California, many European countries and the countries located in the Mediterranean climatic zone.

Preparation

The specific method of preparation of pectin is solely guided by the source of raw material, that is, lemon/orange rind or apple pomace; besides the attempt to prepare either low methoxy group or high methoxy group pectins.

In general, the preserved or freshly obtained lemon peels are gently boiled with approximately 20 times its weight of fresh water maintained duly at 90°C for duration of 30 min. The effective pH (3.5–4.0) must be maintained with food grade lactic acid/citric acid/tartaric acid to achieve maximum extraction. Once the boiling is completed the peels are mildly squeezed to obtain the liquid portion which is then subjected to centrifugation to result into a clear solution. From this resulting solution both proteins and starch contents are suitably removed by enzymatic hydrolysis. The remaining solution is warmed to deactivate the added enzymes. The slightly coloured solution is effectively decolourized with activated carbon or bone charcoal. Finally, the pectin in its purest form is obtained by precipitation with water-miscible organic solvents (e.g. methanol, ethanol, acetone, etc.), washed with small quantities of solvent and dried in a vacuum oven and stored in air-tight containers or poly bags. As Pectin is fairly incompatible with Ca^{2+}, hence due precautions must be taken to avoid the contact of any metallic salts in the course of its preparation.

Morphology

Colour	Cream or yellowish coloured powder
Odour	Odourless
Taste	Mucilaginous
Appearance	It is coarse or fine light powder and hygroscopic in nature. Completely soluble in 20 parts of water, forming a solution containing negatively charged and very much hydrated particles. Dissolves more swiftly in water, if previously moistened with sugar syrup, alcohol and glycerol or if first mixed with three or more parts of sucrose

Chemical Constituents

Pectin is a polysaccharide with a variable molecular weight ranging from 20,000 to 400,000 depending on the number of carbohydrate linkages. The core of the molecule is formed by linked D-polygalacturonate and L-rhamnose residues. The neutral sugars D-galactose, L-arabinose, D-xylose and L-fructose form the side chains on the pectin molecule. Once extracted, pectin occurs as a coarse or fine yellowish powder that is highly water soluble and forms thick colloidal solutions. The parent compound, protopectin, is insoluble, but is readily converted by hydrolysis into pectinic acids, (also known generically as pectins).

Chemical Tests

1. A 10% (w/v) solution gives rise to a solid gel on cooling.
2. A transparent gel or semigel results by the interaction of 5 ml of 1 % solution of pectin with 1 ml of 2 % solution of KOH and subsequently setting aside the mixture at an ambient temperature for 15 min. The resulting gel on acidification with dilute HCl and brisk shaking yields a voluminous and gelatinous colourless precipitate which on warming turns into white and flocculent.

Uses

Pectin is used as an emulsifier, gelling agent and also as a thickening agent. It is a major component of antidiarrhoeal formulation. Pectin is a protective colloid which assists absorption of toxin in the gastrointestinal tract. It is used as haemostatic in cases of haemorrhage. As a thickener it is largely used in the preparation of sauces, jams and ketchups in food industry.

One of the best characterized effects of pectin supplementation is its ability to lower human blood lipoprotein levels. Pectin supplements appear to act as 'enteroabsorbents', protecting against the accumulation of ingested radioactivity.

Toxicology

Pectin is a fermentable fibre that results in the production of short-chain fatty acids and methane. Concomitant administration of pectin with beta-carotene containing foods or supplements can reduce levels of beta-carotene by more than one-half. There is some indication that concomitant ingestion of pectin with high energy diets may reduce the availability of these diets, as demonstrated in a controlled trial of undernourished children; urea production was also shown to be lower in children who ingested pectin with their caloric supplement.

KARAYA GUM

Synonyms

Indian tragacanth, Sterculia gum, Karaya gum, Bassora tragacanth, kadaya, mucara, kadira, katila, kullo.

Biological Source

Gum karaya is a dried, gummy exudates obtained from the tree *Sterculia urens* (Roxburgh), *Sterculia villosa* (Roxburgh), *Sterculia tragacantha* (Lindley) or other species of *Sterculia*, belonging to family Sterculiaceae.

Geographical Source

The *S. urens* is found in India especially in the Gujarat region and in the central provinces.

Collection and Preparation

The gum is obtained from the *Sterculia* species by making incisions and, thereafter, collecting the plant exudates usually after a gap of 24 h. The large irregular masses of gums (tears) which weigh between 250 g and 1 kg approximately are hand picked and dispatched to the various collecting centres. The gum is usually tapped during the dry season spreading over from March to June. Each healthy fully grown tree yields from 1 to 5 kg of gum per year; and such operations may be performed about five times during its lifetime. In short, the large bulky lumps (tears) are broken to small pieces to cause effective drying. The foreign particles, for example, pieces of bark, sand particles and leaves are removed. Thus, purified gum is available in two varieties, namely:

(a) **Granular or Crystal Gum:** Having a particle size ranging between 6 and 30 mesh, and
(b) **Powdered Gum:** Having particle size of 150 mesh

Morphology

Colour	White, pink or brown in colour
Odour	Slight odour resembling acetic acid
Taste	Bland and mucilaginous
Shape and size	Irregular tears or vermiform pieces

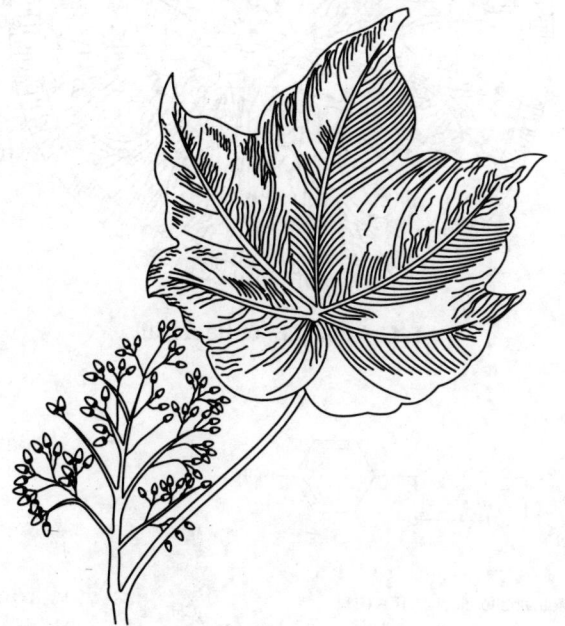

FIG. 14.6 Karaya twig

History

Karaya gum has been used commercially for about 100 years. Its use became widespread during the early 20th century, when it was used as an adulterant or alternative for tragacanth gum. However, experience indicated that karaya possessed certain physiochemical properties that made it more useful than tragacanth; furthermore, karaya gum was less expensive. Traditionally, India is the largest producer and exporter of karaya gum. Increasing amounts are exported by African countries. Currently the gum is used in a variety of products, including cosmetics, hair sprays and lotions, to provide bulk. The bark is astringent.

Chemical Constituents

Karaya gum is partially acetylated polysaccharide containing about 8% acetyl groups and about 37% uronic acid residues. It undergoes hydrolysis in an acidic medium to produce D-galactose, L-rhamnose, D-galacturonic acid and a trisaccharide acidic substance. It contains a branched heteropolysaccharide moiety having a major chain of 1,4-linked α- D-galacturonic acid along with 1,2-linked L-rhamnopyranose units with a short D-glucopyranosyluronic acid containing the side chains attached 1→3 to the main chain, that is, D-galactouronic acid moieties.

Chemical Test

1. To 1 g of powdered Karaya Gum, add 50 ml of water and mix. A viscous solution is produced and it is acidic.
2. Add 0.4 g of powdered Karaya Gum to 10 ml of an ethanol-water mixture (3:2), and mix. The powder is swelling.
3. It readily produces a pink colour with a solution of ruthenium red.

Uses

Karaya gum is not digested or absorbed systemically. Medicinally, karaya gum is an effective bulk laxative, as gum particles absorbs water and swells to 60–100 times their original volume. The mechanism of action is an increase in the volume of the gut contents. Karaya gum should be taken with plenty of fluid and it may take a few days for effects to be noticeable. It also has been used as an adhesive for dental fixtures and ostomy equipment, and as a base for salicylic acid patches. The demulcent properties of the gum make it useful as an ingredient in lozenges to relieve sore throat. A protective coating of karaya gum applied to dentures has been shown to reduce bacterial adhesion by 98%. The use of karaya gum as a carrier for drugs with differing solubility in aqueous medium has been investigated. In pharma industry, it is also used as emulsifier, thickener and stabilizer. Karaya gum is also used in paper and textile industries.

Adulterant and Substitutes

It is used as a substitute for gum tragacanth.

BAEL

Synonyms

Bael fruits, Bel, Indian Bael, Bengal Quince, Belan.

Biological Source

Bael consists of the unripe or half-ripe fruits or their slices or irregular pieces of *Aegle marmelos* Corr., belonging to family Rutaceae (Fig. 14.7).

Geographical Source

Sub-Himalayan tract and throughout India, especially Central and Southern India, Burma, occurring as wild and also cultivated.

Collection

Tree is deciduous about 12 m in height. It is a sacred tree and the leaves known as *Bilipatra* are used for worshipping Lord Shiva. The tree has strong, straight spines, compound

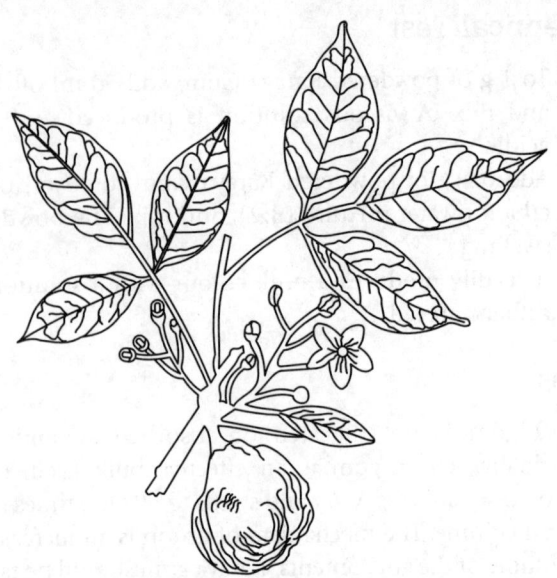

FIG. 14.7. Aegle marmelos

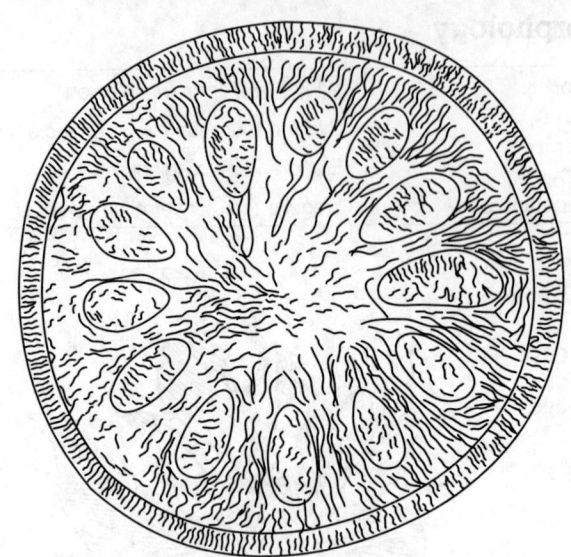

FIG. 14.8. T.S. of Bael fruit

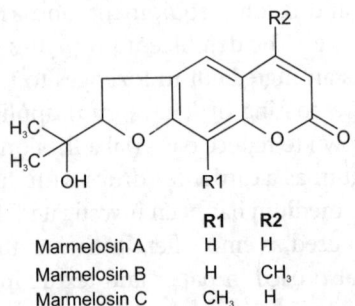

	R1	R2
Marmelosin A	H	H
Marmelosin B	H	CH₃
Marmelosin C	CH₃	H

O-Methylhalfordinol R = CH₃
Isopentylhalfordinol R = CH₂– CH = CH – CH₃

trifoliate leaves and berry fruit. Fruits are collected during April–May. After collection, epicarp removed and usually cut into transverse slices or irregular pieces.

Morphology

Odour	Aromatic
Taste	Mucilaginous
Shape and size	Subspherical berry, 5–10 cm in diameter
Epicarp	Hard, woody, externally reddish-brown, smooth or granular.
Mesocarp and Endocarp	Consist of pulp which is reddish-brown and made up of 10–12 carpels. Each carpel contains several seeds with oblong, flat, multicellular, woolly white hairs. Seeds are surrounded by mucilage.

Chemical Constituents

The chief constituent of the drug is marmelosin A, B and C (0.5%), which is a furocoumarin. Other coumarins are marmesin, psoralin and umbelliferone. The drug also contains carbohydrates (11–17%), protein, volatile oil and tannins. The pulp also contains good amount of vitamins C and A. Two alkaloids O-methylhalfordinol and isopentylhalfordinol have been isolated from fruits. Other

alkaloids reported in the drug are angelenine, marmeline and dictamine.

Uses

Drug is very popular in Ayurveda and is used in diarrhoea and dysentery. Action is attributed to mucilage. Leaves contain alkaloids and are considered useful in diabetes. The oil obtained from seeds possesses antibacterial, antiprotozoal and antifungal properties. The root of *bael* is one of the constituents of well-known Ayurvedic preparation Dasmula.

In large doses it may lead to abortion, therefore, it can be used as abortifacient agent and hence it should not be used in pregnant women.

Substitutes

Mangosteen fruits: Garcinia mangostana Linn. (Guttiferae) is a substitute for this fruit, and it can be identified by the darker rind and the wedge shaped radiate stigmas.

Wood apple: Limonia acidissima Linn. (Rutaceae) is a five lobed fruit with rough exterior part.

Pomegranate rind: Punica granatum Linn. (Punicaceae) contain triangular impressions on the seeds and has astringent taste.

Marketed Products

It is one of the ingredients of the preparations known as Lukol for leucorrhoea; Chyawanprash (Himalaya Drug Company); Isabbael and Bilwadi churna (Baidyanath Company); Madhushantak (Jamuna Pharma) and Sage bilva churn (Sage Herbals).

AGAR

Synonym

Agar-agar, Japanese Isinglass, Vegetable gelatin.

Botanical Source

It is the dried gelatinous substance obtained by extraction with water from *Gelidium amansii* (Fig. 14.9) or various species of red algae like *Gracilaria* and *Pterocladia*, belonging to family Gelidiaceae (*Gelidium* and *Pterocladia*), Gracilariaceae (*Gracilaria*).

Geographical Source

Japan was the only country producing agar before the World War II, but it is now produced in several countries like, Japan: *Gelidium amansii* and other *Gelidium species*, Australia; *Gracilaria confervoides*, New Zealand; *Pterocladia lucida* and other allied species, Korea, South Africa, United States, Chile, Spain and Portugal.

History

The history of agar and agarose extends back to centuries and the utility of the compounds closely follow the emergence and development of the discipline of microbiology. The gel like properties of agar are purported to have been first observed by a Chinese Emperor in the mid sixteenth century. Soon thereafter, a flourishing agar manufacturing industry was established in Japan. The Japanese dominance of the trade in agar only ended with World War II. Following World War II, the manufacturing of agar spread to other countries around the globe. For example, in the United States, the copious sea weed beds found along the Southern California coast has made the San Diego area a hot bed of agar manufacture. Today, the manufacture and sale of agar is lucrative and has spawned a competitive industry.

Collection

The red algae are grown in rocks in shallow water or on the bamboos by placing them in the ocean. Collection of the algae is usually made in summer (May and October). The bamboos are taken out and the seaweeds are stripped off. Algae are dried, beaten with sticks and shaken to remove the sand and shell attached to them. Then the entire material is taken to high altitude, washed with water and bleached by keeping them in trays in the sunlight, sprinkling water and rotating them periodically. The agar is then boiled; one part of algae with 50 parts of water acidified with acetic acid or dilute sulphuric acid. The hot extract is subjected for coarse and fine filtration using cloth to remove the large and small impurities present in them. The filtered extract is then transferred into wooden trough which on cooling forms a jelly like mass. The mass thus obtained is then passed through screw press to obtain strips of agar. These strips contain water and to remove the water present in them, the agar strips are placed in open air to get the benefits of the Japanese climate. During this season, Japan has a very warm day and the nights are very cold with a temperature less than 0°C. As a result of this climate the water present on top of the strips are converted into ice at night, and during day they are reconverted to water and the excess water present in them are removed. Then, these strips are again dried in the sunlight in trays.

Modern method of deep freezing is being utilized in the preparation of agar in recent development of technology. The algae which is collected is washed in running water for a day and then extracted firstly with dilute acid in steam heated digester and then with water for 30 min, the hot solution so obtained is cooled and deep freezed in an ice machine. The water present in the agar is converted to ice and these masses are powdered, melted and filtered in rotary vacuum filter. The moist agar is dried using dry air and powdered agar is obtained.

Morphology

Colour	Yellowish white to grey or colourless
Odour	Slight/odourless
Taste	Mucilaginous
Shape	Strips, flakes or coarse powder
Size	Strips are about 60 cm in length and 4 mm wide. Wide sheets are 50–60 cm long and 10–15 cm wide
Solubility	Insoluble in organic solvents, cold water but soluble in hot water and forms a gelatinous solution after cooling the hot solution.

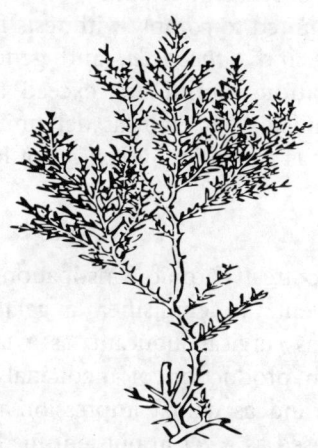

FIG. 14.9 *Gelidium amansii*

Chemical Constituents

Agar is a complex heterosaccharide and contains two different polysaccharides known as agarose and agaropectin. Agarose is neutral galactose polymer and is responsible for the gel property of agar. It consists of D-galactose and L-galactose unit. The structure of agaropectin is not completely known, but it is believed that it consists of sulphonated polysaccharide in which galactose and uronic acid are partly esterified with sulphuric acid. Agaropectin is responsible for the viscosity of agar solution.

Agarose

Chemical Tests

1. Agar responds positively to Fehling's solution test.
2. Agar gives positive test with Molisch reagent.
3. Aqueous solution of agar (1%) is hydrolysed with concentrated HCl by heating for 5–10 min. On addition of barium chloride solution to the reaction mixture, a white precipitate of barium sulphate is formed due to the presence of sulphate ions. This test is absent in case of starch, acacia gum and tragacanth.
4. To agar powder a solution of ruthenium red is added. Red colour is formed indicating mucilage.
5. Agar is warmed in a solution of KOH. A canary yellow colour is formed.
6. An aqueous solution of agar (1%) is prepared in boiling water. On cooling it sets into a jelly.
7. To agar solution an N/20 solution of iodine is added. A deep crimson to brown colour is obtained (distinctive from acacia gum and tragacanth).
8. To a 0.2% solution of agar an aqueous solution of tannic acid is added. No precipitation is formed indicating absence of gelatin.
9. Agar is required to comply with tests for the absence of *E. coli* and *Salmonella*, and general microbial contamination should not exceed a level of 10^3 microorganisms per gram as determined by a plate count. It has a swelling index of not less than 10.

Uses

Agar is used to treat chronic constipation, as a laxative, suspending agent, an emulsifier, a gelating agent for suppositories, as surgical lubricant, as a tablet excipient, disintegrant, in production of medicinal encapsulation and ointment and as dental impression mould base. It is extensively used as a gel in nutrient media for bacterial cultures, as a substitute for gelatin and isinglass, in making emulsions including photographic, gel in cosmetic, as thickening agent in food especially confectionaries and dairy products, in meet canning; sizing for silk and paper; in dying and printing of fabrics and textiles; and in adhesive.

Substitutes and Adulterants

Some of the common adulterants present in agar are gelatin and Danish agar. The presence of gelatin can be detected by addition of equal volume of 1% trinitrophenol and 1% of agar solution; the solution produces turbidity or precipitation. Danish agar has an ash of 16.5–18.5%, it is formed from rhodophyceae indigenous to the Denmark costal region. The Danish agar has a gel strength which is half of its gel strength of Japanese agar.

MANNA

Biological Source

It is saccharine exudation obtained from the stem of *Fraxinus ornus* Linn., belonging to family Oleaceae (Fig. 14.10).

Geographical Source

It is small tree widely found in Mediterranean basin and Southern Europe. It is also reported in Spain and commercially cultivated in Sicily.

Morphology

Colour	Yellowish white
Odour	Agreeable
Taste	Sweet
Shape	Three sided, flakes
Size	Pieces of 10–15 to 2–3 cm.
Extra features	It is very much friable showing crystalline structure and concentric layering. It is soluble in water and insoluble in organic solvents

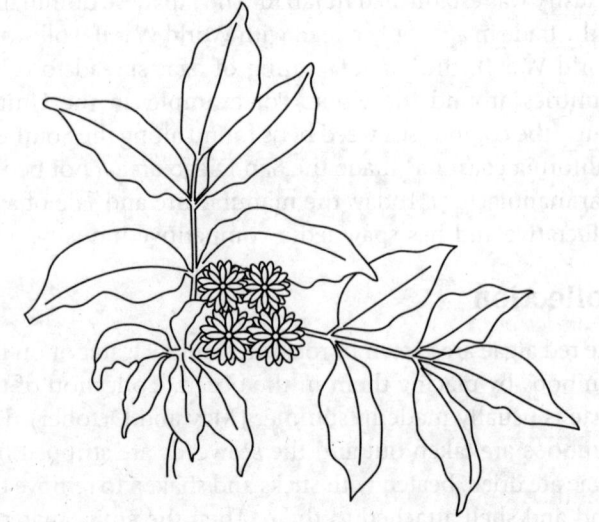

FIG. 14.10 *Fraxinus ornus*

Chemical Constituents

Manna contains 40–60% mannitol, along with 5–15% mannotriose and 10–15% mannotetrose, while dextrose, mucilage and small quantity of a fluorescent substance fraxin are the other contents of manna.

Use

It is used as a laxative.

XANTHAN GUM

Synonyms

Xynthan gum.

Biological Source

Xanthan is a microbial polysaccharide produced from *Xanthomonas campestris*.

Production

One of the latest techniques of biotechnology, that is, recombinant DNA technology has been duly exploited for the commercial production of xanthan gum.

First of all the genomic banks of *Xanthomonas campestris* are meticulously made in *Escherichia coli* by strategically mobilizing the broad-host-range cosmids being used as the vectors. Subsequently, the conjugal transfer of the genes take place from *E. coli* into the nonmucoid *Xanthomonas campestris*. Consequently, the wild type genes are duly separated by virtue of their unique ability to restore mucoid phenotype. As a result, a few of the cloned plasmids incorporated in the wild type strains of *Xanthomonas campestris* shall afford an increased production of xanthan gum.

Interestingly, the commercial xanthan gums are available with different genetically controlled composition, molecular weights and as their respective sodium, potassium or calcium salts.

Morphology

Colour	Cream coloured powder
Odour	Odourless
Solubility	Soluble in cold and hot water giving highly viscous solution, this is stable towards change in pH and also to heat.
Extra features	The aqueous solution of xanthan gum forms films on evaporation. Aqueous solutions are pseudoplastic

Chemical Constituents

Xanthan gum is composed of chiefly D-glucosyl, D-mannosyl and D-glucosyluronic acid residues along with variant quantum of O-acetyl and pyruvic acid acetal. The primary structure essentially comprises of a cellulose backbone with trisaccharide side chains and the repeating moiety being a pentasaccharide.

Uses

Xanthan is found to have very wide range of applications. It is widely used as a stabilizer and suspending agent in emulsion, paints, agricultural and herbicidal sprays. Applications are found in food, pharmaceutical and other industries. Specific applications depend upon the rheological behaviour of xanthan in solution. Synergistic effects are observed in food when xanthan is mixed with galactomannans such as guar gum or locust bean gum. It is used as a viscosity controller in abrasives and adhesives. It finds its valuable applications as gelling agent in explosives and flocculating agent in extraction.

Marketed Products

Xanthan is the only microbial gum that is currently produced on commercial scale by Kelco Inc., San Diego, United States, and by Rhone Poulenc, S.A., Melle, France. It is marketed under the variety of trade names like Keltrol©, Kelzan© or Rhodogel©.

GHATTI GUM

Synonyms

Ghatti, Gutty.

Biological Source

It is the gummy exudates obtained from the tree bark of *Anogeissus latifolia* Wallich, belonging to family Combretaceae (Fig. 14.11).

Geographical Source

It is most commonly found in the forests of the sub-Himalayan tract in Sivalic hills as well as in the mountainous region throughout India at the altitude of 1200 m. It has got this name from its transportation routes, as they are obtained after their travel through mountain 'ghats'.

Cultivation and Collection

Artificial incisions are made on the tree bark in the absence of rain and gum is picked up in the month of April. The gums are graded into different grades depending upon the colour of the gum. The lighter the gum the superior its grade is. About two to three grades of Ghatti are available in the United States. The No. 1 Grade has low levels of ash and high viscosity. Gum is dried under sun for many days and then pulverized. It is then subjected to undergo various processes like sifting, aspiration and density table separation, for the removal of impurities.

Characters

Colour	Best quality is colourless but the inferior are light yellow to dark brown
Odour	Odourless
Taste	Bland
Shape	Translucent round tears or vermiform masses
Size	1 cm diameter
Solubility	Insoluble in ethyl alcohol, about 90% of the gum dissolves in water yielding a colloidal dispersion. The gum when dissolved in alcohol or if the pH of the solution is increased to neutral, it gives solution with high viscosities. It loses its viscosity at high pH

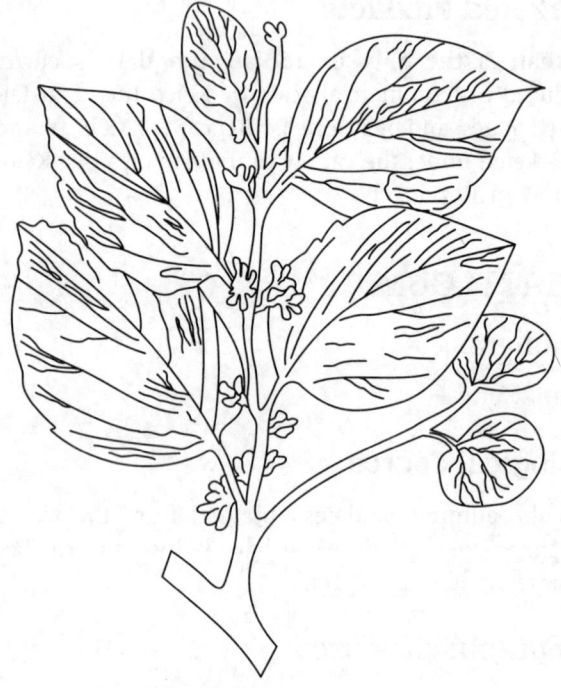

FIG. 14.11 *Anogeissus latifolia* twig

Chemical Constituents

It consists of the calcium salt of a complex high molecular weight polysaccharide made up of sugars and uronic acid units. One of the polysaccharide acid ghattic acid contains mainly arabinose, galactose, mannose, xylose and galacturonic acid. On hydrolysis of gum ghatti, it also affords aldobiouronic acid 6-O-β-D-glucopyranosyl uronic acid and D-galactose which is also found in gum acacia. Complete analysis of ghatti gum shows 26.3% pentosans, 7.6% methyl pentosan, 7.6% galactan, 15.8% moisture, about 3% ash and smaller quantities of ribof

Identification Tests

1. Aqueous solution (5%) of gum ghatti treated with Million's reagent gives fine precipitate.
2. Aqueous solution of gum treated with 2% gelatin solution gives white precipitates.
3. White precipitate is produced with 10% solution of tannic acid.
4. With water the gum forms viscous colourless mucilage which is glairy and ropy.

Uses

Gum ghatti is used as a very good emulsifier, stabilizer and thickener in pharmaceutical, food and also in ceramic industry. It is an efficient binder for the compressed tablets which is comparable with acacia gum and starch paste. It gives stable oil in water emulsion therefore used in the formulation of oil soluble vitamin preparation.

Gum is edible. It is administered as a good tonic to women after child birth. It is extensively use in the pure state in calico printing and in confectionery. It is good stabilizer for ice cream in 0.5% concentration. The gum also finds its applications in the petroleum industry as a drilling mud conditioner.

ISPAGHULA

Synonyms

Ispaghula, Isabgol, Ishabgula, Spongel seeds.

Botanical Source

Ispaghula consists of dried seeds of *Plantago ovata* Forskal, belonging to family Plantaginaceae.

Geographical Source

Ispaghula is an annual herb cultivated in India in Gujarat, Maharashtra, Punjab and in some parts of Rajasthan and Sindh Province of Pakistan. It is cultivated extensively around Sidhpur in north Gujarat.

History

Blonde psyllium (*Plantago ovata*) is a low herbaceous annual plant native to Iran and India, extensively cultivated there and in other countries, including Pakistan (Fig. 14.12). Black psyllium of the *P. afra* species is native to the western Mediterranean region, Northern Africa and Western Asia, now cultivated in Southern France and Spain. Black psyllium of the *P. indica* species is native to Southeastern Europe and Asia. In commerce, blonde psyllium is obtained mainly from India, Pakistan and Iran. Black psyllium is obtained mainly from southern France.

Psyllium has a long history of medical use in both conventional and traditional systems of medicine throughout Asia, Europe and North America. Blonde psyllium is official in the National Pharmacopeias of France, Germany, Great Britain and the United States. Psyllium monographs also appear in the Ayurvedic Pharmacopoeia, British Herbal Pharmacopoeia, British Herbal Compendium, ESCOP Monographs, Commission E Monographs and the German Standard License Monographs. The World Health Organization (WHO) has published a monograph on psyllium seed covering *P. afra*, *P. indica*, *P. ovata* and *P. asiatica* (WHO, 1999). Asian psyllium seed (*P. asiatica* Linn. or *P. depressa* Willd.) is official in the National pharmacopeias of China and Japan.

Cultivation and Collection

Isabgol seeds are sown in the month of November by broadcasting method. Well-drained loamy soil with a pH of 7.5–8.5, cool and dry climate is suitable for its growth. Ammonium sulphate is also added as a fertilizer. Good water supply to the plants is to be provided at 8–10 days interval, seven to eight times. Though ispaghula is not affected by pests or disease, the percentage yield is decreased to great extend due to heavy rainfall or storms. The fruits are collected in the month of March/April after the fruits are completely mature and ripe. The fruits are then dried and the seeds separated.

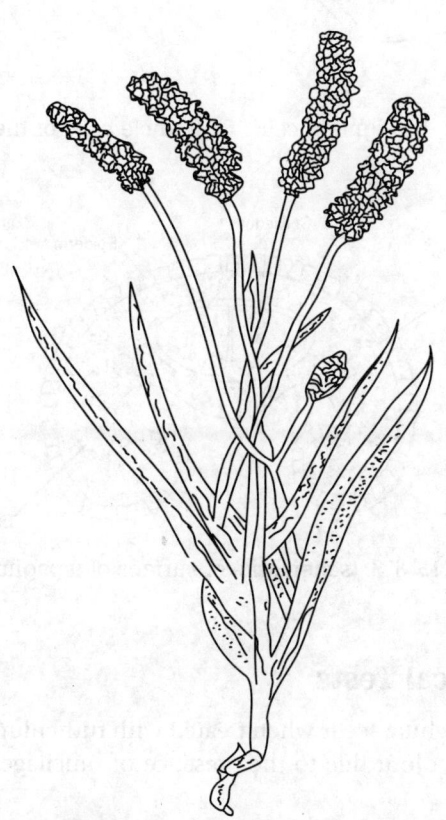

FIG. 14.12 *Plantago ovata* plant

Morphology

Colour	Pinkish grey to brown
Odour	None
Taste	Mucilaginous
Shape	Ovate, boat shaped, cymbiform
Size	1.5–3.5 mm long, 1–1.8 mm wide
Weight of 100 seeds	0.15–0.19 g
Appearance	Seeds are hard, translucent and smooth, the dorsal (convex surface) consist of a small elongated glossy reddish brown spot at the centre while the ventral (concave surface) has a cavity having nil urn covered with a thin whitish membrane

Microscopy

A thin transverse section observed under microscope shows the following characters:

Epidermis: Single layered, thick walled transparent, tangentially elongated cells containing mucilage, which exudes if brought in contact with water.

Pigment Layer: Usually collapsed which is yellow in colour.

Endosperm: Outer layer consists of palisade like cells which are thick walled but inner cells are irregular and are also thick walled consisting of aleurone grains and oil globules.

Embryo: Have two cotyledons, with three to five vascular bundles in each, a portion of raphe remains attached to the seed.

Powder Microscopy

The powder is pale pinkish in colour with mucilaginous taste. Microscopical examination shows fragments of epidermis, composed of large, thin-walled cells filled with mucilage, which swells rapidly in aqueous mounts. Endosperm consists of thick-walled cells with numerous large pits, usually found attached to pigment layer. Pigment cells are thin-walled, indistinct and contain brown pigment. Cells of cotyledons are thin-walled, polygonal to slightly rounded, in surface view; some of them contain oil globules. Cells of radicle are thin-walled, uniformly arranged in layers. Starch grains, simple or compound (four or more components), are present in epidermis and sometimes embedded in mucilage.

Chemical Constituents

Ispaghula seeds contain about 10% mucilage which is present in the epidermis of testa. Mucilage consists of two complex polysaccharides, of which one is soluble in cold water and the other soluble in hot water. Chemically it is pentosan and aldobionic acid. Pentosan on hydrolysis yields xylose and arabinose and aldobionic acid yields

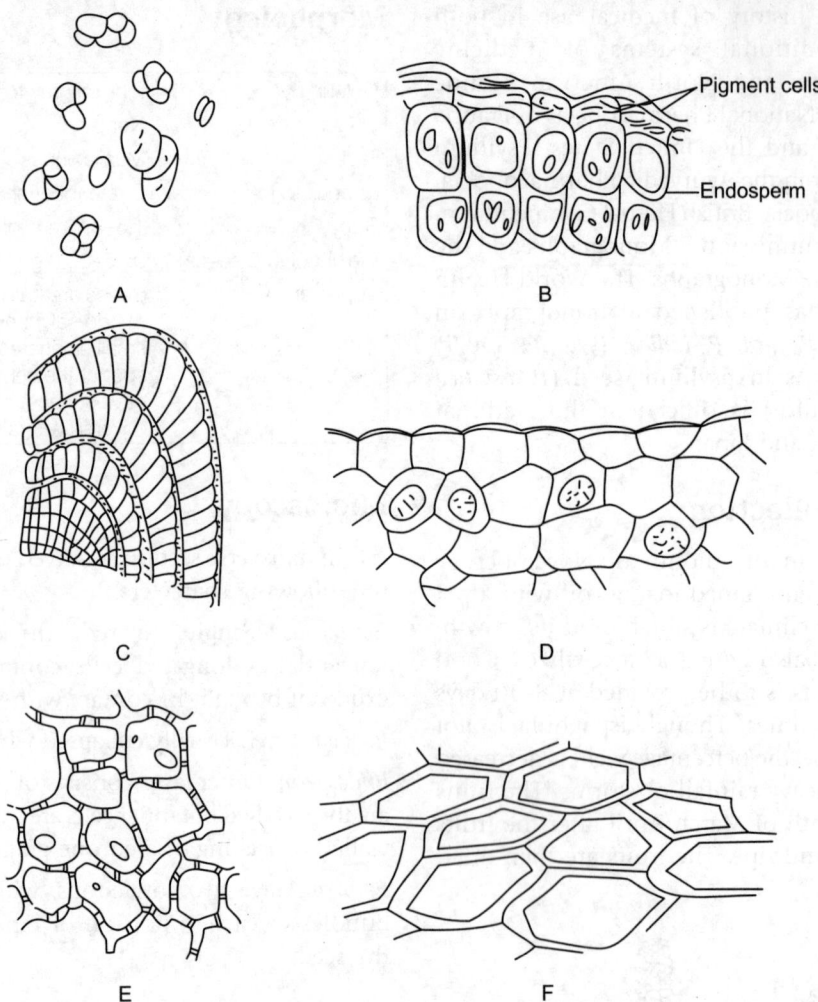

FIG. 14.13 Powder characteristics of Ispaghula seed. (A: Starch granules, B: Pigment cells, C: Radicle cells of the embryo, D: Cells of cotyledon, E: Cells of endosperm, F: Cells of epidermis)

galactouronic acid and rhamnose. Protein and fixed oil are present in endosperm and embryo.

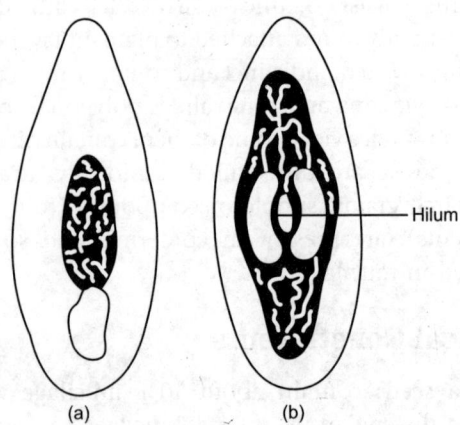

FIG. 14.14 (a) Dorsal and (b) Ventral

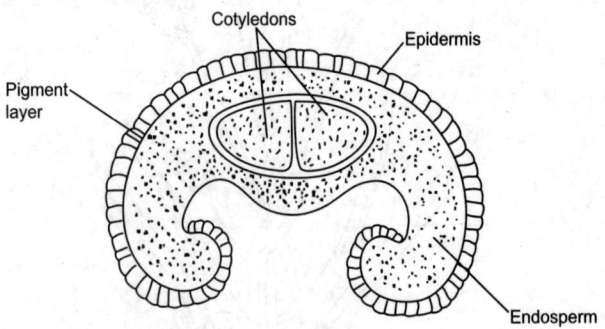

FIG. 14.15 T.S. (schematic) of surface of ispaghula seed

Chemical Tests

1. Ispaghula seeds when treated with ruthenium red give red colour due to the presence of mucilage.

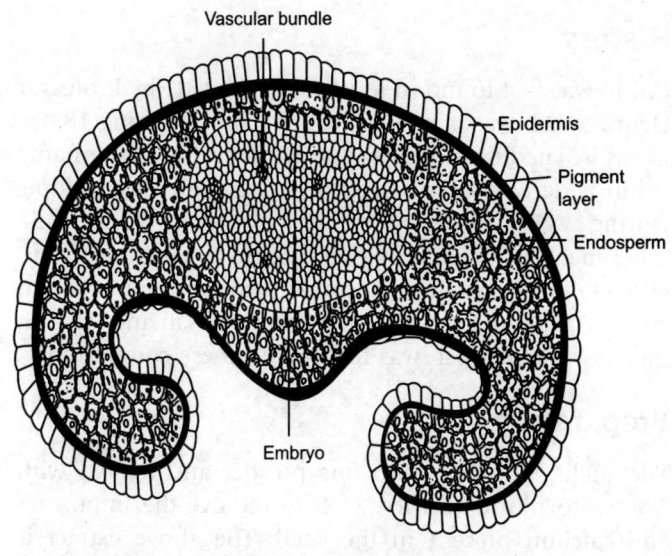

FIG. 14.16 Transverse section of ispaghula seed

2. Add water to few seeds on a slide, mucilage comes out and forms zone surrounding the seeds.
3. *Swelling factor:* Swelling factor is the parameter to determine the purity of seeds. Swelling can be determined quantitatively by swelling factor. 1 g of the drug is put in a measuring cylinder of 25 ml capacity and 20 ml water is added. It is shaken periodically for first 23 h and kept for one more hour. The volume occupied by the drug is called swelling factor. Swelling factor of ispaghula seeds is 10–13.

Uses

Ispaghula seeds are used as an excellent demulcent and bulk laxative in chronic constipation. The laxative activity of ispaghula mucilage is purely mechanical. It is also useful in dysentery, chronic diarrhoea, in cases of duodenal ulcers and piles. It works effectively as a soothing agent. Ispaghula husk is also used for similar purpose.

Substitutes and Adulterants

P. lanceolata Linn., occurring wild in India, is adulterated in ispaghula. Its seeds are oblong elliptical in shape with yellowish brown colour. The seeds of *P. asiatica*, (syn. *P. major* L.), found in Andhra Pradesh and Tamil Nadu, are substituted to ispaghula. It is also adulterated with the seeds of *P. arenaria*. The seeds of *Salvia aegyptica* are frequently mixed which also yield copious mucilage. The seeds of *P. media* L. have different colour and swell very little in water.

P. asiatica contains mucilage which is composed of β-1,4-linked D-xylopyranose residues having three kinds of branches.

Marketed Products

Sat Isabgol, Trifgol by Dabur, Sat-Isabgol by Dr Morepen.

TAMARIND

Synonyms

West Indian Tamarind, *Imli*.

Botanical Source

Tamarind consists of dried ripe fruits (freed from the brittle epicarp) of *Tamarindus indica* Linn., belonging to family Leguminosae (Fig. 14.17).

Geographical Source

West Indies (Barbados), India.

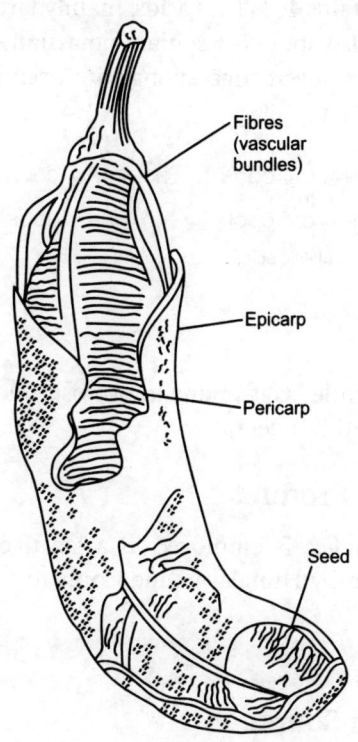

FIG. 14.17 Fruit of tamarind

Collection

Tamarind is a superior indehiscent legume 5–20 cm long and 2 cm in width. Epicarps of the legumes are brittle, rough, brownish and hard. Mesocarp is the pulp and is acidic in nature with fibres which are vascular strands. Endocarp is leathery and encloses three to six seeds.

Dried ripe fruits are collected, epicarp is removed and hot boiling syrup is poured over it for the purpose of preservation. Rarely sugar is also sprinkled in addition to syrup.

In India fruits are collected and epicarp is removed either partially or fully, and 10% salts added as a preservative. Some fermentation takes place and the drug obtains a black colour.

Morphology

Colour	Reddish-brown
Odour	Pleasant and agreeable
Taste	Sweet and acidic
Shape	As firm black cakes which contain fibres, seeds and little epicarp
Size	5–20 cm long and 2 cm in width

Chemical Constituents

The pulp contains 10% fruit acids, mainly tartaric acid and maleic acid, also about 8% sodium potassium tartarate and about 25–40% invert sugar along with pectin. The acidity ranges from 11 to 16%.

```
H — C — COOH        HO — CH — COOH
    ||                    |
H — C — COOH        HO — CH — COOH

   Maleic acid          Tartaric acid
```

Uses

It acts as a gentle laxative due to osmosis and is also used as present acid refrigerant.

Marketed Product

Tamarindus indica is employed as a laxative in Laxa Tea manufactured by Himalaya Drug Company.

CHITIN

Biological Source

It is a nitrogenous polysaccharide consisting of amino and acetyl group found in the exoskeleton of the tarantula. Its a tough semitransparent horny substance—the principal component of the exoskeletons of arthropods and the cell walls of certain fungi. This is the dense substance forming the indigestible outer skeleton of insects, and the material from which the walls of the mycelia are made. This product can be found in crustaceans, such as crabs, lobsters and shrimp. It can also be found in insects, worms and fungus or mushrooms. Depending upon the different place and different creatures, the percentage of chitin content varies.

History

Chitin was first found in Mushrooms in 1811 by Professor Henri, which was later to be called Chitin. During 1830s, it was isolated from insects and named Chitin. The name chitin is derived from Greek meaning tunic or envelope. During 1850s, Professor C. Roughet discovered while experimenting with Chitin that it could be transferred into water-soluble form through some chemical reaction and in late 1870s name Chitin modified to Chitosan and later on much of the research was focused on these compounds.

Preparation

The shells are made into fine powder and treated with 5% hydrochloric acid for 24 h to remove the impurities and calcium present in the shell. The above extract is then treated with proteolytic enzyme like pepsin for the removal of protein from the shell. The product is then bleached with acidified hydrogen peroxide for 4–6 h. It is then deacetylated at 120°C with a mixture containing two parts of potassium hydroxide, one part of ethyl alcohol and one part of ethylene glycol. The process of deacetylation is continued till the test for acetylization gives report of minimum acetyl content. This deacetylated product is known as the chitosan.

Solubility

Insoluble in water, dilute acid, alcohol and organic solvents, Soluble in sulphuric acid and hydrochloric acid.

Chemical Constituents

Chitin mainly consists of the aminosugar N-acetylglucosamine, which is partially deacetylated. The mostly deacetylated form of chitin is called chitosan. Chitin is present in nature usually complexed with other polysaccharides and with proteins.

Chemical Test

1. Chitosan is soaked in iodine solution and to it add 10% sulphuric acid. It gives deep violet colour.

2. Chitosan is dissolved in 50% nitric acid and crystallized for the formation of sphere crystals of chitosanitrate. The crystals when observed under polarized light using crossed nicol, a distinct cross is observed.

Uses

It is used in wound healing preparations, cuts and burns. It is in medicine that the bacteriostatic, immunologic, antitumoural, haemostatic and anticoagulant properties of chitin and its derivatives have been of the greatest use. Due to its biocompatibility with human body tissue, the cicatrizant properties of chitin has demonstrated their effectiveness for all forms of dressings-artificial skin, corneal bandages and suture thread in surgery, as well as for implants or gum cicatrization in bone repair or dental surgery. In dental creams, it keeps the paste healthy and regenerates gums that are in poor condition.

Chitin is also used as a sizing agent for rayon, cotton, wool and even for synthetic fibres. It has adhesivity to glass and plastics. Industrially chitin is used in the process of water treatment by separating organic compounds and heavy metals, and for treating sewage by precipitating certain anionic wastes and capturing pollutants such as DDT and PCBs (polychlorobenzene).

CARRAGEENAN

Synonyms

Carrageenan, Chondrus extract, Irish moss extract.

Biological Source

It is the sulphated polysaccharide obtained from the seaweed called Irish moss, the red algae *Chondrus crispus* Linn., belonging to family Gigartinaceae, class Rhodophyceae (Fig. 14.18).

Geographical Source

France, Denmark and the United States are the major producers of carrageenan in the world market.

Collection and Preparation

In autumn the algae grown on rocks are collected by means of long rakes from tide water. Carrageenan is extracted from many species of red seaweeds. The process begins with harvesting, followed by drying, cleaning, bagging or bailing. In the factory, the seaweeds are sorted, tested for quality and stored. Before being processed, they are hand-inspected, then washed to remove dirt and marine organisms and then subjected to hot alkaline extraction. When the carrageenan is dissolved, it is clarified through conventional filtration and is then concentrated by membrane ultrafiltration. The carrageenan is precipitated by alcohol or potassium chloride to separate it from soluble impurities. This is followed by drying and grinding to appropriate particle size.

Morphology

Colour	Before bleaching purplish red to purplish brown in colour and after bleaching the drug is yellowish white, translucent and horny
Odour	Slight odour
Taste	Mucilaginous or saline taste
Shape	Strips, flakes or coarse powder
Solubility	Swells in cold water and above 75% dissolves in hot water

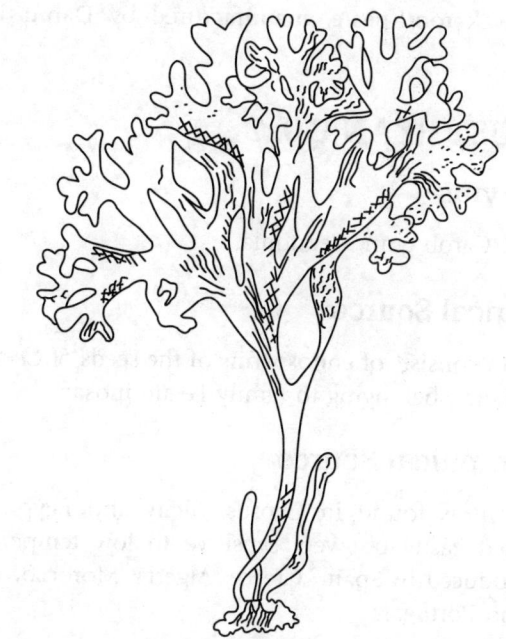

FIG. 14.18 *Chondrus crispus*

Constituents

The constituents of Irish moss are the similar polysaccharides as that of agar. The major constituent is galactans which is known as carrageenan. Carrageenan are classified on the basis of 3,6-anhydro-D-galactose and the position of ester sulphate groups. Three major types of carrageenan are characterized as Kappa, Iota and Lambda-carrageenan. Hydrolysis of the polysaccharides yield galactose, glucose, fructose, arabinose and calcium salt of acid esters of sulphuric acid.

Uses

Carrageenan is used as emulsifying agent, stabilizing agent, solubilizing agent and viscosity builder in food products. Tooth paste, creams, lotions and other cosmetic products are prepared by using carrageenan. In food industry, it is utilized in milk products, ice creams, gels in the concentration of 0.5–1%.

Carrageenan is a popular phlogistic agent for inducing inflammation in the rat paw oedema model for the study of anti-inflammatory activity.

Substitutes and Adulterants

Irish moss is occasionally mixed with seaweeds like *Gigartina stellata* Batt. or *G. pistillata* Lam., which are distinguished stalked cystocarps.

Marketed Product

It is one of the ingredients of the preparations known as Meswak toothpaste, manufactured by Dabur India Limited.

LOCUST BEAN GUM

Synonyms

Arobon, Carob gum, Ceratonia.

Biological Source

This gum consists of endosperms of the seeds of *Ceratonia siliqua* Linn., belonging to family Leguminosae.

Geographical Source

The plant is found in Cyprus, Sicily and Egypt. It is cultivated easily but very sensitive to low temperature. It is produced in Spain, Greece, Algeria, Morocco, Israel, Italy and Portugal.

History

The cultivation of locust bean trees was known before Christian era. Dioscorides referred its curative properties in the first century A.D. In Sicily, the carob trees were probably planted in 16th century. Arabs used carob seed as a unit of weight and it was labelled as carat, which in turn has become unit of weight for precious stones.

Cultivation and Collection

Carob is an evergreen tree growing to a height of about 10 m and has luxuriant perennial foliage. The tree grows on rocky soil and has very long roots that penetrate up to 18–25 m and survive in an area where there is very little rain fall.

It starts bearing fruits only after three years. The plants start flowering in January to March every year, and the fully matured fruits are ready by October–November. The fruits (pods) are harvested by shaking the twigs and picked up from the earth by hand and sent to market.

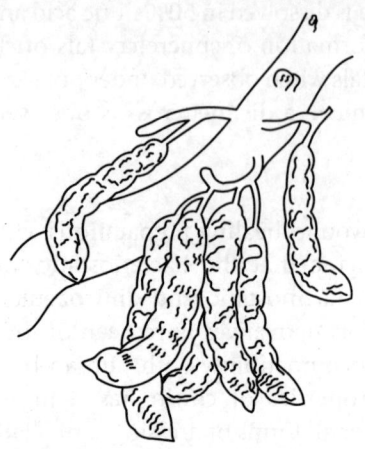

FIG. 14.19 Locust bean branch with pods

The locust bean fruits or carob are dark chocolate coloured, 10–20 cm long, 2.0–5 cm wide and 0.5–1.0 cm thick. The seeds are ovoid dark brown, very hard and weigh 0.21 g or 3.2 grains (i.e. 1 carat). The locust bean tree can be planted or even grafted.

Preparation and Purification of Gum

Locust bean pods consist of 90% of pulp and 8% of kernels (Fig. 14.19). The pods are fed to kibbling machine. The kernels separated consist of 30–33% of husk, germ (about 25%) and endosperm (42–46%). Preparation of high quality gum consists of separation of endosperm from embryo. Successful removal of outer dark coloured husk decides the quality of the gum. Decorticated seeds (dehusked seeds) split lengthwise and are separated from the embryo. The presence of yellow germ (i.e. embryo) increases the rate of fermentation of the gum solutions in further products. Hence, it must be thoroughly removed from the endosperm. It is then pulverized and graded according to the mesh size. The normal mesh sizes available in Italian market are 150, 175 and 200.

Description

Colour	Colourless
Odour	Odourless
Taste	Mucilaginous
Shape	Gum is translucent-white, opaque at the edge, hard, horny and very difficult to break.
Solubility	It is insoluble in alcohol, but is incompletely dispersed in water at room temperature. Most of the gum is dispersed in concentrations up to 5%
Extra features	The gum solutions are pseudoplastic. Gum is a neutral polysaccharide. Hence, pH has little effect on its viscosity in the range of 3–11. The viscosity of 2% dispersion of gum powder in cold water at 25°C is about 1600 centipoises while in hot water dispersed gum, it is about 3200 centipoises

Chemical Constituents

Locust bean gum contains about 88% of D-galacto-D-mannoglycan, 4% pentan, 6% protein, 1% cellulose and 1.0% ash. The ratio of D-galactose to D-mannose is approximately 20:80. Commercial locust bean gum contains no specks and gum particles should not exceed 8–10%. The natural moisture content of gum is about 14.0%.

Identification Test

Locust bean gum mucilage when boiled with 5.0% potassium hydroxide solution becomes clear and shows no yellow colour as in agar and tragacanth or brown colour as in sterculia gum.

Uses

It is useful as a stabilizer, thickner and binder in cosmetics; adsorbent and demulcent therapeutically. It is used as sizing and finishing agent in textiles and also as drilling mud additive. In food industry, it is used as substitute for starch.

STARCH

Synonyms

Amylum.

Biological Source

Starch consists of polysaccharide granules obtained from the grains of maize (*Zea mays* Linn.); rice (*Oryza sativa* Linn.); or wheat (*Triticum aestivum* Linn.); belonging to family Gramineae or from the tubers of potato (*Solanum tuberosum* Linn.), family Solanaceae.

Geographical Source

Most of tropical, as well as, subtropical countries prepare starch commercially.

Preparation of Starch

Depending upon the raw material to be used for processing or type of the starch to be produced, different processes are used for the commercial manufacture of starch.

Potato Starch: The potatoes are washed to remove the earthy matter. They are crushed or cut and converted into slurry. Slurry is filtered to remove the cellular matter. As potatoes do not contain gluten, they are very easy to process further. After filtration, the milky slurry containing starch is purified by centrifugation and washing. Then, it is dried and sent to the market.

Rice Starch: The broken pieces of rice resulted during the polishing are used for processing. The pieces of rice are soaked in water with dilute sodium hydroxide solution (0.5%), which causes softening and dissolution of the gluten. After this, the soaked rice pieces are crushed and starch prepared as described under potato starch.

Maize Starch (corn starch): Maize grains are washed thoroughly with water to remove the adhered organic matter after which they are softened by keeping in warm water for 2–3 days. Sufficient sulphur dioxide is passed to the medium to prevent fermentation. The swollen kernels are passed through attrition mill to break the grains, so as to separate the endosperm and outermost coating of the grains. At this point, special attention is given to separate the germ (embryo). This is effected by addition of water, wherein germs float and are separated. The water which is used to soften the grains dissolves most of the minerals, soluble proteins and carbohydrates from the grains. The water, being rich in all these contents, is used as a culture medium for the production of antibiotics like penicillin (corn steep liquor). The separated germs are used to prepare the germ oil by expression method and are known as corn oil. The oil contains fatty acids like linoleic and linolenic acids and vitamin E. It is used commercially, for the preparation of soap. The starchy material contains gluten; most of this is removed by simple sieving and then by washing. Starch being heavier, settles at the bottom and is followed by gluten. Several treatments with cold water wash the starch effectively, which is then centrifuged or filter-pressed and finally, dried in flash dryers on a moving belt dryer.

Wheat Starch: Wheat being the major article of food is restrictedly used for preparation of starch. In this process, the wheat flour is converted into dough and kept for-a-while. The gluten in the dough swells and the masses are taken to grooved rollers, wherein water is poured over them with constant shaking. The starchy liquid coming out of the rollers is processed conveniently to take out the starch, which is then dried and packed suitably.

Description

Colour	Rice and maize grains are white, while wheat is cream coloured and potato is slightly yellowish
Odour	Odourless
Taste	Mucilaginous
Shape	Starch occurs as fine powder or irregular, angular masses readily reducible to powder

Microscopic Characters (Fig. 14.20)

Rice Starch: The granules are simple or compound. Simple granules are polyhedral, 2–12 µm in diameter. Compound granules are ovoid and 12–30 µm × 7 to 12 µm in size. They may contain 2–150 components.

Wheat Starch: Simple lenticular granules which are circular or oval in shape and 5–50 µm in diameter. Granules contain hilum at the centre and concentric faintly marked striations. Rarely, compound granules with two to four components are also observed.

Maize Starch: Granules are polyhedral or rounded, 5–31 in diameter, with distinct cavity in the centre or two to five rays cleft.

Potato Starch: Generally, found in the form of simple granules, which are subspherical, somewhat flattened irregularly ovoid in shape. Their sizes vary from 30 to 100 µm. Hilum is present near the narrower end with well-marked concentric striations.

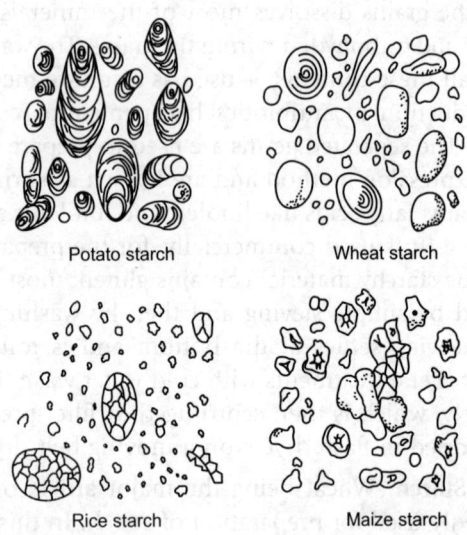

Potato starch   Wheat starch

Rice starch   Maize starch

FIG. 14.20 Starch grains obtained from the different sources

Chemical Constituents

Starch contains chemically two different polysaccharides, such as amylose (β-amylose) and amylopectin (α-amylose), in the proportion of 1:2. Amylose is water soluble and amylopectin is water insoluble, but swells in water and is responsible for the gelatinizing property of the starch. Amylose gives blue colour with iodine, while amylopectin yields bluish black colouration.

Identification Tests

1. Boil 1 g of starch with 15 ml of water and cool. The translucent viscous jelly is produced.
2. The above jelly turns deep blue by the addition of solution of iodine. The blue colour disappears on warming and reappears on cooling.

Uses

Starch is used as a nutritive, demulcent, protective and as an absorbent. Starch is used in the preparation of dusting talcum powder for application over the skin. It is used as antidote in iodine poisoning, as a disintegrating agent in pills and tablets, and as diluent in dry extracts of crude drug. It is a diagnostic aid in the identification of crude drugs. Glycerin of starch is used as an emollient and as a base for suppositories. Starch is also a starting material for the commercial manufacture of liquid glucose, dextrose and dextrin. Starch is industrially used for the sizing of paper and cloth.

Substitutes and Adulterants

Tapioca Starch or Cassava or Brazilian Arrowroot: This starch is obtained from *Manihot esculenta* (Euphorbiaceae) and is used as substitute for starch.

Drugs Containing Alkaloids

CONTENTS

15.1. INTRODUCTION

One of the largest groups of chemicals produced by plants is the alkaloids. Many of these metabolic by-products are derived from amino acids and include an enormous number of bitter, nitrogenous compounds. More than 10,000 different alkaloids have been discovered in species from over 300 plant families. Alkaloids often contain one or more rings of carbon atoms, usually with a nitrogen atom in the ring. The position of the nitrogen atom in the carbon ring varies with different alkaloids and with different plant families. In some alkaloids, such as mescaline, the nitrogen atom is not within a carbon ring. In fact, it is the precise position of the nitrogen atom that affects the properties of these alkaloids. These compounds are renowned for their potent pharmacological activities. Whilst tiny amounts of some can immobilize an elephant or a rhinoceros, others have important clinical use, such as analgesics, antimalarial, antispasmodics, for pupil dilation, treatment of hypertension, mental disorders and tumours.

They are all nitrogen heterocycles which occur mainly in plants as their salts of common carboxylic acids, such as citric, lactic, oxalic, acetic, maleic and tartaric acids as well as fumaric, benzoic, aconitic and veratric acids. Their amine character produce an alkaline solution in water and hence the origin of their name—alkaloids.

Although they undoubtedly existed long before humans, some alkaloids have remarkable structural similarities with neurotransmitters in the central nervous system (CNS) of humans, including dopamine, serotonin and acetylcholine. The amazing effect of these alkaloids on humans has led to the development of powerful painkiller medications, spiritual drugs and serious addictions by people who are ignorant of the properties of these powerful chemicals.

KEY TERMS

15.2. DEFINITION

An alkaloid is a nitrogenous organic molecule that has a pharmacological effect on humans and animals. They are a class of compounds which typically contain nitrogen and have complex ring structures. They occur naturally in seed bearing plants and are found in berries, bark, fruit, roots and leaves. Often, they are bases which have some physiological effect. The name derives from the word alkaline; originally, the term was used to describe any nitrogen-containing base (an amine in modern terms). Alkaloids are found as secondary metabolites in plants (e.g. in Vinca and Datura), animals (e.g. in shellfish) and fungi, and can be extracted from their sources by treatment with acids (usually hydrochloric acid or sulphuric acid, though organic acids, such as maleic acid and citric acid are sometimes used).

Usually alkaloids are derivatives from amino acids. Even though many alkaloids are poisonous (e.g. strychnine or coniine), some are used in medicine as analgesics (pain relievers) or anaesthetics, particularly morphine and codeine. Most alkaloids have a very bitter taste.

15.3. HISTORY

Evidence suggests that alkaloids have been used by humanity for thousands of years. The first civilizations to use them were probably the ancient Sumarians and Egyptians. However, it was not until the early nineteenth century that these compounds were reproducibly isolated and analysed. Advances in analytical separation techniques, such as chromatography and mass spectroscopy, led to the elucidation of the chemical structure of alkaloids. The term for these compounds is thought to have originated from the fact that the alkaloid, morphine, had similar properties to basic salts derived from the alkali ashes of plants thus, it was called a vegetable alkali or alkaloid. Since the first alkaloids were isolated, thousands more have .been identified and classified.

Prior to approximately 300 years ago, malaria was the scourge of Europe, likely having been introduced through the Middle East. Malaria is caused by protozoa of the genus *Plasmodium*, contained as spores in the gut of the Anopheles mosquito, which then spreads the spores to humans when it bites. As the Spanish and Portuguese explorers began to colonize South America, they discovered a cure for malaria known to the native Indians. This was the bark of the Cinchona trees. The use of Cinchona bark to treat malaria was first reported in Europe in 1633, and the first bark reached Rome about 12 years later. Teas made from the bark cured people suffering from malaria, one of the major scourges in Europe at that time, and the bark was known as Jesuit's bark. Because of the philosophical differences between Protestants and Catholics, many Protestants refused to be treated with the bark. One of the most prominent Protestants of the time, Oliver Cromwell, reportedly died of malaria because of this stubbornness.

The French apothecary Derosne probably isolated the alkaloid afterwards known as narcotine in 1803 and the Hanoverian apothecary Serturner further investigated opium and isolated morphine (1806 and 1816). Morphine is the principal alkaloid and was first isolated between 1803 and 1806. It was widely used for pain relief beginning in the 1830s, but was also recognized as being addictive. Isolation of other alkaloids, particularly by Pelletier and Caventou, rapidly followed: strychnine (1817), emetine (1817), brucine (1819), piperine (1819), caffeine (1819), quinine (1820), colchicine (1820) and conine (1826). Coniine was the first alkaloid to have its structure established and to be synthesized, but for others, such as colchicine, it was well over a century before the structures were finally elucidated. In the second half of the twentieth century alkaloids featured strongly in the search for plant drugs with anticancer activity. A notable success was the introduction of catharanthus alkaloids and paclitaxel into medicine and there is much current interest in other alkaloids having anticancer properties as well as those exhibiting antiaging and antiviral possibilities.

15.4. CLASSIFICATION

Alkaloids are generally classified by their common molecular precursors, based on the biological pathway used to construct the molecule. From a structural point of view, alkaloids are divided according to their shapes and origins. There are three main types of alkaloids: (1) true alkaloids, (2) protoalkaloids and (3) pseudoalkaloids. True alkaloids and protoalkaloids are derived from amino acids, whereas pseudoalkaloids are not derived from these compounds.

True Alkaloids

True alkaloids derive from amino acid and they share a heterocyclic ring with nitrogen. These alkaloids are highly reactive substances with biological activity even in low doses. All true alkaloids have a bitter taste and appear as a white solid, with the exception of nicotine which has a brown liquid. True alkaloids form water-soluble salts. Moreover, most of them are well-defined crystalline substances which unite with acids to form salts. True alkaloids may occur in plants (1) in the free state, (2) as salts and (3) as N-oxides. These alkaloids occur in a limited number of species and families, and are those compounds in which decarboxylated amino acids are condensed with a nonnitrogenous structural moiety. The primary precursors of true alkaloids are such amino acids as L-ornithine, L-lysine, L-phenylalanine/L-tyrosine, L-tryptophan and L-histidine.

Examples of true alkaloids include such biologically active alkaloids as cocaine, quinine, dopamine and morphine.

Protoalkaloids

Protoalkaloids are compounds, in which the N atom derived from an amino acid is not a part of the heterocyclic. Such kinds of alkaloid include compounds derived from L-tyrosine and L-tryptophan. Protoalkaloids are those with a closed ring, being perfect but structurally simple alkaloids. They form a minority of all alkaloids. Hordenine, mescaline and yohimbine are good examples of these kinds of alkaloid. Chini et al. have found new alkaloids, stachydrine and 4-hydroxystachydrine, derived from *Boscia angustifolia*, a plant belonging to the Capparidacea family. These alkaloids have a pyrroline nucleus and are basic alkaloids in the genus *Boscia*. The species from this genus have been used in folk medicine in East and South Africa. *Boscia angustifolia* is used for the treatment of mental illness, and occasionally to combat pain and neuralgia.

Pseudoalkaloids

Pseudoalkaloids are compounds, the basic carbon skeletons of which are not derived from amino acids. In reality, pseudoalkaloids are connected with amino acid pathways. They are derived from the precursors or post-cursors (derivatives the indegradation process) of amino acids. They can also result from the amination and trans-amination reactions of the different pathways connected with precursors or post-cursors of amino acids.

These alkaloids can also be derived from nonaminoacid precursors. The N atom is inserted into the molecule at a relatively late stage, for example, in the case of steroidal or terpenoid skeletons. Certainly, the N atom can also be donated by an amino acid source across a trans-amination reaction, if there is a suitable aldehyde or ketone. Pseudoalkaloids can be acetate and phenylalanine derived or terpenoid, as well as steroidal alkaloids. Examples of pseudoalkaloids include such compounds as coniine, capsaicin, ephedrine, solanidine, caffeine and theobromine.

Alkaloids are mainly divided into two categories on the basis of their chemical structure, that is, heterocyclic rings (Table 15.1).

Atypical alkaloids

These are also known as nonheterocyclic alkaloids and contain nitrogen in aliphatic chain.

Typical alkaloids

These are also known as heterocyclic alkaloids and contain nitrogen in heterocyclic ring system.

Table 15.1: Classification of alkaloids

Groups	Example	Source	Uses
1. Nonheterocyclic Alkaloids			
Phenyl ethyl amine alkaloid	Ephedrine, Mescaline, Hordenine	*Ephedra* sp.	Asthma
Tropolone alkaloids	Colchicine	*Colchicum* sp.	Gout
Modified diterpene	Taxol	*Taxus* sp.	Anticancer
2. Heterocyclic Alkaloids			
a. Mononuclear Heterocyclic Alkaloids			
Pyridine	Lobeline	*Lobelia* sp.	Asthma
Piperidine	Piperine	*Piper* sp.	Gonorrhoea, Anti-oxidant
Pyrrole	Hygrine	*Coca* sp.	CNS Stimulant
Pyrrolidine	Nicotine	*Tobacco* sp.	CNS Stimulant
Imidazole	Pilocarpine	*Pilocarpus* sp.	Contraction of pupil
b. Polynuclear Heterocyclic alkaloids			
Isoquinoline	Morphine, papaverine	Opium	Narcotic analgesic
Quinoline	Quinidine, quinidine	Cinchona	Antimalarial
Indole	Ergotamine, reserpine, vincristine, Strychnine	Ergot, Rauwolfia, Vinca, Nux vomica	Oxytocic, Anti-HT, Anticancer, CNS stimulant
Quinazoline	Vasicine	Vasaka	Antitussive
Tropane	Atropine, hyo-scine	Datura, belladona	Parasympatholytic
Purine	Caffeine	Coffee, tea	CNS stimulant
Steroid	Solasodine	*Solanum* sp.	Steroidal precursor
Terpenoid	Aconitine	*Aconite* sp.	Neuralgia

The interrelationship between different ways of classifications can be summarized by the Table 15.2.

15.5. OCCURRENCE IN NATURE

Alkaloids are substances very well known for their biological activity at the beginning of world civilization. They were used in shamanism, in traditional herbal medicine for the cure of diseases and in weapons as toxins during tribal wars and during hunting. They also had, and still have, socio-cultural and personal significance in ethnobotany. Moreover, they have been and continue to be the object of human interest concerning new possibilities for their safe utilization

Table 15.2: Main types of alkaloids and their chemical groups

Alkaloid Type	Precursor Compound	Chemical Group of Alkaloids	Parent Compounds	Examples of Alkaloids
True alkaloids	L-Ornithine	Pyrrolidine alkaloids	Pyrrolidine	Cuscohygrine, Hygrine
		Tropane alkaloids	Tropane	Atropine, Cocaine, Hyoscyamine, Scopolamine/hyoscine
		Pyrrolizidine alkaloids	Pyrrolizidine	Ilamine, Indicine-N-oxide, Meteloidine, Retronecine
	L-Lysine	Piperidine alkaloids	Piperidine	Anaferine, Lobelanine, Lobeline, Pelletierine, Piperidine, Piperine, Pseudopelletierine, Sedamine
		Quinolizidine alkaloids	Quinolizidine	Cytisine, Lupanine, Sparteine
		Indolizidine alkaloids	Indolizidine	Castanospermine, Swansonine
	L-Tyrosine	Phenylethyl-amino alkaloids	Phenylethyl amine	Adrenaline, Anhalamine, Dopamine, Noradrenaline, Tyramine
		Simple tetrahydroisoquinoline Alkaloids	Benzyltetrahydroisoquinoline	Codeine, Morphine, Norcoclaurine, Papaverine, Tetrandrine, Thebaine, Tubocurarine
	L-Tyrosine or L-Phenylalanine	Phenethylisoquinoline alkaloids	Amaryllidaceae alkaloids	Autumnaline, Crinine, Floramultine, Galanthamine, Galanthine, Haemanthamine, Lycorine, Lycorenine, Maritidine, Oxomaritidine, Vittatine
	L-Tryptophan	Indole alkaloids	Indole	
		Simple indole alkaloids		Arundacine, Arundamine, Psilocin, Serotonin, Tryptamine, Zolmitriptan
		Simple β-carboline alkaloids		Elaeagnine, Harmine
		Terpenoid indole alkaloids		Ajmalicine, Catharanthine, Secologanin, Tabersonine
		Quinoline alkaloids	Quinoline	Chloroquinine, Cinchonidine, Quinine, Quinidine
		Pyrroloindole alkaloids	Indole	Yohimbine, Chimonantheine, Corynantheine, Corynantheidine, Corynanthine
		Ergot alkaloids		Ergotamine, Ergocryptine
	L-Histidine	Imidazole alkaloids	Imidazole	Histamine, Pilocarpine, Pilosine
		Manzamine alkaloids	Xestomanzamine	Xestomanzamine-A, Xestomanzamine-B
	L-Arginine	Marine alkaloids	β-carboline	Saxitoxin, Tetrodotoxin
	Anthranilic acid	Quinazoline alkaloids	Quinazoline	Peganine
		Quinoline alkaloids	Quinoline	Acetylfolidine, Acutine, Bucharine, Dictamnine, Dubunidine, Kokusaginine, Maculosine, Perfamine, Perforine, Polifidine, Skimmianine
		Acridone alkaloids	Acridine	Acronycine, Rutacridone
	Nicotinic acid	Pyridine alkaloids	Pyridine/Pyrrolidine	Anabasine, Cassinine, Celapanin, Evoline, Evonoline, Evorine, Maymyrsine, Nicotine, Regelidine, Wilforine
Proto alkaloids	L-Tyrosine	Phenylethyl-amino alkaloids	Phenylethyl-amine	Hordenine, Mescaline

Alkaloid Type	Precursor Compound	Chemical Group of Alkaloids	Parent Compounds	Examples of Alkaloids
	L-Tryptophan	Terpenoid indole alkaloids	Indole	Yohimbine
	L-Ornithine	Pyrrolizidine alkaloids	Pyrrolizidine	4-hydroxy stachydrine Stachydrine
Pseudo alkaloids	Acetate	Piperidine alkaloids	Piperidine	Coniine Coniceine Pinidine
		Sesquiterpene alkaloids	Sesquiterpene	Cassinine Celapanin Evonine Evonoline Evorine Maymyrsine Regelidine Wilforine
	Pyruvic acid	Ephedra alkaloids	Phenyl C	Cathine Cathinone Ephedrine Norephedrine
	Ferulic acid	Aromatic alkaloids	Phenyl	Capsaicin
	Geraniol	Terpenoid alkaloids	Terpenoid	Aconitine Actinidine Atisine Gentianine β-skytanthine
	Saponins	Steroid alkaloids		Cholestane Conessine Jervine Pregnenolone Protoveratrine A Protoveratrine B Solanidine Solasodine
	Adenine/Guanine	Purine alkaloids	Purine	Caffeine Theobromine Theophylline

and ensuing health benefits. Of all secondary compounds, historically and contemporaneously, only alkaloids are molecules of natural origin with highly important benefits and diagnostic uses. They can be characterized as the most useful and also the most dangerous products of nature.

Alkaloids are most abundant in higher plants. At least 25% of higher plants contain these molecules. In effect, this means that on average; at least one in fourth plants contains some alkaloids. In reality, it is not impossible that alkaloids occur more commonly. Using the latest equipment and technology, such slight traces of alkaloids may be detected (e.g. less than 10 gigagrams per kg of plant mass) that these have no real influence on biological receptors and activity. Generally these species are not considered as alkaloid species. Hegnauer has defined alkaloid plants as those species which contain more than 0.01% of alkaloids. This is right from the point of view of the classification. From the genetic point of view, and the genetic mechanism of alkaloid synthesis, it is a real limitation. Paying attention to slight traces of alkaloids in plants, we see the members of the plant family which are relatives. They have a genetically determined alkaloid mechanism with a species expression. Moreover, this expression is also on the hybrid level.

The distribution of alkaloids in nature is restricted to some specific plants, animals or lower plants. The pattern of distribution of compound and its pharmacological activity have a great role in chemotaxonomical classification. Alkaloids are chiefly found to be distributed in angiosperms and to some extent in lower plants (mosses, liverworts) and animals. Nearly about 47–50% of various bacterial species also contain alkaloids, for example, pyocyanine from *Pseudomonas aeruginosa*. Alkaloids are commonly found in the families like, Chenopodiaceae, Lauraceae, Berberidaceae, Menispermaceae, Ranunculaceae, Papaveraceae, Fumariaceae, Leguminosae, Papilionaceae, Rutaceae, Apocynaceae, Loganiaceae, Rubiaceae, Boraginaceae, Convolvulaceae, Solanaceae, Campanulaceae, Compositae, etc. They may be present in any part of the plant like, roots (reserpine from Rauwolfia), aerial parts like (Ephedra), barks (quinine from cinchona), leaves (Cocaine from Coca), seeds (caffeine from Coca seeds) or even in entire plant (vinblastine from Vinca). 300 alkaloids belonging to more than 24 classes are reported to occur in the skins of amphibians.

15.6. PROPERTIES

Although numerous alkaloids exist, they have similar properties when separated. In general, they are colourless, crystalline solids which are basic, have a ring structure, and have definite melting points. They are also derived from plants and have a bitter taste. However, some exceptions are known. For instance, some alkaloids are not basic and others are brightly coloured (betanidine, beriberine, sanguinarine) or liquid (nicotine). Other alkaloids are produced synthetically. Most alkaloids are also chiral molecules which mean they have nonsuperimposable mirror images. This results in isomers that have different chemical properties. For example, one isomer may have a physiological function while the other does not.

Generally free bases of alkaloids are soluble in organic solvents and insoluble in water, where as alkaloidal salts are soluble in water and partially soluble in organic solvents. For example, strychnine hydrochloride is much more soluble in water than strychnine as a base.

15.7. EXTRACTION

The extraction of alkaloids is based on their basic character and solubility profiles. Generally alkaloids are extracted mainly using two methods.

Method A

The powdered material that contains alkaloidal salts is moistened with alkaline substances like sodium bicarbonate, ammonia, calcium hydroxide, etc., which combines with acids, tannins and other phenolic substances and sets free the alkaloids bases. Extraction is then carried out with organic solvents such as ether or petroleum spirit. The concentrated organic liquid is then shaken with aqueous acid and allowed to separate. Alkaloid salts will be present in aqueous liquid, while many impurities remain behind in the organic liquid.

Method B

The collected powdered material is extracted with water or aqueous alcohol containing dilute acid. Chloroform or other organic solvents are added and shaken to remove the pigments and other unwanted materials. The free alkaloids are then precipitated by the addition of excess alkalis like, sodium bicarbonate or ammonia and separated by filtration or by extraction with organic solvents.

Volatile liquid alkaloids (nicotine and coniine) are isolated by distillation. The powdered material that contains alkaloids is extracted with water and the aqueous extract is made alkaline with sodium carbonate or ammonia and the alkaloid is distilled off in steam. This could be collected and purified.

15.8. CHEMICAL TESTS

The chemical tests are performed from neutral or slightly acidic solution of drug.

Dragendorff's Test

Drug solution + Dragendorff's reagent (potassium bismuth iodide), formation of orangish red colour.

Mayer's Test

Drug solution + few drops of Mayer's reagent (potassium mercuric iodide), formation of creamy-white precipitant.

Hager's Test

Drug solution + few drops of Hager's reagent (saturated aq. solution of picric acid), formation of crystalline yellow precipitate.

Wagner's Test

Drug solution + few drops of Wagner's reagent (dilute iodine solution), formulation of reddish-brown precipitate.

Tannic Acid Test

Drug solution + few drops of tannic acid solution, formation of buff coloured precipitate.

Ammonia Reineckate Test

Drug solution + slightly acidified (HCl) saturated solution of ammonia reineckate, formation of pink flocculent precipitate.

15.9. TROPANE ALKALOIDS

The tropane alkaloids, which have the 8-azabicyclo octane nucleus, are commonly found in plants of three families, the Solanaceae, Erythroxylaceae and Convolvulaceae families. Tropane alkaloids are tropene derivatives. Tropane ring is composed of pyrrolidine and piperidine rings. Tropane is 3-hydroxy tropene. There are two stereoisomers of tropene, tropine and pseudotropine. They are esters combined with acids. These esters of tropic acid could be detected by Vitali-Morin reaction. The acids present are tropic acid in atropine and atropic acid formed by the loss of water from tropic acid in apoatropine. Other organic acids like tiglic acid, acetic acid, isobutyric acid and isovaleric acid are also present.

The alkaloids isolated from plants of these families, while having several legitimate medicinal uses, are probably best known for their toxic properties. This can be a major problem since the plants produce very attractive berries which are tempting to small children. As few as three berries of henbane (*Hyoscyamus niger*) or deadly nightshade (*Atropa belladonna*) can cause death in infants. Many of the plants in the Solanaceae family contain tropane alkaloids, which are responsible for the toxic effects of the plants. Cleopatra is reputed to have tested the effects of henbane and deadly nightshade on her slaves to investigate the possibility of using these extracts to commit suicide (she found the toxic effects too painful). The wives of the Roman emperors, Augustus and Claudius, used deadly nightshade to murder large numbers of Romans. The mandrake (*Mandragora officinarum*) was reputed to possess aphrodisiac properties and was prized for these properties. However, the roots also contain large quantities of the tropane alkaloid hyoscine (scopolamine), making the plant highly toxic.

BELLADONNA

Synonyms

Belladonna herb; Belladonna leaf; Deadly night shade leaves; Banewort; Death's herb, Dwale; Poison black cherry; Folia belladonnae.

Biological Source

Belladonna consists of dried leaves and flowering tops of *Atropa belladonna* Linn. (European Belladonna), belonging to family Solanaceae (Fig. 15.1). It contains about 0.35% of total alkaloids calculated as hyoscyamine.

Geographical Source

A. belladonna is cultivated in United States, Canada, UK, Germany and India.

Cultivation and Collection

Plants are cultivated by sowing seeds in nurseries and seedlings are transplanted in April to moist, calcareous and loamy soil. Weeds are removed and manure is applied for proper growth of the crop. During flowering session leaves and flowering tops are cut at least three times in a year at an interval of two months from one to three years old plants. When the plant is four years old, roots are dug out. The collected drug is dried at 40–50°C. Undried leaves deteriorate and give off ammonia. Belladonna plant infected with the fungus *Phytophthora belladonnae* should be destroyed to prevent further infection. Sometimes the leaves are damaged by flea-bettle insect and the roots by a fungus.

Characteristics

The drug contains leaves, smaller stems of about 5 mm diameter, flowers and fruits. Leaves are stalked, brittle, thin, entire, long-pointed, 5–25 cm long, 2.5–12 cm wide, ovate lanceolate, slightly decurrent lamina, margin-entire, apex acuminate, colour dull-green or yellowish-green, surface glabrous, lateral veins join the midrib at an angle of 60°C, curving upwards and are anastomose. The upper side is darker than the lower. Each has a petiole about 0.5–4 cm long and a broadly ovate, slightly decurrent lamina about 5–25 cm long and 2.5–12 cm wide. The margin is entire and the apex acuminate. A few flowers and fruits may be present. If the leaves are broken, they are characterized by the venation and roughness of the surface due to the presence of calcium oxalate in some mesophyll cells which causes minute points on the surface of the leaf on drying. The flowers blooming in June are solitary, shortly stalked, drooping and about 2.5 cm long. The corolla is campanulate, five-lobed and of a dull purplish colour. The five-lobed calyx is persistent, remaining attached to the purplish-black berry. The fruit is bilocular, contains numerous seeds and is about the size of a cherry. A yellow variety of the plant lacks the anthocyanin pigmentation.

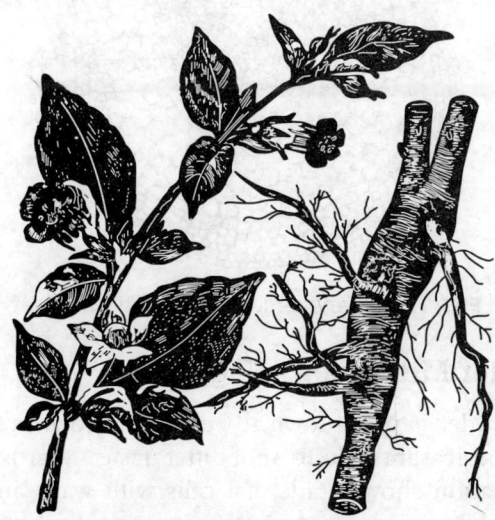

FIG. 15.1 *Atropa belladonna*

Microscopy

A transverse section of the leaf of *A. belladonna* has a bifacial structure. The epidermal cells have-wavy walls and a striated cuticle. Anisocytic type and some of the anomocytic type stomata arc present on both surfaces but are most common on the lower. Hairs are most numerous on young leaves, uniseriate, two- to four-celled clothing hairs; or with a uni-cellular glandular head. Some hair has a short: pedicel and a multicellular glandular head. Certain of the cells of the spongy mesophyll are filled with microsphenoidal (sandy) crystals of calcium oxalate. The midrib is convex above and shows the usual bicollateral vascular bundle. A zone of collenchyma is present in epidermis near midrib.

Chemical Constituents

Belladonna contains 0.3–1.0% total alkaloids, the prominent base is L-hyoscyamine and other components are atropine, apoatropine, as choline, belladonnine, cuscohygrine, chrysatropic acid, volatile bases, such as atroscine, leucatropic acid; phytosterol, N-methylpyrroline, homatropine, hyoscyamine N-oxide, rutin, kaempferol-3-rhamnogalactoside and 7-glucoside, quercetin-7-glucoside, scopoletin, calcium oxalate, 14% acid soluble ash and 4% acid-insoluble ash. Addition of ammonia to the alcoholic solution of scopoletin shows blue fluorescence. This test is useful to detect Belladonna poisoning. Atropine is formed by racemization during the extraction process.

Hyoscyamine

Atropine

Belladonine

Uses

The drug is used as adjunctive therapy in the treatment of peptic ulcer; functional digestive disorders, including spastic, mucous and ulcerative colitis; diarrhoea, diverticulitis and pancreatitis. Due to anticholinergic property, it is used to control excess motor activity of the gastrointestinal tract and spasm of the urinary tract.

Belladonna is anticholinergic, narcotic, sedative, diuretic mydriatic and used as anodyne and to check secretion.

Other uses are similar to hyoscyamus. It relieves spasm of gut or respiratory tract. Consumption of belladonna checks excessive perspiration of patients suffering from tuberculosis. Belladonna acts as a parasympathetic depressant.

Marketed Products

It is one of the ingredients of the preparation known as belladona plaster (Surgi Pharma) for backache, stiffness of muscles and boil, swollen joints.

DATURA HERB

Biological Source

Datura herb consists of the dried leaves and flowering tops of *Datura metel* Linn. and *Datura metel var. fastuosa* belonging to family Solanaceae (Fig. 15.2).

Geographical Source

It is found in India, England and other tropical and subtropical countries.

Characteristics

Datura metel is also an Indian plant and resembles *D. fastuosa*; it differs in that the leaves are heart-shaped, almost entire and downy, and the flowers always white.

D. metel var. fastuosa is known in commerce as black datura. The leaves are ovate and more or less angular, the flowers being mostly purplish, sometimes white. Corolla is double or triple. Outer corolla has five teeth and inner Corolla has six to ten teeth.

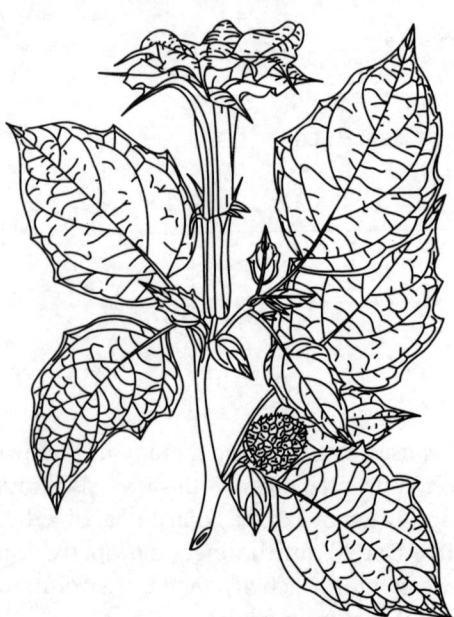

FIG. 15.2 *Datura metel*

Microscopy (Figs. 15.3 and 15.4)

Transverse section shows a bifacial structure. The following characters were observed in the lamina and the midrib region. In the lamina it has the upper epidermis which is single layer, rectangular cells covered with cuticle. Both covering and glandular trichomes are present. The covering trichomes are uniseriate, multicellular, warty and with blunt apex. The glandular trichomes have one stalk consisting of one cell and multicellular head. The mesophyll has spongy parenchyma and palisade parenchyma in it. Palisade cells are radially elongated, single layer and compactly arranged. Spongy parenchyma are several layers, loosely arranged consisting of microsphenoidal crystals and vascular strands. In the midrib, strips of collenchyma appear below the upper and above the lower epidermis followed by the cortical parenchymatous cells containing calcium oxalate. The lower epidermis is similar to that of the upper one but has more number of trichomes and stomata when compared with upper epidermis.

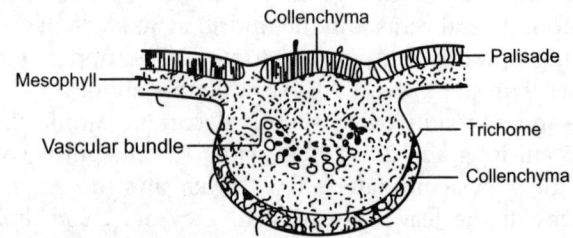

FIG. 15.3 T.S. (schematic) diagram of datura leaf

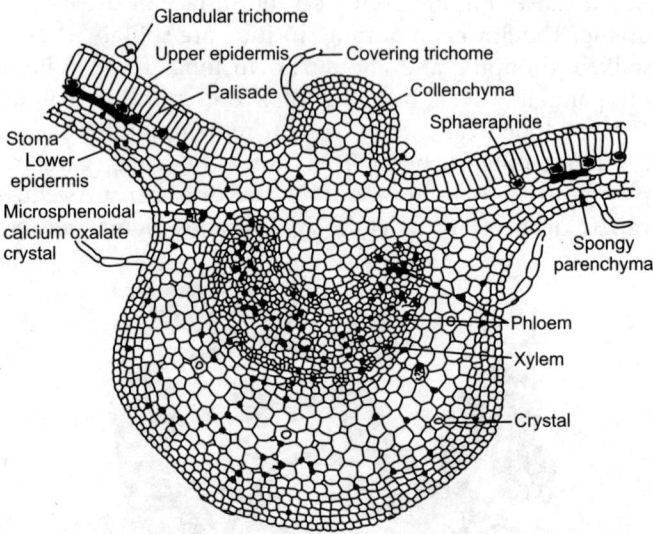

FIG. 15.4 Transverse section of datura leaf

Powder Microscopy (Fig. 15.5)

The powder is pale brown to yellowish brown in colour with unpleasant odour and bitter taste. Microscopical examination shows epidermal cells with wavy anticlinal walls and anisocytic stomata. Covering trichomes are

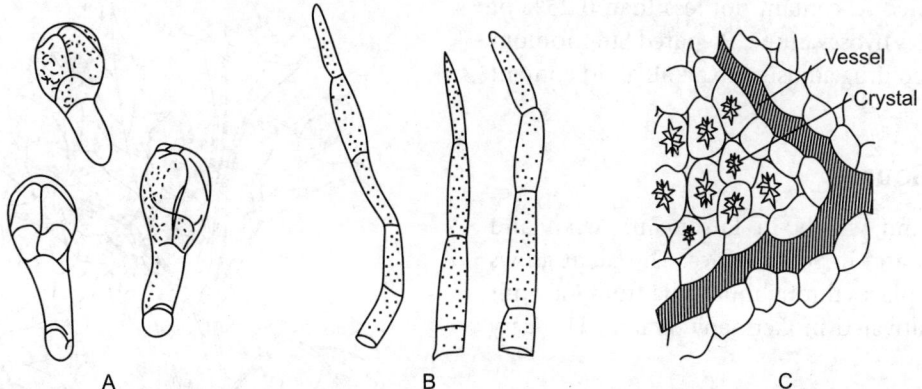

FIG. 15.5 Powder characteristics of datura leaf. (A: Glandular trichome, B: Covering trichome, C: Veinlet with crystal layer)

uniseriate, multicellular and conical. Glandular trichomes have unicellular stalk and uni- or multicellular head. Fragments of vessels with spiral thickening and plenty of calcium oxalate crystals, collenchyma and palisade cells can also be seen (Fig. 15.5).

Chemical Constituents

Datura herb contains up to 0.5% of total alkaloids, among which hyoscine (scopolamine) is the main alkaloid, while L-hyoscyamine (scopoline) and atropine are present in very less quantities.

Scopolamine

Chemical Tests

1. *Vitali-Morin test:* The tropane alkaloid is treated with fuming nitric acid, followed by evaporation to dryness and addition of methanolic potassium hydroxide solution to an acetone solution of nitrated residue. Violet colouration takes place due to tropane derivative.
2. On addition of silver nitrate solution to solution of hyoscine hydrobromide, yellowish white precipitate is formed, which is insoluble in nitric acid, but soluble in dilute ammonia.

Uses

In Ayurveda black datura is considered more efficacious or more toxic. *D. metel* is used in the manufacture of hyoscine or scopolamine. It exhibits parasympatholytic with anticholinergic and CNS depressant effects. The drug is used in cerebral excitement, asthma and in cough. The Rajpoot mothers are said to smear their breasts with the juice of the *D. metel* leaves, to poison their newly born female infants.

Other Species

D. arborea, a South American species (the Tree Datura), growing freely in Chile, contains about 0.44% alkaloid, nearly all hyoscine. A tincture of the flowers is used to induce clairvoyance. *D. quercifolia*, of Mexico, contains 0.4% in the leaves and 0.28% of alkaloids in the seeds, about half hyoscyamine and half hyoscine. *Datura innoxia* is found throughout India. It is a perennial herb with a thick fleshy hairy stem. Leaves are thick and pubescent. Corolla is single, white, 10-toothed and calyx inflated. Fruit is a capsule with prominent spines. Leaves contain both hyoscine and hyoscyamine. *Datura tatula*, Purple Stramonium owes its activity to the same alkaloids as *D. Stramonium*, and its leaves are also much used in the form of cigarettes as a remedy for spasmodic asthma. *D. ferox*, Chinese Datura, is used in homoeopathy.

Marketed Products

It is one of the ingredients of the preparations known as Jatifaladi Bati, Jatyadi tail (Baidyanath) and J.P. Massaj oil, Pain kill oil, J.P. Grace oil (Jamuna Pharma).

STRAMONIUM

Synonyms

Thorn apple leaves; Jimson or Jamestown weed; Dhatura; Stinkweed; Devil's apple; Apple of Peru; Folia stramonii.

Biological Source

Stramonium consists of dried leaves and flowering tops of *Datura stramonium* Linn., or its variety *D. tatula* Linn., belonging to family Solanaceae (Fig. 15.6).

The drug is required to contain not less than 0.25% of alkaloids calculated as hyoscyamine. Prepared Stramonium is the finely powdered drug adjusted to an alkaloid content of 0.23–0.27%.

Geographical Source

Stramonium is found widely in European, Asian and American countries, and in South Africa. The plant grows commonly in waste places throughout India from Kashmir to Malabar. It is cultivated in Germany, France, Hungary and South America.

Cultivation and Collection

Datura prefers a rich calcareous soil. It can be grown from seeds in spring in drills; the plants are later thinned to stand 3 m apart in raws. The plant is sensitive to frost and sheltered situations are preferred for cultivation. Entire plants are cut down when the fruits are mature. Nitrogen manuring, which favours the growth of plants, also flavours alkaloid formation. At the end of August leaves and flowering tops are collected and dried at 45–50°C.

Characteristics

D. stramonium is a bushy annual herb, 1.5 m high, having whitish roots and numerous rootlets. The dried leaves are greyish-green in colour, thin, brittle, twisted, broken, whole leaves 8–25 cm long and 7–15 cm wide; shortly petiolate, ovate or triangular-ovate in shape, acuminate at the apex and have a sinuate-dentate margin. The margin possesses teeth dividing the sinuses; the lateral veins run into the marginal teeth.

Microscopy

A transverse section of a leaf has a bifacial structure; covered with a smooth cuticle and possess both stomata and hairs. Microsphenoidal and prismatic cluster crystals of calcium oxalate are abundant in the mesophyll. The stomata are of the anisocytic and anomocytic types. The epidermal cells have wavy walls. The uniseriate clothing hairs are three- to five-celled, slightly curved and have thin, warty walls. Small glandular hairs with a one- or two-celled pedicel and an oval head of two to seven cells are also present. The midrib has a bicollateral structure and characteristic subepidermal masses of collenchyma on both surfaces. The xylem is a curved arc. Sclerenchyma is absent.

Chemical Constituents

Stramonium contains 0.2–0.6% alkaloids. The main alkaloids are hyoscyamine and hyoscine (scopolamine). It also contains protein albumin and atropine.

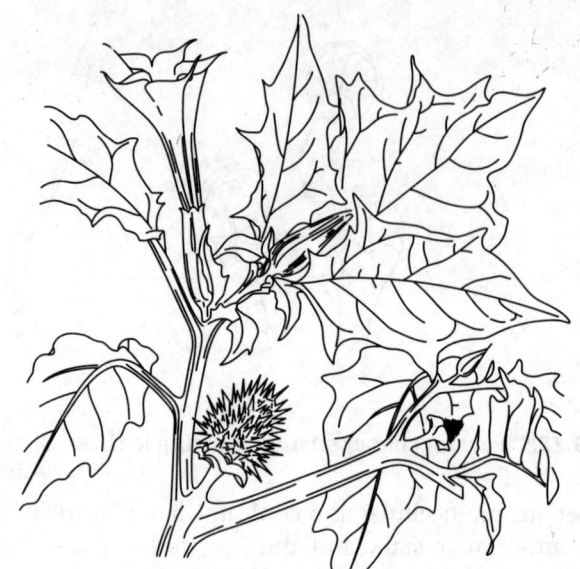

FIG. 15.6 *Datura stramonium*

Atropine is formed from hyoscyamine by racemization. At the time of collection these alkaloids are usually present in the proportion of about two parts of hyoscyamine to one part of hyoscine, but in young plants hyoscine is the predominant alkaloid. The larger stems contain small amount of alkaloid and the official drug should contain not more than 3% stem with a diameter exceeding 5 mm.

Ditigloyl esters of 3,6-dihydroxytropane and 3,6,7-trihydroxytropane have also been isolated from the roots in addition to hyoscine, hyoscyamine, tropine and pseudotropine,

D. stramonium also contains 6-hydroxyhyoscyamine, skimmianine, meteloidine, acetyl derivatives of caffeic, p-coumaric and ferulic acids, β-sitosterol, stigmasterol, campesterol, withanolide I, steroidal glycosides daturataturins A and B; flavonoids chrysins, quercetin and kaempferol and their esters.

Hyoscyamine

Scopolamine

Uses

It is a narcotic, antispasmodic and anodyne drug and used to relieve the spasm of the bronchioles in asthma. The leaves are ingredient of *Pulvis stramonii compositus* and other powders used for the relief of asthma. The leaves may be made into cigarettes or smoked in a pipe to relieve asthma. They are also used in the treatment of parkinsonism, boils, sores and fish bites. The flower juice is used to treat earache.

The fruit juice is applied to the scalp for curing dandruff and falling hair. Stramonium ointment, containing lanolin, yellow wax and petroleum, is employed to cure haemorrhoids.

Marketed Products

It is one of the ingredients of the preparation known as Maharasayan vati (Mahaved healthcare).

HYOSCYAMUS

Synonyms

Common Henbane, Hyoscyamus, Hog's-bean, Jupiter's-bean, Symphonica, Cassilata, Cassilago, Deus Caballinus.

Biological Source

Hyoscyamus consists of the dried leaves and flowering tops of *Hyoscyamus niger* Linn., belonging to family Solanaceae. It contains not less than 0.05% alkaloids, calculated as hyoscyamine (Fig. 15.7).

Geographical Source

It is found throughout Central and Southern Europe and in Western Asia, extending to India and Siberia. As a weed of cultivation it now grows also in North America and Brazil. Apart from these countries, it grows in Scotland, England and Wales and also in Ireland, and has been found wild in 60 British countries.

History

The medicinal uses of Henbane date from Ancients times, being particularly commended by Dioscorides (first century A.D.), who used it to procure sleep and allay pains, and Celsus (same period) and others made use of it for the same purpose, internally and externally. This use is mentioned in a work by Benedictus Crispus (A.D. 681) under the names of Hyoscyamus and Symphonica. There is frequent mention made of it in Anglo Saxon works on medicine of the eleventh century, in which it is named 'Henbell', and in the old glossaries of those days it also appears as Caniculata, Cassilago and Deus Caballinus.

Later it was not used. It was omitted from the London Pharmacopoeia of 1746 and 1788, and only restored in 1809; its reintroduction being chiefly due to experiments and recommendations by Baron Storch, who gave it in the form of an extract, in cases of epilepsy and other nervous and convulsive diseases.

Cultivation and Collection

Drug is usually obtained from cultivated biennial herb. Henbane will grow on most soils, in sandy spots near the sea, on chalky slopes, and in cultivation flourishing in a good loam. It requires a light, moderately rich and well-drained soil for successful growth and an open, sunny situation, but does not want much attention beyond keeping the ground free from weeds. The seed should be sown in the open, early in May or as soon as the ground is warm, as thinly as possible, in rows 2–2.5 feet apart, the seedlings thinned out to 2 feet apart in the rows, as they do not stand transplanting well. In order to more readily ensure germination, it is advisable to soak the seeds in water for 24 h before planting the unfertile seeds will then float on the top of the water and may thus be distinguished. Ripe seed should be grey, and yellowish or brown seeds should be rejected, as they are immature. Let the seeds dry and then sift out the smallest, using only the larger seeds. Only the larger seedlings should be reserved, especially those of a bluish tint. The soil where the crop is to be, must have been well manured, and must be kept moist until the seeds have germinated, and also during May and June of the first year. It is also recommended to sow seeds of biennial Henbane at their natural ripening time, August, in porous soil.

The ground must never be water-logged, drought and late frosts stunt the growth and cause it to blossom too early, and if the climatic conditions are unsuitable, especially in a dry spring and summer, the biennial Henbane will flower in its' first year, while the growth is quite low, but well manured soil may prevent this. Much of the efficacy of Henbane depends upon the time at which it is gathered. The leaves should be collected when the plant is in full

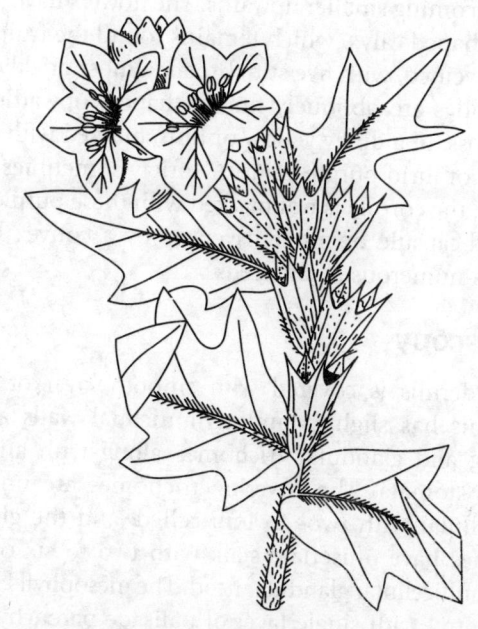

FIG. 15.7 *Hyoscyamus niger*

flower. In the biennial plant, those of the second year are preferred to those of the first; the latter are less clammy and foetid, yield less extractive, and are medicinally considered less efficient. The leaves of the biennial variety are collected in June or the first week of July and those of the annual in August. They are dried at 40–50°C in drying sheds, heated from outside. The dried drug is stored in airtight containers at low temperature, protected from light and moisture.

Characteristics

Both varieties are used in medicine, but the biennial form is the one considered official. The leaves of this biennial plant spread out flat on all sides from the crown of the root like a rosette; they are oblong and egg-shaped, with acute points, stalked and more or less sharply toothed, often more than a foot in length, of a greyish-green colour and covered with sticky hairs. These leaves perish at the appearance of winter. The flowering stem pushes up from the root-crown in the following spring, ultimately reaching from 3 to 4 feet in height, and as it grows, becoming branched and furnished with alternate, oblong, unequally lobed, stalkless leaves, which are stem-clasping and vary considerably in size, but seldom exceed 9–10 inches in length. These leaves are pale green in colour, with a broad conspicuous midrib, and are furnished on both sides (but particularly on the veins of the under surface) with soft, glandular hairs, which secrete a resinous substance that causes the fresh leaves to feel unpleasantly clammy and sticky. Similar hairs occur on the subcylindrical branches.

The flowers are shortly stalked, the lower ones growing in the fork of the branches, the upper ones stalkless, crowded together in one side, leafy spikes, which are rolled back at the top before flowering, the hairy, leafy, coarsely toothed bracts becoming smaller upwards. The flowers have a hairy, pitcher shaped calyx, which remains round the fruit and is strongly veined, with five stiff, broad, almost prickly lobes. The corollas are obliquely funnel-shaped, upwards of an inch across, of a dingy yellow or buff, marked with a close network of lurid purple veins. A variety sometimes occurs in which the corolla is not marked with these purple veins. The seed-capsule opens transversely by a convex lid and contains numerous small seeds.

Microscopy

The epidermis is covered with smooth layer of cuticle. Epidermis has slightly sinuous anticlinal walls and has covering and glandular trichomes along with anisocytic type of stomata. The covering trichomes are uniseriate, multicellular with two- to four-celled, and the glandular trichomes have uniseriate stalk with two to six cells and ovoid multicellular glandular head. The mesophyll is usually dorsiventral with single layer of palisade parenchymatous cells only below the upper epidermis and rarely isobilateral.

A crystal layer is present below the palisade, with tetragonal prisms or clusters of few components. In the midrib region it has long narrow arc of radially arranged xylem above the phloem and an endodermis consisting of starch. The remaining portion is covered with parenchyma with small supernumerary phloem.

The transverse section of stem shows a large central hollow and consists of numerous perimedullary phloem bundles in the pith region. Tetragonal calcium oxalate as prisms or clusters or in microsphenoidal sandy shape is also present in the pith.

Chemical Constituents

The chief constituent of Henbane leaves is the alkaloid Hyoscyamine, together with smaller quantities of Atropine and Hyoscine, also known as Scopolamine. The proportion of alkaloid in the dried drug varies from 0.045% to 0.14%. Other constituents of Henbane are a glucosidal bitter principle called hyoscytricin, choline, mucilage, albumin, calcium oxalate and potassium nitrate. On incineration, the leaves yield about 12% of ash. The chief constituent of the seeds is about 0.5–0.6% of alkaloid, consisting of Hyoscyamine, with a small proportion of Hyoscine, The seeds also contain about 20% of fixed oil.

Hyoscyamine

Scopolamine

Atropine

Uses

It is used as antispasmodic, hypnotic and mild diuretic. The leaves have long been employed as a narcotic medicine. It is similar in action to belladonna and stramonium, though milder in its effects. The drug combines the therapeutic actions of its two alkaloids, hyoscyamine and hyoscine. Because of the presence of the former, it tends to check secretion and to relax spasms of the involuntary muscles, while through the narcotic effects of its hyoscine it lessens pain and exercises a slight somnifacient action. It will also relieve pain in cystitis. It is used to relieve the griping caused by drastic purgatives, and is a common ingredient of aperient pills, especially those containing aloes and colocynth.

Marketed Products

It is one of the ingredients of the preparations known as muscle and joint rub (Himalaya Drug Company), Brahmi vati, Sarpagandhaghan Vati (Dabur) and Zymnet drops (Aimil Pharmaceuticals).

COCA LEAVES

Synonyms

Coca, Cuca, Cocaine, Folium cocae, Peruvian coca, Truxillo coca, Java coca, Bolivian coca.

Biological Source

Coca consists of the dried leaves of various species of *Erythroxylon*, that is, *Erythroxylon coca* Lam (Huanco or Bolivian coca) or *Erythroxylon coca* var. *Spruceanum* (Peruvian, Truxillo or Java coca) also known as *Erythroxylon truxillense* Rusby., belonging to family Erythroxylaceae (Fig. 15.8).

Geographical Source

It is mainly found in Bolivia, Peru, Indonesia, Ceylon, Java and India.

Cultivation

Coca shrubs grow well in the situations similar to tea plantations. It requires rich, light and well-drained soil at an altitude of 1500–6000 m. Cultivation is carried out by sowing seeds. Fertilizers have their effects over these plants. In the second year the leaves will be matured enough to collect in dry weather. The collected leaves are dried in shade and packed.

Characteristics

- *Erythroxylon coca*: Leaves are brownish-green in colour, oval, entire and glabrous, with a bitter taste, 3–8 cm long and 1.5–4 cm wide.
- *Erythroxylon truxillense*: The leaves are much smaller and pale green in colour, elliptical, entire, glaborous, not glossy, with bitter taste.

Microscopy

The epidermis has straight anticlinal walls and stomata present are of the rubiaceous type only on the lower surface. The mesophyll reveals the presence of single layer of palisade parenchyma cells only below the upper epidermis. Prism of calcium oxalate crystals are seen in the spongy

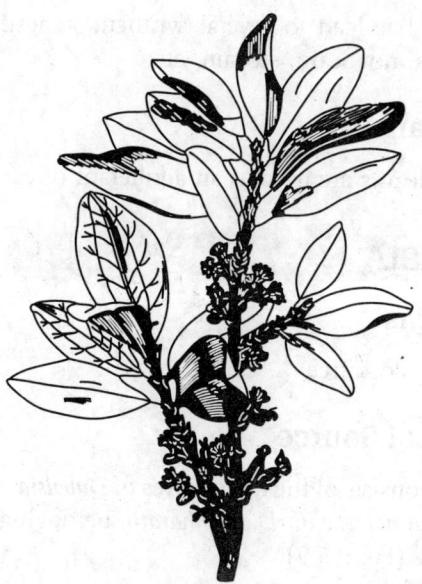

FIG. 15.8 *Erythroxylon coca*

parenchyma. The midrib has vascular bundle composed of xylem and phloem with a band of pericyclic fibres below and few sclerenchyma above. Leaf has an outstanding ridge, filled with collenchyma, presence of lignified idioblasts, and development of sclerenchyma above and below the side veins are its unique characters.

Chemical Constituents

Coca leaves contain the alkaloids Cocaine, Annamyl Cocaine and Truxilline or Cocamine. Truxillo or Peruvian leaves contain more alkaloid than the Bolivian, though the latter are preferred for medicinal purposes. Java Coca contains tropacocaine and four yellow crystalline glucosides in addition to the other constituents.

Cocaine

Uses

The actions of coca depend principally on the alkaloid Cocaine. Cocaine has stimulant action on CNS. The leaves are extensively chewed to relieve hunger and fatigue. Coca alkaloids cause also hallucination. Coca leaves are used as a cerebral and muscle stimulant, especially during convalescence, to relieve nausea, vomiting and pains of the stomach without upsetting the digestion. Cocaine also has local anaesthetic action on skin and mucous membrane; and is used as dental anaesthesia and minor local surgery of ophthalmic, ear, nose and throat. Chemical structure of cocaine has lead to several synthetic anaesthetics like anaesthesia, novocain, stovain, etc.

Adulterant

Jaborandi leaves are used as an adulterant of coca leaves.

DUBOISIA

Synonyms

Corkwood, cork tree.

Biological Source

Duboisia consists of the dried leaves of *Duboisia myoporoides* R., *Duboisia hopwoodii*, *D. leichhardtii*, belonging to family Solanaceae (Fig. 15.9).

Geographical Source

It is mainly found in Australia and Ecuador.

Characteristics

- *Duboisia hopwoodii:* Perennial shrub to 3 m, sometimes as small tree with brown to purplish bark on the young stems and corky older bark. Leaves are narrow, long and alternate to 15 cm, with recurved point and straight margins. Open clusters of white (with purple striped tube) flowers at the end of the branches. Black berry to 6 mm, containing one to two seeds in a dark pulp.
- *Duboisia myoporoides:* Perennial shrub to small tree with corky bark with intensely bitter taste, Leaves alternate pale green 3–10 cm × 1–1.5 cm, tapered at both ends. Open clusters of small white flowers at the end of the branches and black juicy berry, containing a few seeds in a dark pulp.
- *Duboisia leichhardtii:* Perennial shrub to small tree with corky bark with intensely bitter taste, similar to *D. myoporoides*. Leaves narrowly elliptic pale green 4–10 cm × 1–2 cm, tapered at both ends. Open clusters of small white flowers, sometimes tinged with mauve, at the end of the branches. Flowers, late winter to spring. Black juicy berry, containing a few seeds in a dark pulp.

Microscopy *(Duboisia myoporoides)*

The upper epidermis consists of polygonal tabular cells covered with thick and striated cuticle. Stomata are very less with very few near the midrib. The mesophyll has cylindrical palisade cells and just next to it is a row of subrectangular collecting cells and 7 or 8 rows of spongy parenchyma with scattered idioblasts. Each scattered idioblasts consist of small microsphenoidal crystals of calcium oxalate. In the lower epidermis it has numerous stomata which are cruciferous in nature. Scattered glandular trichomes occur on both surfaces

which are about 75–95 µm long and 15–25 µm wide at the head. The midrib has well developed ridge and contains a meristele with xylem and superior supernumerary phloem.

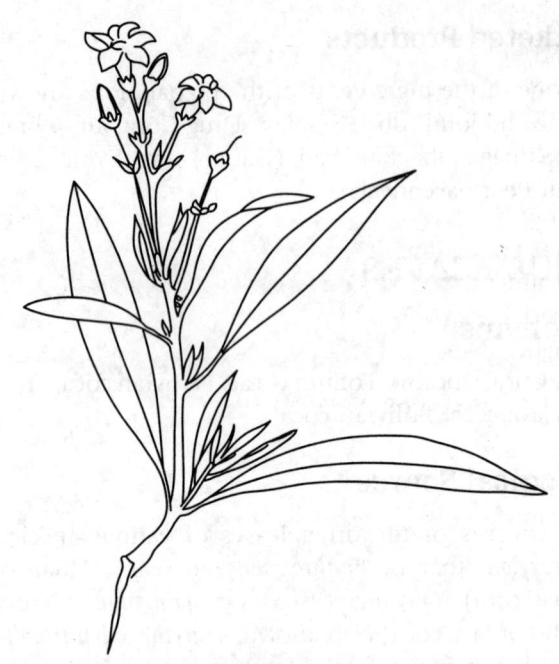

FIG. 15.9 *Duboisia myoporoides*

Chemical Constituents

Duboisia myoporoides is considered as the chief commercial source of scopolamine and atropine. It contains hyoscyamine which is converted to atropine during extraction. Along with it, the drug also contains norhyoscyamine, tigloidine, valtropine, tiglyoxytropine. The synthetic process for scopolamine and atropine is very costly and hence, much reliance is placed on its natural source. Atropine ($C_{17}H_{23}O_3N$) occurs as colourless crystals, with a bitter taste and no odour. It is soluble in chloroform and alcohol. It is a racemic form of hyoscyamine.

The chief constituent of *Duboisia hopwoodii* was found to be nicotine and nonnicotine, with content reportedly up to 25% of the dried weight of the plant material.

Hyoscyamine

Chemical Tests

1. The addition of gold chloride solution to atropine in water and hydrochloric acid gives lemon yellow precipitate.
2. It gives positive Vitali-Morin reaction.

Uses

Duboisia leaves are the main source of atropine and scopolamine. Atropine is the parasympatholytic drug. It also causes stimulant action on central, medullary and higher nerve centres. Atropine has many different therapeutic uses. It is used as an antidote for pilocarpine, physostigmine and other choline esters. It relieves bronchial spasms in asthma. As it suppresses the gastric secretions, it is used in peptic ulcer. It has applications in ophthalmic practice, because of its dilatory effects on pupil of the eye. It is also used to reduce tremor and rigidity in Parkinsonism. Scopolamine is used as treatment for air and sea sickness and in the treatment of stomach ulcers. Sedative, hypnotic and mydriatic (of variable strength), which augments the activity of the respiratory system. Its alkaloid, sulphate of duboisia, is sometimes used as a substitute for atropine. The homoeopaths use the tincture and the alkaloid for paralysis and eye infections; a red spot interfering with vision is an indication for its use. It is antidoted by coffee and lemon juice.

15.10. INDOLE ALKALOIDS

Indole (1-H-indole) is a benzopyrrole in which the benzene and pyrrole rings are through the 2,3-positions of the pyrrole. The indole nucleus is found in a large number of naturally occurring compounds. It is of commercial importance as a component of perfumes. Isoindole (I-H-isoindole), the isomer in which the benzene and pyrrole rings are fused through the 3- and 4-positions of the pyrrole, is not stable. A few of its derivatives are known, the simplest being *N*-methylisoindole.

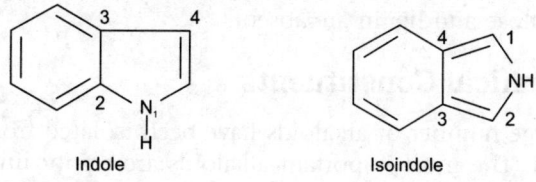

Indole   Isoindole

Indole was first obtained (and its structure elucidated) in 1866 by Adolf von Baeyer. Interest in indole chemistry revived about 1930 when it was discovered that the essential amino acid, tryptophan, the plant growth hormone, heteroauxin and several groups of important alkaloids are indole derivatives. It was shown that 3-methylindole (skatole) is produced with indole during pancreatic digestion or putrefactive decomposition of proteins and, hence, both are found in the intestines and faeces. Interest has centred on medicinal and biochemical aspects of indole chemistry. Serotonin, which has been identified as a metabolite in brain chemistry; the psychotomimetic indoles, psilocin and psilocybin from mushrooms; the tranquilizer reserpine; and the melanin pigments are a few of the compounds that have been studied.

Indole is a colourless crystalline solid (mp 52–54°C, bp 254°C). The heat of combustion at constant volume is 4268 MJ/mol (10–20 kcal/mol). The molecule is planar and has only moderate polarity. Indole has good solubility in a wide range of solvents including petroleum ether, benzene, chloroform and hot water. The solubility in cold water is only 1:540 at 25°C; thus, water is a good solvent for purification by recrystallization. Indole forms salts with high concentrations of both strong bases and strong acids.

The various plants containing indole alkaloids are vinca, ergot, Rauwolfia, nux vomica, physostigma, etc.

ERGOT

Synonyms

Ergot; Rye Ergot; Secale cornutum; Spurred rye; Ergot of rye; Ergota.

Biological Source

Ergot is the dried sclerotium of a fungus, *Claviceps purpurea* Tulasne, belonging to family Clavicipitaceae, developing in the ovary of rye plant, *Secale cereale* (Family Poaceae) (Fig. 15.10).

Ergot should yield about 0.15% of the total alkaloids calculated as ergotoxine and water-soluble alkaloids equivalent to about 0.01% of ergonovine.

Geographical Source

It is mainly found in Czechoslovakia, Hungary, Switzerland, Germany, France, Yugoslavia, Spain, Russia and India. In India ergot is cultivated at Kodaikanal (T.N.).

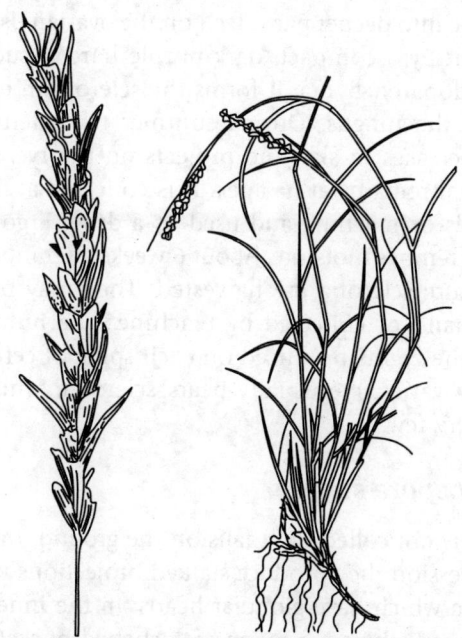

FIG. 15.10 *Claviceps purpurea*

Cultivation and Collection

The life cycle of the fungus, *Claviceps purpurea*, which is a parasite, passes through the following characteristic stages:

1. Sphacelia or honeydew or asexual stage
2. Sclerotium or ascigerous or sexual stage and
3. Ascospore stage.

1. Sphacelia or honeydew or asexual stage

The rye plant becomes infected by the spores of the fungus in the spring session when flowers bloom for about one week. The spores are carried by the wind or by insects to the flowers and collected at the base of the young ovary where moisture is present. There germination of the spores takes place. A filamentous hyphae is formed which enters into the wall of the ovary by enzymatic action. A soft, white mass over the surface of ovary is formed, which is known as sphacelia. A sweet viscous yellowish liquid, known as honeydew, is secreted during the sphacelia stage which contains reducing sugars (reduce Fehling solution). From the ends of some hyphae small oval conidiospores (asexual spore/s) are abstricted which remain suspended on honeydew. The sweet taste of honeydew attracts some insects like ants and weevils. Insects suck the sweet liquid and carry the conidiospores to the plants and spread the fungal infection in the rye plants. Cultured conidiospores are used for the inoculum. Strains capable of producing about 0.35% of selected alkaloids, mainly ergotamine, are now utilized.

2. Sclerotium or ascigerous or sexual stage

During the sphacelia stage the hyphae enter only the outer wall of the ovary. On further development they penetrate into deeper parts, feed on the ovarian tissues and replace it by a compact, dark purple hard tissue known as pseudoparenchyma. It forms the sclerotium or resting state of the fungus. During summer the sclerotium or ergot increases in size and projects on the rye, showing sphacelial remains at its apex. It is collected at this stage by hands or machine and used as a drug. Ergot is then dried to remove moisture. About 6 weeks after inoculation, the mature sclerotia are harvested. They may be picked up by hand or collected by machine. The number and size of the ergots produced on each spike of cereal by *C. purpurea* varies, rye usually bears sclerotia, while wheat bears very few.

3. Ascospore stage

If ergot is not collected, it falls on the ground. In the next spring session they produce stalked projections known as stromata which have globular heads. In the inner surface of the heads there are many flask-shaped pockets known as perithecia. Each of these perithecia contains many sacs (asci) which possesses eight of the thread-like ascospores. These ascospores are carried out by insects or wind to the flowers of the rye as described in the first stage. In this way life cycle of ergot is completed.

The ascospores may be germinated on a nutritive medium to get conidiospore bearing cultures. The suspension of these conidiospores is usually used as a spray to infect rye plants for commercial production of ergot.

Ergot is collected from fields of rye when the sclerotia are fully developed and projecting from the spike, or they are removed from the grain by shifting. The size of the crop varies according to weather conditions. The vegetative phase of the fungus can, like that of other moulds, be cultivated artificially. Under such conditions the typical sclerotia do not develop.

Characteristics

The size of sclerotium (Ergot) is about 1–4 cm long, 2–7 mm broad. Shape is fusiform, slightly curved, subcylindrical, tapering at both ends. The outer surface is dark or violet-black in colour, has longitudinal furrows and sometimes small transverse cracks. The fractured surface shows thin, dark outer layer, a whitish or pinkish-white central zone of pseudoparenchyma in which darker lines radiate from the centre. Odour is characteristic and taste is unpleasant.

Microscopy

Ergot shows an outer zone of purplish-brown, obliterated rectangular cells. The pseudoparenchyma consists of oval or rounded cells containing fixed oil and protein, and with highly refractive walls which give a reaction for chitin. Cellulose and lignin are absent.

Chemical Constituents

A large number of alkaloids have been isolated from the Ergot. The most important alkaloids are ergonovine and ergotamine. On the basis of solubility in water the alkaloids are divided into two groups: water-soluble ergometrine (or ergonovine) group or water-insoluble (ergotamine and ergotoxine) groups as given hereunder:

	Group	Alkaloids
Water-soluble group		
I.	Ergometrine group	Ergometrine, Ergometrinine
Water-insoluble group		
II.	Ergotamine group	Ergotamine, Ergotaminine, Ergosine, Ergosinine
III.	Ergotoxine group	Ergocristine, Ergocristinine, Ergocryptine, Ergocryptinine, Ergocornine, Ertgocorninine

Only the first group, ergometrine group, belongs to water-soluble compounds. Alkaloids of Group II and III

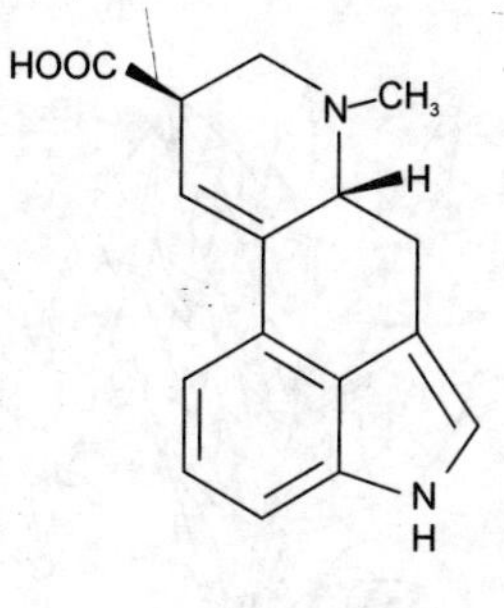

Lysergic acid

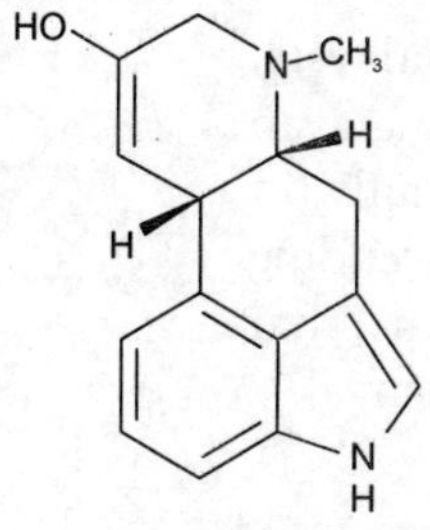

Agroclavine

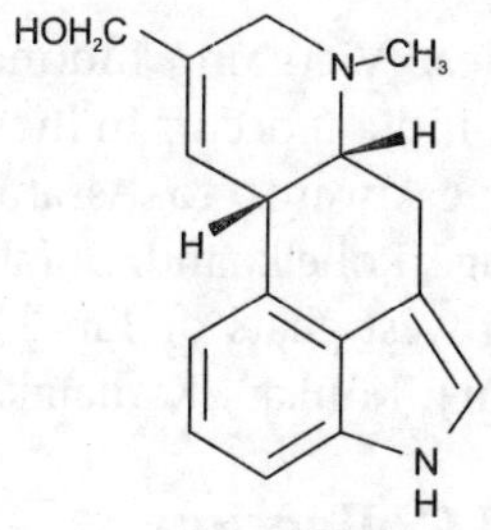

Elymoclavine

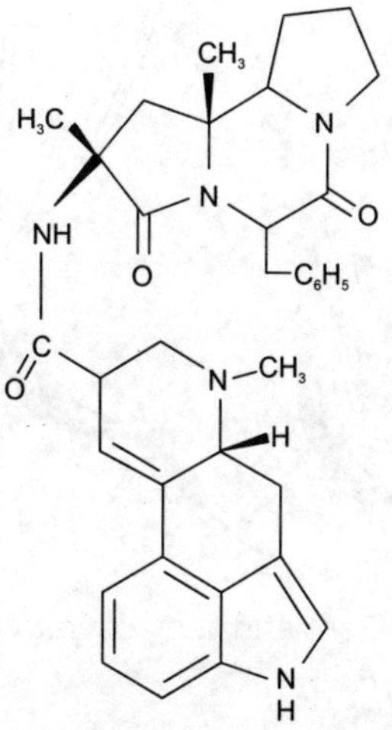

Ergotamine

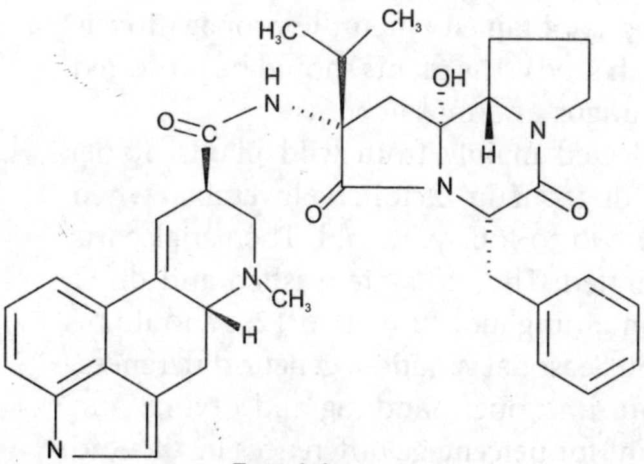

Ergocristine

are polypeptides in which lysergic acid or isolysergic acid is linked to amino acids. Alkaloids obtained from lysergic acid are physiologically active compounds. In the first group, for example, ergometrine alkaloids, lysergic acid or its isomer is linked to an amino alcohol.

The ergot alkaloids (ergolines) can also be divided into two classes (1) the clavine-type alkaloids, which are derivatives of 6,8-dimethyl-ergoline and (2) the lysergic acid derivatives, which are peptide alkaloids and contains the pharmacologically active alkaloids that characterize the ergot sclerotium (ergot). Each active alkaloid occurs with an inactive isomer involving isolysergic acid.

Chemical Tests

1. Ergot under UV light shows a red-coloured fluorescence.
2. Ergot powder is extracted with a mixture of $CHCl_3$ and sodium carbonate. The $CHCl_3$ layer is separated and a mixture of p-dimethylaminobenzaldehyde (0.1 g), H_2SO_4 (35%, v/v, 100 ml) and 5% ferric chloride (1.5 ml) is added. A deep blue colour is produced.

Uses

Ergot is oxytocic, vasoconstrictor and abortifacient and used to assist delivery and to reduce postpartum haemorrhage. Lysergic acid diethylamide (LSD-25), obtained by

partial synthesis from lysergic acid, is a potent specific psychotomimetic. Ergometrine is oxytocic and used in delivery. It stimulates the tone of uterine muscles and prevents postpartum haemorrhage.

Only ergometrine produces an oxytocic effect, ergotoxine and ergotamine having quite a different action. Ergometrine is soluble in water or in dilute alcohol. It is known as ergonovine. Ergotamine and the semisynthetic dihydroergotamine salts are used as specific analgesics for the treatment of migraine. Lysergic acid diethylamide (LSD-25), prepared by partial synthesis from lysergic acid, is a potent specific psychotomimetic.

RAUWOLFIA

Synonyms

Sarpagandha, Chandrika; Chootachand; Indian snake root.

Biological Source

Rauwolfia consists of dried roots of *Rauwolfia serpentina* Benth., belonging to family Apocynaceae (Fig. 15.11).

Geographical Source

It is an erect, evergreen, small shrub native to the Orient and occurs from India to Sumatra. It is also found in Burma,

Thailand, Philippines, Vietnam, Indonesia, Malaysia, Pakistan and Java. In India it occurs in the sub-Himalayan tracts from Sirhind eastwards to Assam, especially in Dehradun, Sivalik range, Rohelkhand, Gorakhpur ascending to 1300 m, east and west ghats of Tamil Nadu, in Bihar (Patna and Bhagalpur), Konkan, Karnataka and Bengal.

Cultivation and Collection

Rauwolfia grows in tropical forests at an altitude of 1200–1300 m at temperature 10–40°C. There should be enough rain or irrigation for its cultivation. The soil should be acidic (pH 4–6), clayey and manure is applied for better crop. Propagation is done by planting seeds, root cuttings or stem cuttings. Better drug is obtained when the propagation is carried out with fresh seeds. The plants should be protected from nematodes, fungus and mosaic virus.

The drug is collected mainly from wild plants. Roots and rhizomes are dug out in October–November when the plant roots are two to four years old. The aerial parts and roots are separated. The roots are washed and dried in air. The roots containing moisture up to 12% should be protected from light. Seasonal variation, genetic differences, geographic location, improper handling and drying, and other factors account for percentage differences in alkaloid amount. Rauwolfia should be packaged and stored in well-closed containers in a cool, dry place that is secure against insect attack.

Characteristics

The roots and rhizomes are almost identical in external characters. The drug occurs in cylindrical or slightly tapering, tortuous pieces, 2–10 cm long, 5–22 mm in diameter. The roots are rarely branched. Rootlets, 0.5–1 mm in diameter, are rare. The outer surface is greyish-yellow, light-brown or brown. Young pieces contain slight wrinkles while old pieces have longitudinal ridges. Circular scars of rootlets are present. Bark exfoliation is present in old samples leaving behind patches of exposed wood. The fracture is short. A narrow, yellowish-brown bark and a dense pale yellow wood are present on the smooth transverse surface at both the ends. Pieces of rhizome closely resemble the root but may be identified by a small central pith. They are attached to them with small pieces of aerial stem. Slight odour is felt in recently dried drug which decreases with age; taste is bitter.

Microscopy (Fig. 15.12)

Transverse section of the root shows a stratified cork, which is divided, into two to eight alternating zones. It consists of one to seven layers of smaller and radially narrower, suberised, nonlignified cells alternating with one to three layers of larger radially broader, lignified cells. The phelloderm is composed of about ten to twelve layers of tangentially

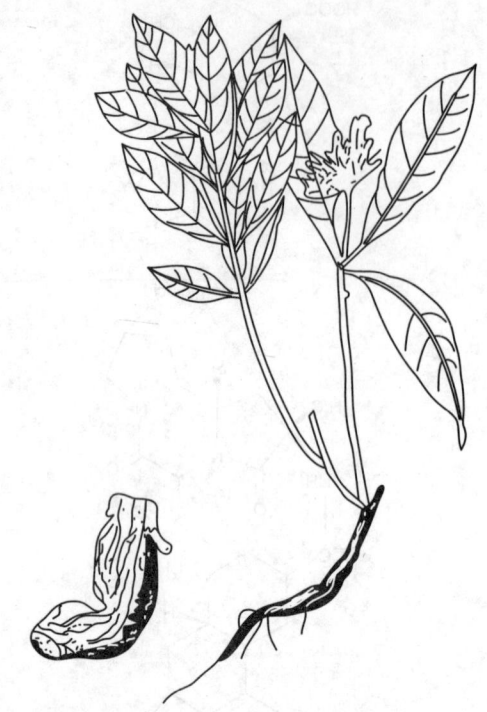

FIG. 15.11 Root and twig of *Rauwolfia serpentina*

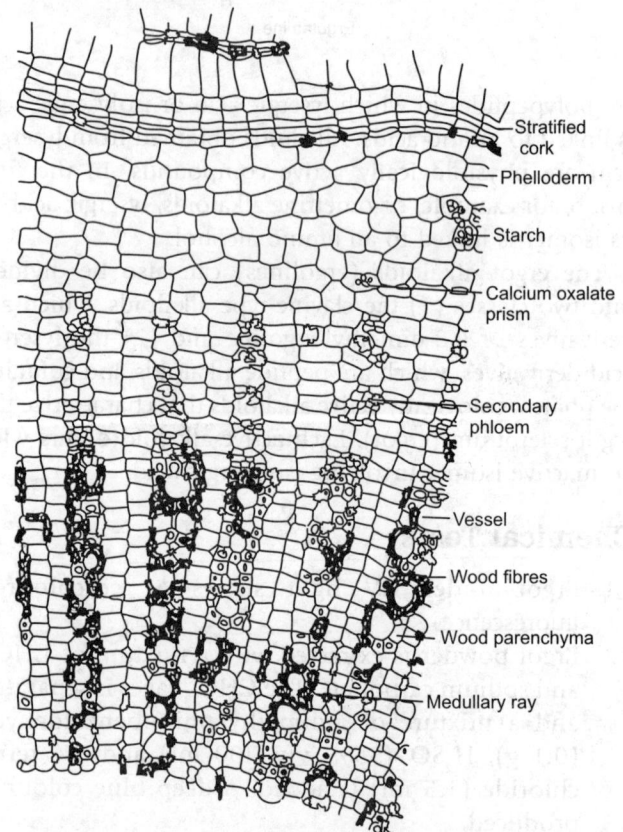

FIG. 15.12 Transverse section of Rauwolfia root

elongated to isodiametric, cellulosic parenchymatous cells. Cells of secondary cortex are parenchymatous and contain starch grains, simple and compound (two to four components), spherical with a distinct hilum in the form of a split. Phloem is narrow and consists of parenchyma with scattered sieve tissue; parenchyma alternate with broader medullary rays composed of large cells and usually two to four cells wide. Xylem is wide, entirely lignified and usually shows two to five annual rings. Medullary rays, one to five cells wide, contain starch grains and alternate with secondary xylem consisting of vessels, tracheids, fibres and parenchyma. Xylem vessels have pitted thickening.

Powder Microscopy (Fig. 15.13)

The powder is pale brownish-yellow in colour with bitter taste. Microscopical examination shows abundant starch grains (4–20–50 μm long), simple and compound (2–4

components), spherical, with a distinct hilum in the form of a split. Fibres are lignified, slightly pitted, found with or without attached vessels and tracheidal vessels. Vessels are lignified, fairly narrow with bordered pits, found usually in groups; and tracheids are pitted with tapered ends. Cork cells are polygonal in surface view. Few irregularly prismatic calcium oxalate crystals are present in small groups in some parenchymatous cells of the phloem.

Chemical Constituents

Rauwolfia contains about 0.7–2.4% total alkaloidal bases from which more than 80 alkaloids have been isolated. The prominent alkaloids isolated from the drug are reserpine, rescinnamine, ψ-reserpine, rescidine, raubescine and deserpidine. The other alkaloidal components are

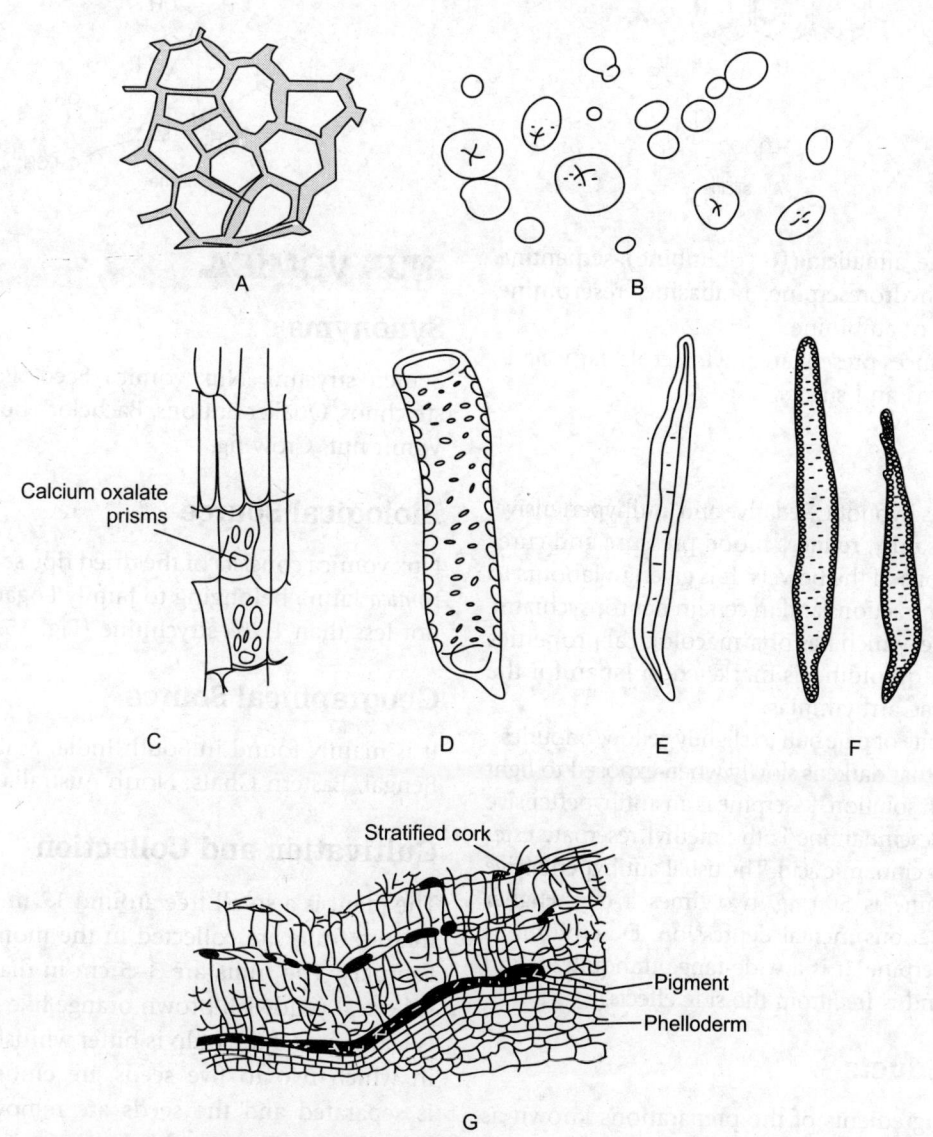

FIG. 15.13 Powder characteristics of Rauwolfia root. (A: Cork cells, B: Starch grains, C: Phloem parenchyma with calcium oxalate crystals, D: Vessel, E: Fibre, F: Tracheids, G: Cork cells)

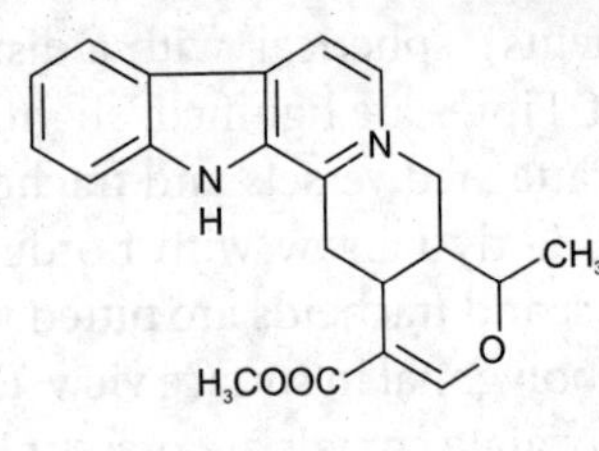

Serpentine

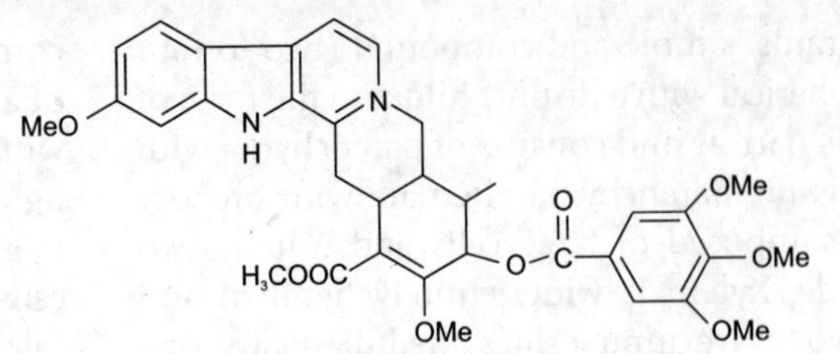

Reserpine

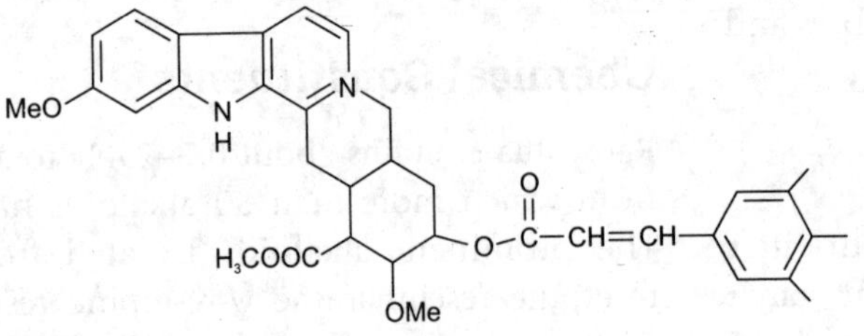

Rescinnamine

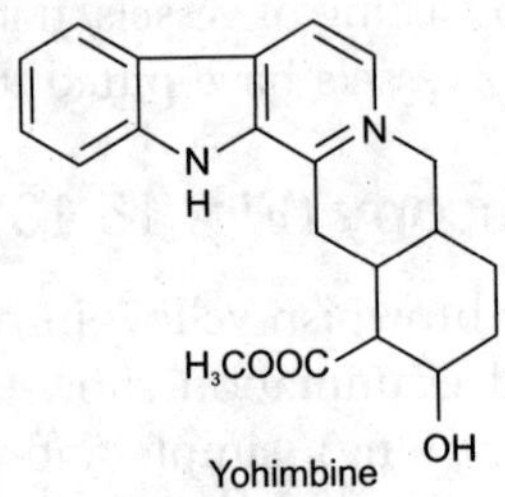

Yohimbine

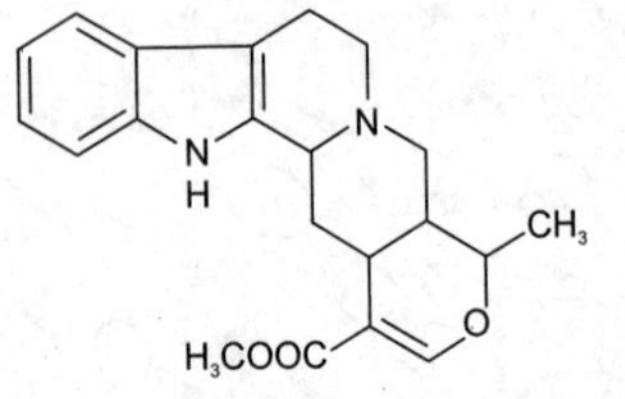

Ajmalicine

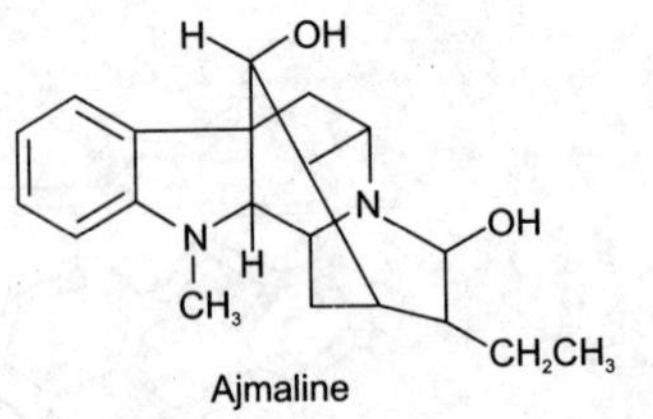

Ajmaline

ajmalinine, ajmaline, ajmalicine (δ-yohimbine), serpentine, serpentinine, tetrahydroreserpine, raubasine, reserpinine, isoajamaline and yohambinine.

The other substances present are phytosterols, fatty acids, unsaturated alcohols and sugars.

Uses

Rauwolfia in used as hypnotic, sedative and antihypertensive. It is specific for insanity, reduces blood pressure and cures pain due to affections of the bowels. It is given in labours to increase uterine contractions and in certain neuropsychiatric disorders. Ajmaline, which has pharmacological properties similar to those of quinidine, is marketed in Japan for the treatment of cardiac arrhythmias.

Reserpine is a white or pale buff to slightly yellow, odourless, crystalline powder that darkens slowly when exposed to light and rapidly when in solution. Reserpine is an antihypertensive and tranquilizer. Rescinnamine is the methyl reserpate ester of 3,4,5-trimethoxy cinnamic acid. The usual antihypertensive dose of rescinnamine is 500 μg, two times a day. Higher doses may cause serious mental depression. Deserpidine is 11-des-methoxyreserpine. It is a wide-range tranquilizer and antihypertensive and is free from the side effects.

Marketed Products

It is one of the ingredients of the preparations known as Confido, Lukol, Serpina (Himalaya Drug Company) and Sarpagandhan bati (Baidyanath).

NUX VOMICA

Synonyms

Semen strychni, Nux vomica Seed, Poison Nut, Semen strychnos, Quaker Buttons, Bachelor's buttons, Dog buttons, Vomit nut, Crow fig.

Biological Source

Nux vomica consists of the dried ripe seeds of *Strychnos nux vomica* Linn., belonging to family Loganiaceae; containing not less than 1.2% strychnine (Fig. 15.14).

Geographical Source

It is mainly found in South India, Malabar Coast, Kerala, Bengal, Eastern Ghats, North Australia and Ceylon.

Cultivation and Collection

The plant is a small tree around 12 m in height. Ripe and mature fruits are collected in the month of November to February. The fruits are 3–5 cm in diameter and are sub-spherical yellowish brown orange like berries. The epicarp is leathery and the pulp is bitter whitish and mucilaginous in which two to five seeds are embedded. The epicarp is separated and the seeds are removed and washed to remove pulp. They are dried on mats in the sun and graded according to size and exported.

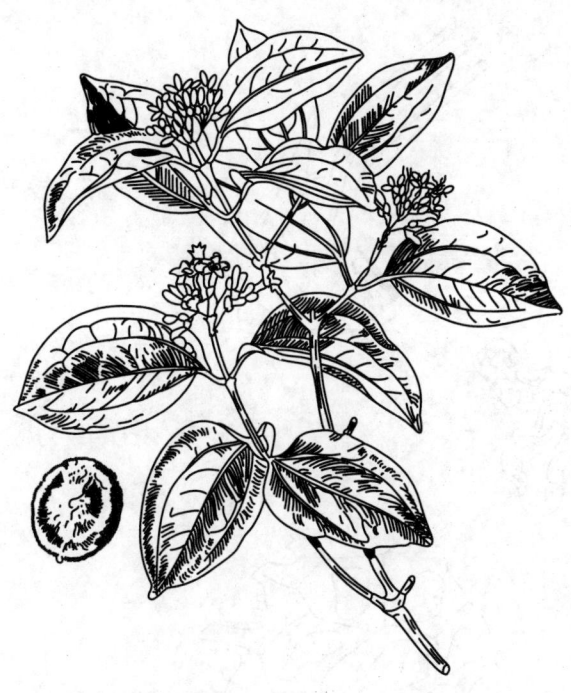

FIG. 15.14 *Strychnos nux vomica*

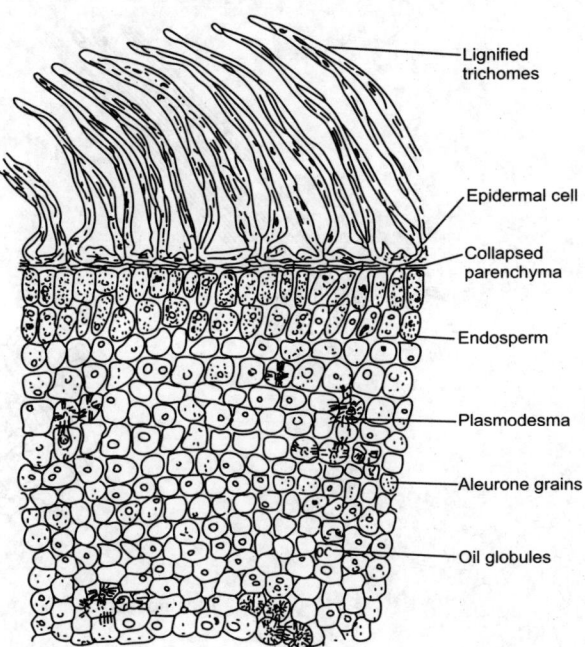

FIG. 15.15 Transverse section of Nux vomica seed

Characteristics

A medium-sized tree with a short, crooked, thick trunk, the wood is white hard; close grained, durable and the root very bitter. Branches irregular, covered with a smooth ash-coloured bark; young shoots deep green, shiny. Leaves opposite, short stalked, oval, shiny, smooth on both sides, about 4 inches long and 3 inches broad. Flowers small, greenish-white, funnel shape, in small terminal cymes, blooming in the cold season and having a disagreeable smell. Fruit, about the size of a large apple with a smooth hard rind or shell which when ripe is a lovely orange colour, rilled with a soft white jelly-like pulp containing five seeds covered with a soft woolly like substance, white and horny internally. Seeds have the shape of flattened disks densely covered with closely appressed satiny hairs, size is 10–30 mm in diameter 3–5 mm thick, radiating from the centre of the flattened sides and giving to the seeds a characteristic sheen; they are very hard, with a dark grey horny endosperm in which the small embryo is embedded; no odour but a very bitter taste.

Microscopy (Fig. 15.15)

Epidermis consists of thick-waved, bent and twisted lignified covering trichomes. The base of the trichome is large thick walled with slit like pits. The upper part of the trichome is nearly at right angle to the base and has wavy walls. Endosperm consists of thick walled isodiametric cells consisting of hemicellulose which swells with water and contains plasmodesma. Aleurone grains and fixed oil are present in endosperm and embryo.

Powder Microscopy (Fig. 15.16)

The powder is yellowish-grey to greenish-grey in colour. Microscopical examination shows epidermis of testa with attached trichomes. Endosperm cells from central region are large and very thick-walled while those from outer part, small and relatively thin-walled. Trichomes are narrow lignified rods running longitudinally. A few fragments of endosperm show faint plasmodesma.

Chemical Constituents

Nux vomica contains the alkaloids, strychnine (1.25%) and brucine (1.5%), also traces of strychnicine, and a glucoside loganin, about 3% fatty matter, caffeotannic acid and a trace of copper. It contains about 2.5–3.5% bitter indole alkaloids. Strychnine is therapeutically active and toxic alkaloid and is located in central portion of endosperm. Brucine is chemically dimethoxystrychnine and is less toxic and has very little physiological action. It is intensely bitter and is used as a standard for determining the bitter value, of many bitter drugs. Brucine is more in the outer part. Vomicine and pseudostrychnine are minor alkaloids.

The seeds also contain chlorogenic acid or caffeotannic acid. Alkaloids are combined with chlorogenic acid or caffeotannic acid. Loganin, a glucoside is also present. Cell walls of endosperm of nux vomica are thick walled and contain reserve material hemicellulose consisting of mannan and galactan which on hydrolysis yield mannose

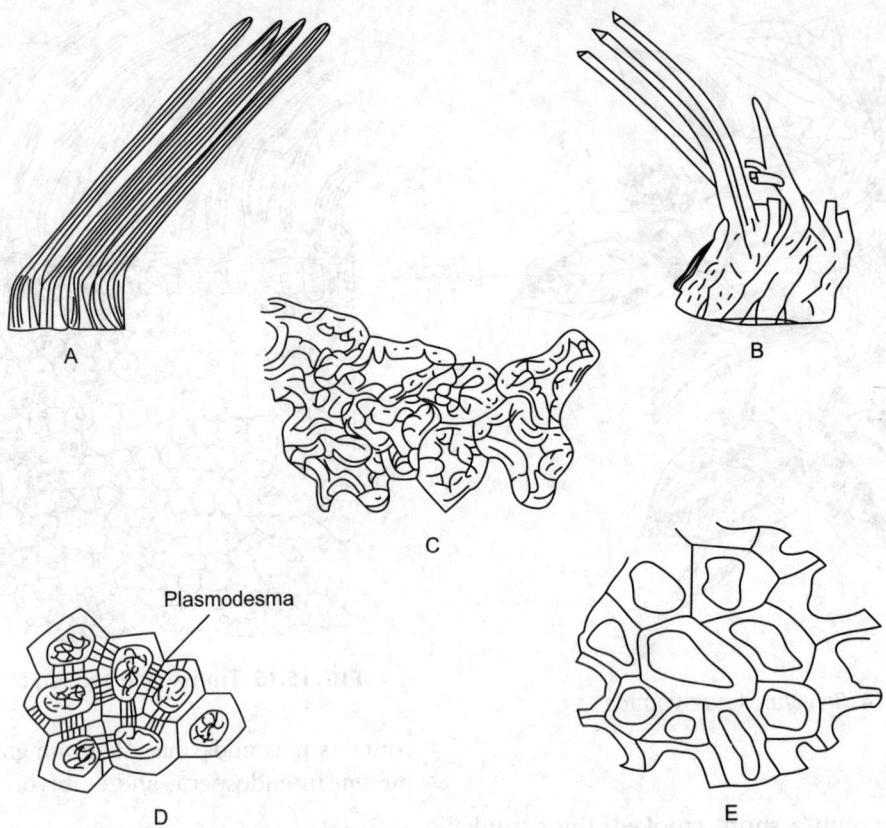

FIG. 15.16 Powder characteristics of Nux vomica seed. (A: Lignified trichomes, B: Epidermis of testa attached withtrichomes, C: Bases of trichomes in surface view, D: Cells of endosperm showing plasmodesma, E: Endosperm cells)

and galactose. Fatty matter is 3% aleurone grains and a trace of copper is present in the endosperm of the seed. The pulp of the fruit contains about 5% of loganin together with the alkaloid strychnicine.

	R1	R2	
Strychnine	H	H	OH
Brucine	OCH₃	OCH₃	Loganin

Chemical Tests

1. *Strychnine Test:* To a section of endosperm add ammonium vanadate and sulphuric acid. Strychnine in the middle portion of endosperm is stained purple.
2. *Potassium Dichromate Test:* Strychnine gives violet colour with potassium dichromate and conc. sulphuric acid.

3. *Brucine Test:* To a thick section add concentrated nitric acid. Outer part of endosperm is stained yellow to orange because of brucine.
4. *Hemicellulose Test:* To a thick section add iodine and sulphuric acid. The cell walls are stained blue.

Uses

The properties of nux vomica are substantially those of the alkaloid strychnine. In the mouth it acts as a bitter, increasing appetite; it stimulates peristalsis, in chronic constipation due to atony of the bowel it is often combined with cascara and other laxatives with good effects. Strychnine, the chief alkaloid constituent of the seeds, also acts as a bitter, increasing the flow of gastric juice; it is rapidly absorbed as it reaches the intestines, after which it exerts its characteristic effects upon the CNS, the movements of respiration are deepened and quickened and the heart slowed through excitation of the vagal centre. Strychnine has a stimulant action on spinal cord and reflex movements are better. It is considered as nervine and sex tonic. The senses of smell, touch, hearing and vision are rendered more acute, it improves the pulse and raises blood pressure and is of great value as a tonic to the circulatory system in cardiac failure. In toxic doses strychnine causes violent tetanus like convulsions and death takes place due to asphyxia and respiratory failure.

Brucine closely resembles strychnine in its action, but is slightly less poisonous; it paralyses the peripheral motor nerves. It is said that the convulsive action characteristic of strychnine is absent in brucine almost entirely. It is used in pruritis and as a local anodyne in inflammations of the external ear. Nux vomica is also known as vomiting nut but it has no vomiting properties. However *Strychnos potatorum* has emetic action.

Marketed Products

It is one of the ingredients of the preparation known as Neo Tablets (Charak Pharma Pvt. Ltd.).

VINCA

Synonyms

Vinca rosea, Catharanthus, Madagascar periwinkle, Barmasi.

Biological Source

Vinca is the dried entire plant of *Catharanthus roseus* Linn., belonging to family Apocynaceae (Fig. 15.17).

Geographical Source

The plant is a native of Madagascar and is found in many tropical and subtropical countries especially in India, Australia, South Africa and North and South America. The plant is cultivated as garden plant in Europe and India.

Cultivation and Collection

The plant is perennial and retains its glossy leaves throughout the winter. The plant prefers light (sandy), medium (loamy) and heavy (clay) soils and can grow in heavy clay soil. The plant prefers acid, neutral and basic (alkaline) soils. It can grow in full shade (deep woodland) semishade (light woodland) or no shade. It requires dry or moist soil and can tolerate drought. It is cultivated either by directly sowing the seeds or sowing the seeds in nursery. Nursery sowing method is found to be economical and the fresh seeds are sown in nursery in the month of February or March. The seedlings attain a height of 5–8 cm after two months and then they are transplanted in to the field at a distance of 45 cm × 30 cm. Proper fertilization and weeding is done timely and leaves are stripped after nine months. In order to collect the whole plant, the stems are first cut about 10 cm above the grounds and the leaves, seeds, stems are separated and dried. The roots are collected by plugging which are later washed and dried under shade and packed.

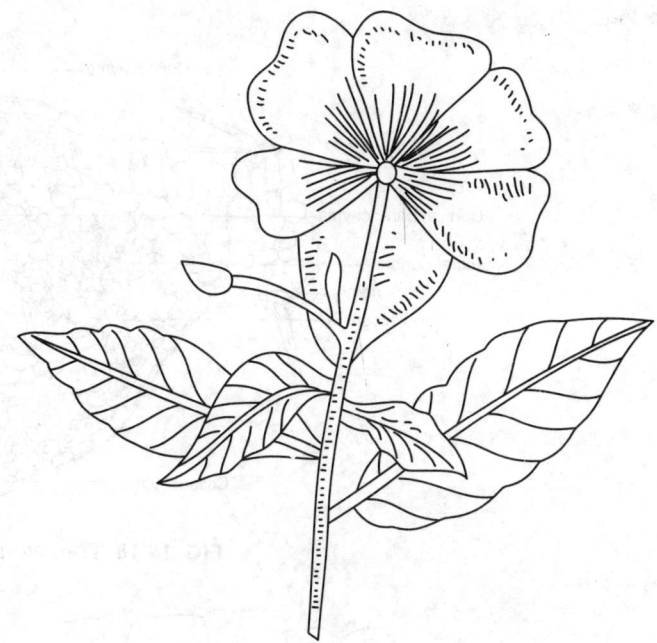

FIG. 15.17 *Catharanthus roseus*

Characteristics

The leaves are green in colour, flowers are either violet, pinkish white or carmine red and roots are pale grey in colour. It has characteristic odour and bitter taste. The flowers are hermaphrodite (have both male and female organs) and are pollinated by bees. Leaves are petiolate, entire margin, ovate or oblong, glossy appearance and with acute apex. Fruit is follicles with numerous black seeds.

Microscopy (Fig. 18.18)

Vinca has dorsiventral leaf structure. Epidermis is a single layer of rectangular cells covered with thick cuticle. It consists of unicellular covering trichome and cruciferous stomata. In the mesophyll region single layer of elongated and closely packed palisade parenchyma cells are present just below the upper epidermis. In the midrib region two to three layers of collenchyma is present, both below the upper epidermis and above the lower epidermis. Vascular bundle consisting of xylem and phloem is present in the middle of midrib region and rest of the intercellular space is covered by five to eight layers of spongy parenchyma. Calcium oxalate crystals are absent.

Powder Microscopy (Fig. 15.19)

The powder is dark green in colour. Microscopical examination shows epidermal cells with straight and wavy anticlinal walls and anomocytic stomata. Fragments of palisade and spongy parenchyma cells, spiral and pitted vessels and collenchymatous cells can also be seen.

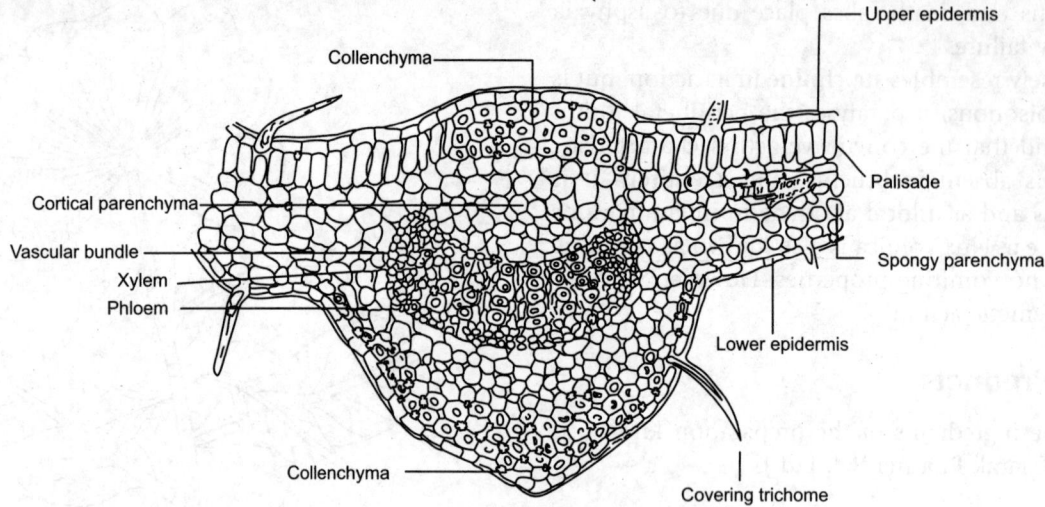

FIG. 15.18 Transverse section of Vinca leaf

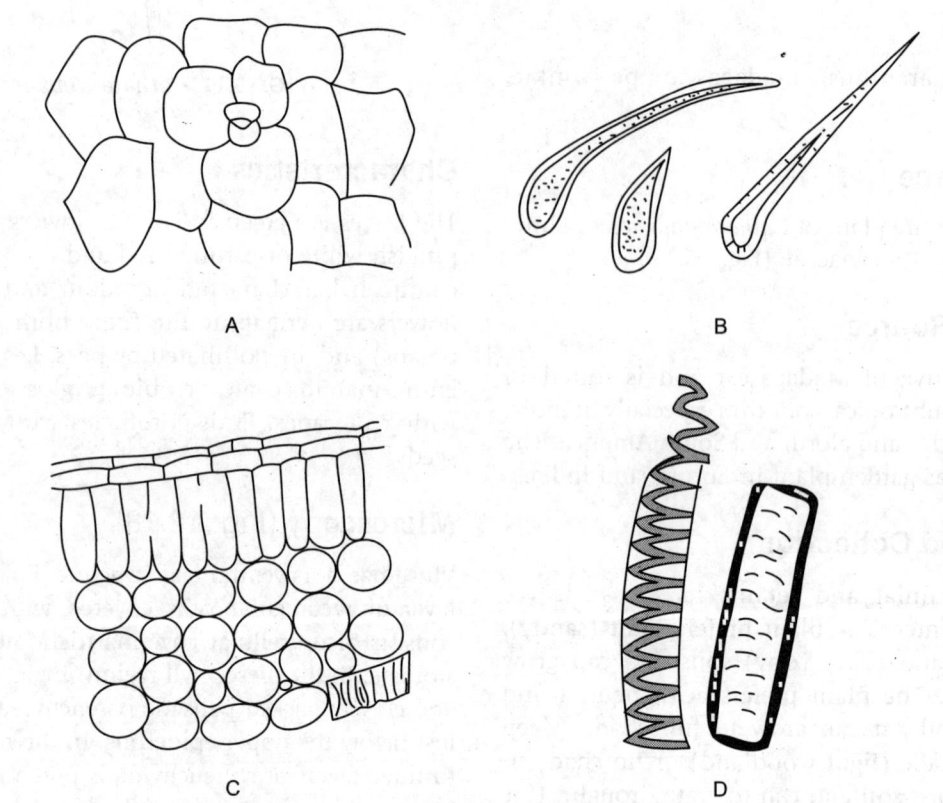

FIG. 15.19 Powder characteristics of Vinca leaf. (A: Epidermal cell, B: Covering trichomes, C: Mesophyll (Palisade and spongy parenchyma), D: Vessels)

Chemical Constituents

Alkaloids are present in entire shrub but leaves and roots contain more alkaloids. About 90 alkaloids have been isolated from Vinca from which some like ajmalicine, serpentine and tetrahydroalstonine are known and are present in other species of Apocynaceae. The important alkaloids in catharanthus are the dimer indole indoline alkaloids vinblastine and vincristine and they possess definite anticancer activity. Vindoline and catharanthine are indole monomeric alkaloids. It also contains monoterpenes, sesquiterpene, indole and indoline glycoside.

Uses

Vinblastine is an antitumour alkaloid used in the treatment of Hodgkin's disease. Vincristine is a cytotoxic compound and used to treat leukaemia in children. Vinca is used in herbal practice for its astringent and tonic properties in menorrhagia and in haemorrhages generally. In cases of

Vinblastine

Vincristine

scurvy and for relaxed sore throat and inflamed tonsils, it may also be used as a gargle. For bleeding piles, it may be applied externally, as well as taken internally. It is also used in the treatment of diabetes.

The flowers of the periwinkle are gently purgative, but lose their effect on drying. If gathered in the spring and made into a syrup, they impart all their virtues, and this, it is stated, is excellent as a gentle laxative for children and also for overcoming chronic constipation in grown persons.

Marketed Products

It is one of the ingredients of the preparation known as cytocristin (Cipla).

PHYSOSTIGMA

Synonyms

Calabar bean, Ordeal bean, Chop nut.

Biological Source

Calabar beans are the dried ripe seeds of *Physostigma venenosum* half containing not less than 0.15% alkaloids, belonging to family Leguminosae (Papilionaecae) (Fig. 15.20).

Geographical Source

The plant is a perennial woody climber and grows in West Africa, Old Calabar, India and Brazil.

History

The plant came into notice in 1846 and was planted in the Edinburgh Botanical Gardens, where it grew into a strong perennial creeper. The natives of Africa employ the bean as an ordeal owing to its very poisonous qualities. They call it esere, and it is given to an accused person to eat. If the prisoner vomits within half an hour he is accounted innocent, but if he succumbs he is found guilty. A draught

of the pounded seeds infused in water is said to have been fatal to a man within an hour.

Characteristics

It is a great twining climber, pinnately trifoliate leaves, pendulous racemes of purplish bean-like flowers; seeds are two or three together in dark brown pods about 6 inches long and kidney-shaped, thick, about 1 inch long, rounded ends, roughish but a little polished, and have a long scar on the edge where adherent to the placenta. The seeds ripen at all seasons.

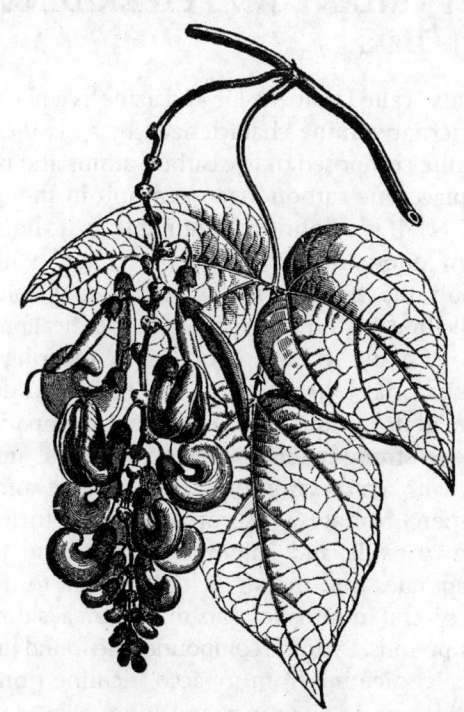

FIG. 15.20 *Physostigma venenosum*

Chemical Constituents

Drug contains 0.1–0.2% indole alkaloids of which half is physostigmine known also as eserine (a crystalline solid, white or pinkish coloured, readily soluble in alcohol, sparingly soluble in water) and is the important alkaloid. The other alkaloids are eseramine, geneserine and physovenine. Physostigmine the major alkaloid is present in cotyledons up to 0.04–0.3%, Physostigmine is methyl carbamide acid ester of eroline. These alkaloids are pyrrolidine-indoline derivatives. Calabar beans also contain stigmasterol.

Physostigmine

Uses

Mainly used for diseases of the eye; it causes rapid contraction of the pupil and disturbed vision. Also used as a stimulant to the unstriped muscles of the intestines in chronic constipation. Its action on the circulation is to slow the pulse and raise blood pressure; it depresses the CNS, causing muscular weakness; it has been employed internally for its depressant action.

15.11. PYRIDINE AND PIPERIDINE ALKALOIDS

Pyridine, also called azabenzene and azine, is a heterocyclic aromatic tertiary amine characterized by a six-membered ring structure composed of five carbon atoms and nitrogen which replace one carbon–hydrogen unit in the benzene ring (C_5H_5N). It is colourless, flammable, toxic liquid with unpleasant odour, miscible with water and with most organic solvents, boils at 115°C. Its aqueous solution is slightly alkaline. Pyridine is a base with chemical properties similar to tertiary amines. Nitrogen in the ring system has an equatorial lone pair of electrons, which does not participate in the aromatic pi-bond. It is incompatible and reactive with strong oxidizers and strong acids, and reacts violently with chlorosulphonic acid, maleic anhydride, oleum, perchromates, β-propiolactone, formamide, chromium trioxide and sulphuric acid. Liquid pyridine easily evaporates into the air. If it is released to the air, it may take several months to years until it breaks down into other compounds. Pyridine compounds are found in nature. For example, nicotine from tobacco, ricinine from castor bean, pyridoxine or vitamin B and P products, etc.

Piperidine, hexa-hydropyridine, is a family of heterocyclic organic compound derived from pyridine through hydrogenation. It has one nitrogen atom in the cycle. It is a clear liquid with pepper-like aroma. It boils at 106°C, soluble in water, alcohol and ether. Piperidine

derivative compounds are used as intermediate to make crystal derivative of aromatic nitrogen compounds containing nuclear atoms. They are used in manufacturing pharmaceuticals.

LOBELIA

Synonyms

Herba lobellae, Indian tobacco, Pukeweed, Asthma Weed.

Biological Source

Lobelia consists of the dried aerial parts of *Lobelia inflata* Linn., belonging to family Lobeliaceae (Fig. 15.21).

Geographical Source

Indigenous to Eastern and Central United States, Canada and India.

Cultivation and Collection

It is an erect annual or biennial herb, 1–2 feet high; lower leaves and also flower are stalked, the latter being pale violet-blue in colour, tinted pale yellow within. Drug is obtained both from cultivated and wild plants. It is propagated using seeds. For cultivation seeds are sown in rich, moist, loamy soil usually in March to April. After sowing, seeds are covered with soil and pressure is applied on them by placing wooden board over them and walking on it. Collection is done in August to September when

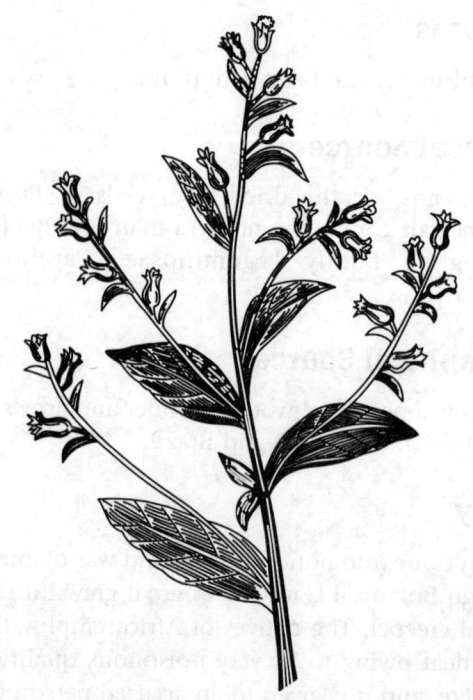

FIG. 15.21 *Lobelia inflata*

capsular fruits get inflated. Aerial parts are collected and dried in the shade to maintain green colour.

Characteristics

Stem is green with purple patches. Upper part of the stem is cylindrical, hairy and having two to three wings. In the lower part it is channeled and neatly glabrous. Leaves are sessile in the upper part and prolate below. Those on the upper part of the stem are small and about 2 cm long. They are ovate, oblong and irregularly toothed. Pedicel of the flower is 3–5 mm long. Flowers are 7 mm long, light blue, having inferior ovary. Calyx consists of five subulate sepals. Corolla is tubular and bilabiate. Stamens are five, epigynous and syngenesious. At the apex of the stamen is tuft of hairs. Fruit is an inferior capsule, 7–8 mm long, and yellowish green in colour and inflated. Capsule is obovate, bilocular and contains about 500 extremely small seeds. Pericarp is thin, membranous and bears 10 ridges. Ridges are joined by horizontal veinlets. Seeds are 0.6–0.7 mm long and 0.25–0.30 mm broad, reddish brown in colour and covered on the outer surface with fine elongated, polygonal, lignified reticulations. It has an irritating odour and taste is unpleasant, acrid and burning.

Microscopy

The epidermis consists of axially elongated cells. Trichomes which are 1200 μm long are present on the epidermis and stomata are parallel to the axis. The cortex region has parenchyma which is round in shape. It has a well developed endodermis composed of large cells. The phloem has a cylindrical net work of laticiferous vessels. It has a large pith taking about one-third to one-half of the diameter of the stem. It has thin walled parenchyma with simple pits which are lignified. In the mesophyll region of the leaf it has the elongated palisade parenchyma cells under the upper epidermis giving it a dorsiventral leaf structure. The epidermis is nearly straight anticlinal walls with thick and striated cuticle. The lower epidermis has abundant stomata. In the midrib region phloem is present which has a well developed laticiferous tissues system. It usually has unicellular and occasionally uniseriate and bicellular conical trichomes which are lignified.

Chemical Constituents

Lobelia contains about 0.4% crystalline alkaloids of which lobeline is the important active alkaloid. Other alkaloids are lobelidine, lobelanidine, lobelanine and isolobinine chemically related to lobeline. Also, gum, resin, chlorophyll, fixed oil, lignin, salts of lime and potassium with ferric oxide are present. Lobelacrine, formerly considered to be the acrid principle, is probably lobelate of lobeline. The seeds contain a much higher percentage of lobeline than the rest of the plant.

Lobeline

Lobelanidine

Uses

It is mainly used as expectorant, diaphoretic, antiasthmatic. It should not be employed as an emetic. Some authorities attach great value to it as an expectorant in bronchitis, others as a valuable counterirritant when combined with other ingredients in ointment form. It is sometimes given in convulsive and inflammatory disorders, such as epilepsy, tetanus, diphtheria and tonsillitis. Lobeline is a respiratory stimulant and is used in asphyxia of the newborn, in gas, alcohol and narcotic poisoning and in drowning in water, electric shock and collapse. It has relaxant and dilatory action and is used in asthma and dyspnoea. Lobelia is also used to discontinue smoking habit. Externally, an infusion has been found useful in ophthalmia, and the tincture can be used as a local application for sprains, bruises or skin diseases, alone, or in powder combined with an equal part of slippery elm bark and weak lye water in a poultice. The oil of Lobelia is valuable in tetanus.

TOBACCO

Synonyms

Tobacco, Tabaci Folia.

Biological Source

It consists of dried leaves of *Nicotiana tobaccum*, belonging to family Solanaceae (Fig. 15.22).

Geographical Source

It is mainly found in India, United States, China, Brazil, Russia, Turkey and Italy.

History

The genus derives its name from Joan Nicot, a Portuguese who introduced the Tobacco plant into France. The specific name being derived from the Haitian word for the pipe in which the herb is smoked.

Cultivation and Collection

Cultivation is done by sowing seeds. Warm climate and well drained fertile land is required for good growth. Transplantation is done when the seedlings are 12 weeks old. Flowering tops are cut in order to enhance growth of foliage. After 70–90 days of transplantation leaves are collected.

Characteristics

Colour	Green or slightly brown
Odour	Characteristic to nicotine
Taste	Bitter
Shape	Ovate, elliptic or lanceolate
Size	60–80 cm in length 35–45 cm in width

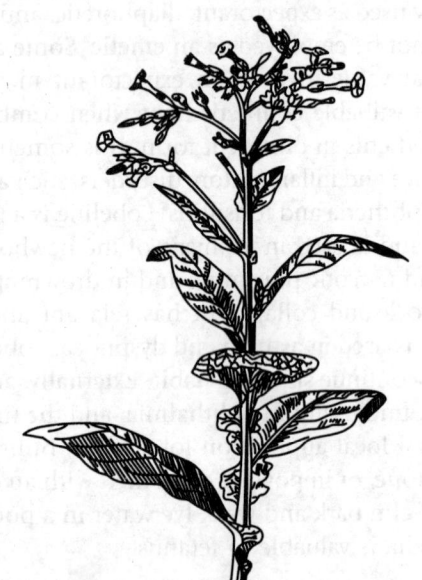

FIG. 15.22 *Nicotiana tobaccum*

Chemical Constituents

The most important constituent is the alkaloids nicotine, nicotianin, nicotinine, nicotine, nicoteline. After leaves are smoked the nicotine decomposes into pyridine, furfurol, collidine, hydrocyanic acid, carbon monoxide, etc. The poisonous effects of tobacco smoke are due to these substances of decomposed nicotine.

Nicotine   Nicotine acid

Uses

Nicotine is very like coniine and lobeline in its pharmacological action, and the pyridines in the smoke modify very slightly its action. It is used as a sedative, diuretic, expectorant, discutient and sialagogue. The leaves in combination with the leaves of belladonna or stramonium make an excellent application for obstinate ulcers, painful tremors and spasmodic affections. Tobacco leaves are made wet and applied for piles. Externally nicotine is an antiseptic. Nicotine exerts stimulant effects on heart and nervous system.

ARECA NUTS

Synonyms

Betal nuts; Pinang; Semina Areacae, Supari (Hindi).

Biological Source

Areca nuts are the seeds of *Areca catechu* Linn., belonging to family Palmaceae (Fig. 15.23).

Geographical Source

The tree is cultivated in tropical India, Sri Lanka, Malay States, South China, East Indies, Philippine Islands and parts of East Africa (including Zanzibar and Tanzania). In India it is cultivated in the coastal regions of southern Maharashtra, Tamil Nadu, Karnataka, Bengal and Assam.

Cultivation and Collection

Areca palm is mostly propagated by seeds. The palm requires a moist tropical climate for luxuriant growth; it is very sensitive to drought. It grows in areas with heavy rainfall in between temperature of 15–38°C. It is cultivated in plains, hill slopes and low lying valleys. The seeds are collected from 25–50-year-old trees.

Areca nut is a handsome palm with a tall, slender stem crowned by large elegant leaves. Each tree contains about 100 fruits per year which are detached by means of bamboo poles and the seeds extracted. The pericarp is fibrous and surrounds a single seed which is easily separated. The seeds are usually boiled in water with the addition of a little lime and dried.

Characteristics

Areca nuts are about 2.5 cm in length, bluntly rounded, conical in shape and 2–3 cm wide at the base. The testa is brown and marked with a network of small depressed lines. The ruminate endosperm is opal-white. Patches of a silvery coat, the inner layer of the pericarp, occasionally adhere to the testa. The deep-brown testa is marked with a network of depressed fissures; the colour of the testa is due to the presence of tannin. In the centre basal part of the endosperm, the small embryo is situated and an external pale area indicated its position. The seed is very hard, has a faint cheese-like odour when broken and an astringent, acrid taste.

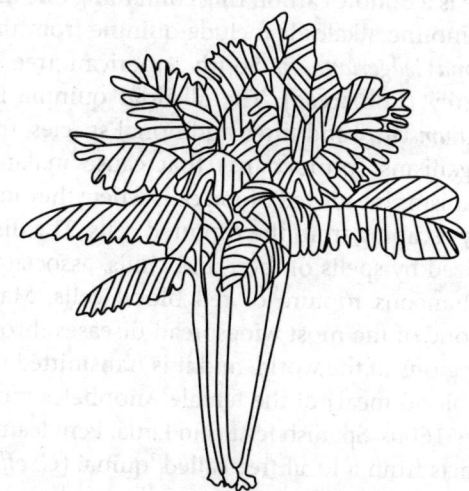

FIG. 15.23 Tree of *Areca catechu*

Chemical Constituents

Areca nut contains a number of alkaloids of a piperidine series, such as arecoline (methyl ester of arecanine), arecaine (*N*-methyl guvacine), guvacine (tetrahydronicitinic acid), arecaidine, guvacoline, arecolidine, leucocyanidine, (+)-catechin, (-)-epicatechin, procyanidins A-1, B-1 and B-2; phthalic, lauric, myristic, palmitic and stearic acids, β-sitosterol and choline. Arecoline is present in about 0.1–0.5% yield and is medicinally important. In addition to alkaloids, areca nuts contain fat (14%) and amorphous red tannin (15%) known as areca red of phlobaphene nature. The fat consists mainly of the glycerides of lauric, myristic and oleic acids.

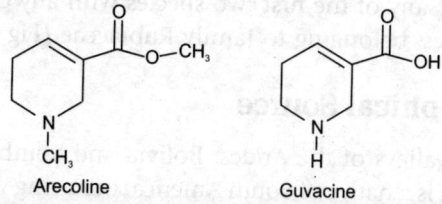

Arecoline   Guvacine

Uses

Powdered Areca is used as anthelmintic, taenifuge and vermifuge for dogs. It has aphrodisiac action and useful in urinary disorders, as nervine tonic and emmenagogue. The chewing of Areca nut may cause mouth cancer.

Substitutes and Adulterants

Nuts from other plants, such as, *Areca caliso*, *A. concinna*, *A. ipot*, *A. laxa*, *A. nagensis*, *A. triandra*, *Caryota cumingii* and *Heterospathe elata* are used as substituents for *Areca* nuts.

Sago palm nuts (*Metroxylon* species), dried tapioca (*Manihot esculenta*) and slices of sweet potato (*Ipomoea* *batatas*) form cheap adulterants that are mixed with slices of Areca nuts and prove a serious menace affecting the industry. Nuts of *Caryota urens*, cut to various shapes and sizes resembling genuine Areca nuts, and coated with concentrated Areca nut extract *kali*, form the principal adulterant. Adulteration above 10% significantly increases the fibre content of the sample, which can be used as a measure of detecting adulteration.

Marketed Products

It is one of the ingredients of the preparations known as Himplasia (Himalaya Drug Company), Khadiradi bati (Baidyanath) and Pigmento (Charak Pharma Pvt. Ltd.).

15.12. IMIDAZOLE ALKALOIDS

Imidazole is a heterocyclic aromatic organic compound. This ring system is present in important biological building blocks such as histidine and histamine. Imidazoles can act as bases (pK_a = 7.0) and as weak acids (pK = 14.5). Imidazole exists in two tautomeric forms with a hydrogen atom moving between the two nitrogens.

The most important plant of this group is *Pilocarpus jaborandi*.

PILOCARPUS

Synonyms

Jaborandi, Arruda do Mato, Arruda brava, Jamguarandi, Juarandi.

Biological Source

The drug consists of the leaves of *Pilocarpus jaborandi*, belonging to family Rutaceae (Fig. 15.24).

Geographical Source

It is indigenous to South America and especially grown in Brazil also it is found in Venezuela, Caribbean islands and Central America.

History

Dr. Coutinho in 1874 sent the plant to Europe from Pernambuco, hence the name Pernambuco jaborandi or *Pilocarpus jaborandi*. Later, Byasson in 1875 showed its alkaloidal nature and further Gerrard and Hardy isolated the main alkaloid pilocarpine.

Characteristics

The shrub grows from 4 to 5 feet high; the bark is smooth and greyish; the flowers are thick, small and reddish-purple in colour, springing from rather thick, separate stalks about 1/4 inch long. The leaves are large compound, pinnate with an odd terminal leaflet, with two to four pairs of leaflets.

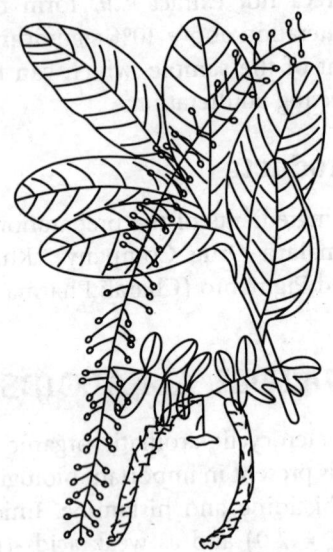

FIG. 15.24 *Pilocarpus jaborandi*

Chemical Constituents

The drug contains imidazole alkaloids among, which pilocarpine is most important. Other alkaloids are isopilocarpine, pilocarpidine, pilosine, pseudopilocarpine and isopilosine. The range of total alkaloids in different species is between 0.5% and 1%.

Pilocarpine   Pilosine

Chemical Test

To the drug containing pilocarpine, small quantities of dilute sulphuric acid, hydrogen peroxide solution, benzene and potassium chromate solution is added and shaken, organic layer gives bluish-violet colour and yellow colour appears in aqueous layer.

Uses

Pilocarpine is antagonistic to atropine, stimulating the nerve endings paralysed by that drug and contracting the pupil of the eye. Its principal use is as a powerful and rapid diaphoretic. It induces also free salivation and excites most gland secretions, some regarding it as a galactagogue. It is also used in ophthalmic practice in the treatment of glaucoma.

15.13. QUINOLINE ALKALOIDS

Quinoline is a double carbon ring containing one nitrogen atom. Quinoline alkaloids include quinine from the bark of *Cinchona ledgeriana*, a South American tree in the coffee family (Rubiaceae). The alkaloid quinine is toxic to *Plasmodium vivax* and three additional species, the one-celled organisms (protozoans) that cause malaria. The microorganisms invade red blood cells where they multiply, eventually escaping from the ruptured cells. The disease is characterized by spells of fever and chills, associated with the simultaneous rupture of red blood cells. Malaria is certainly one of the most widespread diseases throughout tropical regions of the world, and it is transmitted through the bite (blood meal) of the female Anopheles mosquito. During the 1600s, Spanish Jesuits in Lima, Peru learned that bark extracts from a local tree called 'quina' (*C. officinalis*) could cure malaria. They successfully used this extract on Countess Chinchon. Some strains of Plasmodium are resistant to many of the synthetic quinine analogues, so natural: quinine is still used to this day.

CINCHONA

Synonyms

Cortex Cinchonae, Countess, Peruvian or Jesuit's bark, Cinchona

Biological Source

Cinchona is the dried bark of the stem or of the root of *Cinchona calisaya* Wedd., *Cinchona ledgeriana* Moens., *Cinchona officinalis* Linn. and *Cinchona succirubra* Pavon., or hybrids of any of the first two species with any of the last two species, belonging to family Rubiaceae (Fig. 15.25).

Geographical Source

Tropical valleys of the Andes. Bolivia and Southern Peru. Cinchona is a native of South America, occurring wild there. At present, it is mainly cultivated in Indonesia (Java), Zaire, India, Guatemala, Bolivia, Ceylon, etc.

History

The use of cinchona as an antimalarial is reported in 1638, when the wife of Spanish governor was cured by it. Later on the Spanish missionaries passed on the trade of cinchona bark for approximately 200 years.

In 1736 the French botanist for the first time collected a bark from the tree, eventually the demand for the tree was increased and the barks were collected by felling method. Due to the increased demand for the tree, its cultivation was tried in various parts of the world like Europe, Java, India, etc. The cultivation in Europe was totally unsuccessful while the cultivation those species grown in India (*C. succirubra*) and in Java (*C. ledgeriona*) were very successful. Today India exports cinchona for more than one crore.

Cultivation and Collection

Cinchona is propagated by seed sowing method. The seeds with approximately 3 mm long and flat are picked and are used for cultivation. The seeds are sown in boxes and the seedlings are transplanted to nurseries when they reach a height of 5 cm, the nurseries are covered by a roof so as to protect the seedlings from direct sunlight. The seedlings grown in shade till they attain a height of about 25 cm and in between this period they are at least transplanted twice. Cinchona grows well at an altitude of 1500–2000 m above sea level, temperature ranging from 10°C to 30°C and an annual rainfall of 200–400 cm. When the plants are about 1.5 years old they are transplanted to open space at a distance of 1 m into well drained, rich and porous soil.

The plant is allowed to grow till six years and then the first crop is collected by coppicing, uprooting or by felling method. The bark is collected till the plant is 9 years old because the alkaloid content in the bark decreases thereafter. Rainy season is considered suitable for the collection of the bark. The trunks and the branches are beaten to loose the periderm and the bark is removed into small pieces of 45 cm long and 12 cm in width. They are then dried under sun or by artificial heating by providing gentle heat. During drying the barks attain quill shape and the colour changes to red or brownish red.

Characteristics

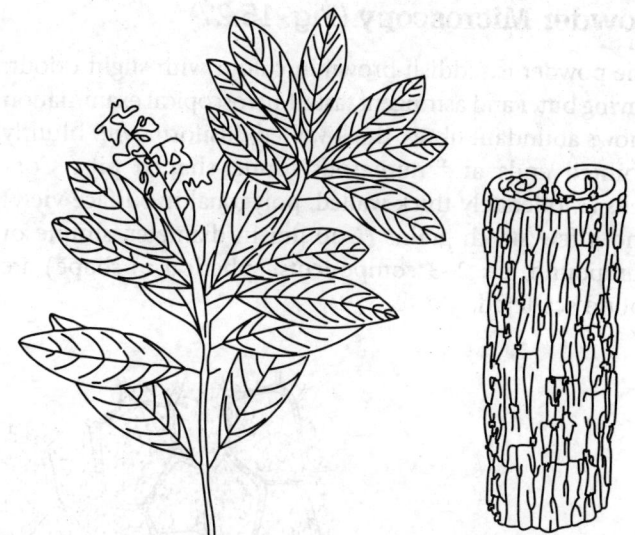

FIG. 15.25 Twig and bark of *Cinchona ledgeriana*

Colour	The outer surface is yellowish to brown, with short fractures and the inner surface varies in all the four species; like *Cinchona calisaya* and *Cinchona ledgeriana* is yellowish, *Cinchona officinalis* is slightly brown and *Cinchona succirubra* is reddish brown
Odour	Distinctive
Taste	Highly bitter and astringent
Shape	Curved, quill or double quill
Size	30 cm long and 2–7 mm thick
Extra features	The outer surface consist of longitudinal and transverse cracks, fissures, ridges

Microscopic Characters (Fig. 15.26)

Transverse section of bark shows cork composed of uniformly arranged several layers of thin-walled cells, containing amorphous reddish-brown matter. Below cork is a region of cortex, composed of tangentially elongated parenchymatous cells with red-brown and thin walls, containing small starch grains. Idioblasts, containing microcrystals of calcium oxalate (2–6 μm long), and secretion cells are scattered in the cortex. Phloem

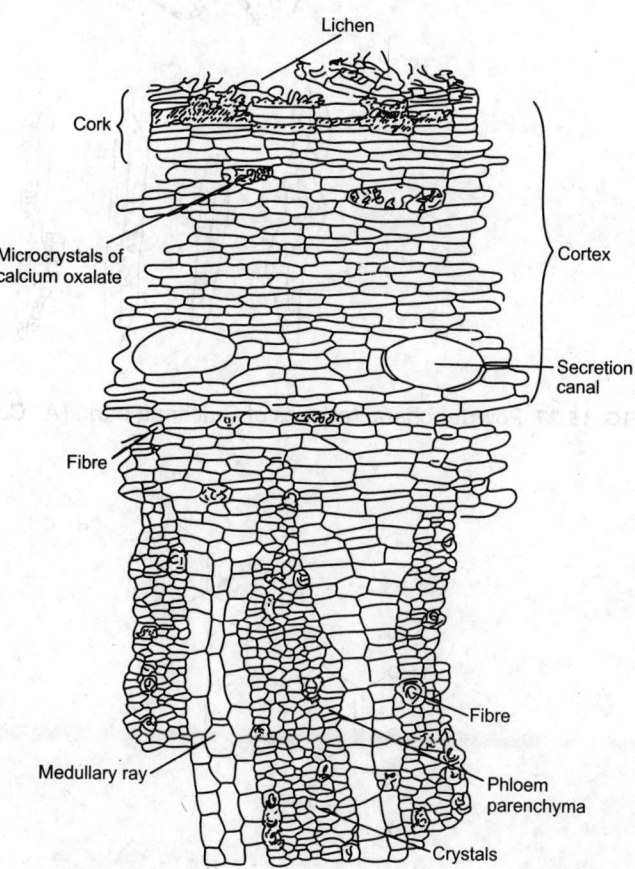

FIG. 15.26 Transverse section of Cinchona bark

consists of compressed and collapsed sieve tubes, phloem parenchyma similar to cortex, and irregularly arranged, large spindle-shaped lignified fibres. Medullary rays are narrow, two to three cells wide and almost straight. Longitudinal section of bark shows brick-shaped cells of medullary rays, longitudinally elongated cells of phloem parenchyma and fibres with conspicuous pits.

Powder Microscopy (Fig. 15.27)

The powder is reddish-brown in colour with slight odour; having bitter and astringent taste. Microscopical examination shows abundant fibres, thick-walled, fusiform with bluntly pointed ends and numerous funnel-shaped pits. Cork cells (moderately thick-walled, polygonal in surface view) and a few starch grains (6-10 μm in diameter, simple or compound, i.e. 2–3 components, spherical in shape) are found scattered.

Chemical Constituents

More than 30 alkaloids have been reported in cinchona. The chiefly identified alkaloids are quinidine, quinine, cinchonine and cinchonidine. These constituents are the stereoisomers of each other like quinine is stereoisomer of quinidine and cinchonine is stereoisomer of cinchonidine. The other constituents available are quiniarnine, cinchotine, hydroquinine, hydrocinchonidine, cinchotannic acid, etc. Quinine and quinidine has a methoxy group in it but

FIG. 15.27 Powder characteristics of Cinchona bark. (A: Cork cells, B: Starch grains, C: Fibres, D: Calcium oxalate crystals)

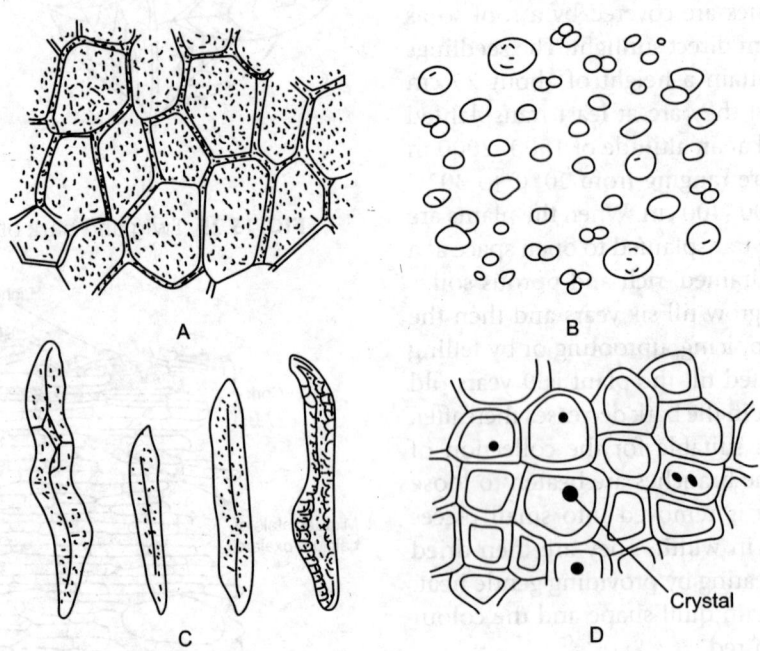

Quinine

Quinidine

Cinchonine

Cinchonidine

cinchonine and cinchonidine do not have a methoxy group. Other than these it also consist of bitter glycoside, starch grains, calcium oxalate crystals and crystalline acid like quinic acid.

Chemical Test

1. *Thalleioquin test:* To the extract of cinchona powder add one drop of dilute sulphuric acid and 1 ml of water. Add bromine water drop wise till the solution acquires permanent yellow colour and add 1 ml of dilute ammonia solution, emerald green colour is produced.
2. The powdered drug when heated with glacial acetic acid in dry test tube, evolves red fumes, which condense in the top portion of the tube.
3. Cinchona bark, when moistened with sulphuric acid and observed under ultraviolet light shows a blue fluorescence due to the methoxy group of quinine and quinidine.

Uses

It is mainly employed as antimalarial drug, but it is also used as analgesic, antipyretic, protoplasmic, bitter stomachic and tonic. Quinidine is cardiac depressant and cinchonidine is used in rheumatism and neuralgia.

Substitutes

Cuprea Bark (*Remijia pedupiculato*); Family: Rubiaceae. It differs in its morphological character with cinchona but consist of constituents like quinine, quinidine, cinchonine, cinchonamine, etc., the other species of *Remijia*, that is, *R. purdieana* (false Cuprea bark) does not contain quinine.

Marketed Products

It is one of the ingredients of the preparations known as Herbipyrin tablet, M.P. 6 Capsules (Vasu Healthcare).

15.14. ISOQUINOLINE ALKALOIDS

Isoquinoline is a double carbon ring containing one nitrogen atom. Plants containing isoquinoline alkaloids are *Argemone* species (Prickly poppy), *Chelidonium* species (Celandine poppy), *Corydalis* species (Fitweed), *Dicentra* species (Dutchman's breeches), *Papaver* species (Poppy) and *Sanguinera* species (Bloodroot).

The isoquinoline alkaloids papaverine, sangumarine, protoverine and chelidonine are GI tract irritants and CNS stimulants. Isoquinoline alkaloids are found in varying quantities in the prickly poppy, bloodroot and celandine poppy. Many have varying degrees of neurological effects, ranging from relaxation and euphoria to seizures. They also cause vasodilation.

Many of these plants have been used in herbal preparations. Scotch broom is smoked for relaxation and has mild sedative-hypnotic effects. Prickly poppy is smoked as a euphoriant. Mescal bean is a hallucinogenic, which is used in Native American rituals and in medicine. *Sanguinaria* species (bloodroot) extract is used commercially as a dental plaque inhibitor. Papaverine, found in prickly poppy and bloodroot, has been used medically as a smooth muscle relaxant. Prickly poppy extracts act as capillary dilators and have been implicated in epidemic glaucoma in India. Celandine extracts are used as treatment of gastric and biliary disorders.

As a group, the isoquinolines have proven to be more poisonous to domestic livestock than to humans. In humans, pediatric poisonings are most common. Most of the isoquinolines are noxious in smell and taste and discourage ingestion, thus human toxicity is rare. Interestingly, some domestic species tolerate ingestion of isoquinoline and other alkaloids, and humans can ingest toxic alkaloids from the milk of poisoned animal and manifest symptoms.

IPECAC

Synonyms

Ipecacuanha, Brazilian or Johore Ipecac, Hippo, Ipecacuanha root, Radix ipecacuanhae.

Biological Source

Ipecac consists of the dried root or rhizome of *Cephaelis ipecacuanha* (Brot.) A. Rich. (Rio or Brazilian Ipecac) or of *Cephaelis acuminata* Karst. (Cartagena, Nicaragua or Panama Ipecac), belonging to family Rubiaceae. It should contain about 2% of ether soluble alkaloids calculated as emetine (Fig. 15.28).

Geographical Source

The plant is indigenous to Brazil and also found in Colombia, Cartagena, Nicaragua, Savantilla, Malaya, Burma, Panama and West Bengal. In India it is cultivated at Mungpoo (Darjeeling), in Nilgiri near Collar and in Sikkim.

Cultivation and Collection

The plant is a low, straggling shrub containing slender rhizome with annulated wiry roots. The roots are smooth, slender and whitish when young, develop on maturation a thick brownish bark with numerous closely placed transverse furrows.

The plant is unusually slow growing. It thrives best in forest areas on sandy loams in humus, potash, magnesia and lime. A maximum rainfall of 90 inch is required throughout the year. A temperature between 15 and 40°C and shaded situations are essential for successful cultivation. Temperature fluctuations should be narrow and the soil should be well drained. Propagation is by stem or root cuttings planted about a foot apart each way. Roots are harvested when the plants are about 2.5 years old and the alkaloid content exceeds 20%. The plant may be dug up at any time of the year; the roots are washed and dried in shade.

Characteristics

The rhizome is thin or sometimes thick and annulated. Rio Ipecac is 5–15 cm long, 6 mm in diameter, shape is cylindrical, slightly, tortuous, external surface is broadly annulated, brick red to brown in colour, the ridges are rounded and encircle the root, fracture of root is short and shows a thick, greyish bark and small dense wood. Odour is slight and taste is bitter and acrid.

Cartagena Ipecac is 4–6.5 mm in diameter, greyish-brown in colour, less crowded and less projecting annulations, has transverse ridges. Half of the portion contains bark.

The Mato Grosso drug occurs in tortuous pieces, up to 15 cm long and 6 mm diameter. The colour of the outer surface varies from a deep brick-red to a very dark brown; the colour is dependent on the type of soil in which the plant has been grown. Most of the roots are annulated externally, and some have a portion of the rhizome and nonannulated roots are also found. The ridges are rounded and completely encircle the root; in some parts the bark has completely separated from the wood.

The fracture shows a thick greyish bark and a small, dense wood, but no pith. The rhizomes have a much thinner bark and definite pith.

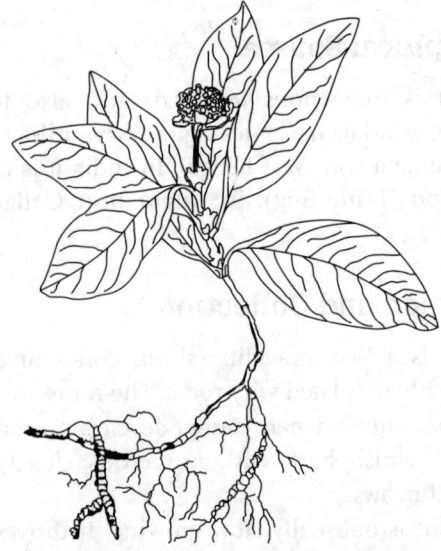

FIG. 15.28 *Cephaelis ipecacuanha*

Microscopy (Fig. 15.29)

A transverse section of the root shows a thin, brown cork, the cells of which contain brown, granular material. There is wide, secondary cortexes (phelloderm), the cells of which are parenchymatous and contain starch in compound grains with from two to eight components, or raphides of calcium oxalate. The individual starch grains are muller shaped. The phloem is parenchymatous, containing no sclerenchymatous cells or fibres. The compact central mass of xylem is composed of small tracheidal vessels, tracheids, substitute fibres, xylem fibres and xylem parenchyma. Starch is present in the xylem parenchyma and in substitute fibres.

The transverse section of ipecacuanha rhizome shows a ring of xylem and large pith. The pericycle contains characteristic sclerenchymatous cells. Spiral vessels occur in the protoxylem. The pith is composed of pitted lignified parenchyma.

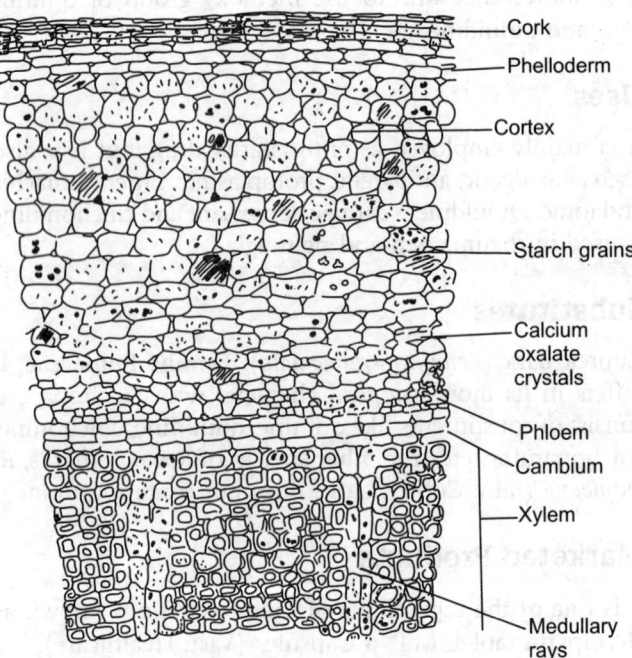

FIG. 15.29 Transverse section of Ipecacuanha root

Powder Microscopy (Fig. 15.30)

The powder is light greyish-fawn in colour with irritating and sternutatory odour and bitter taste. Microscopical examination shows abundant starch grains, mostly compound (2–8 components), spherical-ovoid, with occasional hilum in the form of a cleft. Acicular crystals of calcium oxalate are found scattered or in bundles in phelloderm cells. Fibres are lignified, slightly pitted, elongated with 2–3 transverse septa and tapered ends. Tracheidal vessels and tracheids are lignified, small, bordered pitted, found usually in groups. Cork cells are polygonal in surface view.

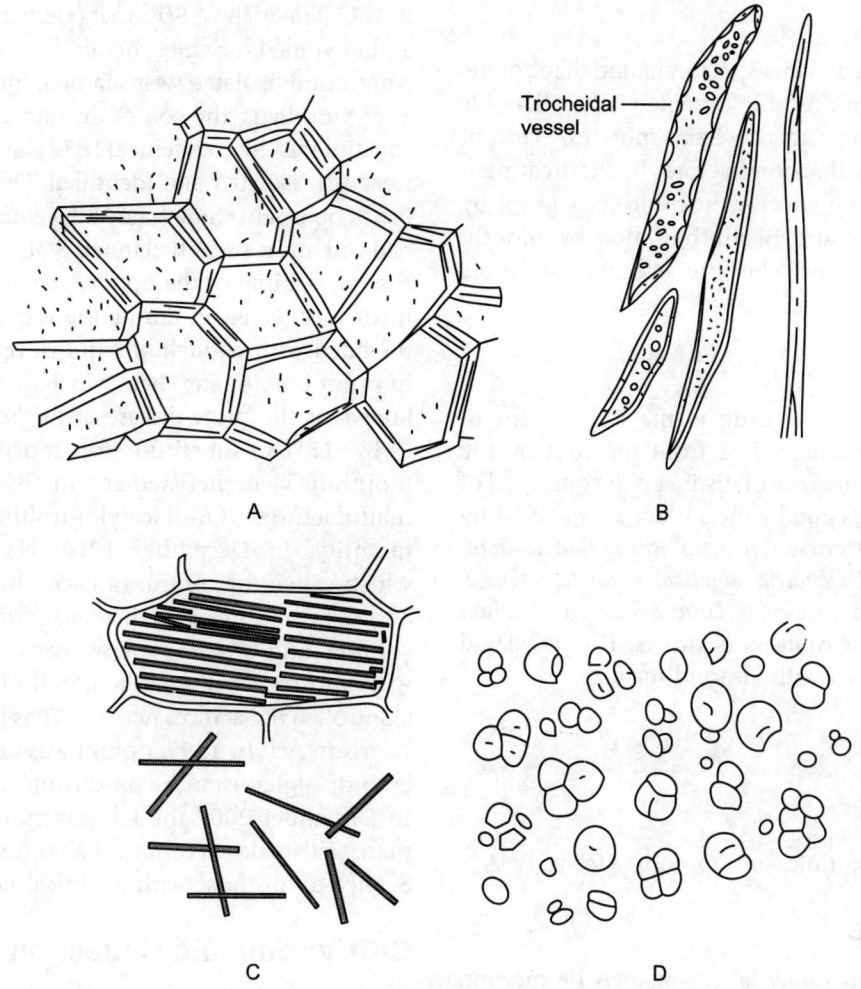

FIG. 15.30 Powder characteristics of Ipecacuanha root. (A: Cork cells, B: Tracheids and Fibre, C: Acicular crystals of calcium oxalate, D: Starch granules)

Chemical Constituents

Ipecac root contains 2–3% of total alkaloids. These include emetine, cephaeline, psychotrine and psychotrine methyl ether. All the alkaloids have isoquinoline ring system and, are present in the bark. Emetine is the active alkaloid and as it does not contain a free phenolic group it is called nonphenolic alkaloid. Emetine base is noncrystalline but its salts are crystalline, Rio ipecac contains slightly more than 2% alkaloids from which emetine are two-thirds and cephaeline is one-third. In Cartagena ipecac, alkaloids are up to 2.2% and emetine is about one-third and cephaeline two-thirds. The other alkaloids are in traces.

Chemical Test of Emetine

1. Powdered drug (0.5 g) is mixed with HCl (20 ml) and water (5 ml), filtered and to the filtrate (2 ml) potassium chloride (0.01) is added. If emetine is present, a yellow colour develops which on standing for 1 hour gradually changes to red.

Emetine

Cephaeline

Uses

Ipecac is emetic and used as an expectorant and diaphoretic and in the treatment of amoebic dysentery. The alkaloids have local irritant action. Emetine has a more expectorant and less emetic action than cephaeline. In the treatment of amoebic dysentery emetine hydrochloride is given by injection and emetine and bismuth iodide by mouth. Psychotrine and its methyl ether are selective inhibitors of human immunodeficiency virus.

Adulterants

The chief adulterant of the drug is the aerial stem of the plant. It can be distinguished from the root by the longitudinal striation, presence of distinct pith composed of cells with lignified walls and by the surface scars. The drug is often substituted by stem and roots of *Richardsonia scabra*, *Cryptocoryne spiralis*, *Psychotria emetica*, *Manettia ignita*, *Hybanthus ipecacuanha*, *Asclepias curassavica*, *Anodendron paniculatum*, *Calotropis gigantea* and others. The powdered drug is often adulterated with almond meal.

OPIUM

Synonyms

Crude Opium, Raw Opium, Gum Opium, Afeem, Post.

Biological Source

Opium is the air dried milky latex obtained by incision from the unripe capsules of *Papaver somniferum* Linn., or its variety *P. album* Decand., belonging to family Papaveraceae (Fig. 15.31).

Opium is required to contain not less than 10% of morphine and not less than 2.0% of codeine. The thebaine content is limited to 3%.

Geographical Source

It is mainly found in Turkey, Russia, Yugoslavia, Tasmania, India, Pakistan, Iran, Afghanistan, China, Burma, Thailand and Laos. In India, Opium is cultivated in M.P. (Neemuch) and U.P. for alkaloidal extraction and seed production.

History

The cultivation of opium dates back to 3400 B.C. in Mesopotamia and by 1300 B.C. Egyptians began the cultivation of opium thebaicum. Hippocrates 'the father of medicine', (460–357 B.C.) prescribed drinking the juice of the white poppy mixed with the seed of nettle and also acknowledged its use as narcotic and styptic in internal diseases. It was Alexander the Great, who introduced opium to India and Persia. During the 17th century tobacco smoking was introduced in China, which resulted in its extensive. In 1800 control on opium supply and prices was brought and in 1805 Friedrich W. Seiturner (German pharmacist) isolated and identified the chief chemical constituent of opium. The compound isolated was named morphium (morphine) after Morpheus, the god of dreams. Eventually many other constituents like codeine (1832) and papaverine (1848) were also isolated and identified. Due to the uncontrolled use of opium in china (late 18th century), the imperial court had to ban its use. The United States in 19th century made easy av lability of the opium preparations and the 'patent medicines'. Later on during the war, the Union Army were provided with enough amount of opium pills, laudanum, morphine sulphate, etc., which made opium addiction known as the 'army disease or the 'soldier's disease'.

By 1870s, substitute for morphine by acetylating morphine were prepared and in 1898 a German company manufactured 3,6-diacetylmorphine (Heroin) in bulk quantity. In December 1914, Harrison Narcotics Act which called for control of each phase of the preparation and distribution of medicinal opium, morphine, heroin, cocaine, and any new derivative with similar properties, was enforced by the United States Congress. The Federal Controlled Substances Act of 1970 is the redefined act of the Harrison Act. In 1999, opium was declared as the Bumper crop of Afghanistan by producing 75% of world's heroin. In December 2002 the UK government under the health plan, will make heroin available free on National Health Service to all those with a clinical need for it.

Cultivation and Collection

Opium is cultivated under license from the government. Its seeds are sown in October or March in alluvial soil. After germination of seeds snow falls. In spring the thin plant attains the height of 15 cm. Fertilizers are used for better crop. The poppy of first crop blossoms in April or May and the capsule mature in June or July. When the capsules are about 4 cm in diameter, the colour changes from green to yellow; they are incised with a knife about 1 mm deep around the circumference between midday and evening. The knife, known as a 'nushtur', bears narrow iron spikes which are drawn down the capsule to produce several longitudinal cuts. The incision must not penetrate into the interior of the capsule otherwise latex will be lost. The latex tube opens into one another. The latex, which is white in the beginning, immediately coagulates and turns brown. Next morning it is removed by scrapping with a knife and transferred to a poppy leaf. Each capsule is cut several times at intervals of two or three days. After collection the latex is placed in a tilted vessel so that the dark fluid which is not required may drain off. By exposure to air the opium acquires a suitable consistency for packing. The dried latex is kneaded into balls, wrapped in poppy leaves and dried in shade. The principal commercial varieties of Opium are Turkish Opium, Indian Opium, Chinese Opium, Yugoslavian Opium and Persian Opium.

Characteristics

Opium occurs in rounded or flattened mass which is 8–15 cm in diameter and weighing from 300 g to 2 kg each. The external surface is pale or chocolate-brown, texture is uniform and slightly granular. It is plastic like when fresh and turns hard and brittle after sometime. Fragment of poppy leaves are present on the upper surface. Internal surface is coarsely granular, reddish-brown, lustrous; odour is characteristic; taste is bitter and distinct. Opium is intended only as a starting material for the manufacture of galenical preparations and is not dispensed as such.

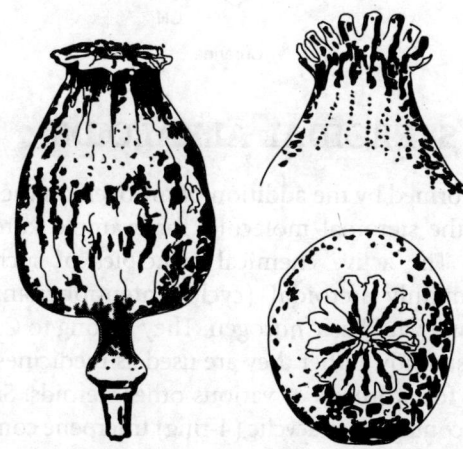

FIG. 15.31 *Papaver somniferum* capsules

Chemical Constituents

Opium contains about 35 alkaloids among which morphine (10–16%) is the most important base. The alkaloids are combined with meconic acid. The other alkaloids isolated from the drug are codeine (0.8–2.5%), narcotine, thebaine (0.5–2%), noscapine (4–8%), narceine and papaverine (0.5–2.5%). Morphine contains a phenanthrene nucleus. The different types of alkaloids isolated are:

1. *Morphine Type:* Morphine, codeine, neopine, pseudo or oxymorphine, thebaine and porphyroxine. Morphine

consists of alkaloids which has phenanthrene nucleus whereas those of the papaverine group has benzylisoquinoline structure. Protopine and hydrocotamine are of different structural types. The morphine molecule has both a phenolic and an alcoholic hydroxyl group and acetylated form is diacetyl morphine or heroin. Codeine is ether of morphine (methyl-morphine). Other morphine ethers which are used medicinally are ethylmorphine and pholcodine.

2. *Phthalide Isoquinoline Type:* Hydrocotarnine, narcotoline, 1-narcotine, noscapine, oxynarcotine, narceine and 5′-O-demethyl-narcotine.
3. *Benzyl Isoquinoline Type:* Papaverine, dl-laudanine, laudanidine, codamine and laudanosine.
4. *Cryptopine Type:* Protopine, cryptopine.
5. *Unknown Constituents:* Aporeine, diodeadine, meconidine, papaveramine and lanthopine.

The drug also contains sugars, sulphates, albuminous compounds, colouring matter and moisture. In addition to these anisaldehyde, vanillin, vanillic acid, β-hydroxystyrene, fumaric acid, lactic acid, benzyl alcohol, 2-hydroxycinchonic acid, phthalic acid, hemipinic acid, meconin and an odorous compound have also been reported.

Chemical Tests

1. Aqueous extract of opium with $FeCl_3$ solution gives deep reddish purple colour which persists on addition of HCl. It indicates the presence of meconic acid.
2. Morphine gives dark violet colour with conc. H_2SO_4 and formaldehyde.

Uses

Opium and morphine have narcotic, analgesic and sedative action and used to relieve pain, diarrhoea dysentery and cough. Poppy capsules are astringent, somniferous, soporific, sedative and narcotic and used as anodyne and emollient. Codeine is mild sedative and is employed in cough mixtures. Noscapine is not narcotic and has cough

Thebaine

Morphine

Codeine

Heroin

Papaverine

suppressant action acting as a central antitussive drug. Papaverine has smooth muscle relaxant action and is used to cure muscle spasms. Opium, morphine and the diacetyl derivative heroin, cause drug addiction.

CURARE

Synonyms

South American arrow poison, Ourari, Urari, Woorari, Wourara, Woorali.

Biological Source

Curare is a crude dried extract from stems of *Strychnos castelnaei* Wedd., *S. toxifiera* Benth, *S. crevauxii* G. Planchon, *S. gubleri* G. Planchon, belonging to family Loganiaceae. The extract is also prepared from *Chondodendron tomentosum* Ruiz et Par and *C. microphylla* (Menispermaceae) (Fig. 15.32).

Characteristics

Earlier curare has been imported in earthen pots and bamboos, now it is being imported in tins. It is dark brown or black in colour. It is odourless and very bitter in taste.

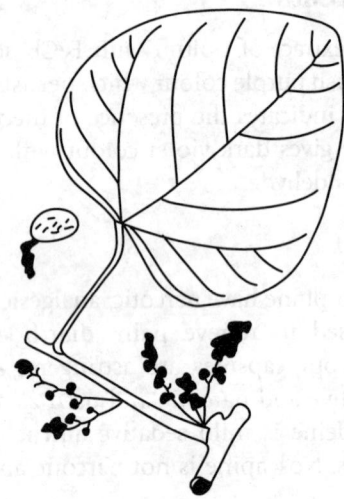

FIG. 15.32 Twig of curare

Chemical Constituents

Curare contains several alkaloids and quaternary compounds. The most important alkaloid is curarine and two quaternary bases, calabashcurarine I and calabashcurarine II. Though the drug contains strychnos, but strychnine is not present.

Uses

Curare has been used in the treatment of hydrophobia, cholera and tetanus. It is used as a source of alkaloids. It has muscular relaxation in surgery and is used to control convulsions of strychnine poisoning and of tetanus.

Curarine

15.15. STEROIDAL ALKALOIDS

They are formed by the addition of nitrogen on the similar point in the steroidal molecule, for example kurchi and veratrum. The active chemical principles of such drugs contain mainly steroidal (cyclopentenophenanthrene) entity, along with basic nitrogen. They belong to C_{21} or C_{27} group of steroids. Either they are used as medicines or as a precursor for synthesis of various other steroids. Steroidal alkaloids contain a tetracyclic (4-ring) triterpene compound called the steroid nucleus or steroidal backbone. Because some steroidal alkaloids contain a sugar molecule, they are also referred to as alkaloidal glycosides (sugar + steroidal alkaloid). Species of nightshades (*Solanum*) in the tomato family (Solanaceae) contain a complex of toxic alkaloidal glycosides (glycoalkaloid). Solanine is an example of a glycoalkaloid. Some of the important drugs under this class are *Solanum* species. Glycoalkaloids, principally solanine and chaconine, are present at variable concentrations in the vegetative organs of *Solanum* species. Glycoalkaloids are synthesized in the leaves and then translocated to the different plant organs. Although a number of factors, both abiotic—such as light, soil type and moisture, fertilization or pesticides and biotic—such as plant age, type of organ (berries, leaves, stems, sprouts and tubers) considered, tuber size or tuber integrity (fracture damages, crushing, splits)—influence glycoalkaloid concentration; the synthesis of these molecules is also largely determined by the genetic constitution of the plant.

One of the most interesting and poisonous steroidal alkaloids is produced by Central and South American poison dart frogs of the genera *Dendrobates* and *Phyllobates*.

VERATRUM

Synonyms

American Hellebore, Green Hellebore, American Veratrum, Indian poke.

Biological Source

Veratrum consists of dried roots and rhizomes of the perennial herbs, *Veratrum viride* Aiton and *Veratrum album* Linn., belonging to family Liliaceae (Fig. 15.33).

Geographical Source

It is mainly found in Canada, United States, Carolina, Tennessee and Georgia.

Cultivation and Collection

American drug is collected in the eastern parts of Canada and the United States and white hellebore in central and southern Europe. The rhizomes are dug in autumn season, cleaned, cut longitudinally and dried.

Characteristics

The entire rhizome is conical, 3–8 cm long and 2–3.5 cm wide; externally brownish-grey. The roots are numerous and almost completely cover the rhizome. Entire roots are up to 8 cm long and 4 mm diameter, light brown to light orange and usually much wrinkled. Odourless, taste, bitter and acrid.

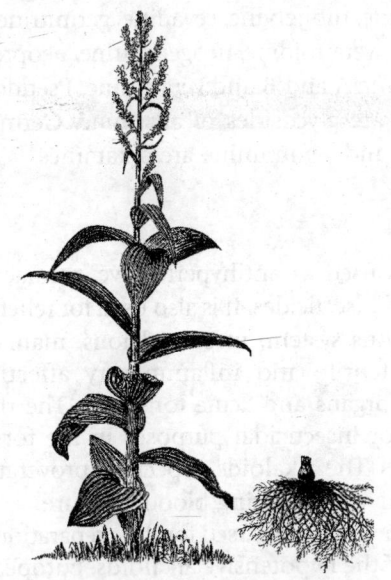

FIG. 15.33 Twig and root of *Veratrum viride*

Chemical Constituents

Various steroidal alkaloids have been isolated from Veratrums. The important alkaloids are jervine,

Protoveratrine A

Protoveratrine B

Jervine

pseudojervine, rubijervine, cevadine, germitrine, germidine, veratralbine, veratroidine, neogermitrine, neoprotoveratrine, protoveratrine A and B and veratridine. Pseudojervine and veratrosine are glycosides of alkamine. Germine, jervine, rubijervine and veratramine are alkamines.

Uses

Veratrum is used as antihypertensive, cardiac depressant, sedative and insecticides. It is also used for relief in irritation of the nervous system, in convulsions, mania, neuralgia, headache, febrile and inflammatory affections of the respiratory organs and acute tonsillitis. The rhizomes are also used for insecticidal purposes in the form of sprays and in dusts. The alkaloids, especially proveratrines A and B, are effective in reducing blood pressure.

American veratrum is used for the preparation of veriloid, a mixture of the hypotensive alkaloids. European veratrum is used for the preparation of the protoveratrines. The drugs are used as insecticides.

KURCHI BARK

Synonyms

Holarrhena, Kurchi (Hindi).

Biological Source

Kurchi bark consists of dried stem bark of *Holarrhena antidysenterica* Wall, belonging to family Apocynaceae (Fig. 15.34).

Geographical Source

The plant is found throughout India, ascending up to 1250 m in the Himalayas, especially in wet forests.

Cultivation and Collection

Kurchi is a deciduous laticiferous shrub or small tree, 9–10 m high. The bark is collected from the tree by making suitable transverse and longitudinal incisions. The alkaloidal content is high soon after the rains when new shoots are produced which declines during winter months.

Characteristics

The pieces of Kurchi bark are small and recurved both longitudinally and transversely. The size and thickness vary from piece to piece. Outer surface is buff to reddish brown and bears numerous prominent circular or transversely elongated horizontal lenticels and longitudinal wrinkles. The thicker pieces are rugose and show numerous yellowish warts; inner surface cinnamon-brown, longitudinally striated, frequently with portions of pale yellow wood attached; fracture is brittle and splintery. The taste is acrid and bitter while the odour is not distinct.

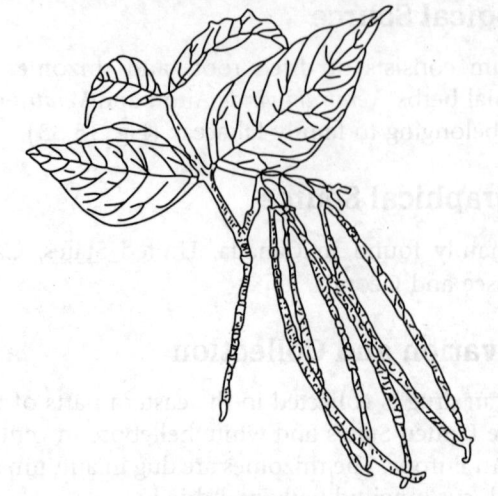

FIG. 15.34 Twig of *Holarrhena antidysenterica*

Microscopy (Figs. 15.35 and 15.36)

Transverse section of bark shows cork composed of uniformly arranged several layers of tangentially elongated cells. Below cork is a broad zone of cortex, composed of thin-walled, irregular, polygonal parenchymatous cells containing starch grains and prismatic calcium oxalate crystals. Groups of sclereids are scattered in the cortex; individual sclereid cells are more or less rounded-oval, thick-walled with numerous pits. Cortex is limited below by a zone of groups of sclereids, which alternate with parenchymatous zone. Phloem consists of phloem parenchyma similar to cortex, traversed longitudinally by medullary rays at regular intervals. Medullary rays are narrow, one to two cells wide and almost straight.

Powder Microscopy (Fig. 15.37)

The powder is light brown in colour with bitter taste. Microscopical examination shows groups of sclereids,

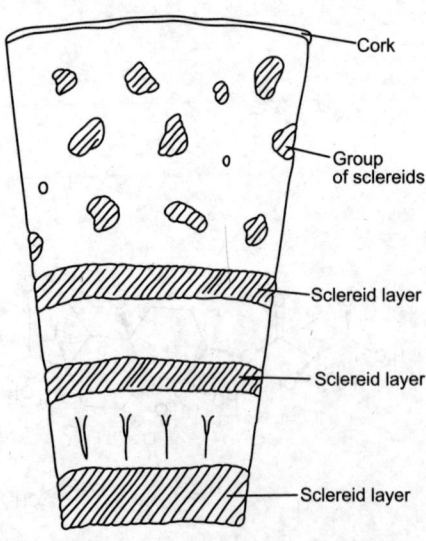

FIG. 15.35 T.S. (schematic) of Kurchi bark

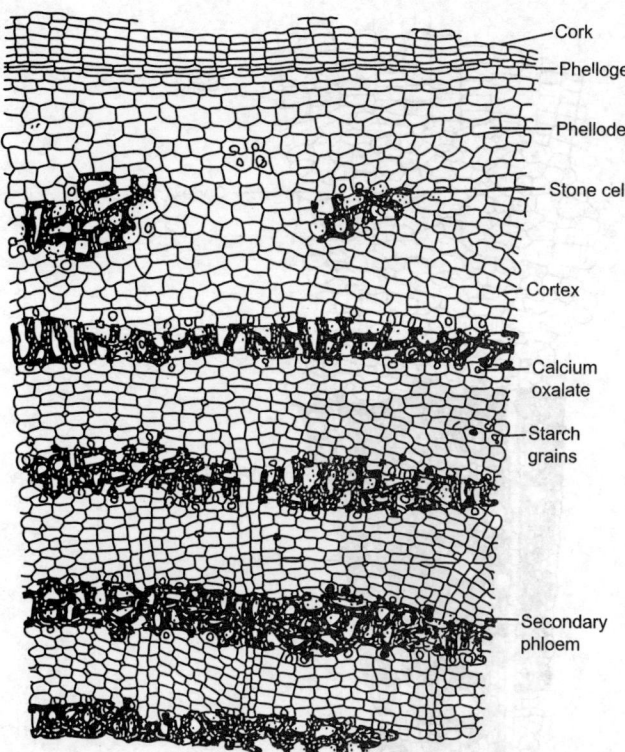

FIG. 15.36 Transverse section of Kurchi bark

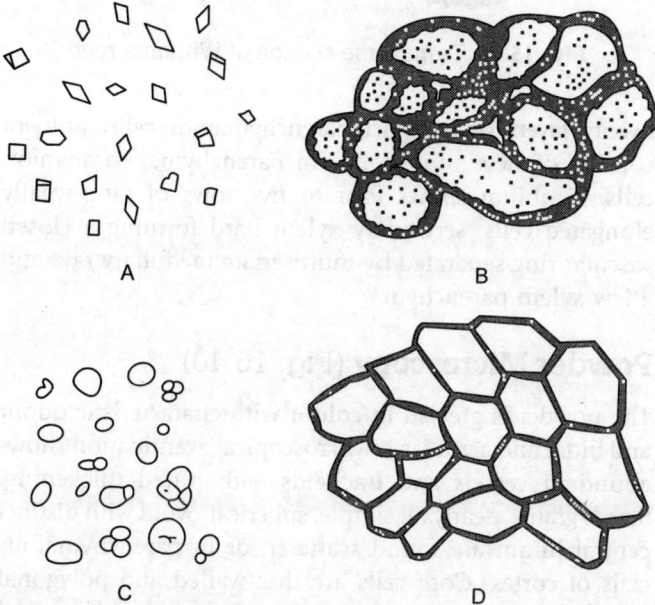

FIG. 15.37 Powder characteristics of Kurchi bark. (A: Prismatic crystals of calcium oxalate, B: Sclereids, C: Starch grains, D: Cork cells in surface view)

composed of thick-walled, densely packed cells with numerous pits. Cork cells are moderately thick-walled and polygonal in surface view. Prismatic crystals of calcium oxalate, small and uniform in size, and starch grains, simple or compound (2–4 components), spherical-ovoid are usually found scattered.

Chemical Constituents

The total alkaloidal constituents of Kurchi bark vary from 1.1% to 4.72%. The main steroidal alkaloid is conessine (20–30%). The other alkaloids isolated include conarrhimine, conimine, conamine, conessimine, isoconessimine, dimethyl conkurchine and holarrhimine. In addition to alkaloids the bark also contains gum, resin, tannin, lupeol and digitenol glycoside holadysone.

Conessine

Uses

The bark is considered to be stomachic, astringent, tonic, antidysenteric, febrifuge and anthelmintic. The dried bark is rubbed over the body in dropsy. Kurchi bark is used to cure amoebic dysentery and diarrhoea.

Marketed Products

It is one of the ingredients of the preparations known as Diarex PFS, Diarex Vet. (Himalaya Drug Company), Mahamanjishthadi kwath, Mahamanjisthadyarishta (Dabur) and Amree plus granules, Purodil capsules (Aimil Pharmaceuticals).

ASHWAGANDHA

Synonyms

Withania root, Ashwagandha, Clustered Winter cherry.

Biological Source

It consists of the dried roots and stem bases of *Withania somnifera* Dunal, belonging to family Solanaceae (Fig. 15.38).

Geographical Source

Withania is widely distributed from southern Europe to India and Africa.

History

The use of ashwagandha in Ayurvedic medicine extends back over 3000–4000 years to the teachings of an esteemed rishi (sage) Punarvasu Atriya. It has been described in the sacred texts of Ayurveda, including the Charaka and Sushruta

Samhita where it is widely extolled as a tonic especially for emaciation in people of all ages including babies, enhancing the reproductive function of both men and women.

Cultivation and Collection

Withania somnifera are propagated by division, cuttings or seed. Seed is the best way to propagate them. Seed sown on moist sand will germinate in 14–21 days at 20°C. *Withania somnifera* need full sun to partial shade with a well-drained slightly alkaline soil mix. Plants do best when the soil pH is 7.5–8.0. Soil mix consisting of two parts sandy loam to one part sand will to better. The plants are allowed to dry thoroughly in between waterings. In containers, too much water causes root rot. Plants are fertilized once during the year with a balanced fertilizer.

Characteristics

A low lying plant, often reaching only 1–2 ft, but occasionally 6 ft. It is a perennial, but can be grown as an annual. Plant and fruits resemble its relatives the ground cherry and Chinese lantern. Young roots are straight, unbranched and conical and in pieces of different lengths. Root thickness varies according to age and usually it is 5–12 mm below crown. Outer surface is buff to yellow and longitudinally wrinkled. Taste is bitter and mucilaginous.

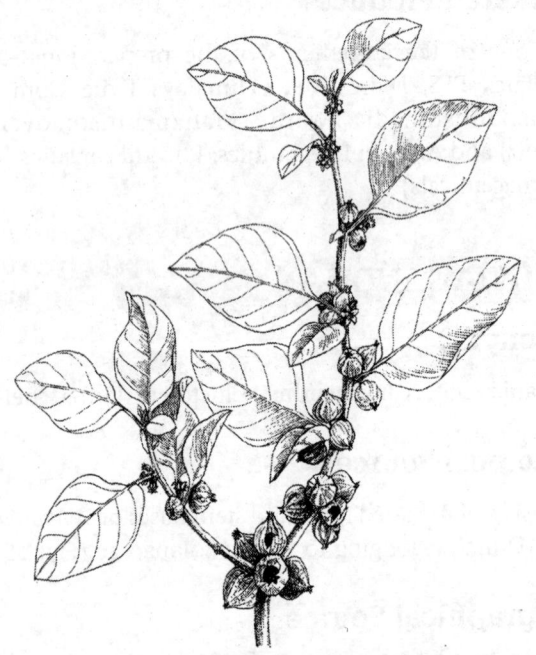

FIG. 15.38 *Withania somnifera*

Microscopy (Fig. 15.39)

Transverse section of root shows cork exfoliated or crushed; when present isodiametric and nonlignified; cork cambium of two to four diffused rows of cells; secondary cortex about

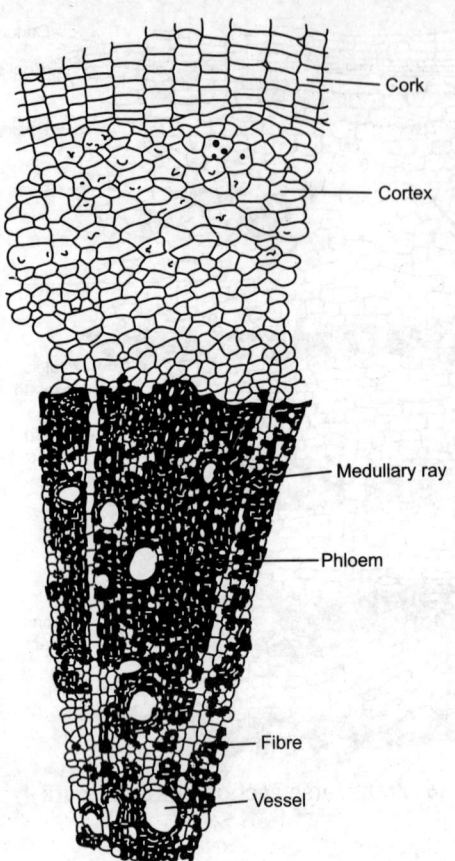

FIG. 15.39 Transverse section of Withania root

twenty layers of compact parenchymatous cells; phloem consists of sieve tubes, phloem parenchyma, companion cells, cambium shows four to five rows of tangentially elongated cells; secondary xylem hard forming a closed vascular ring separated by multiseriate medullary rays and a few xylem parenchyma.

Powder Microscopy (Fig. 15.40)

The powder is greyish in colour with characteristic odour and bitter and acrid taste. Microscopical examination shows abundant vessels and tracheids with pitted thickening. Starch grains, nearly all simple, spherical-ovoid with distinct central hilum are found scattered or in parenchymatous cells of cortex. Cork cells are thin-wailed and polygonal in surface view. Fibres are narrow, elongated with tapered ends.

Chemical Constituents

The plants contain the alkaloid withanine as the main constituent and somniferine, pseudowithanine, tropine and pseudotropine, hygrine, isopellederine, anaferine, anahygrine and steroid lactones. The leaves contain steroid lactone, commonly known as withanolides.

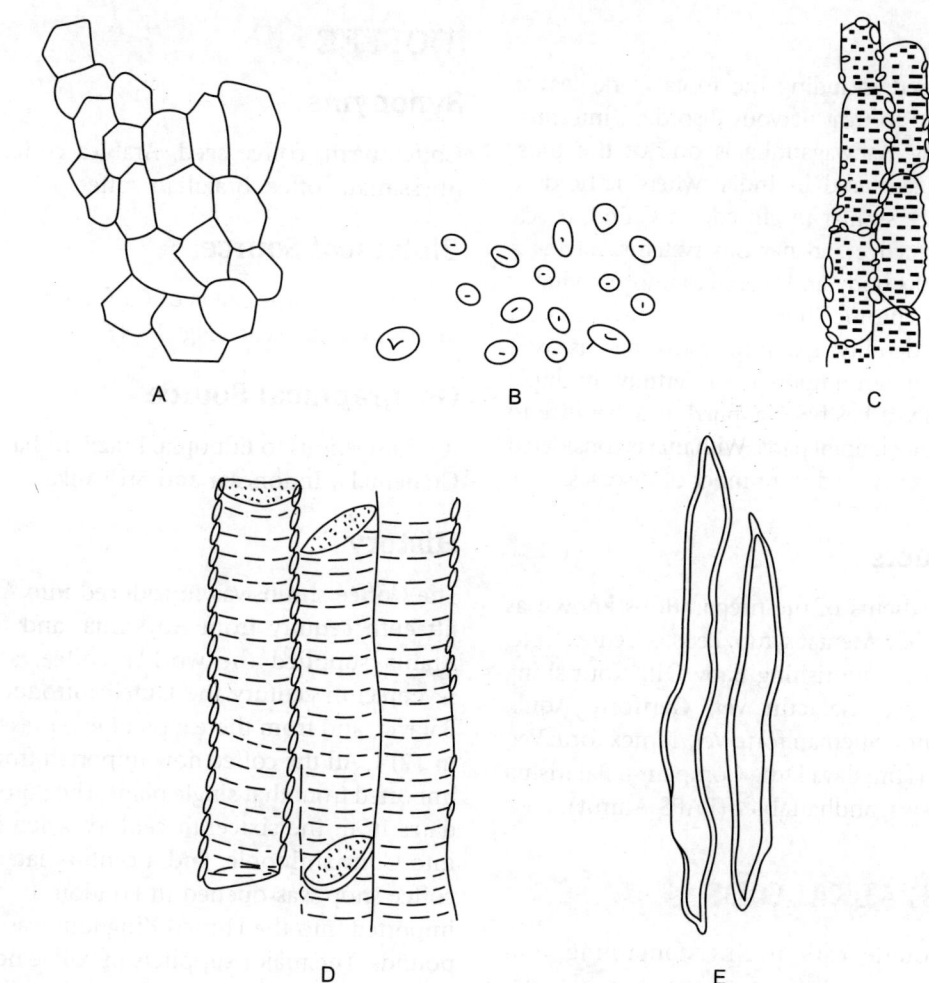

FIG. 15.40 Powder characteristics of Withania root. (A: Cork cells, B: Tracheids, C: Starch grains, D: Vessels, E: Fibres)

Hygrine

Tropine

Withanolide D

Withanolide F

Uses

All plant parts are used including the roots, bark, leaves, fruit and seed are used to treat nervous disorders, intestinal infections and leprosy. Ashwagandha is one of the most widespread tranquillizers used in India, where it holds a position of importance similar to ginseng in China. It acts mainly on the reproductive and nervous systems, having a rejuvenative effect on the body, and is used to improve vitality and aid recovery after chronic illness. It is also used to treat nervous exhaustion, debility, insomnia, wasting diseases, failure to thrive in children, impotence, infertility; multiple sclerosis, etc. Externally it has been applied as a poultice to boils, swellings and other painful parts. Withania is considered as an adaptogen and so is used in number of diseases.

Marketed Products

It is one of the ingredients of the preparations known as Abana, Geriforte, Mentat, Mentat syrup, Reosto, Tentex forte, AntiStress Massage Oil, Nourishing Baby Oil, Nourishing Skin Cream, Anxocare, Galactin Vet, Geriforte Aqua, Geriforte Vet, Immunol, Speman forte Vet, Tentex forte Vet, Ashwagandha tablet (Himalaya Drug Company), Balarishta (Baidyanath) and Aswagandha tablet (BAPS Amrut).

15.16. PURINE ALKALOIDS

Purine contains double carbon ring containing four nitrogen atoms. Purine alkaloids have a molecular structure remarkably similar to the nitrogenous purine base adenine, which is found in DNA, RNA and ATP. Iriosine and xanthosine monophosphate, (IMP and XMP) are two important precursors derived via the primary purine biosynthetic pathway. They have a CNS; stimulant effect, relax bronchial smooth muscles and have a diuretic effect. Mode of action is via inhibition of phosphodiesterase, this increases production of cAMP causing release of adrenaline. These alkaloids are derived from adenine and guanine which are the purine base components of the nucleotides adenosine and guanosine. The nucleotides adenosine and guanosine are derived from IMP and XMP respectively. The purine alkaloids are derived from XMP.

Most notable of the purine alkaloids are the mild stimulants caffeine and the very similar theobromine. Caffeine occurs naturally in many beverage plants, including coffee (*Coffea arabica*) belonging to the family Rubiaceae, tea (*Thea sinensis*) belonging to the tea family (Theaceae), yerba mate (*Ilex paraguariensis*) in the holly family (Aquifoliaceae) and cola (*Cola nitida*) in the chocolate family (Sterculiaceae). The primary source of theobromine is from the seeds of Cacao (*Theobroma cacao*), another member of the chocolate family (Sterculiaceae).

COFFEE

Synonyms

Coffee bean, coffee seed, Arabica coffee, Arabian coffee, Abyssinian coffee, Brazilian coffee.

Biological Source

It is the dried ripe seeds of *Coffea arabica* Linn., belonging to family Rubiaceae (Fig. 15.41).

Geographical Source

It is indigenous to Ethiopia, Brazil, India, Vietnam, Mexico, Guatemala, Indonesia and Sri Lanka.

History

The Coffee shrub was introduced into Arabia early in the fifteenth century from Abyssinia, and for two centuries, Arabia supplied the world's coffee; at the end of the seventeenth century the Dutch introduced the plant into Batavia, and from there a plant was presented to Louis XIV in 1714. All the coffee now imported from Brazil has been imported from that single plant. The European use of coffee dates from the sixteenth century when it was introduced into Constantinople, and a century later in 1652 the first coffee shop was opened in London. In 1858 the quantity imported into the United Kingdom was over sixty million pounds. The major suppliers of coffee nowadays are Brazil and India. Karnataka, Kerala and Tamil Nadu grow large plantation of coffee.

Cultivation and Collection

Propagation is usually by seed; however, budding, grafting and cuttings have been used. Traditional method of plants on virgin soil is to put 20 seeds in each hole, 3.5 × 3.5 m at the beginning of rainy season. Half are eliminated naturally. In Brazil, a more successful method is to raise seedlings in shaded nurseries. At 6–12 months, seedlings are taken to fields, hardened and then planted on contoured fields 2–3 m apart in 3–5 m rows. Holes are prepared 40 × 40 × 40 cm and 4 seedlings placed in each. Plants may be shaded by taller trees or left unshaded.

Average economic age of plants 30–40 years, with some 100 year old plantations still bearing. Trees come into bearing three to four years after planting and are in full bearing at six to eight years. Fruits mature seven to nine months after flowering. Selective picking of ripe red fruits produces highest quality. Crop ripens over a period of several weeks. In Brazil all berries are stripped at one time onto ground cloths, usually in April to June; in Ethiopia, harvest season is October to December after the rainy season. Berries are dried in sun; in some humid areas, artificial heat is used. Depulping after picking is increasingly practiced.

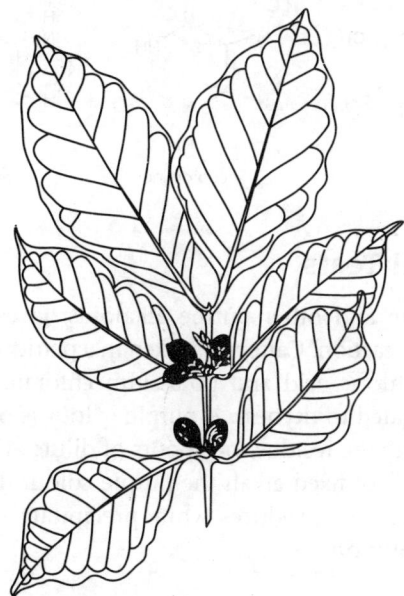

FIG. 15.41 *Coffea arabica*

Characteristics

Evergreen, glabrous shrub or small tree, up to 5-m tall when unpruned. Leaves opposite, dark green, glossy, elliptical, acuminate-tipped, short-petioled, 5–20 cm long, 1.5–7.5 cm broad, usually 10–15 cm long and 6 cm broad. Flowers white, fragrant, in axillary clusters, opening simultaneously 8–12 days after wetting; corolla tubular, 1 cm long, 5-lobed; calyx small, cup-shaped. Fruit a drupe, about 1.5 cm long, oval-elliptic, green when immature, ripening yellow and then crimson, black upon drying, 7–9 months to maturity. Seeds usually 2, ellipsoidal, 8.5–12.5 mm long, inner surface deeply grooved, consisting mainly of green corneous endosperm and small embryo.

Chemical Constituents

The main constituents of coffee are caffeine, tannin, fixed oil and proteins. It contains 2–3% caffeine, 3–5% tannins, 13% proteins and 10–15% fixed oils. In the seeds, caffeine is present as a salt of chlorogenic acid. Also it contains oil and wax.

Caffeine

Chemical Tests

1. Caffeine and other purine alkaloids, gives murexide colour reaction. Caffeine is taken in a petridish to which hydrochloric acid and potassium chlorate crystals are added and heated to dryness. A purple colour is obtained by exposing the residue to vapours of dilute ammonia. In addition of fixed alkali the purple colour disappears.
2. Caffeine also produces white precipitate with tannic acid solution.

Uses

Coffee is widely used as a flavouring agent, as in ice cream, pastries, candies and liquors. Source of caffeine, dried ripe seeds are used as a stimulant, nervine and diuretic, acting on CNS, kidneys, heart and muscles. Very valuable in cases of snake-bite, helping to ward off the terrible coma. It also exerts a soothing action on the vascular system, preventing a too rapid wasting of the tissues of the body; these effects are not only due to the volatile oil but to the caffeine it contains.

TEA

Biological Source

It contains the prepared leaves and leaf buds of *Thea sinensis* (Linne) kuntz., belonging to family Theaceae (Fig. 15.42).

Geographical Source

It is mainly cultivated in India (Assam), Ceylon, Japan and Java.

Cultivation and Collection

It is an evergreen shrub growing to 4 m × 2.5 m at a slow rate. The plant prefers light (sandy) and medium (loamy) soils and requires well-drained soil. The plant prefers acid and neutral soils and can grow in very acid soil. It can grow in semishade (light woodland). It requires moist soil and prefers a pH between 5 and 7. Prefers the partial shade of light woodland or a woodland clearing. It is reported to tolerate an annual rainfall of 70–310 cm, an average annual temperature range of 14–27°C and a pH in the range of 4.5–7.3. It prefers a wet summer and a cool but not very frosty dry winter. Seed can be sown as soon as it is ripe in a green house. Stored seed should be presoaked for 24 h in warm water and the hard covering around the micropyle should be filed down to leave a thin covering. It usually germinates in one to three months. Prick out the seedlings into individual pots when they are large enough to handle and grow them on in light shade in the green house for at least their first winter. Plant them out into their permanent positions when they are more than 15 cm tall and give them some protection from winter cold for their first year or three outdoors. Seedlings take 4–12 years before they start to produce seed.

Characteristics

Leaves are dark green in colour, lanceolate or elliptical, on short stalks, blunt at apex, base tapering, margins shortly serrate, young leaves hairy, older leaves glabrous.

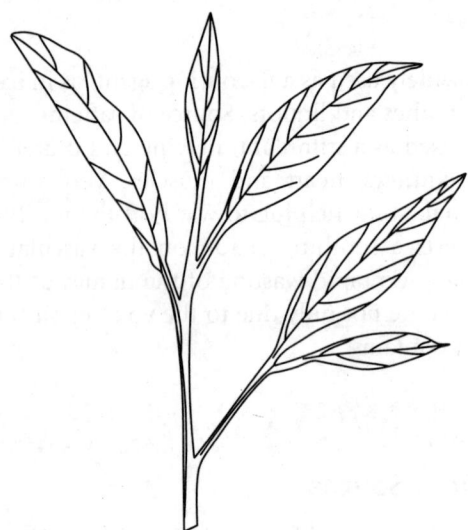

FIG. 15.42 Twig of tea plant

Microscopy

The epidermal cells are made of polygonal cells which are slightly wavy walls. It consist on itself stomata and trichomes. The trichomes are thick walled, unicellular, conical (covering) which arise on the lower surface and in large number in young leaves. The mesophyll region consist of two rows of palisade parenchyma cells and large lignified sclereids which arise at some intervals and are extended across the mesophyll from one epidermis to the other. Cluster crystals of calcium oxalate are scattered in phloem and in parenchyma. In the midrib area a prominent ridge is present both above and below. Vascular bundle consisting of xylem and phloem are present; the entire region being covered by slightly lignified band of pericyclic fibres. The pericyclic fibres are up to four fibres in width at the widest region. The remaining portion is covered with spongy parenchyma with scattered lignified sclereids.

Chemical Constituents

The leaves are a rich source of caffeine (1–5%). It also contains theobromine and theophylline in minor quantities. The colour of tea leaves is due to tannin (10–20% gallotannic acid). The agreeable odour is due to presence of a yellow volatile oil. Tea leaves also contain protein, wax, resin and ash.

Caffeine | Theobromine | Theophyline

Chemical Tests

1. Caffeine and other purine alkaloids, gives murexide colour reaction. Caffeine is taken in a petridish to which hydrochloric acid and potassium chlorate are added and heated to dryness. A purple colour is obtained by exposing the residue to vapours of dilute ammonia. In addition of fixed alkali the purple colour disappears.
2. Caffeine also produces white precipitate with tannic acid solution.

Uses

It is used as stimulant, astringent and also as diuretic.

COCOA

Synonyms

Cocoa seed, cocoa bean, chocolate tree.

Biological Source

It is obtained from seeds of *Theobroma cocoa*, belonging to family Sterculiaceae.

Geographical Source

Cultivated in tropical America, Ceylon, Java, South American countries like Brazil, Ecuador, Guiana and Caribbean islands.

Cultivation and Collection

Cocoa is cultivated up to an altitude of 1000 m. The plant can tolerate a rain fall of 150–500 cm per annum but the rain should be properly distributed. It requires well drained soil, with a capacity to hold moisture. The top soil (15–30 cm) should have sufficient organic matter. Proper irrigation is essential at least for the first two years of cultivation so as to facilitate tap root of the plant to penetrate deep in the soil. Though cocoa plant requires adequate sun light, it cannot tolerate direct sun light. So, permanent evergreen forest trees are developed to provide shade. Coconut or areca nut trees are cultivated in between cocoa plants. Cocoa plants start bearing fruits after three years of planting and survive for 60–70 years. The flowers are small and are succeeded by deep red fruits or orange coloured fruits. The fruits are about 15–20 cm long, containing 40–50 colourless, fleshy seeds embedded in the mucilaginous pulp,

The usual season for gathering the fruit is June and December. When ripe they are cut open and the beans or nuts surrounded by their sweetish acid pulp are allowed to ferment so that they may be more easily separated from the shell. The beans are then usually dried in the sun, though sometimes in a steam drying shed.

Characteristics

The tree is handsome, 12–16 feet high, trunk about 5 feet long, wood light and white coloured, bark brown. Leaves are lanceolate, bright green and entire. Flowers are small reddish and almost odourless. Fruits are yellowish red, smooth; rind flesh coloured; pulp white; when seeds are ripe they rattle in the capsule when shaken; each capsule contains about 25 seeds; if separated from the capsule they soon become infertile, but if kept therein they retain their fertility for a long time.

Chemical Constituents

Cocoa beans mainly contain theobromine and cocoa butter. The percentage of caffeine is less in this, various volatile compounds, polyphenols, together with mucilage, etc., are also present.

Caffeine   Theobromine

Uses

It is used as an ingredient in cosmetic ointments and in pharmacy for coating pills and preparing suppositories. It has excellent emollient properties and is used to soften and protect chapped hands and lips. Theobromine, the alkaloid in the beans, resembles caffeine in its action, but its effect on the CNS is less powerful. It is also used as diuretic. It is also employed in high blood pressure as it dilates the blood vessels. Cocoa is also used as nutritive.

15.17. DITERPENE ALKALOIDS

Diterpene alkaloids are selectively accumulated in plants of the Aconitum, Delphinium, Carrya and Thalictrum genera. The interest in this alkaloids and the area of their application are ever increasing. Diterpene bases are subdivided into two categories: the ones based on C_{19} skeleton and those based on C_{20} skeleton.

ACONITE

Synonyms

Monkshood, Friar's cowl; Mouse-bane; Aconite root; Mithazahar (Hindi); Radix aconiti.

Biological Source

Aconite is the dried roots of *Aconitum napellus* Linn., collected from wild or cultivated plants., belonging to family Ranunculaceae (Fig. 15.43).

Geographical Source

The plant has been originated from the mountainous and temperate regions of Europe. It occurs in Alps and Carpathian mountains, hills of Germany and Himalayas. The greater part of the commercial drug is derived from wild plant grown in central and southern Europe, particularly Spain.

Cultivation and Collection

Aconite is a perennial herb with a fusiform tuberous root. The plant is propagated from the daughter tubers. An apical bud on the apex and six lateral buds on its surface are developed. A lateral shoot bearing a thin lateral root is produced from each lateral bud. The lateral roots are called daughter roots and the main root is known as parent root. The daughter root develops gradually, becomes thick in autumn and buds are produced on its apex and surface.

Daughter roots are painted in soil containing leaf mould and some amount of lime. The roots are collected in autumn. Collection of aconite from wild plants is done during flowering season. Roots are dried at 40–50°C. Thus aconite arises from one or more lateral shoots which develop into conical daughter tubers.

Morphology

Appearance of aconite varies from season to season. Aconite collected in autumn is conical in shape and tapering below. Surface is slightly twisted bearing longitudinal ridges. Some aconites may contain fibrous rootlets or their scars. On the top of parent root some remains of stem base are present which are more shrivelled. An apical bud is present at the apex. The colour is dark-brown. The root is 4–10 cm in length and 1–3 cm in diameter at the crown. Rootlets may be present. The fracture is short and starchy. The fractured surface is five to eight angled, contains stellate cambium and a central pith. The odour is slight. Taste is sweet at first followed by tingling and numbness.

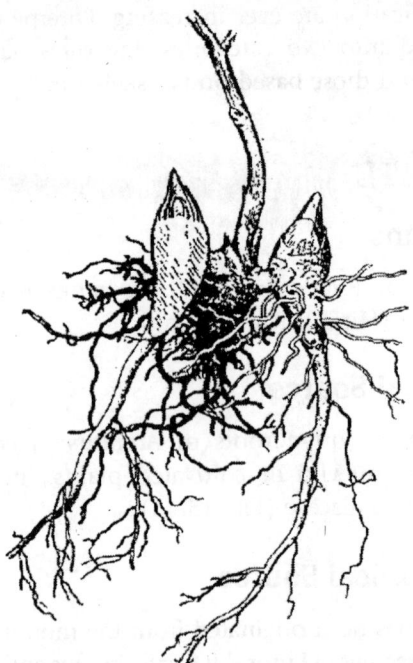

FIG. 15.43 *Aconitum napellus*

Chemical Constituents

Aconite contains aconitine (0.4–0.8%), hypaconitine, mesaconitine, aconine, napelline (isoaconitine, pseudoaconitine), neoline, ephedrine, sparteine, picraconitine, acotinic acid, itaconic acid, succinic acid, malonic acid, fat, starch, aconosine, hokbusine A, senbusines A and C and mesaconitine. The aconitines are diacyl esters of polyhydric amino alcohols and are extremely poisonous. The basic skeleton of aconite alkaloid is consisted of a pentacyclic diterpene.

Uses

It is used externally as a local analgesic in liniments and to treat neuralgia, rheumatism and inflammation. Tincture aconite is antipyretic in small doses. Aconitine in amount 2–3 mg can lead respiratory failure, heart failure and in the end death. The drug is used for the preparation of an antineuralgic liniment.

Marketed Products

It is one of the ingredients of the preparation known as J.P. Painkill oil (Jamuna Pharma).

15.18. AMINO ALKALOIDS

One or more carbon rings with a nitrogen atom on a carbon side chain. One of the most interesting alkaloids in this group is mescaline from *Lophophora williamsii*. Mescaline has a molecular structure that is remarkably similar to the brain neurotransmitter dopamine. It is also structurally similar to the neurohormone norepinephrine (noradrenalin) and to the stimulant amphetamine. In the peyote cactus, mescaline is formed in a complex pathway from the amino acid tyrosine. A similar pathway in humans produces epinephrine (adrenalin) and its demethylated precursor norepinephrine from tyrosine. Dopamine and its precursor L-dopa are also derived from a tyrosine pathway. Mescaline also occurs in several other cactus species, including the commonly cultivated, night-blooming, South American San Pedro cactus (*Trichocereus pachanoi*).

Another alkaloid called ephedrine has a molecular structure similar to that of mescaline. Since ephedrine has a chemical structure similar to epinephrine (adrenalin), it works like a powerful cardiac stimulant that may cause cardiac arrest in infants and heart patients. New synthetic drugs based on the ephedrine/epinephrine ring structure are now marketed as effective and safer bronchodilators. Pseudoephedrine, an isomer of ephedrine, also occurs in species of Ephedra, and may be produced synthetically. Compared to ephedrine, it causes fewer heart symptoms, such as palpitation, but is equally effective as a bronchodilator.

Colchicine is a 3-ring amine alkaloid derived from the corms of *Colchicum autumnale*, a member of the lily family (Liliaceae). Like the anticancer indole alkaloids, vinblastine and vincristine, it is a spindle poison causing depolymerization of mitotic spindles into tubulin subunits. This effectively stops the tumour cells from dividing, thus causing remission of the cancer. It is a powerful inducer of polyploidy because it can stop plant cells from dividing after the chromatids have separated during anaphase of mitosis. It is used as a mutagen.

Aconitine

Hypaconitine

EPHEDRA

Synonyms

Ma Huang.

Biological Source

Ephedra consists of the dried aerial parts of *Ephedra gerardiana* Wall, *Ephedra sinica* Stapf, *Ephedra equisetina* Bunge, *Ephedra nebrodensis* Tineo and other Ephedra species, belonging to family Ephadreaceae (Fig. 15.44).

Geographical Source

It is mainly found in China, India, Nepal, Turkey, Pakistan and Bhutan.

Cultivation and Collection

It is an evergreen shrub growing to 0.6 m × 2 m. The plant prefers light (sandy) and medium (loamy) soils and requires well-drained soil. The plant prefers acid, neutral and basic (alkaline) soils. It cannot grow in the shade. It requires dry or moist soil and can tolerate drought. Seeds are sown as soon as they are ripe in the autumn in a greenhouse. It can also be sown in spring in a greenhouse in sandy compost. Seedlings are transferred into individual pots as soon as they are large enough to handle and grown them for at least their first winter in a greenhouse.

Drug is collected in autumn since it contains maximum percentage of alkaloids. Green slender twigs are collected in autumn, dried and packed loose in bags. Sometimes the twigs are pressed tightly.

Characteristics

Ephedra gerardiana: It consists of cylindrical woody stem that is grey or greenish in colour. Nodes, internodes, scaly leaves and terminal buds are present in the stems. The distance between the internodes is 3–4 cm and the nodes bare the scaly leaves. They are bitter in taste. The plant has stamens and pistils on separate flowers, staminate flowers in catkins and a membraneous perianth, pistillate flowers terminal on axillary stalks, within a two-leaved involucre. Fruit has two carpels with a single seed in each and is a succulent cone, branches slender and erect, small leaves, scale-like, articulated and joined at the base into a sheath.

Ephedra sinica: Thickness of the stem is 4–7 mm branches are 1–2 mm. Length up to 30 cm of branches and 3–6 cm of internodes. The main stem is brown in colour. Leaves are 2–4 mm long, opposite, decussate and subulate. Leaf, base is reddish-brown, apex acute and recurved and lamina white in colour. A pair of sheathing leaves present at the nodes, encircling the stem and fused at the base.

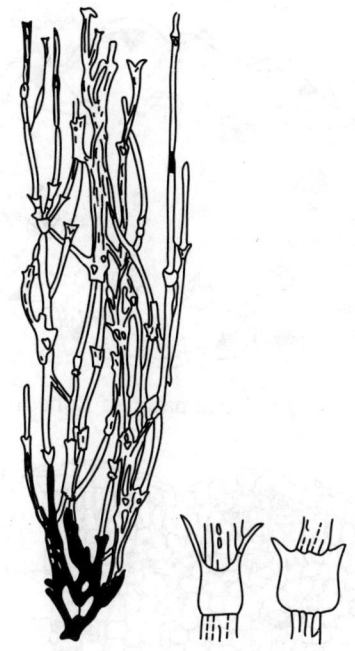

FIG. 15.44 *Ephedra sinica*

Ephedra equisetina: Stems are woodier and more branched 1.5–2 mm. Length 25–200 cm of branches and 1–2.5 cm of internodes, outer surface is grey to pale green and smooth.

Ephedra nebrodensis: The stems are 15–35 cm in length; 1–2 mm thick, cylindrical, greenish-yellow in colour, nodes are brownish and distinct and fractured surface is fibrous in the cortex but pith contains brownish powdery mass. The leaves are brownish to whitish-brown in colour, scaly, connate, opposite and decussate, acute, agreeable and slightly aromatic odour and taste is astringent and bitter.

Microscopy (Figs. 15.45 and 15.46)

Transverse section of the stem shows epidermis, composed of thick-walled, quadrangular cells, covered by thick cuticle. Sunken stomata are present between many vertical ridges. Papillae are present in the ridges. Below the ridges, groups of nonlignified hypodermal fibres (nine to twenty per group) are present. Cortex is composed of chlorenchyma with outer zone of radially elongated cells and inner zone of spongy parenchyma. Cortex also contains few isolated fibres or groups of fibres (two to six per group), which are lignified. Pericycle is composed of groups of lignified fibres outside the phloem region. Vascular bundles are 6–10 in number, radially arranged in the cortex and composed of phloem and xylem. Pith is large with rounded cells, containing dark brown mucilaginous substance in pigment cells.

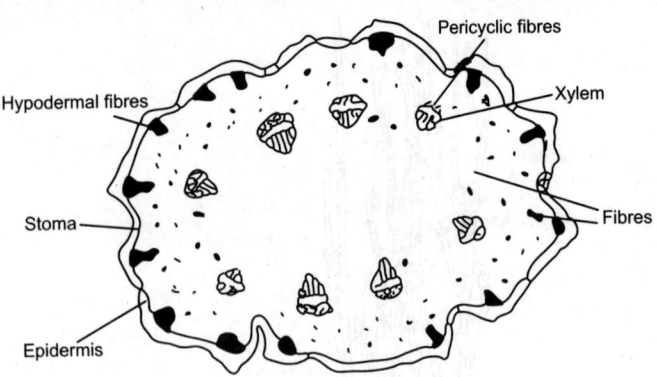

FIG. 15.45 T.S. (schematic) of Ephedra herb

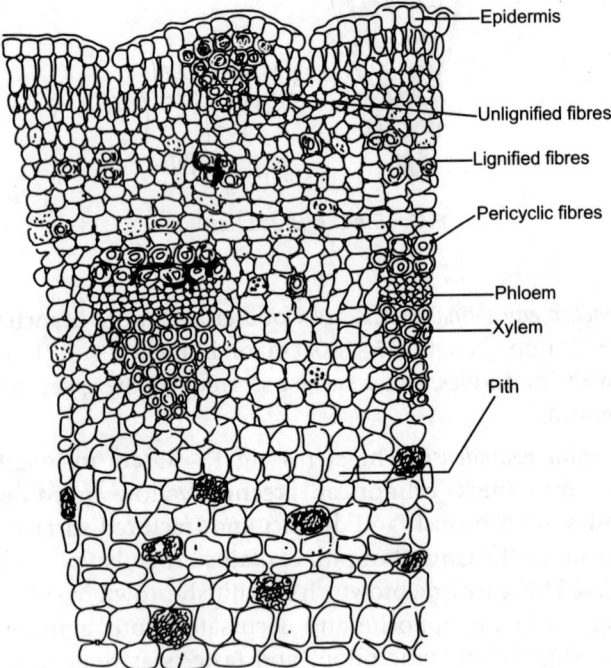

FIG. 15.46 Transverse section of Ephedra herb

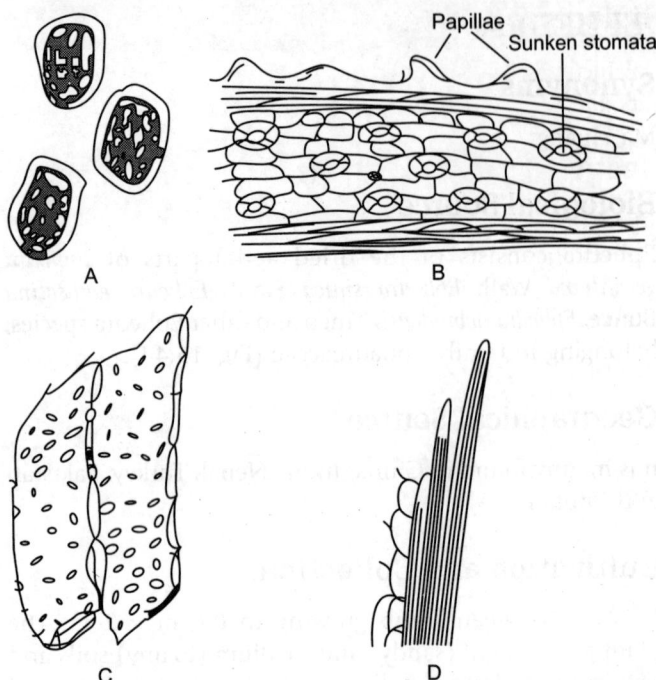

FIG. 15.47 Powder characteristics of Ephedra herb. (A: Isolated masses of pigment, B: Epidermis, C: Fragment of vessels, D: Fibres)

Ephedrine   (+)-Pseudoephedrine

Powder Microscopy (Fig. 15.47)

The powder is pale yellowish brown in colour with characteristic odour and slightly bitter taste. Microscopical examination shows epidermis with sunken stomata and papillae, pitted xylem vessels, elongated fibres tapering at both ends and isolated masses of pigment cells.

Chemical Constituents

Ephedra contains alkaloids ephedrine (water-soluble salt of an alkaloid), pseudoephedrine (analog of ephedrine) and norpseudoephedrine (an analog of ephedrine). The leaves and stems of ephedra also contain many potentially active compounds, such as tannins, saponin, flavone and volatile oils.

Chemical Test

1. To the drug (10 mg) in water (1 ml) dilute HCl (0.2 ml), copper sulphate solution (0.1 ml) and sodium hydroxide solution (2 ml) are added; the liquid turns violet. On adding solvent ether (2 ml) and shaking vigorously, the ethereal layer turns purple and the aqueous layer becomes blue.

Uses

Ephedrine is antiallergenic, antiasthmatic, antispasmodic, decongestant, cough suppressant, stimulant and vasoconstrictor. Pseudoephedrine is decongestant, cough suppressant and norpseudoephedrine is peripheral vasodilator used to treat angina. As a whole it is decongestant; it opens sinuses, increases sweating, dilates bronchioles (antiasthmatic use), diuretic, CNS stimulant, raises blood pressure, alleviates aches and rheumatism, alleviates hay fever/colds, etc.

COLCHICUM

Synonyms

Autumn Crocus, Cigdem, Colquico, Meadow Saffron, Naked Boys, European Colchicum Seed.

Biological Source

Colchicum consists of dried ripe seeds and corms of *Colchicum autumnale* Linn., belonging to family Liliaceae (Fig. 15.48).

Geographical Source

It is mainly found in Central and South Europe, Germany, Greece, Spain, Turkey and England.

Cultivation and Collection

The plant prefers light (sandy), medium (loamy) and heavy (clay) soils and requires well-drained soil. The plant prefers acid, neutral and basic (alkaline) soils. It can grow in semishade or no shade. It requires moist soil. Seed are sown as soon as it is ripe in early summer in a seed bed or a cold frame. Germination can be very slow, taking up to 18 months at 15°C. It is best to sow the seed thinly so that it is not necessary to transplant the seedlings for their first year of growth. Liquid fertilizers are applied during their first summer to ensure they get sufficient nourishment. Seedlings are taken out once they are dormant, putting perhaps two plants per pot, and allowed to grow them in a greenhouse or frame for at least a couple of years. The seedlings take 4–5 years to reach flowering size.

Division of the bulbs in June/July when the leaves have died down. Larger bulbs can be planted out direct into their permanent positions, though it is best to pot up the smaller bulbs and grow them on in a cold frame for a year before planting them out. The plant can be divided every other year if a quick increase is required

The plant bears leaves and capsular fruits in next spring. From June to July brown fruits are collected and placed in muslin bags. During ripening seeds become dark in colour and arc covered by a sweet saccharine secretion. Seeds are separated by sifting. Colchicum seeds are derived from, amphitrophous ovules and have a short raphe. The corms are harvested in mid to late summer when the plant has fully died down. They are dried and used.

Characteristics

Seeds are 2–3 mm in diameter, globular. Outer surface is dark reddish-brown, pitted, very hard. Endosperm is large, hard and oily. It is odourless; bitter and acrid in taste.

The corm or root is usually sold in transverse slices, notched on one side and somewhat reniform in outline, white and starchy internally, about 1/8 inch thick and varying from 3/4 to 1 inch in diameter. Taste sweetish, then bitter and acrid and odour radish-like in fresh root, but lost in drying.

Chemical Constituents

The active principle is said to be an alkaline substance of a very poisonous nature called colchicine. Besides colchicine,

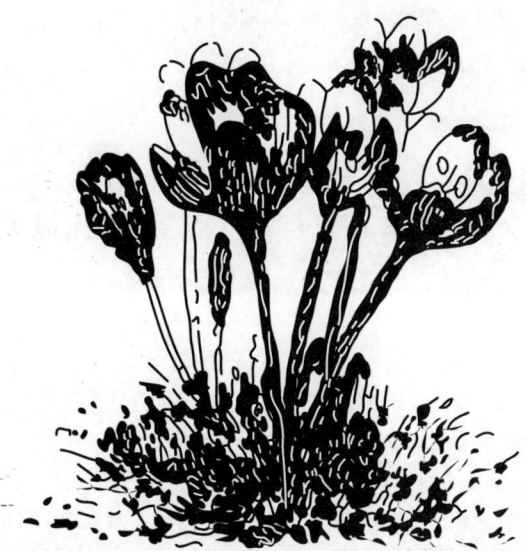

FIG. 15.48 Twig of *Colchicum autumnale*

demecolcine and other alkaloids are present. They also contain resin, called colchicoresin, fixed oil, glucose and starch.

Colchicine

Chemical Test

Colchicum corm with sulphuric acid (70%) or conc. HCl produces yellow colour due to the presence of colchicines.

Uses

Both the corm and the seeds are analgesic, antirheumatic, cathartic and emetic. They are used mainly in the treatment of gout and rheumatic complaints, usually accompanied with an alkaline diuretic. Leukaemia has been successfully treated with autumn crocus, and the plant has also been used with some success to treat Bechet's syndrome, a chronic disease marked by recurring ulcers and leukaemia. A very toxic plant, it should not be prescribed for pregnant women or patients with kidney disease, and should only be used under the supervision of a qualified practitioner.

Marketed Products

It is one of the ingredients of the preparation known as Aujai capsules (Crown Pharma Exports).

Drugs Containing Glycosides

CONTENTS

16.1. INTRODUCTION

A glycoside is any molecule in which a sugar group is bonded through its anomeric carbon to another group via glycosidic bond. A glycosidic bond is a certain type of chemical bond that joins a sugar molecule to another molecule. Specifically, a glycosidic bond is formed between the hemiacetal group of a saccharide (or a molecule derived from a saccharide) and the hydroxyl group of an alcohol. A substance containing a glycosidic bond is a glycoside. The glycone and aglycone portions can be chemically separated by hydrolysis in the presence of acid. There are also numerous enzymes that can form and break glycosidic bonds.

The sugar group is known as the glycone and the nonsugar group as the aglycone or genin part of the glycoside. The glycone can consist of a single sugar group (monosaccharide) or several sugar groups (oligosaccharide). The sugars found in glycosides may be glucose and rhamnose (monosaccharides) or, more rarely, deoxysugars such as the cymarose found in cardiac glycosides.

In plants glycosides are both synthesized and hydrolysed under the influence of more or less specific enzymes. They are crystalline or amorphous substances that are soluble in water or alcohols and insoluble in organic solvents like benzene and ether. The aglycone part is soluble in organic solvents like benzene or ether. They are hydrolysed by water, enzymes and mineral acids. They are optically active. While glycosides do not themselves reduce Fehling's solution, the simple sugars which they produce on hydrolysis will do so with precipitation of red cuprous oxide. The sugars present in glycoside are of two isomeric forms, that is, α form and β form, but all the natural glycosides contain β-type of sugar.

The term 'glycoside' is a very general one which embraces all the many and varied combinations of sugars and aglycones.

16.2. CLASSIFICATION

The glycosides can be classified by the glycone, by the type of glycosidal linkage and by the aglycone.

On the Basis of Glycone

If the glycone group of a glycoside is glucose, then the molecule is a glucoside; if it is fructose, then the molecule is a fructoside; if it is glucuronic acid, then the molecule is a glucuronide, etc.

On the Basis of Glycosidic Linkage

1. **O-glycosides:** Sugar molecule is combined with phenol or –OH group of aglycon, for example, amygdaline, indesine, arbutin, salicin, cardiac glycosides, anthraquinone glycosides like sennosides, etc.
2. **N-glycosides:** Sugar molecule is combined with N of the –NH (amino group) of aglycon, for example, nucleosides.
3. **S-glycosides:** Sugar molecule is combined with the S or SH (thiol group) of aglycon, for example, sinigrin.
4. **C-glycosides:** Sugar molecule is directly attached with C—atom of aglycon, for example, anthraquinone glycosides like aloin, barbaloin, cascaroside and flavan glycosides, etc.

On the Basis of Aglycone

The various classes according to aglycone moiety are given below:

S. No.	Class	Examples
1.	Anthraquinone glycosides	Senna, aloe, rhubarb, etc.
2.	Sterol or cardiac glyco-sides	Digitalis, thevetia, squill, etc.
3.	Saponin glycosides	Dioscorea, liquorice, ginseng, etc.
4.	Cyanogenetic and cyano-phoric glycosides	Bitter almond, Wild cherry bark, etc.
5.	Thiocyanate and isothio-cyanate glycosides	Black mustard
6.	Flavone glycosides	Ginkgo
7.	Aldehyde glycosides	Vanilla
8.	Phenol glycosides	Bearberry
9.	Steroidal glycoalkaloids	Solanum
10.	Bitter and miscellaneous glycosides	Gentian, picrorhiza, chirata, etc.

16.3. DISTRIBUTION OF GLYCOSIDES

Glycosides are the class of compounds abundant in nature. Some plant families containing important glycosides are listed below:

1. Scrophulariaceae (*Digitalis purpurea* and *Digitalis lanata*, *Picrorhiza kurroa*).
2. Apocynaceae (*Nerium oleander* and *Thevetia peruviana*).
3. Liliaceae (*Urginea indica* and *U. maritima*, *Aloe vera*)
4. Leguminosae (*Cassia acutefolia* and *C. angustifolia*, *Glycyrrhiza glabra*, *Psoralea corylifolia*)
5. Dioscoreaceae (*Dioscorea floribunda*)
6. Rosaceae (*Prunus amygdalus*, *Carategus oxycantha*)
7. Cruciferae (*Brassica* sp.)
8. Gentianaceae (Gentian and Chirata)
9. Acanthaceae (Kalmegh)
10. Simarubaceae (Quassia)
11. Umbelliferae (*Ammi majus*, *Ammi visnaga*)
12. Rutaceae: *Citrus* sp. (*Ruta graveolens*)
13. Polygonaceae (*Fagopyrum* sp.)
14. Myrtaceae (*Eucalyptus* sp.)

16.4. CHEMICAL TESTS OF GLYCOSIDES

Glycosides are the compounds with organic molecules having attached glucose or any mono-oligosaccharide unit. Usually, these are crystalline or amorphous solids; optically active, soluble in water and alcohol but insoluble in organic solvents like ether, chloroform and benzene, etc. Generally, aqueous or alcoholic extracts of crude drugs are tested with specific reagents for presence of various types of glycosides.

Chemical Tests for Anthraquinone Glycosides

Borntrager's test

To 1 gm of drug add 5–10 ml of dilute HCl boil on water bath for 10 min and filter. Filtrate was extracted with CCl_4/benzene and add equal amount of ammonia solution to filtrate and shake. Formation of pink or red colour in ammonical layer due to presence of anthraquinone moiety.

Modified Borntrager's test

To 1 gm of drug, add 5 ml dilute HCl followed by 5 ml ferric chloride (5% w/v). Boil for 10 min on water bath, cool and filter, filtrate was extracted with carbon tetrachloride or benzene and add equal volume of ammonia solution, formation of pink to red colour due to presence of anthraquinone moiety. This is used C-type of anthraquinone glycosides.

Chemical Tests for Saponin Glycosides

Haemolysis test

A drop blood on slide was mixed with few drops of aq. saponin solution, RBC's becomes ruptured in presence of saponins.

Foam test

To 1 gm of drug add 10–20 ml of water, shake for few minutes, formation frothing which persists for 60–120 s in presence of saponins.

Chemical Tests for Steroid and Triterpenoid Glycosides

Liebermann–Burchard test

Alcoholic extract of drug was evaporated to dryness and extracted with $CHCl_3$, add few drops of acetic anhydride followed by conc. H_2SO_4 from side wall of test tube to the $CHCl_3$ extract. Formation of violet to blue coloured ring at the junction of two liquid, indicate the presence of steroid moiety.

Salkowski test

Alcoholic extract of drug was evaporated to dryness and extracted with $CHCl_3$, add conc. H_2SO_4 from sidewall of test tube to the $CHCl_3$ extract. Formation of yellow coloured ring at the junction of two liquid, which turns red after 2 min, indicate the presence of steroid moiety.

Antimony trichloride test

Alcoholic extract of drug was evaporated to dryness and extracted with $CHCl_3$, add saturated solution of $SbCl_3$ in $CHCl_3$ containing 20% acetic anhydride. Formation of pink colour on heating indicates presence of steroids and triterpenoids.

Trichloro acetic acid test

Triterpenes on addition of saturated solution of trichloro acetic acid forms coloured precipitate.

Tetranitro methane test

It forms yellow colour with unsaturated steroids and triterpenes.

Zimmermann test

Meta dinitrobenzene solution was added to the alcoholic solution of drug containing alkali, on heating it forms violet colour in presence of keto steroid.

Chemical Tests for Cardiac Glycosides

Keller–Kiliani test

To the alcoholic extract of drug equal volume of water and 0.5 ml of strong lead acetate solution was added, shaked and filtered. Filtrate was extracted with equal volume of chloroform. Chloroform extract was evaporated to dryness and residue was dissolved in 3 ml of glacial acetic acid followed by addition of few drops of $FeCl_3$ solution. The resultant solution was transferred to a test tube containing 2 ml of conc. H_2SO_4. Reddish brown layer is formed, which turns bluish green after standing due to presence of digitoxose.

Legal test

To the alcoholic extract of drug equal volume of water and 0.5 ml of strong lead acetate solution was added, shaked and filtered. Filtrate was extracted with equal volume of chloroform and the chloroform extract was evaporated to dryness. The residue was dissolved in 2 ml of pyridine and sodium nitroprusside 2 ml was added followed by addition of NaOH solution to make alkaline. Formation of pink colour in presence of glycosides or aglycon moiety.

Baljet test

Thick section of leaf of digitalis or the part of drug containing cardiac glycoside, when dipped in sodium picrate solution, it forms yellow to orange colour in presence of aglycones or glycosides.

3,5-Dinitro benzoic acid test

To the alcoholic solution of drug few drops of NaOH followed by 2% solution of 3,5-dinitro benzoic acid was added. Formation of pink colour indicates presence of cardiac glycosides.

Chemical Tests for Coumarin Glycosides

FeCl₃ test

To the concentrated alcoholic extract of drug few drops of alcoholic $FeCl_3$ solution was added. Formation of deep green colour, which turned yellow on addition of conc. HNO_3, indicates presence of coumarins.

Fluorescence test

The alcoholic extract of drug was mixed with 1N NaOH solution (1 ml each). Development of blue-green fluorescence indicates presence of coumarins.

Chemical Tests for Cyanophoric Glycoside

Sodium picrate test

Powdered drug was moistened with water in a conical flask and few drops of conc. sulphuric acid was added. Filter paper impregnated with sodium picrate solution followed by sodium carbonate solution was trapped on the neck of flask using cork. Formation of brick red colour due to volatile HCN in presence of cyanophoric glycosides takes place.

Chemical Tests for Flavonoid Glycosides

Ammonia test

Filter paper dipped in alcoholic solution of drug was exposed to ammonia vapour. Formation of yellow spot on filter paper.

Shinoda test

To the alcoholic extract of drug magnesium turning and dil. HCl was added, formation of red colour indicates the presence of flavonoids. To the alcoholic extract of drug zinc turning and dil. HCl was added, formation of deep red to magenta colour indicates the presence of dihydro flavonoids.

Vanillin HCl test

Vanillin HCl was added to the alcoholic solution of drug, formation of pink colour due to presence of flavonoids.

16.5. ISOLATION

Stas-Otto Method

The general method of extraction of glycosides is outlined here. The drug containing glycoside is finely powdered and the powder is extracted by continuous hot percolation using soxhlet apparatus with alcohol as solvent. During this process, various enzymes present in plant parts are also deactivated due to heating. The thermolabile glycosides, however, should be extracted at temperature preferably below 45°C. The extract is treated with lead acetate to precipitate tannins and thus eliminate nonglycosidal impurities. The excess of lead acetate is precipitated as lead sulphide by passing hydrogen sulphide gas through solution. The extract is filtered, concentrated to get crude glycosides. From the crude extract, the glycosides are obtained in pure form by making use of processes like fractional solubility, fractional crystallization and chromatographic techniques such as preparative thin layer and column chromatography.

The characterization of isolated purified compounds is done by IR, UV, visible, NMR and mass spectrometry and elemental analysis.

16.6. ANTHRACENE GLYCOSIDES

Anthracene glycosides are chiefly found in dicot plants but to some extent it is also found in monocot and lower plants. It consists of glycosides formed from aglycone moieties like anthraquinones, anthranols, anthrones or dimers of anthrones or their derivatives. Anthrones are insoluble in alkali and do not show strong fluorescence with them, while anthranols which are soluble in alkali show strong fluorescence. The reduced anthraquinones are biologically more active. Anthroquinones that are present in fresh drugs are in reduced form, which on long storage get oxidized and hydrolysed. Glycosides of reduced derivatives are more active than oxidized aglycones. This is due to the fact that sugars take the glycosides to the site of action and thus are more active.

Anthraquinone is an aromatic organic compound and a derivative of anthracene. It has the appearance of yellow or light grey to grey-green solid crystalline powder. Its chemical formula is $C_{14}H_8O_2$. It melts at 286°C, boils at 379.8°C. It is insoluble in water or alcohol, but dissolves in nitrobenzene and aniline. It is chemically fairly stable under normal conditions.

Anthraquinone naturally occurs in some plants (e.g. aloe, senna, rhubarb and cascara), fungi, lichens and insects, where it serves as a basic skeleton for their pigments. Natural anthraquinone derivates tend to have laxative effects.

These glycosides are characterized by a chemical test, known as Borntrager test and show the property of microsublimation. Most of the glycosides are O-glycosides and S-glycosides, by

Anthraquinone

Anthrone

Oxanthrone

Anthranol

Dianthranol

their hydrolysis derivatives of 1,8-dihydroxy anthraquinone, anthranol, anthrone or dianthrone are obtained.

The common aglycones are aloe-emodin, emodin, rhein, chrysophanol and physcion which may exist as anthraquinones, anthranols or anthrones. The sugars presents are usually arabinose, rhamnose and glucose.

In the drug originally glycosides of reduced derivatives or their dimers are present. During drying and storage by hydrolysis and oxidation free anthraquinones are produced.

SENNA LEAF

Synonyms

Alexandrian senna, Tinnevelly senna, Folia senna.

Biological Source

Senna leaf consists of the dried leaflets of *Cassia acutifolia* Delile (*C. senna* L.) known as Alexandrian senna and of *C. angustifolia* Vahl., which is commercially known as Tinnevelly senna. It belong family Leguminosae (Fig. 16.1).

Geographical Source

Alexandrian senna is indigenous to South Africa. It widely grows and sometimes is cultivated in Egypt and in the middle upper territories of Nile river. It is also cultivated in Kordofan and Sennar regions of Sudan. Indian or Tinnevelly senna is indigenous to southern Arabia and cultivated largely in Tinnevelly and Ramnathpuram districts of Tamil Nadu. It also grows in Somaliland, Sindh and Punjab region.

Cultivation and Collection

Senna plant is a small shrub of 1–1.5 m height with paripinnate compound leaves. Tinnevelly senna is mostly cultivated in well-ploughed, levelled, rich clayed semi-irrigated land sometimes after paddy crop in South India. Propagation is done by seeds which are rubbed with coarse sand and sown thinly by broadcasting or in rows 30 cm apart, first during February–March and second after rain in July. Seeds germinate on the third day. The crop becomes ready for harvesting after about 2 months but first plucking of leaflets is done after 3 months of sowing when the leaves appears mature, thick and bluish in colour. Second plucking is followed after a month and subsequent pluckings after 4–6 weeks. The plant can survive for two to three years, but it is grown as an annual. After third plucking the plants are uprooted. Plant shows great tolerance for salinity. It sometimes shows die-back symptoms in which the branches or shoots die from the tip inward, which is caused by parasites or environmental conditions. Leaflets of Tinnevelly senna are collected by careful plucking from luxuriantly grown plants and compressed into bales.

Alexandrian senna is obtained almost entirely from the wild and sometimes from the cultivated plants. At the stage of fully formed fruits, branches are cut off and rapidly dried in the sun. Pods and large stalks are first separated by using sieves. Leaves separated from stalks are graded into whole leaves, whole and half leaves and shiftings. Whole leaves and shiftings are generally used for making galenical preparations. The leaves are packed loosely in bales for marketing.

Characteristics

Senna leaflets are 3–5 cm long, 2 cm wide and about 0.5 mm thick. It shows acute apex, entire margin and asymmetric base. Outline is lanceolate to ovate lanceolate. Pubescent lamina is found on both the surfaces. Leaves show greyish green colour for Alexandrian senna and yellowish green for Tinnevelly senna. Leaves of Tinnevelly senna are somewhat larger, less broken and firmer in texture than that of Alexandrian senna. Odour of leaves is slight but characteristic and the taste is bitter, mucilagenous. Both the types of leaflets show impression or transverse markings due to the pressing of midrib. Distingushing characters of Alexandrian and Indian senna are given in Table 16.1.

Table 16.1: Distinguishing characters of Alexandrian and Indian senna

Character	Indian Senna	Alexandrian Senna
Appearance	Generally entire and less broken in good condition	Broken and brittle in nature
Size	2.5–5.0 cm long and 7–9 mm wide	2.4 cm long and 6–12 mm wide.
Shape	Lanceolate	Ovate lanceolate
Apex	Less acute with a sharp spine	Acute with a sharp spine
Margin	Entire, flat	Entire curled
Base	Less asymmetrical	Conspicuously asymmetrical
Veins	Pinnate, distinct towards the under surface and anastomosing towards margin	Pinnate, distinct towards the under surface and anastomosing towards margin
Surface	Transverse and oblique impressions, less pubescent (hairy)	Without transverse and oblique impressions and more pubescent
Texture	Flexible and less brittle	Thin more brittle
Odour	Faint	Faint
Colour	Light green	Light greyish green
Test	Bitter mucilaginous	Bitter mucilaginous
Vein islet number	19–22.5	25–29.5
Stomatal index	14–20	10–15
Palisade ratio	4–12	4.5–18

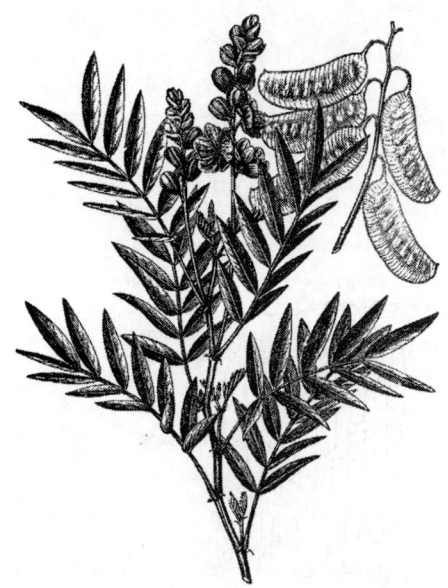

Microscopy (Figs. 16.2 and 16.3)

Being isobilateral leaf, senna shows more or less similar features at both the surfaces of leaf with few differences. Transverse section of leaf shows upper and lower epidermis with straight wall cells, few of which contain mucilage. Paracytic stomata and nonlignified unicellular trichomes are found on both the surfaces. A single layer of palisade parenchyma is observed at both the sides but it is discontinued in the midrib region of lower epidermis due to the zone of collenchymatous tissues. Palisade is followed by spongy mesophyll which contains cluster crystals of calcium oxalate and vascular strands. Midrib shows the vascular bundle containing xylem and phloem,

almost surrounded by lignified pericyclic fibres and a sheath of parenchyma which contains prismatic crystals of calcium oxalate.

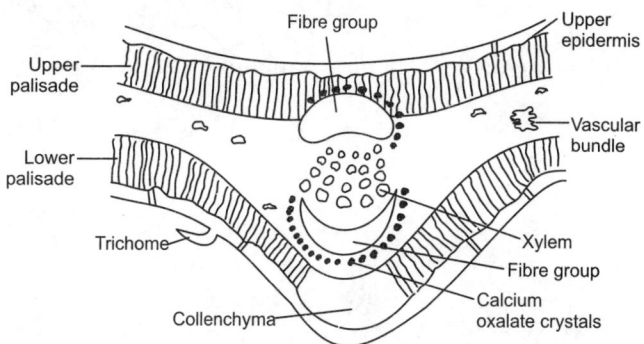

FIG. 16.2 Transverse section of senna leaf (schematic)

Powder Microscopy (Figs. 16.4)

The powder is greyish green or yellowish green in colour, with faint characteristic odour and mucilaginous, bitter taste. Microscopical examination shows epidermal cells with straight anticlinal walls and paracytic stomata. Covering trichomes are unicellular, conical and thick-walled with warty cuticle. Fragments of xylem vessels, fibres surrounded by a calcium oxalate prism sheath, and plenty of cluster and prismatic calcium oxalate crystals are found scattered.

Chemical Constituents

Senna contains sennosides A and B (2.5%) based on the aglycones sennidin A and B, sennosides C and D which are glycosides of heterodianthrones of aloe-emodin and rhein are present. Others include palmidin A, rhein

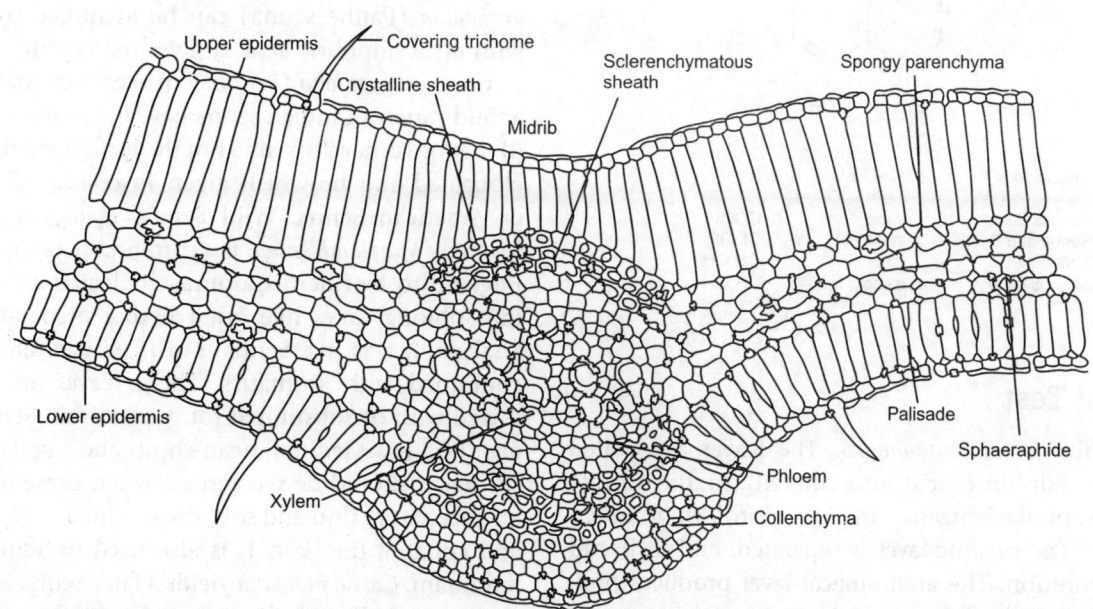

FIG. 16.3 Transverse section of senna leaflet

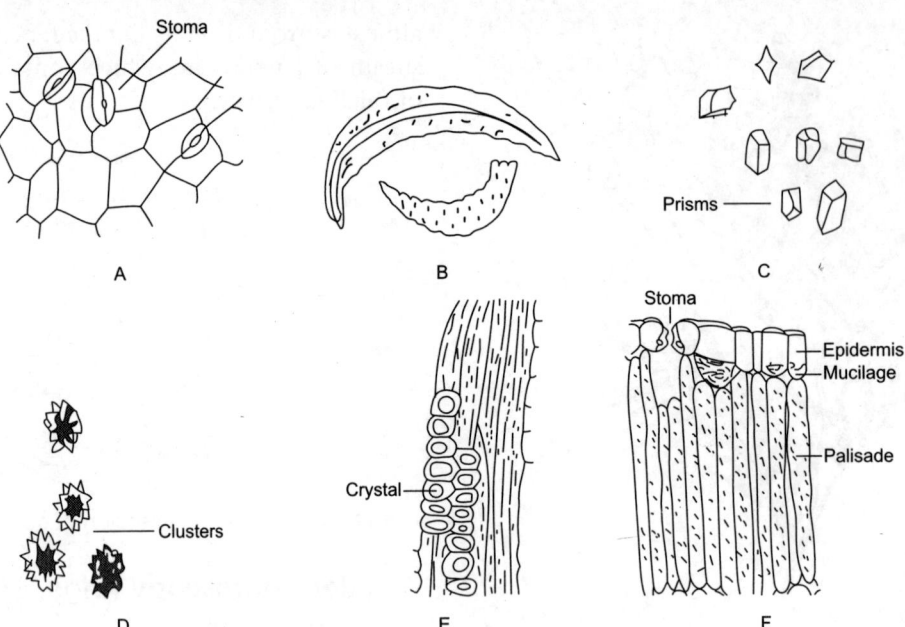

FIG. 16.4 Powder characteristics of Senna leaflets. (A: Epidermal cell, B: Covering trichomes, C: Prismatic crystals of calcium oxalate, D: Cluster crystals of calcium oxalate, E: Portion of fibres with crystal sheath, F: Palisade cells)

anthrone and aloe-emodin glycosides. Senna also contains free chrysophanol, emodin and their glycosides and free aloe-emodin, rhein, their monoanthrones, dianthrones and their glycosides. Mucilage is present in the epidermis of the leaf and gives red colour with ruthenium red.

Glycoside	10 - 10'	R
Sennoside A	trans	COOH
Sennoside B	meso	COOH
Sennoside C	trans	CH_2OH
Sennoside D	meso	CH_2OH

Chemical Test

Borntrager Test for Anthraquinones: The leaves are boiled with dilute sulphuric acid and filtered. To the filtrate organic solvent like benzene, ether or chloroform is added and shaken. The organic layer is separated, and to it add ammonia solution. The ammoniacal layer produces pink to red colour indicating the presence of anthraquinone glycoside.

Uses

Senna leaves are used as laxative. It causes irritation of large intestine and have some griping effect. Thus they are prescribed along with carminatives. Senna is stimulant cathartic and exerts its action by increasing the tone of the smooth muscles in large intestine.

Adulterants

Cassia obovata (Dog Senna): They occur as small pieces with Alexandrian senna but can be easily identified by its obovata shape and obtuse and tapering apex. It has only 1% anthraquinone derivatives. The presence of *Cassia auriculata* (Palthe senna) can be identified by treating it with 80% sulphuric acid. It gives red colour.

Cassia angustifolia (Bombay or Mecca or Arabian senna) a mild variety of Indian senna have the morphology similar to that of Tinnevelly senna but the leaflets are narrow, more elongated and brownish green in colour. *C. marilandica* or American Senna, Wild Senna, *Poinciana pulcherrima,* formerly *Maryland Senna,* is a common perennial from New England to Northern Carolina. Its leaves are compressed into oblong cakes like other herbal preparations of the Shakers. It acts like Senna, but is weaker, and should be combined with aromatics. These leaves are also found mixed with or substituted for Alexandrian Senna. *Coriaria myrtifolia* is a Mediterranean shrub and highly poisonous, so that it should be recognized when present. The leaves are green, very thin and soft, three veined, ovate-lanceolate, and equal at the base. It is also used to adulterate sweet marjoram. *Cassia montana* yields a false Senna from Madras, partly resembling the Tinnevelly Senna, though the colour of the upper surface of the leaves is browner.

Marketed Products

It is one of the ingredients of the preparations known as Constivac, Softovac (Lupin Herbal Laboratory) and Isova powder, Kultab tablet (Vasu Healthcare).

ALOE

Biological Source

Aloe is the dried juice collected by incision, from the bases of the leaves of various species of Aloe. *Aloe perryi* Baker, *Aloe vera* Linn or *Aloe barbadensis* Mil and *Aloe ferox* Miller., belonging to family Liliaceae (Fig. 16.5).

Aloe perryi Baker is found in Socotra and Zanzibar islands and in their neighbouring areas and so the aloes obtained from this species is known as Socotrine or Zanzibar aloe. *Aloe vera* Linn is also known as *Aloe vulgaris* Lamarck or *Aloe barbadensis* Mil. or *Aloe officinalis* Forskal. It was formerly produced on the island of Barbados, where it was largely cultivated, having been introduced at the beginning of the sixteenth century. It is now almost entirely made on the Dutch islands of Curacao, Aruba and Bonaire. The aloes obtained from this species is known as Curacao or Barbados aloe. *Aloe ferox* Miller and hybrids of this species with *Aloe africana* and *Aloe spicata, A. platylepia* and other species of Aloe grows in Cape Colony and so is known as Cape aloe.

Geographical Source

Aloes are indigenous to East and South Africa, but have been introduced into the West Indies and into tropical countries, and will even flourish in the countries bordering on the Mediterranean.

Cultivation and Collection

It is an evergreen perennial growing to 0.8 m × 1 m at a slow rate. The plant prefers light (sandy) and medium (loamy) soils, requires well-drained soil and can grow in nutritionally poor soil. The plant prefers acid, neutral and basic (alkaline) soils. It cannot grow in the shade. It requires dry or moist soil and can tolerate drought. They are xerophytic plant. It can be propagated by seeds. Seeds are sown in the spring in a warm green house. The seed usually germinates in 1–6 months at 16°C. The seedlings are transferred to the pots containing well-drained soil. They are allowed to grow in sunny part for at least their first two winters. The offsets will be available, usually in spring. The plants produce offsets quite freely and they can be divided at any time of the year as long as it is warm enough to encourage fresh root growth to allow reestablishment of the plants. Young offsets are planted in the soil after the rainy season in rows situated at a distance of 60 cm.

In the second year leaves are collected by the natives by protecting their hands because of the spiny nature of leaves. The leaves are cut near the base, kept inside of kerosene tins and taken them to a central place for the preparation of aloe. Juice of aloe is present in parenchymatous cells of pericycle that are mucilage cells. In a single incision mucilage cells exert pressure on pericycle cells and the entire juice from the leaves is drained out.

Preparation of Aloe

Curacao or Barbados aloe

In West Indies the cut leaves are arranged with their cut surface on the inner side, on the sides of V-shaped vessel of about 1–2 m long and the flowing juice is collected in a tin vessel that is placed below the V-shaped vessel. This juice thus collected is concentrated either by spontaneous evaporation, or more generally by boiling until it becomes of the consistency of thick honey. These conditions favours the crystallization of barbaloin and this aloe contains crystals of barbaloin because of the presence of which it becomes opaque and so also known as hepatic or livery aloe. On cooling, it is then poured into gourds, boxes or other convenient receptacles and solidifies.

Socotrine aloe

When it is prepared, it is commonly poured into goat skins, and spontaneous evaporation is allowed for about a month when it becomes viscous pasty mass which are then packed into cases. In European countries it is dried in wooden pans with hot air till moisture is about 10%.

Zanzibar aloe

This aloe is prepared similar to Socotrine aloe. It is packed in skins, of carnivorous animals. This aloe is also known as monkey skin aloe.

Cape aloe

The leaves of the plants from which Cape aloe is obtained are cut off near the stem and arranged around a hole in the ground, in which a sheep skin is spread, with smooth side upwards. When a sufficient quantity of juice has drained from the leaves it is concentrated by heat in iron cauldrons and subsequently poured into boxes or skins in which it solidifies on cooling. Large quantities of the drug are .exported from Cape Town and Mossel Bay.

Characteristics

Curacao aloe

It is usually opaque and varies in colour from bright yellowish or rich reddish brown to black. Sometimes it is vitreous and small fragments are then of a deep garnet-red colour and transparent. It is then known as 'Capey Barbados' and is less valuable, but may become opaque and more valuable by keeping. Curacoa Aloes possesses the nauseous and bitter taste that is characteristic of all Aloes and a disagreeable, penetrating odour. It is almost entirely soluble in 60% alcohol and contains not more than 30% of substances insoluble in water and 12% of moisture. It should not yield more than 3% of ash. The fracture is waxy.

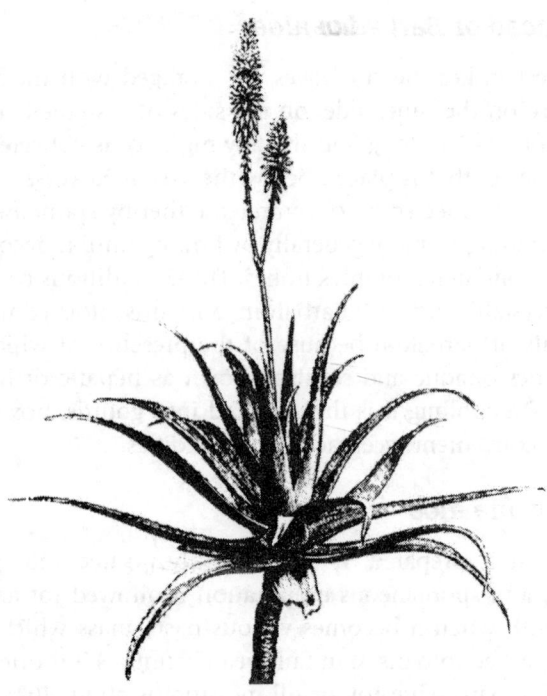

FIG. 16.5 *Aloe vera*

Socotrine aloes

It may be distinguished principally from Curacoa aloes by its different odour. Much of the dry drug is characterized by the presence of small cavities in the fractured surface; it is yellow-brown to dark-brown in colour and opaque. Fracture is irregular and porous and taste is bitter.

Zanziber aloes

Zanzibar aloes often very closely resembles Curacoa in appearance and is usually imported in liver-brown masses which break with a dull, waxy fracture, differing from that of Socotrine aloes in being nearly smooth and even. It has a pleasant odour and bitter taste.

Cape aloes

It forms dark coloured masses which break with a clean glassy fracture and exhibit in their splinters a yellowish, reddish-brown or greenish tinge. Its translucent and glossy appearance are very characteristic and red-currant like odour sufficiently distinguish it from all other varieties of aloes.

Chemical Constituents

The most important constituents of aloes are the three isomers of aloins, barbaloin, β-barboloin and isobarbaloin, which constitute the so-called 'crystalline' aloin, present in the drug at from 10 to 30%. Other constituents are amorphous aloin, resin, emodin and aloe-emodin. Barbaloin is present in all the varieties; it is slightly yellow coloured, bitter, water soluble, crystalline glycoside. Isobarbaloin is a crystalline substance, present in Curacao aloe and in trace amount in Cape aloe and absent in Socotrine and Zanzibar aloe. The chief constituents of Socotrine and Zanzibar aloe are barbaloin and β-barbaloin.

Barbaloin

Aloesin

Aloin

Chemical Tests

Boil 1 gm of drug with 100 ml water, allow it to cool; add 1 gm kieselguhr, stir it well and filter through filter paper.

1. *Borax Test (Schoenteten's Reaction):* Take 10 ml of aloe solution and to it add 0.5 gm of borax and heat; a green coloured fluorescence is produced indicating the presence of aloe-emodin anthranol.

2. *Modified Borntrager's Test:* To 0.1 gm of drug, 5 ml of 5% solution of ferric chloride is added followed by the addition of 5 ml dilute hydrochloric acid. The mixture is heated on water bath for 5–6 min and cooled. An organic solvent (benzene or chloroform) is added and shaken. Separate the organic solvent layer and add an equal volume of dilute ammonia. The ammoniacal layer produces pinkish red colour.

3. *Bromine Test:* To 5 ml of aloe solution, add equal volume of bromine solution; bulky yellow precipitate is formed due to the presence of tetrabromaloin.

4. *Nitrous Acid Test:* To 5 ml of aloe solution, add little of sodium nitrite and few drops of dilute acetic acid;

it produces pink or purplish colour. Zanzibar and Socotrine aloes give negative test.

5. *Nitric Acid Test:* 2 ml of concentrated nitric acid is added to 5 ml of aloe solution; Curacao aloe gives deep reddish-brown colour, Socotrine aloe gives pale yellowish-brown colour, Zanzibar aloe gives yellowish-brown colour and Cape aloe first produces brown colour which on standing changes to green.

6. *Cupraloin Test:* 1 ml of the aloe solution is diluted to 5 ml with water and to it 1 drop of copper sulphate solution is added. Bright yellow colour is produced which on addition of 10 drops of saturated solution of sodium chloride changes to purple and the colour persist if 15–20 drops of 90% alcohol is added. This test is positive for Curacao aloe, faint for Cape aloe and negative for Zanzibar and Socotrine aloes.

Uses

The drug aloes is one of the safest and stimulating purgatives, in higher doses may act as abortifacient. Its action is exerted mainly on the large intestine; also it is useful as a vermifuge. The plant is emmenagogue, emollient, stimulant, stomachic, tonic and vulnerary. Extracts of the plant have antibacterial activity. The clear gel of the leaf makes an excellent treatment for wounds, burns and other skin disorders, placing a protective coat over the affected area, speeding up the rate of healing and reducing the risk of infection. To obtain this gel, the leaves can be cut in half along their length and the inner pulp rubbed over the affected area of skin. This has an immediate soothing effect on all sorts of burns and other skin problems.

Substituents and Adulterants

A. candelabrum (Natal aloes) is dull greenish black to dull brown in colour, opaque. When scraped it gives a pale greyish green or a yellow powder. It can be distinguished as it gives negative test to borax test and produces a deep blue colour. Jafferabad aloes and the Mocha aloes are the other two type of aloe which is used as adulterant.

Marketed Products

It is one of the ingredients of the preparations known as Diabecon, Evecare (Himalaya Drug Company), Mensonorm (Chirayu Pharma) and Kumari Asava (Baidyanath).

RHUBARB

Synonyms

East Indian rhubarb, China rhubarb, Turkey rhubarb.

Biological Source

Rhubarb consists of the peeled dried rhizomes and roots of *Rheum palmatum* Linn., belonging to family Polygonaceae (Fig. 16.6).

Geographical Source

It is mainly found in E. Asia, N.W. China in Yunnan, W. Sichuan, E. Xizang and Gansu, Tibet and India.

Cultivation and Collection

The plant is perennial growing to 3 m × 2 m. The plant prefers medium (loamy) and heavy (clay) soils, requires well-drained soil and can grow in heavy clay soil. The plant prefers acid, neutral and basic soils. Drug is collected from wild plants but is also cultivated to some extent. The plant grows at an altitude of 2500–4000 m. It can grow in semishade or no shade. It requires moist soil. Plants can be grown in quite coarse grass, which can be cut annually in the autumn. Seeds are sown in autumn in a shaded cold frame. The seed can also be sown in spring in a cold frame. When large enough to handle, seedlings are pricked out and transferred into individual pots and allowed to grow them on in the green house or cold frame for their first winter, then they are transplanted out in the spring.

The rootstocks are divided in early spring with a sharp knife, making sure that there is at least one growth bud on each division and the required amount of drugs is collected and the remaining are planted.

Rhizomes are large and roots are thick branched, Drug is collected in autumn in September or October from 6 to 15 years old plants. Rhizomes are dug out, crown and lateral roots are removed and the outer bark is separated by peeling. The rhizomes that are small in size are kept as such or cut into transverse slices and so they are round.

Large rhizomes are made flats by making cut into longitudinal slices. These slices are dried by boring holes in the flat pieces and passing thread through the holes and hanging between shades of trees. In absence of the required climatic conditions the drugs are dried artificially heated stones, which are previously heated by woodfire. Drug dried in this way is called high dried. The drugs that are dried in above said manner exerts an unpleasant odour and darker in colour and is considered inferior. The remaining bark is peeled off and graded according to size, shape and quality.

Characteristics

The leaves of the Turkey rhubarb are palmate and somewhat rough. The root is thick, of an oval shape, sending off long, tapering branches; externally it is brown, internally a deep yellow colour. The stem is erect, round, hollow, jointed, branched towards the top, from 6 to 10 feet high.

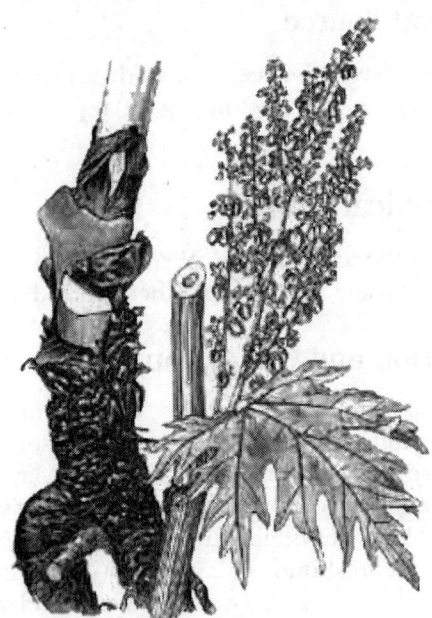

FIG. 16.6 *Rheum palmatum*

This species is distinguished from other rhubarbs by its much larger size, the shape of its leaves, with their oblong, sharpish segments, and the graceful looseness of its little panicles of greenish-white flowers. The first buds which appear in spring are yellow, not red.

Chinese or Turkey rhubarb occurs in commerce in brownish-yellow pieces of various sizes, usually perforated, the holes often containing a portion of the cord used to hang the sections of the root on during drying. The outer surface is generally powdery (the bark having been removed) and shows a network of white lines. The taste is astringent and nauseous, and there is a characteristic odour.

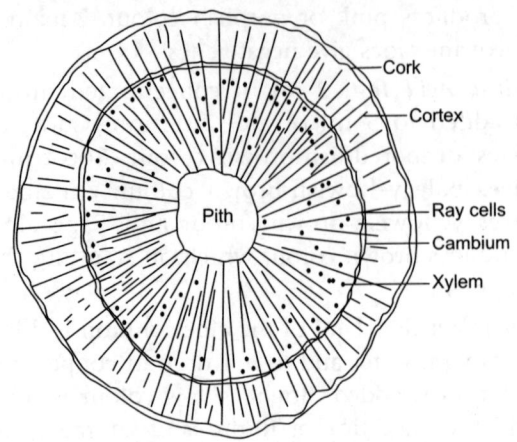

FIG. 16.7 Schematic diagram (T. S.) of rhizome

Microscopy (Figs. 16.7 and 16.8)

Transverse section of the rhizome shows a brown cork composed of usually 10–12 layers of nonlignified, nearly rectangular cells. Cork surrounds a broad cortex, composed of thin-walled, mostly irregularly rounded parenchymatous cells and some of them merge into the secondary phloem tissue, which consists of few layers of cells. Cortex contains starch grains, simple or compound with a distinct central hilum; cluster crystals of calcium oxalate, very large (20–200 µm in diameter), and tannin masses. Cambium is wavy and much compressed. Radial medullary rays are very prominent and consist of 1–2 layers of cells containing yellow masses of anthraquinones. The secondary xylem is composed of thick-walled xylem vessels and xylem parenchyma. Pith is composed of thin-walled parenchymatous cells.

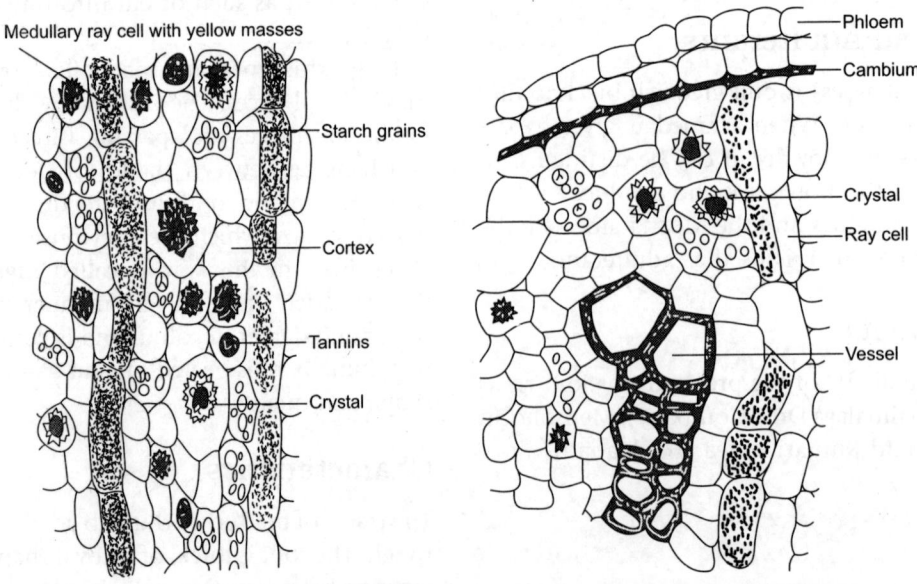

FIG. 16.8 Transverse section through cortex portion and xylem portion

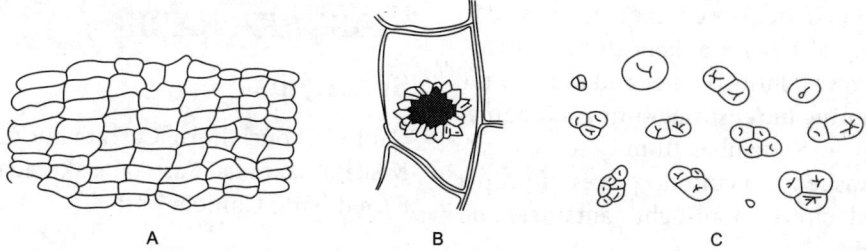

FIG. 16.9 Powder characteristics of Rhubarb rhizome. (A: Cork cells, B: Cluster crystals of calcium oxalate, C: Starch grains)

Powder Microscopy (Fig. 16.9)

The powder is yellowish-brown in colour with aromatic odour and bitter and astringent taste. Microscopical examination shows abundant starch grains (4–30 µm long), compound (2–5 components) or simple, spherical with a distinct central hilum in the form of a cleft or radiating split. Abundant cluster crystals of calcium oxalate (20–200 µm in diameter) are found scattered and in some parenchymatous cells. Cork cells, nearly rectangular in transverse view, thick-walled; abundant parenchyma, thin-walled cells, elongated, filled with starch grains; and abundant vessels, with reticulate thickening are found scattered.

Chemical Constituents

Rhubarb contains free anthraquinones, their glycosides, reduced derivatives, anthrones or dianthrone and heterodianthrones. The anthraquinones of rhubarb are chrysophanol, aloe-emodin, emodin, physcion and rhein. Anthrones or dianthrones are of chrysophanol, emodin and aloe-emodin. Heterodianthrones contain two different molecules of anthrones and they are from above anthrones. It also contains tannoid constituents, starch and calcium oxalate. There are also several resinous matters, one of which, phloretin, is purgative, and mineral compounds are also present. The astringency of rhubarb is due to a peculiar tannic acid (rheo-tannic), which is soluble in water and alcohol.

Rhein

Chrysophanol

Aloe-emodin

Emodin

Chemical Tests

1. Rhubarb powder when treated with ammonia pink colour is produced.
2. With a solution of 5% potassium hydroxide it gives blood red colour.
3. It gives a positive indication with modified Borntrager's test (see under aloes).

Uses

The root is anticholesterolemic, antiseptic, antispasmodic, antitumour, aperient, astringent, cholagogue, demulcent, diuretic, laxative, purgative, stomachic and tonic. The roots contain anthraquinones, which have a purgative effect, and also tannins and bitters, which have an opposite astringent effect. When taken in small doses, it acts as an astringent tonic to the digestive system, whilst larger doses act as a mild laxative. The root is taken internally in the treatment of chronic constipation, diarrhoea, liver and gall bladder complaints, haemorrhoids, menstrual problems and skin eruptions due to an accumulation of toxins. This remedy is not prescribed for pregnant or lactating women, or for patients with intestinal obstruction. Externally, the root is used in the treatment of burns.

Marketed Products

It is one of the ingredients of the preparation known as Diet Master Herb Tea (Health King Enterprise and Balanceuticals Group, Inc.).

Other Rhubarbs

Indian rhubarb

It consists of the dried rhizomes and roots of *R. emodi* and *R. webbianum*. *R. emodi* is a stout herb, 1.5–3.0 m in height, distributed in the Himalayas from Kashmir to Sikkim at altitudes of 3300–5200 m. It is also cultivated in Assam for its leaves consumed as vegetable. Roots are very stout.

The drug is collected from the wild plant, found in the hills of Kangra, Kulu, Kumaun, Nepal and Sikkim. The herb is drought resistant, and can be propagated either through rhizome cuttings or seeds. The plant requires deep, rich soil, mixed with well-rotten manure. The cuttings are planted in early spring at a spacing of 1.2–1.5 m beneath the surface. Aerial portions wither away during winter and die, but the rhizomes regenerate during the ensuring spring. Rhizomes and roots are dug up in September from 3 to 10 years old plants. They are washed and cut into pieces of proper size, kiln- or sun-dried, stored in air-tight containers and protected from sunlight.

Indian rhubarb contains a number of anthraquinone derivatives based on emodin, emodin-3-monomethyl ether (physcion), chrysophanol, aloe-emodin and rhein. These occur free and as quinone, anthrone or dianthrone glycoside. The astringent principle consists of gallic acid, present as glucogallin, along with tannin and catechin. The drug also contains cinnamic and rheinolic acids, volatile oil, starch and calcium oxalate. Free chrysophanic acid, sennoside A and sennoside B are also present. The characteristic odour of the essential oil is due to the presence of eugenol.

R. webbianum contains 1,8-dihydroxy-3-methyl-1,8-dihydroxy-3-hydroxymethyl-, 1,6,8-trihydroxy-3-methyl-anthraquinones and 3′,5-dihydroxy-4-methoxystilbene.

Indian rhubarb is used as a purgative and astringent tonic, in atonic dyspepsia and for cleaning teeth. Powdered roots are sprinkled over ulcers for quick healing.

Chinese rhapontic (Rhapontic rhubarb)

It is obtained from *Rheum rhaponticum*. Its odour is sweet. It consists of untrimmed pieces sometimes split longitudinally. The transverse surface shows a radiate structure, with concentric rings of paler and darker colour and a diffuse ring of star spots. The centre may be hollow. The odour, which is sweetish, differs from that of official rhubarb. Rhapontic rhubarb gives a positive test for anthraquinone derivatives. When the test for absence of rhapontic rhubarb is applied, it gives a distinct blue fluorescence, which may be further intensified by exposure to ammonia vapour.

Rhapontic rhubarb contains a glycoside, rhaponticin, which is a stilbene (diphenylethylene) derivative. Rhaponticin and desoxyrhaponticin (glucoside of 3,5-dihydroxy-4′-methoxystilbene) show the difference in fluorescence between official and rhapontic rhubarbs. Rhapontic rhubarb does contain anthraquinone derivatives, although these differ from those in the official drug. One is the glucoside glucochrysaron. It also contains 3,3′,4′-5-tetrahydroxystilbene.

Test for Rhapontic Rhubarb: An extract of 0.5 g of powder with 10 ml of 45% alcohol for 20 min is prepared. Place one drop of the filtrate on a filter paper. When examined in ultra violet light, the spot shows no blue colour with official rhubarb but a distinct blue fluorescence; if rhapontic rhubarb is present. The colour is intensified by exposure to ammonia vapour. Its alcoholic extract on filter paper shows a distinct blue fluorescence in U.V. light due to rhaponticin.

CASCARA BARK

Synonyms

California buckthorn, Cascara buckthorn, Cascara sagrada, Kaskara sakrada, Kasukarasakurada, Pursh's buckthorn, Sacred bark, Chittem bark.

Biological Source

Cascara is the dried bark of *Rhamnus purshiana* DC., belonging to family Rhamnaceae (Fig. 16.10). It is collected at least one year before use.

Geographical Source

It is indigenous to North America, British Columbia, Canada and Kenya.

Cultivation and Collection

It is an evergreen tree growing to 6–12 m in height. The plant prefers sandy, loamy and clay soils. The plant prefers acid, neutral and basic soils. It can grow in semishade or no shade. It requires moist soil. It is cultivated using different techniques like sowing seeds, cuttings and layering. Seeds are sown in the autumn in a cold frame. Stored seed will require 1–2 months cold stratification at about 5°C and should be sown as early in the year as possible in a cold frame or outdoor seed bed. Seedlings are transferred to the pots and then they are transplanted in late spring or early summer of the following year. Cuttings are carried out using half-ripe wood, July/August. Layering can be done in early spring.

Earlier the barks were collected by felling technique and then by making longitudinal incisions on the trees. To save the destruction of this species nowadays it is collected by coppicing method. So the stump remaining above the soil produces new shoots, which bear leaves, flowers and fruits and seed dispersal takes place and new plants grow. Bark is collected from 9 to 15 years old trees having minimum 10 cm diameter in dry weather after rains in May to August by making suitable transverse and longitudinal incisions. During drying the outer bark is protected from moisture and rains and inner bark is protected from direct sunlight. Moisture leads to mould due to the sunlight bark becomes black colour. After complete drying the bark is made in to small pieces that form squill. It should be harvested in the autumn or spring at least 12 months before it is used medicinally, in order to allow the more violent purgative effect to be modified with age.

Characteristics

The drug mostly occurs in quilled, channelled or incurved of varying lengths and sizes, usually 20 cm long and 1–4 mm thick, smooth or nearly so externally, covered with a greyish-white layer, which is usually easily removed, and frequently marked with spots or patches of adherent lichens. Beneath the surface it is violet-brown, reddish-brown or brownish, and internally a pale yellowish-brown and nearly smooth. Fracture is short and granular in the outer part and fibrous in the phloem. It has no marked odour, but a nauseous, bitter taste. It is frequently also imported in flattened packets, consisting of small pieces of the bark compressed into a more or less compact mass.

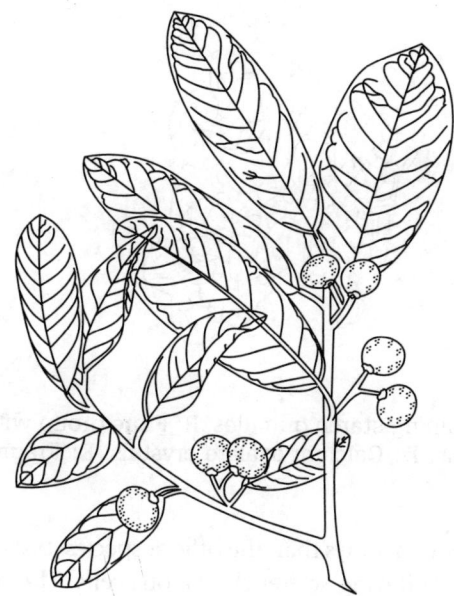

FIG. 16.10 *Rhamnus purshiana*

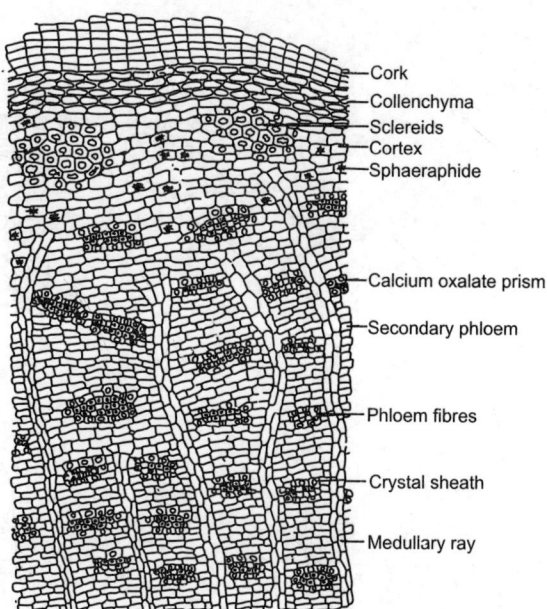

FIG. 16.11 Transverse section of Cascara bark

Microscopy (Fig. 16.11)

The cork consists of numerous layers of small, thin walled flattened, polygonal prisms, arranged in radial rows and having yellowish brown contents. Next to cork few layers of collenchyma cells are present. Groups of irregular thick walled lignified stone cells are in the cortex and 1–5 celled wide phloem rays and tangentially elongated lignified fibres in the phloem. The fibres are crystal fibres and surrounded by parenchyma containing calcium oxalate prisms. Crystal fibres are of diagnostic importance in identification of the powdered drug.

Powder Microscopy (Fig. 16.12)

The powder is yellowish-brown in colour with characteristic odour and intensely bitter and nauseous taste. Microscopical examination shows groups of sclereids, composed of thick-walled, densely packed cells with numerous branching pits, partially surrounded by a sheath of prismatic calcium oxalate crystals. Fibres are abundant, thick-walled, lignified with few pits and each fibre is surrounded by a sheath of prismatic calcium oxalate crystals. Cork cells are thin-walled, polygonal in surface view and filled with reddish-brown contents. Cells of parenchyma and collenchyma of cortex contain cluster crystals of calcium oxalate and starch grains. Phloem parenchymatous cells have uneven thick walls and characteristic swellings in the walls. Cluster and prismatic crystals of calcium oxalate and occasional fragments of mosses composed of thin-walled, elongated cells are found scattered.

Chemical Constituents

Cascara bark contains 80–90% of C-glycosides and 10–20% O-glycosides. The C-glycosides present in cascara are aloin or barbaloin and 11-deoxyaloin or chrysaloin. Cascarosides A and B are the primary glycosides of aloin and cascarosides C and D are primary glycosides of chrysaloin. Cascara also contains chrysaloin and barbaloins, dianthrones of emodin, aloe-emodin, chrysophanol; heterodianthrones like Palmidins A, B and C, free emodin, aloe-emodin and a bitter lactone. Apart from glycosides it also contains fat, starch, glucose, volatile odorous oil, malic and tannic acids.

Fresh cascara bark contains anthranol derivatives which have griping and emetic properties and after storage for one year, anthranol derivatives are oxidized to anthraquinone derivatives and bark loses irritant properties.

Chemical Test

It gives red colour with 5% potassium hydroxide solution.

Uses

Cascara sagrada is widely used as a gentle laxative that restores tone to the bowel muscles and thus makes repeated doses unnecessary. It is considered suitable for delicate

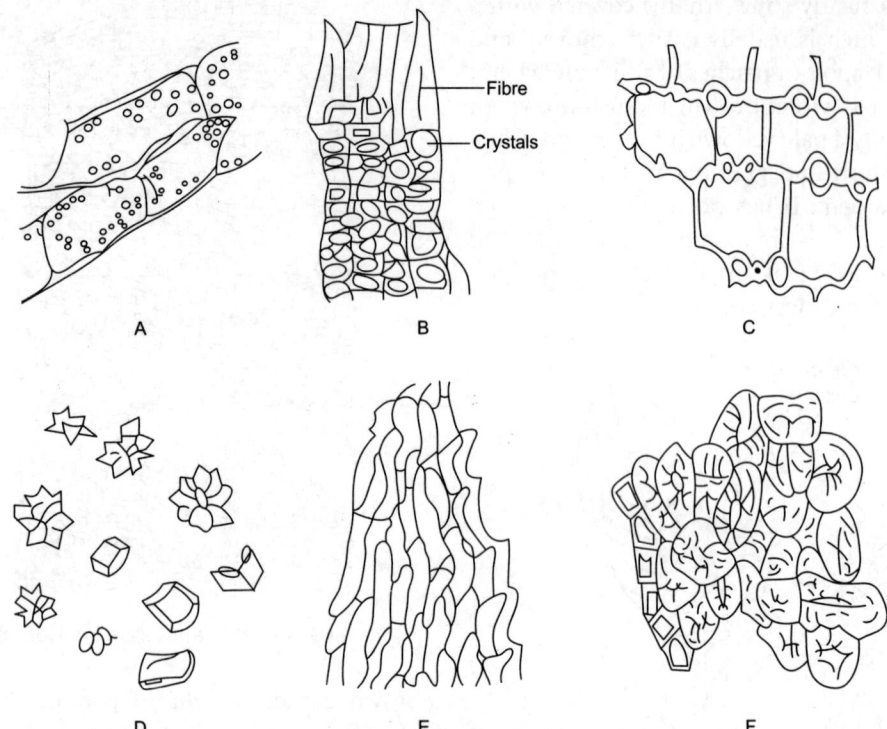

FIG. 16.12 Powder characteristics of Cascara bark. (A: Parenchyma containing starch granules, B: Fibre group with crystal sheath, C: Phloem parenchymatous cells showing swellings in the walls, D: Calcium oxalate crystals, E: Fragment of a moss, F: Sclereids)

Cascaroside A

and elderly persons and is very useful in cases of chronic constipation. The bark also has tonic properties, promoting gastric digestion and appetite. As well as its uses as a laxative, it is taken internally in the treatment of digestive complaints, haemorrhoids, liver problems and jaundice.

Substitutes

These include *R. alnifolia*, which is too rare to be a likely substitute; *R. crocea*, whose bark bears little resemblance to the official drug. *R. californica* is very closely related to *R. purshiana*. It has a more uniform coat of lichens and wider medullary rays than the official species, but resembles the latter in having sclerenchymatous cells. The bark of *R. fallax* has been recorded as a cascara substitute.

Marketed Products

It is one of the ingredients of the preparations known as Herbal Laxative (Trophic Canada Ltd.).

FRANGULA

Synonyms

Buckthorn bark, Alder buckthorn, Black dogwood, Berry alder, Arrow wood, Persian berries.

Biological Source

Frangula bark is the dried bark of *Rhamnus frangula* Linn. belonging to the family *Rhamnaceae*.

Geographical Source

The plant is a shrub, which grows abundantly in Europe, the Mediterranean coast of Africa and Western Asia.

Cultivation and Collection

The preparation of frangula bark resembles to that of cascara bark. Just like the cascara bark, the frangula bark must be aged for at least a period of 1 year before it is used therapeutically so as to permit the reduced forms of the glycosides with harsh action to be oxidized to comparatively milder forms.

Chemical Constituents

The seed, bark and root bark of *Rhamnus species*, specifically in *Alder Buckthorn (Rhamnus alnifolia L'Her.), Rhamnus cathartica L.* and *Rhamnus purshiana DC (Cascara sagrada)* consists of the *two* important glycosides, frangulins A and B, which were initially thought to be isomeric compounds. Later on two more glycosides known as *glucofrangulins A and B* have also been reported. However, the structures of frangulins A and B along with glucofrangulins A and B are given below:

Frangulin A : R = H;
Glucofrangulin A : R = β-D-Glucopyranose

Frangulin B : R = H;
Glucofrangulin B : R = β-D-Glucopyranose

Besides *frangulin* the frangula bark contains emodin and chrysophanic acid.

Substitutes and Adulterants

As the activity of frangula bark corresponds to that of *cascara sagrada*, it finds a good substitute and comparable usage in Europe and the Near East. Interestingly, the drug substances obtained from the ripe and duly dried fruits of *Rhamnus catharticus* Linn. are invariably employed in Europe and the Near East for their recognized cathartic therapeutic activity.

Uses

It is mostly used as a cathartic.

Marketed Products

It is one of the ingredients of the preparation known as *Slimatee* (Goodness Foods) and VIVA Cleanse Tea (Viva).

16.7. STEROL OR CARDIAC GLYCOSIDES

The cardiac glycosides are an important class of naturally occurring drugs whose actions include both beneficial and toxic effects on the heart. Plants containing cardiac steroids have been used as poisons and heart drugs at least since 1500 B.C. Throughout history these plants or their extracts have been variously used as arrow poisons, emetics, diuretics and heart tonics. Cardiac steroids are widely used in the modern treatment of congestive heart failure and for treatment of atrial fibrillation and flutter. Yet their toxicity remains a serious problem. These drugs all act by affecting the availability of intracellular Ca^{+2} for myocardial contraction or increasing the sensitivity of myocardial contractile proteins.

Cardiac glycosides are composed of two structural features: the sugar (glycone) and the nonsugar (aglycone–steroid) moieties.

The steroid nucleus has a unique set of fused ring system that makes the aglycone moiety structurally distinct from the other more common steroid ring systems. The steroid nucleus has hydroxyls at 3- and 14-positions of which the sugar attachment uses the 3-OH group. 14-OH is normally unsubstituted. Many genins have OH groups at 12- and 16-positions. These additional hydroxyl groups influence the partitioning of the cardiac glycosides into the aqueous media and greatly affect the duration of action. The lactone moiety at C-17 position is an important structural feature. The size and degree of unsaturation varies with the source of the glycoside. Normally plant sources provide a five-membered unsaturated lactone while animal sources give a six-membered unsaturated lactone.

One to four sugars are found to be present in most cardiac glycosides attached to the 3β-OH group. The sugars most commonly used include L-rhamnose, D-glucose, D-digitoxose, D-digitalose, D-digginose, D-sarmentose, L-vallarose and D-fructose. These sugars predominantly exist in the cardiac glycosides in the β-conformation. The presence of acetyl group on the sugar affects the lipophilic character and the kinetics of the entire glycoside.

Two classes have been observed in nature—the cardenolides and the bufadienolides.

The cardenolides have an unsaturated butyrolactone ring while the bufadienolides have a pyrone ring. The lactone of cardenolides has a single double bond and is attached at the C-17 position of steroidal nucleus. They are five-membered lactone ring and form a C_{23} steroids (Leguminosae, Cruciferae, Euphorbiaceae, etc.), while the lactone of bufadienolides have two double bond which is attached at the 17 α-position of the steroidal nucleus. They are six-membered lactone ring and form C_{24} steroids (Liliaceae, Ranunculaceae).

Cardenolide

Bufadienolide

DIGITALIS LEAVES

Synonyms

Digitalis, purple foxglove, finger flower, lady's glove, foxglove leaves, Folia Digitalis.

Biological Sources

Digitalis consists of dried leaves of *Digitalis purpurea* Linn., belonging to family Scrophulariaceae (Fig. 16.13).

Geographical Sources

It is mainly found in England, Germany, France, North America, India, Iraq, Japan, Kurdistan, Mexico, Nepal, Spain, Turkey.

Cultivation and Collection

Digitalis is a biennial herb growing wild but good quality of the drug is obtained especially from cultivated plant. The plant will flourish best in well drained loose soil, preferably of siliceous origin, with some slight shade. The plants growing in sunny situations possess the active qualities of the herb in a much greater degree than those shaded by trees, and it has been proved that those grown on a hot, sunny bank, protected by a wood, give the best results.

It grows best when allowed to seed itself, if it is desired to raise it by sown seed, 2 lb of seed to the acre are required. For cultivation special strains of the seeds are selected which would produce disease-resistant plants with maximum activity. Attention is specially paid to the structure of the

soil in seed beds. As the seeds are so small and light, they should be mixed with fine sand in order to ensure even distribution. Before sowing soil is sterilized. They should be thinly covered with soil. The seeds are uncertain in germination, but the seedlings may be readily and safely transplanted in damp weather, and should be pricked out to 6–9 inches apart. Sown in spring, the plant will not blossom till the following year. Seeds must be gathered as soon as ripe. In dry season sufficient water is supplied to the plant. In the first year, a long stalk with rosette of leaves is produced. The flowers of the true medicinal type must be pure, dull pink or magenta, not pale-coloured, white or spotted externally.

Collection of these leaves is carried out from September to November by hand and thus other organic matter and discoloured leaves are avoided. After collection the leaves should be dried as soon as possible at 60°C. By quick drying characteristic green colour of the leaves is maintained. Drying is carried out till moisture is not more than 5%. Leaves are packed under pressure in airtight containers.

Morphology

Colour	Dark greyish green in colour
Odour	Odourless
Taste	Bitter
Shape	Ovatelanceolate to broadly ovate. Leaves have a subacute apex, decurrent base and crenate or dentate margin. The upper surface of leaf is hairy, slightly pubescent, dark green and little wrinkled. The lower surface of leaf is hairy, greyish-green and very pubescent.
Size	10–30 cm long and 4–10 cm wide

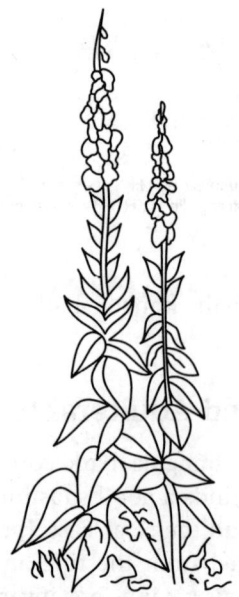

FIG. 16.13 *Digitalis purpurea*

Microscopy (Figs. 16.14 and 16.15)

Digitalis has dorsiventral leaf structure. It has plenty of simple covering and glandular trichomes on both the surfaces. The covering trichomes are uniseriate, usually three to four cells long, having collapsed cells, acute apex and finely warty cuticle. The glandular trichomes have a short, unicellular stalk and bicellular or rarely unicellular head. It has anomocytic or ranunculaceous type of stomata. Trichomes and stomata are more in lower surface. The pericycle is parenchymatous above and collenchymatous below. Calcium oxalate crystals are absent.

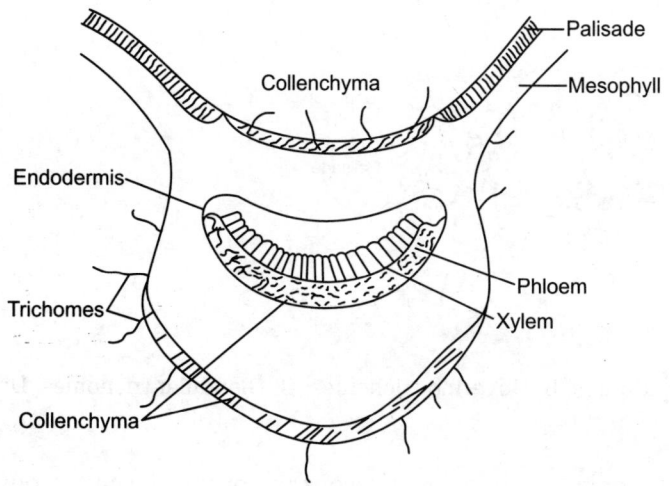

FIG. 16.14 T.S. (schematic) of digitalis leaf

Powder Microscopy (Fig. 16.16)

The powder is pale green in colour with slight odour and bitter taste. Microscopical examination shows epidermal cells with wavy anticlinal walls and numerous stomata on lower epidermis; marginal teeth with water pores; small spiral, annular and reticulate vessels; palisade and spongy parenchyma with chloroplast. Covering trichomes are simple, bluntly pointed uniseriate, multicellular with fine warty walls and occasional collapsed cells. Glandular trichome bears a unicellular or bicellular gland with unicellular or, more rarely, uniseriate, multicellular stalk.

Chemical Constituents

Digitalis leaves contains 0.2–0.45% of both primary and secondary glycosides. Purpurea glycosides A and B and glucogitoloxin are primary glycosides. Because of greater stability of secondary glycosides, and lesser absorption of primary glycosides a higher content of primary glycosides are not considered ideal and secondary glycosides are used. Purpurea glycosides A and B are present in fresh leaves and by their hydrolysis digitoxin and glucose or gitoxin and glucose are obtained respectively. Hydrolysis of purpurea glycosides can take place by digipuridase (enzyme) present in the leaves. Digitoxin yields on hydrolysis digitoxigenin and three digitoxose. By hydrolysis of verodoxin, gitaloxigenin and digitalose are obtained. Digitalis leaves also contains glycosides like odoroside-H, gitaloxin, verodoxin and glucoverodoxin.

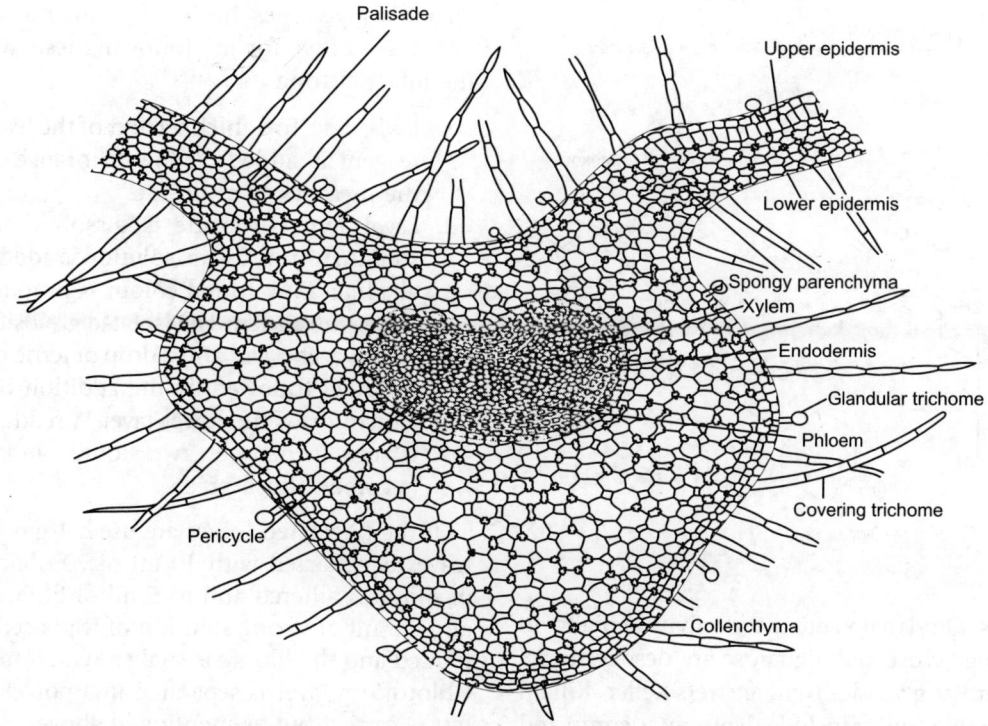

FIG. 16.15 Transverse section of digitalis leaf

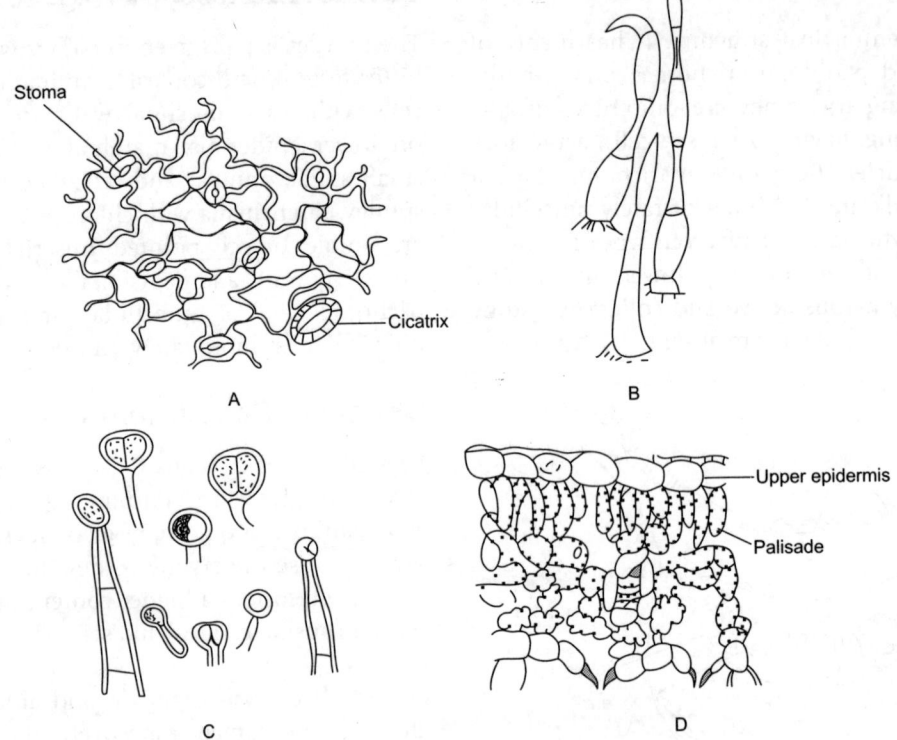

FIG. 16.16 Powder characteristics of digitalis leaf. (A: Lower epidermis, B: Covering trichomes, C: Glandular trichomes, D: Lamina)

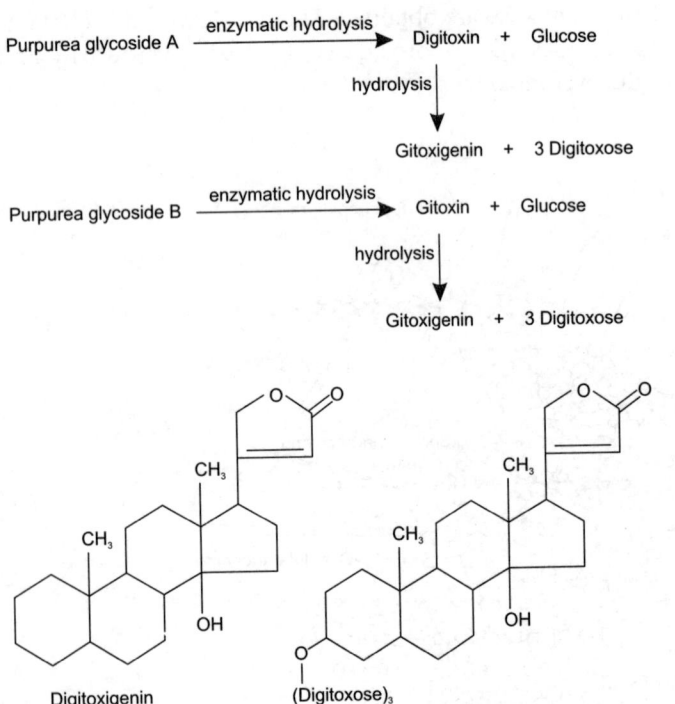

Purpurea glycoside A $\xrightarrow{\text{enzymatic hydrolysis}}$ Digitoxin + Glucose

$\downarrow$ hydrolysis

Gitoxigenin + 3 Digitoxose

Purpurea glycoside B $\xrightarrow{\text{enzymatic hydrolysis}}$ Gitoxin + Glucose

$\downarrow$ hydrolysis

Gitoxigenin + 3 Digitoxose

Digitoxigenin   (Digitoxose)$_3$ Digitoxin

Verodoxin was found to potentiate the activity of digitoxin by synergism. Digitoxose and digitalose are desoxy sugars found only in cardiac glycosides and answers Keller–Kiliani test. The important saponins include digitonin, tigonin and gitonin, and luteolin, a flavone responsible for the colour of the drug are also present in the leaves.

Chemical Tests

Digitalis glycosides having five membered lactone ring answers positive for the following tests which are due to the intact lactone.

1. *Baljet Test:* To a thick section of the leaf sodium picrate reagent is added. Yellow to orange colour indicates the presence of glycoside.
2. *Legal Test:* Glycoside is dissolved in pyridine and sodium nitroprusside solution is added to it and made alkaline. Pink to red colour is produced.
3. *Keller–Kiliani Test:* The isolated glycoside is dissolved in glacial acetic acid and a drop of ferric chloride solution is added followed by the addition of sulphuric acid which forms the lower layer. A reddish-brown colour is seen in between two liquids and the upper layer becomes bluish green.

If the powdered leaves are used, 1 gm of the powdered leaves is extracted with 10 ml of 70% alcohol for couple of minutes, filtered and to 5 ml of filtrate 10 ml of water and 0.5 ml of strong solution of lead acetate is added and filtered and the filtrate is shaken with 5 ml of chloroform. Chloroform layer is separated in a porcelain dish and the test is carried out as mentioned above.

Uses

The foxglove is a widely used herbal medicine with a recognized stimulatory effect upon the heart. It is also used in allopathic medicine in the treatment of heart complaints. It has a profound tonic effect upon a diseased heart, enabling the heart to beat more slowly, powerfully and regularly without requiring more oxygen. At the same time it stimulates the flow of urine which lowers the volume of the blood and lessens the load on the heart. It has also been employed in the treatment of internal haemorrhage, in inflammatory diseases, in delirium tremens, in epilepsy, in acute mania and various other diseases. Digitalis has a cumulative effect in the body, so the dose has to be decided very carefully.

Adulterants

Verbascum thapsus also known as Mullelin leaves. These leaves are covered with large woolly branched candelabra trichomes.

Primula vulgaris (Primrose leaves) can be detected by the presence of long eight- to nine-celled covering trichomes in them.

Symphytum officinale (Comfrey leaves), this leaves contains multicellular trichomes forming hook at the top.

Inula conyza (Ploughman's Spikenard), may be distinguished by their greater roughness, the less-divided margins, the teeth of which have horny points and odour when rubbed.

Marketed Products

It is one of the ingredients of the preparation known as Lanoxin tablets (Glaxo Smith Kline).

DIGITALIS LANATA

Synonym

Grecian Foxglove.

Biological Source

It consists of the dried leaves of *Digitalis lanata* J. F. Ehrh., belonging to family Scrophulariaceae.

Geographical Source

It is mainly found in Central and Southern Europe, England, California and India.

Cultivation and Collection

It is an evergreen biennial/perennial growing to 0.6 m by 0.3 m. The plant prefers light (sandy), medium (loamy) and heavy (clay) soils. The plant prefers acid, neutral and alkaline soils. It can grow in semishade or no shade. It requires dry or moist soil. It grows well even in ordinary garden soil, especially if it is rich in organic matter. It is propagated by seeds. Seed are sown on early spring in a cold frame. The seed usually germinates in 2–4 weeks at 20°C. When they are large enough to handle, seedlings are transplanted into individual pots and planted them out in the summer.

Characteristics

The leaves are sessile, linear-lanceolate, about 30 cm long and 4 cm broad with entire margin and apex is acuminate. The veins leave the midrib at an acute angle. The epidermal cells are beaded with anticlinal walls, has 10–14 celled nonglandular trichomes, and the glandular one.

Chemical Constituents

Digitalis lanata contains cardiac glycosides like lanatoside A, B, C and E. Lanatosides A and B are acetyl derivatives of purpurea glycosides A and B respectively. Hydrolysis of Lanatoside C yields digoxin, a crystalline active glycoside.

Uses

It has gained much importance in recent years because of the less cumulative effect and three to four times greater activity

	R1	R2	R3
Lanatoside A	H	H	CH₃CO
Lanatoside B	H	OH	CH₃CO
Lanatoside C	OH	H	CH₃CO

than *D. purpurea*. They have the same actions as that of the *D. purpurea*. It is the commercial source of digoxin. Employed in the treatment of auricular fibrillation and congestive heart failure. Their use should always be supervised by a qualified practitioner since in excess they cause nausea, vomiting, slow pulse, visual disturbance, anorexia and fainting.

THEVETIA

Synonyms

Yellow oleander, lucky nut tree, trumpet flower.

Biological Source

It is the dried seeds of *Thevetia nerifolia* Juss, Syn. *Thevetia peruviana* Merrill., belonging to family Apocynaceae (Fig. 16.17).

Geographical Source

It is a large, evergreen shrub 450–600 cm tall with scented bright yellow flowers in terminal cymes bears triangular fleshy drupes, containing two to four seeds. Leaves are about 10–15 cm in length, linear acute. It is mainly found in the United States, India and West Indies.

Morphology

Colour	Green to greenish black
Odour	None
Taste	Bitter
Shape	Oblong

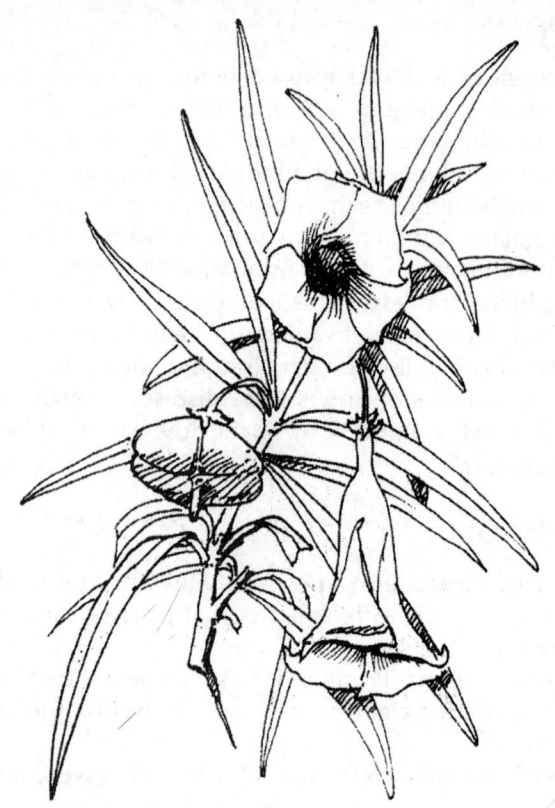

FIG. 16.17 *Thevetia nerifolia*

Chemical Constituents

Thevetia kernels mainly contain cardioactive glycosides, thevetin A, thevetin B (cerebroside), peruvoside, neriifolin, thevenenin (ruvoside), peruvosidic acid (perusitin), etc. The sugar units are L-thevetose and D-glucose.

Thevetin

Peruvoside

Neriifolin

Uses

Roots of these plants are made in to a paste and applied to tumours. Seeds are used in the treatment of rheumatism, dropsy and also used as abortifacient and purgative. They are toxic in nature.

SQUILL

Synonyms

Scillae bulbus, Squill, Scilla bulb, White squill, European scilla, *Urginea scilla, Drimia maritima.*

Biological Source

Squill consists of the dried slices of the bulb of white variety of *Urginea maritima* (Linn.) Baker, belonging to family Liliaceae (Fig. 16.18a and b).

Geographical Source

It is mainly found in Spain, Portugal, Morocco, Algeria, Corsica, southern France, Italy, Malta, Dalmatia, Greece, Syria and Asia.

Cultivation and Collection

The plant prefers light (sandy) and medium (loamy) soils and requires well-drained soil. The plant prefers acid, neutral and basic (alkaline) soils. It cannot grow in the shade. It requires dry or moist soil. The plant can tolerate strong winds but not maritime exposure. Seeds are sown as soon as it is ripe in a greenhouse. The seeds were sown thinly so that the seedlings can be left in the pot for their first growing season. Fertilizers are to be used regularly. Once the plant becomes dormant the young bulbs are divided, placing two to three bulbs in each pot. After an year they are transplanted to the field. Division of offsets is done in late summer when the bulb is dormant. Larger bulbs can be replanted immediately into their permanent positions. It is probably best to pot up smaller bulbs and grow them on in a greenhouse for a year before planting them out when they are dormant in late summer.

The bulb is large and 18–20 cm high with 12 cm to 15 cm in diameter. Bulbs are dug out from the soil in the end of August and external scaly leaves and central portion are removed. The slices are dried completely in the sunlight or by heat of the stove. The drug is stored in airtight and especially in moisture proof containers.

Characteristics

It is a perennial plant with fibrous roots proceeding from the base of a large, tunicated, nearly globular bulb, 4–6 inches long, the outer scales of which are thin and papery, red or orange-brown in colour. The bulb, which is usually

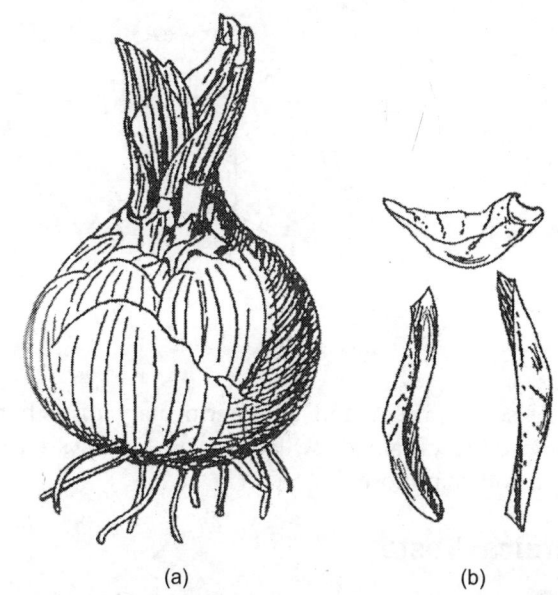

FIG. 16.18 (a) Squill bulb and (b) dried slice of squill bulb

only half immersed in the sand, sends forth several long, lanceolate, pointed, somewhat undulated, shining, dark-green leaves, when fully grown, feet long. From the middle of the leaves, a round, smooth, succulent flower-stem rises, from 1 to 2 feet high, terminating in a long, close spike of whitish flowers, which stand on purplish peduncles, at the base of each, is a narrow, twisted, deciduous floral leaf or bract.

The undried bulb is somewhat pear-shaped, and generally about the size of a man's fist, but often larger, weighing from 1/2 lb to more than 4 lb. It has the usual structure of a bulb, being formed of smooth juicy scales, closely wrapped over one another. It has little odour, but its inner scales have a mucilaginous, bitter, acrid taste, owing to the presence of bitter glucosides. The dried slices are narrow, flattish, curved, yellowish-white or with a roseate hue, according to the variety of squill from which they are obtained, from 1 to 2 inches long, more or less translucent.

Chemical Constituents

Squill contains cardiac glycosides of bufadienolides types, scillaren A and B and enzyme scillatenase. The other constituents present are glucoscillaren A (cardiac glycoside), proscillaridin A, flavonoid, mucilage, volatile substances and sinistrin. The cardiac glycoside (glucoscillaren A) on hydrolysis gives three glucose molecules, two molecules of glucose and a molecule of rhamnose along with scillarenin. Scillaren A is crystalline and responsible for the activity of the drug. Scillaren B is amorphous and its exact chemical structure is not known. Scillaren A on hydrolysis with enzyme yields proscillaridin A and glucose. Proscillaridin A on further acid hydrolysis yields the aglycone scillarenin A and rhamnose. If scillaren A is hydrolysed with acid

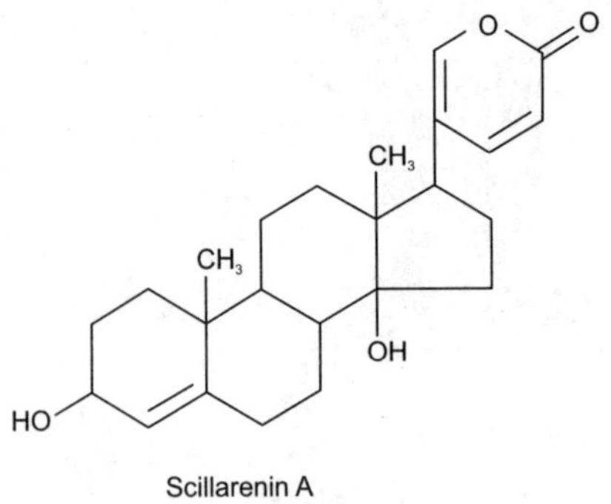

Scillarenin A

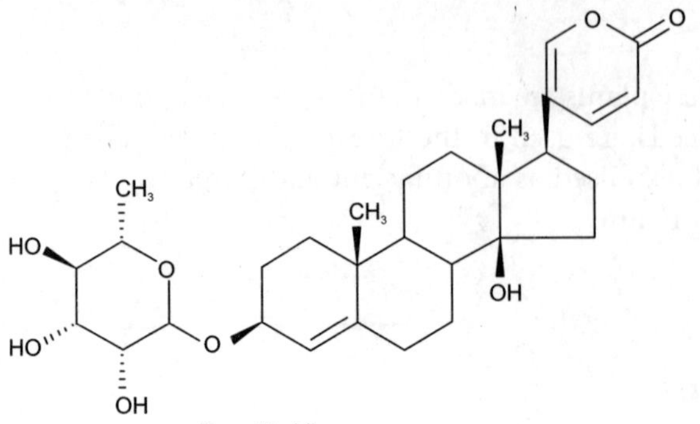

Proscillaridin

directly scillarenin A and an intermediary disaccharide scillabiose are obtained; scillabiose on hydrolysis yields glucose and rhamnose.

Chemical Tests

1. They show negative results for Baljet test and Legal test.
2. The Liebermann's sterol test is positive in squill glycosides.
3. In the mesophyll region of squill, muciage, calcium oxalate and yellow colouring matter xanthoscillide are present. Mucilage does not give colour reaction with ruthenium red but stains red with corallin soda and pale yellow with iodine.

Uses

It is largely used for its stimulating, expectorant and diuretic properties, and is also a cardiac tonic, acting in a similar manner to digitalis, slowing and strengthening the pulse, though more irritating to the gastrointestinal mucous membrane. It is considered most useful in chronic bronchitis, catarrhal affections and asthma. It is a potential substitute for foxglove in aiding a failing heart.

RED SQUILL

Red squill consists of the bulb of *Urginea maritima*. The red species has deep, reddish-brown outer scales and yellowish white inner scales, covered with a pinkish epidermis, intermediate forms also occurring. Red colour is attributed to anthocyanin. There is no much difference in constituents when compared to white squill but it contains scilliroside, a glycoside; which is toxic to rats. No essential difference exists in the medicinal properties of the two kinds. The white and red squills are called chemical races.

INDIAN SQUILL

Synonyms

Sea onion, Urginea, jangli pyaj.

Biological Source

Indian squill consists of dried slices of the bulb of *Urginea indica* Kunth., belonging to family Liliaceae

Geographical Source

It is found throughout India (Western Himalaya, Konkan, Coramandal coast, Bihar, etc.).

Cultivation and Collection

Though it is not been cultivated, it grows well at a temperature of 15–20°C and in sandy soil. The bulbs grow to full size within 5 years. The bulbs are collected after flowering, cut in to small slices and dried under sun.

Morphology

Colour	Slightly yellowish-white
Odour	Slight and characteristic
Taste	Bitter, acrid and mucilaginous
Shape	United in groups which are curved, pear shape
Size	Length 3–5 cm; breadth 0.3–0.8 cm

Microscopy (Fig. 16.19)

A thin transverse section when observed under the microscope shows the following characters. Single layer of polygonal elongated epidermis is present which is covered with the cuticle. Mesophyll region consists of acicular calcium oxalate crystals, mucilage sheath, small round starch grains and vascular bundle (annular and spiral xylem vessels).

Chemical Constituents

Indian squill contains cardiac glycosides, similar to European squill. Mucilage is present in mesophyll cells.

Chemical Tests

1. Mucilage stains reddish purple with iodine water where as European squill does not.
2. Colarin solution stains mesophyll region red.

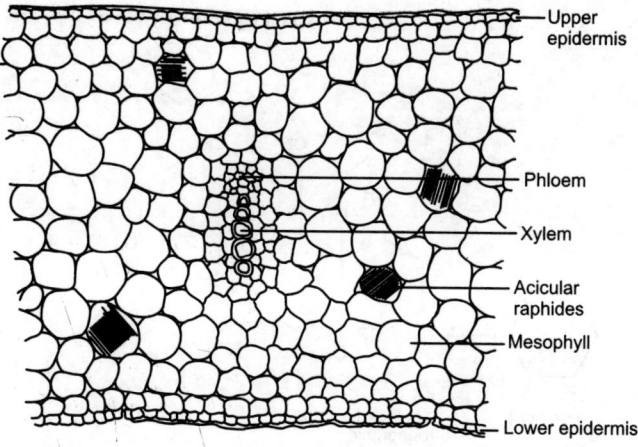

FIG. 16.19 Transverse section of slice of squill bulb

Uses

It is used as cardiotonic, expectorant, stimulant, diuretic, cathartic. It is also a bronchodilator and anticancer agent.

Other Species

Scilla indica Baker (*L. hyacinthina*, Roth.), a native of India and Abyssinia, has a bulb often confused in the Indian bazaars with the preceding, but easily distinguished when entire by being scaly, not tunicated, its cream coloured scales overlapping one another. The bulbs are about the size and shape of a small pear, somewhat smaller than those of *U. indica*. It is considered a better representative of the European squill. It has a nauseous odour and a bitter acrid taste. They are collected soon after the plants have flowered, divested of their dry, outer, membraneous coats, cut into slices and dried.

The chief constituents are bitter principles; similar to the glucosidal substances found in ordinary squill, and needle shaped crystals of calcium oxalate are also present. The drug possesses stimulant, expectorant and diuretic activity.

STROPHANTHUS

Synonyms

Kombe Seeds, Strophanti Semina, Semen Strophanthi, Strophanthus Seeds.

Biological Source

Strophanthus consists of dried ripe seeds of *Strophanthus kombe* Oliv. deprived of their awns belonging to family Apocynaceae.

Geographical Source

It is mainly found in East Africa near lakes of Nyasaland and Tanganyika, Portuguese, Cameroon. The tribal are using this seeds as arrow poison.

Cultivation and Collection

The plants are large, woody climbers, climbing on the large trees in the forests of Africa. Fruit consists of two divergent follicles which are dehiscent and many seeded. Each follicle is 30 cm long, 2.5 cm broad, tapering both at the apex and base. Mature and ripe fruits are collected in the month of June–July. After collection epicarp and fleshy mesocarp are removed and seeds separated from yellow-brown leathery endocarp and awns. Seeds are washed and dried. The seeds are derived from anatropous ovules.

Characteristics

The name *Strophanthus* is derived from the Greek *strophos* (a twisted cord or rope) and *anthos* (a flower), thus expressing the chief peculiarity of its appearance, the limb of the corolla being divided into five, long, tail-like segments.

The official description of the seeds is lance-ovoid, flattened and obtusely edged; from 7 to 20 mm in length, about 4 mm in breadth and about 2 mm in thickness; externally of a light fawn colour with a distinct greenish tinge, silky lustrous form, a dense coating of flat-lying hairs (*S. Kombe*) bearing on one side a ridge running from about the centre to the summit; fracture short and somewhat soft, the fractured surface whitish and oily; odour heavy when the seeds are crushed and moistened; taste very bitter.

Microscopy

Epidermis consists of elongated, polygonal, tabular cells and lignified covering trichomes. Next to epidermis collapsed layer of parenchyma cells are present that contain calcium oxalate crystals. Thin walled endosperm contains aleurone grains and fixed oil.

Chemical Constituents

The drug contains 8–10% cardiac glycosides known as k-strophanthin. k-strophanthin is a mixture of three glycosides, cymarin, k-strophanthin P and k-strophanthoside, which differ only through attached sugars and on hydrolysis yields same aglycone strophanthidin. It contains a sugar cymarose that is methoxy digitoxose which gives positive reaction for Keller–Kiliani test. The drug also contains mucilage, resin, fixed oil, choline, trigonelline and kombic acid—an acid saponin.

Chemical Tests

1. Generally, the strophanthus glycosides exhibit an emerald green colouration on the addition of sulphuric acid.
2. Dissolve about 0.1 g of strophanthin in 5 ml of water and add to it a few drops of ferric chloride solution followed by a 1–2 ml of concentrated sulphuric acid; the appearance of an initial red precipitate that finally turns green within a period of 1–2 hours.

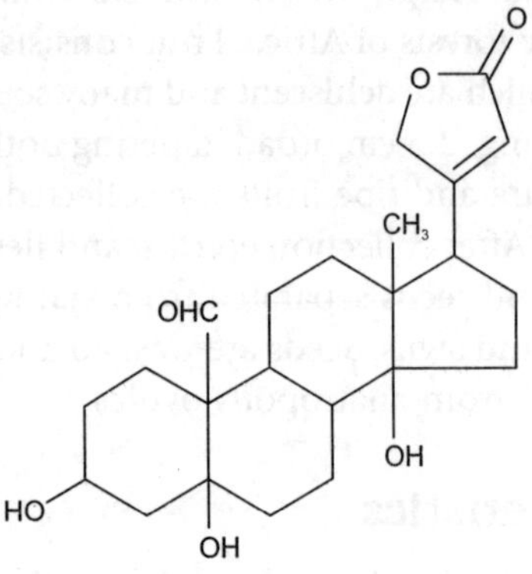

Strophanthidin

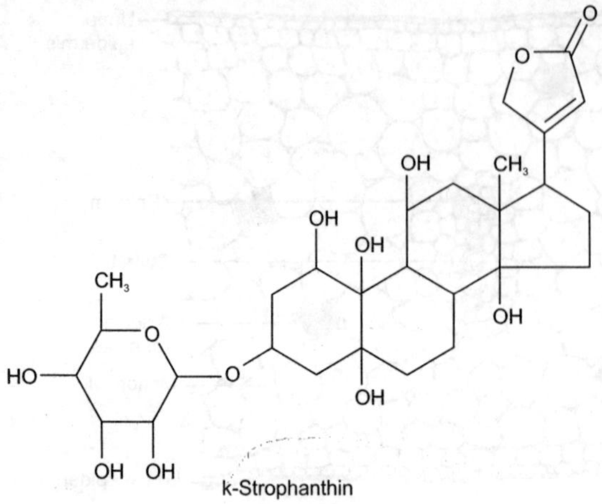

k-Strophanthin

3. To 50 mg of strophanthin add 5 ml of water, shake and add 2 ml of 2% tannic acid solution, the appearance of a distinct precipitate affirms its presence.
4. It shows positive Baljet test, Legal test and Keller–Kiliani test.

Uses

The use of strophanthus in medicine is for its influence on the circulation, especially in cases of chronic heart weakness. As its action is same as that of digitalis, it is often useful as an alternative or adjuvant to the drug. Believed to have greater diuretic power, it is esteemed of greater value in cases complicated with dropsies. Unlike digitalis it has no cumulative property.

Substituents and Adulterants

The *S. kombe* is commonly adulterated with *S. hispidus*, *S. nicholsoni*, *S. gratus*, *S. courmontii*, *S. emini*, *S. sarmentosus*, etc.

S. hispidus has a shape, colour, similar to that of the *S. kombe*, it consist of k-strophanthin. *S. nicholsoni* has a whitish seed; the trichomes form a tangled surface covering. The calcium oxalates are absent in both embryo and the seed coats. *S. gratus* are brown in colour, and has a glabrous appearance to the naked eyes. It reveals the presence of small warty trichomes when observed under the microscope. *S. courmontii* has a brownish tinge and has a similar character to that of the genuine drug. It can be distinguished due to its small size, lanceolate shape and less bitter taste.

OLEANDER

Biological Source

It consists of the dried seeds and leaves of *Nerium indicum* Linn, belonging to family Apocynaceae.

Geographical Source

It is mainly found in the United States, India, West Indies.

Characteristics

Leaves exstipulate, linear, lanceolate 10–20 cm long and up to 2.5 cm wide, thick, dark green and shining above and dotted beneath.

Microscopy

Lamina shows an isobilateral structure, 3–4 layered palisade parenchyma cells below upper and above lower epidermis in the mesophyll, single layer of epidermis covered externally by thick cuticle, epidermal cells elongate to form unicellular, nonlignified and nonglandular hairs; four to seven layers of collenchymatous cells and a wide zone of parenchyma follows the epidermis; parenchymatous cells thin walled, more or less isodiametric with intercellular spaces, some cells contain rosette crystals of calcium oxalate; petiole receives three vascular bundles from stem, central one large and crescent shaped while other two much smaller and somewhat circular present on each side of central vascular bundle. The leaves contain anomocytic type of stomata.

Chemical Constituents

Cardiac glycosides oleandrine, gitoxigenin, neridiginoside, adynerigenin, etc., also it contains terpenoids, sterols, tannins, essential oils.

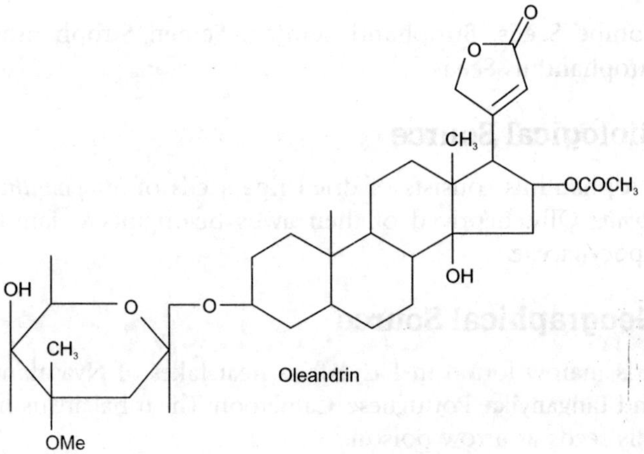

Oleandrin

Uses

Leaves are used in cutaneous eruptions. The paste of the root is applied externally in haemorrhoids and ulcerations.

16.8. SAPONIN GLYCOSIDES

Saponins are glycoside compounds often referred to as a 'natural detergent' because of their foamy texture. They get their name from the soap wort plant (Saponaria), the root of which was used historically as a soap (Latin *sapo*—soap). Foremost among this is the strong tendency to froth formation when shaken with water. The other properties are haemolytic activity, sneezing effect, toxicity, complex formation with cholesterol and antibiotic properties.

Saponins have long been known to have strong biological activity. When studying the effect that saponins have on plants, it has been discovered that saponins are the plants active immune system. They are found in many plants, they consist of a polycyclic aglycone that is either a choline steroid or triterpenoid attached via C_3 and an ether bond to a sugar side chain. The aglycone is referred to as the sapogenin and steroid saponins are called sarsaponins. The ability of a saponin to foam is caused by the combination of the nonpolar sapogenin and the water soluble side chain.

Saponins are bitter and reduce the palatability of livestock feeds. However if they have a triterpenoid aglycone they may instead have a licorice taste as glucuronic acid replaces sugar in triterpenoids. Some saponins reduce the feed intake and growth rate of nonruminant animals while others are not very harmful. For example, the saponins found in oats and spinach increase and accelerate the body's ability to absorb calcium and silicon, thus assisting in digestion. As mentioned earlier they are composed of a steroid (C-27) or triterpenoid (C-30) saponin nucleus with one or more carbohydrate branches.

Steroid Saponins

Steroid saponins are similar to the sapogenins and related to the cardiac glycosides. They have ability to interact medically and beneficially with the cardiac glycosides, sex hormones, Vitamin D and other factors, render these phytochemicals components of great medical significance. Diosgenin is the important steroid sapogenin. Recently from these saponins steroid hormones like progesterone, cortisone, etc., are obtained by partial synthesis and thus their importance has increased considerably. Some of the families with steroidal saponins are Solanaceae, Apocynaceae, Liliaceae, Leguminosae, etc.

Triterpenoid Saponins

Triterpenoid saponins, or sapogenins, are plant glycosides which lather in water and are used in detergents, or as foaming agents or emulsifiers, and have enormous medical implications due to their antifungal, antimicrobial and adaptogenic properties. Triterpene saponins are usually β-amyrin derivatives and some are also α-amyrin and lupeol derivatives. It has a pentacyclic triterpenoid nucleus which is linked with either sugar or uronic acid. Glycyrrhizin, from licorice root, is an example of a saponin used for anti-inflammatory purposes in place of cortisone.

They are commonly available in dicot plants belonging to the family Rubiaceae, Compositae, Rutaceae, Umbelliferae, etc.

Saponins are rarely crystalline and generally amorphous powder with high molecular weight. They carry many asymmetric centres and are optically active. They are generally soluble in water and form colloidal solutions. These are also soluble in ethyl and methyl alcohol and are usually insoluble in organic solvents like petroleum ether, chloroform and acetone, etc. They are bitter in taste and nonalkaline in nature, produce sneezing and have the property of lowering surface tension. They are hydrolysed by acids, alkalies to yield aglycone called sapogenin and one or more molecule of same or different sugars or their oxidation products. They can also be hydrolysed by enzymes, soil bacteria and photolysis. In mild conditions using very dilute acids (0.01–0.1 N), organic acids give rise to partially hydrolysed saponins called prosapogenin.

Saponins are extremely toxic to fishes but do not render them inedible, as saponins are not poisonous to

Tetracyclic triterpenoids
(Steroidal saponins)

Pentacyclic triterpenoids

man when taken orally. Very dilute solution of saponins haemolyses red blood corpuscles. The haemolysis take place due to the formation of complex with the cholesterol of erythrocyte membrane causing its destruction, this is a chief property of saponin, very rarely shown by any other plants product. Saponins accelerate the germination and growth of the seeds. Saponins show fungicidal, bactericidal activity, antiviral activity, antibiotic property, inflammation inhibition activity, spermicidal, antifertility, molluscicidal, etc. Saponins have been reported to possess blood purifying and abortion causing properties, anthelmintic effect, sedative property and antispasmodic effects.

Saponins find wide occurrence in plant kingdom. In a systematic study, 672 triterpenic and 125 steroidal saponins were found in 1730 species belonging to 104 families. In the whole 75% of the families showed the presence of saponins. The wide occurrence and its comparatively higher contents (0.1–30%) in plants, the saponins can be regarded as the most occurring plant materials. Saponins from the different parts of the same plants have found to possess different properties. Saponins may be distributed throughout the plant; their content is affected by variety and stage of growth. Their function in the plant is as storage in form of carbohydrate in the plant and act as immune system of the plant. Saponins have also been identified in the animal kingdom in snake venom, starfish and sea cucumber, etc.

DIOSCOREA

Synonym

Yam.

Biological Source

Dioscorea is the dried rhizome of several species of *Dioscorea* like *D. villosa*, *D. prazeri* Prain and Burk; *D. composite*; *D. spiculiflora*; *D. deltoidea* and *D. floribunda*, belonging to family Dioscoreaceae.

Geographical Source

It is mainly found in North America, Mexico, India (Himalayas from Kashmir and Punjab up to an altitude of 3000 m), Nepal and China.

Cultivation and Collection

It is a perennial climber growing to 3 m. The plant prefers sandy, loamy and clay soils and requires well-drained soil. The plant prefers acid, neutral and basic (alkaline) soils. It can grow in semishade or no shade. It requires moist soil. It can be cultivated in three methods, by sowing seeds or stem cuttings or by tubercles. Seeds are sown in the month of March to April in a sunny position in a warm green

house and only just covered. It germinates in one to three weeks at 20°C. The seedlings are taken out as soon as they are large enough to handle and grown on in a green house for their first year. Transplanted in late spring as the plant comes into new growth. Basal stem cuttings are done in the summer. Division is done in the dormant season, never when in growth. The plant will often produce a number of shoots, the top 5–10 cm of the root below each shoot can be potted up to form a new plant whilst the lower part of the root can possibly be eaten.

Tubercles (baby tubers) are formed in the leaf axils. These are harvested in late summer and early autumn when about the size of a pea and coming away easily from the plant. They should be potted up immediately in individual pots in a greenhouse or cold frame and transplanted out in early summer when in active growth.

Characteristics

The colour of the plant is slightly brown, odourless with bitter taste and vary in size.

Microscopy

The transverse section of the drug when observed under the microscope shows the absence of epidermis, the cork is made up of few layers and next to cork it has cortical parenchymatous tissue with thin wall. The major part of the drug is occupied by stele and consists of collateral type of fibrovascular bundles. The drug has indistinguishable endodermis and pericycle.

Chemical Constituents

The roots contain diosgenin (4–6%) a steroidal sapogenin and its glycoside smilagenin, epismilagenin and beta isomer yammogenin. It also contains sapogenase (enzyme), phenolic compounds and starch (75%).

Diosgenin

Uses

It is a main source of diosgenin. This is widely used in modern medicine in order to manufacture progesterone and other steroid drugs. These are used as contraceptives and in the treatment of various disorders of the genitary organs as well as in a host of other diseases such as asthma and arthritis.

Marketed Products

It is one of the ingredients of the preparations known as Explode (Herbotech Pharmaceuticals).

LIQUORICE

Synonyms

Radix Glycyrrhizae, Sweet liquorice.

Biological Source

Liquorice consists of subterranean peeled and unpeeled stolons, roots and subterranean stems of *Glycyrrhiza glabra* Linn, and other species of *Glycyrrhiza*, belonging to family Leguminosae (Fig. 16.20).

Geographical Source

It is mainly found in China, Europe, India, Iraq, Japan, Kurdistan, Spain, Turkey and the United States.

Cultivation and Collection

Liquorice is often cultivated for its edible root which is widely used in medicine and as flavouring. The plant requires a deep well cultivated fertile moisture-retentive soil for good root production. Prefers a sandy soil with abundant moisture and does not flourish in clay. Slightly alkaline conditions produce the best plants. The plant thrives in a maritime climate. It is propagated using seeds and roots. The seeds are presoaked for 24 h in warm water and then sown in spring or autumn in a greenhouse. The seedlings are individually potted when they are large enough to handle, and grown them for their first winter in a green house. They are transplanted in late spring or early summer when in active growth. Plants are rather slow to grow from seed. The plant parts are procured from old plantations, being waste from the harvesting process, consisting of those side roots or runners which have eyes or buds, cut into sections about 6 inches long. They are dibbled in rows 3 or 4 feet apart, about 4 inches underneath the surface and about 18 inches apart in the rows. In the autumn, the ground is dressed with farmyard manure, about 40 tons to the acre. Plants are slow to settle in and do not produce much growth in their first two years after being moved. The young growth is also very susceptible to damage by slugs and so the plant will require some protection for its first few years. This species has a symbiotic relationship with certain soil bacteria; these bacteria form nodules on the roots and fix atmospheric nitrogen. Some of this nitrogen is utilized by the growing plant but some can also be used by other plants growing nearby.

Harvesting generally occurs in the autumn of the fourth year. The soil is carefully removed from the space between the rows to a depth of 2 or 3 feet as required, thus exposing the roots and rhizomes at the side, the whole being then removed bodily. The earth from the next space is then removed and thrown into the trench thus formed and these operations are repeated continuously. Every portion of the subterranean part of the plant is carefully saved; the drug consists of both runners and roots, the former constituting the major part. The roots are properly washed, trimmed and sorted, and either sold in their entire state or cut into shorter lengths and dried, in the latter case the cortical layer being sometimes removed by scraping. The older or 'hard' runners are sorted out and sold separately; the young, called 'soft,' are reserved for propagation.

Characteristics

Liquorice root is in long, straight, nearly cylindrical, unpeeled pieces, several feet in length, varying in thickness from 1/4 inch to about 1 inch, longitudinally wrinkled, externally greyish brown to dark brown, warty; internally tawny yellow; pliable, tough; texture coarsely fibrous; bark rather thick; wood porous, but dense, in narrow wedges; taste sweet, very slightly acrid. The underground stem which is often present has a similar appearance, but contains thin pith. When peeled, the pieces of root (including runners) are shorter, a pale yellow, slightly fibrous externally, and exhibit no trace of the small dark buds seen on the unpeeled runners here and there. Otherwise it resembles the unpeeled.

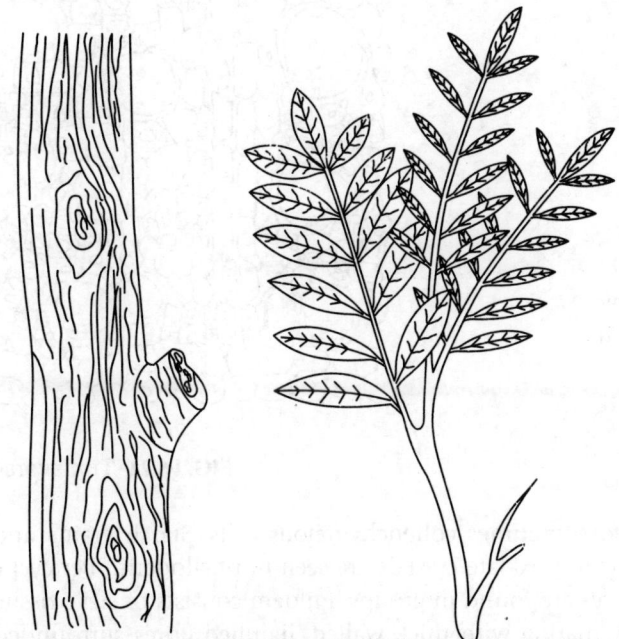

FIG. 16.20 Root and twig of *Glycyrrhiza glabra*

Microscopy (Fig. 16.21)

Cork consists of several rows of radially arranged thin walled tubular cells. Phelloderm is composed of parenchymatous

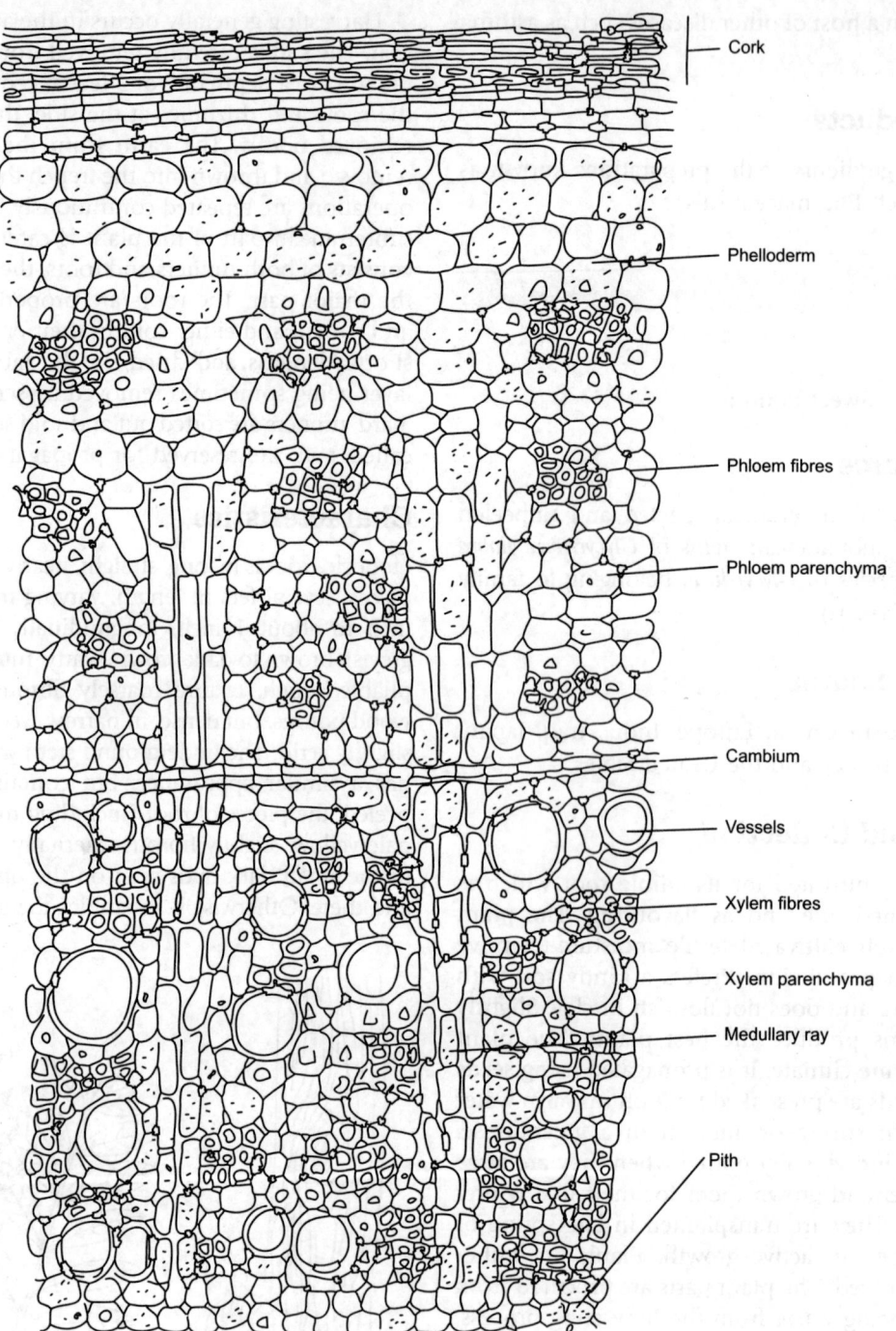

Cork

Phelloderm

Phloem fibres

Phloem parenchyma

Cambium

Vessels

Xylem fibres

Xylem parenchyma

Medullary ray

Pith

FIG. 16.21 Transverse section of liquorice stolon

and sometimes collenchymatous cells. Starch grains and calcium oxalate crystals are seen in phelloderm. Pericyclic fibres are found in groups. Phloem consists of sieve tissue alternating with thick walled, lignified fibres surrounded by a sheath of parenchymatous cells containing prisms of calcium oxalate. Xylem vessels and xylem parenchyma are present. Medullary rays are radially elongated. Pith is present in rhizomes and absent in root.

Powder Microscopy (Fig. 16.22)

The powder is pale,S yellowish-brown in colour with characteristic odour and sweet taste. Microscopical examination shows abundant starch grains (3–20 μm long), simple or compound (2–4 components), slightly flattened, spherical-oval with a slit-shaped hilum. Fibres occur in groups, slightly pitted, surrounded by a sheath

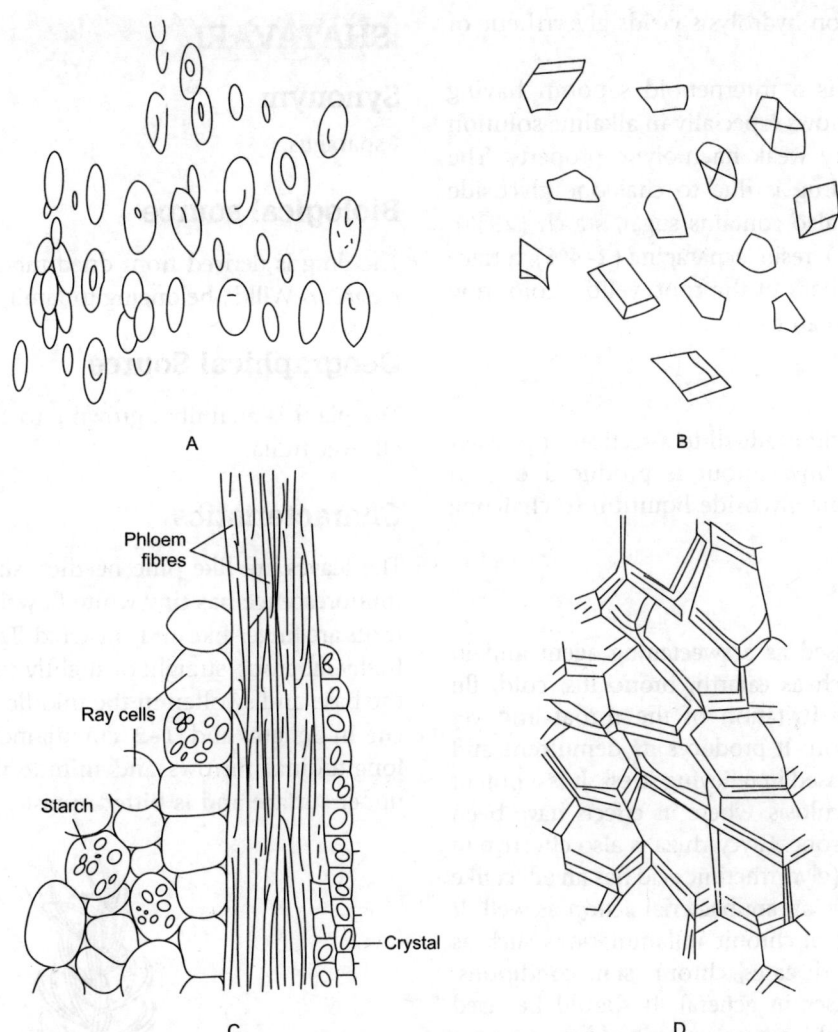

FIG. 16.22 Powder characteristics of liquorice stolon. (A: Starch grains, B: Prismatic calcium oxalate crystals, C: Phloem fibres, D: Cork cells)

Phloem fibres

Ray cells

Starch

Crystal

of prismatic calcium oxalate crystals. Cork cells, thick-walled, polygonal in surface view; abundant parenchyma, thin-walled cells, spherical to rectangular, filled with starch grains; abundant vessels, large and small, bordered pitted; and prismatic calcium oxalate crystals (up to 30 μm long) are found scattered.

Chemical Constituents

The chief constituent of liquorice root is glycyrrhizin (6–8%), obtainable in the form of a sweet, which is 50 times sweeter than sucrose, white crystalline powder, consisting of the calcium and potassium salts of glycyrrhizic

Glycyrrhetinic acid

Glycyrrhetic acid

acid. Glycyrrhizic acid on hydrolysis yields glycyrrhetic or glycyrrhetinic acid.

Glycyrrhizinic acid is a triterpenoid saponin having α-amyrin structure. It shows especially in alkaline solution frothing but it has very weak haemolytic property. The yellow colour of the drug is due to chalcone glycoside isoliquiritin. The drug also contains sugar, starch (29%), gum, protein, fat (0.8%), resin, asparagine (2–4%), a trace of tannin in the outer bark of the root, yellow colouring matter and 0.03% of volatile oil.

Chemical Test

When 80% sulphuric acid is added to a section or powder of the drug orange yellow colour is produced due to transformation of flavone glycoside liquiritin to chalcone glycoside isoliquiritin.

Uses

Glycyrrhiza is widely used as a sweetening agent and in bronchial problems such as catarrh, bronchitis, cold, flu and coughs. It reduces irritation of the throat and yet has an expectorant action. It produces its demulcent and expectorant effects. It is used in relieving stress. It is a potent healing agent for tuberculosis, where its effects have been compared to hydrocortisone. Glycyrrhiza is also effective in helping to reduce fevers (glycyrrhetinic acid has an effect like aspirin), and it may have an antibacterial action as well. It is used in the treatment of chronic inflammations such as arthritis and rheumatic diseases, chronic skin conditions, and autoimmune diseases in general. It should be used in moderation and should not be prescribed for pregnant women or people with high blood pressure, kidney disease or taking digoxin-based medication. Prolonged usage raises the blood pressure and causes water retention. Externally, the root is used in the treatment of herpes, eczema and shingles.

Substitutes and Adulterants

Glycyrrhiza uralansis, also known as Manchurian Liquorice, which is pale chocolate brown in appearance having wavy medullary rays and exfoliated cork, is mostly used as an adulterant for *G. glabra*. This particular species is from sugar, but contains glycyrrhizin. Sometimes, the Russian Liquorice is also used as an adulterant, because the drug is purplish in appearance, has long roots and is without stolons.

Marketed Products

It is one of the ingredients of the preparations known as Herbolex, Koflet, Regurin (Himalaya Drug Company), Jeevani malt (Chirayu Pharma), Eladi Bati, Madhumehari (Baidyanath), J.P. Nikhar oil, J.P. Kasantak (Jamuna Pharma), Respinova (Lupin Herbal Laboratory) and Yastimadhu (Zandu Pharmaceuticals Works Ltd.).

SHATAVARI

Synonym

Asparagus.

Biological source

The drug is derived from dried tuberous roots of *Asparagus racemosus* Willd., belonging to family Liliaceae (Fig. 16.23).

Geographical Source

The plant is a climber growing to 1–2 m in length found all over India.

Characteristics

The leaves are like pine needles, small and uniform. The influorescence has tiny white flowers, in small spikes. The roots are finger-like and clustered. The roots are cylindrical, fleshy raberous, straight or slightly curved, tapering towards the base and swollen in the middle; white to colour, 5–15 cm in length and 1–2 cm diameter, irregular fracture, longitudinal furrows and minute transverse wrinkles on upper surface and is bitter in taste.

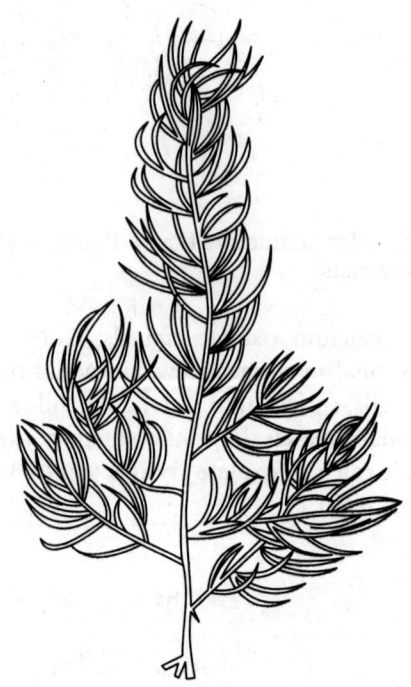

FIG. 16.23 *Asparagus racemosus*

Powder Microscopy (Fig. 16.24)

The powder is white in colour with slight odour. Microscopical examination shows abundant vessels with spiral thickening and tracheids with pitted thickening. Acicular crystals of calcium oxalate are found scattered or usually in bundles in parenchymatous cells of cortex. Cork

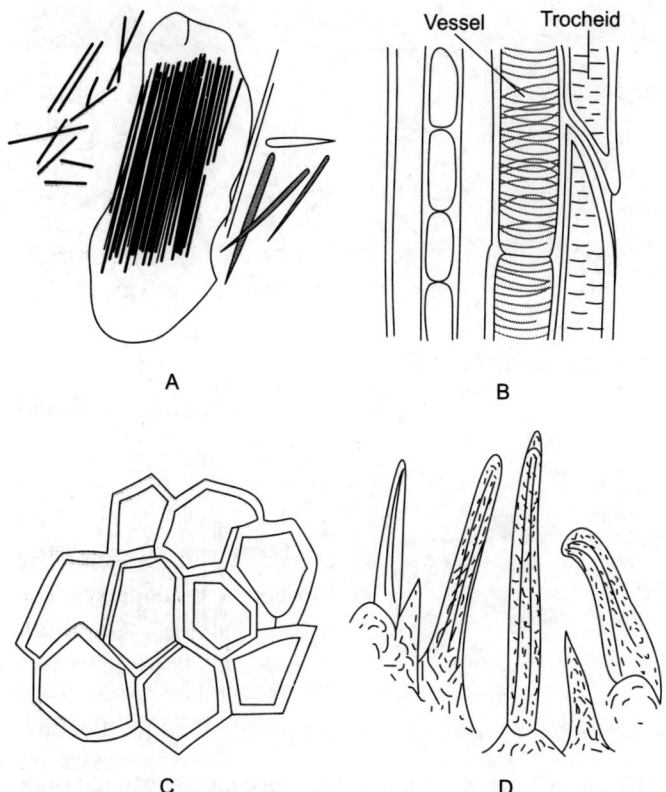

FIG. 16.24 Powder characteristics of asparagus root. (A: Acicular calcium oxalate crystals, B: Vessel and tracheid, C: Cork cell, D: Root hairs)

cells, small root hairs and a few pitted parenchyma of pith region are found in fragments.

Chemical Constituents

The active constituents are steroidal saponins, such as, Shatavarin I-IV (0.1–0.2%). The aglycone unit is sarsapogenin. In shatavarin I three glucose and one rhamnose molecules are attached whereas shatavarin IV possesses two glucose and one rhamnose molecules. The other compounds isolated from *A. racemosus* are β-sitosterol, stigmasterol, their glycosides, sarsasapogenin, spirostanolic acid, furostanolic saponins, 4,6-dihydroxy-2-O-(2′-hydroxy-isobutyl) benzaldehyde, undecanyl cetanoate and polycyclic alkaloid asparagamine A.

Uses

The root is alterative, antispasmodic, aphrodisiac, demulcent, diuretic, galactagogue and refrigerant. It is taken internally in the treatment of infertility, loss of libido, threatened miscarriage, menopausal problems, hyperacidity, stomach ulcers and bronchial infections. Externally it is used to treat stiffness in the joints. The root is used fresh in the treatment of dysentery.

Marketed Products

It is one of the ingredients of the preparations known as K.G. Tone (Aimil), Menosan, Diabecon, Galactin, Abana (Himalaya), Dhatupaushtik churna, Rhuma oil, Brahmi Rasayan, Mahanarayan tel (Baidyanath), J.P. Massaj oil, Painkill oil (Jamuna Pharma), Memoplus, Jeevani malt (Chirayu) and Shatavari kalpa and Satavarex granules (Zandu).

BRAHMI

Synonyms

Indian Pennywort, Mangosteen.

Biological Source

Brahmi is the fresh or dried herb of *Centella asiatica* (L.) (syn. *Hydrocotyl asiatica* Linn.), belonging to family Umbelliferae (Fig. 16.25).

Shatavarin

Geographical Source

The plant is found in swampy areas of India, commonly found as a weed in crop fields and other waste places throughout India up to an altitude of 600 m and also in Pakistan, Sri Lanka and Madagascar.

Characteristics

It is a slender, herbaceous creeper. Stems are long, prostate, filiform, often reddish and with long internodes, rooting at nodes. Leaves are long-petioled, 1.3–6.3 cm in diameter, several from rootstock and 1–3 cm from each node of stem. They are orbicular, reniform, rather broader than long, glabrous on both sides and with numerous slender nerves from a deeply cordate base. Fruit 8 mm long, ovoid, hard with a thick pericarp.

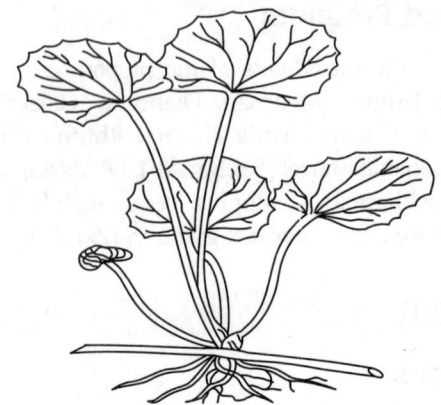

FIG. 16.25 *Centella asiatica*

Microscopy

Root: Outer cork consisting of three- to five-layered, exfoliated rectangular cells, followed by cortex region consisting three or four layers of parenchyma cells containing oval to round, simple, starch grains and microsphenoidal crystals of calcium oxalate; secondary cortex composed of thin walled, oval to polygonal parenchymatous cells. Secretory cells are also present.

Stem: Single layered epidermis composed of round to cubical cells covered by striated cuticle. Two or three layers of collenchymatous cells are found below the epidermis, collenchymatous cells are followed by six to eight layers of thin walled, isodiametric, parenchymatous cells with intercellular space present; vascular bundles collateral, open, arranged in a ring, capped, by patches of sclerenchyma and traversed by wide medullary rays. Resin ducts are also present in parenchymatous cells of cortex; pith consists of isodiametric parenchyma cells with intercellular spaces.

Leaf: Single layered epidermis covered by a thick cuticle, two- or three-layered collenchyma in the midrib region on

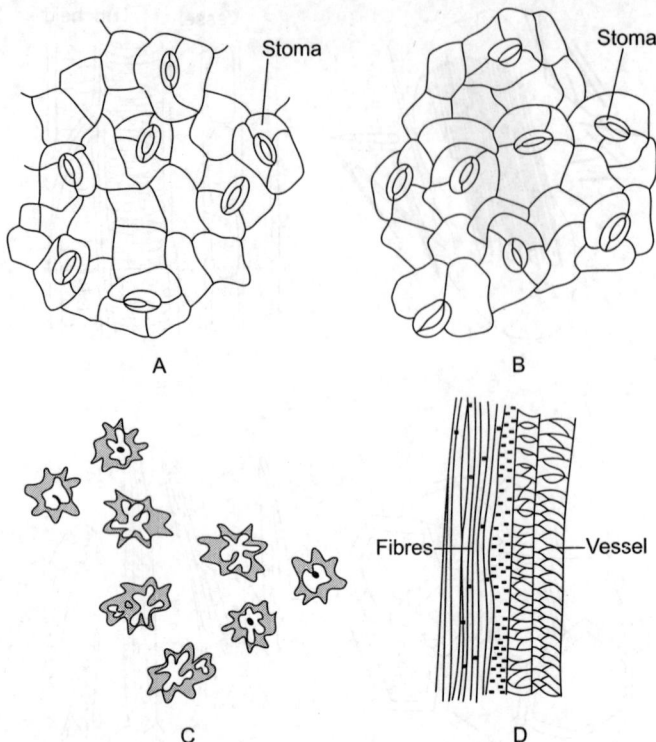

FIG. 16.26 Powder characteristics of centella leaf. (A: Upper epidermis in surface view, B: Lower epidermis in surface view, C: Calcium oxalate crystals, D: Vessels and Fibres)

both surfaces, central zone occupied by vascular bundles, mesophyll consists of two or three layers of palisade cells, five to seven layers of loosely arranged, more or less isodiametric spongy parenchyma cells. Rosette type crystals of calcium oxalate and anisocytic stomata are also present. Few anomocytic stomata are also seen.

Powder Microscopy (Fig. 16.26)

The powder is green in colour. Microscopic examination shows epidermal cells with slightly straight anticlinal walls and characteristic stomata. Fragments of pitted vessels with spiral thickening, cluster of calcium oxalate crystals, collenchyma and palisade cells are found scattered.

Chemical Constituents

The drug contains triterpenoid saponin glycosides, indocentelloside, brahmoside, brahminoside, asiaticosides, thankuniside and isothankuniside. The corresponding trirerpene acids obtained on hydrolysis of the glycosides are indocentoic, brahmic, asiatic, thankunic and isothankunic acids. These acids, except the last two, are also present in free form in the plant from isobrahmic and betulic acids. The presence of mesoinositol, a new oligosaccharide, centellose, kaempferol, quercetin and stigmasterol, have also been reported.

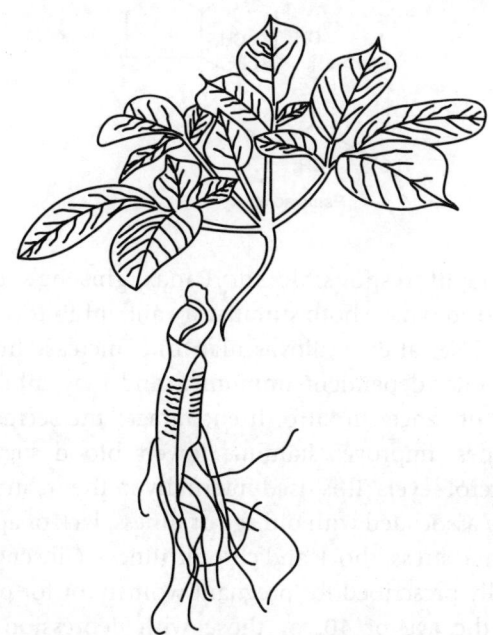

	R1	R2
Asiatic acid	-H	-OH
Madecassic acid	-OH	-OH
Asiaticoside	-H	-O-glu-glu-rha
Madecassoside	-OH	-O-glu-glu-rha

Uses

The plant is used as tonic, in diseases of skin, nerves, blood and also to improve memory. It also strengthens our immune system. Asiaticosides stimulate the reticuloendothelial system where new blood cells are formed and old ones destroyed, fatty materials are stored, iron is metabolized, and immune responses and inflammation occur or begin. The primary mode of action of centella appears to be on the various phases of connective tissue development, which are part of the healing process. Centella also increases keratinization, the process of building more skin in areas of infection such as sores and ulcers. Asiaticosides also stimulate the synthesis of lipids and proteins necessary for healthy skin. Finally centella strengthens veins by repairing the connective tissues surrounding veins and decreasing capillary fragility.

Marketed Products

It is one of the ingredients of the preparations known as Iqmen (Lupin Herbal Lab.) and Abana, Geriforte, Menosan and Mentat (Himalaya Drug Company).

GINSENG

Synonyms

Panax, Asiatic Ginseng, Chinese Ginseng, Ginseng Root, Pannag, Ninjin.

Biological Source

It consists of dried roots of *Panax ginseng* C.A. Mey and other species of Panax like *Panax japonicus* (Japanese Ginseng), *Panax pseudoginseng* (Himalayan Ginseng), *Panax quinquefolius* (American Ginseng), *Panax trifolius* (Dwarf Ginseng) and *Panax vietnamensis* (Vietnamese Ginseng), belonging to family Araliaceae (Fig. 16.27).

Geographical Source

It is mainly found in China, Russia, Korea, Japan, Canada and India.

History

Ancient healers in India, Russia, China and Japan all revered ginseng for its medicinal and health-enhancing properties. In traditional Chinese medicine (TCM), ginseng is used for many purposes, including normalizing blood pressure and blood sugar, as a sexual tonic for both men and women and to strengthen overall health when the body is debilitated.

The botanical name *Panax* comes from the Greek word panacea, meaning 'cure all.' The Chinese name for ginseng, *ren shen*, means 'man root' for its characteristic shape that resembles the trunk, arms and legs of a human being.

FIG. 16.27 *Panax ginseng*

Chemical Constituents

Several saponin glycosides belonging to triterpenoid group, ginsenoside, chikusetsusaponin, panaxoside. More than 13 ginsenosides have been identified. Ginsenosides consists of aglycone dammarol where as panaxosides have oleanolic acid as aglycone. It also contains large amount of starch, gum, some resin and a very small amount of volatile oil.

Uses

The root is adaptogen, alterative, carminative, demulcent, emetic, expectorant, stimulant and tonic. The saponin glycosides, also known as ginsenosides or panaxosides,

Oleanolic acid

Panaxadiol

are thought responsible for Panax ginseng's effects. Ginsenosides have both stimulatory and inhibitory effects on the CNS, alter cardiovascular tone, increase humoral and cellular-dependent immunity, and may inhibit the growth of cancer in vitro. It encourages the secretion of hormones, improves stamina, lowers blood sugar and cholesterol levels. It is used internally in the treatment of debility associated with old age or illness, lack of appetite, insomnia, stress, shock and chronic illness. Ginseng is not normally prescribed for pregnant women, or for patients under the age of 40, or those with depression, acute anxiety or acute inflammatory disease. It is normally only taken for a period of 3 weeks. Excess can cause headaches, restlessness, raised blood pressure and other side effects, especially if it is taken with caffeine, alcohol, turnips and bitter or spicy foods.

Substitutes

Codonopsis tangshen, a bell-flowered plant, used by the poor people in China as a substitute for the costly Ginseng.

Ginseng is sometimes accidentally collected with Senega Root (*Polygala senega*, Linn.) and with Virginian Snake Root (*Aristolochia serpentaria*, Linn.), but it is easily detected, being less wrinkled and twisted and yellower in colour.

Blue Cohosh (*Caulophyllum thalictroides*, Linn.) is often called locally in the United States 'Blue' or 'Yellow Ginseng,' and Fever Root (*Triosteum perfoliatum*, Linn.) also is sometimes given the name of Ginseng.

SENEGA

Synonyms

Snake root, Senegae radix, Seneca, Milkwort, Mountain flax, Rattlesnake root, Radix senegae, Senega root.

Biological Source

Senega consists of dried roots and rootstocks of *Polygala senega* Linn., belonging to family Polygalaceae (Fig. 16.28).

Geographical Source

Grows throughout central and western North America and Canada.

History

The name of the genus, *Polygala*, means 'much milk,' alluding to its own profuse secretions and their effects. 'Senega' is derived from the Seneca tribe of North American Indians, among whom the plant was used as a remedy for snake bites.

Cultivation and Collection

It is a perennial growing to 0.3 m × 0.3 m. Prefers a moderately fertile moisture-retentive well-drained soil, succeeding in full sun if the soil remains moist throughout the growing season, otherwise it is best in semishade. It is propagated by seeds or cuttings. Seeds are sown in spring or autumn in a cold frame. When the seedlings are large enough to handle, they are kept in individual pots and grown them on in the green house for their first winter. They are transplanted in late spring or early summer, after the last expected frosts.

The roots should be gathered when the leaves are dead, and before the first frost. Roots are dug out and the aerial stems attached to them are removed. From carelessness in collection other roots are often found mixed with it, but not for intentional adulteration. However some stem bases persist in the drug. Roots are washed and dried.

Characteristics

The root, varying in colour from light yellowish grey to brownish grey, and in size from the thickness of a straw to that of the little finger, has as its distinguishing mark a projecting line, along its concave side. It is usually twisted,

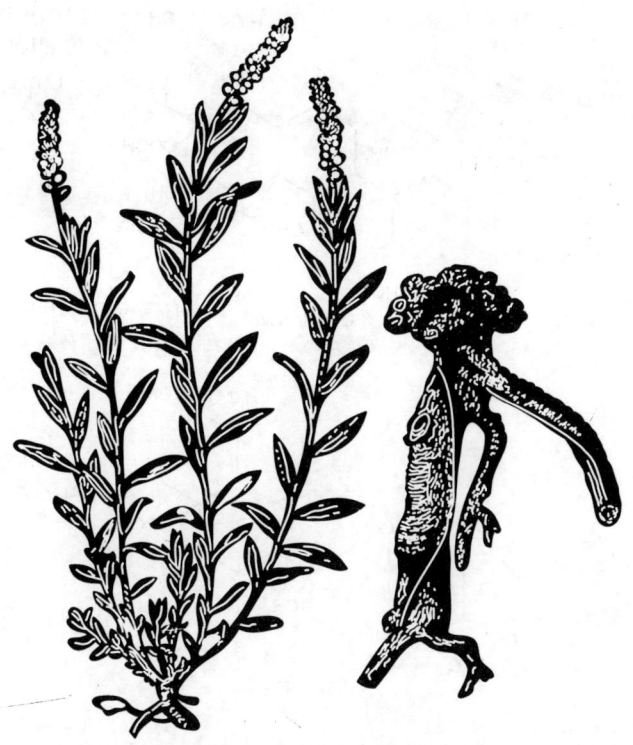

FIG. 16.28 Rootstocks of *Polygala senega*

sometimes almost spiral, and has at its upper end a thick, irregular, knotty crown, showing traces of numerous, wiry stems. It breaks with a short fracture, the wood often showing an abnormal appearance, since one or two wedge-shaped portions may be replaced by parenchymatous tissue, as if a segment of wood had been cut out. The keels are due to the development of the bast, and not to any abnormality in the wood. It taste sweet first and then turns to acrid and have characteristic odour.

Chemical Constituents

The root contains triterpenoid saponins. The active principle, contained in the bark, is senegin. It is a white powder easily soluble in hot water and alcohol, forming a soapy emulsion when mixed with boiling water.

Senega contains 8–10% of a mixture of at least eight different saponins. The main saponin is senegin, which on hydrolysis yields presenegenin, glucose, galactose, rhamnose and xylose. The root contains polygalic acid, virgineic acid, pectic and tannic acids, yellow, bitter, colouring matter, cerin, fixed oil, gum, albumen, woody fibre, salts, alumina, silica, magnesia and iron.

Uses

The root promotes the clearing of phlegm from the bronchial tubes. It is antidote, cathartic, diaphoretic, diuretic, emetic, expectorant, sialagogue and stimulant. It was used by the North American Indians in the treatment of snake bites and has been found used in the treatment of various respiratory problems including pleurisy and pneumonia.

Allied Drugs

Polygala senega var. *latifolia.* (Northern senega), collected in the northwestern states, is considerably larger than the usual variety (Western senega), and darker in colour; it shows the keel less distinctly, but it has a very acrid taste.

QUILLAIA

Synonyms

Quillaia; Soap bark, Quillary bark, Panama bark; China bark, Murillo bark, Panama wood; Cortex quillaiae.

Biological Source

Quillaia bark is the inner dried bark of *Quillaia saponaria* Molina and other species of *Quillaia*, belonging to family Rosaceae (Fig. 16.29).

Geographical Source

Q. saponaria is about 18 m high evergreen, graceful tree found in Peru, Chile, Bolivia, South America and California.

Characteristics

Quillaia bark occurs in flat pieces, about 1 m long, 20 cm wide and 3–10 cm thick. Outer surface is brownish-white, smooth and contains reddish- or blackish-brown patches

H₃C   CH₃

CH₃   CH₃   COO - fructose

rhamnose - xylose - galactose

3,4-dimethoxycinnamic acid

HO   CH₂OH

glucose — O

H₃C   COOH

Senegin

of rhytidome adhere to the outer surface. The rhytidome is made of dead secondary phloem. The inner surface is yellowish-white and smooth. Fracture is splintery. Large crystals of calcium oxalate are present. Odour is sternutatory and taste is acidic and astringent.

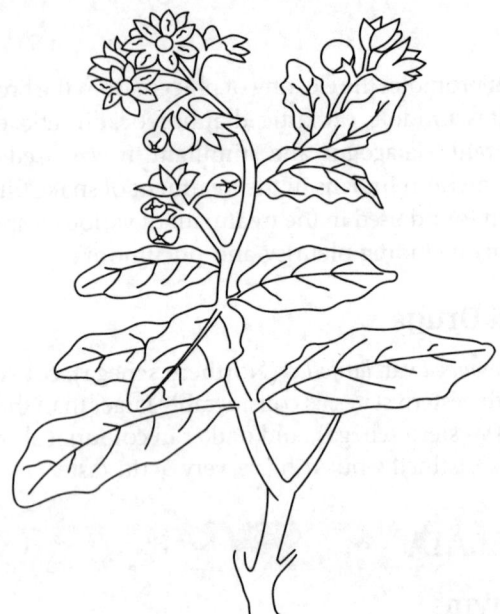

FIG. 16.29 *Quillaia saponaria*

Microscopy

A transverse section of quillaia bark shows alternating bands of lignified and nonlignified phloem. The medullary rays are usually two to four cells wide. The phloem fibres are tortuous and often accompanied by small groups of rectangular sclereids. The parenchyma contains numerous starch grains and calcium oxalate prism.

Chemical Constituents

Quillaia bark contains saponins (10%), quillaic acid, calcium oxalate, starch, sucrose and tannin. Quillaia saponin on hydrolysis forms pentacyclic triterpenoid, quillaic acid (Quillaia sapogenin), a sugar glucuronic acid and gypsogenin.

Chemical Tests

1. Powdered drug on shaking with water produces soap like froth which persists for some time.
2. On addition of a small portion of drug or its alcoholic extract in a drop of blood on a microscopic slide, a haemolytic zone surrounding the drug is formed.

Uses

Quillaia bark is used as an emulsifying agent, for coal tar emulsion, cleaning industrial equipments, washing

Quillaic acid

Gypsogenin

delicate fabrics, to prepare tooth powders, tooth pastes, hair shampoos, hair tonics, tar solutions and metal polishes. It is added in topical preparations for skin disorders, and as a protective agent for cracks, bruises, frostbite and insect bites. The drug is highly irritating and causes nausea and is expectorant on internal consumption. It is diuretic and a cutaneous stimulant.

GOKHRU

Synonym

Caltrops fruit.

Biological Source

In Ayurveda two types of Gokhru are used, that is, Bada and Chota Gokhru. The smaller or Chota Gokhru is the dried ripe seeds of *Tribulus terrestris* Linn., belonging to family Zygophyllaceae (Fig. 16.30).

Geographical Source

The plant is an annual, prostrate herb growing throughout India up to 3500 m in Kashmir.

Characteristics

The fruits are yellowish in colour, globose, 1.2 cm in diameter containing five woody, densely hairy, spiny cocci. Large pointed spines are present in each coccus. Two smaller and shorter spines are directed downwards. Several seeds are present in each coccus.

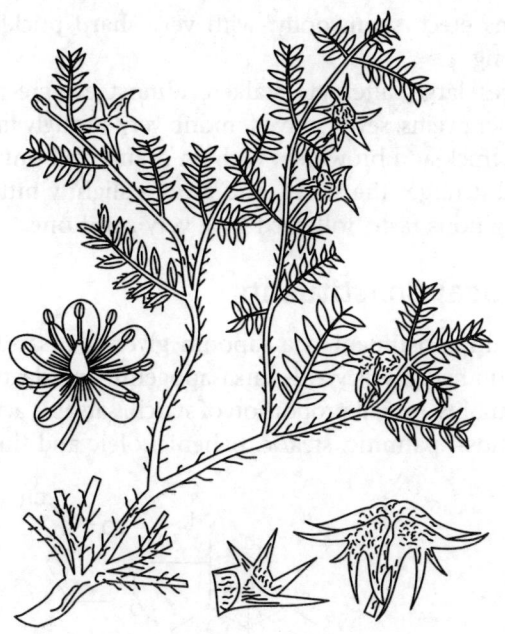

FIG. 16.30 *Tribulus terrestris*

Microscopy

Fruit section shows small rectangular epidermal cells of each coccus. Unicellular trichomes are found on the surface; 6–10 layers of large parenchymatous cells forms mesocarp, next to mesocarp three to four compact layers of small cells are present which contains rosette of calcium oxalate crystals.

Chemical Constituents

The dried fruits of *T. terstris* consist of steroidal saponins as the major constituents. It includes terestrosins A, B, C, D and E, desgalactotigonin, F-gitonin, desglucolanatigonin and gitonin. The hydrolysed extract consists of sapogenins such as diosgenin, chlorogenin, hecogenin and neotigogenin. Certain other steroidal such as terestroside F, tribulosin, trillin, gracillin, dioscin have also been isolated from the aerial parts of the herb. The flavonoid derivatives reported from the fruits includes tribuloside and number of other glycosides of quercetin, kaempferol and isorhamnetin. It also consists of common phytosterols, such as, β-sitosterol, stigmasterol and cinnamic amide derivative, terestiamide.

Uses

The fruit has cooling, anti-inflammatory, antiarthritic, diuretic, tonic, aphrodisiac properties. It is used in building immune system, in painful micturition, calculus affections and impotency. Improves and prolongs the duration of erection. It exerts a stimulating effect on reproductory organs.

Terestrosin A,   R = H
Terestrosin E,   R = OH

Trillin,   R = Glu
Gracillin,   R = Glu-Glu-Rha

Chlorogenin

Tribulosin

Marketed Products

It is one of the ingredients of the preparations known as Bonnisan, Confido, Himplasia, Renalka (Himalaya), Dhatupaushtik churna (Baidyanath), Semento (Aimil) and Body plus capsule (Jay Pranav Ayurvedic Pharmaceuticals).

SARSAPARILLA

Synonyms

Smilax Medica, Red-bearded Sarsaparilla, Radix sarsae, Radix sarsaparillea, Jamaica sarsaparilla.

Biological Source

It consists of dried roots of *Smilax ornata* Hooker., belonging to family Liliaceae (Fig. 16.31).

Characteristics

This plant derived its name from being exported to Europe through Jamaica. The word Sarsaparilla comes from the Spanish *Sana*, meaning a bramble, and *parilla*, a vine, in allusion to the thorny stems of the plant.

It is a large perennial climber, the drugs are found bundles in the market, each bundles consists of numerous long slender roots 3 mm in thickness. They are dark red to brown in colour. They are shrunken and furrowed longitudinally and bear numerous root lets. They are tough and flexible difficult to break. It is odourless and slight bitter in taste.

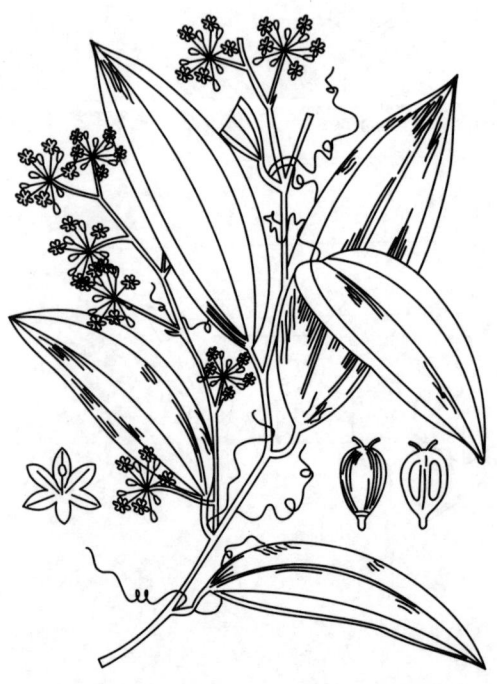

FIG. 16.31 *Smilax ornata*

Stems erect, semiwoody, with very sharp prickles 1/2 inch long.

Leaves large, alternate stalked, almost evergreen with prominent veins, seven nerved midrib very strongly marked. Cortex thick and brownish, with an orange red tint; when chewed it tinges the saliva, and gives a slightly bitter and mucilaginous taste, followed by a very acrid one.

Chemical Constituents

The main constituent is a saponin glycoside, sarsaponin which on hydrolysis yields sarsasapogenin and dextrose. It also contains a small proportion of starch, sarsapic acid, and fatty acids—palmitic, stearic, behenic, oleic and linolic.

Sarsasapogenin

Uses

Used in chronic skin diseases, rheumatism, passive dropsy and in syphilis.

Other Species

Smilax officinalis (Native Jamaica Sarsaparilla) is obtained from the same place and it could be distinguished by colour, size and other characters. It has a twining stem, angular and prickly; young shoots unarmed; leaves ovate, oblong, acute, cordate, smooth, 1 foot long; petioles 1 inch long, having tendrils above the base. It consists of very long roots, with a thick bark, grey or brown colour. The roots bear scattered, stout rootlets. It is odourless and has mucilaginous taste.

Marketed Products

It is one of the ingredients of the preparation known as Purodil Capsules and Syrup (Aimil Pharmaceuticals).

16.9. CYANOGENIC GLYCOSIDES

These are the glycosides which on hydrolysis yields hydrocynic acid (HCN), benzaldehyde and sugars. The medicinal activity of cyanogenetic glycosides is due to presence of hydrocyanic acid and these are the characteristics of family Rosaceae. For examples amygdalin obtained from bitter almond (*Prunus amygdalus*), prunasin obtained from wild cherry bark.

Identification Tests

1. A strip of white filter paper is dipped in 10% aqueous solution of picric acid, drain it and dip in a 10% sodium carbonate solution and drain again. Moisten the powdered drug with water and put into a conical flask. Trap the sodium picrate paper on the neck of flask with cork. Because of volatile hydrocyanic acid, the paper will become brick red colour.
2. When drug treated with 3% aqueous solution of mercurous nitrate reduction to metallic mercury takes place.

ALMOND

Biological Source

Almond oil is a fixed oil obtained by expression from the seeds of *Prunus amygdalus* (Rosaceae) var. dulcis (sweet almonds) or *P. amygdalus* var. amara (bitter almonds) (Fig. 16.32).

Geographical Source

The oil is mainly produced from almonds grown in the countries bordering the Mediterranean (Italy, France, Syria, Spain and North Africa) and Iran.

Characteristics

Almond trees are about 5 m in height. The young fruits have a soft, felt-like pericarp, the inner part of which gradually becomes sclerenchymatous as the fruit ripens to form a pitted endocarp or shell. The shells, consisting mainly of sclerenchymatous cells, are sometimes ground and used to adulterate powdered drugs.

The sweet almond is 2–3 cm in length, rounded at one end and pointed at the other. The bitter almond is 1.5–2 cm in length but of similar breadth to the sweet almond. Both varieties have a thin, cinnamon-brown testa which is easily removed after soaking in warm water. The oily kernel consists of two large, oily planoconvex cotyledons, and a small plumule and radicle, the latter lying at the pointed end of the seed. Some almonds have cotyledons of unequal sizes and are irregularly folded. Bitter almonds are found in samples of sweet almonds; their presence may be detected by the sodium picrate test for cyanogenetic glycosides.

Chemical Constituents

Both varieties of almond contain 40–55% of fixed oil, about 20% of proteins, mucilage and emulsin. The bitter almonds contain in addition 2.5–4.0% of the colourless, crystalline, cyanogenic glycoside, amygdalin.

Almond oil is obtained by grinding the seeds and expressing, them in canvas bags between slightly heated iron plates. The oil is clarified by subsidence and filtration. It is a pale yellow liquid with a slight odour and bland nutty taste. It contains olein, with smaller quantities of the glycosides of linoleic and other acids. Bitter almonds, after maceration on hydrolysis of amygdalin yield a volatile oil that is used as a flavouring agent. Sweet almonds are extensively used as a food, but bitter almonds are not suitable for this purpose.

Essential or volatile oil of almonds is obtained from the cake left after expressing bitter almonds. This is macerated with water for some hours to allow hydrolysis of the amygdalin to take place. The benzaldehyde and hydrocyanic acid are then separated by stem distillation.

Almond oil consists of a mixture of glycerides of oleic (62–86%), linoleic (17%), palmitic (5%), myristic (1%), palmitoleic, margaric, stearic, linolenic, arachidic, gadoleic, behenic and erucic acid. Bitter almond oil contains benzaldehyde and 2–4% of hydrocyanic acid. Purified volatile oil of bitter almonds has all its hydrocyanic acid removed and, therefore, consists mainly of benzaldehyde. The unsaponifiable matter contains β-sitosterol, Δ^5-avenasterol, cholesterol, brassicasterol and tocopherols.

Uses

Expressed almond oil is an emollient and an ingredient in cosmetics. Almond oil is used as a laxative, emollient, in the preparation of toilet articles and as a vehicle for oily injections. The volatile almond oils are used as flavouring agents.

Marketed Products

It is one of the ingredients of the preparations known as Baidyanath lal tail (Baidyanath Company), Himcolin gel, Mentat, Tentex Royal (Himalaya Drug Company) and Sage badam roghan (Sage Herbals).

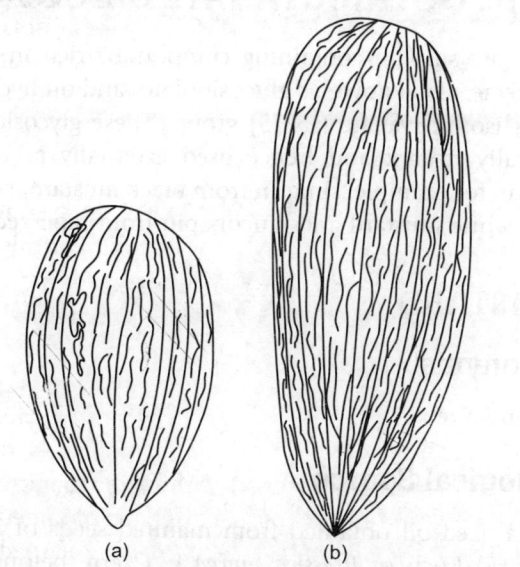

FIG. 16.32 (a) Bitter almond and (b) sweet almond

WILD CHERRY BARK

Synonyms

Virginian Prune, Black Cherry, Virginian Bark, Cortex Pruni.

Biological Source

Wild cherry bark is the dried bark of *Prunus serotina* Ehrhart., belonging to family Rosaceae (Fig. 16.33).

Geographical Source

North America generally, especially in Northern and Central States.

Cultivation and Collection

This tree grows from 50 to 80 feet high, and 2–4 feet in diameter. The bark is collected in autumn from young branches and stem. In some cases cork and cortex are removed after collection, by peeling. If the bark is peeled it is called rossed bark and if not peeled, it is unrossed barks. It is carefully dried and preserved in airtight containers.

Characteristics

The bark is black and rough and separates naturally from the trunk. Leaves deciduous, 3–5 inches long, about 2 inches wide, petioles have two pairs of reddish glands, they are obovate, acuminate, with incurved short teeth, thickish and smooth and glossy on upper surface; flowers bloom in May, and are white, in erect long terminal racemes, with occasional solitary flowers in the axils of the leaves.

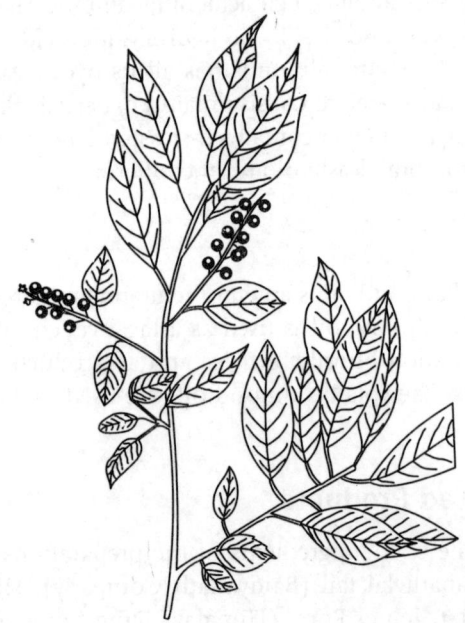

FIG. 16.33 *Prunus serotina*

Fruit about the size of a pea, purply-black, globular drupe, edible with bitterish taste, is ripe in August and September. The root-bark is of most value, but that of the trunk and branches is also utilized. This bark must be freshly collected each season as its properties deteriorate greatly if kept longer than a year. It has a short friable fracture, and in commerce, it is found in varying lengths and widths of 1–8 inches, slightly curved, outer bark removed with a reddish-fawn colour. These fragments easily powder. It has the odour of almonds, which almost disappears on drying, but is renewed by maceration. Its taste is aromatic, prussic and bitter. It imparts its virtues to water or alcohol, boiling impairs its medicinal properties.

Chemical Constituents

It contains prunasin, a cyanogenetic glycoside. Prunasin is hydrolysed in presence of water by prunase enzyme present in the drug into benzaldehyde, glucose and hydrocyanic acid. It further contains coumarin derivative scopoletin. Starch, resin, tannin, gallic acid, fatty matter, lignin, red colouring matter, salts of calcium, potassium and iron, also a volatile oil associated with hydrocyanic acid are present.

Prunasin

Uses

Astringent tonic, pectoral, sedative and expectorant. It has been used in the treatment of bronchitis of various types. It is valuable in catarrh, whooping cough and dyspepsia.

16.10. ISOTHIOCYANATE GLYCOSIDES

These are sulphur-containing compounds rich in family cruciferae, also known as glucosinolates and on hydrolysis yields isothiocyanate (-NCS) group. These glycosides are generally irritant and hence used externally as counter irritant, for example, sinigrin from black mustard, sinalbin from white mustard and gluconapin from rapeseed.

MUSTARD

Synonyms

Sarson ka tel.

Biological Source

It is a fixed oil obtained from matured seeds of *Brassica nigra* (L) Koch or *Brassica juncea* L. Czern, belonging to family Cruciferae (Brassicaceae) (Fig. 16.34).

Geographical Source

It is cultivated in India, China, Canada and England.

Description

It is yellow coloured liquid of strong acrid odour until refined, sp. gr. 0.914–0.923, saponification value 173–184, iodine value 96–194 and unsaponifiable matter 0.9–1.0%.

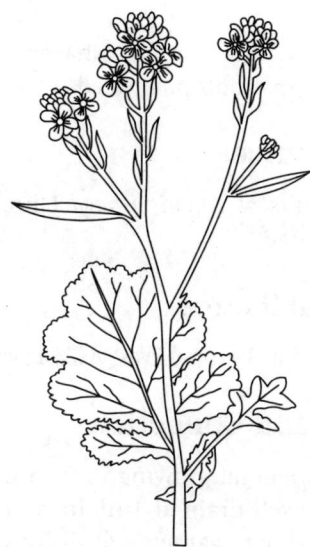

FIG. 16.34 *Brassica nigra*

Chemical Constituents

Mustard oil contains glycerides of arachidic (0.5%), behenic (2–3%), eicosenoic (7–8%), erusic (40–60%), lignoceric (1–2%), linoleic (14–18%), linolenic (6.5–7.0%), oleic (20–22%) and myristic (0.5–10%) acids.

Black mustard seeds contain 35–40% of fixed oil and a glycoside known as sinigrin along with an enzyme myrosin. Allyl isothiocyanate is responsible for the strong acrid smell of volatile oil of mustard produced on hydrolysis of glycoside.

$$CH_2 = CH - CH_2 - C \begin{cases} S \text{ - glucose} \\ N \text{ - } OSO_3K \end{cases} \qquad H_2C = CH - CH_2 - N = C = S$$

Sinigrin   Allyl isothiocyanate

Uses

Fixed oil is used as edible oil after refining, but medicinal properties are due to allyl isothiocyanate, which is a local irritant and emetic. If applied externally, it is rubefacient and vesicant. It is also used as condiment and in manufacture of soap. Refined mustard oil is used in vegetable ghee.

Marketed Products

Dabur mustard oil is the one of the purest mustard oil that has a variety of uses. It is also one of the ingredients of the preparation known as Saaf Organic Eraser Body Oil.

16.11. FLAVONE GLYCOSIDES

These are complex organic compounds containing phenyl-benzopyrone ring system. Flavones are present in plants in a free state or in glycosidal state (O-glycoside or C-glycoside) with its different derivatives like flavane, flavonol, flavonone, isoflavone and chalcones, for example, Rutin, quercitrin, hyperoside, diosmin (buchu leaf), hesperidin (lemon and orange peel) and vitexin (Carategus).

GINKGO

Biological Source

The leaves of Ginkgo are obtained from the dioeceous tree *Ginkgo biloba*, belonging to family Ginkgoaceae (Fig. 16.35).

Geographical Source

It is a native to China and Japan and cultivated ornamentally in many temperate regions.

Characteristics

The leaves are bilobed, each lobe being triangular in outline with a fine radiating, fan-like venation. The leaf is glabrous, petiolate and has an entire margin.

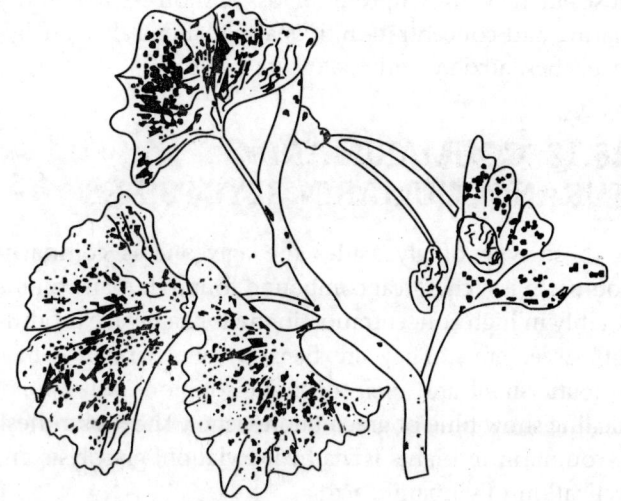

FIG. 16.35 Ginkgo biloba

Chemical Constituents

The diterpene lactones and flavonoids possess therapeutic activity. Five diterpene lactones (ginkgolides A, B, C, J, M) have been characterized; these have a cage structure involving a tertiary butyl group and six 5-membered rings including a spirononane system; a tetrahydrofuran moiety and three lactonic groups. These compounds are platelet-activating factor (PAF) antagonists and as they do not react with any other known receptor, their effect is very specific. A tertiary butyl group is present in the sesquiterpene bilobalide; no PAF-antagonist activity has been demonstrated for this compound.

About 40 flavonoids have now been isolated from the leaves including glycosides of kaempferol, quercetin and isorhamnetin derivatives. The tree also synthesizes a number of biflavonoids based on amentoflavone.

	R1	R2	R3
Ginkgolide A	OH	H	H
Ginkgolide B	OH	OH	H
Ginkgolide C	OH	OH	OH
Ginkgolide J	OH	H	OH
Ginkgolide M	H	OH	OH

Uses

Ginkgo is used as an antiasthmatic and bronchodilator. Extracts of the leaf containing selected constituents are used for improving peripheral and cerebral circulation in those elderly with symptoms of loss of short-term memory, hearing and concentration; it is also claimed that vertigo, headaches, anxiety and apathy are cured.

16.12. COUMARIN AND FURANOCOUMARIN GLYCOSIDES

In these type of glycosides the aglycone is coumarin. Coumarin is a chemical compound found in many plants, notably in high concentration in the tonka bean, woodruff and sweet grass. They are benzopyrone derivative have aromatic smell and their alcoholic solutions when made alkaline show blue or green fluorescence. The biosynthesis of coumarin in plants is via hydroxylation, glycolysis and cyclization of cinnamic acid.

It has clinical value as the precursor for several anticoagulants, notably warfarin. Some naturally occurring coumarin derivatives include umbelliferone (7-hydroxycoumarin), herniarin (7-methoxy-coumarin), psoralen and imperatorin. Coumarins have flavouring property but they cause damage to liver. Coumarin drugs also cause drug interactions with many other drugs. Medicinally, coumarin glycosides have been shown to have haemorrhagic, antifungicidal and antitumour activities.

Furanocoumarins are toxic compounds that consist of a coumarin nucleus bonded to a furan ring. Several plants contain the psoralens that are generally the precursors of furocoumarins. Furanocoumarins are found especially in Rutaceae, Umbelliferae and Leguminosae. They are also produced by some plants, for example, celery and parsnips, in response to fungal infestation.

VISNAGA

Synonyms

Bishop's flower, Greater Ammi, Khaizaran, Khellakraut, Khillah, Pick Tooth, Toothpick weed, Viznaga.

Biological Source

These are the fruits of *Ammi visnaga* Linn., belonging to family Umbelliferae.

Geographical Source

It is mainly found in Europe, West Asia, Egypt, West Africa.

Cultivation and Collection

It is an annual/biennial growing to 0.75 m × 0.4 m. The plant prefers a well-drained soil in a sunny position, succeeding in ordinary garden soil. Tolerates a pH in the range of 6.8–8.3. The seeds are sown in prepared beds on a well drained loamy soil in the month of August. When the plants attain a height of 6–7 cm they are transplanted to open fields. The crop is cut in March–April when the fruits are ripe. The dried plants are thrashed on the floor and the fruits are collected and winnowed.

Characteristics

Fruit, cremocarp, usually separated into its two mericarps, rarely entire, with a part of the pedicel attached. Mericarp, small, ovoid, about 2 mm long and 1 mm broad; crowned with a disc-like nectary, the stylopod; brownish to greenish-brown with a violet tinge (Distinction from *Ammi majus*); externally, glabrous, marked with five distinct, pale brownish, rather broad primary ridges and four inconspicuous dark secondary ridges; internally, the mericarp shows a pericarp with six vittae, four in the dorsal and two in the commissural side, a large oily orthospermous endosperm and a small apical embryo. Carpophore, single, no split; passing at the apex in to the raphe of each mericarp. Odour, slightly aromatic; taste, aromatic, bitter and slightly pungent.

Microscopy

The mericarp is an almost regular pentagon and the seeds are orthospermous. There are five vascular strands and four vittae; on the outer side of each vittae a group of radiating club shaped cells and these cause a slight elevation of the surface over each vitta, thus forming the secondary ridges. It contains a large lacuna on the outer side of each vascular strand in the primary ridges.

Chemical Constituents

The drug contains furanocoumarin compounds. The chief constituents are khellin and visnagin, which are γ-benzopyrone derivatives. Khellol and khellol glucoside are also present. In addition it contains pyranocoumarin esters visnadin, samidin and dihydrosamidin. Fixed oil and proteins are also present.

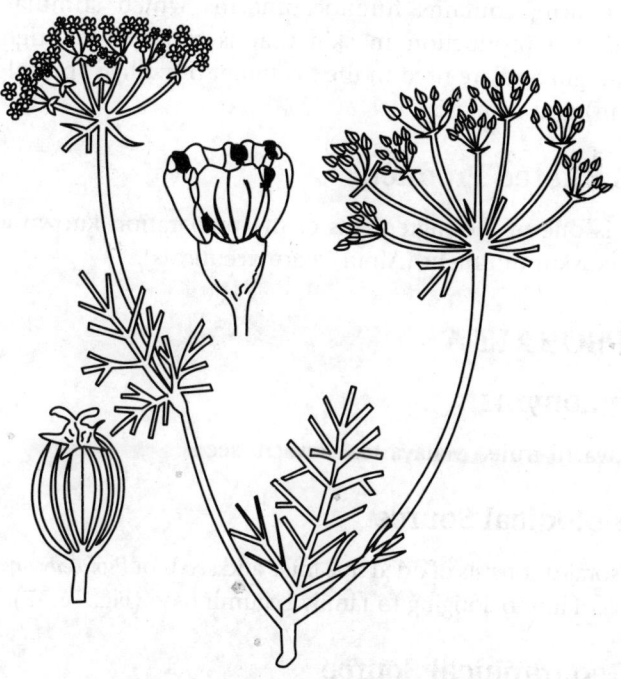

Khellin

Visnagin

Khellol

Chemical Test

The drug when treated with strong mineral acid shows lemon yellow colour while in *Ammi majus* dirty green brown colour is seen.

Uses

Visnaga is an effective muscle relaxant and has been used for centuries to alleviate the excruciating pain of kidney stones. Khellin is used in treatment of asthma. The seeds are diuretic, antiasthmatic and lithontriptic. The seeds have a strongly antispasmodic action on the smaller bronchial muscles; they also dilate the bronchial, urinary and blood vessels without affecting blood pressure.

Marketed Products

It is one of the ingredients of the preparations known as Lukoskin oral drops (Aimil Pharmaceuticals).

AMMI

Synonyms

Bishop's weed, Laceflower, Large Bullwort, Toothpick Arami.

Biological Source

These are the fruits of *Ammi majus* Linn., belonging to family Umbelliferae (Fig. 16.36).

Geographical Source

It is mainly found in Europe, Egypt, West Africa and India.

Cultivation and Collection

The plant prefers sandy, loamy and clay soils. The plant prefers acid, neutral and basic (alkaline) soils. It can grow in semishade or no shade. It requires moist soil. It is propagated using seeds. Before sowing, the seeds are mixed with soil and sown in the month of October. The seeds germinate within a month. It is in flower from June to October, and the seeds ripen from July to October. The fruits are collected when they are immature in April–May and dried.

Characteristics

Fruits are 22.5 mm long and 0.5–1.7 mm broad. *Ammi majus* fruits can be distinguished by the presence of four prominent secondary ridges and by the absence of lacuane outside the vascular bundles, seen in the transverse section of *Ammi visnaga*. Odour, slightly aromatic, terbenthinate; taste, strongly pungent and slightly bitter.

FIG. 16.36 *Ammi majus*

Chemical Constituents

The drug contains furanocoumarins, xanthotoxin (0.4–1.9%), imperatorin, bergapten and isopimpinellin.

Xanthotoxin

Imperatorin

Bergapten

Identification Tests

1. Boil about 1 g of the drug with 10 ml of water for 1 min and strain, add one or two drops of this decoction to 2 ml of a solution of sodium hydroxide, no rose colour is produced (distinction from *Ammi visnaga*).

2. Alcoholic extract of the fruit gives blue fluorescence when examined under UV light.

Uses

The drug contains furanocoumarins which stimulate pigment production in skin that is exposed to bright sunlight and are used in the treatment of vitiligo (piebald skin) and psoriasis.

Marketed Products

It is one of the ingredients of the preparation known as Lukoskin ointment (Aimil Pharmaceuticals).

PSORALEA

Synonyms

Bavachi fruits, Malaya tea, Bavachi seeds.

Biological Source

Psoralea consists of dried ripe fruits and seeds of *Psoralea corylifolia* Linn, belonging to family Leguminosae (Fig. 16.37).

Geographical Source

Psoralea is mainly found in India, China, Sri Lanka, Nepal and Vietnam.

Characteristics

The plant is an annual herb attending to a height of 60 cm to 1 m. The plant contains prominent grooves of glands and white hairs on the stem and branches. Fruits are very small 3–4.5 mm long and 2–3 mm broad. Fruits are dark chocolate to black in colour with pericarp attached to seeds. Fruits are ovate, oblong or bean shaped, compressed, glabrous rounded or mucronate and pitted. Seed is produced from campylotropous ovule and are kidney shaped, 2–4 mm long, 2–3 mm broad, smooth, exalbuminous with straw coloured hard testa. Fruit has no smell, taste is bitter, acrid and unpleasant.

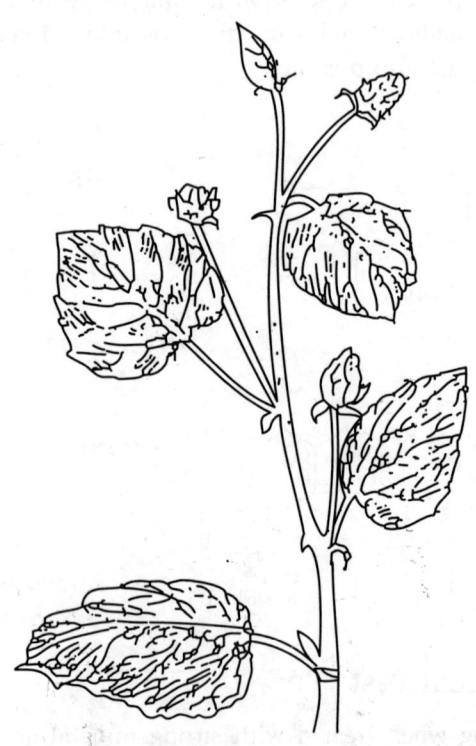

FIG. 16.37 *Psoralea corylifolia*

Microscopy

A thin section of fruit shows pericarp with prominent ridges and depressions, consisting of collapsed parenchyma and large secretory glands containing oleoresinous matter; testa, outer layer of palisade epidermis, layer of bearer cells which are much thickened in the inner tangential and basal radial walls and two to three layers of parenchyma are seen; cotyledons of polyhedral parenchyma and three layers of palisade cells on the axial side are also present.

Chemical Constituents

Psoralea contains coumarin compounds like psoralen, isopsoralen, psoralidin, isopsoralidin, carylifolean, bavachromanol and psoralenol. It also contains fixed oil (10%), essential oil (0.05%) and resin.

The seeds contain flavonoids such as bavachalcone, bavachinin, isobavachalcone, bavachin and isobavachin, etc. The seed oil yielded limonene, β-caryophyllene oxide, 4-terpineol, linalool, geranyl acetate, angelicin, psoralen and bakuchiol.

Psoralen   Psoralidin

Chemical Tests

1. Psoralea dissolved in alcohol and sodium hydroxide solution is added and observed under UV light, yellow fluorescence is observed.
2. Psoralea is dissolved in small amount of alcohol and add 3 times of propylene glycol, 5 times of acetic acid and 40 times of water, a blue fluorescence is observed under UV light.

Uses

The fruits are aphrodisiac, antibacterial and tonic to the genital organs. The seed is anthelmintic, antibacterial, aphrodisiac, astringent, cytotoxic, diaphoretic, diuretic, stimulant, stomachic and tonic. It is used in the treatment of febrile diseases, premature ejaculation, impotence, lower back pains, frequent urination, incontinence, bed wetting, etc. It is also used externally to treat various skin ailments including leprosy, leucoderma and hair loss.

Marketed Products

It is one of the ingredients of the preparations known as Purim, Erina (Himalaya Drug Company), Purodil, Lukoskin (Aimil Pharmaceuticals) and Sage Somaraji oil (Sage Herbals).

16.13. ALDEHYDE GLYCOSIDES

VANILLA

Biological Source

Vanilla (Vanilla Pods) consists of the cured fully grown but unripe fruits of *Vanilla fragrans* (Salis.), belonging to family Orchidaceae.

Geographical Source

Vanilla fragrans is grown in the woods of eastern Mexico, Reunion (or Bourbon), Mauritius, Seychelles, Madagascar, Java, Sri Lanka, Tahiti, Guadeloupe, Martinique and Indonesia. It is cultivated in tropical countries where the temperature does not fall below 18°C and where the humidity is high.

The plants are perennial, climbing, dioecious epiphytes attached to the trunks of trees by means of aerial rootlets.

Cultivation and Collection

The plant is usually propagated by means of cuttings and, after two or three years, reaches the flowering stage. The cuttings attach to trees (e.g. *Casuarina equisetifolia*) where they strike roots on the bark; it continues to bear fruit for 30 or 40 years. The flowers, approximately 30 on each plant, are hand pollinated, thus producing larger and better fruits.

The fruits are collected as they ripen to a yellow colour, 6–10 months after pollination, and are cured by dipping in warm water and repeated sweating between woollen blankets in the sun during the day and packing in wool-covered boxes at night. The characteristic colour and odour of the commercial drug are only developed as a result of enzyme action during the curing. Curing consists of slow drying in sheds with carefully regulated temperatures. This requires about 2 months, during which the pods lose from 70 to 80% of their original weight and take on the characteristic colour and odour of the commercial drug. The pods are then graded, tied into bundles of about 50–75 and sealed in tin containers for shipment.

Characteristics

Vanilla pods are 15–25 cm long, 8–10 mm diameter and somewhat flattened. The surface is longitudinally wrinkled, dark brown to violet-black in colour and frequently covered with needle shaped crystals of vanillin ('frosted'). The fruits are very pliable and have a very characteristic odour and taste.

Chemical Constituents

Green vanilla contains glycosides, namely glucovanillin (vanilloside) and glucovanillic alcohol. During the curing these are acted upon by an oxidizing and a hydrolysing enzyme which occur in all parts of the plant. Glucovanillic alcohol yields on hydrolysis glucose and vanillic alcohol; the latter compound is then by oxidation converted into vanillic aldehyde (vanillin). Glucovanillin yields on hydrolysis glucose and vanillin.

The vanilla species differ in their relative contents of anisyl alcohol, anisaldehyde, anisyl ethers, anisic acid esters, piperonal and p-hydroxybenzoic acid. These minor components, together with the two diastereoisomeric vitispiranes, add to the flavour of the pods.

Vanillin   Piperonal

Uses

Vanilla pods are widely used in confectionery and in perfumery.

16.14. PHENOL GLYCOSIDES

BEARBERRY

Synonyms

Uva ursi, Bearberry leaves, Busserole.

Biological Source

These are the dried leaves of *Arctostaphylos uva-ursi* (Linne) Sprengel, belonging to family Ericaceae.

Geographical Source

It is found in different parts of Central and North Europe, North America, Canada and Scotland.

Characteristics

Leaves are spatula like, 2–2.5 cm in size tapering towards base, with short stalk or petiole. Fruits are scarlet red with calyx at base. The leaves are collected in April to June and dried under sun. They show olive green upper surface and pale colour on lower surface. They are small coriaceous, shining leaves. They have astringent and bitter taste, without any specific odour.

Chemical Constituents

The leaves contain a glycoside called arbutin which contains phenolic aglycone. The leaves also contain methyl arbutin, quercetin, ursone, iriodoids, quinones, tannins (6–10%), gallic acid, ursolic acid, α-amyrin, β-amyrin and terpenoids.

Uses

The leaves have diuretic and astringent properties. As an infusion, it is used in urethritis and cystitis.

16.15. STEROIDAL GLYCOSIDES

SOLANUM

Biological Source

It consists of dried berries of *Solanum khasianum* C.B. Clarke, belonging to family Solanaceae.

Geographical Source

The plant is found widely growing at various altitudes in India right from coastal region up to 2000 m. It is found in hilly regions of Assam, Manipur, Sikkim, Nilgiri, Central India and also in Myanmar and China. Nowadays it is cultivated on commercial scales in Maharashtra.

Cultivation and Collection

In view of its solasodine content, it has commercial significance. Solasodine, a steroidal glycoalkaloid, has similar applications as that of diosgenin. The cultivation of this plant is scientifically studied and the observations of those trials are given here in brief. The seeds are used for propagation, either through nursery beds or by direct broadcasting. In February, the seeds are sown in nursery beds. The seed beds are covered with sand or farmyard manures and weeding is done periodically. When the seedlings show sufficient growth, they are transplanted into open fields. The raising in nurseries is preferred to direct broadcasting. The plant grows in various climatic and agricultural conditions. The well drained soil and sunny atmosphere are preferred. The seedlings are transplanted in moist soil at 50 x 50 cm distance. Urea, potash and superphosphate are given as fertilizers. In the initial period, irrigation is done once in a week and then in later stages as per requirement. After 6 months, the plants are harvested for collection of berries. They are immediately dried in shade or artificially at low temperature to reduce the large content of moisture.

Characteristics

It bears yellowish to greenish berries which are globose and 2.5 cm in diameter with compressed smooth brown seeds.

Chemical Constituents

The berries contain about 3% of steroidal glycoalkaloid called solasodine. A new glycoalkaloid solakhasianin having rhamnose and galactose as sugar components have been isolated. Mucilage surrounding part of the seeds contain highest amount of alkaloid. Immatured and over-ripe fruits contain negligible content of alkaloid, while it is maximum when fruits change colour from green to yellow. Colour change of fruits takes place about two months after setting the fruits to the plants. The berries also contain 8–10% of greenish-yellow fixed oil.

Uses

Solasodine is used as a precursor for steroidal synthesis. Like diosgenin, it is first converted to 16-dehydro-pregnenelone acetate. The latter is a precursor for steroids, like corticosteroids, pregnane and androstanes. All of these are useful as sex hormones, oral contraceptives, etc.

16.16. BITTER AND MISCELLANEOUS GLYCOSIDES

Bitter glycosides are a class of compounds that plays an important role in the digestive process. Bitter drugs and bitter constituents are used since a very early period as stomachics, febrifuges, and bitter tonics and in digestive disturbances.

The bitterness of food on the tongue plays a very important role as the taste of bitter foods stimulates the appetite and triggers the secretion of digestive juices in the stomach, which in turn improves the break down of food. Bitters begin by stimulating the taste buds. This triggers off a reflex nerve action which increases the flow of saliva and stomach enzymes. At the same time, the hormone gastrin is secreted by the walls of the stomach. This improves the digestive process, by improving the passage of food from the stomach to the intestines. The sum total of this is an improvement in the digestive function of the stomach and small intestines. Bitters can also be very useful to improve immune disorders resulting from food intolerance or dietary antigen leakage, protect gut tissue (by increasing the tone of the gastroesophageal sphincter thereby preventing reflux of corrosive stomach contents into the oesophagus in 'heart burn', hiatus hernia or oesophageal inflammation), promote bile flow (thereby providing for increased ability of the liver to remove a toxic load from incomplete digestion and also provide for better digestion in the duodenum and small intestine), and enhance pancreatic function (normalizing hormone secretions to moderate excessive swings in blood–sugar levels).

Examples of bitter digestives are blessed thistle, barberry bark, goldenseal, dandelion, hops flowers, yellow dock and gentian root. Bitter drugs preparations should be taken before or during meals otherwise they cause digestive disturbances like diarrhoea, and pain in the stomach.

GENTIAN

Synonyms

Gentian Root, Yellow Gentian Root.

Biological Source

Gentian consists of dried unfermented rhizomes and roots of *Gentiana lutea* Linn., belonging to family Gentianaceae (Fig. 16.38).

Geographical Source

Mountainous regions of Central and south Europe, of France and Switzerland, of Spain and Portugal, the Pyrenees, Sardinia and Corsica, the Apennines, the Mountains of Auvergne, the Jura, the lower slopes of the Vosges, the Black Forest and throughout the chain of the Alps as far as Bosnia and the Balkan States.

Cultivation and Collection

It is a perennial plant growing to 1.2 m × 0.6 m. For cultivation, a strong loamy soil is most suitable, the deeper the better, as the stout roots descend a long way down into the soil. Plenty of moisture is also desirable and a position where there is shelter from cold winds and exposure to sunshine. Old plants have large crowns, which may be divided for the purpose of propagation, but growing it on a large scale, seeds would be the best method. It is advantageous to keep the seed at about 10°C for a few days after sowing, to enable the seed to imbibe moisture. Following this with a period of at least 5–6 weeks with temperatures falling between 0 and –5°C will usually produce reasonable germination. They could be sown in a frame, or in a nursery bed in a sheltered part of the garden and the young seedlings transplanted. They take about three years to grow to flowering size. It is, however, likely that the roots are richest in medicinal properties before the plants have flowered.

Collection is done from two to five years old plants in spring. The rhizome and roots collected and dried. When fresh, they are yellowish-white externally, but gradually become darker by slow drying. Slow drying is employed to prevent deterioration in colour and to improve the aroma. Occasionally the roots are longitudinally sliced and quickly dried, the drug being then pale in colour and unusually bitter in taste.

Characteristics

When fresh, they are yellowish-white externally, but gradually become darker by slow drying. Slow drying is employed to prevent deterioration in colour and to improve the aroma. Occasionally the roots are longitudinally sliced and quickly dried; the drug being then pale in colour and unusually bitter in taste, but this variety is not official.

The dried root as it occurs in commerce is brown and cylindrical, 1 foot or more in length, or broken up into shorter pieces, usually 1/2 inch to 1 inch in diameter, rather soft and spongy, with a thick reddish bark, tough and flexible, and of an orange-brown colour internally. The upper portion is marked with numerous rings, the lower longitudinally wrinkled. The root has a strong, disagreeable odour and the taste is slightly sweet at first, but afterwards very bitter.

Microscopy

The transverse section of root shows triarch primary xylem at the centre, where each primary bundle is represented by one to three very small vessels. The secondary xylem is very wide with parenchymatous and medullary rays not clearly marked. The drug also shows reticulately thickened

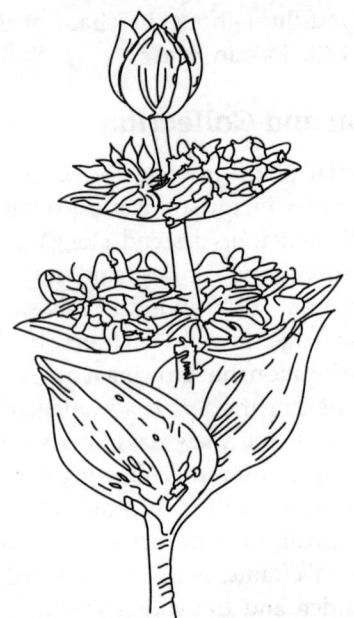

FIG. 16.38 *Gentiana lutea*

Gentianine

Gentiopicrin

xylem vessels very few being annular or spiral, scattered throughout the parenchyma of the xylem. Secondary phloem is wide and composed chiefly of parenchyma, with groups of sieve-tissue. The phloems are surrounded by a narrow parenchymatous phelloderm and externally are several rows of polygonal tabular, thin walled cork cells. Parenchyma cells in all regions of the root contain scattered needles of calcium oxalate crystals, about 3–6 μm long and 0.5–1.1 μm wide, also small prismatic crystals.

Chemical Constituents

Gentian contains bitter glycosides. The dried gentian root contains gentinin and gentiamarin, bitter glucosides, together with gentianic acid (gentisin), the latter being physiologically inactive. Gentiopicrin, another bitter glucoside, a pale yellow crystalline substance, occurs in the fresh root, and may be isolated from it by treatment with boiling alcohol. Gentinin, crystalline glycoside is not a pure chemical substance, but a mixture of gentiopicrin and a colouring substance gentisin (gentianine) or gentlanic acid. Gentian contains a bitter trisaccharide, gentianose which on hydrolysis yields two molecules of glucose and one molecule of fructose. The saccharine constituents of gentian are dextrose, laevulose, sucrose and gentianose, a crystallizable, fermentable sugar. It is free from starch and yields from 3 to 4% ash.

Uses

Gentian root has a long history of use as an herbal bitter in the treatment of digestive disorders. It contains some of the most bitter compounds known and is used as a scientific basis for measuring bitterness. It is useful in states of exhaustion from chronic disease and in all cases of debility,

weakness of the digestive system and lack of appetite. It is one of the best strengthened of the human system, stimulating the liver, gall bladder and digestive system, and is an excellent tonic to combine with a purgative in order to prevent its debilitating effects.

It is also used as anthelmintic, anti-inflammatory, antiseptic, bitter tonic, cholagogue, emmenagogue, and febrifuge, refrigerant and stomachic. It is taken internally in the treatment of liver complaints, indigestion, gastric infections and anorexia. It should not be prescribed for patients with gastric or duodenal ulcers.

PICRORHIZA

Synonyms

Kami, Kuru (Hindi), Katvee.

Biological Source

It consists of dried rhizome of *Picrorhiza kurroa* Royle ex Benth., cut into small pieces and freed from attached rootlets, belonging to family Scrophulariaceae (Fig. 16.39).

Geographical Source

The plant is common on the alpine Himalayas from Kashmir to Sikkim between 3000 and 5000 m.

Characteristics

It is a low, hairy herb with a perennial woody bitter rhizome, 15–25 cm long, covered with dry leaf-bases. It occurs as pieces, 2–4 cm long and 0.3–1.0 cm in diameter. Scales at distant intervals are present; frequently small protuberances, which probably represent accessory buds, are observed both at the rhizomes and the stolones.

The drug consists of small pieces. Colour is greyish-brown, light, cylindrical, straight or slightly curved, often with remains of aerial stem which is very dark brown and wrinkled longitudinally, upper and lower surfaces bear a few small root scars, numerous scale leaves and thin scars; odour slightly unpleasant; taste very bitter.

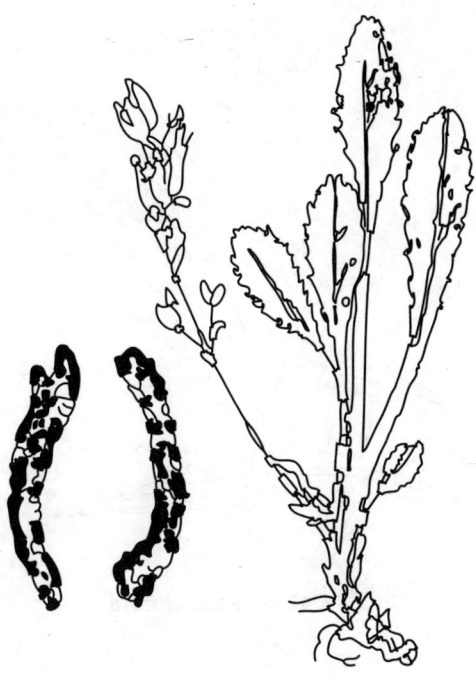

FIG. 16.39 *Picrorhiza kurroa*

Microscopy (Fig. 16.40)

Transverse section of the rhizome shows cork composed of several layers of uniformly arranged, tightly packed, thin-walled cells. Cork surrounds a broad cortex, composed of thin-walled; mostly irregularly rounded-oval parenchymatous cells and some of them merge into the secondary phloem tissue, which consists of sieve tubes, companion cells and

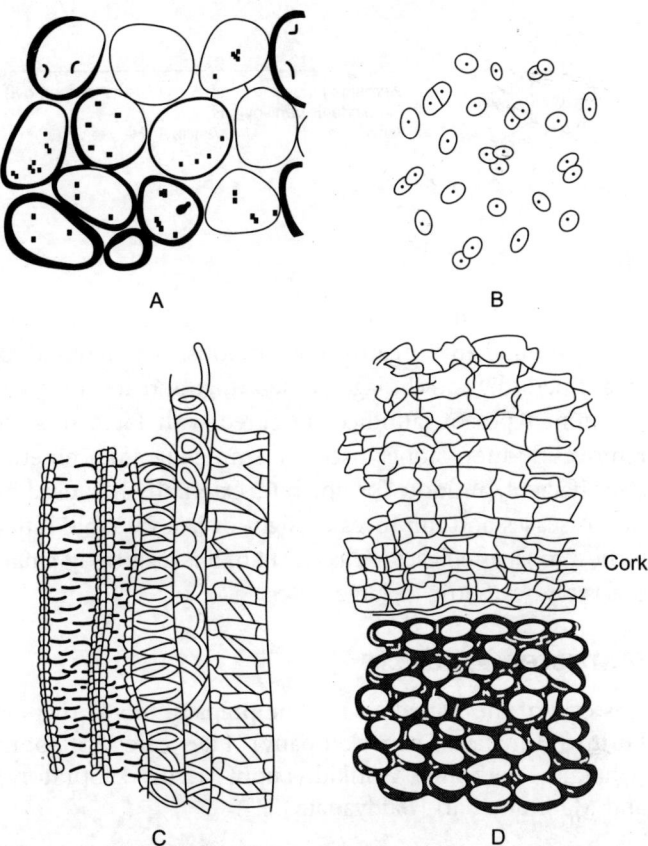

FIG. 16.41 Powder characteristics of Picrorhiza rhizome. (A: Pith cells with pitted wall, B: Starch grains, C: Vessels, D: Part of cork and cortex)

parenchyma. Cambium is narrow and wavy consisting of several layers of compressed cells. The secondary xylem is composed of thick-walled vessels with annular, spiral or reticulate thickening, tracheids and fibres. Pith is composed of thin-walled parenchymatous cells.

Powder Microscopy (Fig. 16.41)

The powder is greyish-brown in colour with bitter taste. Microscopical examination shows pith cells with numerous pits, and fragments of cork cells with associated cortex. Starch grains, simple or compound (2–3 components) with distinct central hilum and fragments of vessels with annular, spiral or reticulate thickening are found scattered.

Chemical Constituents

The active constituent of picrorhiza is picrorhizin, a glucoside which yields picrorhizetin and dextrose on hydrolysis. It also contains kutkin, a glucosidal bitter principle, picroside-I, picroside-II, picroside-III, D-mannitol, vanillic acid, kurrin, kutkiol, kutkisterol, apocynin, vernicoside, apocynin, kutkoside, 6-feruloyl catapol, veronicoside, minecoside, picein, androsin, β-D-6-cinnamoylglucose, arvenin III, phenolic glycosides picein and androsin and seven cucurbitacin glycoside.

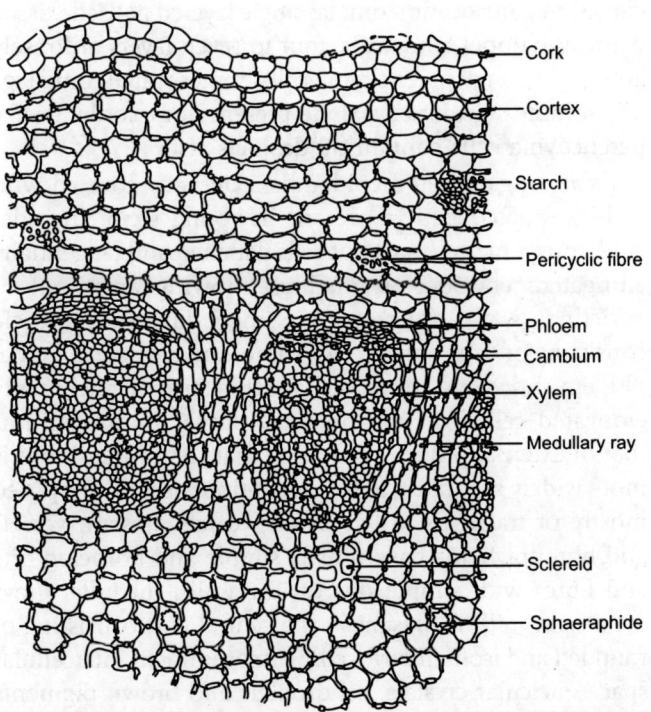

Cork
Cortex
Starch
Pericyclic fibre
Phloem
Cambium
Xylem
Medullary ray
Sclereid
Sphaeraphide

FIG. 16.40 Transverse section of Picrorhiza rhizome

	R₁	R₂	R₃
Picroside I	H	H	trans (cinnamoyl)
Picroside II	Vanilloyl	H	H
Kutkoside	H	Vanilloyl	H

Uses

Picrorhiza is bitter, cathartic, stomachic, used in fever and dyspepsia and in purgative preparations. It is reputed as an antiperiodic and cholagogue, febrifuge and antimalarial. Different types of jaundice are cured with Picrorhiza. It removes kidney stone, used as emmenagogue, emetic, abortifacient, antidote for dog bite; externally it is used in skin diseases and improves eyesight. It is a valuable bitter tonic almost as efficacious as Gentian. It is laxative in small doses and cathartic in large doses.

Marketed Products

It is one of the ingredients of the preparations known as Purim (Himalaya Drug Company), Piles care, Aptizoom (Charak), Herbohep, Aptikid (Lupin Herbal Laboratory) and Madhumehari (Baidyanath).

CHIRATA

Synonyms

Indian Gentian, Indian Balmony, Chirayta, *Ophelia chirata*, *Swertia chirayita*.

Biological Source

Chirata consists of the entire herb of *Swertia chirata* Buch-Ham, belonging to family Gentianaceae. It contains not less than 1.3% bitter constituent (Fig. 16.42).

Geographical Source

It is mainly found in India, Nepal and Bhutan.

Characteristics

It is an annual, about 3 feet high; branching stem, upper part of the stem is yellow to brown, thinner and 2 mm broad. The lower part is purplish or brown to dark brown; 6 mm broad cylindrical and exfoliated at some places showing dull wood. Leaves are smooth entire, opposite, very acute, lanceolate dark brown up to 8 cm long, 1.5–2 cm broad. Flowers numerous; peduncles yellow; one-celled capsule. Rhizome is angular to 5 cm long, pale yellow to brown in colour and covered with dense scale leaves. Root is primary, 5–10 cm long, light brown, oblique somewhat twisted, tapering, longitudinally wrinkled and with transverse ridges. Drug has no odour but taste is very bitter.

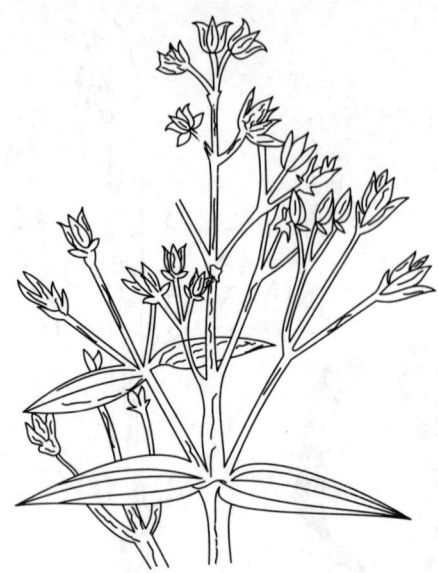

FIG. 16.42 *Swertia chirata*

Microscopy

Root: 2–4 layers of cork; cortex region consists of 4–12 layers of thickwalled, parenchymatous cells with sinuous walls; secondary phloem composed of thin walled sieve tubes, companion cells and phloem parenchyma; secondary xylem composed of lignified and thick walled vessels, parenchyma, tracheids and xylem fibres; minute acicular crystals present in abundance in secondary cortex and phloem region; resin are also present as dark brown mass in secondary cortex cells.

Leaf: single layered epidermis covered with a thick, striated cuticle and anisocytic stomata; single layered palisade tissue below the upper epidermis, four to seven layers of loosely arranged spongy parenchyma cells in mesophyll, mucilage and minute acicular crystal are present in mesophyll cells; parenchyma cells contain oil droplets also.

Stem: single layered epidermis, externally covered with a thick striated cuticle present in young stem, in older epidermis remains intact but cells flattened and tangentially elongated; endodermis distinct, showing anticlinal or periclinal walls, followed by single layered pericycle consisting of thin walled cells; cambium, between external phloem and xylem composed of a thin strip of tangentially elongated cells, internal phloem, similar in structure as that of external phloem excepting that sieve tube strand is more widely separated; xylem is continuous and composed mostly of tracheids, a few xylem vessels present; vessels and fibre tracheids have mostly simple and bordered pits and fibres with simple pits on the walls; medullary rays are absent; pith is present in the central part consisting of rounded and isodiametric cells with prominent intercellular spaces; acicular crystals, oil droplets and brown pigments are also present.

Chemical Constituents

Chirata contains chiritin, gentiopicrin and amarogentin. Amarogentin is phenol carboxylic acid ester of sweroside a substance related to gentiopicrin. Ophelic acid a non crystalline bitter substance is present. It also contains gentianine and gentiocrucine.

O — Glucose — O

Amarogentin

Uses

It is an important ingredient in the well known ayurvedic preparations Mahasudarshan churna and Sudarshan churna used successfully in chronic fever. The whole plant is an extremely bitter tonic digestive herb that lowers fevers and is stimulant. The herb has a beneficial effect on the liver, promoting the flow of bile; it also cures constipation and is useful for treating dyspepsia.

Marketed Products

It is one of the ingredients of the preparations known ad Diabecon (Himalaya), Mehmudgar bati (Baidyanath), Sabaigo (Aimil Company), J.P. Liver syrup (Jaumana Pharma), Fever end syrup (Chirayu), Sage Chirata (Sage Herbals) and Safi (Hamdard Laboratories).

QUASSIA

Synonyms

Lignum quassiae, Bitter Wood, Jamaica Quassia, Bitter Ash.

Biological Source

Quassia is dried wood of the stem of *Aeschrion excelsa* (*Picroena excelsa* Lindl or *Picrasma excelsa* (S.W.) Planchon), belonging to family Simarubaceae (Fig. 16.43).

Geographical Source

It is indigenous to West Indies, Jamaica, Barbados, Martinique and St. Vincent.

Cultivation and Collection

It is a tree growing 50–100 feet, erect stem over 3 feet in diameter. The stem is cut and small branches are separated. Main trunk and large branches are cut in to small pieces, sewed and logs and billets prepared. Bark is removed from logs and billets and shavings, raspings and chips made and then dried immediately to prevent the growth of moulds.

Characteristics

It is in the form of chips or raspings. Chips are poanoconvex, has no smell but an intense bitter taste. They have false annual rings breaking easily longitudinally. Colour is white, but changes to yellow on contact with the air. Cork easily detaches from phloem. Sometimes black markings are present because of mould.

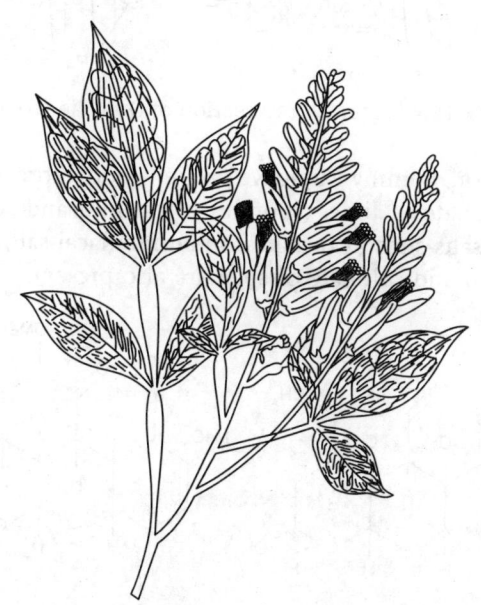

FIG. 16.43 *Picrasma excelsa*

Microscopy (Fig. 16.44)

Wood consists of medullary rays, parenchyma and vessels. The whole drug is stained red with phloroglucinol and hydrochloric acid due to the presence of lignin in the cell wall. Medullary rays are one to five seriate but usually triseriate. Cells of medullary rays are radially elongated and their cell walls are pitted. Vessels are thick walled and are border pitted. Fibres are also present in the wood; they are long; tapering, thick walled with oblique shaped pits. Prismatic type of calcium oxalate is present in cells of medullary rays and parenchyma.

Chemical Constituents

Quassia contains bitter amaroid compounds like quassin, isoquassin (picrasmin), neoquassin and 18-hydroxy quassin.

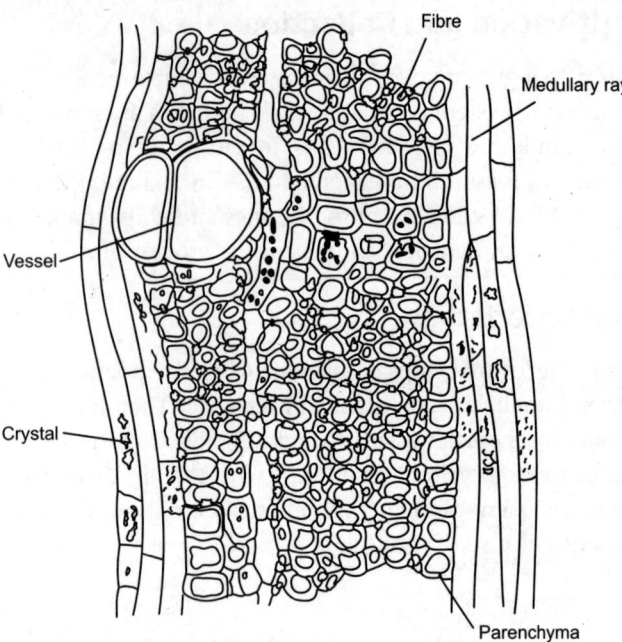

FIG. 16.44 Transverse section of Quassia wood

Volatile oil, gummy extractive pectin, woody fibre, tartrate and sulphate of lime, chlorides of calcium and sodium, various salts such as oxalate and ammoniacal salt, nitrate of potash and sulphate of soda are also present.

Neoquassin   Quassin

Uses

Quassia wood is a pure bitter tonic and stomachic; it is also a vermicide and slight narcotic; it acts on flies and some of the higher animals as a narcotic poison. It is a valuable remedy in convalescence, after acute disease and in debility and atonic dyspepsia; an antispasmodic in fever. In small doses Quassia increases the appetite.

Allied Drugs

Quassia amara, or Surinam Quassia (Simarubaceae), is in much smaller billets than the Jamaica Quassia, and is used in its place on the continent, and is easily recognized from the Jamaica one, which it closely resembles, by its medullary rays, which are only one cell wide, and contain no calcium oxalate.

KALMEGH

Synonyms

Andrographis, King of bitters, Chiretta; Bengal Chirata; Green Chirata; Kiryet (Hindi).

Biological Source

Kalmegh consists of leaves or entire aerial part of *Andrographis paniculata* Nees., belonging to family Acanthaceae (Fig. 16.45).

Geographical source

It grows abundantly in southeastern Asia: India (and Sri Lanka), Pakistan and Indonesia but it is cultivated extensively in China and Thailand, the East and West Indies, and Mauritius.

Cultivation and Collection

It is normally grown from seeds ubiquitously in its native areas where it grows in pine, evergreen and deciduous forest areas, and along roads and in villages. In India, it is cultivated during rainy phase of summer season (Kharif) crop. Any soil having fair amount of organic matter is suitable for commercial cultivation of this crop. About 400 g seed are sufficient for one hectare. The spacing is maintained 30 cm × 15 cm. No major insect and disease infestation has been reported. The plants at flowering stage (90–120 days after sowing) are cut at the base leaving 10–15 cm stem for plant regeneration. About 50–60 days after first harvest, final harvest is performed. In Indian condition, the yield varies between 2000–2500 kg dry herb/hectare.

Characteristics

The stem is erect, greenish brown, woody, 30–100 cm in height, and quadrangular particularly in the upper regions with four bulges arising on the four corners. The leaves are dark green, lanceolate, with a small winged petiole, 7 cm long, 2–5 cm broad; margin is entire, lamina glabrous, apex acuminate, slightly waxy and base tapering. The midrib varies in outline at different regions of the leaf. Stem branching is profuse which bears small arid solitary flowers. The dried drug is odourless and taste is extremely bitter.

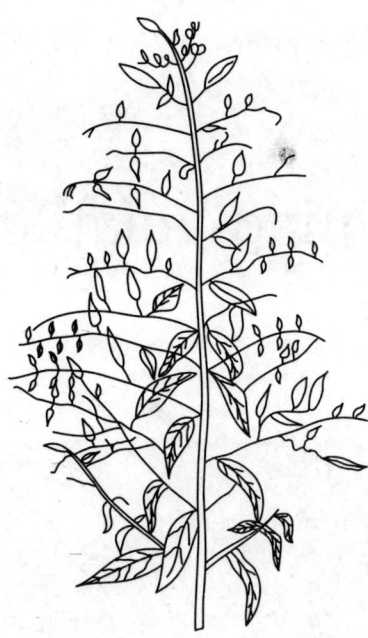

FIG. 16.45 *Andrographis paniculata*

Chemical Constituents

The plant possesses kalmeghin, a bitter crystalline diterpene lactone, such as, andrographolide flavonoids and phenols. The lactones isolated from Kalmegh are andrographolide, 14-deoxy-ll-oxo-andrographolide, 14-deoxy-11,12-didehydroandrographolide, 14-deoxyandrographolide and neoandrographolide.

The leaves contain β-sitosterol glucoside, caffeic, chlorogenic and dicaffeoylquinic acids, carvacrol, eugenol, myristic acid, hentriacontane, tritriacontane, oroxylin A, wogonin, andrograpanin, 14-deoxy-12-methoxyandrographolide, andrographidines A-F and stigmasterol.

Andrographolide

Andrographiside

Uses

Kalmegh has febrifuge, tonic, alterative, anthelmintic, astringent, anodyne, alexipharmic and cholagogue properties. It is useful in debility, cholera, diabetes, swelling, itches, consumption, influenza, piles, gonorrhoea, bronchitis, dysentery, dyspepsia, fever and in weakness. A decoction of the plant is used as a blood purifier and as a cure for torpid and jaundice. The pills prepared from macerated leaves and certain spices (e.g. cardamom, clove and cinnamon) are given for stomach ailments of infants.

Marketed Products

It is one of the ingredients of the preparations known as Purim, Acne-n-pimple cream (Himalaya Drug Company), Herbohep (Lupin Herbal Laboratory), Sage Liverex (Sage Herbals) and Purodil syrup (Aimil Pharmaceuticals).

Drugs Containing Volatile Oils

CONTENTS

17.1. INTRODUCTION

Volatile oils are odorous volatile principles of plant and animal source, evaporate when exposed to air at ordinary temperature, and hence known as volatile or ethereal oils. These represent essence of active constituents of the plant and hence also known as essential oils. In most instances the volatile oil pre-exists in the plant and is usually contained in some special secretory tissues, for example, the oil ducts of umbelliferous fruits, the oil cells or oil glands occurring in the subepidermal tissue of the lemon and orange, mesophyll of eucalyptus leaves, trichomes of several plants, etc.

In few cases the volatile oil does not pre-exist, but is formed by the decomposition of a glycoside. For example, whole black mustard seeds are odourless, but upon crushing the seeds and adding water to it a strong odour is evolved. This is due to allyl isothiocyanate (the main constituent of essential oil of mustard) formed by decomposition of a glycoside, sinigrin, by an enzyme, myrosin. Glycoside and enzyme are contained in different cells of the seed tissue and are unable to react until the seeds are crushed with water present, so that the cell contents can intermingle.

Volatile oils are freely soluble in ether and in chloroform and fairly soluble in alcohol; they are insoluble in water. The volatile oils dissolve many of the proximate principles of plant and animal tissues, such as the fixed oils and fats, resins, camphor, and many of the alkaloids when in the free state.

These are chemically derived from terpenes (mainly mono and sesqui terpenes) and their oxygenated derivatives. These are soluble in alcohol and other organic solvents, practically insoluble in water, lighter than water (clove oil heavier), possess characteristic odour, have high refraction index, and most of them are optically active. Volatile oils are colourless liquids, but when exposed to air and direct sunlight these become darker due to oxidation. Unlike fixed oils, volatile oils neither leave permanent grease spot on filter paper nor saponified with alkalis.

17.2. CLASSIFICATION OF VOLATILE OILS

Volatile oils are classified on the basis of functional groups present as given in Table 17.1.

Table 17.1 Classification of volatile oil

Groups	Drugs
Hydrocarbons	Turpentine oil
Alcohols	Peppermint oil, pudina, sandalwood oil, etc.
Aldehydes	Cymbopogon sp., lemongrass oil, cinnamon, cassia and saffron
Ketones	Camphor, caraway and dill, jatamansi, fennel, etc.
Phenols	Clove, ajowan, tulsi, etc.
Phenolic ethers	Nutmeg, calamus, etc.
Oxides	Eucalyptus, cardamom and chenopodium oil
Esters	Valerian, rosemary oil, garlic, gaultheria oil, etc.

17.3. EXTRACTION OF VOLATILE OILS

Volatile oils are prepared by means of several techniques and those techniques are discussed below:

Extraction by Distillation

The distillation is carried out either by water or steam. The volatile oils from fresh materials are separated by hydrodistillation, and volatile oils from air dried parts are separated by steam distillation. However it is better to use fresh materials in either case.

Extraction by Scarification

This method is used for the preparation of oil of lemon, oil of orange and oil of bergamot. These oils are found in large oil glands just below the surface in the peel of the fruit. The two principal methods of scarification are the sponge and the ecuelle method.

(a) *Sponge Process:* In this process the contents of the fruit are removed after making longitudinal or transverse cut, and the peel is been immersed in water for a short period of time. Then it is ready for expression. The operator takes a sponge in one hand and with the other presses the softener peel against the sponge, so that the oil glands burst open and the sponge absorbs the exuded oil, which is transferred to a collecting vessel. The turbid liquid consisting of oil and water is allowed to stand for a short time, whereupon the oil separates from water and is collected. The whole of the above process is carried out in cool, darkened rooms to minimize the harmful effects of heat and light on the oil.

(b) *Ecuelle Process:* In this process, the rinds are ruptured mechanically using numerous pointed projections with a rotary movement and the oil is collected.

Extraction by Nonvolatile Solvent

A nonvolatile solvent, for example, a fine quality of either lard or olive oil, is used in this process. After saturation with the floral oil the lard or olive oil is sometimes used as a flavouring base for the preparation of pomades, brilliantine, etc., or converted to a triple extract. In the latter instance the lard or oil is agitated with two or three successive portions of alcohol, which dissolve the odorous substances. The mixed alcoholic solutions so obtained constitute the 'triple extract' of commerce.

There are three chief methods that come under this; they are enfleurage, maceration and a spraying process.

(a) *Enfleurage:* In this a fatty layer is prepared using lard and the flower petals are spreaded over it, after the imbibitions is over the fatty layer is replaced with fresh petals. After the saturation of fatty layer the odorous principles are removed by treating with alcohol and a triple extract then prepared. When oil is used as a solvent the flowers are placed on an oil-soaked cloth supported by a metal grid enclosed in a frame. Fresh flowers are added as required, and finally the oil is expressed from the cloths. It may then be used as perfumed oil, or extracted with alcohol to produce a triple extract.

(b) *Maceration:* This is also used to extract the volatile matters of flowers. The lard or oil is heated over a water bath, a charge of flowers added and the mixture stirred continuously for some time. The exhausted flowers are removed, pressed, the expressed fluid returned to the hot fat, fresh flowers, added and the process continued until defined weights of flowers and solvent have been used. Again, a triple extract is prepared by extracting the perfumed lard or oil with alcohol.

(c) *Spraying:* In this process a current of warm air is sprayed through a column of the flowers. Then oil or melted fat is sprayed over this oil-laden air which absorbs and dissolves most of the perfume, the collected oil or fat is then extracted with alcohol as described above.

Extraction by Volatile Solvent

In this the flowers are extracted by using the solvent light petroleum and the latter is distilled off at a low temperature, leaving behind the volatile oil.

17.4. TERPENOIDS

There are many different classes of naturally occurring compounds. Terpenoids also form a group of naturally occurring compounds majority of which occur in plants, a few of them have also been obtained from other sources. Terpenoids are volatile substances which give plants and flowers their fragrance. They occur widely in the leaves and fruits of higher plants, conifers, citrus and eucalyptus.

The term 'terpene' was given to the compounds isolated from turpentine, a volatile liquid isolated from pine trees. The simpler mono and sesquiterpenes is the chief constituent of the essential oils obtained from sap and tissues of certain plant and trees. The di- and triterpenoids are not steam volatile. They are obtained from plant and tree gums and resins. Tetraterpenoids form a separate group of compounds called 'carotenoids'.

The term 'terpene' was originally employed to describe a mixture of isomeric hydrocarbons of the molecular formula $C_{10}H_{16}$ occurring in the essential oils obtained from sap and tissue of plants and trees. But there is a tendency to use more general term 'terpenoids', which includes hydrocarbons and their oxygenated derivatives. However, the term terpene is being used these days by some authors to represent terpenoids.

According to modern definition, 'Terpenoids are the hydrocarbons of plant origin of the general formula $(C_5H_8)_n$ as well as their oxygenated, hydrogenated and dehydrogenated derivatives.'

Isoprene Rule

Thermal decomposition of terpenoids gives isoprene as one of the product. Otto Wallach pointed out that terpenoids can be built up of isoprene unit. Isoprene rule states that the terpenoid molecules are constructed from two or more isoprene unit.

isoprene unit   tail   head

Special Isoprene Rule

It states that the terpenoid molecules are constructed of two or more isoprene units joined in a 'head to tail' fashion.

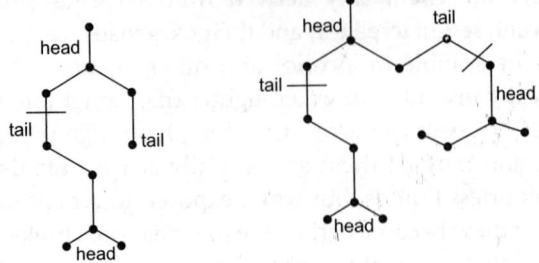

Examples

Myrcene
(monoterpene)

Farnesol
(sesquiterpene)

HOH₂C

But this rule can only be used as guiding principle and not as a fixed rule. For example carotenoids are joined tail to tail at their central, and there are also some terpenoids whose carbon content is not a multiple of five.

17.5. CLASSIFICATION OF TERPENOIDS

Most natural terpenoid hydrocarbons have the general formula $(C_5H_8)_n$. They can be classified on the basis of number of carbon atoms present in the structure (Table 17.2).

Table 17.2 Classification of Terpenoids

S. no.	Number of carbon atoms	Value of n	Class
1.	10	2	Monoterpenoids ($C_{10}H_{16}$)
2.	15	3	Sesquiterpenoids ($C_{15}H_{24}$)
3.	20	4	Diterpenoids ($C_{20}H_{32}$)
4.	25	5	Sesterpenoids ($C_{25}H_{40}$)
5.	30	6	Triterpenoids ($C_{30}H_{48}$)
6.	40	8	Tetraterpenoids ($C_{40}H_{64}$)
7.	>40	>8	Polyterpenoids ($C_5H_8)_n$

Each class can be further subdivided into subclasses according to the number of rings present in the structure.

1. *Acyclic Terpenoids:* They contain open structure.
2. *Monocyclic Terpenoids:* They contain one ring in the structure.
3. *Bicyclic Terpenoids:* They contain two rings in the structure.

4. *Tricyclic Terpenoids:* They contain three rings in the structure.
5. *Tetracyclic Terpenoids:* They contain four rings in the structure.

17.6. EVALUATION OF VOLATILE OILS

Product from different manufacturers varies considerably, since it is inherently difficult to control all the factors that affect a plants chemical composition. Environmental conditions such as sunlight and rainfall, as well as manufacturing process can create substantial variability in essential oil quality. Various procedures are given for the evaluation of essential oils. Preliminary examinations like odour, taste and colour. Physical measurements, which includes optical rotation, relative density and refractive index. Chromatographic techniques are used to determine the proportions of individual components of certain oils. The ketone and aldehyde content of oils are determined by reaction with hydroxylamine hydrochloride (oxime formation) and titration of the liberated acid. The oil, which passes the above examinations, would be having good quality and therapeutic value.

17.7. CHEMICAL TESTS

Natural drugs containing volatile oils can be tested by following chemical tests:

1. Thin section of drug on treatment with alcoholic solution of Sudan III develops red colour in the presence of volatile oils.
2. Thin section of drug is treated with tincture of alkana, which produces red colour that indicates the presence of volatile oils in natural drugs.

17.8. STORAGE OF VOLATILE OILS

Volatile oils are liable to oxidation on storage in presence of air, moisture and light. The oxidation is followed by the change in colour, increase in viscosity and change in odour. Hence, volatile oils must be stored in well-closed completely filled containers and away from light in cool places.

17.9. PHARMACEUTICAL APPLICATIONS

Volatile oils are used as flavouring agent, perfuming agent in pharmaceutical formulations, foods, beverages and in cosmetic industries. These are also used as important medicinal agent for therapeutic purposes like:

1. Carminative (e.g. Umbilliferous fruits)
2. Anthelmintic (e.g. Chenopodium oil)
3. Diuretics (e.g. Juniper)
4. Antiseptic (e.g. Eucalyptus)
5. Counter irritant (e.g. Oil of winter green)
6. Local anaesthetic (e.g. Clove)
7. Sedative (e.g. Jatamansi)
8. Local irritant (e.g. Turpentine)
9. Insect repellent (e.g. Citronella)
10. Source of vitamin A (e.g. Lemongrass)

17.10. VOLATILE OILS CONTAINING HYDROCARBONS

Hydrocarbons are present in all volatile oils. Limonene is the most widely distributed of the monocyclic terpenes. It occurs in Citrus, Mint, Myristica, Caraway, Thyme, Cardamom, Coriander and many other oils. Another monocyclic hydrocarbon monoterpene is *p*-cymene, present in Coriander, Thyme, Cinnamon and Myristica oils. Pinene, a dicyclic monoterpene, is also widely distributed. It occurs in many conifer oils and in Lemon, Anise, Eucalyptus, Thyme, Fennel, Coriander, Orange flower and Myristica oils. Sabinene, a dicyclic monoterpene of the thujane class, present in cardamom and lemon oils. Acyclic monoterpene myrcene occurs in Myricia, Lemon and Myristica. Cadinene occurring in juniper tar, is a sesquiterpene hydrocarbon. β-Caryophyllene is a sesquiterpene found in Wormwood, Peppermint, Cinnamon and Clove oils.

A volatile oil drug composed mainly of hydrocarbons is turpentine oil.

TURPENTINE OIL

Synonyms

Oleum terebinthinae, rectified oil of turpentine.

Botanical Source

Turpentine oil is the volatile oil obtained by the distillation of oleoresin from *Pinus longifolia* Roxb. and various species of Pinus, belonging to family Pinaceae.

Geographical Source

Pinus longifolia is cultivated in India and Pakistan, the other species are cultivated in the United States, France, Europe and Russia.

Collection and Preparation

The oleoresins which are collected are transferred to copper stills, water is added and heated. The impurities like woody debris, sand and other particles float on the surface of water which is skimmed off. The clarified resin is then subjected to distillation for obtaining the oil. The oil obtained is then treated with aqueous solution of sodium hydroxide. The treatment with sodium hydroxide removes the traces of phenols, cresol and resin acids. This oil which is produced is called the rectified turpentine oil.

Characteristics

Turpentine oil is a colourless to slightly yellowish transparent liquid with a strong characteristic odour and bitter, pungent taste. It is soluble in alcohol, insoluble in water, and miscible with glacial acetic acid, ether, chloroform and fixed oil. Turpentine oil should be stored in air-tight containers and in a cool place.

Chemical Constituents

Oil of turpentine contains more than 40 terpenes; the chief terpenes are α- and β- pinene with small quantity of camphene, limonene, etc.

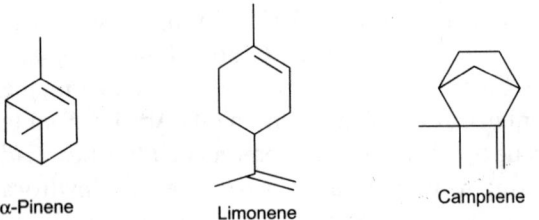

α-Pinene   Limonene   Camphene

Uses

Turpentine oil is used as counterirritant, rubefacient, in swelling, neuralgia, as mild antiseptic, as an expectorant in chronic bronchitis, as diuretic, and urinary antiseptic. When taken internally it causes irritation of kidney also. In industries it is used in the preparation of disinfectants, insecticides, paints, varnishes and pine oil.

Adulterants

The common adulterants are resin oil, wood turpentine and petroleum jelly. The last adulterant is detected by low weight per ml of the oil and resin oil forms a stain of fatty matters on staining on a paper.

Marketed Products

It is one of the ingredients of the preparations known as Rumalaya gel and Pain balm (Himalaya Drug Company).

17.11. VOLATILE OILS CONTAINING ALCOHOLS

Alcohols found in volatile oils are classified as: (1) acyclic alcohols, (2) monocyclic alcohols and (3) dicyclic alcohols. Methyl, ethyl, isobutyl, isoamyl, hexyl and the higher aliphatic alcohols occur in volatile oils. They are soluble in water, hence, they are washed away in the process of steam distillation. Many natural oils contain acyclic alcohols, geraniol, linalool and citronellol. The important monocyclic alcohols are menthol (from peppermint) and α-terpineol; borneol is a dicyclic terpene alcohol from borneo camphor; sesquiterpene alcohols include zingiberol, santalols and artemisin.

The important alcohol volatile oil containing drugs are peppermint, cardamom oil, coriander oil, rose oil, orange flower oil, juniper oil and pine oil.

PEPPERMINT

Synonym

Brandy mint.

Botanical Source

It is the oil obtained by the distillation of *Mentha piperita*, belonging to family Labiatae (Fig. 17.1).

Geographical Source

It is mainly found in Europe, United States and also in damp places of England.

Cultivation and Collection

Peppermint thrives best in a fairly warm, preferably moist climate, with well-drained, deep soils rich in humus. Peppermint will grow successfully, if once started into growth and carefully cultivated. The usual method of cultivation is to dig runners in the early spring and lay them in shallow trenches, 3 feet apart in well-prepared soil. The growing crop is kept well-cultivated and absolutely free from weeds and in the summer when the plant is in full bloom, the mint is cut by hand and distilled in straw. A part of the exhausted herb is dried and used for cattle food.

Characteristics

The leaves are shortly and distinctly stalked, 2 inches long and 3/4 to 1.5 inches broad. The margins are finely toothed, with smooth upper and lower surfaces The stems are 2–4 feet high, frequently purplish in colour. The flowers are reddish-violet in colour, present in the axils of the upper leaves, forming loose, interrupted spikes. The plant has a characteristic odour and if applied to the tongue has a hot, aromatic taste at first and afterwards produces a sensation of cold in the mouth caused by menthol present in it. Oil is colourless, yellowish or greenish liquid, with penetrating odour and a burning, camphorescent taste. On storage it becomes thick and reddish but increases the mellowness even if it is stored for 14 years.

Chemical Constituents

The chief constituent of peppermint oil is menthol, along with other constituents like menthyl acetate, isovalerate, menthone, cineol, inactive pinene, limonene and other less important bodies. Menthol separates on cooling it to a low temperature (–22°C). The flavouring properties of the oil are due to both the ester and alcoholic constituents, whereas the medicinal value is attributed only due to the alcoholic components. The English oil contains 60–70% of menthol, the Japanese oil containing 85% and the American has only about 50%.

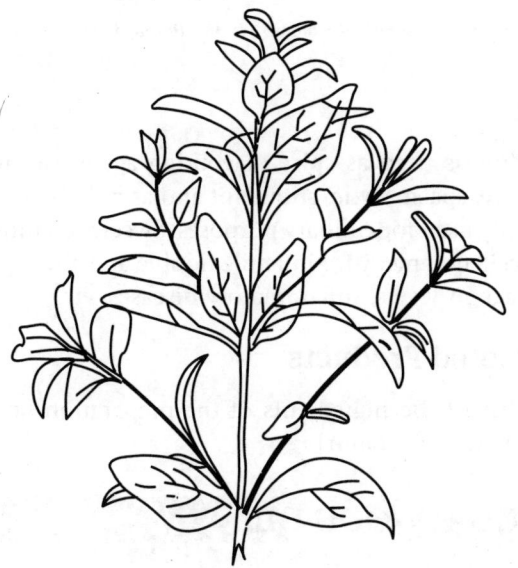

FIG. 17.1 *Mentha piperita*

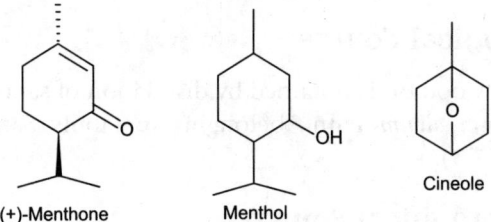

(+)-Menthone   Menthol   Cineole

Uses

It is stimulant, stomachic, carminative, inflatulence and colic; in some dyspepsia, sudden pains, for cramp in the abdomen and also in cholera and diarrhoea. Oil of peppermint allays sickness and nausea, as infants cordial. Peppermint is good to aid in raising internal heat and inducing perspiration. It is also used in cases of hysteria and nervous disorders.

Adulterants

Camphor oil, cedarwood oil and oil of African copaiba are occasionally used as an adulterant of peppermint oil, the oil is also adulterated with one-third part of rectified spirit. If adulterated with rectified spirit it can be identified by agitating it with water which produces milkiness. Rosemary oil and turpentine oil are also sometimes used as adulterants.

Marketed Products

It is one of the ingredients of the preparation known as Dabur lal tooth powder (Dabur).

PUDINA

Synonyms

Spearmint, Garden mint, Mackerel mint, Our lady's mint, Green mint, Sage of Bethlehem.

Biological Source

Pudina consists of dried leaves and flowering tops of *Mentha spicata* Linn., belonging to family Labiatae (Fig. 17.2).

Geographical Source

It is originally a native of the Mediterranean region and was later introduced into Britain.

History

Mint is mentioned in all early mediaeval lists of plants; it was grown in English gardens and cultivated in the Convent gardens during the ninth century. The Ancients believed that mint would prevent the coagulation of milk, to scent their bath water and as a restorative, as we use smelling salts today. Mint was so universally esteemed, that it was found wild in nearly all the countries to which civilization has extended. In America for 200 years, the mint was known as an escape from gardens, growing in all moist soils and proving on occasion troublesome like a weed. In the fourteenth century, mint was used for whitening the teeth, and its distilled oil is still used to flavour toothpastes, and in America, it is used especially, to flavour chewing gums, confectionery and also perfume soap.

Cultivation and Collection

Mint does well in almost all soil (though in dry, sandy soils it is occasionally difficult to grow) but should be planted in the cool and damp condition. As the plant is perennial, creeping stems propagations are used by lilting the roots in February or March, the stems are divided into small pieces and planted in shallow trenches, covering with 2 inches of soil. The distance between each plant is six inches within the rows and 8 inches between the rows. Cuttings can be taken at almost, any time during the summer and the young shoots are chosen for cutting. Good topdressing of soil is to be done, to obtain good mint or the plantation should be remade every three years. For liberal topdressing of short, decayed manure, such as an old hotbed or mushroom beds are added. When it commences to grow, or better still, perhaps, after the first or second cutting, will ensure luxuriant growth. When the plants are breaking into bloom, the stalks should be cut a few inches above the root, on a dry day (after the dew has disappeared) and before the hot sun takes any oil from the leaves. All discoloured and insect-eaten leaves should be removed and the stem tied loosely into bunches and hung to dry on strings in the usual manner directed for bunched herb. The bunches should be nearly equal in length and uniform in size to facilitate packing, if intended for sale and placed when dry in airtight boxes to prevent reabsorption of moisture. The leaves may also be stripped from the stems as soon as thoroughly dried and rubbed through a fine sieve, so as to free it from stalks as much as possible, or pounded in a mortar and then powdered, stored in stoppered bottles or tins rendered airtight.

Characteristics

From creeping rootstocks, erect, square stems rise to a height of about 2 feet, with very short-stalked, lance-shaped, acute-pointed, wrinkled, bright green leaves. It has fine-toothed edges and smooth surfaces, the ribs very prominent on the lower surface. Leaves are sessile, lanceolate to oblong, acute apex and coarsely dentate margin. The flowers are densely arranged in whorls in the axils of the upper leaves, forming slender, cylindrical, tapering spikes, pinkish in colour. The plant has characteristic taste and odour.

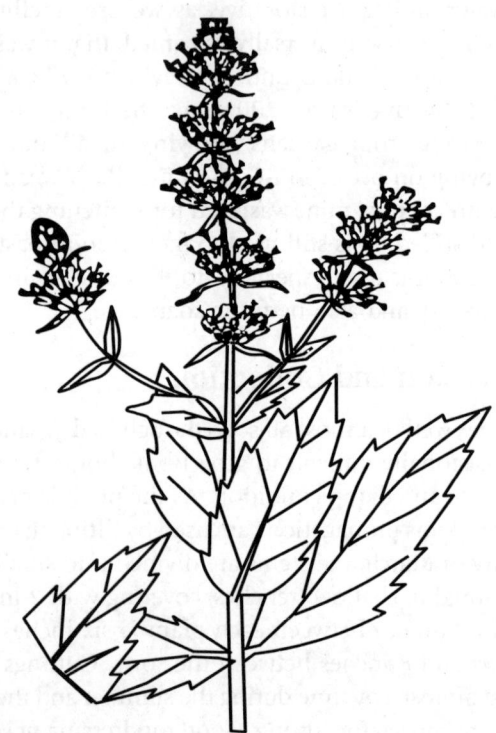

FIG. 17.2 *Mentha spicata*

Chemical Constituents

It contains about 0.5% volatile oil containing carvone. It also contains limonene, phellandrene, dihydrocarveol acetate, esters of acetic, butyric and caproic or caprylic acids. The drug also contains resin and tannins.

Carvone   (-)-α-Phellandrene   (+)-β-Phellandrene   Limonene

Uses

The drug is used as spice, flavouring agent, carminative, digestive, spasmolytic, stimulant and as a diuretic. Pudina is chiefly used for culinary purposes. Sweetened infusion is an excellent remedy for infantile trouble and also a pleasant beverage in fevers, inflammatory diseases, etc.

Marketed Products

It is one of the ingredients of the preparation known as Rheumatil gel (Dabur).

SANDALWOOD OIL

Synonyms

Chandan oil, sandal oil, yellow sandalwood oil, liginum.

Biological Source

Sandalwood oil is obtained by distillation of sandalwood, *Santalum album* Linn., belonging to family Santalaceae (Fig. 17.3).

Geographical Source

Sandal is a small to medium-sized, evergreen semiparasitic tree found in the dry regions of peninsular India from Vindhya Mountains southwards, especially in Mysore and Tamil Nadu. It has also been introduced in Rajasthan, parts of U.P., M.P. and Orissa.

Cultivation

Sandal tree grows mostly on red, ferruginous loam overlying metamorphic rocks, chiefly gneiss, and tolerates shallow, rocky ground and stony or gravelly soils, avoiding saline and calcareous situations. It is not found on the black-cotton soil. The growth is luxuriant on rich and fairly moist soils, such as garden loam and on well-drained deep alluvium along the river banks, but the heartwood from these trees is deficient in oil. The trees grown on poor soils, particularly on stony or gravelly soil, produce more highly scented wood, giving a better yield of the oil.

It reproduces from seeds dispersed by birds. Germination is profuse in the forests immediately after the monsoons. For artificial regeneration, it is necessary to provide suitable climatic and ecological conditions. For procuring seeds, the fruits are collected during January–March. Germination is up to 80%. Just after the first monsoon showers, the sandal seeds are dibbled and protected by thorny bushes. The seeds germinate in about 8–14 days. The seedlings grow rapidly, that is, up to 20–30 cm high, at the end of the first year.

Characteristics

Sandalwood oil is viscous, yellowish liquid having a peculiar, heavy, sweet and very lasting odour. It has sp. gr. 0.97–0.98, viscosity 1.5 and acid value 0.5–0.8.

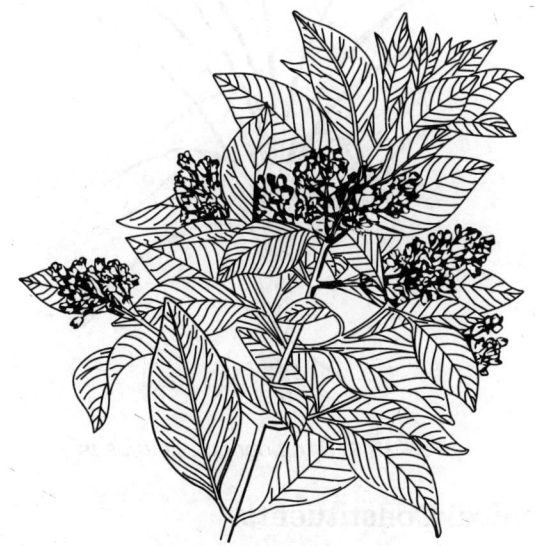

FIG. 17.3 *Santalum album*

Microscopy (Fig. 17.4)

Transverse section of wood shows alternating lighter and darker zones. The xylem consists of vessels and fibres. Vessels are large and usually occur single extending from one medullary ray to the next. Fibres are densely packed with interspersed air space termed as lacunae and constitute bulk of wood. Medullary rays are very fine, usually two cells wide and closed together. Volatile oil is deposited in the heartwood and is found in all the elements of the wood; it is not secreted by or contained in any particular cells or glands.

Chemical Constituents

The main odorous and medicinal constituent of sandalwood is santalol. This primary sesquiterpene alcohol forms more than 90% of the oil and is present as a mixture

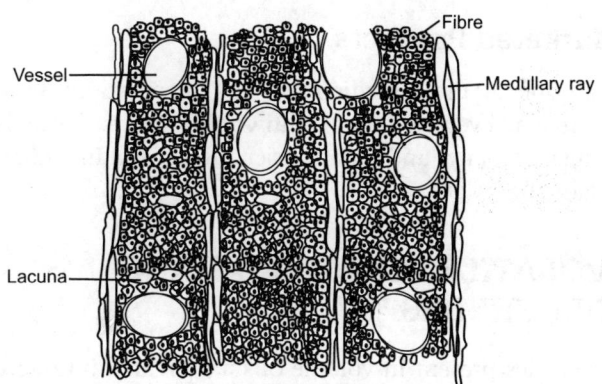

FIG. 17.4 Transverse section of sandalwood

of two isomers, α-santalol and β-santalol, the former predominating. The other constituents reported are hydrocarbons santene, nor-tricycloekasantalene, α- and β-santalenes.

β-Santalol

Uses

Sandalwood oil is highly used in perfumery creations and finds an important place in soaps, face creams and toilet powders. A chemoprotective action on liver carcinogenesis in mice has been demonstrated.

Substitutes and Adulterants

Oil from several plant sources are either used as substitutes for or as adulterants of natural sandalwood oil. Oil obtained from the Australian plant *Fusanus spicatus (Eucarya spicata)* is used as a substitute for genuine sandalwood oil. Wood and oil of *Santalum yasi* have a feeble odour which is not delicate like that of Indian sandalwood oil. East Africa markets the wood and oil derived from *Osyris tenuifolia*, the wood is similar to sandal and is used as an adulterant. An oil from Mauritius possesses most of the characteristics of the Indian oil. In West Indies, oil derived from *Amyris balsamifera* Linn. is marketed as a cheap substitute for Indian sandalwood oil. In India, the wood of *Erythroxylum monogynum* Roxb. is used as an adulterant. The wood of *Mansonia gagei* Drum, resembles sandalwood closely in its physical and other characteristics. Another species, which is common in southern India and used as an adulterant, is *Ximenia americana* Linn. The oil is adulterated with polyethylene glycols.

Marketed Products

It is one of the ingredients of the preparations known as Abana, Evecare, Lukol, Antiwrinkle cream (Himalaya Drug Company) and Mahamarichadi tail, Brahma rasayan (Dabur).

VOLATILE OILS CONTAINING ALDEHYDES

Aldehydes present in volatile oils are divided into acyclic and cyclic. The acyclic aldehydes are citral, which is a 3:1 mixture of geranial to neral, and citronellal, the aldehyde corresponding to citronellol. The cyclic aldehydes are safranal, phellandral, photocitral A and myrtenal. The aromatic aldehydes include cinnamaldehyde and vanillin.

The important drugs in this class are cinnamon, orange oil, lemon peel, lemon oil and citronella oil.

LEMONGRASS OIL

Synonyms

East India lemongrass, Malabar or Cochin lemongrass.

Biological Source

Lemongrass oil is obtained form *Cymbopogon flexuosus* Stapf. (syn. *Andropogon nardus* var. *flexuosus* Hack.), belonging to family Poaceae. It contains not less than 75% of aldehydes calculated as citral (Fig. 17.5).

Geographical Source

Lemongrass is indigenous to India and is found in Tinnevelli, Travancore and Cochin. Two principal varieties of lemongrass are recognized as the red-stemmed variety, the true *C. flexuosus*, which is a source of East Indian lemongrass oil and the white-stemmed variety which is designated as *C. flexuosus* var. *albescens*. The oil from the latter is low in aldehyde content and is slightly soluble in 70% alcohol.

Cultivation

Lemongrass grows best in well-drained sandy loam or in light sandy soil. Dark, heavy, rich soil, gives a higher yield of grass, but the oil obtained from it has lower citral content. Warmth and sunshine favour oil development. The grass grown on lower slopes, less exposed to heavy rains, is rich in oil content. The grass is cultivated in forest clearings or on hill slopes at an altitude of about 700 m. The ground is ploughed in March–April and seeds are sown at random. The grasses come up with the first shower of the monsoon. Weeding is carried out systematically in the plantation. Protection against grazing is necessary. The grass is ready

for cutting at the end of May or early in June and may be harvested every 35–40 days till November or December. The citral content of the oil is high (83%) when it is obtained from grass harvested during September–December. After cutting, the stubbles are burnt before the sporadic April monsoon shower. Fresh shoots come up from the roots with the start of regular monsoon, and the grass is ready for harvesting by the end of May. Plantations are renewed every six to eight years.

Characteristics

A light-coloured oil, rich in citral content, is obtained by steam distillation. The yield varies from 0.25 to 0.5% per acre.

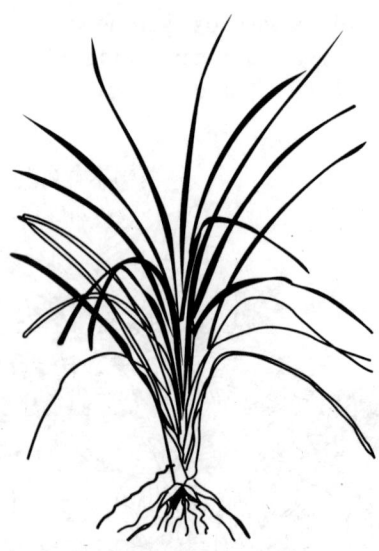

FIG. 17.5 *Cymbopogon flexuosus*

Chemical Constituents

Lemongrass oil is the principal source of citral (68–85%) from which ionone is derived. The oil also contains methyl heptanone, decyl aldehyde, geraniol, linalool, limonene, dipentene, citronellal, triacontane, triacontanol, intermedeol, isointermedeol, α- and β-pinene, car-3-ene, myrcene, ocimene, β-phellandrene, α-terpinene, *p*-cymene, terpinolene, methyl heptenone, geranyl acetate, β-caryophyllene, β-selinene, β-, γ- and δ-elemenes, α- and β-bisabolene, α-curcumene, γ- and δ-cadinene, methyl eugenol, elemol, β -caryophyllene oxide, eugenol, β-eudesmol, elemicin, farnesol, juniper camphor, geraniol, anisaldehyde, terpinen-4-ol, α - and β-terpineol, and borneol.

Citral

Citronellal

Uses

The oil is used in perfumery, soaps and cosmetics, and as a mosquito repellent. Lonones obtained from citral are required for synthetic violet perfumes.

Marketed Products

It is one of the ingredients of the preparation known as Sage lion balm (Sage Herbals).

LEMON PEEL

Synonym

Fructus Limonis.

Biological Source

Lemon peel is obtained from the fresh ripe fruit of *Citrus limon* (L.) Burm. f. (*C medico* var. *limon* Linn.), belonging to family Rutaceae.

Geographical Source

It is cultivated in California. West Indies, Italy, Spain, Sicily, Portugal, Florida, California, Jamaica and Australia; grown all over India, particularly in home gardens and small-sized orchards.

Collection

Lemon plant is a small, 3–5 m high, evergreen thorny tree with shining leaves. Fruits are collected before their green colour changes to yellow in January, August and November. The outer dark yellow peel is removed with a sharp knife. Dried lemon peel is spiral, 20 cm long, 1.5 cm wide, 2–3 mm thick, outer surface is rough and yellow, inner surface is pithy and white. Odour is strong and aromatic, taste is aromatic and bitter.

Chemical Constituents

Lemon peel contains volatile oil (2.5%), vitamin C, hesperidin and other flavone glycosides, mucilage, pectin and calcium oxalate. The important constituents of the volatile oil are limonene (90%), citronellal, geranyl acetate, α-pinene, camphene, linalool, terpineol, methyl heptenone, octyl and nonyl aldehydes, γ-terpinene, β-pinene, neral and geranial.

The peels also contain flavonoids eriocitrin, epigenin, luteolin, chrysoeriol, quercetin, isorhamnetin, limocitrin, limocitrol, isolimocitrol, hesperidin; coumarins scopoletin and umbelliferone; sinapic acid and β-coumaric acid.

Uses

Lemon peel is used as a flavouring agent, perfumery, stomachic and carminative. The oil, externally, is a strong rubefacient and if taken internally in small doses has stimulating and carminative properties.

Marketed Products

It is one of the ingredients of the preparations known as Protein shampoo (Himalaya Drug Company), Pancha Nimba churna (Zaipa Pharmaceuticals) and Ultra Doux conditioner (Garnier).

BITTER ORANGE PEEL

Synonyms

Citrus vulgaris, *Citrus bigaradia*, *Citrus aurantium amara*, Bigarade orange, Bitter orange, Seville orange, (Sweet) Portugal orange, China orange, *Citrus dulcis*, Cortex aurantii amar L, Seville orange peel.

Biological Sources

The orange peel is the fresh or dried outer part of the pericarp of *Citrus aurantium* Linn, belonging to family Rutaceae (Fig. 17.6).

Geographical Source

It is mainly cultivated in India, China, Spain, Madeira, Sicily, Malla and Morocco.

Cultivation and Collection

The tree requires a dry soil. It bears flowers after three years of grafting and the yield is increasing every year till it reaches its maximum, at about twenty years. A full grown tree yield on an average 50–60 lb of blossoms. One hundred orange trees, at the age of 10 years, will occupy nearly an acre of land and will produce about 2200 lb of orange flowers in a season. May is the flowering season, and the flowers are gathered two or three times a week, after sunrise. When the autumn is mild and atmospheric conditions are favourable, flowering takes place in October, and this supplementary harvest continues until January or till flowering is stopped. The autumn flowers have much less perfume than those of the spring, and their value is also one-half the price of May flowers. The Bitter Orange and Edible Orange trees

Hesperidin

resemble each other, but their leafstalks show a marked difference. The Bitter Orange is broadened out in the shape of a heart. The yield of oil is greatly influenced by the temperature and atmospheric conditions prevailing at the time of gathering. Such as damp, cool and changeable weather, considerable diminution is experienced. The dried orange peel is prepared by cutting with hand taking care that oil glands are not ruptured. Orange peel is dried in shade and stored in airtight containers at low temperature.

Characteristics

It is a small tree with a smooth, greyish brown bark and branches that spread into a regular hemisphere. The leaves are oval, alternate, evergreen, size ranging from 3 to 4 inches long, rarely with a spine in the axil. They are glossy, dark green on the upper surface, and lighter beneath. The calyx is cup-shaped and the thick, fleshy petals, five in number, are intensely white and curl back. The fruit is earth-shaped, a little rougher and darker than the common, sweet orange: the flowers are more strongly scented, and the glands in the rind are concave instead of convex. The dried peel is brittle and hard, dark orange red in colour, the surface is rough with oil glands which are slightly raised. The inner surface is yellowish white with pithy on them. It has an aromatic odour, bitter and aromatic taste. The oil of Bitter Orange peel is pale yellow liquid; it is soluble in four volumes of alcohol. Neutral to litmus paper and specific gravity at 25°C is 0.842–0.848.

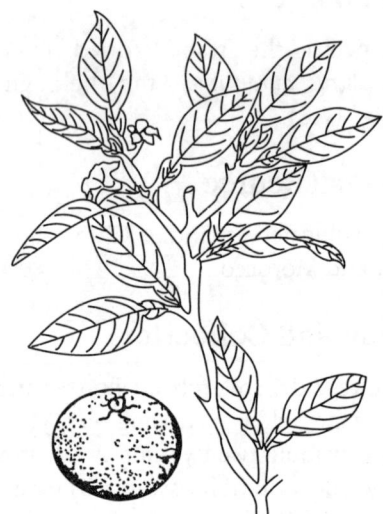

FIG. 17.6 *Citrus aurantium*

Chemical Constituents

Bitter orange peel contains of 1–2.5% volatile oil. The principle component of volatile oil is 90% limonene and small quantities of aldehydes citral, citronellal, bitter amorphous glycoside like aurantiamarin and it's acid; hesperidin, isohesperidin, vitamin C and Pectin.

Citronellal

Uses

It is used as aromatic, stomachic, carminative and flavouring agent, it is used particularly in fish liver oil preparations and liver extract. The oil is used chiefly as a flavouring agent, used in the oil of turpentine in chronic bronchitis. It is nonirritant to the kidneys and pleasant to take.

Marketed Products

It is one of the ingredients of the preparations known as Dabur Vatika Body and Bounce Shampoo (Dabur).

CINNAMON

Synonyms

Cortex cinnamomi, Ceylon cinnamon, Saigon cinnamon, Chinese cassia, *Cinnamomum aromaticum*, *Cinnamomum laurus*.

Biological Source

Cinnamon is the dried inner bark of the coppiced shoots of *Cinnamomum zeylanicum* Nees., belonging to family Lauraceae (Fig. 17.7).

Geographical Sources

Cinnamomum zeylanicum is widely cultivated in Ceylon, Java, Sumatra, West Indies, Brazil, Mauritius, Jamaica and India.

Cultivation and Collection

Cinnamon is cultivated by seed propagation method, about four to five seeds are placed in each hole at 2 m distance between the plants. The tree grows best in almost pure requiring only 1% of vegetable substance. It prefers shelter and constant rain of 75″ to rainfall. Cinnamon is an evergreen tree grows from 20 to 30 feet high, has thick scabrous bark, strong branches. The field is kept away from weeds and the plant is coppiced few inches above the ground, leaving five to six straight shoots on them. The bark is loosened and the longitudinal incisions are made using copper or brass knife. The barks arc stripped off and made into bundles and wrapped in Coir. The bundles are kept aside for about 2 hours to facilitate fermentation due to enzymatic action. The fermentation helps in the loosening of the outer layer up to pericycle. Each strip is taken and then they are scraped using a knife to separate the cork. The pieces are dried and they are categorized and packed one inside the other. Then compound quills are made by packing the small, quills into larger ones. They are cut into pieces of 1 m length and dried first under shade and later under sun. During drying, the original pale colour changes to brown due to the presence of some phlobatannins in the bark.

Characteristics

Cinnamon are either in single- or double-compound quills, with a size of 1 m length, 0.5 mm thickness and 6 to 10 mm diameter. The outer surface has yellowish brown colour having longitudinal lines of pericyclic fibre and scars and holes representing the position of leaves or the lateral shoots. The inner surface is darker than the outer. Cinnamon has a fragrant perfume; taste aromatic and sweet.

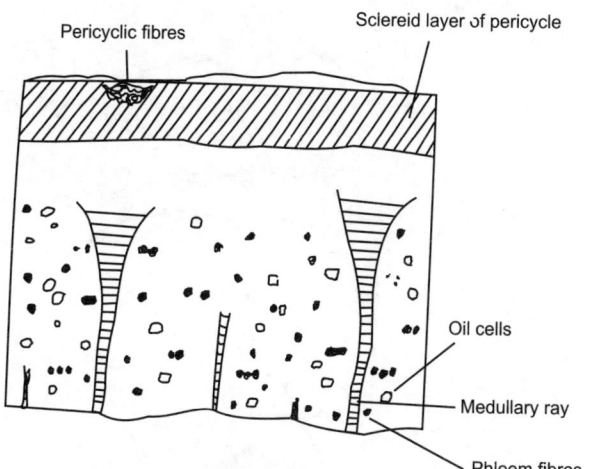

FIG. 17.8 T.S. (schematic) of cinnamon bark

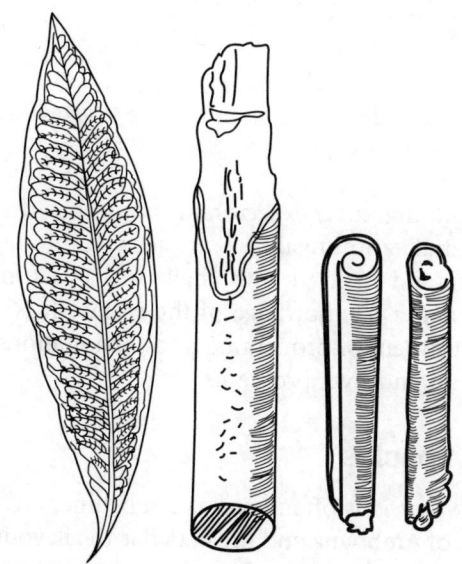

FIG. 17.7 Leaf and bark of *Cinnamomum zeylanicum*

Microscopy (Figs. 17.8 and 17.9)

The transverse section shows the presence of three to four layers of sclereids which are horse shoe shaped consisting of starch grains. The pericyclic fibres (6–15) are present on the outer margin. It consists of sieve tubes which are completely collapsed and are arranged tangentially; lignified phloem fibres, arranged as tangential rows of four to five cells; biseriate medullary rays with needle-shaped calcium oxalate crystals; longitudinally elongated idioblast consisting of volatile oil; subrectangular parenchyma cells with starch grains and calcium oxalate crystals.

Powder Microscopy (Fig. 17.10)

The powder is reddish-brown in colour with fragrant, pleasant and aromatic odour and taste. Microscopical examination shows abundant sclereids, lignified with

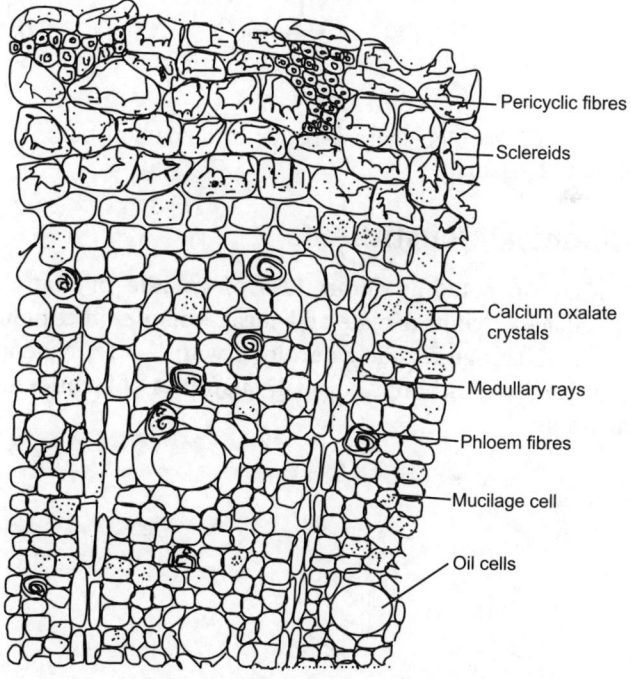

FIG. 17.9 Transverse section of cinnamon bark

U-shaped thickening, more or less isodiametric cells with numerous pits and striations. Fibres are abundant, thick-walled, lignified with few slit-shaped pits, found singly or associated with sclereids of the pericycle or oil cells. Oil cells are large, ovoid, thin-walled and occur singly, usually found associated with phloem elements. Abundant starch grains (individual grain up to 10 μm in diameter), simple or compound (2–4 components), spherical-ovoid with rounded or slit shaped hilum, are found scattered and in parenchyma and sclereids. Fragments of medullary ray cells containing minute acicular crystals of calcium oxalate, occasional fragments of cork cells, thin-walled, polygonal in surface view and minute acicular crystals of calcium oxalate (5–8 μm long) are found scattered.

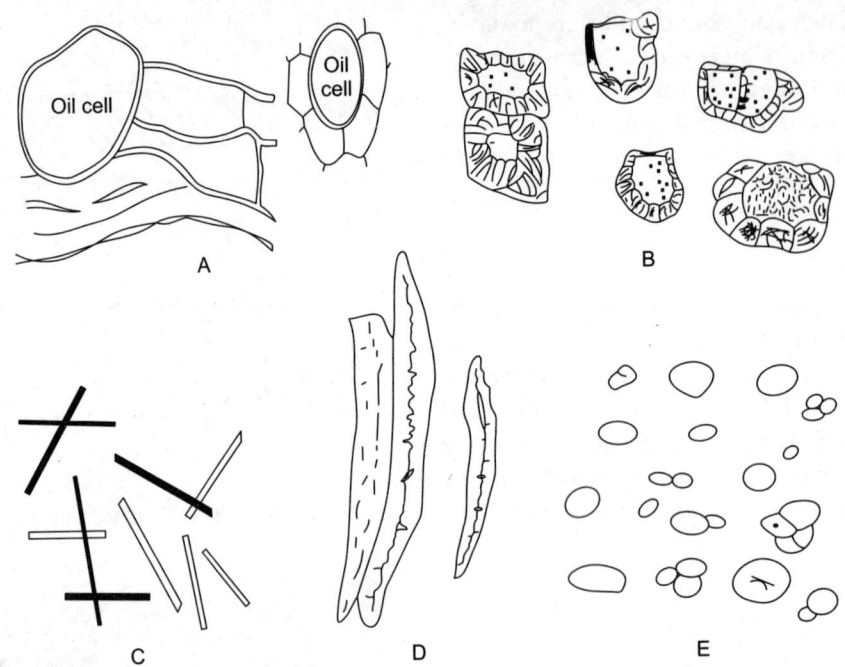

FIG. 17.10 Powder characteristics of cinnamon bark. (A: Oil cells, B: Sclereids, C: Calcium oxalate crystals, D: Fibres, E: Starch grains)

Chemical Constituents

Cinnamon contains about 10% of volatile oil, tannin, mucilage, calcium oxalate and sugar. Volatile oil contains 50–65% cinnamic aldehyde, along with 5–10% eugenol, terpene hydrocarbons and small quantities of ketones and alcohols.

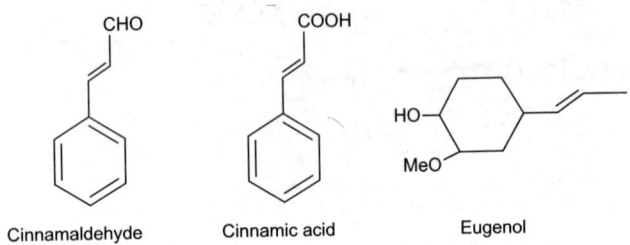

Cinnamaldehyde   Cinnamic acid   Eugenol

Chemical Tests

1. A drop of volatile oil is dissolved in 5 ml of alcohol and to it a drop of ferric chloride is added. A pale green colour is produced. Cinnamic aldehyde gives brown colour with ferric chloride, whereas eugenol gives blue colour.
2. The alcoholic extract is treated with phenylhydrazine hydrochloride, it produces red colour due to the formation of phenylhydrazone of cinnamic aldehyde.

Uses

It is used as an alterative, aromatic, carminative, flavouring agent, analgesic, antiseptic, antirheumatic, antispasmodic, demulcent, digestive, expectorant, stomachic, diaphoretic, antibacterial, antifungal, etc. It stops vomiting, relieves flatulence and is given with chalk and as astringents for diarrhoea and haemorrhage of the womb. It is also used in the treatment of bronchitis, colds, palpitations, nausea, congestion and liver problems.

Other Species

Cinnamon cassia is often used as a substituent. *C. culiawan* is native of Amboyna and the bark has the flavour of clove, *C. iners*, *Cassia burmarin*, *Saigon cinnamon* and *C. nitidum* are also used.

Marketed Products

It is one of the ingredients of the preparations known as Rumalaya gel, Koflet lozenges, Chyavanprash (Himalaya Drug Company), Garbhapal ras, Sutsekhar ras (Dabur) and Sage Staminex capsules (Sage Herbals).

CASSIA BARK

Synonym

Chinese cinnamon, *Cassia lignea*, Bastard cinnamon, *Cassia aromaticum*, Canton cassia.

Biological Source

Cassia is the dried stem bark of *Cinnamomum cassia* Blume, belonging to family Lauraceae.

Geographical Source

It is indigenous to China, Cochin and Assam. It is also cultivated in Ceylon, Japan, Sumatra, Java, Mexico and America.

Cultivation

The collection is done from cultivated plants. The trees are allowed to grow for 6 years and then the branches which are about 3 cm thick and 40 cm long are cut. The twigs and leaves are stripped off, then two longitudinal slits and three to four transverse ring cuts are made. The barks are stripped off. Then cork and some parts of outer cortex are peeled off by running a small plane over it. The bark is then dried, packed in bundles of 30–40 cm long weighing ½ kg and exported.

Characteristics

The barks are either channelled pieces or as single quills; the size of drug ranging from 6 to 40 cm long, 1 to 2 cm in width and 1 to 3 mm in thickness. The fractures are short. The outer surface is dark reddish-brown, smooth with rather rough patches of grey cork. The inner, surface has fine striations. The flavour is more pungent, less sweet, and delicate and slightly bitter than that of cinnamon. The bark may be distinguished from that of cinnamon, because they are thicker, coarser, darker and dull.

Microscopy

Periderm is the outer layer; cork consists of few layers of both thin-walled and thick-walled cells. The inner thick-walled cells are lignified. Cortex consists of 10–15 layers of parenchyma with sclereids isolated or in groups and starch grains. A well-developed belt of sclereids occur between the primary and secondary phloem. Cassia has the lignified and pitted sclereids as its characteristic feature. The secondary phloem consist of phloem parenchyma which is thin-walled, containing abundant starch; isolated or group of phloem fibres embedded in phloem parenchyma and one- to three-celled medullary rays consisting of the starch and acicular raphides.

Chemical Constituents

Cassia bark yields 1–2% of volatile oil. It also has about 80% cinnamyl acetate, cinnamic acid, caryophyllene, phenylpropyl acetate, orthocumaric aldehyde, coumarin, tannic acid and starch. Eugenol is absent. The value of the drug depends on the percentage of cinnamic aldehyde present in it.

Uses

Cassia is used as carminative, mildly astringent, stomachic, decreasing the milk secretion, and emmenagogue. It is used

Cinnamic acid

Caryophyllene

in uterine haemorrhage, menorrhagia, diarrhoea, nausea and vomiting. The cassia oil is a powerful germicide, local stimulant also prescribed in flatulent colic and gastric debility.

Chemical Test

1. Cassia gives a deep blue black colour when a drop of tincture of iodine is mixed with fluid ounce of a decoction of the powder.
2. The cheaper cassia can be distinguished by the greater quantity of mucilage present, which can be extracted by cold water.
3. Cassia oil contains coumarin which gives strong green-blue fluorescence on addition of alkali.

Other Species

Cassia burmannii Blume or the Java or Batavia cinnamon; they have a slightly aromatic odour and aromatic and mucilaginous taste; it can be distinguished by the presence of tabular crystals of calcium oxalate which are not found in other cinnamon barks. C. inners, C. lignea, C. sintok, C. obtusifolium, C. culilawan, C. loureirii, C. pauciflorum, C. inserta, C. nitidum are some of the commonly available species of cinnamon.

Marketed Products

It is one of the ingredients of the preparations known as Diakof, Koflex, Abana (Himalaya Drug Company), Shukra Matrika Bati (Baidyanath) and Madhudoshantak (Jamuna Pharma).

CITRONELLA OIL

Synonyms

Citronella grass, Nardus, Manna grass, Nard grass.

Biological Source

It is the oil obtained by the steam distillation of fresh leaves of Cymbopogon nardus (L.) Rendle, belonging to family Poaceae.

Geographical Source

Citronella is native to Southeast Asia and grown commercially in Sri Lanka, India, Burma, Indonesia and

Java. In South Florida and southern California it is grown as an ornamental.

Cultivation and Collection

It is propagated by seed. It needs a long, warm season and may not survive cool damp winters. They are sown in summer at an altitude of 2000–3000 m above sea level. It requires an annual rainfall of not less than 750 mm. The crop requires proper irrigation and gets ready for harvest after eight months of growth.

Characteristics

It is a tall, tufted perennial, clump-forming tropical grass with narrow leaf blades. They grow to a height of 5–6 ft. The leaves are greyish green, flat, about 3 ft long, and 1 inch wide. Citronella oil has a slightly sweet, lemony smell. It is pale greenish yellow in colour.

Chemical Constituents

Citronella grass contains of volatile oil. The main chemical components of citronella oil are citronellic acid, geraniol, nerol, citral, borneol, camphene, citronellol, citronellal, dipentene and limonene. It consist about 3.0% limonene; 35.3% citronellal; 12.0% citronellol, 24.9% geraniol, 4.3% citronellyl acetate, 6.3% geranyl acetate and 0.8% linalool.

Geraniol   Citral   Citronellal   Linalool

Uses

Citronella grass is the source of the commercial citronella oil, used in perfumery, as an insect repellent. Citronella oil is antiseptic, deodorant, tonic, insecticide, diaphoretic, parasitic, bactericidal and stimulant. Citronella oil can be mixed with other vegetable oils and used in massage on skin for an insect repellent.

SAFFRON

Synonyms

Crocus, Spanish saffron, French saffron.

Biological Source

Saffron is the dried stigma and styletops of *Crocus sativus* Linn., belonging to family Iridaceae (Fig. 17.11).

Geographical Source

The plant is native of south Europe and is found in Spain, France, Macedonia, Italy, Austria, China, Germany, Switzerland and Iran. In India, the plant is cultivated in Kashmir.

Cultivation and Collection

The plant is a small, perennial herb, 6–10 cm high. The corms are planted in July–August in well prepared soil. In the following year flowering takes place. Each corm is replaced by daughter corms. The flowers are collected early in the morning. The style of each flower is separated just below the stigma and dried by artificial heat for 30–45 min. The drug is coated and stored in dry place. About 1 kg of dried drug is collected from nearly 100,000 flowers. Saffron thrives well in cold regions with warm or subtropical climate. It requires a rich, well-drained, sandy or loamy soil. The plant is propagated by bulbs. No manure is applied or irrigation is given once the plants are established. The bulbs continue to live for 10 or 15 years, new bulbs being produced annually and the old ones rotting away. The plants flower in October–December, heavy rains during this period are harmful. Styles and stigmas are separated and dried in the sun or over low heat on sieves in earthen pots. The tripartite stigmas plucked from fleshly collected flowers and dried in the sun constitute saffron of the best quantity.

Characteristics

Saffron is flattish-tubular, almost thread-like stigmas which are about 3 cm long with slender funnel having dentate or fimbricate rim. Colour is reddish-brown with some yellowish pieces of tops of styles. Odour is strong, peculiar and aromatic; taste is aromatic and bitter.

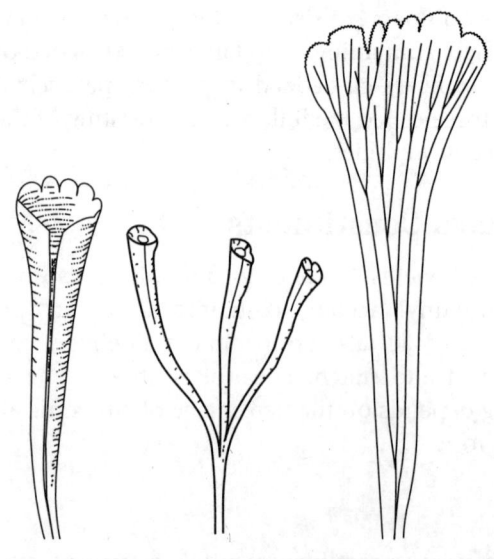

FIG. 17.11 *Crocus sativus*

Chemical Constituents

The drug contains volatile oil (1.3%), fixed oil, and wax. Crocin is the chief colouring principle in saffron. On hydrolysis, it yields digentiobiose and the carotenoid pigment crocetin. Saffron possesses a number of carotenoid coloured compounds such as ester of crocin (a coloured glycoside), picrocrocin (a colourless bitter glycoside), crocetin (an aromatic compound), gentiobiose, α- and γ-carotenes, lycopene, zeaxanthin, crocin-1, crocin-2, crocin-3, crocin-4, mono- and digentiobiosyl and glucosyl esters of crocetin; β-sitosterol, ursolic, oleanolic, palmitoleic, oleic, linoleic and linolenic acids (in bulbs).

Crocin

Crocetin

Chemical Tests

1. Add a drop of sulphuric acid to dry stigma. It turns blue, gradually changing to purple and finally purplish-red.
2. Saffron imparts yellowish orange brown colour with water.

Uses

Saffron is used in fevers, cold, melancholia and enlargement of the liver; as colouring and flavouring agent, catarrhal, snake bite, cosmetic pharmaceutical preparations; and as spice. Saffron has stimulant, stomachic, tonic, aphrodisiac, emmenagogue, sedative and spasmolytic properties.

Adulterant

Saffron is frequently adulterated with styles, anthers and parts of carolla of saffron. Exhausted saffron, flowers and floral parts of some Compositae like calendula species and *Carthamus tinctorius*, com silk, and various materials coloured with coal tar dyes are also used as adulterants. Water, oil or glycerin is added to increase the weight. Coke saffron of commerce often contains safflower florets with adhesive sugary substances.

Marketed Products

It is one of the ingredients of the preparations known as Tentex forte, Speman forte (Himalaya Drug Company), J.P. Nikhar oil (Jamuna Pharma) and Amyron (Aimil Pharmaceuticals).

VOLATILE OILS CONTAINING KETONES

Ketones present in volatile oils are divided into (1) monocyclic terpene ketones, for example, menthone, carvone, piperitone, pulegone and diosphenol; (2) dicyclic ketones, including camphor, fenchone and thujone; and (3) acyclic ketone, for example, artemisia ketone and tagetone.

The important drugs in this category are camphor, caraway, dill, fennel and jatamansi.

CAMPHOR

Synonyms

Gum camphor, Japan camphor.

Biological Source

Camphor is a solid ketone, obtained from the volatile oil of *Cinnamomum camphora* (L.) Nees et Eber, belonging to family Lauraceae (Fig. 17.12). Synthetic camphor, which is optically inactive, is prepared from turpentine and would probably have completely replaced the natural product.

Geographical Source

The plant is a big tree native to Eastern Asia. It is found widely in Mediterranean region, Sri Lanka, Egypt, South Africa, Java, Sumatra, Brazil, Jamaica, Florida, Formosa, Japan, South China, India and California. In India, the tree is planted in gardens up to 1300 m height in the Northwest Himalayas. It is successfully cultivated at Dehradun, Saharanpur, Calcutta, Nilgiris and Mysore.

Preparation

Old trees possess high concentration of camphor. The small wood chips are treated with steam. Camphor is sublimed and liquid volatile oil passed away into the receiver. Excess of camphor is obtained from the volatile oil. Camphor is purified by treating it with lime and charcoal and resublimation into large chambers to form flowers of camphor. The collected camphor is made into blocks by hydraulic pressure.

The specific rotation of natural camphor is +41° to +43°. The synthetic camphor is optically inactive.

Characteristics

Natural camphor is colourless translucent mass with crystalline fracture, rhombohedral crystals from alcohol, cubic crystals by-melting and chilling. Odour is characteristic, and taste is pungent and aromatic which is followed by cold sensation. It evaporates at room temperature and pressure, m.p. 180°, very volatile in steam. At 25°, 1 g dissolves in about 800 ml water (giving a colloidal solution), in 1 ml alcohol, 1 ml ether, 0.5 ml chloroform, 0.4 ml benzene, 0.4 ml acetone, 1.5 ml of turpentine oil and 0.5 ml glacial acetic acid. Camphor has a peculiar tenacity and cannot be powdered in a mortar unless it is moistened with an organic solvent.

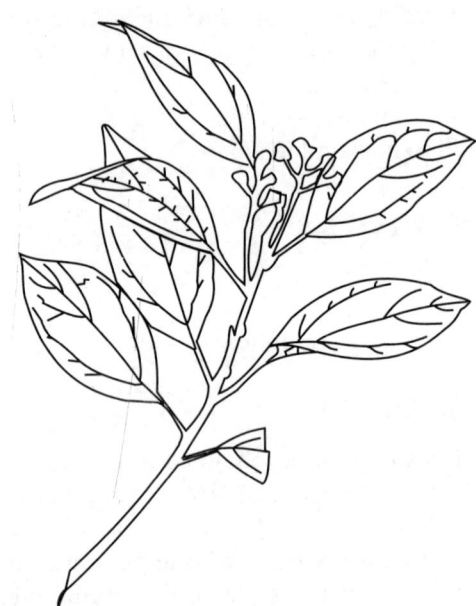

FIG. 17.12 *Cinnamomum camphora*

Chemical Constituents

Camphor oil contains camphor, cineole, pinene, camphene, phellandrene, limonene and diterpenes. Camphor is entirely a monoterpenic ketone. Its basic carbon framework is related to borneol.

Camphor

Uses

Camphor is used externally as a rubefacient, counterirritant and internally as a stimulant, carminative and antiseptic. It is a topical antipruritic and anti-infective, used as 1–3% in skin medicaments and in cosmetic. It is also used to manufacture some plastics, celluloid, in lacquers, varnishes, explosives, pyrotechnics, as moth repellent and in embalming fluids.

Allied drugs

Borneo camphor, obtained from *Dryobalanops aromatica* (Dipterocarpaceae), and Ngai camphor, obtained from *Blumea balsamifera* (Asteraceae), are used in China and Japan. In California levorotatory camphor is produced from species of *Artemisia* (Asteraceae).

Marketed Products

It is one of the ingredients of the preparations known as Ophthacare, Pilex, Rumalaya (Himalaya Drug Company) and Dabur balm (Dabur).

CARAWAY

Synonyms

Caraway fruits, Fructus carvi, Carum, Caraway seed.

Biological Source

Caraway consists of the dried ripe fruits of *Carum carvi* Linn., belonging to family Umbelliferae (Fig. 17.3).

Geographical Source

It is cultivated widely in northern and central parts of Europe, Turkey in Asia, India and North Africa. It is also available in Canada, the United States, Morocco, Germany, Russia, Norway and Sweden.

History

The use of caraway is well-known in classic days and it is believed that its use originated with the ancient Arabs, the ancient Arabs called the 'seeds' *Karawya* and so the origin of our word Caraway and the Latin name *Cam*, According to Pliny the name Carvi was derived from Caria, in Asia Minor, where according to him the plant was originally found. In old Spanish the name of caraway occurs as *Alcaravea*. The use of caraway was also quite popular during the Middle Ages and in Shakespeare's times.

Cultivation

The plant is an erect biennial herb. It prefers loamy soil. About five seeds are sown in March or April in drills, 1 ft apart. The plants when strong enough are thinned out to about 8 inches in the rows. Proper manure and weeding is done. When the oldest fruits are mature and ripe, the plant is cut and the Caraways are separated by thrashing. They are then dried either on trays in the sun or by very gentle heat over a stove with occasional shaking.

Characteristics

The fruits which are incorrectly called seeds are laterally compressed, translucent, slightly curved and somewhat horny in nature. They are yellowish brown in colour with five distinct ridges. The fruits are of 4–7 mm long, 1 mm broad and thick. They evolve a pleasant, aromatic odour when bruised and have an agreeable taste.

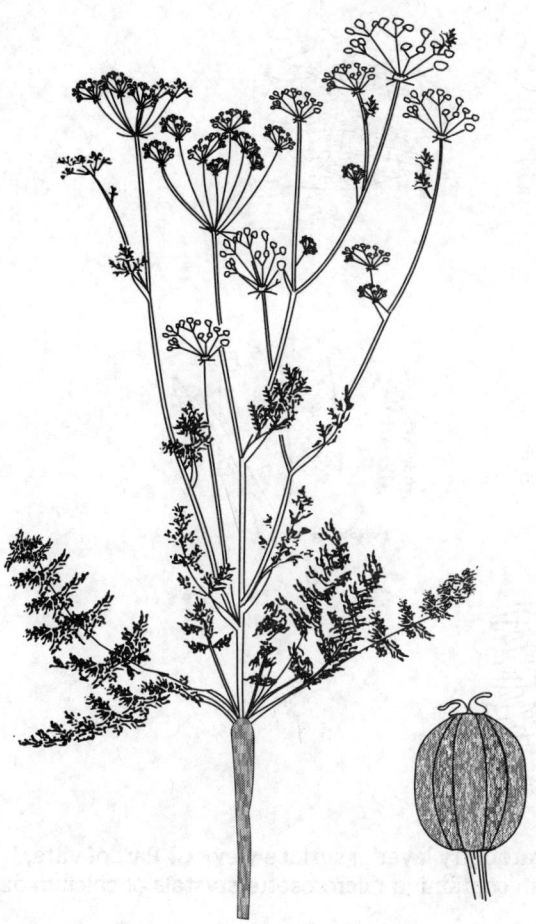

FIG. 17.13 *Carum carvi*

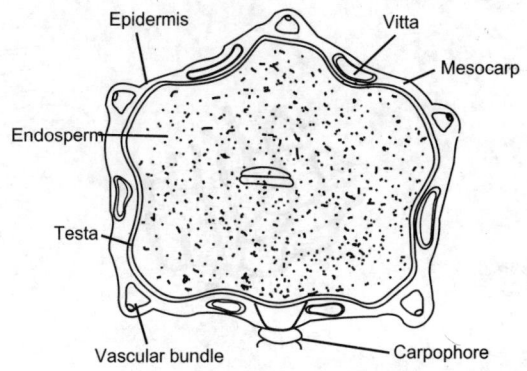

FIG. 17.14 T.S. (schematic) of caraway fruit

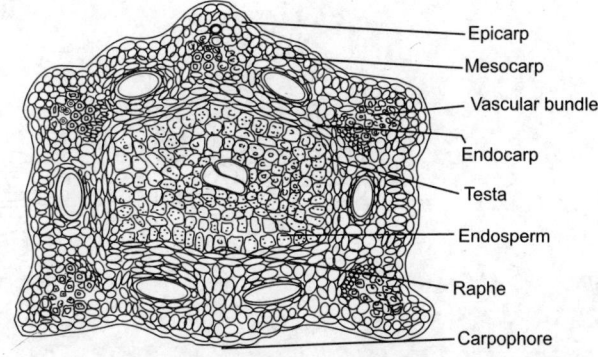

FIG. 17.15 Transverse section of caraway fruit (mericarp)

Microscopy (Figs. 17.14 and 17.15)

Dorsal region consist of four vittae and the commissural surface has two vittae and a carpophore. The epicarp has polygonal tubular cells along with few stomata which are covered with cuticle. The mesocarp consists of rounded parenchyma cells, with scattered sclereids. The endocarp has elongated subrectangular cells, whereas the endosperm is made of thick-walled cellulosic parenchyma cells consisting of oil globules, calcium oxalate crystals and aleurone grains.

Powder Microscopy (Fig. 17.16)

The powder is dark brown in colour with characteristic aromatic odour and taste. Microscopical examinations shows groups of sclereids of mesocarp in a single layer, composed of thick-walled, rectangular to subrectangular pitted cells. Fragment of vitta, composed of thin-walled polygonal cells with transverse septa, is visible in surface view. Epicarp consists of thin-walled, cells with slightly straight anticlinal walls and frequent stomata, parallel to the long axes of epidermal cells. Endocarp, i.e. parquetry layer, is composed of considerably elongated, thin-walled cells with their long axes parallel to one another. Endosperm cells contain microrosette crystals of calcium oxalate, aleurone

grains and oil globules. A few lignified fragments of vascular tissue, i.e. fibres and vessels are found scattered.

Chemical Constituents

Caraway grown in more northerly altitudes are richer in essential oil than that grown in southern regions and similarly if caraway is grown in full sun a greater percentage and richer oil is obtained. It has 4–7% volatile oil which consists of about 60% carvone alone with dihydrocarvone, carveol, carvacrol and terpene limonene. The chief constituent of the oil is a hydrocarbon termed carvene and an oxygenated oil carvol.

Carvone   Carvacrol

Uses

Both fruit and oil possess aromatic, stimulant, flavouring agent and carminative. It is recommended in dyspepsia, as a tonic; as stomachic, for flatulent indigestion, as a excellent vehicle for children's medicine and also as a spice.

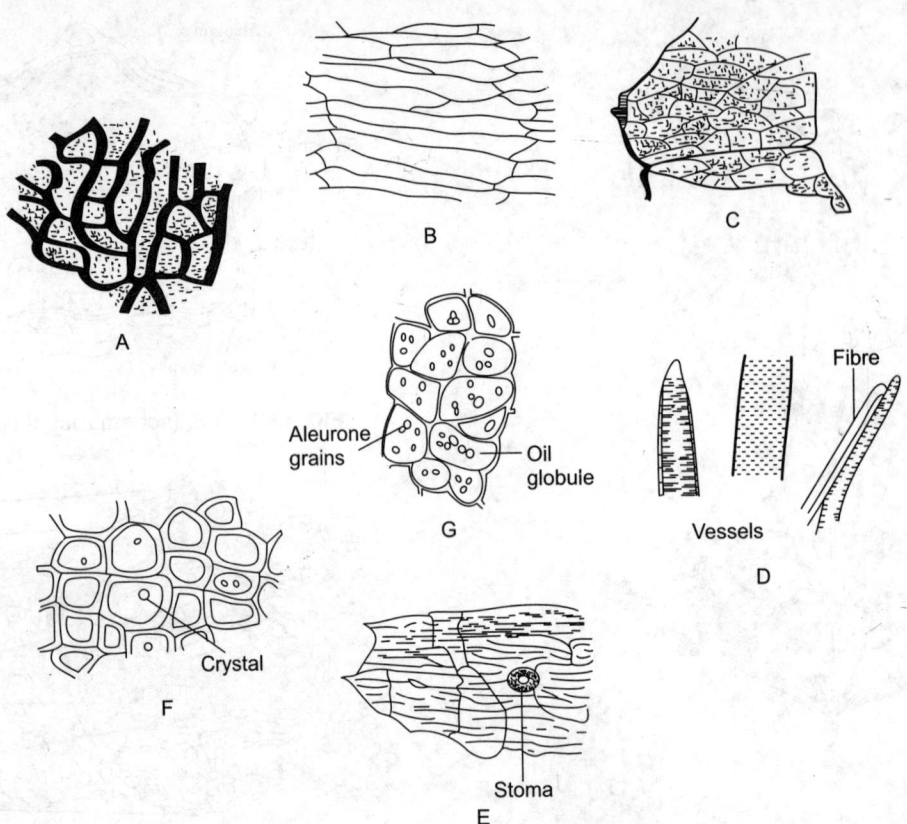

FIG. 17.16 Powder characteristics of caraway fruit. (A: Sclereids, B: Parquetry layer in surface view, C: Part of vitta, D: Vessels and fibre, E: Epidermis of pericarp in surface view, F: Endosperm containing microrosette crystals of calcium oxalate, G: Fragment of endosperm)

Allied Drug

Cuminum cyminum is commonly used in many parts of country. The volatile oil content is only about 3–4%.

Marketed Products

It is one of the ingredients of the preparations known as Gripe water (Himalaya Drug Company) and Sage Baby oil (Sage Herbals).

CORIANDER

Synonyms

Fructus coriandri, Coriander fruits, Cilantro, Chinese parsley.

Biological Source

Coriander consists of dried ripe fruits of *Coriandrum sativum* Linn., belonging to family Umbelliferae (Fig. 17.17).

Geographical Sources

Cultivated in Central and Eastern Europe, particularly in Russia, Hungary, in Africa and India. In India it is cultivated in Maharashtra, U.P., Rajasthan, Jammu and Kashmir. It is also found in a antiwild state in the east of England.

Cultivation and Collection

The coriander seeds are sown in dry weather either in March or in early autumn. Shallow drills, about 1/2 inch deep and 8 inches apart are made and the seeds are sown in it, the rate of germination is slow. The plants are annual herb, which grow to a height of 1–3 feet high, slender and branched. The flowers are in shortly stalked umbels with five to ten rays. The seeds fall as soon as ripe and when the seeds are ripe (about August), the disagreeable odour is produced. Plant is then cut down with sickles; the fruits are collected and dried. During drying fruits develop aromatic smell and the unpleasant odour disappears.

Characteristics

The fruit is a cremocarp, subspherical in shape, Yellowish-brown in colour. The size of the fruit is 3–4 mm in diameter, with aromatic odour, and spicy, aromatic taste.

Microscopy (Fig. 17.18)

The transverse section of coriander shows the presence of a dorsal surface and a commissural surface. The dorsal surface

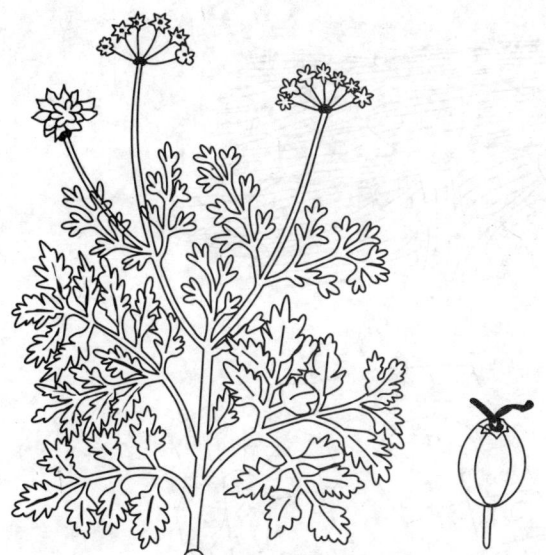

FIG. 17.17 *Coriandrum sativum*

consists of two vittae and a carpophore. The dorsal surface has five primary ridges and four secondary ridges. The epicarp consists of a single row of small thick-walled cells with calcium oxalate crystals. The mesocarp has an outer loosely arranged tangentially elongated parenchyma cells and the middle layer consisting of sclerenchyma. The middle layer is again divided into; the outer region of sclerenchyma is represented by longitudinally running fibres, whereas the inner region has tangentionally running fibres. The vascular bundles are present below the primary ridges. The inner layer has polygonal, irregularly arranged parenchyma cells. The endocarp has the parquetry arrangement. In the testa

it has single-layered, yellowish cells, and the endosperm is thick, polygonal, colourless parenchyma with fixed oil and aleurone grains.

Powder Microscopy (Fig. 17.19)

The powder is greenish to light brown in colour with characteristic, aromatic odour and spicy taste. Microscopical examination shows abundant sclerenchyma of mesocarp, composed of thick-walled, fusiform, pitted cells. Sclerenchyma exhibits a characteristic appearance of sinuous rows, crossing at right angles because of more longitudinally directed arrangement of their cells or fibres in primary ridges and their tangentially directed arrangement in secondary ridges, which can be easily seen in transverse section of pericarp. Epicarp consists of thin-walled, polygonal cells with straight anticlinal walls, infrequent stomata and a small prismatic calcium oxalate crystal per cell. Endocarp (parquetry layer) is composed of elongated, thin-walled cells, arranged in groups with very slight differences in orientation of their long axes and straight anticlinal walls. Endosperm cells contain microrosette crystals of calcium oxalate (3–10 μm) and oil globules.

Chemical Constituents

Coriander consist of about 1% of volatile oil, the chief volatile components are D-(+)-linalool (coriandrol), along with other constituents like borneol, *p*-cymene, camphor, geraniol, limonene and alpha-pinenes. The fruits also contain fatty oil and hydroxycoumarins. The fatty oils include acids of petroselinic acid, oleic acid, linolenic acid,

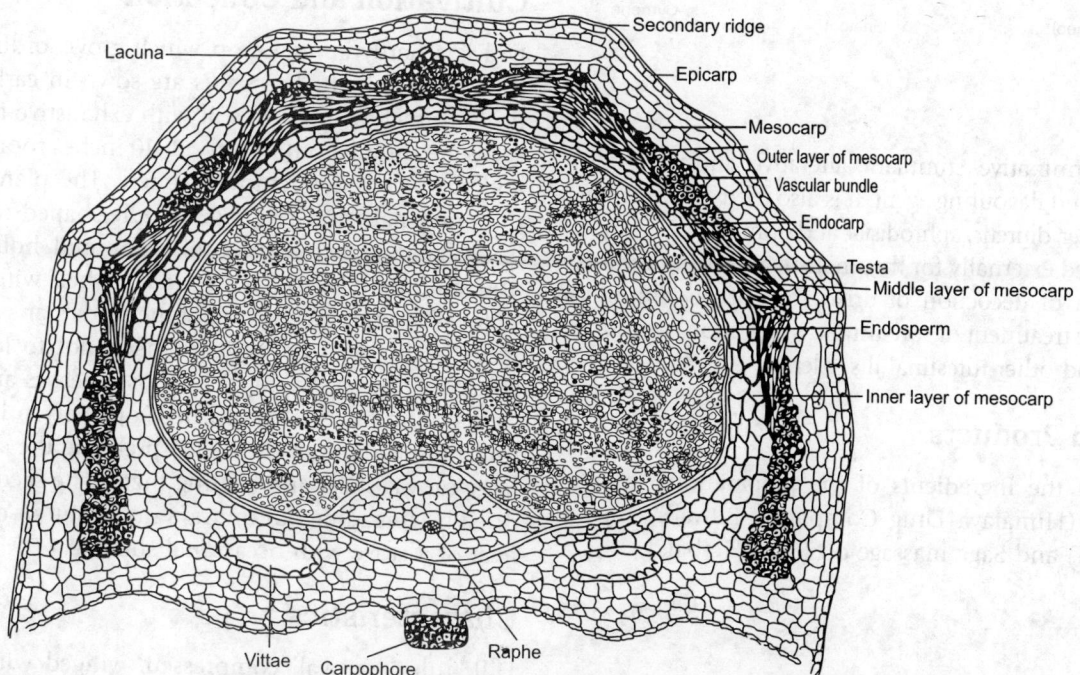

FIG. 17.18 Transverse section of coriander fruit (mericarp)

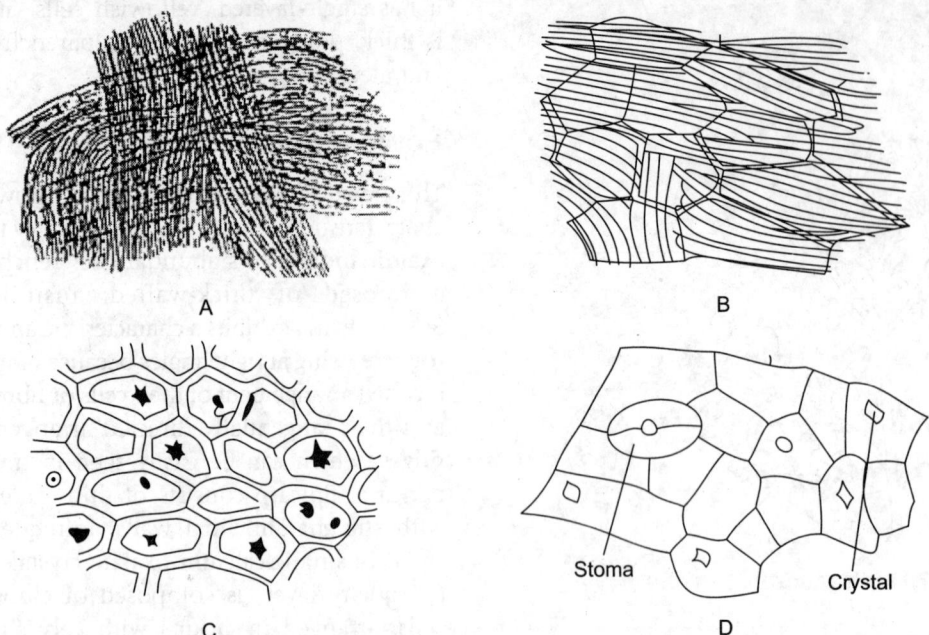

FIG. 17.19 Powder characteristics of coriander fruit (A: Sclerenchymatous fibres, B: Parquetry layer, C: Endosperm containing microrosette crystals of calcium oxalate, D: Epidermis of pericarp)

whereas the hydroxycoumarins include the umbelliferone and scopoletin.

Borneol   Linalool   *p*-Cymene

Uses

Aromatic, carminative, stimulant, alterative, antispasmodic, diaphoretic and flavouring agent. It is also used as refrigerant, tonic, appetizer, diuretic, aphrodisiac and stomachic. Coriander can be applied externally for rheumatism and painful joints. The infusion of decoction of dried fruit of cardamom is useful for the treatment of sore-throat, indigestion, vomiting, flatulence and other intestinal disorders.

Marketed Products

It is one of the ingredients of the preparations known as Cystone (Himalaya Drug Company), Bilwadi churna (Baidyanath) and Sage massage oil (Sage Herbals).

DILL

Synonyms

Fructus anethi, Anethum, European dill.

Biological Source

Dill consists of the dried ripe fruits of *Anethum graveolens* Linn., belonging to family Umbelliferae (Fig. 17.20).

Geographical Source

It is native of the Mediterranean region and Southern Russia. Also grown in Italy, Spain and Portugal.

Cultivation and Collection

Dill is a hardy annual crop which grows ordinarily from 2 to 2.5 feet high. The seeds are sown in early spring in drills 10 inches apart on soil with exhaustive fertility. The seeds are thinned out to leave 8–10 inches room each way, and the weeds are removed timely. The plant has more than one stalk and its long, spindle-shaped root, growth is upright, its stems smooth, shiny and hollow and in mid summer it bears flat terminal umbels with numerous yellow flowers. The mowing of the seeds starts as the lower seeds begin; with proper care taken not to loose any of the seeds due to shaking. The loose sheaves are built into stacks of about 20 sheaves, tied together. In hot weather, thrashing is done in the field, spreading the sheaves on a large canvas sheet and beating them. The seeds are finally dried by spreading out on trays in the sun or on moderate heat of a stove with occasional shaking.

Characteristics

Dill fruits are oval, compressed, winged with 4 mm in length, about one-tenth inch wide and 1 mm thick. The fruits are yellowish or slightly brown having with three

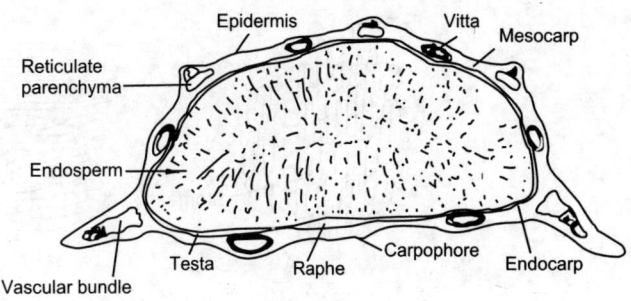

FIG. 17.21 T.S. (schematic) of dill fruit

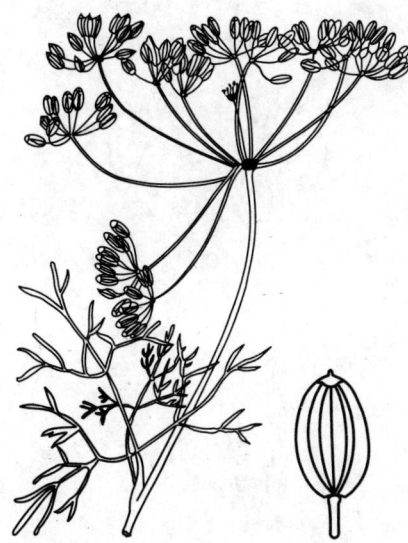

FIG. 17.20 *Anethum graveolens*

longitudinal ridges on the back and three dark lines or oil cells (vittae) between them and two on the flat surface. The taste of the fruits somewhat resembles caraway (aromatic and characteristic). The seeds are small in size, flat and lighter than caraway and have a pleasant aromatic odour.

Microscopy (Figs. 17.21 and 17.22)

Dill has six vittae, of which four are present on the outer surface and two on the commissural surface. Five vascular strands are present in each of the primary ridge. Thin-walled epicarp is present and the mesocarp has rounded parenchyma. The endosperm has thick-walled, elongated cells with parquetry arrangement. Testa is brown in colour and the endosperm has thick-walled cellulosic parenchymatous cells with aleuron grains and oil globules.

Powder Microscopy (Fig. 17.23)

The powder is dark brown in colour with characteristic, aromatic odour and taste. Microscopical examination

shows groups of sclereids of mesocarp, composed of thick-walled, square to rectangular, pitted cells. Fragment of vitta, composed of thin-walled polygonal cells with transverse septa, is visible in surface view. Epicarp consists of thin-walled cells with more straight anticlinal walls and infrequent stomata. Endocarp (parquetry layer) is composed of considerably elongated, thin-walled cells with their long axes parallel to one another and wavy anticlinal walls. Endosperm cells contain microrosette crystals of calcium oxalate. A few fragments of vascular tissue (fibres and vessels), either free or associated with reticulate parenchyma, are found scattered.

Chemical Constituents

The fruit yields about 3.5% of the essential oil, about 20% of fixed oil and protein. The essential oil is an aromatic liquid consisting of a mixture of paraffin hydrocarbon and 40–60% of D-carvone along with D-limonene and other terpenes.

Carvone

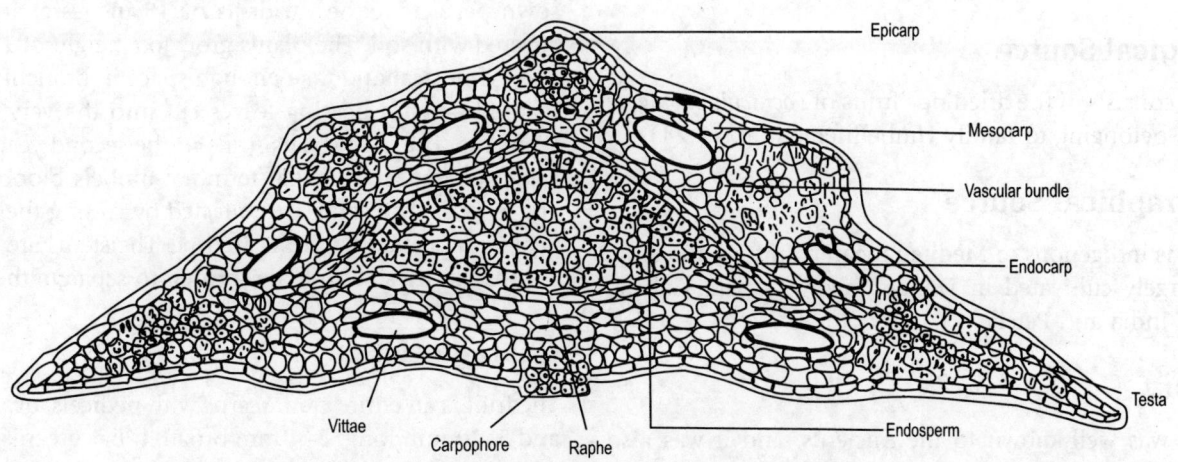

FIG. 17.22 Transverse section of dill fruit (mericarp)

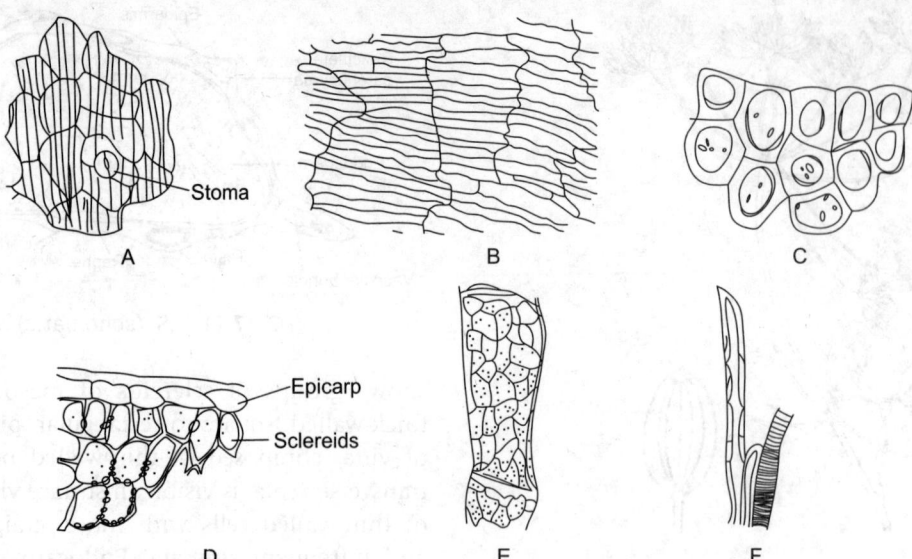

FIG. 17.23 Powder characteristics of dill fruit (A: Epidermis of pericarp, B: Parquetry layer, C: Endosperm containing micro-rosette crystals of calcium oxalate, D: Part of epicarp and mesocarp, E: Part of vitta, F: Element of fibrovascular tissue)

Uses

Dill fruit and oil of dill possess stimulant, aromatic, carminative and stomachic, with considerable medicinal value. Oil of dill is used in mixtures, preparation of dill water is used in the flatulence of infants and also as a vehicle for children's medicine. Oil of dill is employed for perfuming soaps.

Marketed Products

It is one of the ingredients of the preparations known as Woodward's gripe water.

FENNEL

Synonyms

Fructus foeniculi, Fennel fruit, Fenkel, Florence fennel, Sweet fennel, Wild fennel, Large fennel.

Biological Source

Fennel consists of the dried ripe fruits of *Foeniculum vulgare* Miller., belonging to family Umbelliferae (Fig. 17.24).

Geographical Source

Fennel is indigenous to Mediterranean countries and Asia; it is largely cultivated in France, Saxony, Japan, Galicia, Russia, India and Persia.

History

Fennel was well-known to the Ancients, and it was also cultivated by the ancient Romans for its aromatic fruits and edible shoots. It is reported that during third-century B.C. Hippocrates prescribed fennel for the treatment of infant colic, and later on after 400 years Dioscorides called fennel as an appetite suppressant and recommended the seeds for nursing mothers to increase milk secretion. Pliny suggested that fennel cured eye problems and jaundice. Fennel seeds are commonly taken after meals to prevent gas and stomach upset. The use of fennel shoots and seeds are mentioned in ancient record of Spanish agriculture dating A.D. 961.

Cultivation and Collection

Fennel, a hardy, beautiful plant, perennial, umbelliferous herb, with yellow flowers and feathery leaves, grows wild in many parts of the world. Fennel is propagated by seeds during April in ordinary soil. Fennel requires abundance sun light and is adapted to dry in sunny situations, it does not call for heavily manured ground but it will yield more on well-drained calcareous soil. About 4½–5 lb of seed are sown per acre, either in drills or 15 inches apart, evenly covered with soil. The plants grow to a height of 2 m, erect and cylindrical and take enough space in branching. Most of the branches bearing leaves cut into the very finest of segments. The plant bears fruits in the second year and the bright golden flowers, flat terminal umbels bloom in July and August. The fruits are collected by cutting the stems in September, when the fruits are ripe. The stems are dried on sheaves under sun and later beaten to separate the fruits.

Characteristics

The fruit is an entire cremocarps with pedicels, oval-oblong and 5–10 mm long, 2–4 mm broad. It has greenish-brown to yellowish brown colour with five prominent primary ridges and a bifid stylopod at the apex.

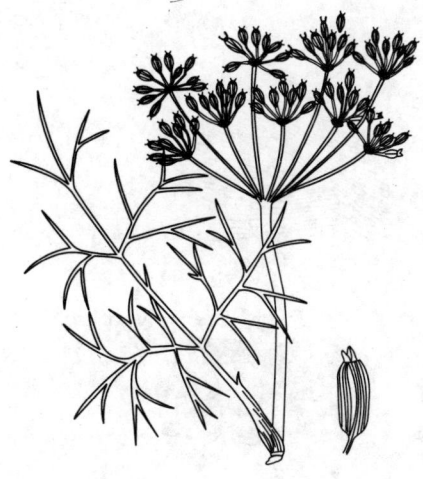

FIG. 17.24 *Foeniculum vulgare*

walled, wide polyhedral, colourless cells. Cells contain fixed oil, aleurone grains and rosette crystals of calcium oxalate.

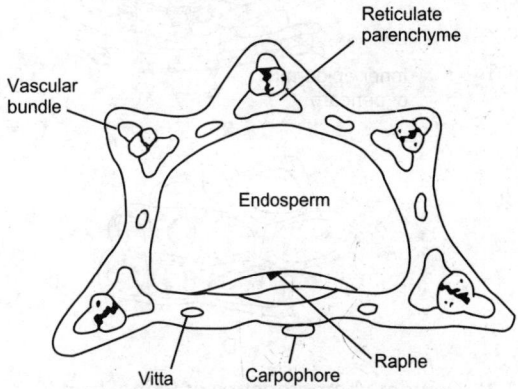

FIG. 17.25 T.S. (schematic) of fennel fruit

Microscopy (Figs. 17.25 and 17.26)

The transverse section of mericarp region of fennel shows two prominent surfaces, the dorsal and the commissural surface. The commissural surface has a carpophore and two vittae, and the dorsal surface has a total of five ridges. The mericarp is divided into pericarp, consisting of the epicarp and mesocarp; the testa and the endocarp. Epicarp consists of polygonal cells of epidermis which are tangentially elongated and covered by the cuticle. Mesocarp has parenchyma cells with five bicollateral vascular bundles; below each primary ridge a lignified reticulate parenchyma surrounds the vascular bundles. There are four vittae on dorsal surface and two vittae on commissural or the ventral surface. Inner epidermis or endocarp shows parquetry arrangement (a group of four to five cells arranged parallelly at acute angles with groups of similar cells in different direction). Testa is a single-layered tangentially elongated cell with yellowish colour. Endosperm consists of thick-

Powder Microscopy (Fig. 17.27)

The powder is pale green in colour with pleasant, aromatic odour and taste. Microscopical examination shows reticulate parenchyma of mesocarp, composed of thick-walled, lignified and ovoid to elongated-rectangular, pitted cells. Fragment of vitta, composed of thin-walled polygonal cells is visible in surface view. Epicarp consists of thin-walled, cells with straight anticlinal walls and a few stomata. Endocarp (parquetry layer) is composed of elongated, thin-walled, lignified cells, arranged in groups of 6 or more cells, with their long axes parallel to one another and straight anticlinal walls. Endosperm cells contain microrosette crystals of calcium oxalate and aleurone grains. A few fragments of vascular tissue (fibres and vessels), either isolated or associated with reticulate parenchyma, are found scattered.

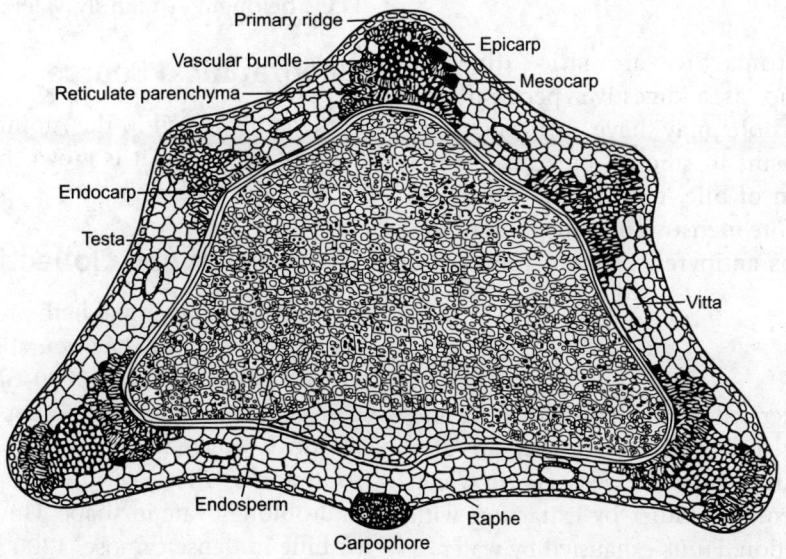

FIG. 17.26 Transverse section of fennel fruit (Mericarp)

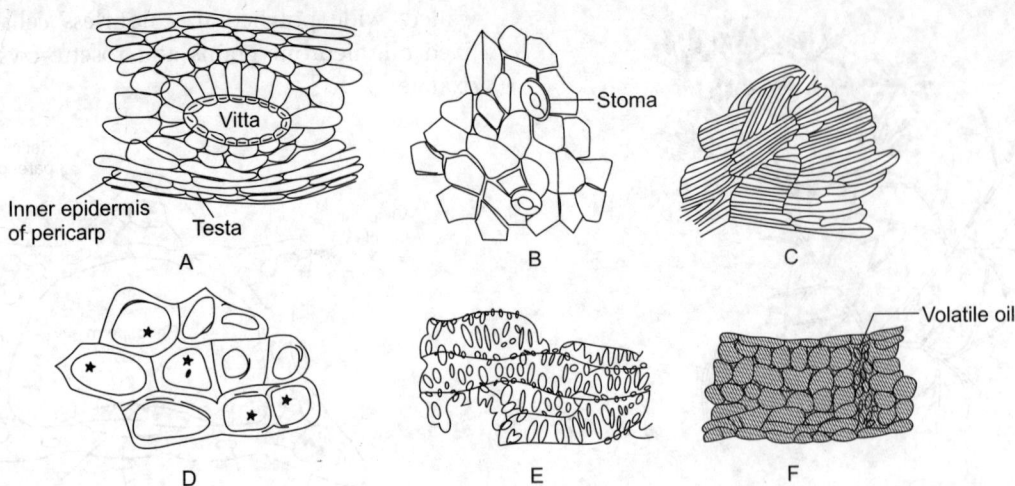

FIG. 17.27 Powder characteristics of fennel fruit. (A: Pericarp showing vitta, B: Epidermis of pericarp, C: Parquetry layer, D: Endosperm containing microrosettecrystals of calcium oxalate, E: Reticulate parenchyma, F: Part of vitta)

Chemical Constituents

The best varieties of Fennel contain 4–5% of volatile oil. The primary constituents of volatile oil are 50–60% of anethole, a phenolic ester; and 18–22% of fenchone, a ketone. Fenchone is chemically a bicyclic monoterpene which is a colourless liquid and the odour and taste is pungent and camphoraceous. The oil of fennel has β-pinene, anisic acid, phellandrene and anisic aldehyde. Fennel also contains about 20% fixed oil and 20% proteins.

Fenchone

Anethole

Uses

Fennel is used as stomachic, aromatic, diuretic, carminative, diaphoretic, as a digestive, pectoral and flavouring agent. Anethole may have oestrogen-like activity and inhibit spasms in smooth muscles. Fennel can increase production of bile, used in the treatment of infant colic, to promote menstruation in women, can increase lactation, act as antipyretic, antimicrobial and anti-inflammatory.

Adulterants

Fennel is generally adulterated with exhausted fennel and due to improper caring during harvesting they are also adulterated with sand, dirt, stem, weed seeds, etc., in which part of volatile oil is removed either by extraction with alcohol or steam distillation. Fruits exhausted by water or steam are darker in colour, contain less essential oil and sink in water, but those exhausted by alcohol still hold 1 to 2% of oil in them.

Marketed Products

It is one of the ingredients of the preparations known as Abana, Shahicool, Anxocare (Himalaya Drug Company), Aptikid (Lubin Herbal Laboratory), Jatiphaladi bati (Baidyanath), Hajmola and Janma Ghunti (Dabur).

JATAMANSI

Synonyms

Indian spike nard, Nard.

Biological Source

Jatamansi consists of dried rhizomes of *Nardostachys jatamansi* D.C., belonging to family Valerianaceae (Fig. 17.28).

Geographical Source

It is mainly found in the Alpine Himalayas at an altitude of 3000–5000 m. It is grown from Nepal to Sikkim and in Bhutan.

Cultivation and Collection

Jatamansi is a perennial herb propagated by cuttings of the underground parts. The favourable altitude for the luxurious growth of the plant is 3000–5000 m. The rhizomes are collected from the wild-grown plants only. The plant is about 10–60 cm in height and with stout and long woody root stocks. The leaves of the plant are sessile, very few and oblong-ovate in shape. Flowers are rosy, slightly pink or blue in dense cymose. 1300 kg/ha of drug is produced after cultivation.

Characteristics

The rhizomes are dark grey in colour and are crowned with reddish-brown tufted fibres, it has a highly agreeable and aromatic odour and acrid, slightly bitter and aromatic taste. The rhizomes are 2.5–7.5 cm in length and having elongated and cylindrical shape. The fibres present on the rhizomes are the remaining of leaf bases. Rhizomes break easily and internally they are reddish-brown in colour.

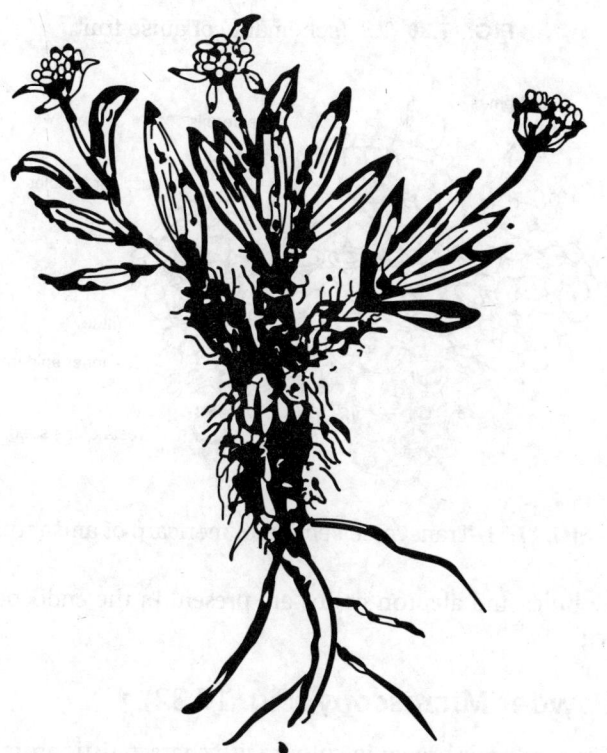

FIG. 17.28 *Nardostachys jatamansi*

Chemical Constituents

Jatamansi contains 1–2% of pale yellow volatile oil, resin, sugar, starch and bitter principle, an alcohol and its isovaleric ester. It also contains jatamansic acid and ketones jatamansone and nardostachone.

Jatamansone

Nardostachone

Chemical Test

Add 2 g of powder to 5 ml of 80% alcohol and shake for ten minutes and filter it. Place one drop of filtrate on filter paper, dry it and examine under UV light. It shows bluish white fluorescence.

Uses

Jatamansi is used as a sedative, antispasmodic, diuretic, emmenagogue and stomachic. It is stimulant in small doses and also useful in epilepsy, hysteria and palpitation of heart. The oil possess antiarrhythmic activity and also used as a flavouring agent in the preparation of medicinal oil. The oil is used as hair tonic, since it is reported to promote the growth of hair and it also imparts blackness to the hair.

Marketed Products

It is one of the ingredients of the preparations known as Abana, Rumalaya gel, Mentat, Anxocare (Himalaya Drug Company), Dasmularishta and Mahamarichadi tail (Dabur).

ANISE

Synonyms

Anise, Anise fruits, Aniseed, Sweet cumin, Star anise, Chinese anise.

Biological Source

Anise consists of dried ripe fruits of *Pimpinella anisum* Linn., belonging to family Umbelliferae (Fig. 17.29).

Geographical Source

Anise is native of Egypt, Greece, Crete, and Asia Minor and at present is cultivated in European countries like Spain, North Africa, Italy, Malta, Russia, Germany, Bulgaria and Mexico.

History

Anise has been in use since the fourteenth century, The ancient Greeks, including Hippocrates, prescribed Anise for coughs. In Virgil's time, the Ancient Romans used Anise in a special cake (Mustacae) which prevents indigestion. Historically, Anise was used due to the flavour, its ability to promote digestion; it acted as an aphrodisiac, for infant colic, etc. Early English herbalists recommended Anise for hiccups, for promoting lactation, in headache, as breath freshener, in asthma, bronchitis, insomnia, nausea, lice, infant colic, cholera, and even in cancer. Anise is one of the herbs that were supposed to avert the evil eye.

Cultivation and Collection

The prorogation is done using seeds; the seeds are sown in dry, light soil, on a warm, sunny border during early April. The plant flowers in July and ripen in autumn. Once the fruits are ripened the plants are cut down and the seeds thrashed out.

Characteristics

Anise is a delicate, white-flowered umbelliferous annual herb which grows to about 18 inches high, with secondary feather-like leaflets of bright green colour. Anise is an entire cremocarp and the pedicel is attached. It has greyish brown colour, ovoid-conical shape. The size of fruit varies from 3 to 5 mm long and 1.5 to 2 mm broad. Due to the presence of short, conical epidermal trichomes the fruits exhibit a rough texture. It has sweet and aromatic odour and taste.

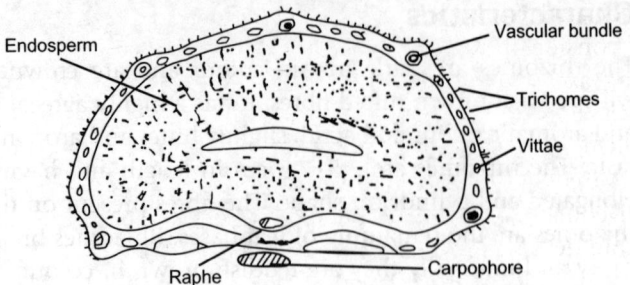

FIG. 17.30 T.S. (schematic) of anise fruit

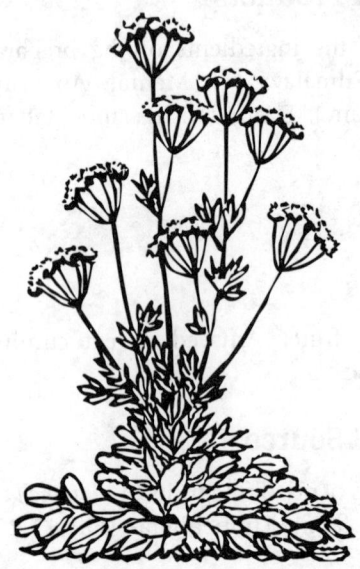

FIG. 17.29 *Pimpinella anisum*

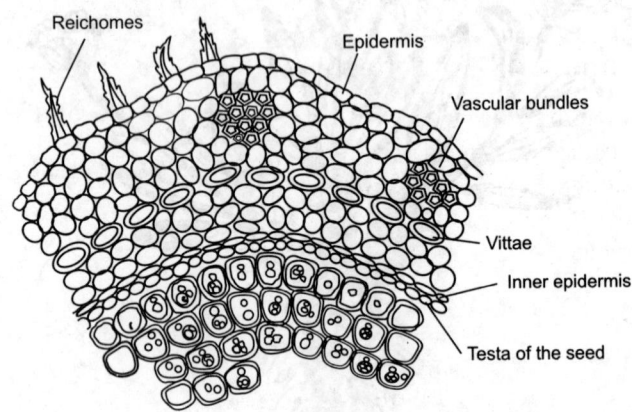

FIG. 17.31 Transverse section of mericarp of anise fruit

globules and aleuron grains are present in the endosperm region.

Microscopy (Figs. 17.30 and 17.31)

Anise has two vittae on the ventral surface and about 20–40 vittae on the dorsal surface. Below the primary ridges it has the vascular strands, the epicarp consists of short, conical, epidermal trichomes. Mesocarp has rounded parenchyma cells showing the parquetry arrangement. Testa is single-layered cell with thin, brown-coloured cells, abundant oil

Powder Microscopy (Fig. 17.32)

The powder is brown in colour with characteristic aromatic odour and taste. Microscopical examination shows groups of sclereids of mesocarp in single layer, composed of thick-walled, square to rectangular, pitted cells. Fragments of vittae composed of thin-walled polygonal cells with some transverse septa are frequently branched and usually found

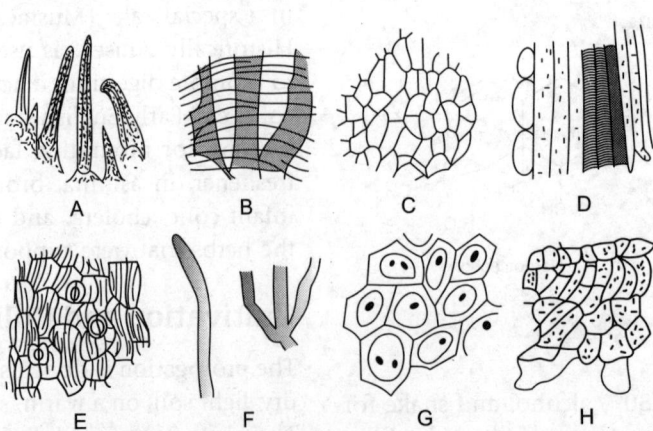

FIG. 17.32 Powder characteristics of anise fruit (A: Covering trichomes, B: Branching vittae and parquetry layer, C: Testa, D: Fibrovascular tissue, E: Epidermal cell of pericarp, F: Unbranched and branched vittae, G: Micro rosette crystals of calcium oxalate, H: A group of sclereids).

associated with parquetry layer. Endocarp is composed of considerably elongated, thin-walled, cells with their long axes parallel to one another, known as parquetry layer. Epicarp (epidermis of pericarp) consists of thick-walled, elongated cells with more straight anticlinal walls and frequent stomata. Covering trichomes are conical, unicellular, thick-walled, slightly curved and are usually found detached from epicarp. Testa is composed of single layer of polygonal cells with thin, slightly beaded walls. Endosperm cells contain microrosette crystals of calcium oxalate. A few fragments of lignified vascular tissue (fibres and vessels) of mesocarp are found scattered.

Chemical Constituents

Anise fruit consist of 2.5–3.5% of a fragrant, syrupy, volatile oil. The chief aromatic component of the essential oil is trans-anethole, present to about 90% along with estragole, anisic acid, anisaldehyde, anise ketone, β-caryophylline, linalool; polymers of anethole, dianethole and photoanethole. It consists of coumarins (umbelliferone, scopoletin), flavonoid glycosides (rutin, isovitexin and quercetin) and phenylpropanoids. Other constituents of the fruit are lipids, fatty acids, sterols, proteins and carbohydrates.

CH = CH - CH₃ / OMe — Anethole

CHO / OMe — Anisaldehyde

COOH / OMe — Anisic acid

Uses

Anise is used as expectorant, carminative, aromatic, antimicrobial and antispasmodic. It can enhance the memory, increases lactation. It is used in the treatment of bronchitis, asthma, relieves menopausal discomforts, in whooping cough, externally in scabies, flatulent colic of infants, overcomes nausea, and as a digestive.

CUMMIN/CUMIN

Synonyms

Jira, cumin fruit.

Biological Source

It consists of dried ripe fruits of *Cuminum cyminum* Linn., belonging to family Umbelliferae (Fig. 17.33).

Geographical Source

It is indigenous to Nile territory. It is cultivated in Morocco, Sicily, India, Syria and China. In India, except Assam and West Bengal, it is cultivated in all states. About 90% of the world production is from India, and most of it comes from Rajasthan and Gujarat.

Characteristics

It is brown-coloured, ridges are light in colour, characteristic and aromatic odour and having characteristic and aromatic taste. It is 4–6 mm in length and about 2 mm thick, elongated and tapering at both ends. Each mericarp is having fine longitudinal ridges. Alternating with these are secondary ridges which are flat and bear conspicuous emergences.

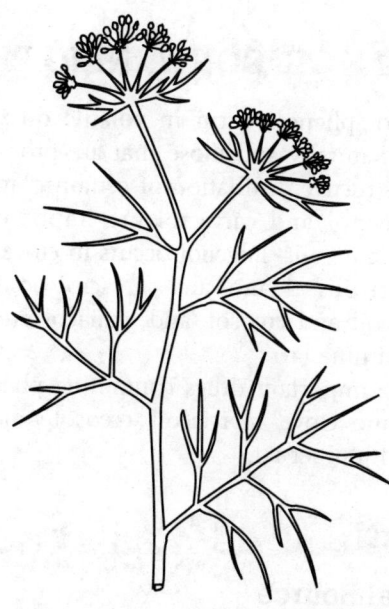

FIG. 17.33 *Cuminum cyminum*

Microscopy

The transverse section of mericarp exhibits an oily endosperm and six vittae, of which four are on dorsal surface and two on ventral surface. The large pluriserial hairs, characteristic to it, are present.

Chemical Constituents

Cumin fruits contain 2.5–4% volatile oil, 10% fixed oil and proteins. Volatile oil mainly consists of 30–50% cuminaldehyde, small quantities of α-pinene, β-pinene, phellandrene, cuminic alcohol, hydrated cuminaldehyde and hydrocuminine.

CHO / H₃C CH₃ — Cuminaldehyde

Uses

Cumin fruits are used as carminative, stimulant and in diarrhoea. The oil of cumin is used to flavour curries and other culinary preparations, confectionary, beverages and cordials.

Marketed Products

It is one of the ingredients of the preparations known as Lukol (Himalaya Drug Company), Hajmola (Dabur), K.G. Tone (Aimil Pharmaceuticals) and M2-tone syrup (Charak Pharma Pvt. Ltd.).

VOLATILE OIL CONTAINING PHENOL

Two kinds of phenols occur in volatile oils: those that are present naturally and those that are produced as the result of destructive distillation of certain plant products. Eugenol, thymol and carvacrol are important phenols found in volatile oils. Eugenol occurs in clove oil, myrcia oil and other oils; thymol and carvacrol occur in thyme oil, ajowan oil and creosol; and guaiacol are present in creosote and pine tar.

The more important drugs containing phenol volatile oils are thyme, clove, myrcia oil, creosote, ajowan, tulsi, pine tar and juniper tar.

AJOWAN

Biological Source

Ajowan is the dried ripe seeds of *Trachyspermum ammi* (L.) Sprague, belonging to family Apiaceae (Fig. 17.34).

Geographical Source

It is a native of Egypt and grown through out India, Mediterranean region and in south-west Asian countries such as Iraq, Iran, Afghanistan and Pakistan.

Cultivation and Collection

Ajowan is an erect, glabrous or minutely pubescent, branched annual herb, up to 90 cm tall. The crop is grown in cold weather, both as a dry crop and under irrigation. It grows on all kinds of soil, but does well on loams or clayey loams. Seeds are sown broadcast in the moist soil from September to November. Germination takes in 5–15 days, depending upon climatic conditions. First irrigation should be light. The flowering takes place in about two months. The harvesting period is February or March. The fruits become ready for harvesting when the flower heads turn brown. The plants then pulled out by the roots and dried. The dried fruits are separated by carefully rubbing with hands or feet.

Characteristics

The drug occurs as entire cremocarps or separated mericarps. Cremocarps are ovoid-cordate to ovate, laterally compressed; 1.7–3.0 mm long; 1.5–2.4 mm broad, dirty yellow to yellowish brown in colour and half to two-thirds apical portion has slight purplish tinge. At the top of the cremocarp is a bifid stylopod surrounded by five minute sepals. Each mericarp shows five light-coloured ridges and is covered with light yellow protuberances. The drug has an agreeable odour and aromatic and warming taste.

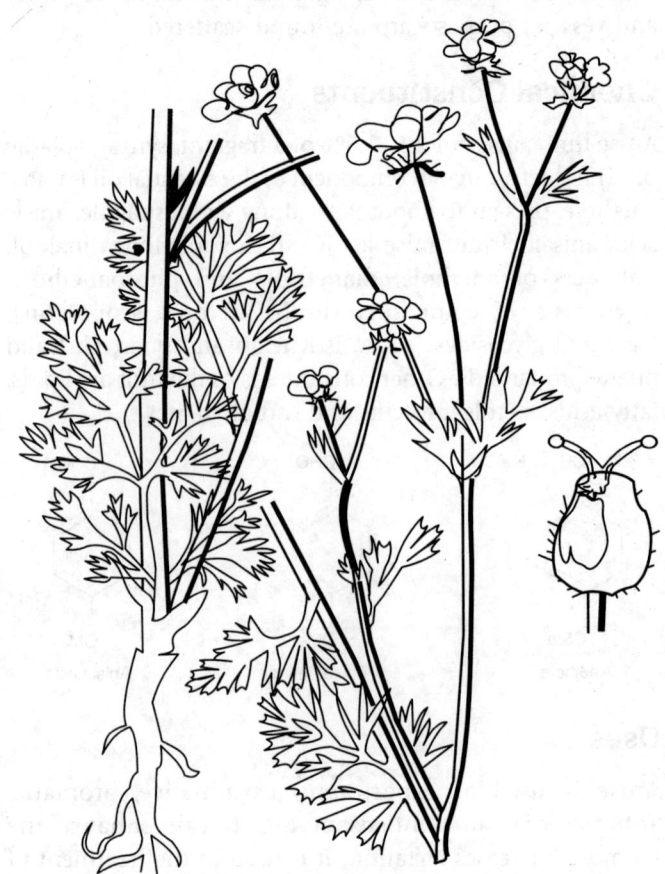

FIG. 17.34 *Trachyspermum ammi*

Chemical Constituents

Ajowan contains an essential oil (2–3.5%), protein (17.1%) and fat (21.8%). Ajowan oil is a colourless or brownish yellow liquid possessing a characteristic odour of thymol and a sharp taste. The principal constituents of the oil are phenol, mainly thymol (35–60%), carvacrol, *p*-cymene, γ-terpinene, α- and β-pinenes, and dipentene. The fatty oil is composed of palmitic, petroselinic, oleic, linoleic and 5,6-octa-decanoic acids.

Uses

Ajowan is widely used as a spice in curries; in pickles, certain types of biscuits, confectionery and in beverages. It is valued for its antispasmodic, stimulant, tonic and carminative properties. It is given in flatulence, atonic dyspepsia, diarrhoea and cholera. It is used most frequently in conjunction with asafoetida, myrobalans and rock salt. Ajowan is also effective in relaxed sore throat and in bronchitis, and often constitutes an ingredient of cough mixture.

Ajowan oil is used as an antiseptic, aromatic, carminative, for perfuming disinfectant soaps, and as an insecticide. The oil is useful as an expectorant in emphysema, bronchial pneumonia and some other respiratory ailments.

Marketed Products

It is one of the ingredients of the preparation known as Aptikid (Lubin Herbal Laboratory).

TULSI

Synonyms

Sacred basil, Holy basil.

Biological Source

Tulsi consists of fresh and dried leaves of *Ocimum sanctum* Linn., belonging to family Labiatae (Fig. 17.35).

Geographical Source

It is a herbaceous, much branched annual plant found throughout India, it is considered as sacred by Hindus. The plant is commonly cultivated in garden and also grown near temples. It is propagated by seeds. Tulsi, nowadays, is cultivated commercially for its volatile oil.

Characteristics

It is much branched small herb and 30–75 cm in height. All parts of tulsi are used in medicine, especially fresh and dried leaves. Leaves are oblong, acute with entire or serrate margin, pubescent on both sides and minutely gland-dotted, The leaves are green in colour with aromatic flavour and slightly pungent taste. Flowers are purplish in colour in the form of racemes. Nutlets are subglobose, slightly compressed, pale brown or red in colour. Seeds are reddish-black and subglobose.

Microscopy (Fig. 17.36)

Tulsi leaf is dorsiventral. Stomata are of diacytic type, particularly abundant on lower surface. Epidermal cells are wavy walled with thin cuticle. A single layer of elongated palisade cells is present below upper epidermis. Mesophyll consists of four to six layers of spongy parenchymatous cells with intercellular spaces and oil glands. Leaf bears both covering and glandular trichomes; covering trichomes, uniseriate, multicellular and often very long (100–400 μm).

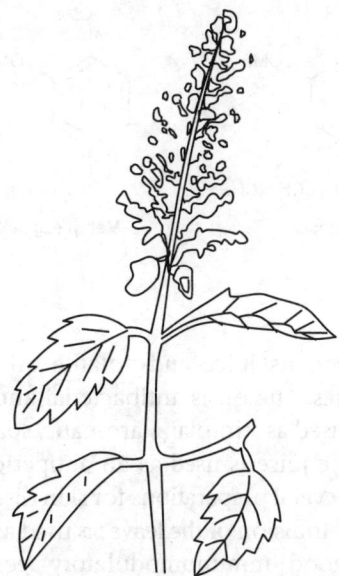

FIG. 17.35 *Ocimum sanctum*

Glandular trichomes are sessile with radiate head composed of eight cells with common cuticle forming a bladder, typical labiate type trichomes. A few glandular trichomes with unicellular stalk and a spherical unicellular head also occur. The midrib region shows collenchymatous cells below both upper and lower epidermis. Xylem bundles are arranged in an arc. The phloem is arranged on the dorsal side of xylem.

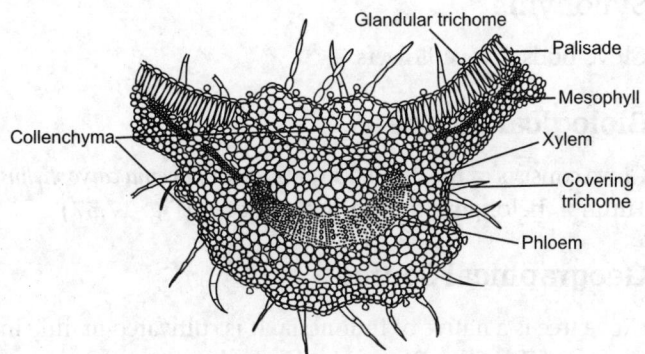

FIG. 17.36 Transverse section of tulsi leaf

Chemical Constituents

Tulsi leaves contain bright, yellow coloured and pleasant volatile oil (0.1–0.9%). The oil content of the drug varies depending upon the type, the place of cultivation and season of its collection. The oil is collected by steam distillation method from the leaves and flowering tops. It contains approximately 70% eugenol, carvacrol (3%) and eugenol-methyl-ether (20%). It also contains caryophyllin. Seeds contain fixed oil with good drying properties. The plant is also reported to contain alkaloids, glycosides, saponin, tannins, an appreciable amount of vitamin C and traces of maleic, citric and tartaric acid.

Eugenol

Methyl eugenol

Uses

The fresh leaves, its juice and volatile oil are used for various purposes. The oil is antibacterial and insecticidal. The leaves are used as stimulant, aromatic, spasmolytic and diaphoretic. The juice is used as an antiperiodic and as a constituent of several preparations for skin diseases and also to cure earache. Infusion of the leaves is used as a stomachic. The drug is a good immunomodulatory agent.

Marketed Products

It is one of the ingredients of the preparations known as Abana, Diabecon, Diakof, Koflet (Himalaya Drug Company), Respinova (Lupin Herbal Laboratory), Amulcure (Aimil Pharmaceuticals), Nomarks (Nyle Herbals), Sualin (Hamdard) and Kofol syrup (Charak Pharma Pvt. Ltd.).

CLOVE

Synonyms

Clove buds, Clove flowers.

Biological Source

Clove consists of the dried flower buds of *Eugenia caryophyllus* Thumb., belonging to family Myrtaceae (Fig. 17.37).

Geographical Source

Clove tree is a native of Indonesia. It is cultivated mainly in Islands of Zanzibar, Pemba, Brazil, Amboiana and Sumatra. It is also found in Madagascar, Penang, Mauritius, West Indies, India and Ceylon.

Cultivation and Collection

Clove tree is evergreen and 10–20 m in height. The plant requires moist, warm and equable climate with well-distributed rainfall. It is propagated by means of seeds. The seeds are sown in well-drained suitable soil at a distance of about 25 cm. The plants should be protected against pests and plant diseases. Initially it has to be protected from sunlight by growing inside a green house or by constructing frames about 1 m high tend covering them with banana leaves. As the banana leaves decay gradually more and more sunlight falls on the young seedlings and the seeds are able to bear full sunlight when they are about 9 months old. The seedlings when become 1 m high, they are transplanted into open spaces at a distance of 6 m just before the rainy season. The young clove trees are protected from sun even for a longer period by planting banana trees in between. The drug can be collected every year starting from 6 years old till they are 70 years old.

Clove buds change the colour as they mature. At the start of the rainy season long greenish buds appear which change to a lovely rosy peach colour and as the corolla fades the calyx turns yellow and then red. The buds are collected during dry weather in the month of August to December. The collection is done either by climbing on the tree or by using some ladders or with the help of mobile platforms. In some places the trees are even beaten using bamboo sticks for the collection of the bud. The drugs which are collected are then separated from the stalks and then placed on coconut mats for drying under sun. The buds loose about 70% of its weight, whereas drying and change their colour to dark reddish-brown. The dried clove is graded and packed.

Characteristics

Clove is reddish-brown in colour, with an upper crown and a hypanthium. The hypanthium is subcylindrical and tapering at the end. The hypanthium is 10–13 mm long, 4 mm wide and 2 mm thick, and has schizolysigenous oil glands and an ovary which is bilocular. The Crown region consists of the calyx, corolla, style and stamens. Calyx has four thick sepals. Corolla is also known as head, crown or cap; it is dome shaped and has four pale yellow coloured petals which are imbricate, immature and membranous. The ovary consists of abundant ovules. Clove has strong spicy, aromatic odour, and pungent and aromatic taste.

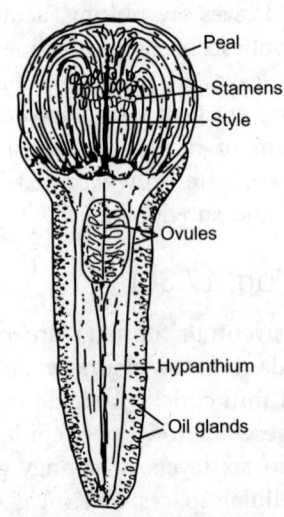

FIG. 17.37 Clove bud

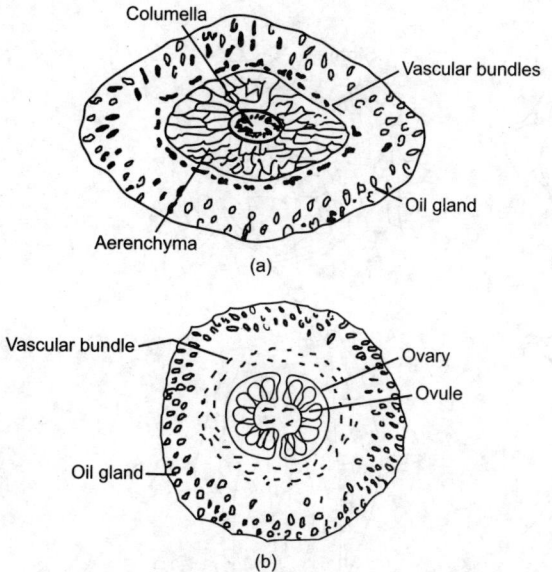

FIG. 17.38 (a) T.S. passing through hypanthium. (b) T.S. passing through ovary

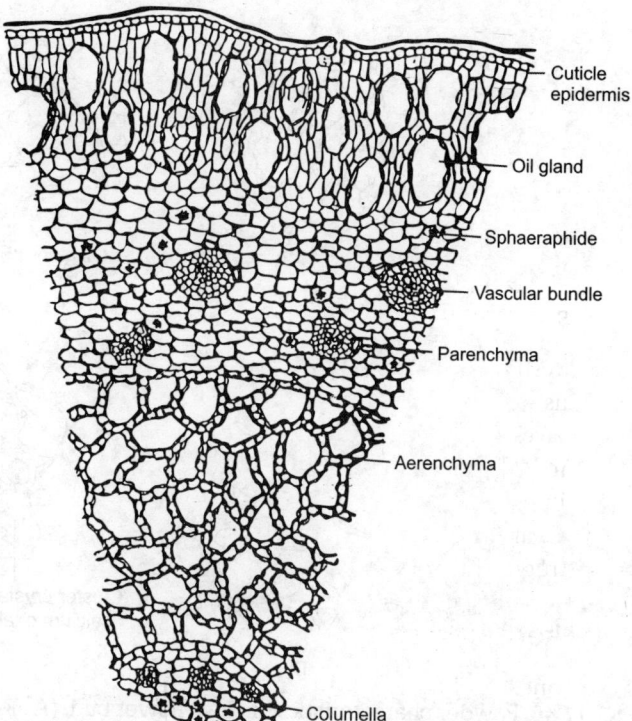

FIG. 17.39 Transverse section of clove flower bud

Microscopy (Figs. 17.38 and 17.39)

The transverse section should be taken through the short upper portion which has the bilocular ovary and also through the hypanthium region. The transverse section through the hypanthium shows the following characters. It has a single layer of epidermis covered with thick cuticle. The epidermis has ranunculaceous stomata. The cortex has three distinct region: the peripheral region with two to three layers of schizolysigenous oil glands, embedded in parenchymatous cells. The middle layer has few layers of bicollateral vascular bundle. In the inner portion it has loosely arranged aerenchyma cells. The central cylinder contains thick-walled parenchyma with a ring of bicollateral vascular bundles and abundant sphaeraphides. The T.S. through ovary region shows the presence of an ovary with numerous ovules in it.

Powder Microscopy (Fig. 17.40)

The powder is dark brown in colour with spicy odour and pungent taste. Microscopical examination shows epidermis of hypanthium, composed of small polygonal cells with numerous anomocytic stomata. Parenchyma of hypanthium showing oil gland is composed of unevenly thickened cells with numerous cluster crystals of calcium oxalate. Filament of anther is composed of epidermis, longitudinally elongated cells with striated cuticle; a thin-walled parenchyma containing cluster crystals of calcium oxalate; and a central vascular strand containing small lignified vessels. Anther lobe is composed of fibrous layer of small, lignified cells, appearing as closely packed longitudinal bands. Fragments of parenchyma of petals containing oil gland, calcium oxalate clusters and

vascular tissues; pollen grains, biconvex with rounded, triangular outline; fibres, either single or in groups, short and broad with bluntly pointed ends are found scattered.

Chemical Constituents

Clove contains 14–21% of volatile oil. The other constituents present are the eugenol, acetyl eugenol, gallotannic acid and two crystalline principles; α- and β- caryophyllenes, methyl furfural, gum, resin and fibre. Caryophyllin is odourless component and appears to be a phytosterol, whereas eugenol is a colourless liquid. Clove oil has 60–90% eugenol, which is the cause of its anaesthetic and antiseptic properties.

Eugenol

Caryophyllene

Chemical Tests

1. To a thick section through hypanthium of clove, add 50% potassium hydroxide solution; it produces needle-shaped crystals of potassium eugenate.

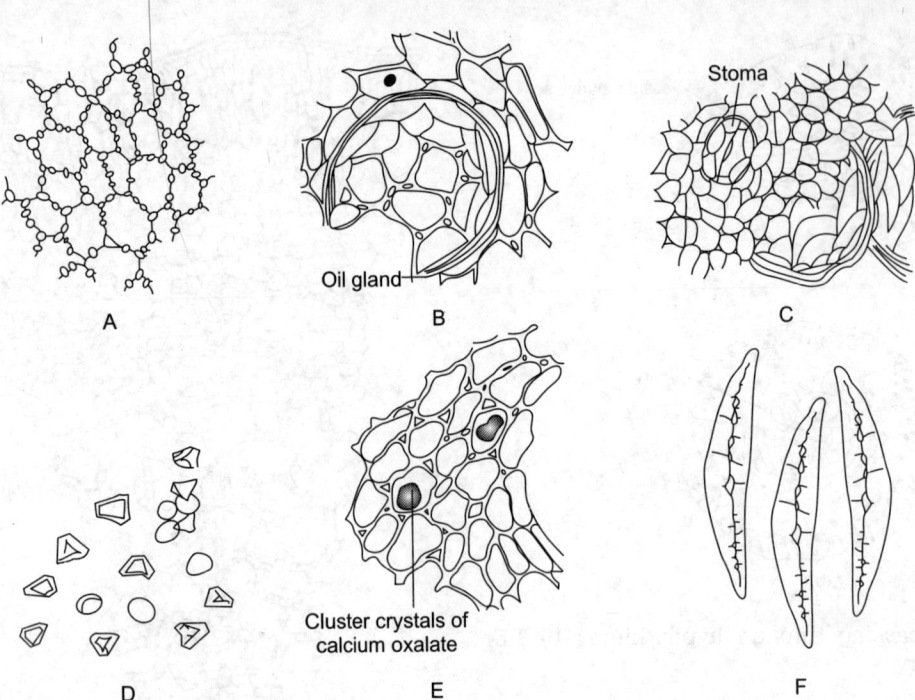

FIG. 17.40 Powder characteristics of clove flower bud. (A: Fibrous layer of the anther, B: Parenchyma of the hypanthium showing an oil gland, C: Epidermis of the hypanthium, D: Mature pollen grains, E: Cluster crystals of calcium oxalate, F: Fibres)

2. A drop of clove oil is dissolved in 5 ml alcohol and a drop of ferric chloride solution is added; due to the phenolic OH group of eugenol, a blue colour is seen.

3. To a drop of chloroform extract of clove add a drop of 30% aqueous solution of sodium hydroxide saturated with sodium bromide; Needle and pear shaped crystals of sodium eugenate arranged in rosette are produced immediately.

Uses

Clove is used as an antiseptic, stimulant, carminative, aromatic, and as a flavouring agent. It is also used as anodyne, antiemetic. Dentists use clove oil as an oral anaesthetic and to disinfect the root canals. Clove kills intestinal parasites and exhibits broad antimicrobial properties against fungi and bacteria and so it is used in the treatment of diarrhoea, intestinal worms and other digestive ailments. Clove oil can stop toothache. A few drops of the oil in water will stop vomiting, eating cloves is said to be aphrodisiac. Eugenol is also used as local anaesthetic in small doses. The oil stimulates peristalsis; it is a strong germicide, also a stimulating expectorant in bronchial problems. The infusion and Clove water are good vehicles for alkalies and aromatics.

Adulterants

The clove is generally adulterated by exhausted clove, clove fruits, blown cloves and clove stalks. The exhausted cloves are those from which volatile oil is either partially or completely removed by distillation. Exhausted cloves are darker in colour and can be identified as they float on freshly boiled and cooled water. Clove fruits are dark brown in colour and have less volatile oil content. These can be identified by the presence of starch present in the seed of the fruit. Blown Cloves are entirely developed clove flowers from which corolla and stamens get separated. While separation, sometimes the stalks are incompletely removed and the percentage of volatile oil in clove stalk is only 5%. As clove stalks contain prism type of calcium oxalate crystals and thick-walled stone cells which are absent in clove the clove stalk can also be detected.

Marketed Products

It is one of the ingredients of the preparation known as Himsagar tail (Dabur).

VOLATILE OIL CONTAINING ETHER

A number of phenolic ethers occur in volatile oils, for example, anethole from anise and fennel, safrole from sassafras and nutmeg. Derivatives of safrole are also often found in volatile oils; for example, myristicin (methoxysafrole) in nutmeg.

NUTMEG

Synonyms

Semen myristicae, Myristica, Nux moschata, *Myristica aromata.*

Biological Source

Nutmeg is the kernel of the dried ripe seed of *Myristica fragrans* Houtt., belonging to family Myristicaceae (Fig. 17.41).

Geographical Source

A native of Molucca islands in Indonesia. It is also cultivated in West Indies, Banda Islands, Archipelago, Malayan, Sumatra and Guiana.

Cultivation, Collection and Preparation

Nutmeg grows well in well-drained loamy soil, in hot and humid climate but requires protection from wind. It is cultivated using seeds and they are protected from wind using banana plantation in between. Nutmeg is a dioecious tree bearing male and female flowers separately. As the drug is obtained only from female plant, the male trees are removed with a proportion of 1:7 (one male for seven female plants). The tree is about 25 feet high, has a greyish-brown smooth bark, abounding in a yellow juice. The branches spread in whorls. Male flowers have three to five more on a peduncle, female are similar to that of the male but their pedicel is solitary. The tree does not flower till it is nine years old, but once it starts to flower it continues to do so for 75 years without any attention. The fruits are harvested twice or thrice a year, that is, in July or August the next in November and finally in March or April. The fruit is collected in the morning by means of a barb attached to a long stick. Fruit is a pendulous, globose drupe, consisting of a pericarp with light yellow colour with the mace arillus covering the hard endocarp. The arillus are stripped off and forms a mace. The arillus when fresh is a brilliant scarlet and when dry becomes more horny, brittle and yellowish-brown in colour. Seeds are dried in trays kept at a height of about 3 m on charcoal fire during night, and during day they are kept under sun to have a continuous drying process. The testa is removed by cracking the seeds using a wooden mallet and the kernels are removed. The drug is graded and packed.

Characteristics

Nutmeg is the kernels consisting of outer and inner perisperm, endosperm and embryo; it has an ovoid or broadly elongated shape with a size of 2–3 cm length and 1.5–2 cm wide. The kernels are greyish brown in colour, with numerous reddish brown spots on them. One end of the nutmeg has a small depression indicating the position of micropyle and slightly by its side it has the position of hilum. The line of raphe extends to opposite end of the kernel to the depression called chalaza. The embryo is present in a small cavity inside the endosperm.

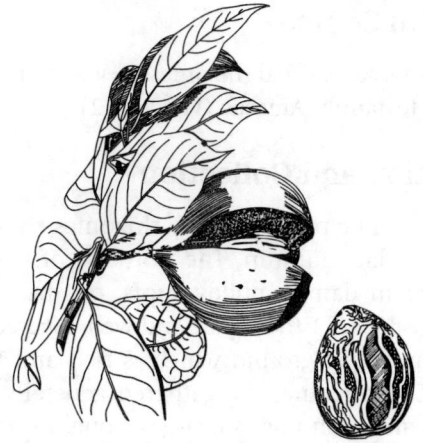

FIG. 17.41 *Myristica fragrans*

Chemical Constituents

Nutmeg contains of 5–15% volatile oil, lignin, stearin, starch, gum, colouring matter, and 0.08% of an acid substance. The volatile oil contains clemicine, myristicin, geraniol, borneol, pinene, camphene and dipentene. It also contains eugenol, safrole, *p*-cymene and isoeugenol in small quantity.

Borneol   α-Pinene   Geraniol   Myristicin

Uses

Nutmeg is aromatic, carminative, flavouring agent. Both nutmeg and mace are used for flatulence, in allay nausea and vomiting. Graded nutmeg along with lard is used in ointment for piles. It has narcotic action and peripherally it irritates and produces anaesthetics action, since it irritates intestine and uterus it can cause abortion. Oil of nutmeg is used to conceal the taste of various drugs and as a local stimulant to the gastrointestinal tract.

Marketed Products

It is one of the ingredients of the preparations known as Diakof, Geriforte, Mentat, Lukol (Himalaya Drug Company) and Kumaryasava (Dabur).

CALAMUS

Synonyms

Sweet Flag, Sweet cane, Sweet root, Sweet grass, Sweet rush, Cinnamon sedge, Myrtle grass, Myrtle flag, Myrtle sedge, Sweet myrtle Beewort, Calamus rhizome, Sweet segg.

Biological Source

Calamus consists of dried rhizomes of *Acorus calamus* Linn., belonging to family Araceae (Fig. 17.42).

Cultivation and Collection

The plants can be propagated by rhizomes either in early spring or in late autumn. The portions of the rhizome are planted in damp, muddy spots, on the margins of water. They are set 1 foot apart and well-covered. It grows very well in moist ground which is rich and frequently watered. The rhizomes are gathered generally after two or three years when they are large enough. It is collected in late autumn or early spring.

Characteristics

It is a semiaquatic perennial plant. The plant grows from 60 to 100 cm tall. The stem is triangular and sprouts from a horizontal, round rootstock, which has the thickness of a thumb. The leaves are yellowish-green, 2–3 feet in length, oblong, sword-shaped, tapering into a long, acute point, often undulate on the margins and arranged in two rows. The rhizome has an intensely aromatic fragrance and a tangy, pungent and bitter taste. The flowers are small dice-shaped, slim, conical spadix, greenish in colour appear from May to July. Fruits are berries, full of mucus, which falls when ripe into the water or to the ground. Rhizomes are about 20 cm long, 1–2 cm in diameter, either peeled or unpeeled, reddish grey in colour, soft, porous, with longitudinal furrows. On the lower surface there are small root scars which are slightly raised.

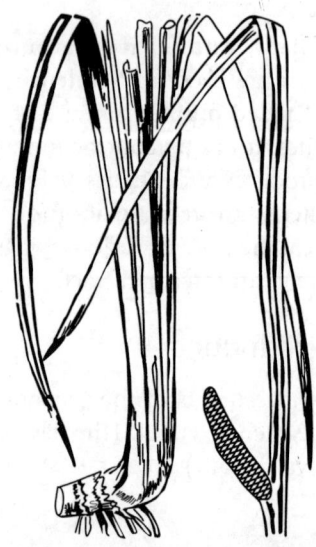

FIG. 17.42 *Acorus calamus*

Chemical Constituents

The dried rhizome contains about 1.5–2.7% of a neutral, yellow, aromatic, essential oil. The fresh aerial parts yield about 0.12% of the volatile oil, whereas the unpeeled roots yield the maximum of 1.5–3.5%. The constituents present in calamus are acorin a volatile essential oil, amorphous, which is semifluid, resinous, neutral in reaction, bitter and aromatic, and soluble in alcohol, chloroform and ether; acoretin or choline is a bitter principle with resinous nature; a crystalline alkaloid soluble in alcohol and chloroform, Calamine; along with other constituents like bitter glucoside, starch, mucilage and traces of tannin. The volatile oil is yellowish-brown in colour and is composed of asaryl aldehyde, heptylic and palmitic acid, eugenol, esters of acetic and palmitic acids, pinene, camphene, sesquiterpene, calamene and a small quantity of phenol, methyl eugenol, cilamenenol and calameone.

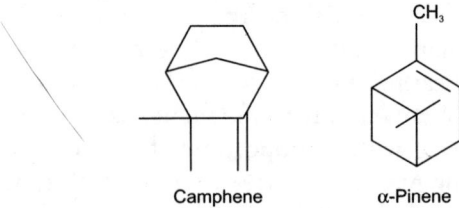

Camphene   α-Pinene

Uses

Calamus is an aromatic, bitter stomachic, carminative, appetizer, digestive, spasmolytic, stomach tonic, nervine sedative and antiperiodic. The volatile oil is aromatic, expectorant and antiseptic, as a flavouring agent, in perfumery. The dried root and rhizomes are chewed to relieve dyspepsia, bronchitis and also chewed to clear the voice.

Marketed Products

It is one of the ingredients of the preparations known as Abana, Mentat, Anxocare Pain massage oil (Himalaya Drug Company) and Mahamarichadi tail, Brahma rasayan (Dabur).

VOLATILE OIL CONTAINING OXIDES

Cineole (eucalyptol) is found in Eucalyptus, Cajuput and other volatile oil-yielding drugs. The presence of limonene-1,2-epoxide, pinene oxides, ascaridole (chenopodium oil) and ascaridole epoxide is also reported.

CHENOPODIUM OIL

Synonyms

Herba sancti mariae, Jesuit's tea, Mexican tea.

Biological Source

Chenopodium oil is the volatile oil obtained by the distillation from the fresh aerial parts of *Chenopodium ambrosioides* Linn, belonging to family Chenopodiaceae (Fig. 17.43).

Geographical Source

It is indigenous to Mexico and South America. It is also cultivated in New England, Europe, Missouri, Austria and eastern United States.

Cultivation and Collection

It is grown in manured soils. The plant flower from July to September, and the fruits ripen successively through the autumn and are collected in October. The fruits contain volatile oil (1–4%).

Characteristics

Chenopodium ambrosioides is stout, erect, angular and grooved stem growing to a height of about 2 feet. The leaves are slightly petiolate, oblong-lanceolate, toothed. It has small, very numerous flowers with yellowish-green colour; calyx has five-cleft, lobes ovate, pointed, five stamens, ovary covered on the top with small, oblong, stalked glands and two to three styles. The fruit is completely enclosed in the calyx, and the seed are smooth, shining and brownish-black in colour. The globular fruit are not larger than the head of a pin with greenish yellow or brown colour. Fruit has strong odour resembling somewhat that of eucalyptus with pungent and bitter taste. The oil is colourless or yellowish, when freshly distilled, becoming deeper yellow and finally brownish on long storage. It has a peculiar, penetrating, somewhat camphoraceous odour, and a pungent, bitter taste. Crushed fruits yield 0.6–1.0% of oil.

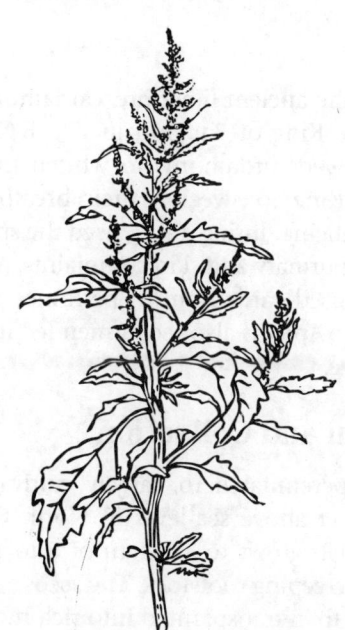

FIG. 17.43 *Chenopodium ambrosioides*

Chemical Constituents

Ascaridole, a terpene peroxide, to the high percentage of 60–70%, an unstable substance is present in the oil. It also contains *p*-cymene, α-perpinene, probably dihydro-*p*-cymene, and possibly sylvestrene. Betzine, choline, glycol and safrole have also been reported.

p-Cymene   Ascaridole

Uses

Chenopodium oil is used as anthelmintic especially in tapeworm, round worms and hook worms. It is also used as active purgative, in the treatment of malaria, hysteria and other nervous diseases. It is employed in veterinary practice in a worm mixture for dogs, in combination with oil of turpentine, oil of aniseed, castor oil and olive oil.

EUCALYPTUS OIL

Synonyms

Eucalyptus, Stringy Bark Tree, Blue gum, Blue Gum Tree.

Biological Source

Eucalyptus oil is the essential oil obtained by the distillation of fresh leaves of *Eucalyptus globulus* and other species like *E. polybractea*, *E. viminalis* and *E. smithii*, belonging to family Myrtaceae.

Geographical Source

It is mainly found in Australia, Tasmania, United States, Spain, Portugal, Brazil, North and South Africa, India, France and Southern Europe.

History

Eucalyptus globulus has been used since a long time for intermittent fever. The leaves and their preparations have been successfully used as a tonic, stimulant, stomachic, in dyspepsia, in catarrh of the stomach, in typhoid fever, in asthma, in whooping cough, etc. More recently it has been recommended as a diuretic in the treatment of dropsy.

Characteristics

Eucalyptus is a tall, evergreen tree, the trunk, which grows to 300 feet high or more, is covered with peeling papery bark. The leaves on the young plant, up to five years old, are opposite, sessile, soft, oblong, pointed and a hoary blue colour. The mature leaves are alternate, petioled, leathery, and shaped like a scimitar. The flowers are solitary and white, without any petals.

Eucalyptus oil is a colourless or straw-coloured fluid, with a characteristic odour and taste, soluble in its own weight of alcohol. According to the British Pharmacopoeia Eucalyptus oil should contain not less than 55%, by volume of Eucalyptol, have a specific gravity 0.910–0.930, and optical rotation –10 degrees to 10 degrees.

Microscopy (Fig. 17.44)

Eucalyptus leaf is isobilateral. Stomata are of anomocytic type and sunken, on both surfaces. Epidermal cells are polygonal with thick cuticle; anticlinal walls are straight on both surfaces. There are three to four layers of elongated palisade cells below each epidermis. Between these palisade regions, two to three layers of spongy parenchyma occur and some of its cells contain cluster and prismatic calcium oxalate crystals. Palisade regions exhibit large subglobular oleoresin cavities. The midrib region shows no collenchymatous cells. Transverse section through the midrib region shows nearly uninterrupted arc of lignified pericyclic fibres just outside the vascular bundle.

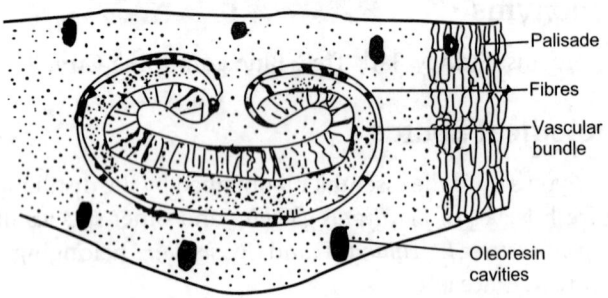

FIG. 17.44 T.S. (schematic) of eucalyptus leaf

Chemical Constituents

Eucalyptus oil contains volatile oil of which 70–85% is 1,8-cineole also known as eucalyptol. The other constituents present are *p*-cymene, α-pinene; small quantity of sesquiterpenes like ledol, aromadendrene; aldehydes, ketones and alcohols. It also has polyphenolic acids like ferulic acid, caffeic acid, gallic acid; flavonoids such as eucalyptin, hyperoside and rutin.

p-Cymene   Cineole   α-Pinene

Uses

The oil is used as stimulant, antiseptic, flavouring agent, aromatic, deodorant, expectorant, antimicrobial, febrifuge, diuretic and antispasmodic. It is also used in the treatment of lung diseases, sore throat, cold, as a vapour bath for asthma and various respiratory ailments and in bronchitis.

Marketed Products

It is one of the ingredients of the preparations known as Cold Balm, Muscle and Joint Rub, Canisep, Erina-EP, Scavon Vet. (Himalaya Drug Company).

CARDAMOM

Synonyms

Cardamom fruit, Cardamom seed, Cardamomi semina, Malabar cardamoms, Capalaga, Gujatatti elachi, Ilachi, Ailum.

Biological Source

Cardamom consists of the dried ripe seeds of *Elettaria cardamomum* Maton., belonging to family Zingiberaceae.

Geographical Source

It is cultivated in South India and Ceylon. Like Mysore, Kerala, etc.

History

According to the ancient literature, cardamom grew in the gardens of the King of Babylon in 720 B.C. The ancient Egyptians chewed cardamoms to whiten their teeth and at the same time to sweeten their breath. The Indian Ayurvedic medicine during 4 B.C. used the spice to remove fat and to treat urinary and skin complaints. Ancient Greeks and Romans used cardamom in perfumes and a famous Roman epicure Apicius also recommended it to counteract overindulgence.

Cultivation and Collection

It is a large perennial herb, largely cultivated in forests 2500–5000 feet above sea-level in North Canara, Coorg and Wayanad. It grows to a height of 6 to 10 feet from a thumb-thick, creeping rootstock. The seeds are first sown in nurseries and then transplanted into rich moist soil, when the seedlings are a year old or about 30 cm. Small crops are obtained after the third year till six to seven years.

It flowers in April and May and the fruit gathering lasts in dry weather for three months, starting in October when the colour turns from green to yellow. (The methods of cultivating and preparing vary in different districts) The collected fruits are washed to remove the impurities like sand, and the fruits are dried quickly by putting them on trays in thin layers, exposed to sunlight, with occasional sprinkling of water and dried.

Characteristics

Cardamom has simple, erect stems, the leaves are lanceolate, upper surface is dark green and glabrous, whereas it is light green and silky below. The small, yellowish flowers grow in loose racemes on prostrate flower stems. The fruit is a three-celled capsule holding up to 18 seeds. The fruit is an inferior trilocular three-angled capsule, 1–2 cm long, greenish to pale buff or yellow in colour. They have an ovoid or oblong shape, rounded at the base; the base has the remains of stalk or the perianth. Seeds are derived from anatropous ovules and the seeds are attached in double rows with axile placentation and the membraneous septa. The seeds are about 1/5 of an inch long, angular, wrinkled and whitish inside. They should be powdered only when wanted for use, as they lose their aromatic properties.

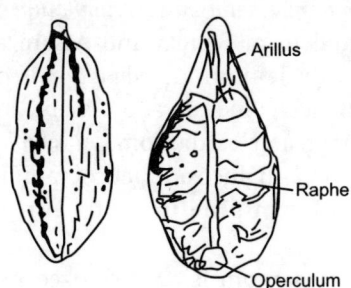

FIG. 17.45 Cardamom seeds covered by arillus

Microscopy (Figs. 17.46 and 17.47)

There is a very thin membraneous arillus, enveloping the seed and composed of several layers of collapsed cells, yellow in colour and containing oil (Fig. 17.45). The brownish testa is composed of an outer epidermis consisting of a single layer of cells rectangular in transverse section, longitudinally elongated and with parenchymatous end walls in surface view; light yellow in colour and having slightly thick end walls; a single layer of large parenchymatous cells containing volatile oil. In the region of the raphe there are two layers of oil cells separated by the raphe meristele; several layers of small flattened parenchymatous cells, and an inner epidermis of sclerenchymatous cells, radially elongated, with anticlinal and inner walls very strongly thickened and reddish-brown in colour. The operculum or embryonic cap is composed of two or three layers of these sclerenchymatous cells. The micropyle is a narrow canal passing through the operculum.

Within the testa is a well-developed perisperm composed of parenchymatous cells packed with minute globular starch grains, and containing in the centre of each cell a small prismatic crystal of calcium oxalate. The perisperm encircles the endosperm and embryo, both composed of thin-walled cells rich in protein.

Cardamom pericarps or husks is identified in the form of powder by the pitted fibres and spiral vessels of the fibrovascular bundles and by the abundant, empty parenchymatous cells.

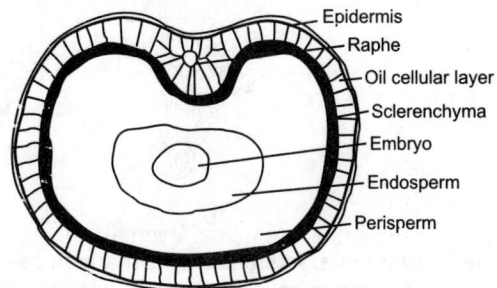

FIG. 17.46 T.S. (schematic) of cardamom seed

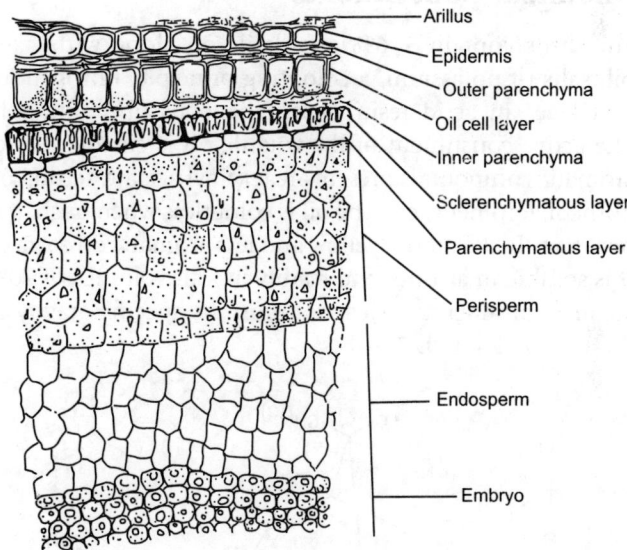

FIG. 17.47 Transverse section of cardamom seed

Powder Microscopy (Fig. 17.48)

The seed powder is greyish-brown in colour with aromatic odour and taste. Microscopical examination shows fragments of the arillus, composed of a few layers of collapsed, thin-walled cells containing oil globules, perisperm of thin-walled parenchyma and thick-walled sclerenchymatous layer with tapered cell walls towards outside, giving funnel shaped lumen. Abundant starch grains and prismatic calcium oxalate crystals are found scattered and in the perisperm cells. Small, lignified vessels, spirally thickened in groups with parenchyma can also be seen.

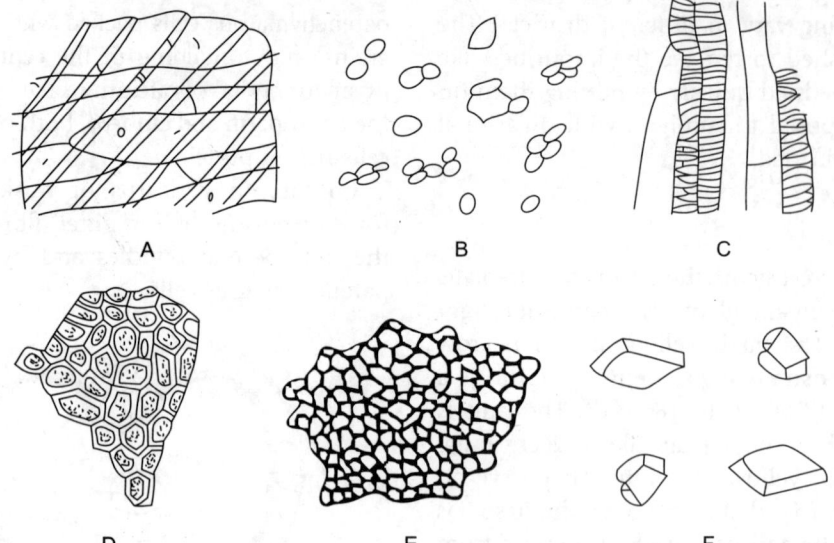

FIG. 17.48 Powder characteristics of cardamom seed. (A: Portion of arillus, B: Starch grains, C: Vessels, D: Sclerenchymatous layer, E: Perisperm cells, F: Calcium oxalate crystals)

Chemical Constituents

The seeds contain 3–6% of volatile oil along with fixed oil, salts of potassium, a colouring principle, nitrogenous mucilage, an acrid resin, starch, ligneous fibre and ash. The active constituent of the volatile oil is cineole. Other aromatic compounds present are terpinyl acetate, terpineol, borneol, terpinene, etc. The oil is colourless when fresh, but becomes thicker, more yellow and less aromatic on storage. It is soluble in alcohol and readily in four volumes of 70% alcohol, producing a clear solution. Its specific gravity at 25°C is 0.924–0.927.

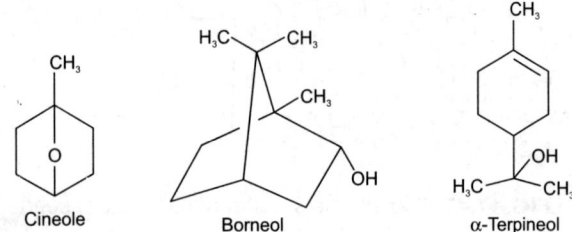

Cineole   Borneol   α-Terpineol

Uses

Cardamom is used as an aromatic, carminative, stimulant, stomachic, expectorant, diaphoretic, digestive, appetizer and flavouring agent. It is used in the treatment of respiratory disorders like asthma, bronchitis, cough, nausea, vomiting, indigestion, headache, diarrhoea, colds, for flatulence, also used as a spice in cooking.

Allied Drug

1. *Elettaria cardamomum* var. *major*: This species is the source of the long wild native cardamom of Sri Lanka.

They are 4 cm long, pericarp is dark brown and coarsely striated. Its volatile oil is used in liquors.

2. *Amomum aromaticum* and *A. subulatum*: *A. aromaticum* is obtained from Bengal and Assam and is known as Bengal cardamom. *A. subulatum* is obtained from Nepal, Bengal, Sikkim and Assam, and known as Nepal or greater cardamom. *A. subulatum* contains petunidin-3,5-diglucoside, leucocyanidin-3-glucoside, cardamonin, alpinetin and aurone glucoside subulin.

3. Malabar cardamom is characterized by a short leafy shoot, 3 m in height, the fruit shape is roundish or elongated, smaller than the Mysore cardamom.

4. Mysore cardamom is a robust with leafy stem, up to 5 m high. Mysore cardamom fruits are elongated, 2–5 cm long, yellowish green when ripe, slightly arched and darkish brown when dry; seeds are numerous, large and less aromatic.

5. Mangalore cardamom resembles the Malabar but is more globular and has a rougher pericarp.

Adulteration

Cardamom fruits are often adulterated with orange seeds and unroasted coffee grains. The adulterants of seeds are small pebbles and seeds of *Amomum* spp. Powdered seeds are adulterated with the powder of husks.

Marketed Products

It is one of the ingredients of the preparations known as Koflet, Renalka syrup, Mentat and Anxocare (Himalaya Drug Company).

VOLATILE OIL CONTAINING ESTER

The most common esters are of terpineol, borneol and geraniol. The perfumes are aged to undergo esterification, thus improving bouquet. Allyl isothiocyanate in mustard oil and methyl salicylate in wintergreen oil are also esters.

The drugs are Lavender oil, dwarf pine needle oil, mustard oil and Gaultheria oil, garlic, Valerian and Rosemary oil.

GARLIC

Synonyms

Allium; Lasan (Hindi).

Biological Source

Garlic is the ripe bulb of *Allium sativum* Linn., belonging to family Liliaceae (Fig. 17.49).

Geographical Source

Garlic occurs in central Asia, southern Europe and United States. It is widely cultivated in India.

Cultivation and Collection

The cultivation of garlic is similar to that of onion. It is generally grown as an irrigated crop throughout the year. It can be grown under a wide range of climatic conditions but it succeeds best in mild climates without extremes of heat and cold. It is grown on a wide variety of soils. It requires a rich well-drained clay loam to grow well. The land is well ploughed to a fine tilth, beds and channels are made. Garlic is planted during October–November in plains and during February–March in the hills. The cloves are separated and pressed lightly into the soil. Garlic requires heavy manuring.

Characteristics

It is a perennial herb having bulbs with several cloves, enclosed in a silky white or pink membraneous envelope.

Chemical Constituents

Allicin, a yellow liquid responsible for the odour of garlic, is the active principle of the drug. It is miscible with alcohol, ether and benzene, and decomposes on distilling. The other constituents reported in garlic are alliin, volatile and fatty oils, mucilage and albumin. Alliin, another active principle, is odourless, crystallized from water acetone and practically insoluble in absolute alcohol, chloroform, acetone, ether and benzene. Upon cleavage by the specific enzyme alliinase, an odour of garlic develops, and the fission products show antibacterial action similar to allicin.

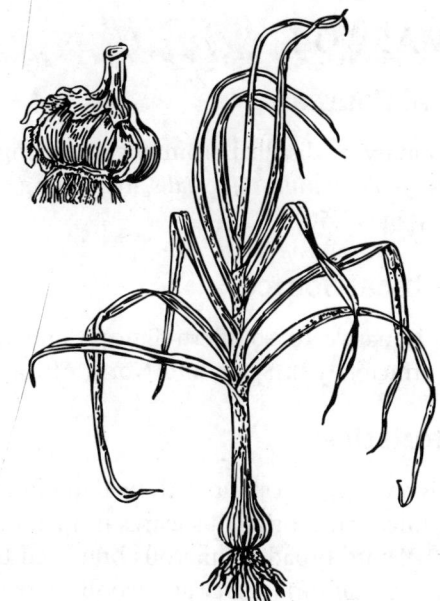

FIG. 17.49 Allium sativum

Essential oil (0.06–0.1%) contains allyl propyl disulphide, diallyl disulphide and allicin. γ-Glutamyl peptides are isolated from the garlic. The amino acids present in the bulb are leucine, methionine, S-propyl-L-cysteine, S-propenyl-L-cysteine, S-methyl cysteine, S-allyl cysteine sulphoxide (alliin), S-ethyl cysteine sulphoxide and S-butyl-cysteine sulphoxide.

$$CH_2 = CH - CH_2 - S - S - CH_2 - CH = CH_2$$
$$\underset{O}{\overset{\|}{}}$$
Allicin

$$CH_2 = CH - CH_2 - S - CH_2 - \underset{\underset{NH_2}{|}}{CH} - COOH$$
Alliin

Uses

Garlic is carminative, aphrodisiac, expectorant, stimulant, and used in fevers, coughs, febrifuge in intermittent fevers, respiratory diseases such as chronic bronchitis, bronchial asthma, whooping cough and tuberculosis. It is also used in atherosclerosis and hypertension.

In Germany, garlic is consumed as a complement in the diet of hyperlipidemic patients and for the prophylaxis of the vascular changes induced by ageing. The garlic can cause gastrointestinal distress and alters breath and skin odour. Garlic or its constituents exhibit various biological activities, such as antibacterial, antifungal, antiviral, antitumour and antidiabetic effects.

Marketed Products

It is one of the ingredients of the preparations known as Lasuna (Himalaya Drug Company) and Lashunadi bati (Baidyanath).

ROSEMARY OIL

Biological Source

Oil of rosemary is distilled from the flowering tops of leafy twigs of *Rosmarinus officinalis*, belonging to family Lamiaceae (Fig. 17.50).

Geographical Source

The plant is native to southern Europe and the oil is produced principally in Spain and North Africa.

Characteristics

Rosemary is an evergreen shrub with rigid, opposite, sessile, persistent, linear and coriaceous leaves from about 3.5 cm long and 2–4 mm broad. Numerous branched trichomes make the lower leaf surface grey and woolly; typical labiate glandular hairs contain the volatile oil.

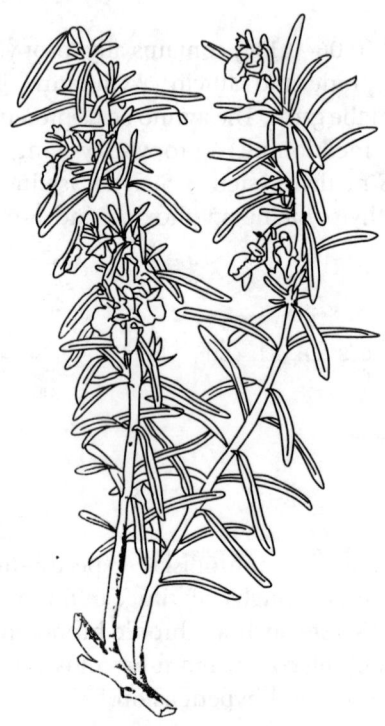

FIG. 17.50 *Rosmarinus officinalis*

Chemical Constituents

The fresh material yields about 1–2% of volatile oil containing 0.8–6% of esters and 8–20% of alcohols. The principal constituents are 1,8-cineole, borneol, camphor, bornyl acetate and monoterpene hydrocarbons. Rosemary leaves also contain the triterpene alcohols α- and β-amyrins, rosmarinic acid, rofficerone caffeic acid, chlorogenic acid, α-hydroxydihydrocaffeic acid, glycosides of luteolin and diosmetin, carnosolic acid, carnosol, rosmanol, epirosmanol and isorosmanol.

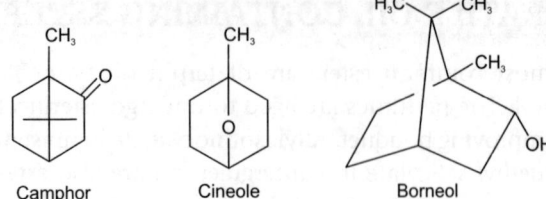

Camphor   Cineole   Borneol

Uses

The oil is mainly used in the perfumery industry. It is a component of soap liniment and is frequently used in aromatherapy. The oil is also used for gastrointestinal disturbances, to enhance urinary and digestive elimination function and as a choleretic or cholagogue. Topically, it is applied to clear nasal passages, for colds, as a mouthwash and for rheumatic ailments. Rosemary extracts are used in food technology as antioxidants and preservatives.

Cornosolic acid, a diterpene isolated from *R. officinalis*, shows a strong inhibition of HIV-1-protease activity. It shows cytotoxicity at the dose which is close to effective antiviral dose.

Adulteration

Adulteration of the oil with Spanish eucalyptus oil, camphor oil and turpentine fractions is common.

Marketed Products

It is one of the ingredients of the preparations known as Anti-Dandruff Hair Oil, Anti-Dandruff Shampoo, Protein Shampoo for oily/greasy hair and Erina Plus (Himalaya Drug Company).

GAULTHERIA OIL

Synonyms

Canada tea, Checker berry, Wintergreen oil.

Biological Source

It is the volatile oil obtained by the distillation of dried leaves of *Gaultheria procumbens* Linn., belonging to family Ericaceae (Fig. 17.51).

Geographical Source

It is mainly found in Northern United States from Georgia to Newfoundland, Canada, etc.

Characteristics

It is small indigenous shrubby, creeping, evergreen in nature. It grows to about 5–6 inches high. It is found in large patches on sandy, barren plains and also on mountainous tracts. The leaves are petiolate, oval, shiny, coriaceous, the upper side bright green and the lower paler. The drooping white flowers are produced at the base of the leaves in June or July, followed by the formation of fleshy bright red coloured berries. The berries are sweet in taste formed by the enlargement of the calyx. The odour is peculiar and aromatic, and the taste of the whole plant is astringent.

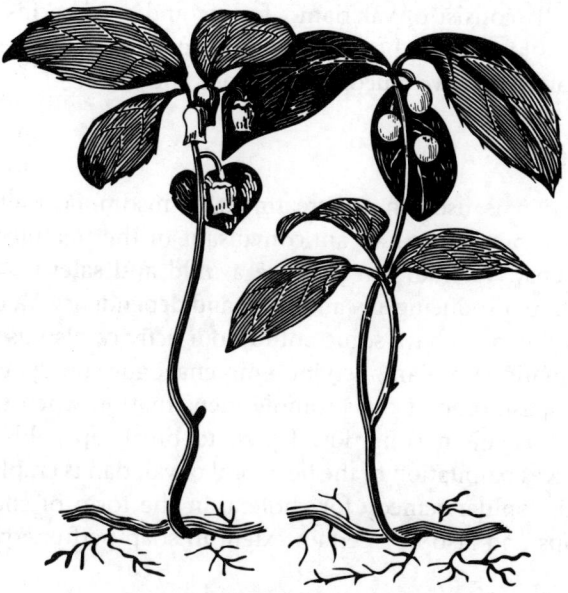

FIG. 17.51 *Gaultheria procumbens*

Chemical Constituents

The volatile oil contains 99% methyl salicylate, along with other components like gaultherilene and an aldehyde or ketone, a secondary alcohol and an ester. The characteristic odour of the oil is due to the alcohol and ester. The oil does not occur crudely in the plant, but is a nonodorous glucoside, produced by the fermentation of (between water and gaultherin) leaves for twelve to twenty-four hours.

Gaultherin

Uses

It is used as tonic, stimulant, antiseptic, astringent, diuretic, emmenagogue, aromatic. Useful as a diuretic, it stimulate stomach, heart and respiration; in chronic inflammatory rheumatism, rheumatic fever, skin diseases, sciatica; for dropsy, gonorrhoea, stomach trouble, bladder troubles and

obstruction in the bowels. The oil is a flavouring agent for tooth powders, liquid dentrifices, pastes, etc., especially if combined with menthol and eucalyptus.

Marketed Products

It is one of the ingredients of the preparations known as Rheumatil gel and Dabur balm (Dabur).

VALERIAN

Synonyms

European valerian, English valerian, German valerian, Valeriana rhizome.

Biological Source

Valerian consists of the dried roots and rhizomes of *Valeriana wallichi* Linn., belonging to family Valerianaceae (Fig. 17.52).

Geographical Source

It is indigenous to Britain and also found in Holland, France, Japan, Belgium and Germany.

Cultivation and Collection

Valerian does well in all ordinary soils, but prefers rich, heavy loam, well-supplied with moisture. Preference is given in collecting root offsets. The daughter plants and young flowering plants, which develop towards the end of summer, at the end of slender runners given off by the perennial rhizomes of old plants. They are set 1 foot apart in rows, 2 or 3 feet apart in soil pretreated with farmyard manure, and after planting it is supplied with liquid manure timely along with plenty of water. Weeding requires considerable attention.

Seed propagation is also done. The seeds are either sown when ripe in cold frames or in open in March in gentle heat. Transplantation if required is done in May to permanent quarters. But to ensure the best alkaloidal percentage, it is best to transplant and cultivate the daughter plants of the wild Valerian. The flowering tops are cut off so as to enabling the better growth of the rhizome. Many of the young plants do not flower in the first year, but produce a luxuriant crop of leaves and yield rhizome of good quality in the autumn. In late September or in early October, all the tops are cut off and the rhizomes are harvested. Large rhizomes are cut into transverse or longitudinal slices and dried as quickly as possible at low temperature.

Characteristics

The drug are found either entire or sliced erect rhizome, which is dark yellowish-brown externally. It has a size of

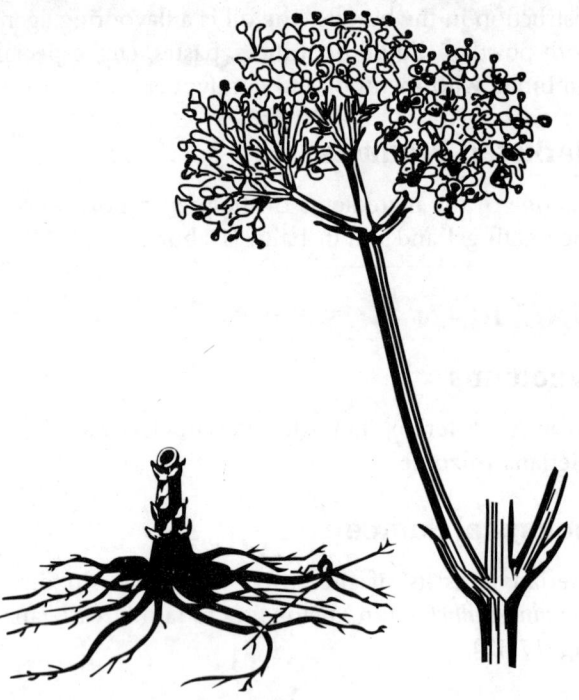

FIG. 17.52 *Valeriana wallichi*

about 1 inch long and ½ inch thick, having numerous slender brittle roots from 2½–4 inches long and few short, slender, lateral branches are also present. The rootstocks are sometimes crowned with the remains of flowering stems and leafscales are usually firm, horny and whitish or yellowish internally. A transverse section shows irregular outline and exhibits a comparatively narrow bark, separated by a dark line from an irregular circle of wood bundles of varying size.

Chemical Constituents

The chief constituent of Valerian is a yellowish-green to brownish-yellow oil, present in the dried root to the extent of 0.5–2%. Oil is contained in the subepidermal layer of cells consist of valerianic, formic and acetic acids; the alcohol known as borneol and pinene. Fresh rhizomes are reported to have glucoside, alkaloid and resin.

Uses

Valerian is used in the treatment of insomnia, hysteria, blood pressure, as an anticonvulsant in the treatment of epilepsy. Valerian can produce a mild and safer sedative without producing any addiction and dependency. Valerian has shown to have some antitumour activity, also used as aromatic, stimulant, nervine, emmenagogue, anodyne and antispasmodic. It can promote menstruation when taken hot. Useful in colic, low fevers, to break up colds and relieves palpitation of the heart. Oil of valerian is employed as a popular remedy for cholera, in the form of cholera drops and also to a certain extent in soap perfumery.

Marketed Products

It is one of the ingredients of the preparations known as Mentat, Anxocare (Himalaya Drug Company) and Saptagun taila (Baidyanath).

Valerenic acid

Valtrate

Borneol

CHAPTER 18

Drugs Containing Resins

CONTENTS

- Definition
- Classification
- Chemical Composition
- Isolation
- Asafoetida
- Balsam of Peru
- Balsam of Tolu
- Cannabis

- Capsicum
- Colocynth
- Colophony
- Ginger
- Guggul
- Ipomoea
- Jalap
- Kaladana

- Male Fern
- Myrrh
- Podophyllum
- Indian Podophyllum
- Siam Benzoin
- Sumatra Benzoin
- Storax
- Turmeric

18.1. DEFINITION

Resin can be defined as the complex amorphous product of more or less solid characteristics which on heating first sets softened and then melt. Resins are produced and stored in the schizogenous or schizolysigenous glands or cavities of the plants. Isolated resin products which come as an unorganized crude drug in the market are more or less solid, hard, transparent, or translucent materials. Resins are insoluble in most polar and nonpolar solvents like water and petroleum ether, respectively, but dissolve completely in alcohol, solvent ether, benzene or chloroform.

18.2. CLASSIFICATION

Resins are classified mostly on the basis of two important features, that is, on the basis of their chemical nature and secondly as per their association with the other group of compounds like essential oils and gums.

Chemical classification of resins categorizes these products according to their active functional groups as given below:

Resin Acids

Resin acids are the carboxylic acid group containing resinous substances which may or may not have association with phenolic compounds. These compounds are found in free states or as the esters derivatives. Being acidic compounds they are soluble in aqueous solution of alkalies producing frothy solution. Resin acids can be derivatized to their metallic salts known as resinates, which finds their use in soap, paints and varnish industries. The abietic acid and commiphoric acid present in colophony and myrrh respectively are the examples of resin acids.

Resin Esters

Resin esters are the esters of the resin acids or the other aromatic acids like benzoic, cinnamic, salicylic acids, etc. They are sometimes converted to their free acids by the treatment with caustic alkali. Dragon's blood and benzoin are the common resin ester containing drugs.

Resin Alcohols

Resin alcohols or resinols are the complex alcoholic compounds of high molecular weight. Like resin acids they are found as free alcohols or as esters of benzoic, salicylic and cinnamic acids. They are insoluble in aqueous alkali solution but are soluble in alcohol and ether. Resinols are present in benzoin as benzoresinol and in storax as storesinol.

Resin Phenols

Resin phenols or resinotannols are also high molecular weight compounds which occur in free states or as esters. Due to phenolic group they form phenoxoids and become soluble in aqueous alkali solution. However they are insoluble in water but dissolve in alcohol and ether. Resinotannols gives a positive reaction with ferric chloride. The resinotannol are found in balsam of Peru as peruresinotannol, in Tolu balsam as toluresinotannol and in benzoin as siaresinotannols.

Glucoresins

Resins sometimes get combined with sugars by glycosylation and produce glucoresins. Glycoresins can be hydrolysed by acidic hydrolysis to the glycone and aglycone.

Resenes

Chemically inert resin products are generally termed as resenes. They are generally found in free state and never form esters or other derivatives. Resenes are soluble in benzene, chloroform and to some extent in petroleum ether. Resenes are insoluble in water. Asafoetida is an example of resene-containing drug, which contains drug about 50% of asaresene B.

Accordingly, other simple classification based on the association of resin with gums and/or volatile oils is given below.

Oleoresins

Oleoresins are the homogenous mixture of resin with volatile oils. The oleoresins posses an essence due to volatile oils. A trace amount of gummy material may sometimes be found in oleoresins. Turpentine, ginger, copaiba, Canada resin are few important examples of oleoresins.

Gum Resins

Gum resins are the naturally occurring mixture of resins with gums. Due to solubility in water, gums can be easily separated out from resin by dissolving the gum in water. Ammoniacum is an example of natural gum resin.

Oleogum Resins

Oleogum resins are the naturally occurring mixtures of resin, volatile oil and gum. The example includes gum myrrh, asafoetida, gamboge, etc. Oleogum resins oozes out from the incisions made in the bark and hardens.

Balsams

Balsams are the naturally occurring resinous mixtures which contain a high proportion of aromatic balsamic acids such as benzoic acid, cinnamic acid and their esters. Balsams containing free acids are partially soluble in hot water. Some important balsams containing drugs are balsam of Peru, balsam of Tolu, benzoin and storax. The oleogum resin containing drugs like copaiba and Canada are sometimes wrongly referred to as balsams.

18.3. CHEMICAL COMPOSITION

The chemical composition of the resin is generally quite complex and diverse in its nature. It can be a complex mixture of acids, alcohols, phenols, esters, glycosides or hydrocarbons. When the resins are associated with volatile oils, contains the components like monoterpenoids, sesquiterpenonoids and diterpenoids. The gums which are associated with resins are similar to acacia gum which sometimes possesses smaller quantities of oxidase enzymes. Resins can be of the physiological origin such as the secretions of the ducts. They can also be pathological products which are exuded through the incisions made on the plant.

18.4. ISOLATION

The process of the isolation of resin from crude drug can be a difficult task due to the presence of various combinations. However the most generalized technique can be the extraction of the drug with alcoholic solvents and then subsequent precipitation of resin by adding concentrated alcoholic extract to a large proportion of water. The method of distillation or hydrodistillation can be used for the separation of volatile oils from resin. This process is used largely for the separation of resin from turpentine.

ASAFOETIDA

Synonyms

Devil's dung; food of the gods; asafoda; asant; hing (Hindi).

Biological Source

Asafoetida is an oleo-gum resin obtained as an exudation by incision of the decapitated rhizome and roots of *Ferula asafoetida* L, *F. foetida*, Royel, *F. rubricaulis* Boiss, and some other species of Ferula, belonging to family Apiaceae (Fig. 18.1).

Geographical Source

The plant grows in Iran, Turkestan and Afghanistan (Karam and Chagai districts).

Collection

The plant is a perennial branching, 3 m high herb possessing large schizogenous ducts and lysigenous cavities containing milky liquid. Upon exudation and drying of the liquid, Asafoetida is obtained. For the collection of the drug the upper part of the root is laid bare and the stem cut off close to the crown in March–April. The exposed surface is covered by a dome-shaped structure made of twigs and earth. After separating each slice, exudation of oleo-gum-resin, present as whitish gummy resinous emulsion in the schizogenous ducts of the cortex of the stem, takes place. It hardens on the cut surface which is collected, packed in tin-line cases and exported. Removal of the exudation and exposure of fresh surface proceeds until the root is exhausted. The yield is usually soft enough to agglomerate into masses when packed.

Characteristics

Asafoetida occurs as a soft solid mass or irregular lumps or 'tears', sometimes almost semiliquid. Tears are rounded or flattened and about 5–30 mm in diameter, greyish-white or dull yellow or reddish brown in colour.

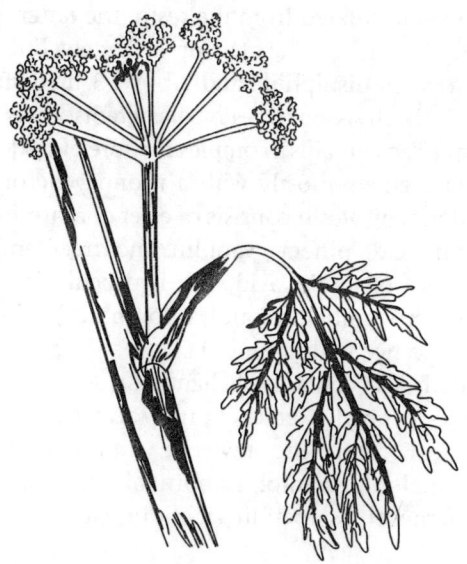

FIG. 18.1 *Ferula asafoetida*

Asafoetida mass is mixed with fruits, fragments of root, sand and other impurities. Asafoetida has a strong garlic-like (alliaceous) odour and a bitter, acrid and alliaceous taste. When triturated with water, it makes a milky emulsion. It should not have more than 50% of matter insoluble in alcohol (90%) and not more than 15% of ash.

Chemical Constituents

Asafoetida contains volatile oil (4–20%), resin (40–65%) and gum (25%). The garlic-like odour of the oil is due to the presence of sulphur compounds. The main constituent of the oil is isobutyl propanyl disulphide ($C_6H_{16}S_2$). The three sulphur compounds, such as 1-methylpropyl-1-propenyl disulphide, 1-(methylthio)-propyl-1-pro-penyl disulphide and 1-methyl-propyl 3-(methylthio)-2-propenyl disulphide

Umbellic acid

Umbelliferone

Foetidin

Asafoetidin

Ferulic acid

have also been isolated from the resin; the latter two have pesticidal properties. The flavour is largely due to R-2-butyl-l-propenyl disulphide and 2-butyl-3-methylthioallyl disulphide (both as mixtures of diastereoisomers).

The drug also contains a complex mixture of sesquiterpene umbelliferyl ethers mostly with a monocyclic or bicyclic terpenoid moiety. Resin consists of ester of asaresinotannol and ferulic acid, pinene, vanillin and free ferulic acid. On treatment of ferulic acid with hydrochloric acid, it is converted into umbelliferone (a coumarin) which gives blue fluorescence with ammonia.

Asafoetida also contains phellandrene, sec-butylpropenyl disulphide, geranyl acetate, bornyl acetate, α-terpineol, myristic acid, camphene, myrcene, limonene, fenchone, eugenol, linalool, geraniol, isoborneol, borneol, guaiacol, cadinol, farnesol, asafoetidin, foetidin, etc.

Chemical Tests

1. On trituration with water it produces a milky emulsion.
2. The drug (0.5 g) is boiled with hydrochloric acid (5 ml) for sometime. It is filtered and ammonia is added to the filtrate. A blue fluorescence is obtained.
3. To the fractured surface add 50% nitric acid. Green colour is produced.
4. To the fractured surface of the drug, add sulphuric acid (1 drop). A red colour is obtained which changes to violet on washing with water.

Uses

Asafoetida is used as carminative, expectorant, antispasmodic and laxative as well as externally to prevent bandage chewing by dogs; for flavouring curries, sauces and pickles; as an enema for intestinal flatulence, in hysterical and epileptic affections, in cholera, asthma, whooping cough and chronic bronchitis.

Adulteration

Asafoetida is adulterated with gum Arabic, other gum-resins, rosin, gypsum, red clay, chalk, barley or wheat flour and slices of potatoes.

Allied Drugs

Galbanum and ammoniacum are oleo-gum-resins obtained, respectively, from *Ferula galbaniflua* and *Dorema ammoniacum*. Galbanum contains umbelliferone and umbelliferone ethers, up to 30% of volatile oil containing numerous mono- and sesquiterpenes, azulenes, and sulphur-containing esters. Ammoniacum contains free salicylic acid but no umbelliferone. The major phenolic constituent is ammoresinol. An epimeric mixture of prenylated chromandiones termed ammodoremin

is also present. The volatile oil (0.5%) contains various terpenoids with ferulene as the major component.

Marketed Products

It is one of the ingredients of the preparation known as Madhudoshantak (Jamuna Pharma).

BALSAM OF PERU

Synonyms

Peruvian balsam; Indian balsam; China oil; Black balsam; Honduras balsam; Surnam balsam; Peru balsam; Balsamum peruvianum.

Biological Source

Peru balsam is obtained by incision of the stem of *Myroxylon balsamum* var. *pereirae* (Royle) Klotsch at high temperature, belonging to family Papilionaceae (Fig. 18.2).

Geographical Source

The plant is most widely found in Colombia, Venezuela, Central America (San Salvador), in forests near Pacific coast and cultivated in West Indies, Cuba, Florida and Sri Lanka.

Collection

M. pereirae is a large tree, about 25 m in height. Peru balsam is a pathological resin and is formed when the plant is injured. The 10-year-old tree is beaten on four sides in November or December. The cracked bark is scorched with torch to separate it from the trunk. Within a week the bark is dropped from trunk and the balsam begins to flow from the exposed wood. The injured part is covered with cloths or rags in which the resin is absorbed. When the cloths are saturated with exudates, they are removed from time to time and boiled with water. On cooling the water extracted balsam is settled out which is removed, strained, packed in tin cans and exported to get balsamo de trapo.

The balsam produced in the bark is obtained by boiling the bark in water and is known as tacuasonte (prepared without fire) or balsamo de cascara (balsam of the bark). By the removal of narrow strips of bark and the replacement of scorching with the use of a hot iron the tree recovers in six months. The drug is chiefly exported from Acajutla (San Salvador) and Belize (British Honduras) in tin container holding about 27 kg.

Characteristics

Fresh Peru balsam is a soft, yellow, viscous syrupy liquid or semisolid. On keeping it becomes dark brown, or nearly black, brittle solid. It softens on heating in which crystals of cinnamic acid may be visible under microscope, it does not stick, has an empyreumatic, aromatic, vanilla-like odour and a bitter, acrid, persistent taste. It is insoluble in water and olive oil but soluble in alcohol, chloroform and glacial acetic acid, usually with a slight opalescense.

The solution in alcohol (90%) becomes turbid on the addition of further solvent. The relative density, 1.14–1.17, is a good indication of purity, and if abnormal indicates adulteration with fixed oils, alcohol and kerosene.

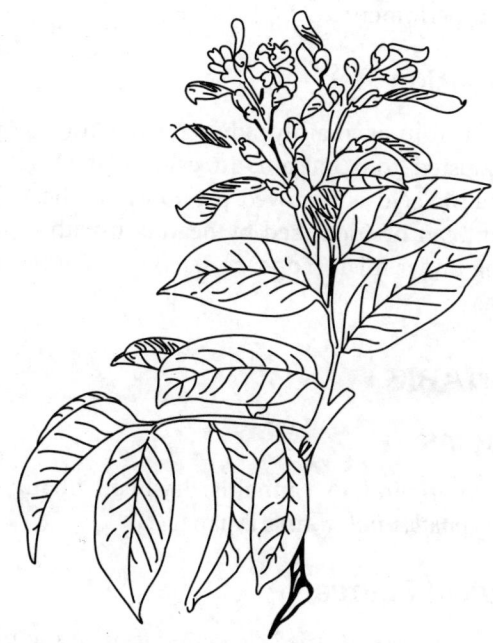

FIG. 18.2 *Myroxylon balsamum* var. *pereirae*

Chemical Constituents

The drug contains balsamic esters (45–70%) like benzyl cinnamate (cinnamein) (50–60%), benzyl benzoate, cinnamyl cinnamate (styracin), resin (28%) consisting of peruresinotannol combined with cinnamic and benzoic acids, alcohols [nerolidol (peruviol), farnesol and benzyl alcohol], and small amounts of vanillin and free cinnamic acid.

Benzyl cinnamate

CH = CH - COOH

Cinnamic acid

Chemical Tests

1. Its alcoholic solution gives green colour with ferric chloride.
2. TLC of its ethyl acetate shows two main spots of benzylic esters under UV light.

3. TLC sprayed with phosphomolybdic acid shows the presence of nerolidol.
4. It reacts with potassium permanganate to yield benzaldehyde.

Uses

Peru balsam is used as miticide, to aid in healing of indolent wounds, as scabicide and parasiticide, in skin catarrh, diarrhoea, ulcer therapy, as local protectant and rubefacient. It is an antiseptic and vulnerary and as a stimulating expectorant. It is also employed in perfumery and some chocolate flavourings, also in making of odours.

Peruvian balsam is topically used as an antiseptic to treat burns, frostbites, cracks, erythema, pruritus, ulcers and wounds. Its suppositories are used to cure pain, pruritus, piles and other anal disorders. It is an ingredient in cosmetic and hygiene products (soups, creams, lotions, detergents) and in fixative. It can cause contact dermatitis in some people.

Marketed Products

It is one of the ingredients of the preparation known as Aubrey Organics Natural Sun SPF 12 Vitamin C Enriched.

BALSAM OF TOLU

Synonyms

Tolu balsam; Thomas balsam; opobalsam; resin tolu; balsam of Tolu; Balsamum tolutanum.

Biological Source

Tolu balsam is obtained by incision of stem of *Myroxylon balsamum* (L.) Harms, belonging to family Papilionaceae (Fig. 18.3).

Geographical Source

The plant grows in Colombia (near lower Magdalena and Canca rivers), West Indies, Cuba, Venezuela and Peru. The trees are cultivated in the West Indies.

Collection

Tolu Balsam is a pathological resin and is formed in trunk tissues as a result of injuries. It is collected all the year except the period of heavy rains by making V-shaped incisions in the bark and sap wood. Calabash cups are placed to receive the flow of balsam. Many other incisions are made on higher portion on the trees. Collected balsam is transferred into larger tin containers and exported.

Characteristics

Tolu balsam occurs as soft, yellowish-brown or brown, semisolid, or plastic solid, transparent in thin layers, brittle when old, dried or kept in cold, odour aromatic, and taste is aromatic, vanilla-like and slightly pungent. It is insoluble in water and petroleum ether; soluble in alcohol, benzene, chloroform, ether, glacial acetic acid, and partially soluble in carbon disulphide and NaOH solution. On keeping it turns to a brown, brittle solid. It softens on warming. Under microscopical examination shows crystals of cinnamic acid, amorphous resin and vegetable debris.

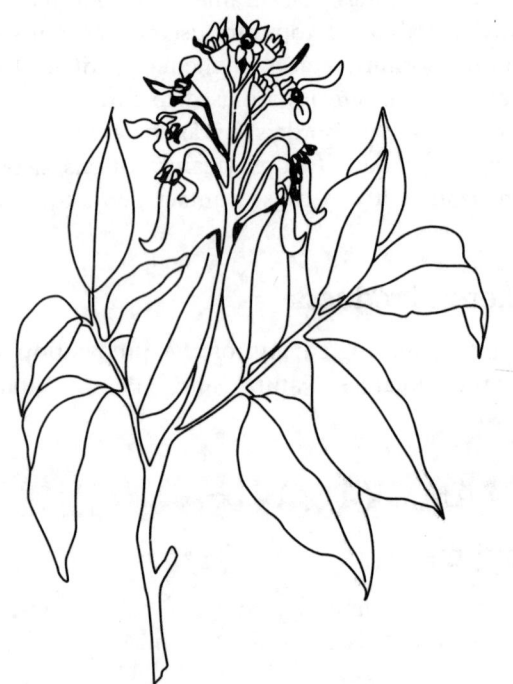

FIG. 18.3 *Myroxylon balsamum* (L.) Harms

Chemical Tests

1. Alcoholic solution of Tolu balsam (1 g) gives green colour with ferric chloride due to toluresinotannols.
2. Alcoholic solution of Tolu balsam is acidic to litmus paper.
3. To filtered solution of Tolu balsam (1 g) in water (5 ml) aqueous potassium permanganate solution is added and heated for 5–10 min. Odour of benzaldehyde is produced due to oxidation of cinnamic acid.

Chemical Constituents

Tolu Balsam contains resin (80%) which is a mixture of resin alcohols combined with cinnamic and benzoic acids. The aromatic acids are also present in free state in proportions 8–15%. The other constituents reported in the drug are benzyl benzoate, benzyl cinnamate, vanillin, styrene, eugenol, ferulic acid, 1,2-diphenylethane (bibenzyl), mono- and sesquiterpene hydrocarbons, alcohols, and triterpenoids. Tolu balsam contains 35–50% of total balsamic acids calculated on the dry alcohol-soluble matter.

Uses

Balsam of Tolu is used as an expectorant, stimulant and antiseptic. It is an ingredient of cough mixtures and compound benzoin tincture. It is also used as a pleasant flavouring agent in medicinal syrups, confectionery, chewing gums and perfumery.

Adulteration

Balsam of Tolu is mainly adulterated with colophony and exhausted tolu balsam. In exhausted tolu balsam, the cinnamic acid is removed previously by heating. The adulterant can be identified by heating it with water and observing under microscope; crystals of cinnamic acid are not seen.

CANNABIS

Synonyms

Indian hemp, Indian cannabis, hashish, bhang, ganja, charas, *Cannabis indica*, marihuana.

Biological Source

Cannabis consists of dried flowering tops of the pistillate plants of *Cannabis sativa* Linn., belonging to family Cannabinaceae (Fig. 18.4).

Geographical Source

Cannabis occurs in India, Bangladesh, Pakistan, Iran, Central America, United States, East Africa, South Africa and Asia Minor.

Cultivation and Collection

Cannabis is an annual dioecious herb, which is cultivated by seed sowing method. The seeds are sown on seedbeds in the month of August and after a month the seedlings are transplanted into the open field. The male plants, which have attained the maturity, are taken and shaken over the female plants so as to facilitate pollination. The flowering tops of female plants are collected in February or March. They are made into bundles and treated under the foot to form flat masses. The flat masses are dried under the shade to obtain 'ganja'. In India the tops are treated to form rounded masses called as 'ganja'.

Cannabis Products

The following products are prepared from Cannabis.

Ganja: It contains up to 10% of its fruits, large foliage leaves and stems over 3 cm. It is known as *Flat* or *Bombay ganja* when 30 cm long pieces of the herb are made into bundles and pressed. *Round* or *Bengal ganja* is prepared by rolling the wilted tops between the hands. Ganja is legally produced only by a few licensed growers in Bengal and southern India. The seeds are sown in rows about 1.3 m apart and male plants are discarded. The resinous tops of the unfertilized plants are cut about 5 months after sowing and pressed into cakes. The yield is nearly 120 kg per acre.

Bhang or Hashish: It consists of the larger leaves and twigs of both male and female plants. It is smoked with or without tobacco. It is unfit for medicinal use owing to deficiency of resin. It is also taken in the form of an electuary made by digestion with melted butter.

Charas: It is the crude resin obtained by rubbing the tops between the hands and beating them on a piece of cloth. This is an inferior product. It may be collected by beating the flowering tops in coarse cotton cloths spread on the ground. A greenish-brown soft mass adheres, and may be purified by pressing it through the cloths. The resin is scraped off. It is mixed with many smoking mixtures.

Morphology

Cannabis occurs in flattened, rough, dull dusky green masses. The dried resin is hard, brittle and does not stick. The flat-ganja is flattened mass of a dull green colour. The odour is very marked in the fresh drug and becomes faint afterwards; taste is slightly bitter.

The flat- or Bombay ganja occurs in agglutinated flattened masses of a dull green or greenish-brown colour. The resin is not sticky but hard and brittle; the odour, which is very marked in the fresh drug, is faint. The drug has a slightly bitter taste. The lower digitate leaves of the plant are not found in the drug. The thin, longitudinally furrowed stems bear simple or lobed; stipulate bracts which subtend the bracteoles, enclosing the pistil late flowers. The bracts are stipulate and the lamina may be simple or three-lobed. The bracteole enclosing each flower is simple.

Microscopy

The resin is secreted by numerous glandular hairs. The head is usually eight-celled and the pedicel multiseriate

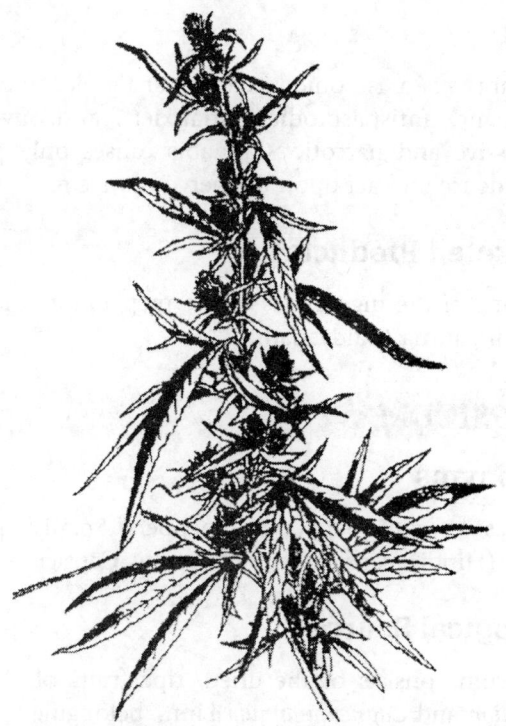

FIG. 18.4 *Cannabis sativa*

or unicellular. Corrigan and Lynch, a reagent consisting of vanillin in ethanolic sulphuric acid, stains the cannabis glands a deep reddish-purple. Abundant conical, curved, unicellular hairs are also found, many having cystoliths of calcium carbonate in their enlarged bases. These cystolith hairs are not confined solely to the genus Cannabis. Cluster crystals of calcium oxalate are abundant, particularly in the bracteoles.

Chemical Constituents

Cannabis consist of 15–20% resin, the resins are amorphous, semisolid, brown coloured, soluble in ether, alcohol and carbon disulphide. The most important active constituents present in cannabis are: cannabidiol, cannabidiolic acid, cannabinol, cannabichromene and *trans*-tetrahydrocannbinol. Cannabis also contains cannabidiolic acid, cannabidiol A9, tetrahydrocannabinol, cannabinol A9, tetrahydrocannabinol (THC), volatile oil, trigonelline and cholene.

Δ^8-Tetrahydrocannabinol

Cannabinol

Cannabidiol

Uses

Cannabis resin is tonic, sedative, analgesic, intoxicant, stomachic, antispasmodic, antianxiety, anticonvulsant, antitussive and narcotic. Cannabis causes only pshycic dependence and act upon the nervous system.

Marketed Products

It is one of the ingredients of the preparation known as Bilwadi churna (Baidyanath).

CAPSICUM

Synonyms

Chillies, cayenne pepper, red peppers, Spanish pepper, mirch (Hindi), capsicum fruits, Fructus Capsici.

Biological Source

Capsicum consists of the dried, ripe fruits of *Capsicum minimum* and *Capsicum annum* Linn., belonging to family Solanaceae (Fig. 18.5).

Geographical Source

Capsicum is native of America and cultivated in tropical regions of India, Japan, southern Europe, Mexico, Africa (Kenya, Tanzania and Sierra Leone) and Sri Lanka.

Cultivation and Collection

Capsicum is cultivated mostly as a rainfed crop. In the Gangetic area, it is a cold weather crop. The crop is raised on a variety of soils, for example, ordinary red loams, black soils and clayey loams. Good drainage is essential and water logging is detrimental. Seedlings are first raised in a nursery. Seeds obtained from selected pods and mixed with ashes are sown by broadcasting. Germination occurs in about a week. The field is ploughed and manured with compost. The field is irrigated once a day until the plants are established. Flowering starts when the plants are 2.5–3.5 months old. Dew and heavy rain at flowering time are injurious. Ripe and nearly ripe fruits are picked at intervals of 5, 10 and 20 days.

The fruits are picked as they become fully ripe. The quality of the drug is in part determined by its colour. The unripe fruits fade to pale buff upon drying. The fruits are dried in sun, graded by colour; occasionally oil is rubbed on the fruits to give glossiness to the pericarps. Most of the calices and pedicels are removed.

Characteristics

Capsicum is 5–12 cm long, 2–4 cm wide, globular, ovoid, or oblong in shape, pericarp is shrivelled, orange or red in

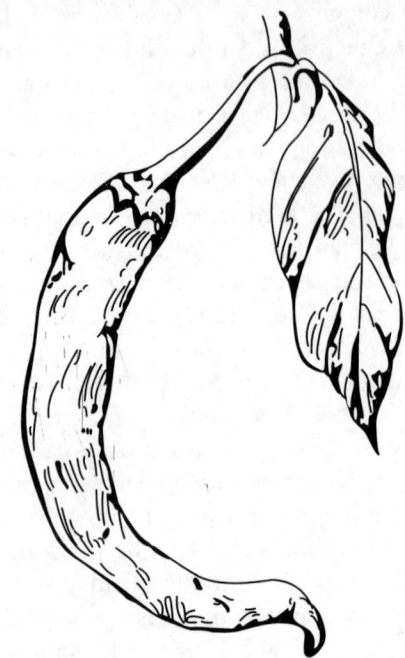

FIG. 18.5 Capsicum fruit

colour, pedicel is prominent and bent. The calyx is toothed. The amount of calices and pedicels should not exceed beyond 3%. Internally the fruits are divided into two halve parts by a membranous dissepiment to which the seeds are attached. The seeds are reniform, flattened, 3–4 mm long, with a coiled embryo and oily endosperm. Capsicum has characteristic odour and an intense pungent taste.

Chemical Constituents

Capsicum contains fixed oils (4–16%), oleoresin, carotenoids, capsacutin, capsico (a volatile alkaloid), thiamine, volatile oil (1.5%) and ascorbic acid (0.2%). The resin contains an extremely pungent principle, capsaicin, (decylenic vanillyl amide) (about 0.5%). Capsaicin retains its characteristic pungency in a dilution of 1 part in 10 million parts with water. Capsanthin is the main carotenoid of red fruits. It also occurs as monoester and diester along with cryptocapsin. Other carotenoids include zeaxanthin, capsorubrin, rubixanthin, phylofluene, capsanthin-5,6-epoxide, capsanthin-3,6-epoxide, lutein, cryptoxanthin, α- and β-carotenes, capsorubin, and few xanthophylls. The carbohydrates reported in chilies are fructose, galactose, sucrose, etc. Tocopherol (vitamin E) is present in trace amounts (~2.4 mg/100 g).

Uses

Capsicum has been used externally as stimulant, counter irritant, rubefacient, in sore throat, scarlatina, hoarseness and yellow fever; internally it is used as carminative, stomachic, dyspepsia and flatulence. In the form of ointment, plaster and medicated wool it is used for the

Capsaicin

Capsanthin

relief of rheumatism and lumbago. Capsaicin is used for the treatment of migraine and cluster headache, and for some patients with neurogenic ladder dysfunction.

Allied Drugs

Japanese Chillies (*C. frutescens*) are about 3–4 cm long. They are usually free from pedicels and calices and have a bright red pericarp. They possess about one-quarter of the pungency of the African Chillies.

Bombay Capsicums (*C. annuum*). The pericarp is thicker and tougher than in the chillies, and the pedicel is frequently bent. They are much less pungent than African chillies.

Natal Capsicums are larger than the Bombay variety, being up to 8 cm long. They have a very bright red, transparent pericarp. They are much less pungent than chillies.

Marketed Products

It is one of the ingredients of the preparations known as Deepact (Lupin Herbal Laboratory) and Capsigyl-D (Shalaks), a topical antirheumatic cream.

COLOCYNTH

Synonyms

Bitter apple, Fructus colocynthidis, Colocynthis.

Biological Source

Colocynth is the dried pithy pulp of the ripe fruits of *Citrullus colocynthis* Schrader, belonging to family Cucurbitaceae (Fig. 18.6).

Geographical Source

Cultivated in Asia, Africa, South Europe; mainly in Syria, Cyprus and Egypt. In India, it is cultivated in Gujarat, Punjab, Tamil Nadu, etc.

Collection

The plant is perennial prostrate herb. It is rarely cultivated. The fruits are fleshy in nature and are collected in autumn, when they are ripe. The ripe fruits are yellow in colour. The fruits are peeled using a knife and dried under the sun or artificially.

Description

The fleshy fruits are 5–8 cm in diameter, subspherical berry, almost white, and the density is very less. On the outer surface it has rind and impressions of the knife. Three splits of placenta, which run from centre to periphery is seen if the fruit is cut transversely. It has two groups of seeds near the periphery and the remaining portion filled with pithy parenchyma. It has characteristic odour and intense bitter taste.

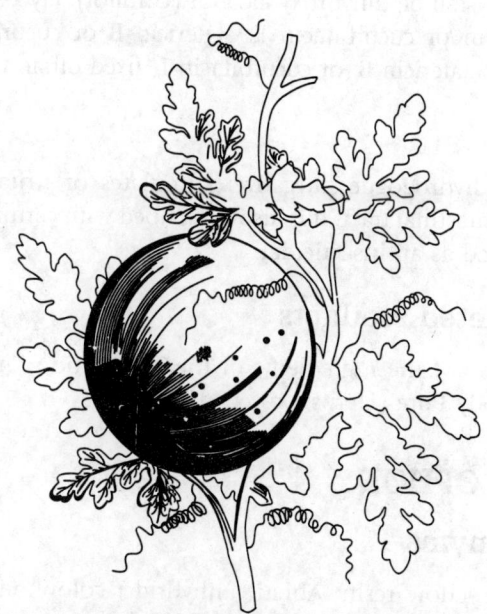

FIG. 18.6 *Citrullus colocynthis*

Cucurbitacin E

Cucurbitacin L

Microscopy

The epicarp has the epidermis made of the polygonal cells, which are covered by a thick cuticle. The cuticle consists of few large stomata. Below the epidermis it has thin-walled parenchymatous cells and thick layer of lignified sclerenchymatous tissues. Sclereides are of three layers and the outermost layer is more lignified than the inner layer of sclereides. The pulp consists of large parenchyma cells with intercellular space and few narrow vascular strands which are scattered. The seeds consist of palisade epidermis of polygonal prismatic cells. The testa consists of thick sclerenchyma which is eight- to ten-celled thick, whereas a collapsed parenchyma is four- to five-celled thick. The embryo consists of thin cellulosic parenchyma containing aleurone grains and fixed oil.

Chemical Constituents

Alkaloid is the main constituent present in the pulp of colocynth. Colocynth also contains amorphous resins that are ether and chloroform soluble. The other constituents are a crystalline dihydroxy alcohol (citrullol), glycosides of α-elaterin or cucurbitacin E, elatericin B or cucurbitacin, dihydroelatericin B, or cucurbitacin L, fixed oil and starch.

Uses

It is a hydrogogue purgative; stimulates or irritates the gastrointestinal tract. It is also prescribed with carminatives and used as an insecticidal.

Marketed Products

It is one of the ingredients of the preparation known as The Body Pure (HerbsForever Inc.).

COLOPHONY

Synonyms

Rosin, yellow resin; Abietic anhydride; colophony resin; amber resin; resin; coloponium.

Biological Source

Colophony is a solid residue left after distilling off the volatile oil from the oleoresin obtained from *Pinus palustris* (long leaf pine) and other species of *Pinus* such as *P. pinaster*, *P. halepensis*, *P. massoniana*, *P. tabuliformis*, *P. carribacea* var., belonging to family Pinaceae (Fig. 18.7).

Geographical Source

The genus *Pinus* is widely found in United States, France, Italy, Portugal, Spain, Greece, New Zealand, China, India (Himalayan region) and Pakistan. Colophony is chiefly produced in the United States contributing about 80% of world supply. Other countries producing the resin are China, France, Spain, India, Greece, Morocco, Honduras, Poland and Russia.

Collection

The collection of the oleoresin is very laborous procedure. Although colophony is a normal (physiological) resin of *Pinus* species, its amount is increased by injuring the plant. For its collection a few-feet long groove or blaze is made in the bark with the help of knife or some other instrument. A metal or earthenware cup is attached below the groove by nails. The cup is adjusted accordingly when the size of groove increases. The resin is taken out at different intervals and sent for further processing.

Cup and Gutter Method

This method is used in America, European countries, India and Pakistan. The 60–100 cm long blaze or longitudinal groove is cut with a suitable instrument. It is enlarged at intervals and in about four years is about 4 m long. The metal or earthenware cups are attached to the trunk by nails and one or two strips of galvanized iron are placed above each to direct the flow of oleoresin. As the grooves are lengthened the cups are moved higher up the tree and new grooves are started when the old ones become exhausted or collection is difficult. The cups are emptied at intervals and the oleoresin sent to the distillery. Trees can be tapped by this method for about 40 years.

Preparation

The crude oleoresin arrives at the distillery in barrels. It is mixed with about 20% by weight of turpentine in a heated stainless steel vessel and allowed to stand to separate water and other impurities. The diluted oleoresin is then transferred to copper or stainless steel stills and the turpentine is removed by steam distillation. When distillation is complete the molten resin is run through wire strainers into barrels, in which it cools and is exported.

The resin obtained from trees during their first year of tapping is of a lighter colour than that obtained later on. The following grades of American rosin are recognized: B, FF (for wood rosin only), D, E, F, G, H, I, K, L, M, N, WG (window-glass), WW (water-white), and the extra-white X grades and American and Portuguese qualities (XA, XB, XC). A great deal of the American tall oil rosin is now paler than grade X. Grade B is almost black.

Characters

Colophony occurs as translucent, hard, shiny, sharp, pale yellow to amber fragments, fracture brittle at ordinary temperature, burns with smoky flame, slight turpentine-like odour and taste, melts readily on heating, density 1.07–1.09. Acid number is not less than 150. It is insoluble in water but freely soluble in alcohol, benzene, ether, glacial acetic acid, oils, carbon disulphide and alkali solutions.

Chemical Constituents

Colophony contains resin acids (about 90%), resenes and fatty acid esters. Of the resin acids about 90% are isomeric α-, β- and γ-abietic acids; the other 10% is a mixture of dihydroabietic acid and dehydroabietic acid. Before distillation, the resin contains excess amounts of (+) and (-) pimaric acids. During distillation the (-) pimaric acid is converted into abietic acid while (+) pimaric acid is stable. The other constituents of colophony are sipinic acid and a hydrocarbon.

Abietic acid

Pimaric acid

Chemical Tests

1. To a solution of powdered resin (0.1 g) in acetic acid (10 ml) one drop of conc. sulphuric acid is added in

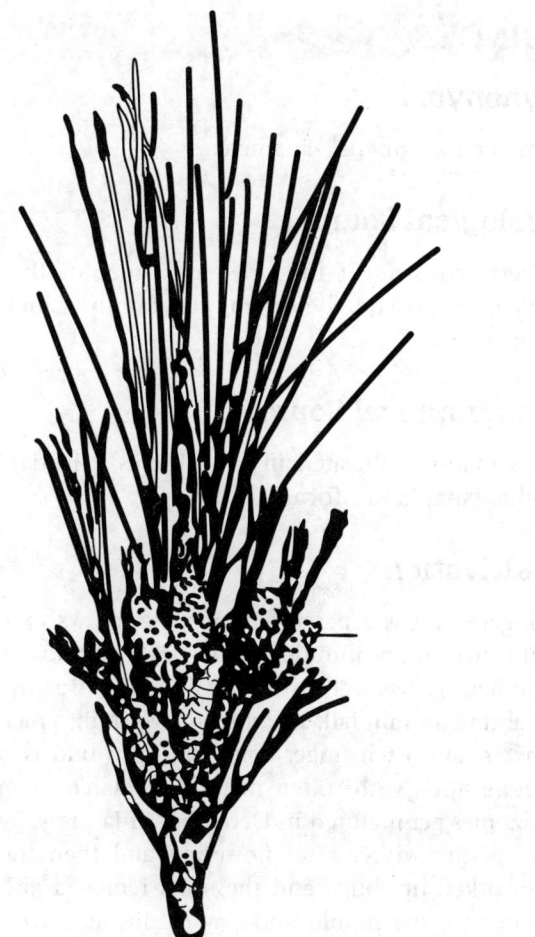

FIG. 18.7 *Pinus palustris*

a dry test tube. A purple colour, readily changing to violet, is formed.
2. To a petroleum ether solution of powdered colophony twice its volume of dilute solution of copper acetate is shaken. The colour of the petroleum ether layer changes to emerald-green due to formation of copper salt of abietic acid.
3. To alcoholic solution of colophony sufficient water is added. It becomes milky white due to precipitation of chemical compounds.
4. Alcoholic solution of colophony turns blue litmus to red due to the presence of diterpenic acids.

Uses

Colophony is used as stiffening agent in ointments, adhesives, plasters and cerates and as a diuretic in veterinary medicine. Commercially it is used to manufacture varnishes, printing inks, cements, soap, sealing wax, wood polishes, floor coverings, paper, plastics, fireworks, tree wax, rosin oil and for water proofing cardboard.

The abietic acids show antimicrobial, antiulcer and cardiovascular activity; some have filmogenic, surfactant and antifeedant properties.

GINGER

Synonyms

Rhizoma zingiberis, Zingibere.

Biological Source

Ginger consists of the dried rhizomes of the *Zingiber officinale* Roscoe, belonging to family Zingiberaceae (Fig. 18.8).

Geographical Source

It is mainly cultivated in West Indies, Nigeria, Jamaica, India, Japan and Africa.

Cultivation

Ginger plant is a perennial herb that grows to 1 m. It is cultivated at an altitude of 600–1500 m above sea level. The herb grows well in well-drained rich, loamy soil and in abundant rain fall. The rhizome is cut into pieces called fingers, and each finger consisting of a bud is placed in a hole filled with rotten manure in March or April. The rhizomes get matured in December or January. By January the plants wither after flowering and then the flowers are forked up, buds and the roots removed and washed to remove the mould and clay or dirt attached to them. The rhizomes are socked in water overnight and the next morning they are scraped with a knife to remove the outer cork and little of parenchyma. They are washed again and then dried under sun for a week. The rhizomes are turned by the sides at regular intervals to facilitate proper drying. This is the 'unbleached Jamaica' or the uncoated ginger. The coated or the unpeeled variety is prepared by dropping the rhizome for few minutes in boiling water, and then skin is removed such that the layer on the flat surface is removed but not in the grooves between the branches. The 'bleached' or 'limed' is prepared by treating it with sulphuric acid or chlorine or dusting it with calcium sulphate or calcium carbonate.

Characteristics

The rhizomes are 5–15 cm long, 3–6 cm wide and about 1.5 cm thick. The Jamaica ginger occurs as branches. It has a sympodial branching and the outer surface has buff yellow colour with longitudinally striated fibres. Small circular depressions at the portion of the buds are seen and fractured surface shows narrow bark, a well-developed endodermis, and a wide stele, with scattered small yellowish points of secretion cells and greyish points of fibrovascular bundles. The ginger has agreeable and aromatic odour and pungent and agreeable taste.

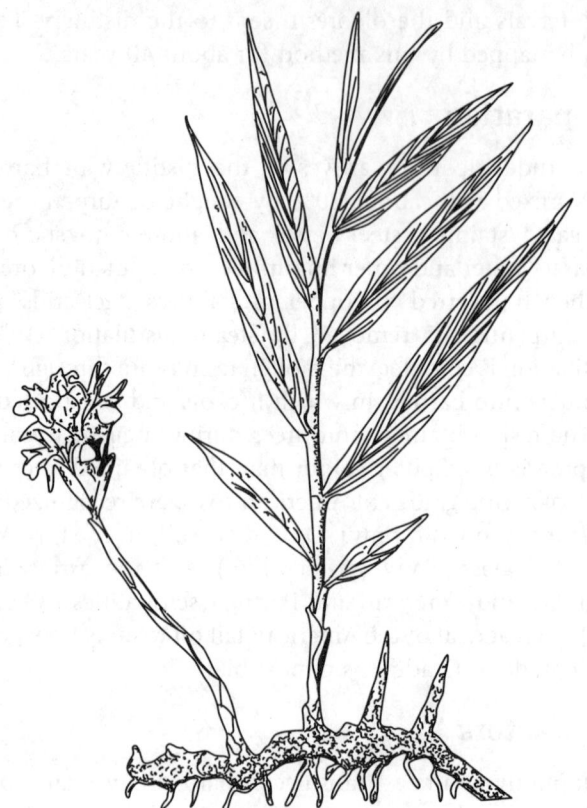

FIG. 18.8 *Zingiber officinale*

Microscopy (Fig. 18.9a and b)

The cork is the outermost layer with irregular parenchymatous cells and dark brown colour. The inner cork is few layered, colourless parenchymatous cells arranged in radial rows. Cork is absent in Jamaica ginger. Phellogen is indistinct and the cortex consists of thin-walled rounded parenchyma with intercellular spaces consisting of abundant starch grains. The starch grains are simple, ovate or sac shaped. Numerous yellowish brown oleoresin are also present along with the collateral fibro vascular bundles. The endodermis is distinct without starch and consists of single layer of tangentially elongated cells containing suberin. Just below the endodermis it has the ground tissue, a ring of narrow zone of vascular bundle which is not covered with sclerenchymatous fibres. The ground tissues contain the large parenchymatous cells rich in starch, oleoresin, fibrovascular bundles. The phloem has well-developed sieve elements, and the xylem consist of vessels, tracheids either annual or spiral, or reticular in nature without lignin. The fibres are unlignified, pitted and separate.

Powder Microscopy (Fig. 18.10)

The powder is pale yellow to cream in colour with agreeable aromatic odour and pungent taste. Microscopical examination shows abundant starch grains, simple and sac-

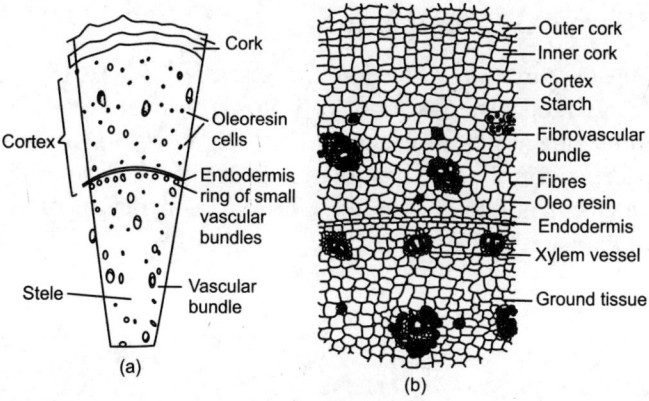

FIG. 18.9 (a) Schematic diagram (T.S.) and (b) Transverse section of ginger rhizome

for the aromatic odour and the pungency of the drug is due to the yellowish oily body called gingerol which is odourless. Volatile oil is composed of sesquiterpene hydrocarbon like α-zingiberol, α-sesquiterpene alcohol α-bisabolene, α-farnesene, α-sesquiphellandrene. Less pungent components like gingerone and shogaol are also present. Shogal is formed by the dehydration of gingerol and is not present in fresh rhizome.

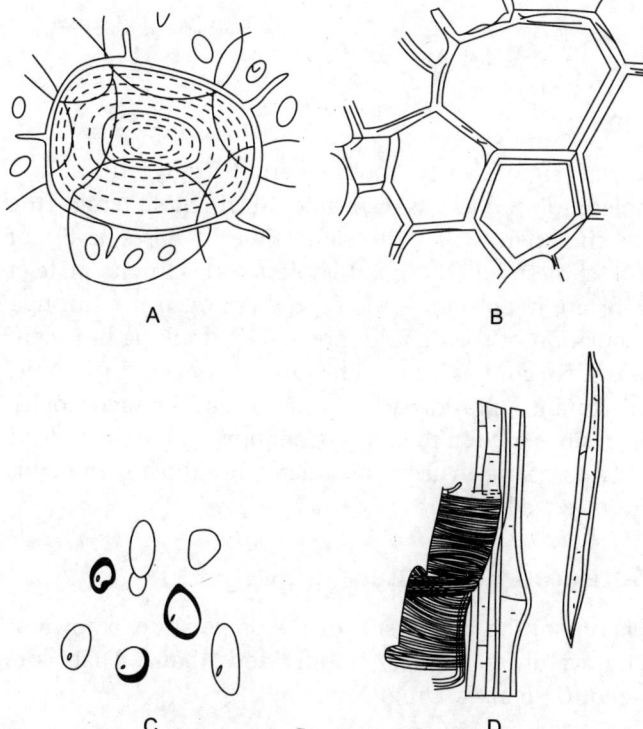

FIG. 18-10 Powder characteristics of ginger rhizome. (A: Oleo-resin cell, B: Cork cells, C: Starch grains, D: Portion of septate fibres with attached vessels)

shaped with a distinct eccentric hilum. Fibres are very large, pitted, slightly lignified, found with or without attached vessels of reticulate thickening. Oleoresin cells, ovoid-spherical; cork cells, polygonal in surface view, thick-walled; and abundant parenchyma, thin-walled cells, spherical-oval, are found scattered.

Chemical Constituents

Ginger contains 1–2% volatile oil, 5–8% pungent resinous mass and starch. The volatile oil is responsible

Gingerols (*n* = 0,2,3,4,5,7,9)

Zingerone

Shogaols (*n* = 4,5,7,9,10)

Uses

Ginger is used as an antiemetic, positive inotropic, spasmolytic, aromatic stimulant, carminative, condiment and flavouring agent. It is prescribed in dyspepsia, flatulent colic, vomiting spasms, as an adjunct to many tonic and stimulating remedies, for painful affections of the stomach, cold, cough and asthma. Sore throat, hoarseness and loss of voice are benefitted by chewing a piece of ginger.

Adulteration

Ginger may be adulterated by addition of 'wormy' drug or 'spent ginger' which has been exhausted in the extraction of resins and volatile oil. This adulteration may be detected by the official standards, for alcohol-soluble portion, water-soluble portion, total ash and water-soluble ash. Sometimes pungency of exhausted ginger is increased by the addition of capsicum.

Marketed Products

It is one of the ingredients of the preparations known as Pain kill oil, J.P. Liver syrup (Jamuna Pharma), Abana, Gasex (Himalaya Drug Company), Hajmola (Dabur), Strepsils (Boots Piramal Healthcare) and Sage Massaj oil (Sage Herbals).

GUGGUL

Synonyms

Gumgugul, Salai-gogil.

Biological Source

Guggal is a gum resin obtained by incision of the bark of *Commiphora mukul* (H. and S.) Engl., belonging to family Burseraceae (Fig. 18.11).

Geographical Source

The tree is a small, thorny plant distributed throughout India.

Collection

Guggal tree is a small thorny tree 4–6 feet tall branches slightly ascending. It is sometimes planted in hedges. The tree remains without any foliage for most of the year. It has ash-coloured bark, and comes off in rough flakes, exposing the innerbark, which also peels off. The tree exudes a yellowish resin called gum guggul or guggulu that has a balsamic odour. Each plant yields about one kilogram of the product, which is collected in cold season.

Characteristics

Guggal occurs as viscid, brown tears; or in fragment pieces, mixed with stem, piece of bark; golden yellow to brown in colour. With water it forms a milk emulsion. It has a balsamic odour and taste is bitter, aromatic.

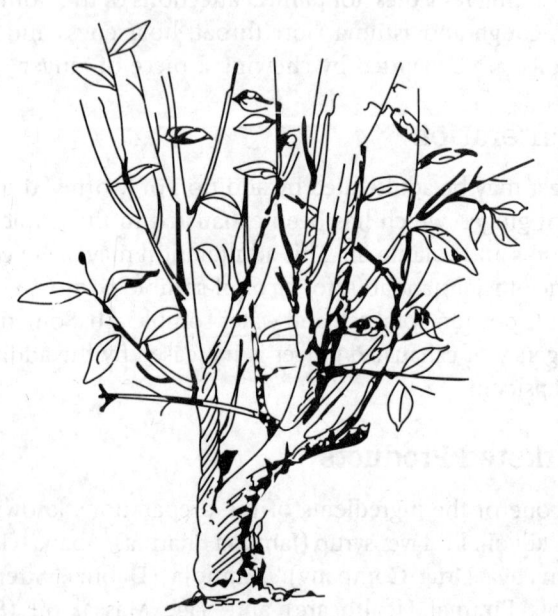

FIG. 18.11 *Commiphora mukul*

Chemical Constituents

Guggal contains gum (32%), essential oil (1.45%), sterols (guggulsterols I to VI, β-sitosterol, cholesterol, *Z*- and *E*-guggulsterone), sugars (sucrose, fructose), amino acids, α-camphorene, cembrene, allylcembrol, flavonoids (quercetin and its glycosides), ellagic acid, myricyl alcohol, aliphatic tetrols, etc.

Z-guggulsterone   E-guggulsterone

Uses

Guggal significantly lowers serum triglycerides and cholesterol as well as LDL and VLDL cholesterols (the bad cholesterols). At the same time, it raises levels of HDL cholesterol (the good cholesterol), inhibits platelet aggregation and may increase thermogenesis through stimulation of the thyroid, potentially resulting in weight loss. Also gum is astringent, aritirheumatic, antiseptic, expectorant, aphrodisiac, demulcent and emmenagogue. The resin is used in the form of a lotion for indolent ulcers and as a gargle in teeth disorders, tonsillitis, pharyngitis and ulcerated throat.

Marketed Products

It is one of the ingredients of the preparations known as Arogyavardhini Gutika (Dabur) and Abana, Diabecon, Diakof (Himalaya Drug Company).

IPOMOEA

Synonyms

Radix ipomoeae, Orizaba jalap root, Mexican scammony root, Mexican scammony, Ipomoea radix.

Biological Source

Ipomoea consists of the dried tuberous roots of *Ipomoea orizabensis* Ledenois., belonging to family Convolvulacae.

Geographical Source

It is mainly found in Mexico (Orizabs), Mexican Andes.

Collection

Ipomoea is perennial climbing twinner. It produces a large, woody and tuberous root. The roots are dug, washed, cut into slices and dried.

Characteristics

Ipomoea roots are large and fusiform, with 3–10 cm thick and about 20 cm long. They occur as irregular pieces, greyish brown in colour, with slight odour and slight acrid taste.

Microscopy

The cork is thin-walled cells, which is lignified. The parenchyma consists of numerous latex cells, starch grains and calcium oxalate crystals. The starch occurs in group of two to six compounds, the calcium oxalate present is of prismatic type. In the middle it has the primary xylem surrounded by the secondary xylem. The vascular bundles are also present in numerous amounts.

Chemical Constituents

Ipomoea consist of 10–20% resin, volatile oil and some fatty acids. The resin has an ether soluble portion and ether insoluble portion. Both the portions contain jalapin; a mixture of acidic glycosides. Ether soluble portion has jalapinolic acid, whereas in ether insoluble part it has hydroxy fatty acids, that is, ipurolic acid and convolvullinic acid.

Uses

Ipomoea resin is strong cathartic.

JALAP

Synonyms

Radix jalapae, Jalap root, Vera cruz or Mexican Jalap.

Biological Source

Jalap consists of dried tuberous roots or tubercles of *Ipomoea purga* Hayne, belonging to family Convolvulaceae.

Geographical Source

It is mainly found in Mexican Andes, India, West Indies and South America.

Collection

The plant is large and twinning perennial herb, and it produces thin horizontal slender runners. Adventitious roots (fusiform or napiform roots) are produced from the nodes of the runners. Some of the roots remain thin but few of them swell due to the storage of starch. These roots are collected after the rainy season, that is, in May. As a result of unfavourable environmental conditions they are dried by woodfire in nets. Since the drug is artificially dried it gains a smoky odour. Some slits are also made on the drug to facilitate the escape of the moisture.

Characteristics

Jalap is cylindrical, fusiform or napiform, irregularly oblong about 5–10 cm long and 2–10 cm wide. It is hard, resinous, compact and heavy. The outer surface is dark brown in colour with furrows and wrinkles and internally it is yellowish grey in colour. Odour is smoky and taste is sweet and starchy in the beginning and later it is acrid.

Microscopy

Cork is the outermost layer consisting of tabular polygonal cells which are brown in colour. Just below the cork it has the secondary phloem. The secondary phloem is formed by the circular cambium and is about 2 mm wide. Inside the cambium it has the secondary xylem. The secondary xylem has vessels, which are either in small groups or scattered. Latex cells are present in the phloem tissues arranged longitudinally and form a dark and resinous point scattered in the drug. The parenchymatous cells contain starch which are simple, rounded or in groups of two to four. Small prism types of calcium oxalate crystals are present in the parenchyma and very few sclerenchymatous cells are seen in the phelloderm region.

Chemical Constituents

Jalap contains 8–12% of glycosidal resin and the other constituents are mannitol, sugar, β-methyl-aesculetin, phytosterin, ipurganol, starch and calcium oxalate. Jalap resin is the resinous constituent that has a soluble portion and an insoluble portion when dissolved in ether. The soluble portion constitutes to 10%, whereas the remaining is the insoluble portion. Ether insoluble portion is called convolvulin and the ether soluble portion is called julapin. Convolvulin is a substance with some 18 hydroxyl groups esterified with valeric, tiglic and exogonic acids. Exogonic acid is 3,6-6,9-dioxidodecanoic acid.

Exogonic acid

Uses

Jalap can stimulate the intestinal secretion; it act as laxative in small doses and purgative in large doses; and it is also used as hydragogue cathartic.

KALADANA

Synonyms

Mirchi (Hindi), Krishna bija (Sanskrit).

Biological Source

Kaladana consists of the dried ripe seeds of *Ipomoea hederacea* L., belonging to family Convolvulaceae (Fig. 18.12).

Geographical Source

It grows throughout India both cultivated and apparently wild, up to 2000 m in the Himalayas.

Characteristics

The seeds are 5–6 mm long, 3.7 mm wide, triangular, brownish black in colour. Each seed has two flat faces joining at an angle of 60°–80°. At the base of joint there is a cordate hilum. Testa is dull black, hard, smooth and glabrous. Taste is first sweetish then acrid.

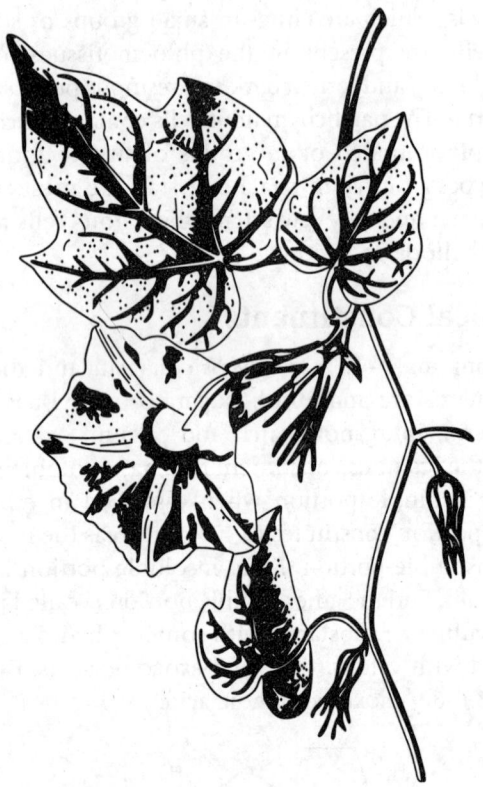

FIG. 18.12 *Ipomoea hederacea*

Chemical Constituents

Drug contains resin (about 15%), mucilage, fixed oil and saponin. Hydrolysis of the resin affords hydroxypalmitic acid and sugar. Lysergol, hederaceterpenol, hederaceteriol, hederaterpenoside, β-sitosterol glucopyranoside and chanoclavine are also present in Kaladana.

The seed oil is composed of glycerides of palmitic, stearic (20.3%), arachidic, oleic (43.9%), linoleic (14.5%) and linolenic acids.

Uses

Kaladana is used as purgative and substituted for Jalap.

MALE FERN

Synonyms

Filix Mass, Rhizoma Filicis Maris.

Biological Source

Male fern consists of the dried rhizomes and its surrounding frond bases of *Dryopteris filix-mas* (Linn.) Schoot, belonging to family Polypodiaceae (Fig. 18.13).

Geographical Source

D. filix-mas is a fern that grows abundantly in Europe especially in England and Germany. In India it grows in Kashmir, Himachal Pradesh and Sikkim at the altitude of 5000–10000 feet in the Himalayas.

Collection and Preparation

The male fern plant is identified on the basis of its oblique rhizomes surrounded by numerous frond bases. The fronds bear numerous long pinnae containing several pairs of pinnules. The plant is dug up in the late autumn. It is washed thoroughly with water. The roots, fronds and the other dead parts are removed, and the trimmed rhizomes are dried. Longer rhizomes are longitudinally cut into two halves for faster and efficient drying.

Characteristics

The dried male fern rhizomes are ovoid or cylindrical pieces, about 7–25 cm long and 3–4 cm thick. The outer surface is mostly covered by fronds which are directed towards the apex. Each frond base is about 45 cm long and is thickly covered with numerous brownish seals called as ramenta. The rhizomes break with a short fracture showing green surface. The rhizomes are brownish black in colour with little odour but sweet, bitter and extremely nauseating taste. The drug should be stored in dry places protected from light.

Microscopy

The transverse section of male fern rhizome with frond bases shows the presence of ground tissue consisting polygonal parenchyma along with abundant starch grains. The hypodermis consists of two to three rows of brownish nonlignified sclerenchymatous fibres. Meristemes possesses

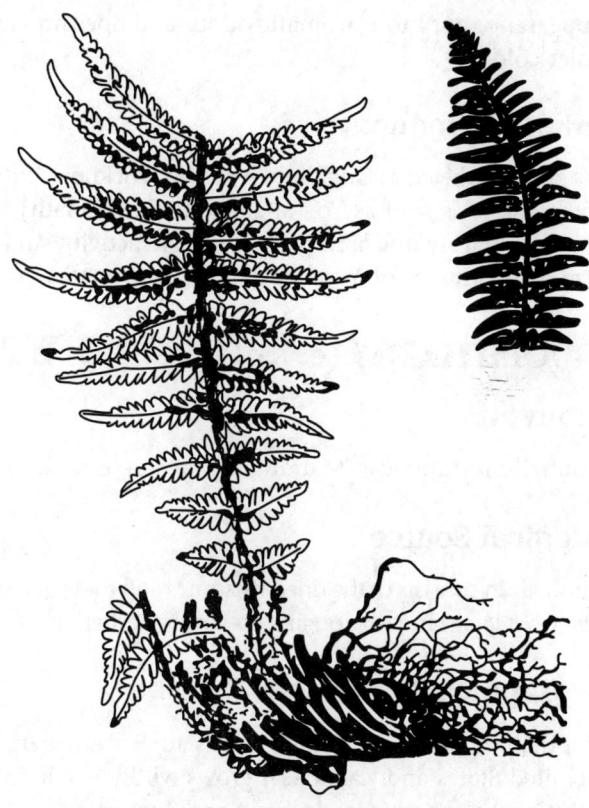

FIG. 18.13 *Dryopteris filix-mas*

large tracheids. The ramenta are made up of twin-cell marginal projections.

Chemical Constituents

Male fern rhizomes contain about 5% of yellow resinous substances responsible for its anthelmintic activity. The major constituents of oleoresin are phloroglucinol derivatives of mono- to tetracyclic compounds. The monocyclic derivatives are butyryl phloroglucinol, aspidinol and acylfilicinic acids. These compounds may condense with each other to produce bicyclic compounds such as albaspidin and flavaspidic acid or tricyclic compounds like filicic acid.

Uses

Male fern extract and the resin are used as a potent taenicide. It kills the worm and expels it out. Considerable care has to be undertaken during its use. Large doses acts as irritant poison. Its absorption from gastrointestinal tract may cause blindness.

Marketed Products

It is one of the ingredients of the preparation known as Paratrex (Global Healing Centre).

MYRRH

Synonyms

Gum-resin Myrrh, Gum Myrrh, Arabian or Somali Myrrh, Myrrha.

Biological Source

Myrrh is an oleo gum-resin obtained from the stem of *Commiphora molmol* Eng. or *C. abyssinica* or other species of Commiphora, belonging to family Burseraceae (Fig. 18.14).

Geographical Source

It grows in Arabian peninsula, Ethiopia, Nubia and Somaliland.

Collection

Myrrh plants are small trees up to 10 m in height. They have the phloem parenchyma and closely associated ducts containing a yellowish granular liquid. The tissues between these ducts often collapse, thereby producing large cavities similarly filled, that is, schizogenous ducts become lysigenous cavities. The gum-resin exudes spontaneously or by incising the bark. The yellowish-white, viscous fluid is solidified readily to produce reddish-brown masses which are collected by the natives.

Characteristics

Myrrh occurs as irregular masses or tears weighing up to 250 g. The outer surface is powdery and reddish-brown in colour. The drug breaks and is powdered readily. Fractured surface is rich brown and oily. Odour is aromatic and taste is aromatic, bitter and acrid.

Aspidinol

Acylfilicinic acid
$(R = CH_3; C_2H_5; C_3H_7)$

Albaspidin

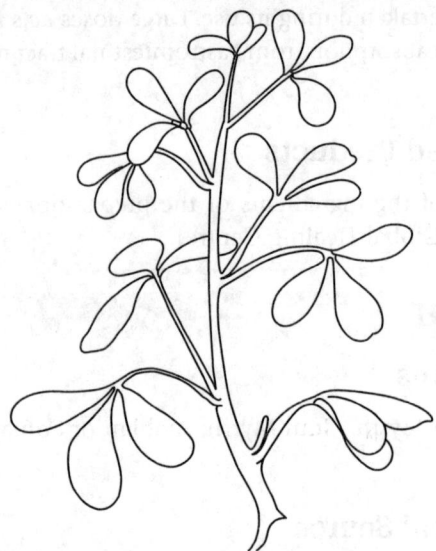

FIG. 18.14 *Commiphora molmol*

Chemical Constituents

Myrrh contains resin (25–40%), gum (57–61%) and volatile oil (7–17%). Large portion of the resin is ether-soluble containing α-, β- and γ-commiphoric acids, resenes, the esters of another resin acid and two phenolic compounds. The volatile oil is a mixture of cuminic aldehyde, eugenol, cresol, pinene, limonene, dipentene and two sesquiterpenes. The disagreeable odour of the oil is due to mainly the disulphide. The gum contains proteins (18%) and carbohydrate (64%) which is a mixture of galactose, arabinose, glucuronic acid and an oxidase enzyme.

Chemical Tests

1. A yellow brown emulsion is produced on trituration with water.
2. Ethereal solution of Myrrh turns red on treatment with bromine vapours. The solution becomes purple with nitric acid.

Uses

Myrrh is used as carminative and in incense and perfumes. It has local stimulant and antiseptic properties and is utilized in tooth powder and as mouth wash. Topically it is astringent to mucous membranes. It is used in a tincture, paint, gargle and rinse due to its disinfecting, deodourizing, and in inflammatory conditions of the mouth and throat. Alcoholic extracts are used as fixatives in the perfumery industry.

Allied Drugs

Four different varieties of bdellium are present. Of these, perfumed or scented bdellium or bissabol is obtained from *C. erythaea* var. *glabrescens*. It resembles soft myrrh in appearance but more aromatic odour and does not give a violet colour.

Marketed Products

It has been marketed as Gugulipid by CDRI, Lucknow, India. In ayurveda, it is sold as Yograj guggulu (Baidyanath) for anti-inflammatory and antihyperlipidemic activity, and it is also a constituent of Madhumehari (Baidyanath).

PODOPHYLLUM

Synonyms

Podophyllum, American Mandrake, May-apple root.

Biological Source

Podophyllum consists of the dried rhizomes and roots of *Podophyllum peltatum* Linn., belonging to family Berberidaceae.

Geographical Source

Podophyllum peltatum is indigenous to Eastern part of the United States and Canada. It grows wildly in Virginia, North Carolina, Kentucky, Indiana and Tennessee.

Collection and Preparation

Podophyllum is a perennial herb which grows wildly in moist and shady places. Most of the drug is collected from the wild plant in autumn. However, the cultivation of podophyllum has been found to be profitable in the area of its occurrence. The rhizomes are dug up, washed with water to remove soil and cut into smaller pieces. The adventitious roots present on the rhizomes are removed. The drug is dried in the sun.

Characteristics

Podophyllum rhizomes come in the form of subcylindrical pieces of 5–20 cm length and 5–6 mm thickness at the internode and about 15 mm at the node. The pieces show occasional branching. It shows the scars of aerial stems and adventitious roots. The outer surface is smooth or wrinkled and dark reddish brown. It shows slight but characteristic odour and bitter, acrid taste. The rhizome breaks with a short, horny fracture. The transversely cut surface show white starchy circles with radially elongated vascular bundles.

Microscopy

A transverse section of the podophyllum rhizome shows darker epidermis and one- or two-layered cork made up of dead cells. The outer cortical zone is made up of thin-walled parenchyma and collenchymatous tissues, whereas the inner cortex consists of a ring of smaller vascular bundles. Central pith is parenchymatous with narrow stone cells. Certain parenchymatous cells of the nodal region shows cluster crystals of calcium oxalate and most of the cells show the presence of starch grains.

Chemical Constituents

Podophyllum rhizomes contain 2–8% resinous material termed as podophyllin. The major constituents of podophyllum resin are the lignan derivatives which are characterized as podophyllotoxin, α- and β-peltatin. The lignans are found in the form of glycosides and also as their free aglycones. It also contains desmethyl podophyllotoxin, deoxypodophyllotoxin, podophyllotoxone, a flavonoid quercetin and starch.

Compound	R1	R2	R3
Podophyllotoxin	H	OH	CH₃
Desmethyl podophyllotoxin	H	OH	H
Deoxypodophyllotoxin	H	H	CH₃
Podophyllotoxone	H	= O	CH₃
α-Peltatin	OH	H	H
β-Peltatin	OH	H	CH₃

Uses

Podophyllum resin or podophyllin shows cytotoxic activity. It is used for the treatment of venereal and other warts. Podophyllotoxin is semisynthetically converted to a potent anticancer agent etoposide which is mainly used for the treatment of lung and testicular cancer. Podophyllum resin is a strong gastrointestinal irritant. It acts as a drastic purgative in moderate doses but it has been mostly replaced by other purgative drugs.

INDIAN PODOPHYLLUM

Synonyms

Rhizoma Podophylli Indici, Indian podophyllum.

Biological Source

Indian podophyllum consists of the dried pieces of rhizomes and roots of *Podophyllum hexandrum* Royle, belonging to family Berberidaceae (Fig. 18.15).

Geographical Source

The plant grows abundantly in the higher slopes of the Himalayas in India and Pakistan. It is also found in Afghanistan and Tibet.

Collection and Preparation

The plants which grow as a perennial herb are dug up in the autumn. The rhizomes are generally collected from above two years old plant. The rhizomes are washed with water, cut into small pieces and dried in the sun.

Characteristics

Indian podophyllum rhizomes are subcylindrical, flattened pieces with a very short internode as compared to American podophyllum. The pieces are about 2–4 cm long and 1–2 cm in diameter, it shows the scars due to cutting of branches and roots. Rhizomes are brownish coloured with characteristic odour and acrid, bitter taste. It breaks with horny fracture but very hard. The transversely cut surface shows a ring of vascular bundle and central pith.

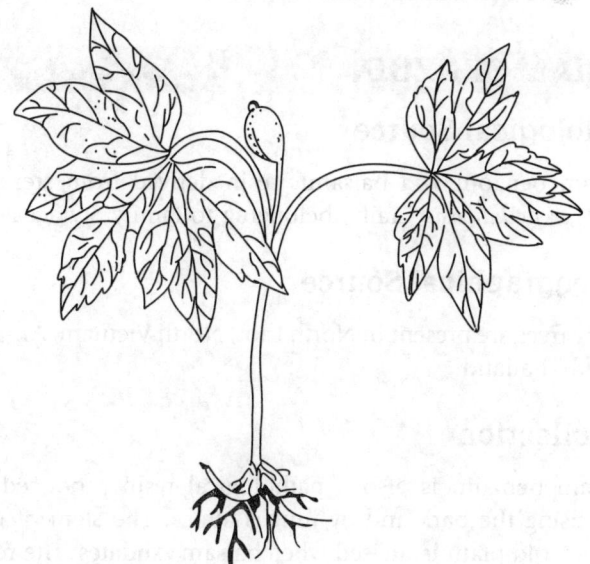

FIG. 18.15 *Podophyllum hexandrum*

Microscopy

A transverse section of the Indian podophyllum rhizome shows the thin-walled, tubular cork. Cortex is made up of cellular parenchyma containing large number of starch grains and cluster crystals of calcium oxalate. The vascular bundles are arranged in a ring with phloem on the outer side and a bit irregular xylem at the inner side. In certain regions fibrovascular bundles are found entering the aerial stem. The central pith shows the crystals of calcium oxalate. The major distinguishing features in *P. hexandrum* and *P. peltatum* are the size of the starch grain and the crystals of calcium oxalate.

Chemical Constituents

The most of the chemical constituents of Indian podophyllum are similar to that of *P. peltatum*. Podophyllum resin present to the extent of 6–12% which contains about 40% podophyllotoxin.

Chemical Tests

The reaction of podophyllum resin alcoholic extract with strong solution of copper acetate develops brown precipitate for Indian podophyllum, whereas American drug produces green colour without precipitate.

Uses

P. hexandrum closely resembles *P. peltatum* in its pharmacological activity. It is largely used for the preparation of podophyllum resin.

Marketed Products

It is one of the ingredients of the preparation known as Podowart (Shalaks Pharmaceuticals).

SIAM BENZOIN

Biological Source

Siam benzoin is a balsamic resin derived from stem of *Styrax tonkinensis* Craib., belonging to family Styraceae.

Geographical Source

The trees are present in North Laos, North Vietnam, Annam and Thailand.

Collection

Siam benzoin is also a pathological resin produced by incising the bark and by fungus attack. The stem of 6–8 years old plant is incised when balsam exudates. The resin is obtained in the form of liquid which is solidified.

Characteristics

Siam benzoin occurs as tears or in blocks of variable sizes and reddish brown externally, but milky-white or opaque internally. Matrix is glassy, reddish-brown, resinous, brittle but softening on chewing and become plastic-like on chewing. It has vanilla-like odour and a balsamic taste.

Chemical Constituents

The principal constituent of Siam benzoin is coniferyl benzoate (60–80%) (3-methoxy-4-hydroxycinnamyl alcohol). Other constituents are free benzoic acid (10%), triterpene siaresinolic acid (6%), vanillin and benzyl cinnamate.

Chemical Tests

1. Heat Sumatra benzoin (5 g) with 10% aqueous potassium permanganate solution. A bitter almond-like odour is produced due to oxidation of cinnamic acid present in Sumatra benzoin. This test is negative in case of Siam Benzoin.
2. To a petroleum ether solution of benzoin (0.2 g), two to three drops of sulphuric acid are added in a China dish. Sumatra benzoin produces reddish-brown colour, whereas Siam benzoin shows purple-red colour on rotating the dish.
3. To alcoholic solution of benzoin ferric chloride solution is added. A green colour is produced in Siam benzoin due to the presence of phenolic compound coniferyl benzoate. This test is negative in case of Sumatra benzoin which does not contain sufficient amount of phenolic constituents.

Uses

Siam benzoin acts as antiseptic, culinary and expectorant; it is used to prepare benzoinated lard, cosmetics, fixatives and in perfumery. It is superior to the Sumatra Benzoin with respect to antioxidative effect in lard and other fats.

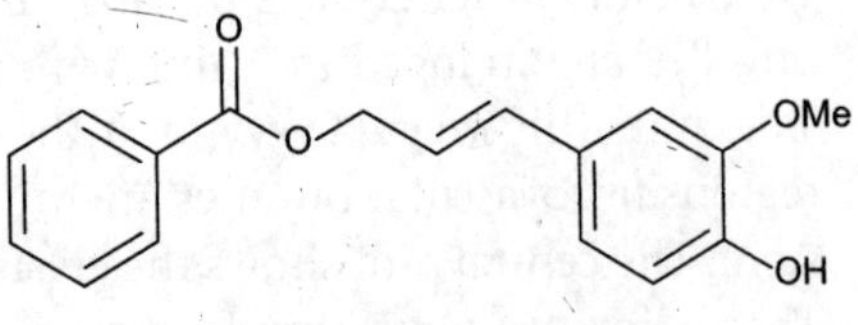

Coniferyl benzoate

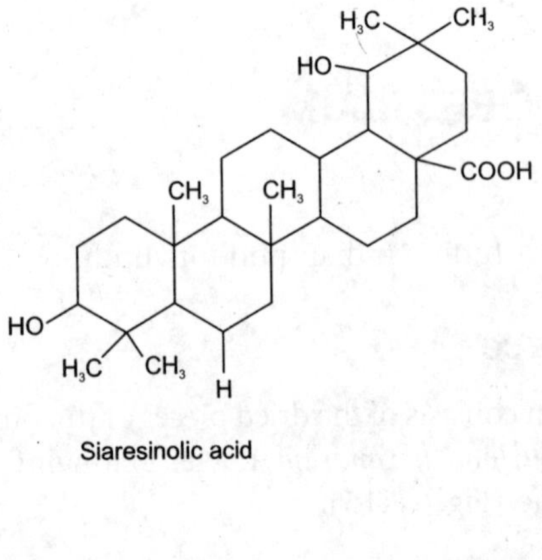

Siaresinolic acid

Marketed Products

It is one of the ingredients of the preparation known as Friar's balsam.

SUMATRA BENZOIN

Synonyms

Gum Benjamin, Benzoinum, Benzoin, Luban (Hindi).

Biological Source

Sumatra benzoin is obtained from the incised stem of *Styrax benzoin* Dryander and *Styrax parallelo-neurus* Perkins., belonging to family Styraceae (Fig. 18.16). It contains about 25% of total balsamic acids, calculated as cinnamic acid.

Geographical Source

The trees are found in Sumatra, Malacca, Malaya, Java and Borneo.

Collection

The plants are medium-sized trees. Sumatra benzoin is a pathological resin which is formed by making incision and by attack of fungi. In Sumatra the seeds are sown in rice fields. The rice plants provide protection to benzoin plants during first year. After harvesting of the rice crop the trees are allowed to grow. When they are 7 years old, three triangular wounds are made in a vertical row. Tapping consists of making in each trunk three lines of incisions which are gradually lengthened. The first triangular wounds are made in a vertical row about 40 cm apart, the bark between the wounds being then scraped smooth. The first secretion is very sticky and is rejected. After making further cuts, each about 4 cm above the preceding ones, a harder secretion is obtained. Further incisions are made at three-monthly intervals, and the secretion becomes crystalline. About 6 weeks after each fresh tapping the product is scraped off, the outer layer (finest quality) being kept separate from the next layer (intermediate quality). About 2 weeks later the strip is scraped again, giving a lower quality darker in colour and containing fragments of bark. Fresh incisions are then made, and the above process is repeated. Second exudation is milky white and is used for medicinal purpose. The stem is incised four times during one year. AH types of exudations are sent to industry for further processing. A single tree yields about 10 kg of resin per year and is completely exhausted by the 19th year of its life.

Characteristics

Sumatra benzoin occurs in brittle masses consisting of opaque, whitish or reddish tears embedded in a translucent, reddish-brown or greyish-brown, resinous matrix. Odour,

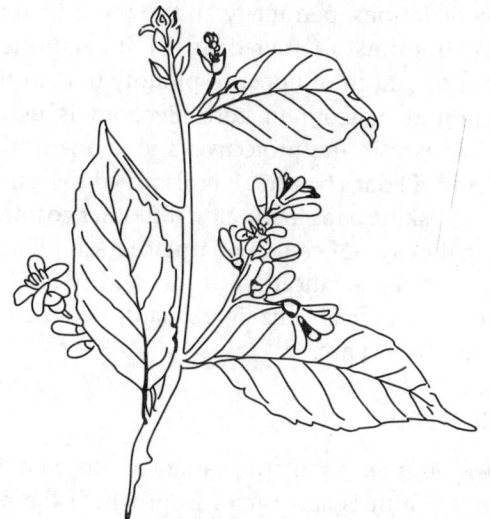

FIG. 18.16 *Styrax benzoin*

agreeable and balsamic, taste, slightly acrid. Siamese benzoin occurs in tears or in blocks. The tears are of variable size and flattened; they are yellowish-brown or reddish-brown externally, but milky-white and opaque internally. The block form consists of small tears embedded in a glassy, reddish-brown, resinous matrix. It has a vanilla-like odour and a balsamic taste.

When heated, benzoin evolves white fumes of cinnamic and benzoic acids which readily condense on a cool surface as a crystalline sublimate.

Chemical Constituents

Sumatra benzoin consists of free balsamic acid (cinnamic and benzoic acids) (25%) and their esters. The amount of cinnamic acid is usually double that of benzoic acid. It also contains triterpenic acids like siaresinolic acid (19-hydroxy-oleanolic acid) and sumaresinolic acid (6-hydroxy-oleanolic acid); traces of vanillin, phenylpropyl cinnamate, cinnamyl cinnamate and phenylethylene.

Siaresinolic acid

Uses

Sumatra benzoin possesses expectorant, antiseptic, carminative, stimulant and diuretic properties. It is used in cosmetic lotions, perfumery and to prepare compound benzoin. It forms an ingredient of inhalations in the treatment of catarrh of upper respiratory tract in the form of compound benzoin tincture. Benzoin is used as an external antiseptic and protective, and is one of the main ingredients of Friar's balsam. It is also used to fix the odour of incenses, skin-soaps, perfumes and other cosmetics and for fixing the taste of certain pharmaceutical preparations. Benzoin retards rancification of fats and is used for this purpose in the official benzoinated lard, also used in food, drinks and in incense.

Allied Drug

Palembang benzoin, an interior variety produced in Sumatra is collected from isolated trees from which the resin has not been stripped for some time. It is very light in weight and breaking with an irregular porous fracture. It consists of reddish-brown resin, with only a few very small tears embedded in it. *Palembang benzoin* is used as a source of natural benzoic acid.

STORAX

Synonyms

Styrax, Sweet oriental gum, Prepared Storax, Liquid Storax, Styrax preparatus.

Biological Source

Storax is a balsam obtained from the trunk of *Liquidambar orientalis* Miller, commercially known as Levant Storax, or of *Liquidambar styraciflua* Linn, known as American Storax, belonging to family Hamamelidaceae (Fig. 18.17).

Geographical Source

Levant Storax is a native to Asia Minor and Southwest of Turkey. American Storax is produced chiefly in Honduras; found along the Atlantic coast from Connecticut to Central America.

Collection

Levant Storax and American Storax are medium-sized trees attaining the height of 15–40 m, respectively. Levant Storax is a pathological resin. In the early summer the bark of three to four years old tree is injured by bruising. Cambium is activated to produce new wood with balsam secreting ducts. The bark is gradually saturated with balsam which is peeled off. The pieces of bark are pressed to get the product. The bark is boiled in hot water and repressed. The crude balsam is poured into casks or cans and exported.

American Storax exudes into natural spaces present in between the bark and the wood. The presence of balsam in spaces may be detected by excrescences on the outside of the bark. From these pockets the balsam is tapped with gutters into containers which are exported in tin cans.

Storax is purified by dissolving the crude balsam in alcohol, filtering and evaporating the solvent under low temperature not to lose volatile compounds. The alcohol insoluble part consists of vegetable debris and a resin.

Characteristics

Levent Storax is a viscous, semiliquid, greyish, sticky, opaque mass which deposits as a dark-brown, heavier, oleoresinous product on standing. American Storax is a semisolid, sometimes solid mass softened by warming, becoming hard, opaque and darker coloured. Storax is transparent in thin layers, has characteristic taste and odour, and is denser than water. It is insoluble in water; almost completely soluble in warm alcohol, ether, acetone and carbon disulphide. Odour is agreeable and taste is balsamic.

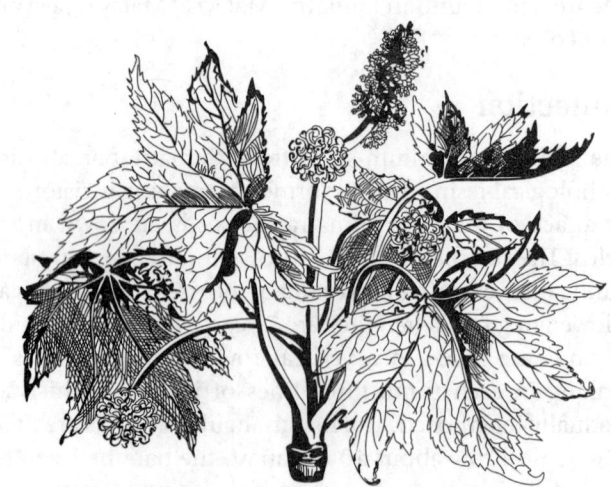

FIG. 18.17 *Liquidambar orientalis*

Chemical Constituents

Storax is rich in two resin alcohol (50%): α-storesin and β-storesin and balsamic acids (30–47%). The alcohols occur partly free and partly as esters of cinnamic acid (10–20%). Storax also contains cinnamyl cinnamate or styracin (5–10%), phenyl-propyl cinnamate (10%); ethyl cinnamate, benzyl cinnamate, free cinnamic acid (5–15%), styrene, traces of vanillin and volatile oil (0.5–1%). Steam distillation of Storax yields a pale yellow or dark brown oil (0.5–1.0%) known as oil of Storax. It has a pleasant but peculiar odour.

Uses

Storax is used as a stimulant, expectorant, parasiticide, topical protectant and an antiseptic. Pharmaceutical preparations like compound benzoin tincture, Friars' balsam and benzoin inhalation are also prepared from Storax.

TURMERIC

Synonyms

Saffron Indian, haldi (Hindi), Curcuma, Rhizoma curcumae.

Biological Source

Turmeric is the dried rhizome of *Curcuma longa* Linn. (syn. *C. domestica* Valeton)., belonging to family Zingiberaceae (Fig. 18.18).

Geographical Source

The plant is a native to southern Asia and is cultivated extensively in temperate regions. It is grown on a larger scale in India, China, East Indies, Pakistan and Malaya.

Cultivation

Turmeric plant is a perennial herb, 60–90 cm high with a short stem and tufted leaves; the rhizomes, which are short and thick, constitute the turmeric of commerce. The crop requires a hot and moist climate, a liberal water supply and a well-drained soil. It thrives on any soil-loamy or alluvial, but the soil should be loose and friable. The field should be well prepared by ploughing and turning over to a depth of about 30 cm and liberally manured with farmyard and green manures. Sets or fingers of the previous crop with one or two buds are planted 7 cm deep at distance of 30–37 cm from April to August. The crop is ready for harvesting in about 9–10 months when the lower leaves turn yellow. The rhizomes are carefully dug up with hard picks, washed and dried.

Characteristics

The primary rhizomes are ovate or pear-shaped, oblong or pyriform or cylindrical, and often short branched. The rhizomes are known as 'bulb' or 'round' turmeric. The secondary, more cylindrical, lateral branched, tapering on both ends, rhizomes are 4–7 cm long and 1–1.5 cm wide and called as 'fingers'. The bulbous and finger-shaped parts are separated and the long fingers are broken into convenient bits. They are freed from adhering dirt and fibrous roots and subjected to curing and polishing process. The curing consists of cooking the rhizomes along with few leaves in water until they become soft. The cooked rhizomes are cooled, dried in open air with intermittent turning over and rubbed on a rough surface. Colour is deep yellow to orange, with root scar and encircling ridge-like rings or annulations, the latter from the scar of leaf base. Fracture is horny and the cut surface is waxy and resinous in appearance. Outer surface is deep yellow to brown and longitudinally wrinkled. Taste is aromatic, pungent and bitter; odour is distinct.

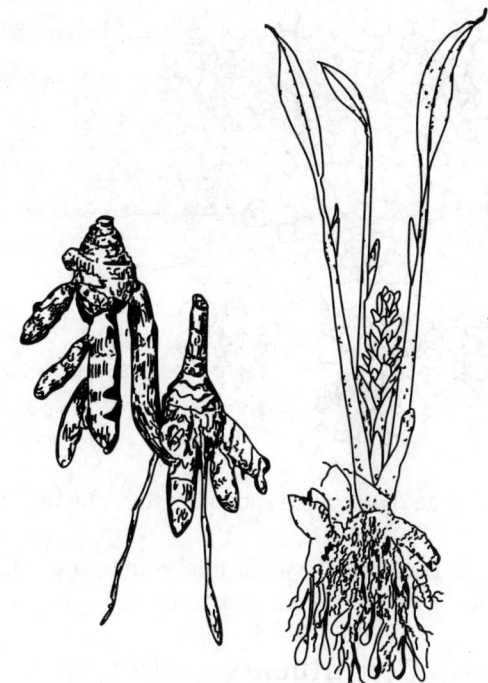

FIG. 18.18 Rhizomes and whole plant of turmeric

Microscopy (Figs. 18.19 and 18.20)

The transverse section of the rhizome is characterized by the presence of mostly thin-walled rounded parenchyma cells, scattered vascular bundles, definite endodermis, few layers of cork developed under the epidermis and scattered oleoresin cells with brownish contents. The epidermis is consisted of thick-walled cells, cubical in shape, of various dimensions. The cork cambium is developed from the subepidermal layers and even after the development of the cork, the epidermis is retained. Cork is generally composed of four to six layers of thin-walled brick-shaped parenchymatous cells. The parenchyma of the pith and cortex contains grains altered to a paste, in which sometimes long lens shaped unaltered starch grains of 4–15 μm diameter are found. Oil cells have suberised walls and contain either orange-yellow globules of a volatile oil or amorphous resinous masses. Cortical vascular bundles are scattered and are of a collateral type. The vascular bundles in the pith region are mostly scattered and they form discontinuous ring just under the endodermis.

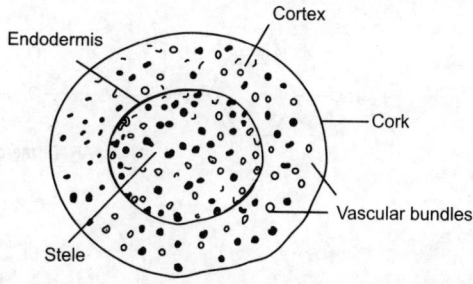

FIG. 18.19 T.S. (schematic) of turmeric rhizome

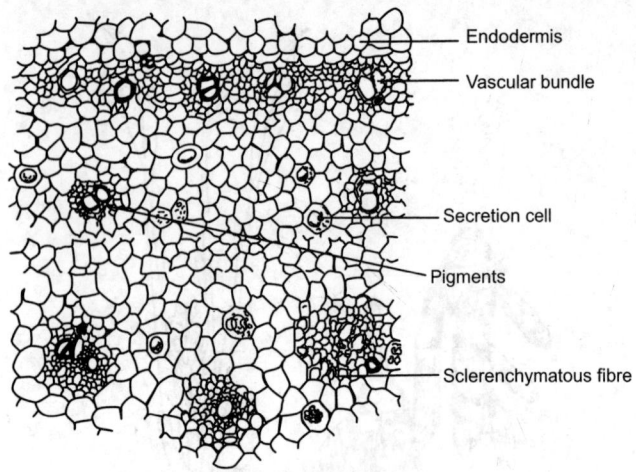

FIG. 18.20 Transverse section of turmeric rhizome

The vessels have mainly spiral thickenings and only a few have reticulate and annular structure.

Chemical Constituents

Turmeric contains yellow colouring matter called as curcuminoids (5%) and essential oil (6%). The chief constituent of the colouring matter is curcumin I (60%) in addition with small quantities of curcumin III, curcumin II and dihydrocurcumin. The volatile oil contains mono- and sesquiterpenes like zingiberene (25%), α-phellandrene, sabinene, turmerone, arturmerone, borneol and cineole.

Choleretic action of the essential oil is attributed to β-tolylmethyl carbinol.

The volatile oil also contains α- and β-pinene, camphene, limonene, terpinene, terpinolene, caryophyllene, linalool, isoborneol, camphor, eugenol, curdione, curzerenone, curlone, AR-curcumenes, β-curcumene, γ-curcumene. α- and β-turmerones and curzerenone.

Chemical Tests

1. Turmeric powder on treatment with concentrated sulphuric acid forms red colour.
2. On addition of alkali solution to turmeric powder red to violet colour is produced.
3. With acetic anhydride and concentrated sulphuric acid turmeric gives violet colour. Under UV light this colour is seen as an intense red fluorescence.
4. A paper containing turmeric extract produces a green colour with borax solution.
5. On addition of boric acid a reddish-brown colour is formed which, on addition of alkalies, changes to greenish-blue.
6. A piece of filter paper is impregnated with an alcohol extract, dried and then moistened with boric acid solution slightly acidified with hydrochloric acid, and redried. Pink or brownish-red colour is developed on the filter paper which becomes deep blue on addition of alkali.

Curcumin-I

Demethoxycurcumin

Bisdemethoxycurcumin

AR-Turmerone

(-)- Zingiberene

Uses

Turmeric is used as aromatic, anti-inflammatory, stomachic, uretic, anodyne for biliary calculus, stimulant, tonic, carminative, blood purifier, antiperiodic, alterative, spice, colouring agent for ointments and a common household remedy for cold and cough. Externally, it is used in the form of a cream to improve complexion. Dye-stuff acts as a cholagogue causing the contraction of the gall bladder. It is also used in menstrual pains. Curcumin has choleretic and cholagogue action and is used in liver diseases. Curcumin is a nontoxic authorized colour, heat resistant and sensitive to changes in pH. Curcuminoids have antiphlogistic activity which is due to inhibition of leukotriene biosynthesis.

Ar-Turmerone has antisnake venom activity and blocks the haemorrhagic effect of venom.

Adulteration

The genuine drug is adulterated with the rhizomes of *Acorus calamus*.

Marketed Products

It is one of the ingredients of the preparations known as J.P. Nikhar oil, J.P. Kasantak (Jamuna Pharma), Diabecon, Purian (Himalaya Drug Company) and Respinova (Lupin Herbal Laboratory).

CHAPTER 19

Drugs Containing Lipids

CONTENTS

- Introduction
- Fixed Oils and Fats
- Waxes
- Almond Oil
- Arachis Oil
- Castor Oil
- Chaulmoogra Oil
- Coconut Oil
- Cod Liver Oil
- Corn Oil
- Cottonseed Oil
- Linseed Oil
- Mustard Oil
- Olive Oil
- Rice Bran Oil
- Safflower Oil
- Sesame Oil
- Shark Liver Oil
- Beeswax
- Carnauba Wax
- Cocoa Butter
- Kokum
- Lanolin
- Lard

19.1. INTRODUCTION

The lipids are a large and diverse group of naturally occurring organic compounds that are related by their solubility in nonpolar organic solvents (e.g. ether, chloroform, acetone and benzene) and are generally insoluble in water. There is great structural variety among the lipids and comprise of fixed oils, fats and waxes. The lipids of physiological importance for humans have the following major functions:

1. They serve as structural components of biological membranes.
2. They provide energy reserves, predominantly in the form of triacylglycerols.
3. Both lipids and lipid derivatives serve as vitamins and hormones.
4. Lipophilic bile acids aid in lipid solubilization.

19.2. FIXED OILS AND FATS

Fixed oils and fats are obtained from plants or animal. They are rich in calories and in plant source, they are present mostly in the seeds, as reserve substances and in animals they are present in subcutaneous and retroperitoneal tissues. They differ only according to their melting point and chemically they belong to the same group. If a substance is liquid at 15.5–16.5°C it is called fixed oil and solid or semisolid at the above temperature, it is called fat. They are made from two kinds of molecules: glycerol (a type of alcohol with a hydroxyl group on each of its three carbons) and three fatty acids joined by dehydration synthesis. Since there are three fatty acids attached, these are known as triglycerides. These fatty acids may be saturated, monounsaturated or polyunsaturated. The terms saturated, monounsaturated and polyunsaturated refer to the number of hydrogens attached to the hydrocarbon tails of the fatty acids as compared to the number of double bonds between carbon atoms in the tail. Fats, which are mostly from animal sources, have all single bonds between the carbons in their fatty acid tails, thus all the carbons are also bonded to the maximum number of hydrogens possible. Since the fatty acids in these triglycerides contain the maximum possible amount of hydrogens, these would be called saturated fats. The hydrocarbon chains in these fatty acids are, thus, fairly straight and can pack closely together, making these fats solid at room temperature. Oils, mostly from plant sources, have some double bonds between some of the carbons in the hydrocarbon tail, causing bends or 'kinks' in the shape of the molecules. Because some of the carbons share double bonds, they are not bonded to as many hydrogens as they could if they weren't double bonded to each other. Therefore these oils are called unsaturated fats. Because of the kinks in the hydrocarbon tails, unsaturated fats can't pack as closely together, making them liquid at room temperature.

Examples of saturated and unsaturated fatty acids are given in Table 19.1.

Table 19.1 Examples of saturated and unsaturated fatty acids

Fatty acid	Source
Saturated fatty acids	
Butyric acid	Butter fat
Lauric acid	Coconut oil
Myristic acid	Palm oil
Palmitic acid	Arachis oil, sesame oil
Stearic acid	Arachis oil
Arachidic acid	Mustard oil
Unsaturated fatty acids	
Linolenic acid	Linseed oil
Linoleic acid	Sesame oil, sunflower oil
Arachidonic acid	Arachis oil
Oleic acid	Safflower oil, corn oil

Fixed oils and fats are insoluble in water and alcohol and are soluble in lipid solvents like light petroleum, ether, chloroform and benzene. Only exception in this solubility is castor oil that is soluble in alcohol because of its hydroxy group of ricinoleic acid. They float in water since their specific gravity is less than one. They produce a permanent translucent stain on the paper and are called fixed oils. Fixed oils and fats cannot be distilled without their decomposition.

Analytical Parameters for Fats and Oils

Following are the parameters used to analyse the fats and oils.

1. **Iodine value:** The iodine value is the mass of iodine in grams that is consumed by 100 g of fats or oil. A iodine solution is violet in colour and any chemical group in the substance that reacts with iodine will make the colour disappear at a precise concentration. The amount of iodine solution thus required to keep the solution violet is a measure of the amount of iodine sensitive reactive groups. It is a measure of the extent of unsaturation and higher the iodine value, the more chance for rancidity.

2. **Saponification value:** The saponification value is the number of milligrams of potassium hydroxide required to saponify 1 g of fat under the conditions specified. It is a measure of the average molecular weight of all the fatty acids present.

3. **Hydroxyl value:** The hydroxyl value is the number of mg of potassium hydroxide (KOH) required to neutralize acetic acid combined to hydroxyl groups, when 1 g of a sample is acetylated.

4. **Ester value:** The ester value is the number of mg of potassium hydroxide (KOH) required to saponify the ester contained in 1 g of a sample.

5. **Unsaponifiable matter:** The principle is the saponification of the fat or oil by boiling under reflux with an ethanolic potassium hydroxide solution. Unsaponifiable matter is then extracted from the soap solution by diethyl ether. The solvent is evaporated and then the residue is dried and weighed.

6. **Acid value:** It is the amount of free acid present in fat as measured by the milligrams of potassium hydroxide needed to neutralize it. As the glycerides in fat slowly-decompose the acid value increases.

7. **Peroxide value:** One of the most widely used tests for oxidative rancidity; peroxide value is a measure of the concentration of peroxides and hydroperoxides formed in the initial stages of lipid oxidation. Milliequivalents of peroxide per kg of fat are measured by titration with iodide ion. Peroxide values are not static and care must be taken in handling and testing samples. It is difficult to provide a specific guideline relating peroxide value to rancidity. High peroxide values are a definite indication of a rancid fat, but moderate values may be the result of depletion of peroxides after reaching high concentrations.

19.3. WAXES

Waxes are esters of long-chain fatty acids and alcohols. The fatty acids are same in wax and fats, but the difference being saponification. Waxes are saponified only by alcoholic alkali but the fats may be saponified either by alcoholic alkali or by aqueous alkali. Along with fatty acids it also contains monohydroxy alcohols of high molecular weight especially cetyl alcohol, melissyl alcohol and myricyl alcohol. Sometimes cholesterol or phytosterols are also present.

As such they are not suitable as food because hydrolysing enzymes of wax are not present in system. Waxes are widely distributed in nature. The leaves and fruits of many plants have waxy coatings, which may protect them from dehydration and small predators. The feathers of birds and the fur of some animals have similar coatings which serve as a water repellent.

Spermaceti, beeswax, carnauba wax, etc., are the examples of waxes.

ALMOND OIL

Biological Source

Almond oil is a fixed oil obtained by expression from the seeds of *Prunus amygdalus* (Rosaceae) var. dulcis (sweet almonds) or *P. amygdalus var. amara* (bitter almonds) (Fig. 19.1a and b).

Geographical Source

The oil is mainly produced from almonds grown in the countries bordering the Mediterranean (Italy, France, Syria, Spain and North Africa) and Iran.

Characteristics

Almond trees are about 5 m in height. The young fruits have a soft, felt-like pericarp, the inner part of which gradually becomes sclerenchymatous as the fruit ripens to form a pitted endocarp or shell. The shells, consisting mainly of sclerenchymatous cells, are sometimes ground and used to adulterate powdered drugs.

The sweet almond is 2–3 cm in length, rounded at one end and pointed at the other. The bitter almond is 1.5–2 cm in length but of similar breadth to the sweet almond. Both varieties have a thin, cinnamon-brown testa which is easily removed after soaking in warm water. The oily kernel consists of two large, oily planoconvex cotyledons, and a small plumule and radicle, the latter lying at the pointed end of the seed. Some almonds have cotyledons of unequal sizes and are irregularly folded. Bitter almonds are found in samples of sweet almonds; their presence may be detected by the sodium picrate test for cyanogenic glycosides.

Chemical Constituents

Both varieties of almond contain 40–55% of fixed oil, about 20% of proteins, mucilage and emulsin. The bitter almonds contain in addition 2.5–4.0% of the colourless, crystalline, cyanogenic glycoside amygdalin.

Almond oil is obtained by grinding the seeds and expressing, them in canvas bags between slightly heated iron plates. The oil is clarified by subsidence and filtration. It is a pale yellow liquid with a slight odour and bland nutty taste. It contains olein, with smaller quantities of the glycosides of linoleic and other acids. Bitter almonds,

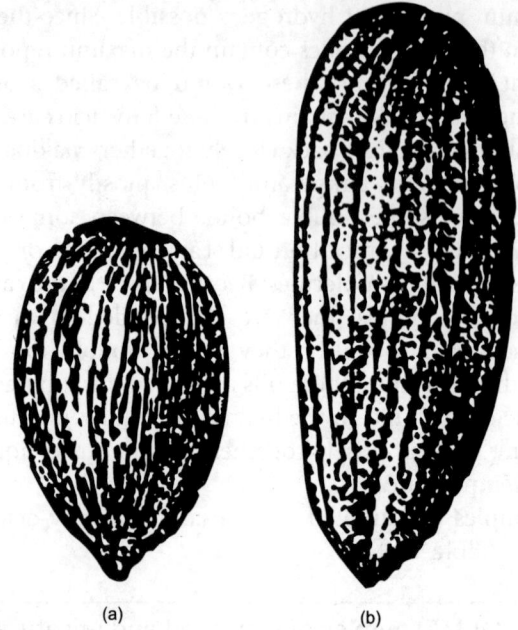

FIG. 19.1 (a) Bitter almond and (b) sweet almond

after maceration on hydrolysis of amygdalin yield a volatile oil that is used as a flavouring agent. Sweet almonds are extensively used as a food, but bitter almonds are not suitable for this purpose.

Essential or volatile oil of almonds is obtained from the cake left after expressing bitter almonds. This is macerated with water for some hours to allow hydrolysis of the amygdalin to take place. The benzaldehyde and hydrocyanic acid are then separated by stem distillation.

Almond oil consists of a mixture of glycerides of oleic (62–86%), linoleic (17%), palmitic (5%), myristic (1%), palmitoleic, margaric, stearic, linolenic, arachidic, gadoleic, behenic and erucic acid. Bitter almond oil contains benzaldehyde and 2–4% of hydrocyanic acid. Purified volatile oil of bitter almonds has all its hydrocyanic acid removed and, therefore, consists mainly of benzaldehyde. The unsaponifiable matter contains β-sitosterol, Δ^5-avenasterol, cholesterol, brassicasterol and tocopherols.

Uses

Expressed almond oil is an emollient and an ingredient in cosmetics. Almond oil is used as a laxative, emollient, in the preparation of toilet articles and as a vehicle for oily injections. The volatile almond oils are used as flavouring agents.

Marketed Products

It is one of the ingredients of the preparations known as Baidyanath lal tel (Baidyanath Company), Himcolin gel, Mentat, Tentex Royal (Himalaya Drug Company) and Sage badam roghan (Sage Herbals).

ARACHIS OIL

Synonyms

Groundnut oil, monkey nut oil, peanut oil, katchung oil, earth-nut oil.

Biological Source

Arachis oil is obtained by expression of shelled and skinned seeds of *Arachis hypogaea* Linn., belonging to family Papilionaceae (Fig. 19.2).

Geographical Source

South America (Brazil) is the original home of ground nut and now found in South and Central America, Peru, Argentina, Nigeria, Australia, India, Gambia and other reasonably warm regions of all countries.

Characteristics

Groundnut plant is a small, prostrate, diffuse, erect, branched, annual herb, 30–60 cm in height, leaves alternate with adnate stipules and yellow papilionaceous flowers. After fertilization, the pedicel elongates rapidly and enters the ground, where the ovary begins to develop into a pod maturing in about two months. Pods or nuts are cylindrical, hard, reticulated, indehiscent and inflated, 2.5–5.0 cm long, one to three seeded, with pericarp constricted between the seeds. The seeds are covered by a light or deep reddish brown seeds coat, and consisting of two white fleshy cotyledons rich in oil and proteins.

Fruits are dug out by raking the plants from the soil, seeds are separated by machine and expressed in a hydraulic press at ordinary temperature. The remaining oil of cakes is removed by solvent extraction. The two oil fractions are combined and purified.

Cultivation

Groundnut is predominantly a crop of the tropical and subtropical countries, up to an elevation of 1160 m. It requires plenty of sunlight, timely and evenly distributed rainfall (50–125 cm) during its growth and a long season for its maturation and harvesting. It also requires a high temperature (21–26°C) particularly during the nights to induce early flowering. The plant does not stand frost, long and severe drought and water stagnation. Groundnut seeds are sown from April–May to June–July. It requires light, well-drained, loose, friable soil. No regular manuring is done by the growers, and the plant is benefitted from green manuring.

Groundnut is susceptible to infection by several fungi, bacteria and viruses. Some important diseases in India are tikka leaf spot, collar rot, dry root rot, stem rot, rust, bud necrosis and yellow mould.

Groundnut oil is a nondrying oil belonging to the oleolinoleic acid group of oils. It is pale-yellow in colour or almost colourless liquid with a nutty odour and bland taste. Clouds are formed in the oil at low room temperature. It has acid value 0.08–6, saponification value 188–195, iodine value 84–102, thiocyanogen value 67–73 and hydroxyl value 2.5–9.5. It is very slowly thickens and becomes rancid on prolonged exposure to air. It is miscible with solvent ether, petroleum ether, chloroform, carbon disulphide, benzene and very slightly soluble in alcohol.

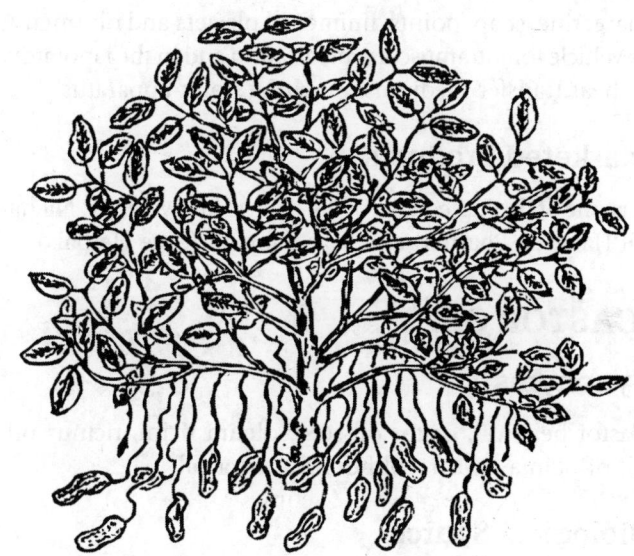

FIG. 19.2 *Arachis hypogaea*

Chemical Constituents

The important constituents of the glycerides of groundnut oil are the fatty acids palmitic (8.3%), stearic (3.1%), oleic (56%), linoleic (26%), arachidic (24%), eicosenoic, behenic (3.1%) and lignoceric (1.1%) acids. Myristic, hexacosanoic, erucic, caprylic, lauric and trace amounts of odd carbon fatty acids are also present. The principal glycerides of the oil are triolein (11%), dioleolinolein (21%), saturated oleolinoleins (22%), dilinoleoolein (12%), saturated diolein (15%) and saturated dilinoleoolein (6%).

The yellow colour of the oil is due to the presence of carotenoid pigments, chiefly β-carotene and lutein. The unsaponifiable matter consists of sterols, (campesterol, stigmasterol, β-sitosterol and cholesterol), sterol glycosides β-sitosterol-D-glycoside and others) and triterpenoid alcohols (β-amyrin, cycloartenol and 24-methylene cycloartenol). Tocopherols occur free in groundnut oil. Squalene, an unsaturated hydrocarbon, occurs in extremely small amounts in the unsaponifiable fraction. Two other unsaturated hydrocarbons, hypogene and arachidene, have also been reported.

The kernels contain fixed oil (40–50%), proteins (26.2%), water (1.8%), carbohydrates (20.6%), ash and high concentration of thiamine. The chief proteins are arachin and conarchin, both are globulins of different solubility. The vitamin content of groundnut is moderate, the largest being in the episperm.

Uses

Groundnut oil is used as an edible oil, in control of pasture bloat, as a substitute for olive oil, as a solvent in pharmaceutical aid, in hydrogenated state as shortening, in mayonnaise, in confections; for the manufacture of margarine, soap, points, liniments, plasters and ointments, as vehicle for intramuscular medication and in the laboratory as heat transfer medium in melting point apparatus.

Marketed Products

It is one of the ingredients of the hair oil known as J.P. Nikhar oil (Jamuna Pharma) and Sage baby oil (Sage Herbals).

CASTOR OIL

Synonyms

Castor bean oil, castor oil seed, oleum ricini, ricinus oil, oil of palma christi, cold-drawn castor oil.

Biological Source

Castor oil is the fixed oil obtained by cold expression of the seeds of *Ricinus communis* Linn., belonging to family Euphorbiaceae (Fig. 19.3).

Geographical Source

It is mainly found in India, Brazil, America, China, Thailand; in India it is cultivated in Gujarat, Andhra Pradesh and Karnataka.

Preparation

Castor oil is obtained from castor seeds. The oil is obtained by two ways; either after the removal of the seed coat or with the seed coat. Seed coats are removed by crushing the seeds under the grooved rollers and then they are subjected to a current of air to blow the testas. The kernels are fed in oil expellers and at room temperature they are expressed with 1–2 tons pressure per square inch till about 30% oil is obtained. The oil is filtered, steamed 80–100°C to facilitate the coagulation and precipitation of poisonous principle ricin, proteins and enzyme lipase present in it. Oil is then filtered and this oil with 1% acidity is used for medical purpose.

The oil cake which remains contains of ricin, lipase and about 20% oil. The cake is grounded, steamed to 40–80°C

and a pressure of 3 tons pressure per sq. inch is applied. This yields the second quality of oil with 5% acidity and is used for industrial purpose.

The residual cake which remains after the expression of the second quality oil still contains about 8–10% oil. This oil is obtained by subjecting it to extraction in soxhlet with lipid solvents. This oil obtained is also used in industry. The residual cake is used as manure and not fed to animal due to the presence of ricin. The cake is also used for the production of lipase.

Characteristics

Medicinal or the first grade or pale pressed castor oil is colourless or slightly yellow coloured. It is a viscid liquid which has slight odour with slightly acrid taste. Castor oil is soluble in absolute alcohol in all proportions; specific gravity is 0.958–0.969, refractive index at 40°C is 1.4695–1.4730, acid value not more than 2, saponification value 177–187 and acetyl value is about 150.

Chemical Constituents

Castor oil consists of glyceride of ricinoleic acid, isoricinoleic, stearic and dihydroxy stearic acids. Ricinoleic acid is responsible for laxative property. Castor oil also contains vitamin F. 90% of the fatty acid content is ricinoleic acid. The ricinoleic acid is an 18-carbon acid having a double bond in the 9–10 position and a hydroxyl group on the 12th carbon. This combination of hydroxyl group and unsaturation occurs only in castor oil.

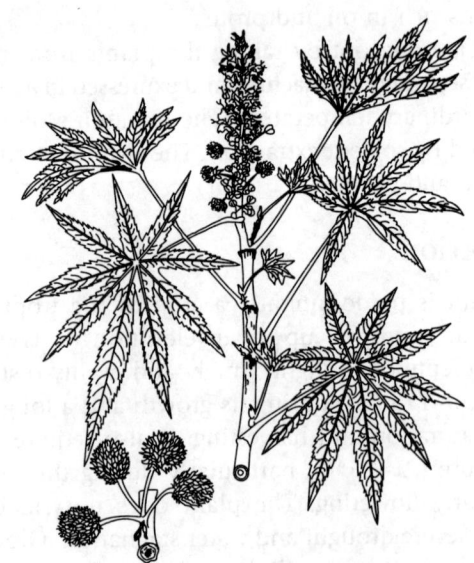

FIG. 19.3 *Ricinus communis*

Identification Tests

1. About 5 ml of light petroleum (50–60°C) when mixed with 10 ml of castor oil at 15.5°C shows a clear solution, but if the amount of light petroleum

is increased to 15 ml, the mixture becomes turbid. This test is not shown by other oils.

Uses

Castor oil is mild purgative, fungistatic, used as an ointment base, as plasticizer, wetting agents, as a lubricating agent. Ricinoleic acid is used in contraceptive creams and jellies; it is also used as an emollient in the preparation of lipsticks, in tooth formulation, as an ingredient in hair oil. The dehydrated oil is used in the manufacture of linoleum and alkyl resin. The main use of castor oil is the industrial production of coatings, also employed to make pharmaceuticals and cosmetics in the textile and leather industries and for manufacturing plastics and fibres.

Marketed Products

It is one of the ingredients of the preparations known as lip balm and muscle and joint rub (Himalaya Drug Company).

CHAULMOOGRA OIL

Synonyms

Hydnocarpus oil, gynocardia oil.

Biological Source

Chaulmoogra oil is the fixed oil obtained by cold expression from ripe seeds of *Taraktogenos kurzii* King, [syn. *Hydnocarpus kurzii* (King) Warb.], *Hydnocarpus wightiana* Blume, *H. anthelminticta* Pierre, *H. heterophylla* and other species of Hydnocarpus, belonging to family Flacourtiaceae (Fig. 19.4).

Geographical Source

The plants are tall trees, up to 17 m high, with narrow crown of hanging branches; native to Burma, Thailand, eastern India and Indo-China.

Characteristics

The oil is yellow or brownish yellow. Below 25°C it is a soft solid. It has peculiar odour and sharp taste. It is soluble in benzene, chloroform, ether, petrol; slightly soluble in cold alcohol; almost entirely soluble in hot alcohol and carbon disulphide.

Chemical Constituents

Chaulmoogra oil contains glycerides of cyclopentenyl fatty acids like hydnocarpic acid (48%), chaulmoogric acid (27%), gorlic acid with small amounts of glycerides of palmitic

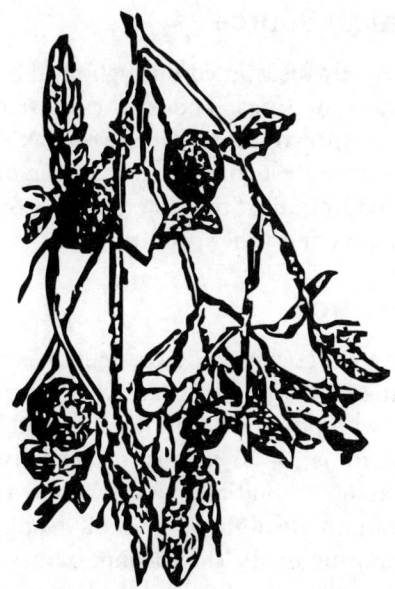

FIG. 19.4 *Hydnocarpus kurzii*

acid (6%) and oleic acid (12%). The cyclic acids are formed during last 3–4 months of maturation of the fruit and are strongly bactericidal towards the Micrococcus of leprosy.

The seeds of *H. wightiana* contain a flavonolignan hydnocarpin, isohydnocarpin, methoxy hydnocarpin, apigenin, luteolin, chrysoeriol, hydnowightin, epivolkenin and cyclopentenoid cyanohydrin glycosides.

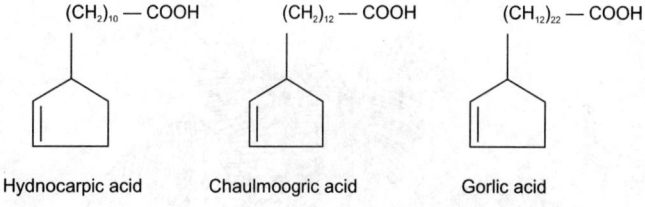

Hydnocarpic acid   Chaulmoogric acid   Gorlic acid

Uses

The oil is useful in leprosy and many other skin diseases. The cyclopentenyl fatty acids of the oil exhibit specific toxicity for *Mycobacterium leprae* and *M. tuberculosis*. The oil has now been replaced by the ethyl esters and salts of hydnocarpic and chaulmoogric acids. At present organic sulphones have replaced chaulmoogra oil in therapeutic use.

COCONUT OIL

Synonyms

Coconut oil, coconut butter, copra oil.

Biological Source

Coconut oil is the oil expressed from the dried solid part of endosperm of coconut, *Cocos nucifera* L., belonging to family Palmae (Fig. 19.5).

Geographical Source

Coconut is widely distributed throughout the world. It is largely cultivated in African and southeast Asian countries. Coconut also known as copra is a dietary as well as industrial product throughout the world. Large quantity of oil is produced in India, Sri Lanka Malaysia, South Africa, China, Indonesia and other countries.

Characteristics

In temperate region below 23°C coconut oil is concrete oil. Coconut butter is a white or pearl white unctuous mass, odourless or with peculiar coconut odour and bland taste. Its melting point is 23–26°C. It is soluble in two volumes of alcohol at 60°C but highly soluble in chloroform, ether and carbon disulphide. The oil readily becomes rancid on exposure to air. The coconut oil has the highest saponification value, 250–264 and the lowest iodine value, 7–10 among the vegetable oils in common use.

Chemical Composition

Coconut obtained from the hard, dried endocarp consists of a mixture of triglycerides of saturated fatty acids. The oil contains about 95% of saturated fatty acids with 8 and 10 carbon atoms. It shows the presence of caprylic acid, 2%; capric acid, 50–80%; lauric acid, 3%; and myristic acid about 1%.

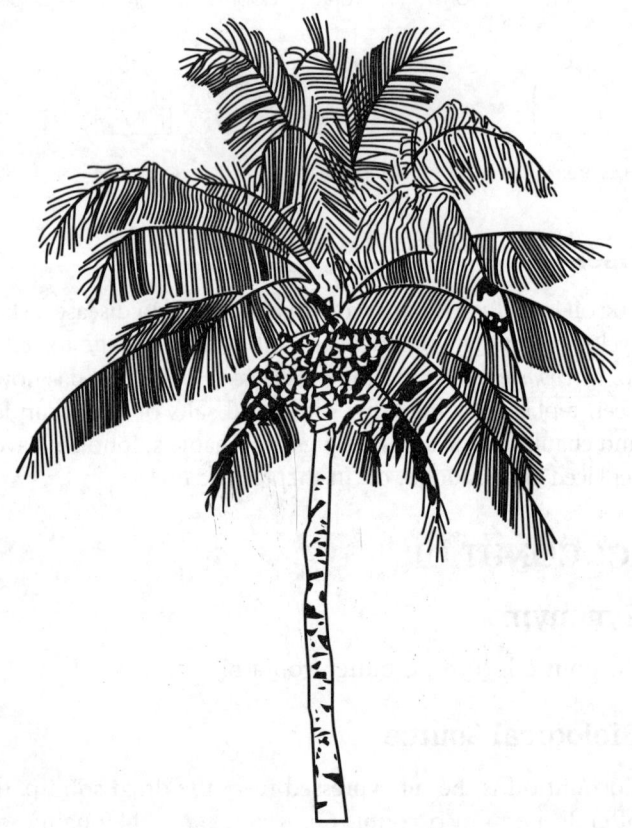

FIG. 19.5 Coconut tree

Uses

Coconut oil is used as dietary products in many areas of the world. In European pharmacopoeia, fractionated coconut oil is known as 'thin vegetable oil'. It is useful as a nonaqueous medium for the oral administration of some medicaments. Fractionated coconut oil is used as a basis for the preparation of oral suspension of drugs unstable in aqueous media. Diets based on medium chain triglycerides including preparations made from coconut oil are used in conditions associated with mal absorption of fat such as cystic fibrosis, enteritis and steatorrhoea. Abdominal pain and diarrhoea have been reported in patients taking diet based on medium chain triglycerides.

Marketed Products

It is one of the ingredients of the preparations known as Lip balm and Evecare (Himalaya Drug Company).

COD LIVER OIL

Biological Source

It is processed from fresh liver of cod fish, *Gadus morrhua* and other species of Gadus, belonging to family Gadidae (Fig. 19.6).

Geographical Source

It is mainly found in Scotland, Norway, Germany, Iceland and Denmark.

Preparation

The liver is cleaned and minced into small pieces and heated to 80°C in a vat by admitting steam for half an hour. The enzyme lipase is destroyed at temperature above 70°C. The oil is removed and put in tin drums which are encased with wooden barrels. The barrels are kept inside the snow and the oil is cooled to –2 to –5°C, the slow cooling process precipitates the palmitin, which is separated by filtration. The oil obtained is medicinal oil. The residual cake formed after the medicinal oil is subjected to heating at higher temperature to obtain oil with inferior quality and brown colour.

Characteristics

The oil is pale yellow in colour; it has fishy odour and taste. Cod liver oil is slightly soluble in alcohol and fully soluble in chloroform, ether, carbon disulphide and petroleum ether. Specific gravity: 0.922–0.929, refractive index: 1.475–1.4745, acid value is less than 2, iodine value 155–173. The oil should be stored in well-filled airtight containers, protected from light and kept in a cool place.

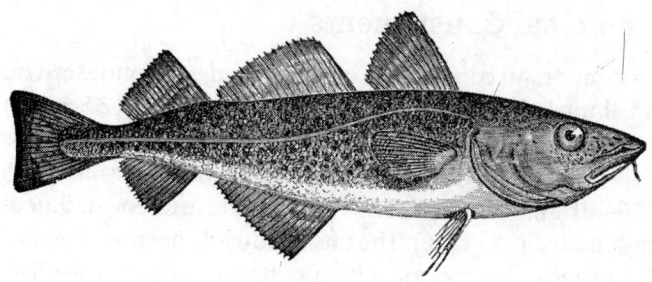

FIG. 19.6 Cod fish (*Gadus morrhua*)

Chemical Constituents

The cod liver oil contains glycerides esters of saturated acids of linoleic, oleic, myristic, gadoleic, palmitic and other acids. The oil has vitamin A and vitamin D. Cod liver oil also contains about 1% unsaponifiable matter; like cholesterol, fatty alcohol, squalene, α-glyceryl esters, etc.

Vitamin D3

Uses

Oil is used as source of vitamins, in treatment of rickets, tuberculosis and also as a nutritive.

CORN OIL

Synonyms

Corn oil, maize oil.

Biological Source

Corn oil is a fixed oil obtained by expression of the embryos of *Zea mays* L., belonging to family Graminae (Fig. 19.7).

Geographical Source

Corn is cultivated throughout the world. The major producers of corn are United States, Canada, Russia, Argentina, Brazil, France, Mexico, Thailand and India. Corn oil is generally obtained as a by-product during the production of maize starch from the maize germs. The

French pharmacopoeia specifies that the corn oil should be obtained from the germs or caryopsis which remains after the removal of major part of the cotyledon.

Characteristics

Refined corn oil is a clear to light golden yellow coloured liquid with a faint characteristic odour and taste. It is slightly soluble in alcohol, miscible with chloroform, ether and light petroleum. Weight per ml is 0.915–0.923 g. It can be sterilized by maintaining at 150°C for 1 hr and stored in a cool place in well-filled airtight containers protected from light. Acid value is 2–6, saponification value is 187–96 and iodine value is 100–133.

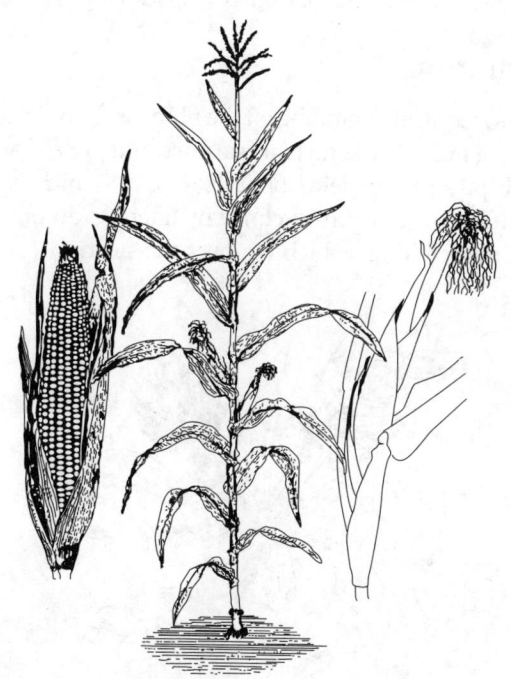

FIG. 19.7 *Zea mays*

Chemical Constituents

Dried corn embryo yields around 20% of fixed oil. The fatty acid composition of the corn oil indicates the presence of palmitic, 8–13%; stearic, 1–4.5%; oleic, 24–33%; linoleic 55–62%; linolenic 0.5–1.5% about 0.5% of arachidic, gadoleic and behenic acids. It shows the presence of about 0.8–2% of unsaponifiable matter containing major proportion of β-sitosterol and campesterol.

Uses

Maize oil shows the properties similar to those of olive oil. As the oil consists of higher contents of unsaturated acids, it is regarded as of value in diets designed to limit blood cholesterol level in patients with hypercholesterolemia, particularly following cardiac infarction. The oil has also indicated good results in the patients with coronary heart disease and diabetes. It is used in place of other vegetable oils, in pharmaceuticals and cosmetic preparations.

Marketed Products

Esoban ointment containing maize oil is used for dermatitis and allergic skin conditions.

COTTONSEED OIL

Biological Source

Cottonseed oil is a refined fixed oil obtained by expression of seeds of *Gossypium herbaceum* Linn, belonging to family Malvaceae, in hydraulic or other presses (Fig. 19.8).

Preparation

The cottonseed, after ginning off the fibres, is decorticated and cleaned of hulls. The kernels are steamed and pressed at about 1500 lb pressure to yield about 30% of oil which is turbid and reddish in colour. It is refined by filtering, decolourizing and 'winter chilling', which removes the stearin.

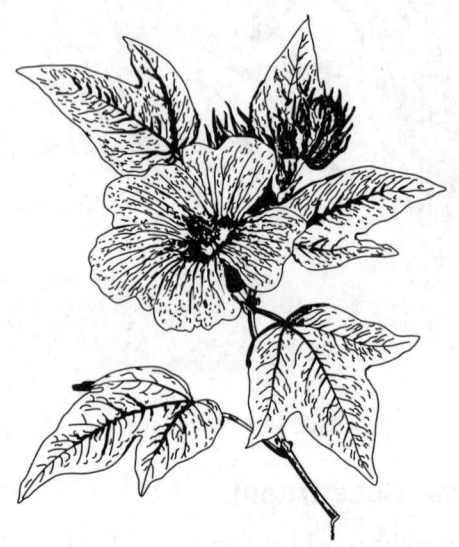

FIG. 19.8 *Gossypium herbaceum*

Characteristics

The crude oil is amber to deep red or black in colour with a characteristic odour, sp. gr. 0.92, saponification value 192–200, iodine value 100–115 and unsaponifiable matter 0.6–2.0%. Refined cottonseed oil is pale yellow in colour with a bland nutty taste and nearly odourless. The oil is a semidrying substance. On cooling a sediment of olein or liquid glycerides separates out which may be collected by the filtration in the cooled condition. When used to adulterate other oils its presence may be detected by the test for semidrying. Cottonseed oil is graded on the basis of its acidity; refining loses flavour. Refined oil is graded according to the colour, odour and flavour.

Chemical Constituents

The important constituents of the glycerides of cottonseed oil are linoleic (45–50%), oleic (23–29%), palmitic (20–33%), myristic (1.5–3.5%), stearic (1.1–2.7%) and arachidic acids (1.0%). The glycerides present are palmito-oleolinoleins (35–40%), palmitodioleins (20%) and trioleo- or lineodisaturated (12–13%). The unsaponifiable fraction contains β-sitosterol, ergosterol, vitamin E and tocopherols. The phosphatides present are lecithin (29%) and cephalins (71%). The minor constituents present in the oil are free fatty acids (0.3–5.6%), gossypol (0.05%), raffinose, pentosans, resins, wax, proteoses, peptones, phospholipids, inosite phosphates, phytosteroline, xanthophyll, chlorophyll and mucilage substances.

Cottonseed cake contains about 0.6% of a toxic principle, gossypol, which occurs in secretory cavities in all parts of the plant. It is present in cold-pressed oil and can be removed by treatment with alkalies.

Gossypol

Uses

Cottonseed oil is used as a solvent for injections and for edible purposes. The oil possesses emollient properties and is used in liniments, in several pharmaceutical preparations, as a substitute of olive oil and in large doses as lubricant cathartic. Low-grade oil is used in the manufacture of soaps, lubricants, sulphonated oils and protective coatings.

Marketed Products

It is one of the ingredients of the preparation known as J.P. Massaj oil (Jamuna Pharma).

LINSEED OIL

Synonyms

Flax seed, alsi (Hindi).

Biological Source

Linseed is the dried, ripe seed of *Linum usitatissimum* Linn. Linseed oil is obtained by expression of linseeds, belonging to family Linaceae.

Geographical Source

Linseed is cultivated in many subtropical countries such as South America, India, United States, Canada, England, Russia, Greece, Italy, Spain and Algeria.

Collection

Linseed in an erect annual herb, 60–120 cm high with sky-blue flowers and a globular capsule. The plant is cultivated for its seeds and fibre (flax). A moderate rainfall is best suited for its growth. It grows in almost all types of soils where sufficient moisture is available, but thrives best in heavy soils with high moisture retaining capacity. As a mixed crop it is sown either on the margins of fields or in rows alternating with the other crop. Nitrogenous fertilizers yield better crop. The crop is harvested in February and March before the capsules are dried. Plants are cut close to the ground, dried in the field and threshed to separate seeds.

Morphology of Seeds (Fig. 19.9a and b)

The seeds are oval, flattened, elongated, 4–6 mm long and 2–3 mm wide. Testa is glossy, smooth, reddish-brown with minutely pitted surface. Seeds are rounded at one end. The other end is obliquely pointed where the hilum and micropyle are present in a slight depression. Raphe is present along one edge. Endosperm is narrow and encircles the embryo. It consists of two thick flattened, plano-convex cotyledons and a radicle. The seeds art odourless but possess an oily and mucilaginous taste.

Microscopical Characters (Figs. 19.10 and 19.11)

Under microscope the testa shows a mucilage-containing outer epidermis; one or two layers of collenchyma or 'round cells'; a single layer of sclerenchyma; the hyaline layers or 'cross-cells' composed in the ripe seed of obliterated parenchymatous cells; and an innermost layer of pigment cells. The outer epidermis is composed of cells, rectangular or five-sided in surface view, which swell up in water and become mucilaginous. The outer cell walls, when swollen in water, show an outer solid stratified layer. The radial layers or 'round cells' are cylindrical in shape and show distinct triangular intercellular air spaces. The sclerenchymatous layer is composed of elongated cells, up to 250 μm in length, with lignified pitted walls. The hyaline layers are attached to portions of the sclerenchymatous layer in the powdered drug. The pigment layer is composed of cells with thickened pitted walls and containing amorphous reddish-brown contents. The cells of the endosperm and cotyledons are polygonal with thickened walls, and contain numerous aleurone grains and globules of fixed oil.

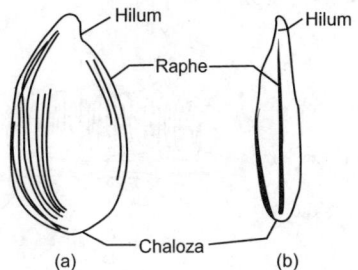

FIG. 19.9 (a) External surface of seed and (b) lateral view of seed

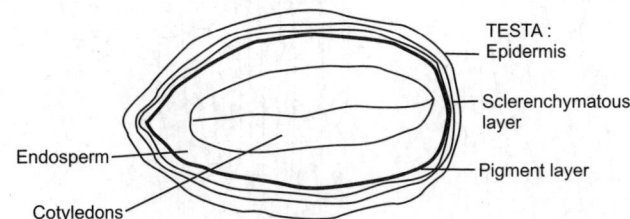

FIG. 19.10 T.S. (schematic) of seed

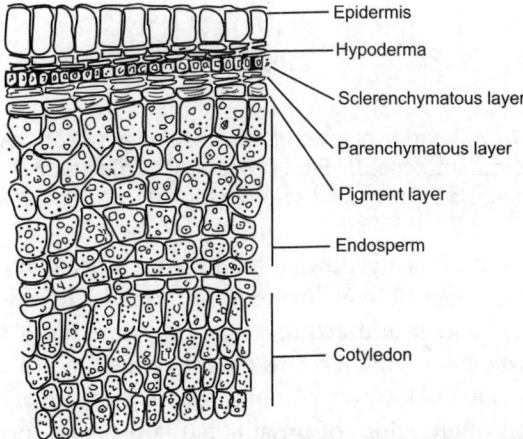

FIG. 19.11 Transverse section of linseed seed

Powder Microscopy (Fig. 19.12)

The powder is yellowish-brown in colour with darker brown fragments. Microscopical examination shows pigment cells of testa, with thick, pitted walls, in groups or isolated masses. Longitudinally elongated cells of sclerenchyma with lignified pitted walls are composed of both thin-walled and thick-walled cells. Part of testa in sectional view shows hypodermal cells, nearly rounded with slightly thickened walls. Hyaline layer is attached to sclerenchyma and pigment layer.

Preparation

The dried seeds are crushed in rollers, moistened and heated to 80–90°C in steam to soften the seed tissues. They are then pressed through hot hydraulic press at a high pressure. The oil so obtained is treated with alkali to separate free fatty acids and bleached with fuller's earth or charcoal. On cooling the oil waxy substances are removed.

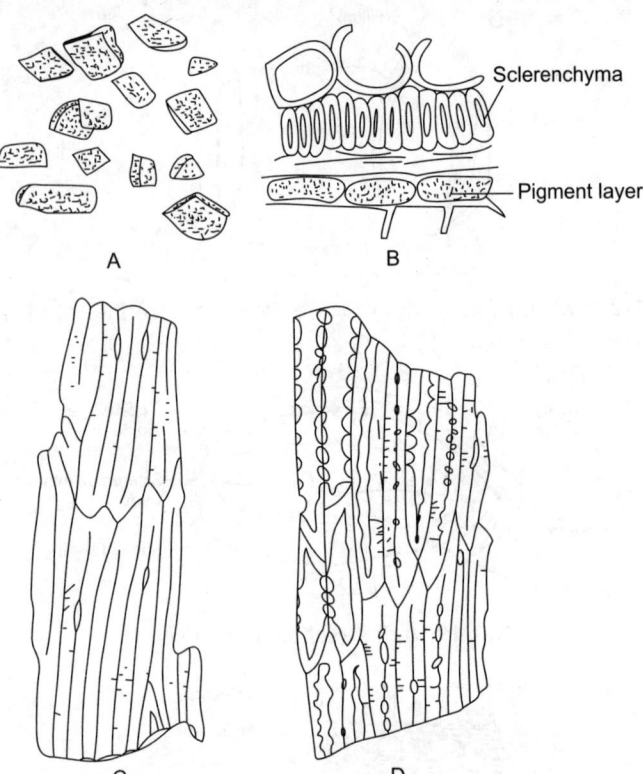

FIG. 19.12 Powder characteristics of linseed seed. (A: Isolated pigment cells, B: Part of testa, C: Thick-walled sclerenchyma, D: Thin-walled sclerenchyma)

Linseed oil is a yellowish liquid, with a peculiar odour and bland taste. On exposure to air it gradually thickens, becomes darker and acquires a more pronounced odour and taste. On drying it forms a hard varnish. It has a high iodine value (~170) which indicates the presence of excess amount of glycerides of unsaturated fatty acids. The oil is slightly soluble in alcohol, miscible with chloroform, ether, petroleum ether, carbon disulphide and turpentine oil. It has density 0.925–0.935, viscosity 1.47, congealing point ~20°C, saponification number 187–195, refractive index 1.47–1.48 and unsaponifiable matters not over 1.5%. A water-soluble resinous matter with antioxidant properties has been isolated from the oil.

Chemical Constituents

Linseed contains fixed oil (30–40%), mucilage (6–10%), protein (25%) (linin and colinin), small amount of enzyme lipase and linamarin which is a cyanogenic glycoside. The carbohydrates present are sucrose, raffinose, cellulose and mucilage. Linamarin is a glucose either of acetone cyanohydrin and is identical to phaseolunatin. Unripe seeds contain starch which is converted to mucilage on ripening the seeds. The mucilage can be fractionated into a neutral fraction a remified, arabinoxylan composed of D-xylose, L-arabinose, D-glucose and D-galactose; and an acidic fraction mainly composed of L-rhamnose and D-galactose. Mucilage

swells with water and forms red colour with ruthenium red. Linamarin on hydrolysis yields acetone, hydrocyanic acid and glucose. The other constituents are phytin, lecithin, wax, resin, pigments, malic acid, cyanogenic glycosides, linustatin, neolinustatin, and secoisolariciresinol and phenylpropanoid glucoside linusitamarin.

On hydrolysis, linseed oil produces unsaturated acids like linolenic acid (30–50%), linoleic acid (23–24%), oleic acid (10–18%) together with saturated acids-myristic, stearic and palmitic (5–11%).

Uses

Linseed is used as demulcent and in form of poultices for gouty and rheumatic swellings. Internally it is used for gonorrhoea and irritation of the genitourinary system. Linseed oil has emollient, expectorant, diuretic, demulcent, and laxative properties and is utilized externally in lotions and liniments. Nonstaining iodine ointment soap, linoleum, greases, polishes, polymers, varnishes, paints, putty, oil cloths, printing inks, artificial rubber, tracing cloth, tanning and enamelling leather, etc., are also prepared from linseed oil.

The mucilaginous infusion is used internally as a demulcent in colds, coughs, bronchial affections, inflammation of the urinary tract, gonorrhoea and diarrhoea.

Adulterants

When market price is high, linseed oil is adulterated with vegetable oils, such as rape, cottonseed, soya bean, sunflower, safflower and candlenut, as well as with rosin and mineral and fish oils. Boiled linseed oil is more frequently adulterated than raw oil.

Admixture of rape and mustard oils may be detected by the presence of erucic acid; the adulterants lower the saponification value. Fish oil may be detected by the odour produced on heating and by melting points of ether insoluble bromides. Rosin and mineral oils increase the proportion of unsaponifiable matter.

Marketed Products

It is one of the ingredients of the preparations known as Canisep and Scavon (Himalaya Drug Company).

MUSTARD OIL

Synonyms

Sarson ka tel.

Biological Source

It is a fixed oil obtained from matured seeds of *Brassica nigra* (L) Koch or *Brassica juncea* L. Czern, belonging to family Cruciferae (Brassicaceae) (Fig. 19.13).

Geographical Source

It is cultivated in India, China, Canada and England.

Description

It is yellow coloured liquid of strong acrid odour until refined, sp. gr. 0.914–0.923, saponification value 173–184, iodine value 96–194 and unsaponifiable matter 0.9–1.0%.

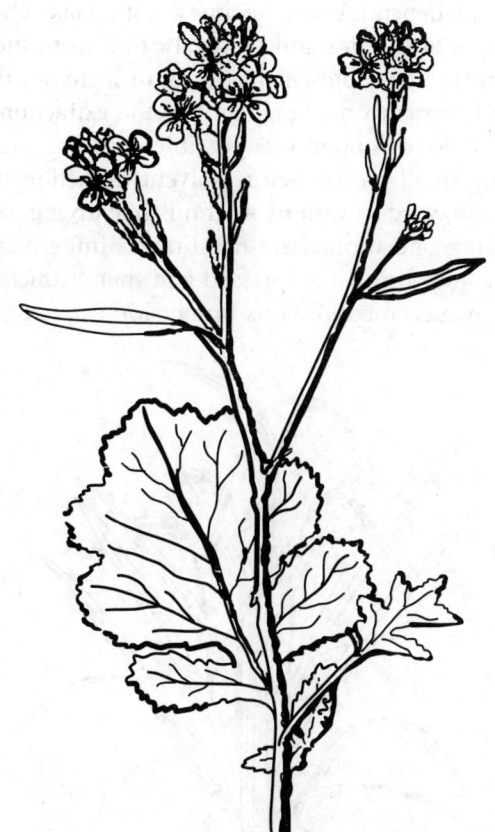

FIG. 19.13 *Brassica nigra*

Chemical Constituents

Mustard oil contains glycerides of arachidic (0.5%), behenic (2–3%), eicosenoic (7–8%), erucic (40–60%), lignoceric (1–2%), linoleic (14–18%), linolenic (6.5–7.0%), oleic (20–22%) and myristic (0.5–10%) acids.

Black mustard seeds contain 35–40% of fixed oil and a glycoside known as sinigrin along with an enzyme myrosin. Allyl isothiocyanate is responsible for the strong acrid smell of volatile oil of mustard produced on hydrolysis of glycoside.

Uses

Fixed oil is used as edible oil after refining, but medicinal properties are due to allyl isothiocyanate, which is a local irritant and emetic. If applied externally, it is rubefacient and vesicant. It is also used as condiment and in manufacture of soap. Refined mustard oil is used in vegetable ghee.

Marketed Products

Dabur mustard oil is the one of the purest mustard oil that has a variety of uses. It is also one of the ingredients of the preparation known as Saaf Organic Eraser Body Oil.

OLIVE OIL

Synonyms

Salad oil, sweet oil, oleum olivae.

Biological Source

Olive oil is a fixed oil obtained by expression of the ripe fruits of *Olea europaea* Linn. or Indian olive (*O. ferruginea*), belonging to family Oleaceae (Fig. 19.14).

Geographical Source

Olive is a native of Palestine and produced extensively in the countries adjoining the Mediterranean Sea. Spain being the largest producer. It is also grown in the south western United States and many other subtropical localities.

Collection and Preparation

The olive is an evergreen tree, up to 12 m in height which produces drupaceous fruits about 2–3 cm in length, purplish in colour when ripe. The fruits are collected from November to April. After grinding, the pulp is introduced into coarse, grass baskets and placed in a screw press. The oil coming out is collected into tubes containing water and the upper layer is skimmed off. The product is called as Virgin oil obtained by gently pressing the peeled pulp freed from the endocarp. The marc is then treated with water and again expressed to yield second grade of edible oil. Finally, the pulp is mixed with hot water and pressed again for technical oil. The pulp may be extracted with carbon disulphide to obtain 'sulphur' olive oil of inferior quality. The yield is from 15 to 40%. If the fruit is not fully mature, the yield of the oil is poor and its taste is bitter.

Characteristics

Olive oil is a pale yellow or light greenish-yellow due to presence of chlorophyll or carotenes, nondrying oily liquid with a pleasanting delicate flavour. Taste is bland becoming cloudy and at 0°C it usually forms a whitish granular mass. It becomes faintly acrid. It is miscible with ether, chloroform and carbon disulphide, and is slightly soluble in alcohol. Upon cooling at +5 to 10°, it becomes cloudy and at 0°C usually forms a whitish granular mass. It becomes rancid on exposure to air. It has specific gravity of 0.914–0.919, acid value 0.2–2.8, saponification value 187–196 and iodine value 79–90.

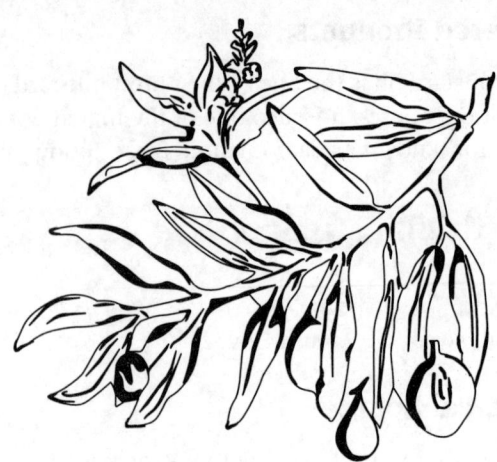

FIG. 19.14 *Olea europaea*

Chemical Constituents

Olive oil contains mixed glycerides of oleic acid (56–85%), palmitic (7–20%), linoleic (3–20%), stearic (1–5%), arachidic (0.9%), palmitoleic (3%), linolenic, eicosenoic, gadoleic and lignoceric acids. The minor constituents are squalene up to 0.7%, phytosterol and tocopherols about 0.2%. Italy–Spain type olive oil is higher in oleic acid and Greece–Tunisia type oil has higher levels of linoleic acid.

Identification Tests

Under UV radiation it gives deep golden-yellow colour, while refined oil gives pale blue fluorescence. Decolourization with charcoal removes fluorescence.

Uses

Olive oil is used in the manufacture of pharmaceutical preparations, soaps, textile lubricants, sulphonated oils, liniments, cosmetics, plasters; as food in salads; and for cooking and baking. It has demulcent, emollient, choleretic or cholagogue and laxative properties. It is a good solvent for parenteral preparations.

Marketed Products

It is one of the ingredients of the preparation known as Figaro oil.

RICE BRAN OIL

Synonym

Rice oil.

Biological Source

Rice bran oil is the oil obtained from the rice bran of the seeds of *Oryza sativa* Linn., belonging to family Graminae (Fig. 19.15).

Preparation

Rice bran is the cuticle present between the rice and the husk of the paddy; consists of embryo and endosperm of the seeds. Rice bran is the by product in rice mill during dehusking of paddy. Rice bran has 15% of fixed oil and the oil is obtained by solvent extraction method. The rice bran oil obtained from fresh brans are of good quality and has good taste and low free fatty acid content. The quality of rice bran oil depends upon the time duration taken between the milling of the rice and removal of oil from the bran. The enzyme lipase present in rice bran increases the free fatty acid content on storage and so the extraction of oil should be done as rapidly as possible. Rice bran occurs as extremely small pieces. Before solvent extraction the rice bran is subjected to various methods like drying, cooking and flaking operations. The rice bran is impermeable to solvents, and so it is first pressed and then extracted with solvent in special continuous immersion extractors.

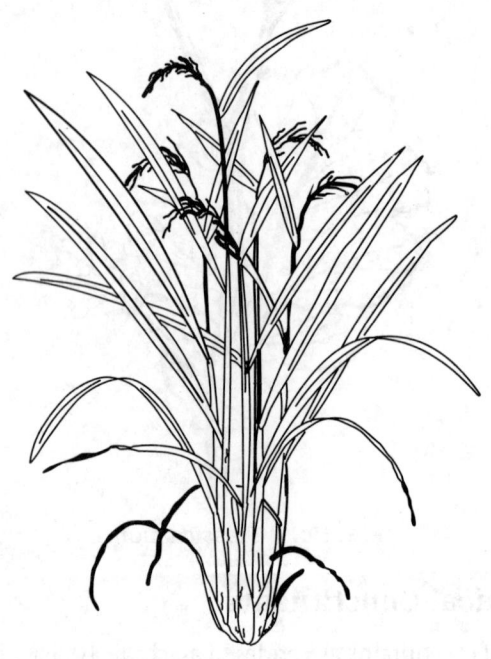

FIG. 19.15 *Oryza sativa*

Characteristics

It is a golden yellow oil, insoluble in water but soluble in common fat solvents and is not affected till heating to 160°C. Specific gravity of 0.916–0.921, iodine value: 99–108, acid value is 04–05, refractive index: 1.470–1.473, and saponification value: 181–189.

Chemical Constituents

Rice bran oil contains both saturated and unsaturated fatty acids. It has 80–85% of unsaturated and 20–25% of saturated fatty acids as glycerides. The chief fatty acids are oleic acid constituting to 40–50%, linoleic acid constituting to 30–40% and palmitic acids which constitutes 12–18%. It is rich in gamma-oryzanol, which will protect and replenish your skin. Rice bran oil also contains squalene and antioxidants like tocopherols.

Uses

It is used as antioxidants, as emollient, used in the manufacture of cosmetics and even as edible oil and in preparation of vegetable ghee. It is a powerful skin protectant. Rice bran oil can be an effective substitute for lanolin. Rice bran oil is used in formulations where softening and moisturizing properties are needed. It is good for mature, delicate or sensitive skin. Rice bran oil is especially good for face and hair formulations or baby formulations.

Marketed Products

It is one of the ingredients of the preparation known as Rice bran scrub.

SAFFLOWER OIL

Biological Source

It is a fixed oil obtained from the ripe and dry seeds of *Carthamus tinctorius* Linn., belonging to family Compositae (Fig. 19.16).

Geographical Source

This is one of the most ancient crops cultivated in Egypt as a dye-yielding herb. Now, it is cultivated as an oil seed plant and regarded as substitute for sunflower. It is cultivated in Russia, Mexico, India, United States, Ethiopia and Australia.

Method of Preparation

For expression of oil, the seeds from promising varieties in India are selected, cleaned and further processed. About 1000 seeds of safflower weigh 20–50 g. The seeds normally contain 35–38% of fixed oil. The oil is prepared by expression in expellers or with the help of hydraulic presses. The oil is filtered and further purified. The seed meal or round seeds are subjected to cooking by means of open steam, which ensures maximum yield of oil. The filtered and decolourized oil is packed into suitable containers.

Characteristics

It is a clear, faint yellowish liquid with characteristic odour and taste. The oil thickens and becomes rancid on exposure to air. Safflower oil is slightly soluble in alcohol and freely soluble in ether, chloroform, benzene and petroleum ether.

Specific gravity 0.9211–0.9215, acid value 01–9, refractive index 1.472–1.475 and saponifiction value 188–194.

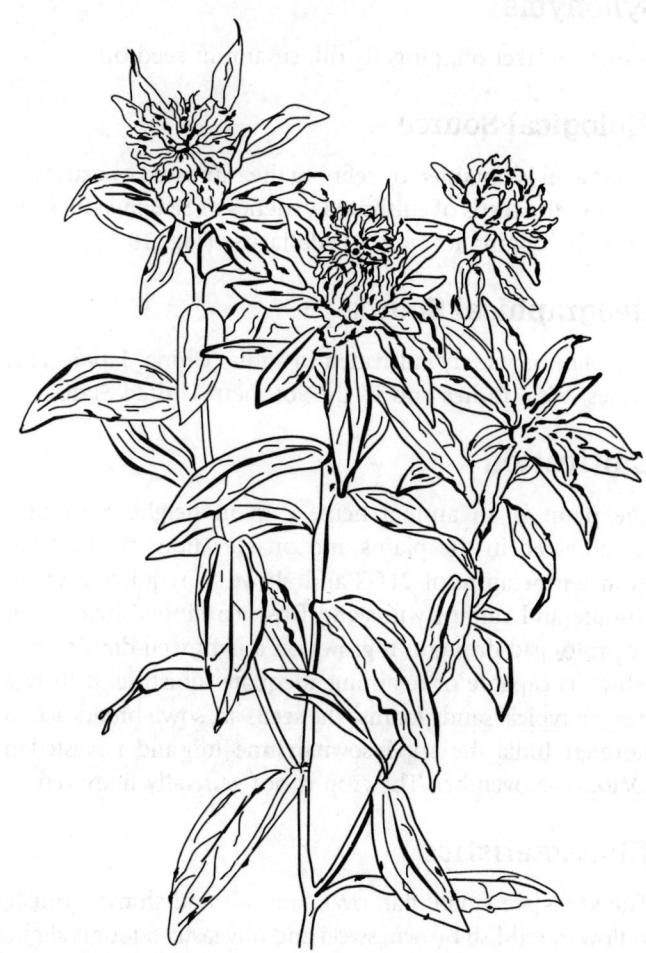

FIG. 19.16 *Carthamus tinctorius*

Chemical Constituents

Safflower oil contains glycerides of palmitic (6.5%), stearic (3.0%), arachidic (0.296%), oleic (13%), linoleic (76–79%) and linolenic acids (90.15%). The polyunsaturated fatty acid content of the oil is highest (75%) and is said to be responsible to control cholesterol level in the blood, and thereby, reduces incidence of heart attacks.

Uses

The edible oil is used in the manufacture of oleomargarine, as a dietary supplement in hypercholesterolemia and also in treatment of atherosclerosis. Due to its high linoleic acid content, it is consumed for preparation of vegetable ghee. Industrially, it is used for preparation of soft-soap varnishes, linoleum and water-proofing material.

Marketed Products

It is one of the ingredients of the preparation known as Saaf Organic Eraser Body Oil.

SESAME OIL

Synonyms

Benne oil, teel oil, gingelly oil, sesamum seed oil.

Biological Source

Sesame oil is obtained by refining the expressed or extracted oil from the seeds of cultivated varieties of *Sesamum indicum* Linn., belonging to family Pedaliaceae (Fig. 19.17).

Geographical Source

The plant is widely cultivated in India, China, Japan, East Indies, West Indies and in the southern United States.

Cultivation

The plant is an annual herb, 1 m in height. Sesamum is cultivated in the plains and on elevations up to 1200 m at temperature of 21°C and above. It requires a warm climate and cannot withstand frost, continued heavy rain or prolonged drought. It grows on a light well-drained soil which is capable of retaining adequate moisture. It thrives best on typical sandy loams. The seeds are sown broadcast. In northern India, the crop is sown in June–July and harvested in October–November. The crop is not generally manured.

Characteristics

The seeds are small, flat, oval, smooth and shiny; whitish, yellow or reddish brown; sweet and oily taste; odour is slight. They are pointed at one end where hilum is located, raphe runs as a line from hilum, along the centre of one flat face to the broader end. The endosperm is present as a thin layer around the embryo. The seeds contain fixed oil (45–55%), proteins (aleurone, 22%) and mucilage (4%).

Preparation

The oil is expressed by hydraulic or low and medium-powered screw presses. A good yield of the oil is obtained by three successive expression. Prior to processing in the screw press, the seed is subjected to a cooking process. If

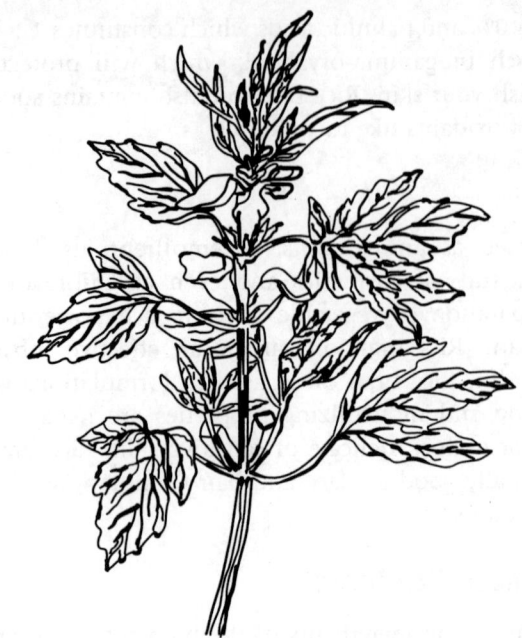

FIG. 19.17 *Sesamum indicum*

live steam is used for cooking, the cuticles separate partly from the kernels and the mixture of kernels, cuticles and seed slips in the cage and lumpy material is obtained instead of a firm cake. If the seed is heated in cooker without the addition of steam or water, and water is added at the point of entry of dried seed into the screw press cage, the efficiency of oil extraction is greatly enhanced. Alkali refining, bleaching, hydrogenation and decolourization of sesame oil can be affected with very little loss.

The sesame oil (40–50%) is pale yellow liquid, almost odourless, bland taste, saponification number 188–193, iodine number 103–122, soluble in chloroform, solvent and petroleum ethers, carbon disulphide; slightly soluble in alcohol and insoluble in water.

Chemical Constituents

Sesame oil consists of a mixture of glycerides of oleic (43%), linoleic (43%), palmitic (9%), stearic (4%), arachidic, hexadecenoic, lignoceric and myristic acids. It also contains the lignan sesamin (1%), the related sesamolin and vitamins A and E. During industrial refining, sesemolin is

Sesamin

Sesamolin

readily converted into antioxidant phenols sesamol and sesamolinol.

The seeds also contain a lignan sesamolinol, γ-tocopherol, sesaminol, pinoresmol, its glycosides, sesaminol glucosides VI, VII and VIII, triglucoside KP3, carbohydrates (20%), proteins (20–25%), sterols (campesterol, stigmasterol, β-sitosterol and Δ^5-avenasterol), γ- and δ-tocopherols.

Chemical Tests

1. *Baudouin Test:* Sesamol forms pink colour when the oil (2 ml) is shaken with concentrated hydrochloric acid (1 ml) containing 1% sucrose.
2. *Villavecchia Test:* Furfural may be used in place of sucrose and this modified test is widely used to detect Sesame oil in other oils and fats. The presence of sesamolin or free sesamol is responsible for this colour which is not found in other vegetable oils.

Uses

Sesame oil is used as demulcent, in dysentery and urinary complaints, as a solvent for injection of steroids, antibiotics and hormones, as mild laxative, nutritive, emollient, in manufacture of oleomargarine, cosmetics, iodized oil, antiacids and ointment. It is injectable as a vehicle for fat soluble substances. The oil is also used in insecticidal sprays. Sesamolin, present in the unsaponifiable fraction of the oil, is an effective synergist for pyrethrum insecticides. An extract enriched in lignans as an antioxidant and radical scavenger is used in cosmetic industry.

Marketed Products

It is one of the ingredients of the preparations known as Saaf Organic Eraser Body Oil and Dabur Lal tel (Dabur).

SHARK LIVER OIL

Synonyms

Oleum selachoide.

Biological Source

Shark liver oil is the fixed oil obtained from the fresh and healthy livers of shark fish *Hypoprion brevirostris*, belonging to family Carcharhinidae (Fig. 19.18).

Geographical Source

Shark is found on seacoasts of many European countries and in India in Tamil Nadu, Maharashtra and Kerala.

Preparation

Livers are removed from the fish, cleaned thoroughly, freed from fatty substances and attached tissues like gallbladders. Then the livers are heated in water at about 80°C. The oil exudes, floats on the top, and is separated, washed and water is removed. The dehydrated oil is cooled to separate stearin. The suspended materials are removed by centrifugation. The oil is supplemented with vitamins A and D in desired amount.

Characteristics

Shark liver oil is pale yellow to brownish yellow, viscous liquid with fishy odour and bland taste. It is insoluble in water, sparingly soluble in alcohol and freely miscible in nonpolar solvents such as petroleum ether, chloroform and benzene. Its acid value is about 2, saponification value 150–200 and iodine value 160–350.

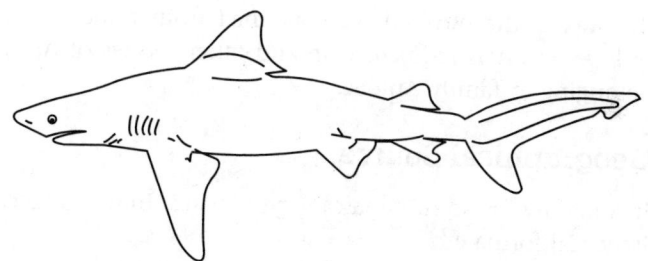

FIG. 19.18 Shark fish *Hypoprion brevirostris*

Chemical Constituents

The active principle of Shark liver oil is vitamin A which varies from 15,000 to 30,000 I.U. per g of the oil. It contains glycerides of saturated and unsaturated fatty acids.

Vitamin A

Chemical Tests

1. A solution of shark liver oil (1 drop) in chloroform (1 ml) is treated with sulphuric acid (1 drop). A violet colour changing to purple or brown is formed due to the presence of vitamin A.
2. Shark liver oil (1 ml) is dissolved in chloroform (10 ml). Few drops of saturated solution of antimony trichloride in chloroform are added to the solution. A blue colour is formed due to the presence of vitamin A.

Uses

Shark liver oil is used to treat xerophthalmia (abnormal dryness of the surface of conjunctiva) occurring due to deficiency of vitamin A. The oil is nutritive and used as a tonic.

Marketed Products

It is one of the ingredients of the preparation known as Shark liver oil softgels (Now Foods).

BEESWAX

Synonyms

White beeswax, yellow beeswax, cera alba and cera flava.

Biological Source

Beeswax is the purified wax obtained from honeycomb of hive bee, *Apis mellifera* Linn and other species of Apis, belonging to family Apidae.

Geographical Source

It is mainly found in Jamaica, Egypt, Africa, India, France, Italy, California etc.

Preparation

The worker bee secretes the wax due to the ability of maintaining a high temperature and the wax is secreted in the last four segments of abdomen on the ventral surface. Just below the sterna it has a smooth layer of cells form the chitinous area that secretes the wax. The chitinous area has small pores through, which the wax exudes out. The wax is passed to the front leg and later to the mouth; in the mouth it gets mixed with the saliva, which is then built on the comb. This wax forms a capping on the honey cells. Wax forms about 1/8th part of the honeycomb. After removal of honey, honeycomb or the capping is melted in boiling water. On cooling the melted wax gets solidified and floats on the surface of water while the impurities settle below and honey leftovers get dissolved in water. The pure wax is then poured into earthen vessels wiped with damp cloth and the wax so obtained is yellow beeswax.

White beeswax is obtained from yellow beeswax. The yellow beeswax is runned on a thin stream of spinning wet drum, from which long ribbon like strips are scrapped off. The ribbon strips are placed on cloth in thin layers, rotated from time to time and bleached in sunlight till the outer layer becomes white. White beeswax is obtained by treating yellow beeswax chemically with potassium permanganate, chromic acid or chlorine or charcoal.

Characterisitics

Yellow wax or cera flava is yellowish to greyish brown coloured solid, with agreeable, honey-like odour and a faint, characteristic taste. When cold, it is somewhat brittle and when broken, shows presence of a dull, granular, noncrystalline fracture. Yellow wax is insoluble in water and sparingly soluble in cold alcohol. It is completely soluble in chloroform, ether and fixed or volatile oils, partly soluble in cold benzene or carbon disulphide and completely soluble in these liquids at about 30°C.

White wax is less unctuous to the touch; it is yellow, soft and ductile at 35°C, and fusible at 65°C. A yellowish-white solid, somewhat translucent in thin layers. It has a faint, characteristic odour which is free from rancidity and tasteless. It is insoluble in water, soluble in chloroform, ether, fixed oil and volatile oils (hot turpentine oil) and sparingly soluble in alcohol. It is not affected by the acids at ordinary temperatures, but is converted into a black mass when boiled with concentrated sulphuric acid.

Chemical Constituents

Beeswax contains myricin, which is melissyl palmitate; melting point 64°C, free cerotic acid ($C_{26}H_{52}O_2$), myricyl alcohol ($C_{30}H_{61}OH$) is liberated when myricyl palmitate is saponified. Melissic acid, some unsaturated acids of the oleic series, ceryl alcohol and 12–13% higher hydrocarbons are present.

Uses

Beeswax is used in the preparation of ointments, plaster and polishes.

Adulterants

Beeswax is adulterated by solid paraffin, ceresin, carnauba wax, or other fats and waxes of animal or mineral origin. Spermaceti and lard render wax softer and less cohesive, of a smoother and less granular fracture and different odour when heated. The melting point and specific gravity are lowered by tallow, suet, lard and especially by paraffin. Ceresin, a principle obtained from ozokerite is also employed as an adulterant. In yellow wax the iodine value is also of use as a test for detection of adulterants but in white wax the bleaching process has altered the bodies which absorb the iodine.

Marketed Products

It is one of the ingredients of the preparations known as Saaf Organic Eraser Body Oil and Jatyadi tel (Dabur).

CARNAUBA WAX

Synonym

Brazil wax.

Biological Source

It is an exudates from pores of the leaves of the Brazilian wax-palm tree *Copernicia prunifera* and *C. cerifera*, belonging to family Palmae (Fig. 19.19).

Geographical Source

Brazilian wax trees are found in North Brazil to Argentina in South America.

Preparation

The leaves of Brazilian wax-palm are collected, dried and then spread on cloth. By brushing and beating, the wax is separated. It is then melted, processed further to purify and poured into the moulds.

Characteristics

It is hard greenish solid wax with crystalline fracture. It has sharp characteristic odour and bland taste. It is soluble in fat solvents.

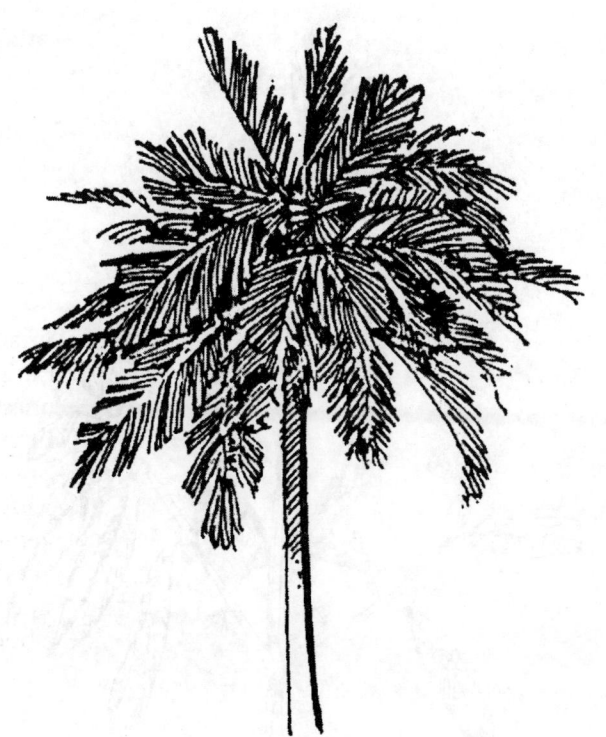

FIG. 19.19 *Copernicia prunifera*

Chemical Constituents

It contains esters of hydroxylated fatty acids, that is, carnaubic and cerotic acid and myricyl cerotate.

Uses

Carnauba wax is used for preparation of cosmetic products, depilatories and deodorant sticks. It is also used for tablet coating. High-quality shoe polishes and automobile waxes are other products made from carnauba wax.

COCOA BUTTER

Synonyms

Theobroma oil, cacao butter, cocoa beans, semina theobromatis.

Biological Source

It is obtained from roasted seeds of *Theobroma cacao* Linn., belonging to family Sterculiaceae (Fig. 19.20).

Geographical Source

Cocoa is cultivated in Brazil, Sri Lanka, Philippines, Curacao, Mexico, West Africa (Ghana, Nigeria) and some parts of India.

Preparation

Cocoa seeds contain nearly 50% of cocoa butter. The seeds are separated from pods and are allowed to ferment. Fermentation process takes place at 30–40°C in tubes, boxes or in the cavities made in the earth for three to six days and during fermentation the colour of the seeds changes from white to dark reddish brown due to enzymatic reaction. If the seeds are not subjected for the process of fermentation and dried in sun, then they are more astringent, bitter tasting and of less value. After fermentation, the seeds are roasted at 100–140°C to remove the acetic acid and water present in the seeds and facilitate removal of seed coat also. The seeds are cooled immediately and are fed into nibbling machine to remove the shells followed by winnowing. The kernels are then fed into hot rollers which yield a pasty mass containing cocoa butter. The pasty mass is further purified to give cocoa butter

Characteristics

Cocoa butter is yellowish white solid and brittle below 25°C. It has pleasant chocolate odour and taste. It is insoluble in water but soluble in chloroform, petroleum ether, ether and benzene. Specific gravity ranges from 0.858

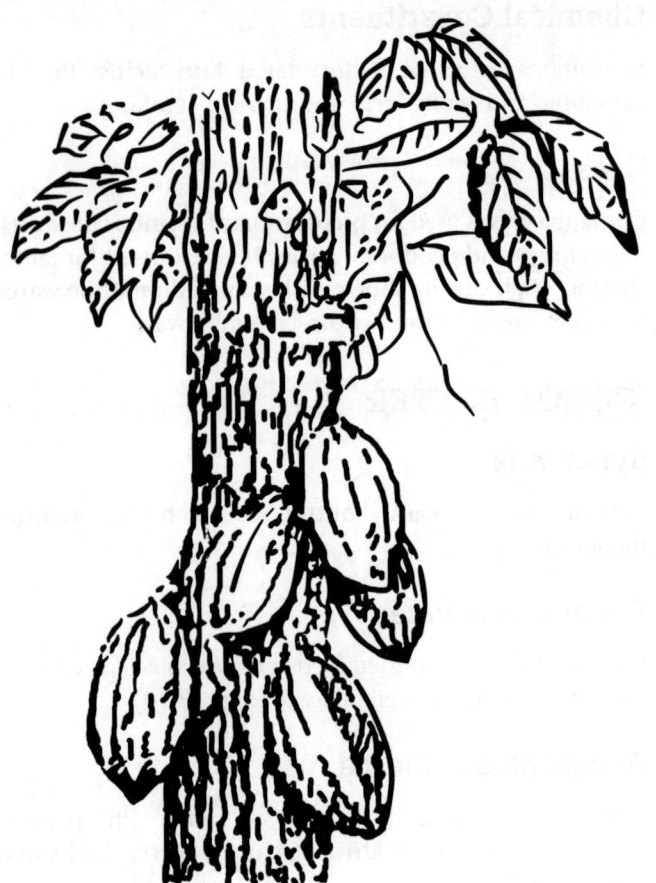

FIG. 19.20 *Theobroma cacao*

to 0.864, melting point between 30°C and 35°C, refractive index varies from 1.4637 to 1.4578, saponification value is 188–195 and iodine value 35–40.

Chemical Constituents

It consists of glycerides of stearic (34%), palmitic (25%), oleic (37%) acids, and small amount of linoleic acids and arachidic acid. Glyceride structure is responsible for nongreasiness of product.

Uses

It is used as an emollient, as a base for suppositories and ointments, manufacture of creams and toilet soaps. It reduces the formation of stretch marks during pregnancy by keeping the skin supple. It is used as an ingredient in lotion bars, lip balms, body butters, soaps and belly balms for expectant mothers.

KOKUM

Synonyms

Goa butter, kokum butter, kokum oil, mangosteen oil.

Biological Source

Kokum is the fat obtained by expression from the seeds of *Garcinia indica* or *G. purpurea*, belonging to family Guttiferae (Fig. 19.21).

Geographical Source

The trees are grown in Thailand, Cambodia, China and India. In India it is cultivated in Malabar, Konkan, Western Ghats and Canara.

Preparation

Fruits are collected, dried and seeds are separated. The kernels from the seeds are churned and it is then boiled with water. The melted fat is separated by skimming process and washed with hot water. Then the fat is decolourized.

Characteristics

Kokum is light grey to yellow in colour, very mild odour, with sweet sour taste. The marketed kokum have an egg shape. Butter is solid at room temperature, but melts readily on contact with the skin with melting point 39–42°C. Refractive index varies from 1.4565 to 1.4575, saponification value is 185–190 and acid value not more than 3.

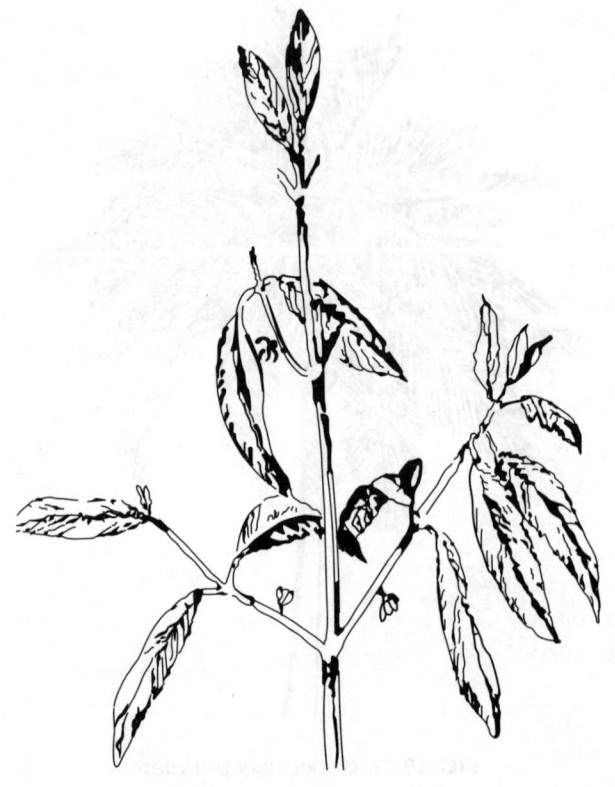

FIG. 19.21 *Garcinia indica*

Chemical Constituents

Seeds contain 30% fat. Kokum consists of glyceride of stearic acid (55%), oleic acids (40%), palmitic acid (2.5%), hydroxyl capric acid (10%) and linoleic acid (1.5%).

Uses

Kokum butter is used as nutritive, demulcent, astringent, emollient, in dysentery and mucous diarrhoea. It is also used in skin diseases, has wound healing property, as a base in ointment, suppository, creams, lotions, balms and make-up foundations.

Marketed Products

It is one of the ingredients of the preparation known as Bioslim (Sunova Pharma Pvt. Ltd.).

LANOLIN

Synonyms

Wool fat, Oesipos, Agnin, Alapurin, anhydrous lanolin, Adeps lanae, Laniol.

Biological Source

Lanolin is the fat-like purified secretion of the sebaceous glands which is deposited into the wool fibres of sheep, *Ovis aries* Linn., belonging to family Bovidae.

Preparation

Wool is cut and washed with a soap or alkali. An emulsion of wool fat, called as wool grease, takes place in water. Raw lanolin is separated by cracking the emulsion with sulphuric acid. Wool grease floats on the upper layer and fatty acids are dissolved in the lower layer. Lanolin is purified by treating with sodium peroxide and bleaching with reagents.

Characteristics

Lanolin is a yellowish white, tenacious, unctuous mass; odour is slight and characteristic. Practically, it is insoluble in water, but soluble in chloroform or ether with the separation of the water. It melts in between 34 and 40°C. On heating it forms two layers in the beginning, continuous heating removes water. Lanolin is not saponified by an aqueous alkali. However, saponification takes place with alcoholic solution of alkali.

Anhydrous lanolin is a yellowish tenacious, semisolid fat with slight odour. Practically it is insoluble in water but mixes with about twice its weight of water without separation. It is sparingly soluble in cold, more in hot alcohol, freely soluble in benzene, chloroform, ether, carbon disulphide, acetone and petroleum ether.

Chemical Constituents

Lanolin is a complex mixture of esters and polyesters of 33 high molecular weight alcohols, and 36 fatty acids. The alcohols are of three types: aliphatic alcohols, steroid alcohols and triterpenoid alcohols. The acids are also of three types: saturated nonhydroxylated acids, unsaturated nonhydroxylated acids and hydroxylated acids. Liquid lanolin is rich in low molecular weight, branched aliphatic acids and alcohols, whereas waxy lanolin is rich in high molecular weight, straight-chain acids and alcohols.

The chief constituents of lanolin are cholesterol, isocholesterol, unsaturated monohydric alcohols of the formula $C_{27}H_{45}OH$, both free and combined with lanoceric ($C_{30}H_{60}O_4$), lanopalmitic ($C_{16}H_{22}O_3$), carnaubic and other fatty acids. Lanolin also contains esters of oleic and myristic acids, aliphatic alcohols, such as cetyl, ceryl and carnaubyl alcohols, lanosterol and agnosterol.

Cholesterol

Identification Tests

Dissolve 0.5 g of lanolin in chloroform, and to it add 1 ml of acetic anhydride and two drops of sulphuric acid. A deep green colour is produced, indicating the presence of cholesterol.

Uses

Lanolin is used as an emollient, as water absorbable ointment base in many skin creams and cosmetic and for hoof dressing. Wool fat is readily absorbed through skin and helps in increasing the absorption of active ingredients incorporated in the ointment. However, it may act as an allergenic contactant in hypersensitive persons.

LARD

Biological Source

It is the purified internal fat obtained from the abdomen of the hog *Sus scrofa* Linn., belonging to family Suidae.

Preparation

The abdominal fat consists of omentum and parts of peritoneum. They are obtained in the form of flat, leafy masses called the 'flare'. The fats are washed to remove the salts or the preservatives used during storage and they are hung in a current of air for drying. The omentum and parts of peritoneum are minced to break the membranous vesicles and to liberate the lard inside then It is then heated to 50–55°C, not more than 57°C to melt the lard. The melted lard is then separated by passing through muslin cloth and cooled with proper stirring. If the lard is not stirred properly it can result in the crystallization. Entrapping of air should be avoided to prevent the lard from becoming rancid on storage.

Characteristics

It is a soft, creamy, white, solid or semisolid homogeneous fat with butter-like consistency. Lard has slight fatty odour but not rancid, cool in nature and sweet taste. It is insoluble in alcohol and soluble in benzene, ether, carbon disulphide and chloroform. Refractive index varies from 1.4520 to 1.4550, saponification value is 192–198, acid value is not more than 2, melting point 34–41°C, specific gravity between 0.934 and 0.938 and iodine value 52–56.

Chemical Constituents

Lard consists of about 60% olein and 40% of stearin and palmitin mixture. The oil separated at 0°C is called the lard oil. About 100 grams of lard contains 900 calories, 95 mg cholesterol, 39 g saturated fat, 45 g monounsaturated fatty acids, 11 g polyunsaturated fatty acids, 0.6 mg vitamin E, 0.1 mg zinc and 0.2 mg selenium.

Uses

It is used as an ointment base and in formulations where more effective absorption is preferred. It is used in difficult bowel movements, dryness in the internal organs like dry cough, skin, eyes, nose and stool. Lard is also used in food manufacturing. Pure lard is especially useful for cooking since it produces very little smoke when heated and has a distinct and pleasant taste when combined with other foods.

Drugs Containing Tannins

CONTENTS

20.1. INTRODUCTION

The name *tannin* is derived from the French *tanin* (tanning substance) and is used for a range of natural polyphenols. Tannins are complex organic, nonnitrogenous plant products, which generally have astringent properties. These compounds comprise a large group of compounds that are widely distributed in the plant kingdom. The term *tannin* was first used by Seguin in 1796 to denote substances which have the ability to combine with animal hides to convert them into leather which is known as tanning of the hide. According to this, tannins are substances which are detected by a tanning test due to its absorption on standard hide powder. The test is known as Goldbeater's skin test.

20.2. CLASSIFICATION

The tannin compounds can be divided into two major groups on the basis of Goldbeater's skin test. A group of tannins showing the positive tanning test may be regarded as true tannins, whereas those, which are partly retained by the hide powder and fail to give the test, are called as pseudotannins.

Most of the true tannins are high molecular weight compounds. These compounds are complex polyphenolics, which are produced by polymerization of simple polyphenols. They may form complex glycosides or remains as such which may be observed by their typical hydrolytic reaction with the mineral acids and enzymes. Two major chemical classes of tannins are usually recognized based on this hydrolytic reaction and nature of phenolic nuclei involved in the tannins structure. The first class is referred to as hydrolysable tannins, whereas the other class is termed as condensed tannins.

Hydrolysable Tannins

As the name implies, these tannins are hydrolysable by mineral acids or enzymes such as tannase. Their structures involve several molecules of polyphenolic acids such as gallic,

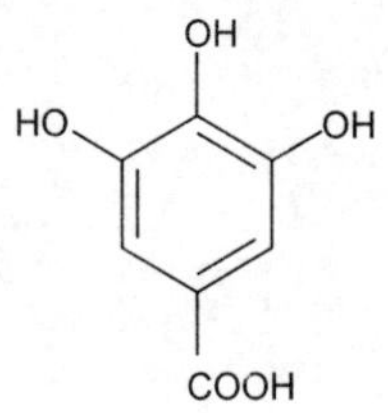

Gallic acid

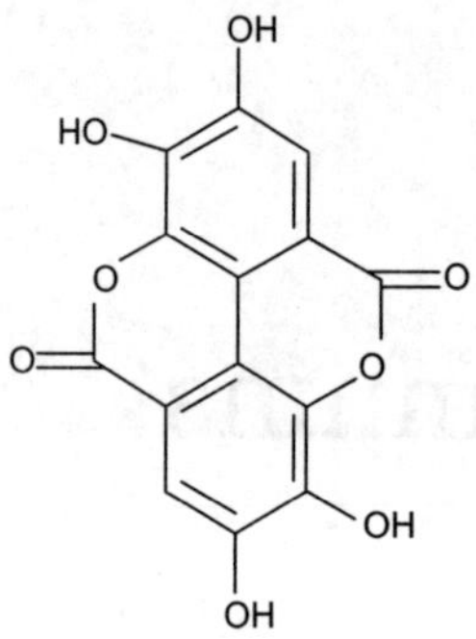

Ellagic acid

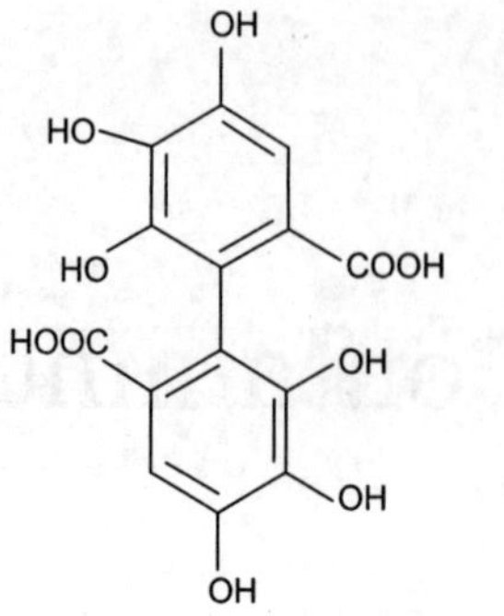

Hexahydroxydiphenic acid

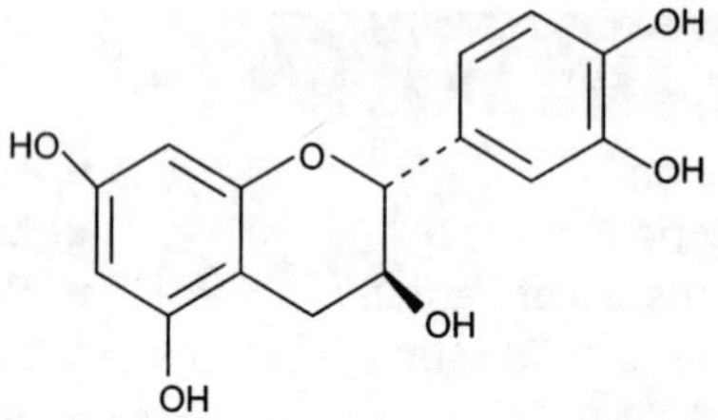

Catechin

Leucoanthocyanidin

hexahydrodiphenic or ellagic acids, bounded through ester linkages to a central glucose molecule. On the basis of the phenolic acids produced after the hydrolysis, they are further categorized under gallotannins composed of gallic acid or ellagitannins which contains hexahydrodiphenic acid which after intraesterification produces ellagic acid.

Hydrolysable tannins are sometimes referred to as pyrogallol tannins as the components of phenolic acids on dry distillation are converted to pyrogallol derivatives. The hydrolysable tannins are soluble in water, and their solution produces blue colour with ferric chloride.

Nonhydrolysable or Condensed Tannins

Condensed tannins, unlike the previously explained group are not readily hydrolysable to simpler molecules with mineral acids and enzymes, thus they are also referred to as nonhydrolysable tannins. The term proanthocyanidins is sometimes alternatively used for these tannins. The compounds containing condensed tannins contain only phenolic nuclei which are biosynthetically related to flavonoids. Catechin which is found in tannins is flavan-3-ol, whereas leucoanthocyanidins are flavan-3,4-diol structures. These phenolics are frequently linked to carbohydrates or protein molecules to produce more complex tannin compounds. When treated with acids or enzymes, they tend to polymerize yielding insoluble red coloured products known as phlobaphens. The phlobaphens give characteristic red colour to many drugs such as cinchona and wild cherry bark. On dry distillation, they yield catechol derivatives. Condensed tannins are also soluble in water and produces green colour with ferric chloride.

The families of the plants rich in both of the above groups of tannins include Rosaceae, Geraniaceae, Leguminosae, Combretaceae, Rubiaceae, Polygonaceae, Theaceae, etc. The members of families Cruciferae and Papaveraceae on the other hand are totally devoid of tannins. In the plants in which tannins are present, they exert an inhibitory effect on many enzymes due to their nature of protein precipitation and therefore contribute a protective function in barks and heartwood.

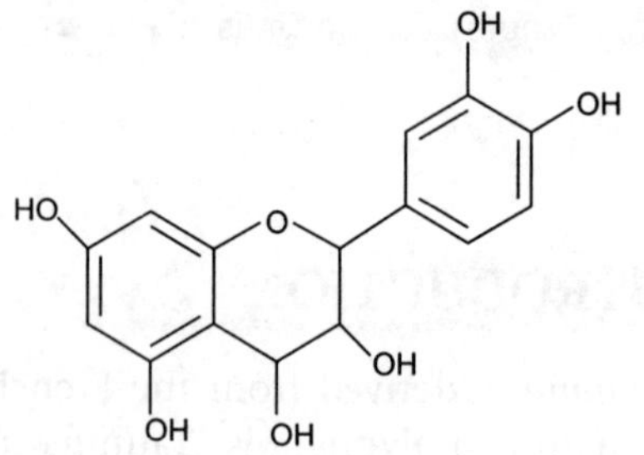

Pseudotannins

Pseudotannins are simple phenolic compounds of lower molecular weight. They do not respond to the tanning reaction of Goldbeater's skin test. Gallic acid, chlorogenic acid or the simple phenolics such as catechin are pseudotannins which are abundantly found in plants, especially in dead tissues and dying cells.

20.3. CHARACTERISTICS OF TANNINS

1. Tannins are colloidal solutions with water.
2. Noncrystalline substance.
3. Soluble in water (exception of some high molecular weight structures), alcohol, dilute alkali and glycerin.
4. Sparingly soluble in ethyl acetate.
5. Insoluble in organic solvents, except acetone.
6. Molecular weight ranging from 500 to >20,000.
7. Oligomeric compounds with multiple structure units with free phenolic groups.
8. Can bind with proteins and form insoluble or soluble tannin—protein complexes.

20.4. BIOSYNTHESIS OF TANNINS

Tannins belong to the phenolics class of secondary metabolites. All phenolic compounds; either primary or secondary are in one way or another formed through shikimic acid pathway (phenylpropanoid pathway). Other phenolics such as isoflavones, coumarins, lignins and aromatic amino acids (tryptophan, phenylalanine and tyrosine) are also formed by the same pathway. Hydrolysable tannins (HTs) and condensed tannins (proanthocyanidins) are the two main categories of tannins that impact animal nutrition.

Common tannins are formed as follows:

- Gallic acid is derived from quinic acid.
- Ellagotannins are formed from hexahydroxydiphenic acid esters by the oxidative coupling of neighbouring gallic acid units attached to a D-glucose core.
- Further oxidative coupling forms the hydrolysable tannin polymers.
- Proanthocyanidin (PA) biosynthetic precursors are the leucocyanidins (flavan-3,4-diol and flavan-4-ol) which on autoxidation, in the absence of heat, form anthocyanidin and 3-deoxyanthocianidin, which, in turn, polymerize to form PAs.

20.5. CHEMICAL TESTS

1. *Goldbeater's Skin Test*: Goldbeater's skin is a membrane produced from the intestine of Ox. It behaves just like untanned animal hide. A piece of goldbeaters skin previously soaked in 2% hydrochloric acid and washed with distilled water is placed in a solution of tannin for 5 minutes. It is then washed with distilled water and transferred to 1% ferrous sulphate solution. A change of the colour of the goldbeater's skin to brown or black indicates the presence of tannin. Hydrolysable and condensed tannins both give the positive goldbeater's test, whereas pseudotannins show very little colour or negative test.
2. *Phenazone Test:* To 5 ml of aqueous solution of tannin containing drug, add 0.5 g of sodium acid phosphate. Warm the solution, cool and filter. Add 2% phenazone solution to the filtrate. All tannins are precipitated as bulky, coloured precipitate.
3. *Gelatin Test:* To a 1% gelatine solution, add little 10% sodium chloride. If a 1% solution of tannin is added to the gelatine solution, tannins cause precipitation of gelatine from solution.
4. *Test for Catechin* (*Matchstick Test*): Catechin test is the modification of the well-known phloroglucinol test for lignin. Matchstick contains lignin. Dip a matchstick in the dilute extract of the drug, dry, moisten it with concentrated hydrochloric acid and warm it near a flame. Catechin in the presence of acid produces phloroglucinol which stains the lignified wood pink or red.
5. *Test for Chlorogenic Acid*: A dilute solution of chlorogenic acid containing extract, if treated with aqueous ammonia and exposed to air, slowly turns green indicating the presence of chlorogenic acid.
6. *Vanillin-Hydrochloric Acid Test:* Drug shows pink or red colour with a mixture of vanillin: alcohol:dilute HCl in the ratio 1:10:10. The reaction produces phloroglucinol which along with vanillin gives pink or red colour.

20.6. ISOLATION

Both hydrolysable and condensed tannins are highly soluble in water and alcohol but insoluble in organic solvents such as solvent ether, chloroform and benzene. Tannin compounds can be easily extracted by water or alcohol. The general method for the extraction of tannic acid from various galls is either with water-saturated ether, or with mixture of water, alcohol and ether. In such cases, free acids such as Gallic and ellagic acid go along with ether, whereas true tannin gets extracted in water. If the drug consists of chlorophyll or pigment, it may be removed by ether. After extraction, the aqueous and ethereal layers are separately concentrated, dried and subjected to further isolation and purification using various separation techniques of chromatography.

20.7. MEDICINAL PROPERTIES AND USES

Tannins occur in crude drugs either as major active constituent as in oak bark, hamamelis leaves, bearberry leaves, etc., or as a subsidiary component as in clove, cinnamon, peppermint or garden sage. In many cases, they synergistically increase the effectiveness of active principles. Tannins are medicinally significant due to their astringent properties. They promote rapid healing and the formation of new tissues on wounds and inflamed mucosa. Tannins are used in the treatment of varicose ulcers, haemorrhoids, minor burns, frostbite, as well as inflammation of gums. Internally tannins are administered in cases of diarrhoea, intestinal catarrh and in cases of heavy metal poisoning as an antidote. In recent years, these compounds have demonstrated their antiviral activities for treatment of viral diseases including AIDS. Tannins are used as mordant in dyeing, manufacture of ink, sizing paper and silk, and for printing fabrics. It is used along with gelatine and albumin for manufacture of imitation horn and tortoise shell. They are widely used in the leather industry for conversion of hide into leather, the process being known as tanning. Tannins are also used for clarifying beer or wine, in photography or as a coagulant in rubber manufacture. Tannins are used for the manufacture of gallic acid and pyrogallol, and sometimes as a reagent in analytical chemistry.

20.8. HYDROLYSABLE TANNINS

MYROBALAN

Synonyms

Chebulic myrobalan, harde, haritaki.

Biological Sources

Myrobalan is the mature dried fruits of *Terminalia chebula*, belonging to family Combretaceae (Fig. 20.1).

Geographical Source

Myrobalan trees are found at an elevation of 300–900 m in North India, Satpura ranges of Madhya Pradesh, Maharashtra and Panchamahal district in Gujarat. It is also found in Myanmar and Sri Lanka.

Collection and Preparation

T. chebula is a moderate-sized or large deciduous tree attaining a height of 25–30 m. The plant lacks natural regeneration. The plant requires direct overhead light and cannot tolerate shady situations. It is a frost and draught resistant tree. The fruits ripen from November to March depending upon the locality, and fall soon after ripening. The mature fruits are collected from January to April by shaking the trees, and then drying by spreading in thin layers preferably in shades. The dried myrobalan fruits are graded under different trade names (Fig. 20.2). Gradation is done on the basis of fruits colour, solidness and freedom from insect attack.

Characteristics

Colour	Yellowish brown to brown
Odour	Slight odour
Taste	Mucilaginous
Shape	Astringent and slightly bitter
Size	2–3 cm long and 1.5–3 cm wide
Solubility	Ovate with longitudinal wrinkles
Extra features	Fruits are drupe. It is hard and stony with four to six longitudinal ribs. Seeds are pale yellow in colour and 1.6–2.3 cm long

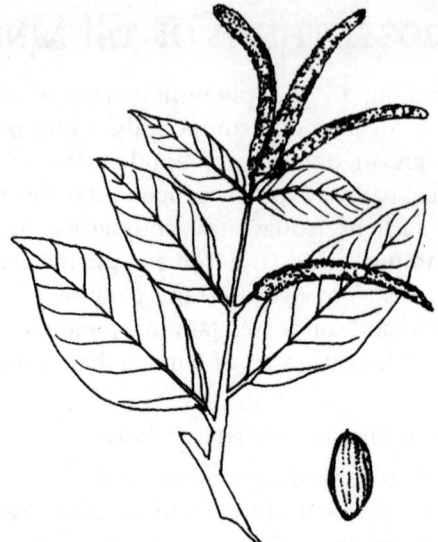

FIG. 20.1 *Terminalia chebula*

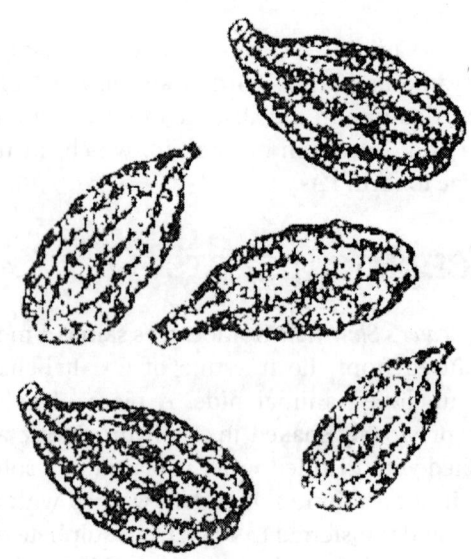

FIG. 20.2 Myrobalan fruits

Chemical Constituents

Myrobalan contains about 30% of the hydrolysable tannins, which consists of chebulinic acid, chebulagic acid and D-galloyl glucose. It contains free tannic acid, gallic acid, ellagic acid and resin myrobalanin. Anthraquinone glycosides, sennosides have been reported in myrobalan.

Chebulic acid

Uses

Myrobalan is reputed in Indian system of medicine as a drug for various types of diseases. Because of antiseptic and healing properties of tannins, it is used externally in chronic ulcers, wounds, piles and as stomachic. It is one of the drugs of the well-known preparation 'Triphala'. It has purgative properties. Fine powder of myrobalan is used in dental preparations. Commercially, it is used in dyeing and tanning industry and also in treatment of water used for locomotives.

Marketed Products

It is one of the ingredients of the preparation known as Constivac (Lupin Herbal Laboratory), a bowel regulator and relieves constipation. Also, it is one of the ingredients of the preparations known as Pilect (Aimil Pharmaceuticals), Abana, Bonnisan, Geriforte, Koflet, Menosan (Himalaya Drug Company), Haritakh churna, Triphala churna, Tentex forte (Baidyanath Company).

BAHERA

Synonyms

Beleric myrobalan, baheda, bibhitak.

Biological Source

It consists of dried ripe fruits of the plant *Terminalia belerica* Linn, belonging to family Combretaceae (Fig. 20.3).

Geographical Source

The tree is found in all decidous forests of India, up to an altitude of 1000 m. It is found in abundance in Madhya Pradesh, Uttar Pradesh, Punjab, Maharashtra, and also in Sri Lanka and Malaya.

Cultivation and Collection

Cultivation of the drug, though not done on commercial scale, can be carried out by sowing the seeds. The seeds can retain the viability for a year and their rate of germination is about 80%. The plant can also be raised by transplantation. It takes about 15–30 days for germination of seed. Maximum height of the plant is about 40 m and the girth is 2–3 m. The stem of the plant is straight the leaves are broadly elliptic and clustered towards the end of the branches. Flowers are simple, solitary and in auxiliary spikes.

Morphology

Colour	Fruits are dark brown to black
Odour	None

Taste	Astringent
Shape	Strips, flakes or coarse powder
Size	1.3–2 cm in length
Shape	Fruits are globular and obscurely five-angled

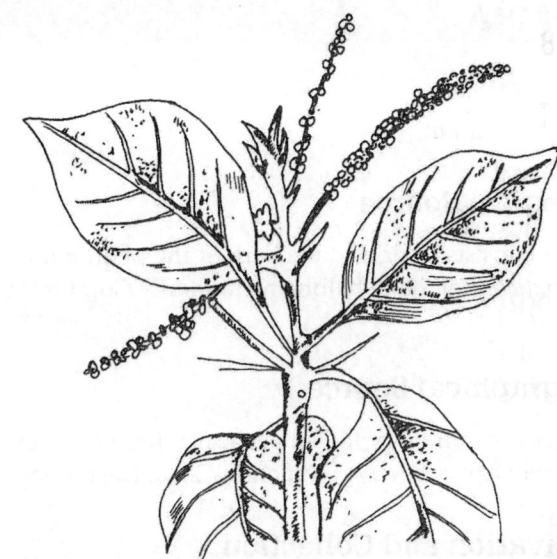

FIG. 20.3 *Terminalia belerica*

Microscopy

Transverse section shows an outer epicarp consisting of a layer of epidermis, most of the epidermal cells elongate to form hair like protuberance with swollen base; next to epidermis it contains a zone of parenchymatous cells, slightly tangentially elongated and irregularly arranged. Stone cells of varying shape and size are present in between these parenchymatous cells. Mesocarp traversed in various directions by numerous vascular bundles collateral, endarch; simple starch grains and rosettes of calcium oxalate crystals are present in parenchymatous cells.

Chemical Constituents

The fruits contain about 20–30% of tannins and 40–45% water-soluble extractives. It contains colouring matter. It contains gallic acid, ellagic acid, phyllemblin, ethyl gallate and galloyl glucose. The seeds contain nonedible oil. The plant produces a gum. It also contains most of the sugars as reported in myrobalan.

Uses

Bahera is used as an astringent and in the treatment of dyspepsia and diarrhoea. It is a constituent of triphala. The purgative property of half ripe fruit is due to the presence of fixed oil. The oil on hydrolysis yields an irritant recipe. Gum is used as a demulcent and purgative. Oil is used for the manufacture of soap.

Marketed Products

It is the chief component of the preparation known as Sage triphala syrup (Sage Herbals), for relieving habitual constipation.

ARJUNA

Synonyms

Arjun bark, arjun.

Biological Source

Arjuna consists of dried stem bark of the plant known as *Terminalia arjuna* Rob, belonging to family Combretaceae (Fig. 20.4).

Geographical Source

The tree is common in Indian peninsula. It is grown by the side of streams and very common in Chota Nagpur region.

Cultivation and Collection

Arjuna is found as naturally growing plant in the dense forests. It is very common in Baitul in Madhya Pradesh and also in Dehradun. Arjuna can be successfully raised by sowing seeds or by means of stumps. The seeds take about 21 days for germination. It needs moist fertile alluvial loam and rainfall in the range of 75–190 cm. It grows satisfactorily up to 45°C. The bark is also collected from wild growing plants, and it is reported that yield per tree varies from 9 to 55 kg.

Morphology (Fig. 20.5)

Colour	Colour of the outer side, as well as, inner side of bark is greyish-brown
Odour	None
Taste	Astringent

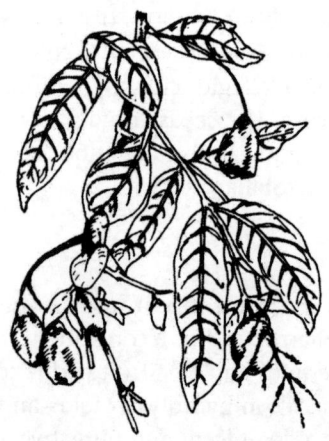

FIG. 20.4 *Terminalia arjuna*

Shape	Flats
Size	The pieces of various sizes, about 15 × 10 × 1 cm
Extra features	The presence of the cork is not reported in the commercial drug. As arjuna is collected from the old trees, the cork gets removed due to exfoliation. The appearance of the transversely cut surface is dark brown with characteristic greyish shining patches

Microscopy (Figs. 20.6 and 20.7)

Transverse section of fresh bark shows cork composed of uniformly arranged several layers of small, tangentially elongated cells. Below cork is a region of cortex, composed of thin-walled, more or less brick-shaped parenchymatous cells containing cluster crystals of calcium oxalate. A few groups of sclerenchymatous pericyclic fibres are scattered in the cortex. Secondary phloem consists of phloem parenchyma composed of thin-walled, polygonal cells with wavy walls containing cluster crystals of calcium oxalate and pigmented cells. Phloem fibres, composed of sclerenchymatous cells, occur in groups and are scattered in the form of patches in parenchyma. Narrow and almost straight medullary rays are also present.

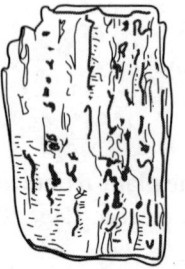
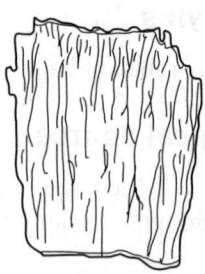

Outer surface of bark   Inner surface of bark

FIG. 20.5 Morphology of Arjuna bark

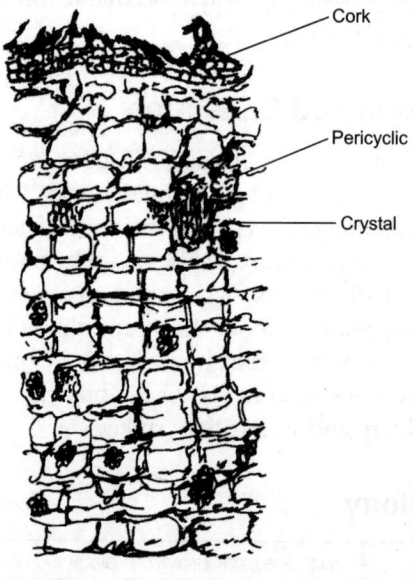

FIG. 20.6 T.S. of the outer part of the bark

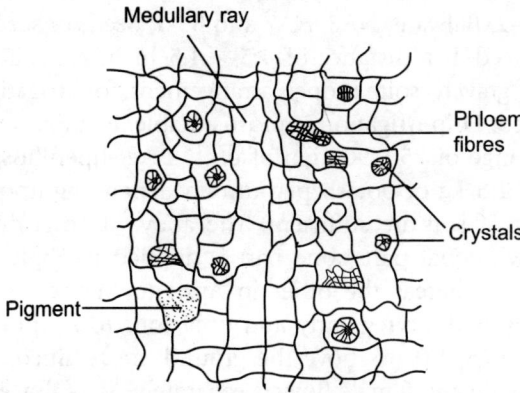

FIG. 20.7 T.S. of the inner part of bark

Powder microscopy (Fig. 20.8)

The powder is pinkish or reddish brown in colour, having an astringent taste. Microscopical examination shows thick-walled fibres with somewhat tapered ends. Cork cells are moderately thick-walled, polygonal in surface view. Cluster crystals of calcium oxalate, starch grains (simple or compound with distinct central hilum) and fragments of parenchymatous pigmented cells are found scattered.

Chemical Constituents

The dry bark from the stem contains about 20–24% of tannin, whereas that of the bark obtained from the lower branches is up to 15–18%. The tannins present in arjuna bark are of mixed type consisting of both hydrolysable and condensed tannins. The tannins are reported to be present are (+) catechol, (+) gallocatechol, epicatechol, epigallocatechol and ellagic acid. The flavonoids such as arjunolone, arjunone and baicalein have been reported from the stem bark. The triterpenoid compounds arjunetin,

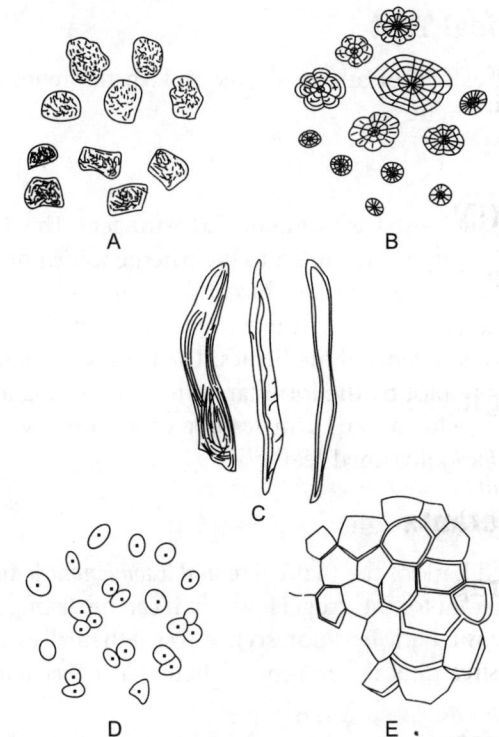

FIG. 20.8 Powder characteristics of arjuna bark. (A: Isolated masses of pigment, B: Cluster of calcium oxalate crystals, C: Fibres, D: Starch grains, E: Cork in surface view)

arjungenin, arjunglucoside I and II, and terminoic acid have also been reported from the bark. The root contains number of triterpenoids such as arjunoside I and II, terminic acid, oleanolic acid, arjunic acid, arjunolic acid, etc. The fruits also contain 7–20% of tannins. A pentacyclic triterpenic glycoside arjunoglucoside III has been reported from the fruits along with hentriacontane, myristyl oleate and arachidic stearate.

Arjunolone

Arjunone

Arjunglucoside III

Terminoic acid

Chemical Test

Ethereal extract of arjuna shows pinkish fluorence under ultraviolet light.

Uses

Arjuna bark is used as a diuretic and astringent. The diuretic properties can be attributed to the triterpenoids present in fruits. It causes decrease in blood pressure and heart rate. It is used in the treatment of various heart diseases in indigenous systems of medicines. The bark was extensively used in the past by the local tanneries for tanning animal hides. It yields a very firm leather of a colour which is similar babool tanned leather.

Adulterants

The dried bark of the plant *Terminalia tomentosa* is used as an adulterant for the drug. However, it can be distinguished from arjuna bark by fluorescence test. Ethereal extract of arjuna gives pink fluorescence, whereas *T. tomentosa* gives pale blue.

Marketed Products

It is one of the ingredients of the preparations known as Abana, Geriforte, Liv 52, Mentat (Himalaya Drug Company), Arjun Ghrita, Arjun churna (Baidyanath Company) and Madhudoshantak (Jamuna Pharma).

AMLA

Synonyms

Emblica, Indian goose berry, amla.

Biological Source

This consists of dried, as well as fresh fruits of the plant *Emblica officinalis* Gaertn. (*Phyllanthus emblica* Linn.), belonging to family Euphorbiaceae (Fig. 20.9).

Geographical Source

It is a small- or medium-sized tree found in all deciduous forests of India. It is also found in Sri Lanka and Myanmar. The leaves are feathery with small oblong pinnately arranged leaflets. The tree is characteristic greenish-grey and with smooth bark.

Cultivation and Collection

It is grown by seed germination. It can also be propagated by budding or cutting. It does not tolerate the frost or drought. It is normally found up to an altitude of 1500 m. Commercially, it is collected from wild-grown plants.

Nowadays, the newly released varieties are selected for better yield. These are known as Banarasi, Kanchan, Anand-2, Balwant, NA6, NA7 and B5-1. Seeds or seedlings are placed at a distance of 4.5 × 4.5 m in red loamy or coarse gravely soil. Proper arrangement for irrigation is required, Drip irrigation is most suitable. Fertilizers in the dose range of 750–900 gm of urea, 1 kg superphosphate and 1–1.5 kg of potash per annum depending upon the quality of soil are sufficient. The above dose is divided into two equal parts, one part is applied in September/ October, whereas the other in April to May every year. Pruning is done regularly and only four to six branches about 0.75–1.0 m above the ground are retained. Plant bears male and female flowers separately. Male flowers are reported in the axil of the leaf, in bunches, whereas female flowers in the axil of the branches are solitary. The extent of fertilization is 25–30% of flowers. Cultivated plants bear comparatively large fruits. The tree flowers in hot season and the fruits ripen during the winter.

Morphology

Colour	Green changing to light yellow or brick red when matured
Odour	None
Taste	Sore and astringent
Shape	The fruits are depressed, globose
Size	1.5–2.5 cm in diameter
Extra features	Fruits are fleshy obscurely four-lobed with 6-trygonus seeds. They are very hard and smooth in appearance

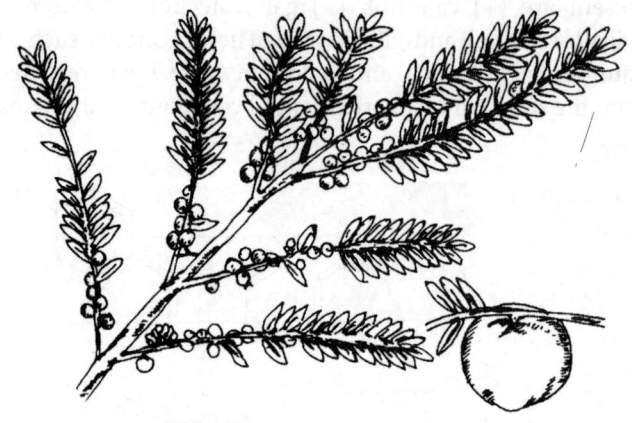

FIG. 20.9 Twig of *Emblica officinalis*

Microscopy

Fruit shows an epicarp consisting of epidermis with a thick cuticle and two to four layers of hypodermis; the cells in hypodermis is tangentially elongated, thick-walled, smaller in dimension than epidermal cells; mesocarp consists of thin-walled isodiametric parenchymatous cells; several collateral fibrovascular bundles scattered throughout mesocarp; xylem composed of tracheal elements, fibre

Vitamin C   Gallic acid   Ellagic acid

tracheids and xylem fibres; tracheal elements, show reticulate, scalariform and spiral thickenings; mesocarp also contains large aggregates of numerous irregular silica crystals.

Chemical Constituents

It is highly nutritious and is an important dietary source of vitamin C, minerals, and amino acids. The edible fruit tissue contains protein concentration 3-fold and ascorbic acid concentration 160-fold compared to that of the apple. The fruit also contains considerably higher concentration of most minerals and amino acids than apples. The pulpy portion of fruit, dried and freed from the nuts contains: gallic acid 1.32%, tannin, sugar 36.10%; gum 13.75%; albumin 13.08%; crude cellulose 17.08%; mineral matter 4.12%; and moisture 3.83%. Tannins are the mixture of gallic acid, ellagic acid and phyllemblin. The alkaloidal constituents such as phyllantidine and phyllantine have also been reported in the fruits. An immature fruit contains indoleacetic acid and four other auxins—a1, a3, a4 and a5 and two growth inhibitors R_1 and R_2.

Chemical Tests

1. Alcoholic or aqueous extract of the drug gives blue colour with ferric chloride solution.
2. To aqueous extract add gelatine and sodium chloride milky white colour is produced.
3. To the aqueous extract of amla add lead acetate remove precipitate by filtration. To the filtrate add solution of 2:6 dichlorophenol—indophenol, colour disappears.

Uses

The fruits are diuretic, acrid, cooling, refrigerant and laxative. Dried fruit is useful in haemorrhage, diarrhoea, diabetes and dysentery. They are useful in the disorders associated with the digestive system and are also prescribed in the treatment of jaundice and coughs. It has antioxidant, antibacterial, antifungal, and antiviral activities. Amla is one of the three ingredients of the famous ayurvedic preparation, triphala, which is given to treat chronic dysentery, biliousness and other disorders, and it is also an ingredient in chyavanprash.

Marketed Products

It is the chief component of the preparation known as Jeevani malt (Chirayu Pharma), Triphala churna (Zandu) and Chyavanprash (Dabur).

NUTGALLS

Synonyms

Nutgalls, blue galls, Turkish galls.

Biological Source

Nutgall consists of the pathological outgrowth obtained from the young twigs of the dyers oak, *Quercus infectoria* Olivier, belonging to family Fagaceae. Outgrowth is caused by the puncture of ovums of insect *Cynips tinctoria* or *Adleria gallaetinctoriae* Olivier, family Cynipidae (Fig. 20.10).

Geographical Source

Oak galls are obtained principally from Asiatic Turkey. Dyers oak is found in Turkey, Syria, Iran, Cyprus and Greece.

Collection and Preparation

Larvae of the insect *C. tinctoria* after emerging from the eggs, pierces the delicate epidermis near the growing point of the twigs where the eggs are deposited by the insect. The gall begins to enlarge, when the chrysalis stage is reached, starch disappears from the neighbourhood of insect and is replaced by gallic acid, whereas central cells consist of tannic acid. The insect passes through the larval and pupal stages. If the galls are not collected and dried at this stage the mature insect comes out of the gall and escapes, and during this stage galls changes the colour from a bluish grey, through olive green to almost white. After the escape of the insect, a central cavity is formed, and the tannic acid is oxidized in the presence of moisture and air. The more porous gall is the white gall of commerce.

In Asiatic Turkey, galls are collected before the escape of the insect in the months of August and September. After drying, they are sorted out according to colour into three grades, that is, blue, green, and white and exported.

Characteristics

Colour	Brown to greenish black or yellow
Odour	Odourless
Taste	Astringent
Shape	Round or globular
Size	1–3 cm in diameter

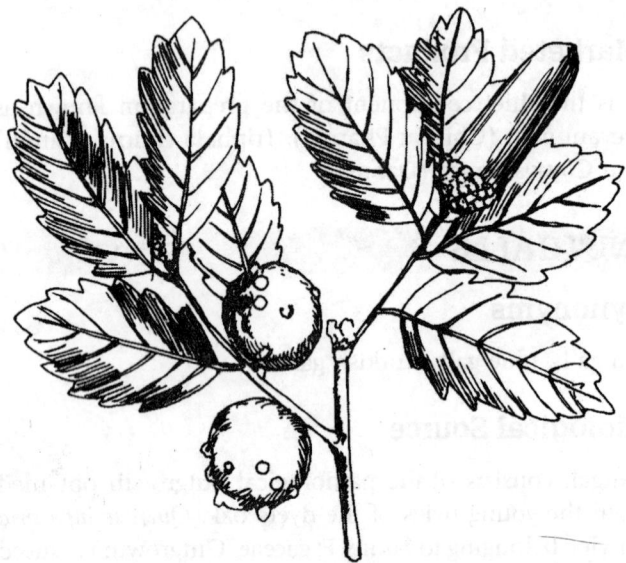

FIG. 20.10 Twigs of *Quercus infectoria*

Microscopy

A transverse section through a nutgall show thin walled parenchymatous outer zone, which is quite larger as compared to inner zone. Parenchyma is followed by a ring of sclerenchyma composed of one or two layers of suberised cells. Inner zone is made up of thick walled parenchyma, which surrounds central cavity. Cells of parenchyma show the presence of numerous starch grains, calcium oxalate clusters and rosettes and tannins. Parenchyma also shows the bodies of lignified tissues, which stains with phloroglucinol and hydrochloric acid.

Chemical Constituents

Nutgalls contains about 50–70% tannin mainly gallotannic acid which is official tannic acid. It also consists of 2–4% gallic acid, ellagic acid, sitosterol, methyl belulate and methyl oleanolate which are methyl esters of betulic and oleanolic acid. Recently few more compounds such as nyctanthic acid, roburic acid and syringic acids have been reported from galls. It contains abundant starch.

Tannic acid of commerce is a hydrolysable tannin which yields gallic acid and glucose. The molecule of tannic acid may contain the gallic acid up to pentagalloyl glucose. It is isolated by fermentation and subsequent extraction of galls with water-saturated ether.

Uses

Nutgall is the major source of tannic acid, which is largely used in tanning and dyeing industry and for the manufacture of ink. It is used medicinally as a local astringent in ointments and suppositories.

Allied Drugs

Various types of galls are produced on plants by insects of the genera *Cynips* and *Aphis*. Chinese and Japanese galls are of commercial interest. These galls are formed on *Rhus chinensis* Mill, family Anacardiaceae by an aphis, *Schlectendalia chinensis*. These galls are knotty, grey, irregular and breaks easily to show irregular cavities. They contain 57–77% of tannins. These drugs have been used in China and Japan since time immemorial as astringent and styptic.

TANNIC ACID

Tannic acid is not a single constituent but a type of hydrolysable tannin that contains several units of gallic or ellagic acids esterified with the glucosyl OH to produce complex tannin compounds. Its exact composition varies according to its source. Turkish galls have a maximum complexity of hexa or heptagalloyl glucose, whereas Chinese galls are octa or nonagalloyl glucose, which affords methylgallate and pentagalloyl glucose on hydrolysis.

Tannic acid is extracted with a mixture of water, alcohol and ether. The extracted liquid separates into two layers. The aqueous lower layer contains gallotannins, whereas the ethereal layer contains free gallic acid and other similar compounds. Aqueous and ethereal extracts are treated separately for further purification.

Tannic acid occurs as amorphous powder containing brownish spongy masses. It has a faint odour and strong astringent taste. It is soluble in water, alcohol and acetone but insoluble in organic solvents.

Tannic acid has strong astringent properties. It is used as an antidote in cases of alkaloidal poisoning as it precipitates alkaloids as tannate salts. It finds its uses in tanning, dyeing industries and for ink manufacture. Its preparation can be used topically for the treatment of bedsores and minor ulcerations. It is utilized in the laboratory as a reagent for detection of gelatine and proteins.

20.9. CONDENSED TANNINS

ASHOKA

Synonyms

Ashoka, ashoka bark.

Biological Source

Ashoka consists of dried stem bark of the plant *Saraca indica* Linn., belonging to family Leguminosae (Fig. 20.11).

Geographical Source

It is distributed in South Asia, that is, in Malaysia, Indonesia, Sri Lanka and India.

Cultivation and Collection

It is one of the most sacred trees of the Hindus. It is frequently grown as an ornamental and avenue tree in India. It is not found to be cultivated on commercial scale. It can be easily propagated from seeds. It is found growing suitably at an altitude of 750 m in the Himalayas, Khasi, Garo and Lushai hills. It is an evergreen tree, bearing dark red-coloured flowers reaching a maximum height of 9 m. Bark is collected from the plant by making transverse and longitudinal incisions.

Morphology

Colour	Outer side is dark brown or almost black with warty surface. Internally, it is reddish brown with fine longitudinal striations
Odour	None
Taste	Astringent and bitter
Shape	It occurs in the form of channels of various sizes
Size	Up to 50 cm length and 1 cm in thickness
Extra features	The bark is marked by bluish and ash white patches of lichens

Microscopy (Figs. 20.12 and 20.13)

Transverse section of bark shows cork cells, cork cambium and phelloderm constituting periderm of bark. Pericycle is composed of sclereids (stone cells), parenchyma and scattered pericyclic fibres. Sclereids usually occur as densely packed zones, composed of thick-walled, tangentially elongated cells, which alternate with parenchyma. Parenchymatous cells are thick-walled, oval containing prismatic crystals of calcium oxalate. Sheath of prismatic crystals of calcium oxalate surrounds zone of sclereids. Secondary phloem is a wide region consisting of phloem parenchyma, traversed longitudinally by medullary rays and phloem fibres. Cells of phloem parenchyma contain prismatic crystals of calcium

oxalate similar to that of parenchyma of Pericycle. Phloem fibres are arranged in small concentric groups of more than three on the radial rows of phloem elements. Medullary rays become much wider, dilated, and funnel shaped on reaching pericycle.

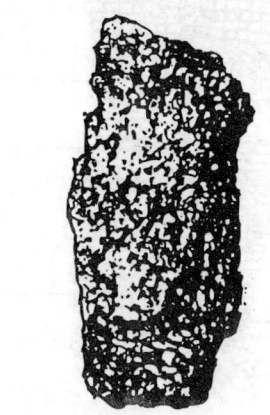

FIG. 20.11 Ashoka bark

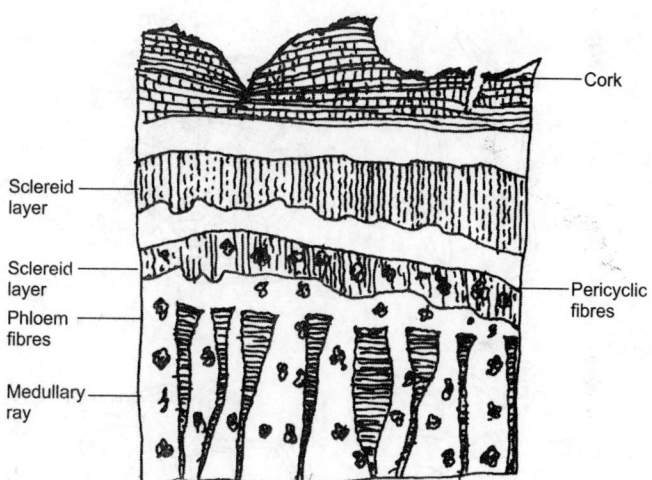

FIG. 20.12 T.S. (schematic) of Ashoka bark

Powder Microscopy (Fig. 20.14)

The powder is rusty brown in colour with astringent taste. Microscopical examination shows groups of sclereids, composed of thick-walled, densely packed cells with numerous pits, found isolated or associated with sheath of prismatic crystals of calcium oxalate. Cork cells are moderately thick-walled and polygonal in surface view. Prismatic crystals of calcium oxalate, small and uniform in size and fibres with tapered ends are usually found scattered.

Chemical Constituents

Ashoka stem bark contains about 6% of tannins and anthocyanin derivatives which includes leucopelargonidin-3-O-β-D-glucoside, leucopelargonidin and leucocyanidin.

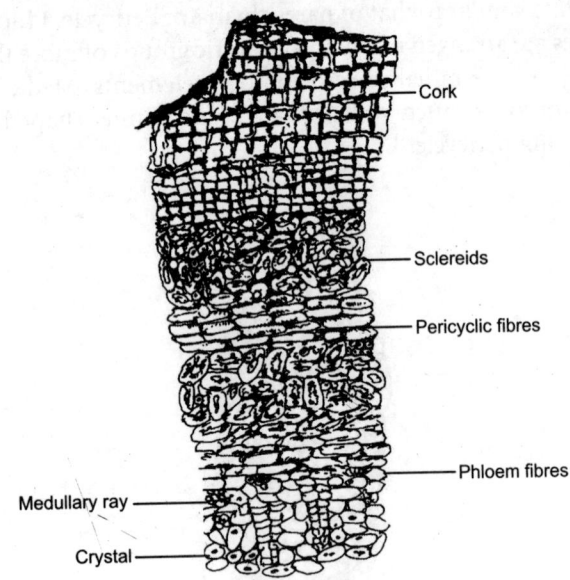

FIG. 20.13 Transverse section of Ashoka bark

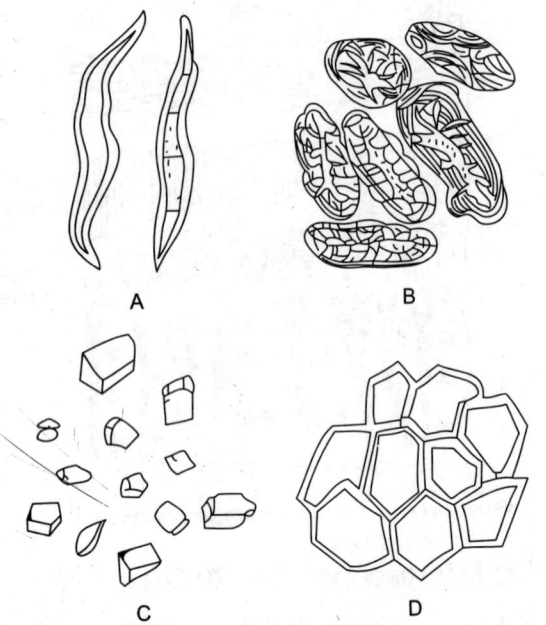

FIG. 20.14 Powder characteristics of Ashoka bark. (A: Fibres, B: Sclereids, C: Calcium oxalate crystals, D: Cork in surface view)

It also contains waxy substance constituted of long chain alkanes, esters, alcohols and *n*-octacosanol. The steroidal components present in the bark includes 24-methylcholest-5-en-3-β-ol, (ZZE)-24-ethylcholesta-5,22-dien-3-β-ol, 24-ethylcholest-5-en-3-β-ol and β-sitosterol.

The root bark contains (−) epicatechin, procyanidin B$_2$ and 11′-deoxyprocyanidin B. The pods consists of (+) catechol, (−) epicatechol and leucocyanidin. The flowers are reported to have various anthocyanin pigments, kaempferol, quercetin and its glycoside, gallic acid and β-sitosterol.

Leucocyanidin R = OH
Leucopelargonidin R = H

24-Methylcholest-5-en-3β-ol

Chemical Tests

1. Powdered bark, when treated with saturated picric acid solution, remains brown for 10 minutes and then slowly turns to orange yellow.
2. Powdered bark gives a deep chocolate colour with 5% KOH solution.

Uses

It is used as uterine tonic and also a sedative. It stimulates the uterus by the prolonged and frequent uterine contractions. It is also suggested in all cases of uterine bleeding, where ergot can also be used. It is reported to have a stimulant effect on the endometrium and ovarian tissue and useful in menorrhagia.

Adulterants

Bark of *Polyalthia longifolia* is generally used as an adulterant.

Marketed Products

It is the chief component of the preparation known as Pmensa (Lupin Herbal Laboratory) for symptomatic relief in painful and psychological symptoms associated with premenstrual syndrome. It is also an important ingredient of the preparation known as Femiplex (Charak Pharma Pvt. Ltd.) and Ashokarishta (Baidyanath).

PALE CATECHU

Synonyms

Gambier, pale catechu, catechu.

Biological Source

Gambier or pale catechu is a dried aqueous extract produced from the leaves and young twigs of *Uncaria gambir* Roxburgh., belonging to family Rubiaceae (Fig. 20.15).

Geographical Source

U. gambier is a native of erstwhile Malaya. It is cultivated in Indonesia, Malaysia, Sumatra, Bornea and Singapore at elevation up to 150 m. The plant is used mostly for the production of the drug, which is marketed through Singapore.

Cultivation, Collection and Preparation

Propagation of *U. gambier* is done by seeds. Seeds are sown in the nursery to raise the seedlings, which after about 9 months are planted out in the clearing about 3 m apart. Leaves and young shoots are collected as a first crop during second year's growth. Later the crop is taken every year. The plant continues to give sufficient leaves and twigs up to 20 years, but the maximum yield is obtained during eighth year of growth.

The collected leaves and twigs are transported to the factory as loose material. The material is put into large drums with about three quarters of boiling water. It is boiled for about three hours with intermittent stirring. The marc is subsequently removed by large wooden forks and lodged on surface to drain the liquor back to the vessels. It is pressed and washed. The washing is added to the extract. The combined total aqueous extract is then concentrated for one and half-hour till it becomes thick, yellowish-green paste. It is transferred from the vessels to wooden tubs, stirred while it is hot and cooling in a stream of water to crystallize tannins. Semicrystallized paste is again transferred to wooden trays in which it sets. They are cut into cubes by wooden knife and dried in sum. The drug is also made into large blocks in kerosene tins.

Morphology

Colour	Dull reddish brown colour externally and pale brown to buff colour internally
Odour	Odourless
Taste	At first it is bitter and astringent but later it is sweet
Shape	Strips, flakes or coarse powder
Size	Pale catechu comes in the form of cubes or rectangular blocks of 2–4 cm length
Shape	Regular cubes or as rectangular blocks

Microscopy

The powdered drug, if mounted in the solution of lactophenol or water, shows the small circular crystals of catechu under microscope. The water insoluble part of the pale catechu

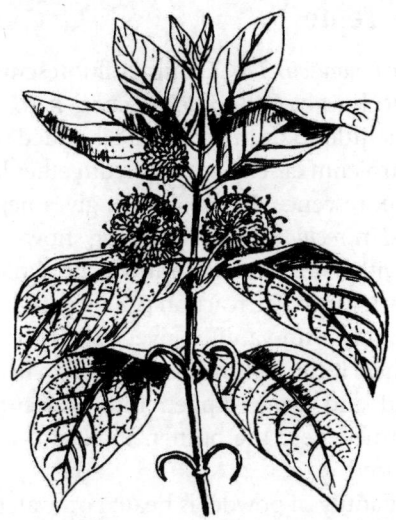

FIG. 20.15 *Uncaria gambir* flowering branch

under the microscope exhibits epidermal pieces, unicellular hairs, cork tissues, lignified fibres, etc. Alcohol insoluble part shows the absence of starch. The pale catechu from Indonesia is reported to have minute starch grains.

Chemical Constituents

Pale catechu contain from about 7 to 30% of pseudotannin catechin and 22 to 55% of a phlobatannin catechutannic acid. Both of the about component constitute over 60% of the drug. It also contains catechu red, gambier fluorescin and quercetin. It contains indole alkaloid up to 0.05%, which includes gambirtannin and its derivatives. Gambirtannin gives a strong fluorescence under UV light. Catechin forms white, needle like crystals, which dissolves in alcohol and hot water. Catechutannic acid gives green colour with ferric chloride.

Catechin

Gambirtannin

Chemical Tests

1. *Gambier Fluorescin Test:* Gambier fluorescin present in pale catechu gives the fluorescence. If to its alcohol extract, a little sodium hydroxide is added and shaken with petroleum ether. The petroleum ether layer shows green fluorescence. Black catechu gives negative test.
2. *Vanillin-Hydrochloric Acid Test:* Drug shows pink or red colour with a mixture of vanillin:alcohol:dilute HCl in the ratio 1:10:10. The reaction produces phloroglucinol which along with vanillin gives pink or red colour.
3. A matchstick dipped in decoction of pale catechu is air dried and again dipped into concentrated HCl and warmed near the burner. Pink or purple colour is produced.
4. Small quantity of powder is heated on water bath with 5 ml chloroform and filtered. The filtrate is evaporated in white porcelain dish on a water bath. A greenish-yellow residue is produced due to the presence of chlorophyll in the drug. Black catechu gives this test negative due to the absence of chlorophyll.

Uses

Pale catechu is medicinally used as local astringent. In diarrhoea, it is used as general astringent. It is largely used in various countries of east for chewing with betel leaf. Large proportion of gambier is used in dyeing and tanning industries. It is used for tanning of animal hides to convert it to leather.

BLACK CATECHU

Synonym

Cutch, black catechu, kattha.

Biological Source

Black catechu is the dried aqueous extract prepared from the heartwood of *Acacia catechu* Willdenow, belonging to family, Leguminosae (Fig. 20.16).

Geographical Source

A. catechu is common throughout the tract from Punjab to Assam ascending to an altitude of 300 m. It is also quite common in drier regions of peninsula such as Madhya Pradesh, Maharashtra, Gujarat, Rajasthan, Bihar and Tamil Nadu.

History

Possibly, the use of black catechu could be traced back in history from the time of chewing betel leaf, in which it has been used as adjuvant. In old days, it was used by women

as a colouring agent for the feet. Since 15th century, this natural material has been exported to Europe. The old information about catechu is by a Portuguese writer Garcia de Orta in 1574. Dr. Wrath first used the scientific process to extract catechu, and showed that catechu consists of two parts, such as, kattha and cutch.

Collection and Preparation

A. catechu is a medium-sized tree with thorns. For preparation of the drug the tree is cut off from the ground. The main trunk and branches are cleared of foliage and thorns. The bark is stripped off, and the heartwood is made into chips. Heartwood is boiled in water in large earthen pots. The decoction is then strained and boiled in an iron pot with continuous stirring till it forms the syrupy mass. When the extract is cool enough, it is spread in the shallow wooden trays and kept for over night. When sufficiently dry, it is cut into pieces. Since the decoction is concentrated in iron vessels, the colour of the catechu becomes darker due to its reaction with iron salts. If the syrupy extract is stirred during cooling, it develops the shining crystals of catechin and produces translucent black catechu. Nowadays stainless steel vessels are used for the manufacture of catechu that produces a lighter coloured product.

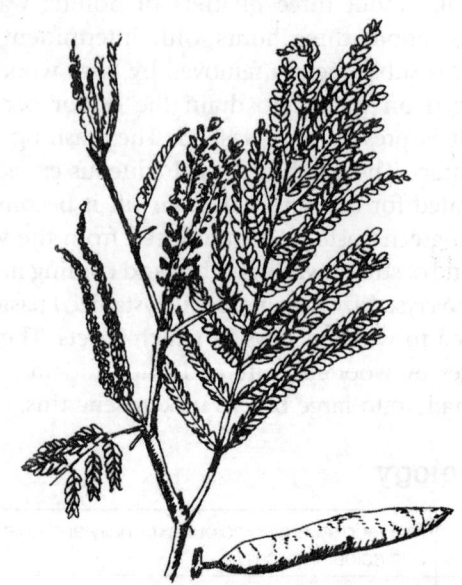

FIG. 20.16 Twig of black catechu

Morphology

Colour	Black or brownish black mass
Odour	Odourless
Taste	Astringent and subsequently sweet taste
Size	Irregular mass
Extra features	Outer surface is firm and brittle. When broken the fractured surface appears glassy with small cavities

Microscopy

A transverse section of *A. catechu* heartwood shows numerous uniseriate and biseriate medullary rays, with vessels occurring isolated or in small groups of two or four. Xylem fibres with narrow lumen occupy major portion of wood and xylem parenchyma is usually predominantly paratracheal, forming a sheath around vessels. Wood consists of crystal fibres having prismatic crystals of calcium oxalate. A few tracheids with scalariform thickening and some cells including vessels are also present.

Chemical Constituents

Cutch or black catechu resembles pale catechu or gambier in its composition. It contains about 2–12% of catechin and about 25–33% of phlobatannin catechutannic acid. The principle fraction of cutch has been identified as a mixture of catechin isomers which includes (–)epicatechin, catechin, DL-acacatechin, L-acacatechin and D-isoacacatechin. It also contains 20–30% gummy matter, catechin red, quercetin and querecitin. It yields 2–3% of ash.

Catechin

Catechol

Chemical Tests

1. Because of the presence of catechin, black catechu gives pink or red colour with vanillin and HCl.
2. Catechin when treated with HCl produces phlorogucinol, which burns along with lignin to give purple or magenta colour. For this purpose, tannin extract is taken on match stick dipped in HCl and heated near the flame.
3. Lime water when added to aqueous extract of black catechu gives brown colour, which turns to red precipitate on standing for some time.
4. Green colour is produced when ferric ammonium sulphate is added to dilute solution of black catechu. By the addition of sodium hydroxide, the green colour turns to purple.

Uses

Cutch is used in medicine as astringent. It cures troubles of mouth, diseases of the throat and diarrhoea. It also increases appetite. In India and eastern countries, it is used in betel leaves for chewing. In dyeing industries, cutch is used for dyeing fabrics brown or black. It is also used in calico printing.

Marketed Products

It is one of the ingredients of the preparation known as Koflet lozenge (Himalaya Drug Company) as cough expectorant, and Gum tone (Charak Pharma Pvt. Ltd.).

PTEROCARPUS

Synonyms

Bijasal, Indian kino tree, Malbar kino.

Biological Source

It consists of dried juice obtained by making vertical incisions to the stem bark of the plant *Pterocarpus marsupium* Linn., belonging to family Leguminosae (Fig. 20.17).

Geographical Distribution

It is found in hilly regions of Gujarat, Madhya Pradesh, Uttar Pradesh, Bihar and Orissa. It is also found in forests of Karnal, Kerala, West Bengal and Assam.

Morphology

Colour	Ruby-red
Odour	Odourless
Taste	Astringent
Shape	Angular grains
Size	3 to 5 to 10 mm granules
Solubility	It is partly soluble in water (about 80—90%), completely soluble in alcohol (90%)
Extra features	The pieces of kino are angular, glistening, transparent, breaking with vitreous fracture

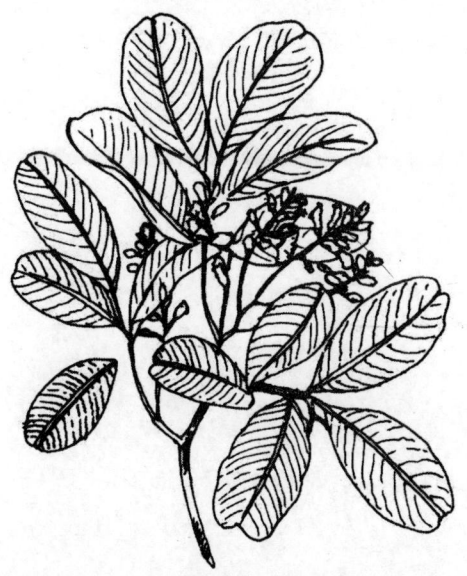

FIG. 20.17 *Pterocarpus marsupium*

Chemical Constituents

Kino contains about 70–80% of kinotannic acid, kino-red, *k*-pyrocatechin (catechol), resin and gallic acid. Kinotannic acid is glucosidal tannin, whereas kino-red is anhydride of kinoin. Kinoin is an insoluble phlobaphene and is produced by the action of oxydase enzyme. It is darker in colour than kinotannic acid.

Chemical Tests

1. When the solution of drug is treated with ferrous sulphate, green colour is produced.
2. With alkali (like potassium hydroxide) violet colour is produced.
3. With mineral acid, a precipitate is obtained.

Uses

Kino is used as powerful astringent and also in the treatment of diarrhoea and dysentery, passive haemorrhage, toothache and diabetes. It is used in dyeing, tanning and printing. The aqueous infusion of the wood is considered to be of much use in diabetes. The alcoholic, as well as, aqueous extracts of heartwood are known to possess hypoglycaemic action. The cups made of wood are available with Khadi and Gramodyog commission for treatment of diabetes.

Marketed Products

It is the one of the components of the preparation known as Gludibit (Lupin Herbal Laboratory) and Diabecon (Himalaya Drug Company) for diabetes mellitus.

Enzymes and Protein Drugs

CONTENTS

21.1. ENZYMES

Enzymes are organic catalysts produced in the body by living organisms. They perform many complex chemical reactions that make up life processes. Enzymes are lifeless and when isolated, they still exert their characteristic catalytic effect. Their chemical composition varies, and they do show several common properties. They are colloids, soluble in water and dilute alcohol but are precipitated by concentrated alcohol. Most enzymes act best at temperatures between 35 and 40°C; temperatures above 65°C, especially in the presence of moisture, destroy them, whereas their activity is negligible at 0°C. Certain heavy metals, formaldehyde and free iodine retard the enzymes activity. Their activity is markedly affected by the pH of the medium in which they act or by the presence of other substances in this medium. They are highly selective in their action.

The enzymes are proteins having molecular weight from about 13,000 to 840,000. At present they are divided according to their action by a complex system established by the Commission on Enzymes of the International Union of Biochemistry. Six major classes are recognized; each has 4–13 subclasses, and each enzyme is assigned a systematic code number (B.C.) composed of 4 digits. The major classes are given in table 21.1.

Enzymes are found in combination with inorganic or organic substances that have an important part in the catalytic action. If these are nonprotein organic compounds, they are known as coenzymes. If they are inorganic ions, they are referred to as activators. Coenzymes are integral components of a large number of enzyme systems. Several vitamins (thiamine, riboflavin, nicotinic acid) have a coenzymatic function.

Enzymes are obtained from plant and animal cells and many have been purified. They are used as therapeutic agents and as controlling factors in certain chemical reactions in industry. Pepsin, pancreatin and papain are used therapeutically as digestants. Hyaluronidase facilitates the diffusion of injected fluids. Streptokinase and streptodornase dissolve clotted blood and purulent accumulations. Zymase and rennin are used in the fermentation and cheese industries; and penicillinase inactivates the various penicillins.

KEY TERMS

Table 21.1 International classification of enzymes

No.	Class	Type of reaction catalysed	Examples
1.	Oxi-doreductases	Transfer of electrons (hydride ions or H atoms)	Dehydrogenases, oxidases
2.	Transferases	Group transfer reactions	Transaminase, kinases
3.	Hydrolases	Hydrolysis reactions (transfer of functional groups to water)	Estrases, digestive enzymes
4.	Lyases	Addition of groups to double bonds or formation of double bonds by removal of groups	Phosphohexoisomerase, fumarase
5.	Isomerases	Transfer of groups within molecules to yield isomeric forms	Decarboxylases, aldolases
6.	Ligases	Formation of C–C, C–S, C–O and C–N bonds by condensation reactions coupled to ATP cleavage	Citric acid synthetase

The names used to designate enzymes usually end in -*ase* or -*in*. The important enzymes are given hereunder.

Properties of Enzymes

1. Enzymes are sensitive to heat and are denatured by excess heat or cold, i.e. their active site becomes permanently warped, thus the enzyme is unable to form an enzyme substrate complex. This is what happens when you fry an egg, the egg white (augmentin, a type of protein, not an enzyme), is denatured.
2. Enzymes are created in cells but are capable of functioning out side of the cell. This allows the enzymes to be immobilized, without killing them.
3. Enzymes are sensitive to pH, the rate at which they can conduct reaction is dependent upon the pH of where the reaction is taking place, for example, pepsin in the stomach has an optimum pH of about 2, whereas salivary amylase has an optimum pH of about 7.
4. Enzymes are reusable and some enzymes are capable of catalysing many hundreds of thousands of reactions, for example, catalase working on hydrogen peroxide, try putting some liver into hydrogen peroxide.
5. Enzymes will only catalyse one reaction, for example, invertase will only produce glucose and fructose, when a glucose solution is passed over beads of enzyme.
6. Enzymes are capable of working in reverse, this act as a cut off point for the amount of product being produced. If there are excess reactants, the reaction will keep going and be reversed, so that there is no overload or build up of product.

DIASTASE

Synonym

Amylase.

Biological Source

It is an amylolytic enzymes present in the saliva (salivary diastase or ptyalin and pancreatic diastase or amylopsin) found in the digestive tract of animals and also in malt extract. Diastase hydrolyses starch, glycogen and dextrin to form in all three instances glucose, maltose and the limit dextrin. Salivary amylase is known as ptyalin; although humans have this enzyme in their saliva, some mammals, such as horses, dogs and cats, do not. Ptyalin begins polysaccharide digestion in the mouth; the process is completed in the small intestine by the pancreatic amylase, sometimes called amylopsin. The amylase of malt digests barley starch to the disaccharides that are attacked by yeast in the fermentation process.

Description

Colour	Yellowish white
Odour	Characteristic
Nature	Amorphous powder
Solubility	Forms a colloidal solution with water, it precipitates in alcohol
Extra features	Thermolabile and denatures at a temperature above 45°C and a pH less than 4. Best active at temperature 35–40°C and pH of 6–7

Uses

It is used as a digestant, used in the production of predigested starchy foods and also for the conversion of starch to fermentable sugars in fermentation.

PEPSIN

Biological Source

It is the enzyme prepared from the mucous membrane of the stomach of various animals like pig, sheep or calf. The commonly used species of pig is *Sus scrofa* Linn, belonging to family Suidae.

The stomach consists of an outer muscular layer and an inner mucous layer. The inner surface is covered with a single layer of epithelial cells which also lines the piths present on them. The piths are about 0.2 mm in diameter, and each pith has two to three narrow tubular ducts opening at the base. The epithelial layer is made of either the parietal cell or the central cell. The central cells are mainly covered with almost cubical shape and secrete pepsinogen and rennin zymogen, whereas the parietal cells are round or oval shaped cells, and they secrete the hydrochloric acid to activate the zymogen to produce rennin and pepsin. Pepsin is the first in a series of enzymes that digest proteins. Pepsin binds with protein chains and breaks it up into small pieces. Pepsin cleaves proteins preferentially at carboxylic groups of aromatic amino acids such as phenylalanine and tyrosine but does not cleave at bonds containing amino acids like valine or alanine. Pepsin mainly cleaves C-terminal to F, L and E, and it does not cleave at V-, A- or G-terminals. Structurally, the active site is located in a deep cleft within the molecule. Optimal activity of pepsin is at pH of 1.8 –3.5, depending on the isoform. They are reversibly inactivated at about pH 5 and irreversibly inactivated at pH 7–8.

Preparation

The mucous membrane is separated from the stomach either by the process of stripping or it is scrapped off, and it is placed in acidified water for autolysis at 37°C for 2 hours. The liquid obtained after autolysis consist of both pepsin and peptone. It is then filtered and sodium or ammonium salts are added to the liquid till it is half saturated. At this point only the pepsin separates out, and the peptone remains in the solution. The precipitates are collected and subjected to dialysis for the separation of salts. Remaining amount of pepsin if any in the aqueous solution is precipitated by the addition of alcohol into it. The pepsin is collected and dried at low temperature.

Description

Pepsin occurs in pale yellow colour, they are odourless or with very faint odour, translucent grains and slightly bitter in taste. It is soluble in dilute acids, water and physiological salt (NaCl) solution. It is best active at a temperature of 40°C with pH 2–4. Pepsin is unstable above pH 6. The enzyme gets denatured at a temperature of 70°C and in the presence of alcohol and sodium chloride. Pepsin can be stored for 1–2 years at 2–8°C.

Uses

It is used in the deficiency of gastric secretion. Pepsin is also used in the laboratory analysis of various proteins; in the preparation of cheese, and other protein-containing foods.

PANCREATIN

Pancreatin is a digestive enzyme extracted from the pancreas of certain animals like hog, *Sus scrofa* (Suidae) or ox, *Bos taurus* (Bovidae) that is used to supplement loss of or low digestive enzymes, often used in people with cystic fibrosis. It is also known as pancreatinum and pancreatic enzymes.

Pancreatin is made up of the pancreatic enzymes trypsin, amylase and lipase. Pancreatin is very similar to another enzyme known as pancrelipase. The primary difference between these two enzymes is that pancrelipase contains more active lipase enzyme than pancreatin. The trypsin found in pancreatin works to hydrolyse proteins to oligopeptides, amylase hydrolyses starches to oligosaccharides and the disaccharide maltose, and lipase hydrolyses triglycerides to fatty acids and glycerols.

Pancreatin is an effective enzyme supplement for replacing missing pancreatic enzymes used in a number of essential body processes.

Pancreatin enzymes have two important functions in the body: digestion of foods and routine cancer eradication. Pancreatin is a mix of many different enzymes and those involved in the digestion of proteins are also used to help eliminate cancers that occur. Cancer is often a disease of protein metabolism because the pancreatin enzyme cancer defence mechanism can be overwhelmed by consuming protein rich foods at inappropriate times or in excessive amounts. The body needs a time span each day approaching 12 hours or more without protein consumption for its pancreatin cancer defence mechanism to work optimally. Pancreatin enzymes can be made ineffective by contact with acids or alcohols. A diet comprised mostly of refined foods and meats may result in an acidic body chemistry that depletes these enzymes. Cancer, once established, ensures its survival by continuously generating acid as it inefficiently metabolizes food. Consuming alcoholic beverages can also interfere with the defence mechanism. Many popular cosmetics that contain acids or alcohols are a special concern for skin cancer. Mercury leakage from amalgam tooth fillings is also debilitating too many enzyme functions. It has also been claimed to help with food allergies, celiac disease, autoimmune disease, cancer and weight loss.

TRYPSIN

Biological Source

Trypsin is a proteolytic enzyme produced by Ox pancreas, *Bos taurus*, belonging to family Bovidae.

It is one of the three principal digestive proteinases which along with other proteinases like pepsin and chymotrypsin break the dietary protein molecules to their amino acids and peptide component. Trypsin cleaves proteins at the carboxyl side like 'C-terminals' of the basic amino acids lysine and arginine. Trypsin is an endopeptidase which cleavage occurs within the polypeptide chain and not the terminal amino acids located at the ends of polypeptides. The aspartate residue located in trypsin is responsible for attracting and stabilizing positively charged lysine and/or arginine.

Production

Trypsin is produced by pancreas in the form of trypsinogen. Trypsin is then transported to the small intestine, where the proteins are cleaved into polypeptides and amino acids. As trypsin is an autocatalytic enzyme, it by itself catalyses the conversion of trypsinogen to trypsin. Another enzyme (enterokinase) is also required in small amount to catalyse the initial reaction of trypsinogen to trypsin.

Process of digestion by trypsin gets started in stomach and is continued to the small intestine where the environment is slightly alkaline. Trypsin has maximum enzymatic activity at pH 8.

Chemical Composition

It has a similar structure as that of other pancreatic proteinase like chymotrypsin and also has the similar mechanisms of action. They differ only in their specificity. Trypsin is active against peptide bonds in protein molecules that have carboxyl groups donated by amino acids like the arginine and lysine, whereas chymotrypsin are active against the carboxyl group denoted by tyrosine, phenylalanine, tryptophan, methionine and leucine. Trypsin is considered the exceptional of all other proteolytic enzyme due to its attack on restricted number of chemical bonds. Trypsin is widely employed as a reagent for the orderly and unambiguous cleavage of proteins in which amino-acid sequence is to be determined.

Uses

In a tissue culture lab, trypsin is used to resuspend cells adherent to the petri dish wall during the process of harvesting cells. It is also used to harvest corn and oats. Trypsin is vital in a cow's diet, without it they would not be able to digest the grass they eat.

HYALURONIDASE

Synonym

Spreading factor, hyalase.

Biological Source

Hyaluronidase is an enzyme product prepared from mammalian testes which shows the capability of hydrolysing hyaluronic acid like mucopolysaccharides. Skin is considered as the largest store of hyaluronidase in the body.

Preparation

Hyaluronidase enzyme is found in type-II *Pneumococci*, in group A and C haemolytic *streptococci*, *S. aureus* and *Clostridium welchii*. Hyaluronidase manufacturers define their product in terms of turbidity reducing (TR) units or

in viscosity units. Prepared solution for injection usually contains 150 TR units or 500 viscosity units dissolved in 1 ml. of isotonic NaCl solution.

Characteristics

Hyaluronidase for injection consists of not more than 0.25 μg of tyrosine for each USP hyaluronidase unit. Due to its action on hyaluronic acid, it promotes diffusion and hastens absorption of subcutaneous infusions. It depolymerises and catalyses hyaluronic acid and similar hexosamine-containing polysaccharides.

Chemical Constituents

Hyaluronidases are a group of enzymes such as 4-lycanohydrolase, hyaluronate 3-glycanohydrolase and hyaluronate lyase. They are mucopeptides composed of alternating *N*-acetylglucosamine and glucuronic acid residues. Hyaluronidases catalyse the breakdown of hyaluronic acid.

Uses

Hyaluronidase for injection is used in the conditions of hypodermoclysis. It is used as a spreading and diffusing agent. It promotes diffusion, absorption and reabsorption.

UROKINASE

Synonym

Uroquinase.

Biological Source

Urokinase is serine protease enzyme isolated from human urine and from human kidney cells by tissue culture or by recombinant DNA technology.

Preparation

Urokinase is a fibrinolytic enzyme produced by recombinant DNA using genetically manipulated *E. coli* cells. It is produced firstly as prourokinase q.v. and then converted to active form by plasmin or kallikrein. Urokinase used medicinally is also purified directly from human urine. It binds to a range of adsorbents such as silica gel or kaolin which can be use to initially concentrate and purify the product. It can be further purified by precipitation with sodium chloride or ethanol or by chromatography. Human urokinase needs sterile filtration, a septic filling and freeze drying.

Characteristics

Urokinase enzyme occurs in two different forms as single and double polypeptide chain forms. It has a half-life of

10–16 minutes after intravenous administration. These enzymes act on an endogenous fibrinolytic system.

Chemical Constituents

Urokinase enzymes are serine proteases that occur as a single low molecular weight (33 kDa) and double, high molecular weight (54 kDa) polypeptide chain forms. They differ in molecular weight considerably. A single chain is produced by recombinant DNA technique and is known as SCUPA.

Uses

Urokinase is used in the treatment of pulmonary embolism, coronary artery thrombosis and for restoring the potency of intravenous catheters. It is generally administered intravenously in a dose of 4400 units/kg body weight per hour for twelve hours.

STREPTOKINASE

Synonym

Plasminokinase.

Biological Source

Estreptokinase, plasminokinase is a purified bacterial protein produced from the strains of group C β-haemolytic *S. griseus*.

Preparation

Streptokinase is a bacterial derived enzyme of serine protease group. The ancestral protease activity lies within the first 230 amino-acid residues at the N-terminal part of the protein that evolves from serine protease due to the replacement of histamine at 57th amino acid by glycine. The amino terminal residue polypeptide chain shows sequence homology to serine protease. Duplication and fusion of gene generate an ancestral streptokinase gene. Streptokinase is produced by fermentation using streptococcal culture and is isolated from the culture filtrate. It is produced in the form of a lyophilized powder in sterile vials containing 250,000 to 750,000 IUs.

Characteristics

Streptokinase is a bacterial protein with half-life of 23 minutes. Its anisolylated plasminogen activator complex (APSAC) has a higher half-life of six hours.

Chemical Constituents

Streptokinase is the purified bacterial protein with about 484 amino-acid residues.

Uses

Streptokinase is the first available agent for dissolving blood clots. It binds to plasminogen in a 1:1 ratio and changes molecular conformation. Thus, the complex formed becomes an active enzyme and promotes the activity of fibrinolytic enzyme plasmin. Plasmin breaks fibrin clots. Anistreptase or the anisolylated plasminogen streptokinase activator complex (APSAC) can also be used in a similar way for degrading blood clots. Streptokinase and anistreptase are both used in the treatment of pulmonary embolism, venous, and arterial thrombosis and coronary artery thrombosis. It is also sometimes administered along with heparin to counter act a paradoxical increase in local thrombin.

BROMELIN

Synonyms

Bromelin, bromelain.

Biological Source

Bromelin is a mixture of proteolytic enzymes isolated from the juice of *Ananas comosus* (pineapple), belonging to family Bromeliaceae (Fig. 21.1).

Geographical Source

Pineapple is a native of tropical America. It is grown in almost all parts of the world including India, China, Thailand, United States, Brazil, Philippines, Mexico, Hawaii and Taiwan.

Cultivation, Collection and Preparation

Bromelin is found in pineapple fruit juice and stem. Pineapple is perennial, and it does not have a natural period of dormancy. It is propagated through suckers, slips and crowns. In India it is planted in August, the plant generally flowers in February–March, and the fruit ripens during July–October.

The fruits must be left on the plant to ripen for the full flavour to develop. Dark green unripe fruits gradually change to yellow and finally to deep orange. The fruits are cut off. The enzyme bromelin does not disappear as the fruit ripens. The enzyme from fruit and stem are known as fruit bromelin and stem bromelin, respectively. It is isolated from pineapple juice by precipitation with acetone and also with ammonium sulphide.

Characteristics

The optimum pH of bromelain is 5.0–8.0. In solution pH below 3.0 and above 9.5 inactivates the enzyme. The optimum temperature is between 50 and 60°C, still it is effective between 20 and 65°C too. The moisture content should not exceed 6%. It is obtained in light brown-coloured powder.

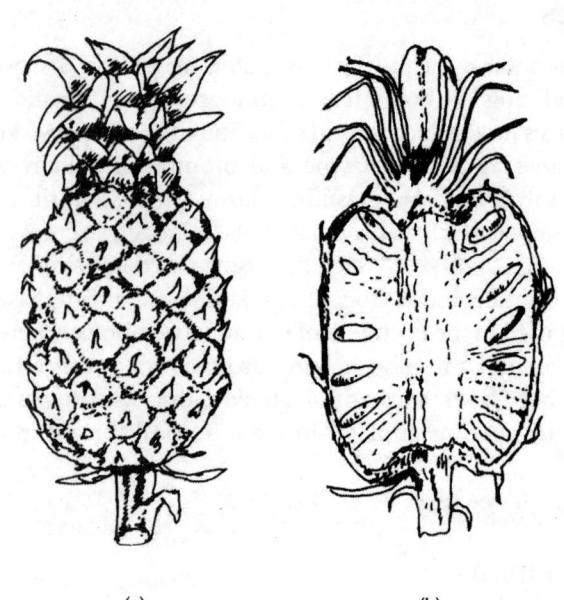

FIG. 21.1 (a) Whole fruit and (b) T.S. of fruit of *Ananas comosus*

Chemical Constituents

Bromelain is not a single substance, but rather a collection of enzymes and other compounds. It is a mixture of sulphur-containing protein-digesting enzymes, called proteolytic enzymes or proteases. It also contains several other substances in smaller quantities, including peroxidase, acid phosphatase, protease inhibitors and calcium.

Uses

Bromelain is an effective fibrinolytic agent; bromelain inhibits platelet aggregation and seems to have both direct as well as indirect actions involving other enzyme systems in exerting its anti-inflammatory effect. Antibiotic potentiation is one of the primary uses of bromelain in several foreign countries; it can modify the permeability of organs and tissues to different drugs. The potentiation of antibiotics and other medicines by bromelain may be due to enhanced absorption, as well as increased permeability of the diseased tissue which enhances the access of the antibiotic to the site of the infection. It is also thought that the use of bromelain may provide a similar access to specific and nonspecific components of the immune system, therefore, enhancing the body's utilization of its own healing resources. Bromelain has been used successfully as a digestive enzyme following pancreatectomy, in cases of exocrine pancreas insufficiency and in other intestinal disorders. Research has indicated that bromelain prevents or minimizes the severity of angina pectoris and transient ischemic attacks (TIA); it is useful in the prevention and treatment of thrombosis

and thrombophlebitis. If administered for prolonged time periods, bromelain also exerts an antihypertensive effect in experimental animals. It may even be useful in the treatment of AIDS to stop the spread of HIV. It has no major side effects, except for possible allergic reactions.

SERRATIOPEPTIDASE

Synonym

Serrapeptase, serratiopeptidase.

Biological Source

Serratiopeptidase is a proteolytic enzyme isolated from nonpathogenic enterobacteria *Serratia* E 15. It is also produced by the larval form of the silk moth.

Preparation

Serratiopeptidase is produced by fermentation technology by using nonpathogenic enterobacteria species such as *Serratia* E 15. The larvae of silk moth produce this enzyme in their intestine to break down cocoon walls. It can thus be obtained from the silk moth larvae.

Characteristics

Serratiopeptidase is very much vulnerable to degradation in the acidic pH. When consumed in unprotected tablet or capsule, it is destroyed by acid in stomach. However enteric coated tablets facilitate its absorption through intestine. One unit of the enzyme hydrolyses casein to produce colour equivalent to 1.0 µmol of tyrosine per minute at pH 7.5 and 35°C.

Chemical Constituents

Serratiopeptidase is a proteolytic enzyme of protease type XXVI. The preparation contains 7.1 units/mg solid.

Uses

Serratiopeptidase is the most widely prescribed anti-inflammatory enzyme in developed countries and also in India. It eliminates inflammatory oedema and swelling, accelerate liquefaction of pus and sputum, and enhance the action of antibodies. It is also used as a fast wound healing agent. It is proving to be a superior alternative to the nonsteroidal anti-inflammatory drugs traditionally used to treat rheumatoid arthritis and osteoarthritis. It has wide ranging applications in trauma surgery, plastic surgery, respiratory medicine, obstetric and gynaecology.

PAPAIN

Synonyms

Papayotin, vegetable pepsin, tromasin, arbuz.

Biological Source

Papain is the dried and purified latex of the green fruits and leaves of *Carica papaya* L., belonging to family Caricaceae (Fig. 21.2).

The plant is cultivated in Sri Lanka, Tanzania, Hawaii and Florida. The plant is 5–6 m in height bearing fruits of about 30 cm length and a weight up to 5 kg. The epicarp adheres to the orange-coloured, fleshy sarcocarp, which surrounds the central cavity. This cavity contains a mass of nearly black seeds.

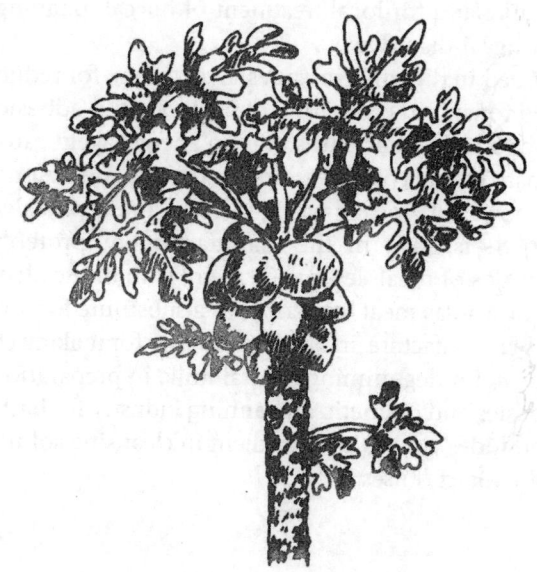

FIG. 21.2 Plant of *Carica papaya*

Preparation

It is distributed throughout the plant, but mostly concentrated in the latex of the fruit.

The latex is obtained by making two to four longitudinal incisions, about 1/8 inch deep, on the surface on four sides of nearly mature but green fruits while still on the tree. The incisions are made early in the morning, at intervals of three to seven days. The latex flows freely for a few seconds but soon coagulates. The exudate is collected in nonmetallic containers. The latex is dried as soon as possible after collection. Rapid drying or exposure to sun or higher temperature above 38°C produce dark colour product with weak in proteolytic activity. The use of artificial heat yields the better grade of crude papain. The final product should be creamy white and friable. It is sealed in air-tight containers to prevent loss of activity. If 10% common salt or 1% solution of formaldehyde is added before drying, the product retains its activity for many months.

Fully grown fruits give more latex of high enzyme potency than smaller or immature fruits. The yield of papain varies from 20 to 250 g per tree. The yield of commercial papain from latex is about 20%.

Characteristics

Papain occurs as white or greyish-white, slightly hygroscopic powder. It is incompletely soluble in water and glycerol. It may digest about 35 times its weight of lean meat. Best grades render digestion of 200–300 times their weight of coagulated egg albumin in alkaline media. A temperature range of 60–90°C is favourable for the digestive process with 65°C the optimum point. Best pH is 5.0, but it functions also in neutral or alkaline media. It is activated by reduction (HCN and H_2S) and inactivated by oxidation (H_2O_2, iodoacetate).

Chemical Constituents

Papain contains several enzymes such as proteolytic enzymes peptidase I capable of converting proteins into dipeptides and polypeptides, rennin-like enzyme, clotting enzyme similar to pectase and an enzyme having a feeble activity on fats.

The enzymes, papain, papaya proteinase and chymopapain, have been isolated in crystalline form from the latex. Papain is atypical protein digesting enzyme with isoelectric point. It contains 15.5% nitrogen and 1.2% sulphur. Crystalline papain is most stable in the pH range 5–7 and is rapidly destroyed at 30°C below pH 2.5 and above pH 12. Papain is a protein of 212 amino acids and having a molecular weight of about 23,000 daltons. It is resistant to heat, inactivated by metal ions, oxidants and reagents which react with thiols, and is an endopeptidase activated by thiols and reducing moieties, for example, cysteine, thiosulphate and glutathione.

The leaves possess dehydrocarpaines I and II, fatty acids, carpaine, pseudocarpaine and carotenoids.

The fruits yield lauric, myristoleic, palmitoleic and arachidic acids, malonated benzyl-*p-o*-glucosides, 2-phenyl ethyl glucoside and 4-hydroxy-phenyl-2-ethyl glucoside.

Uses

Papain is used to prevent adhesions; in infected wounds; internally as protein digestant, as anathematic (nematode), to relieve the symptoms of episiotomy (incision of vulva), in meat industry for tenderizing beef, for treatment of dyspepsia, intestinal and gastric disorders, and diphtheria, for dissolving diphtheria membrane; in surgery to reduce incidence of blood clots where thromboplasma is undesirable and for local treatment of buccal, pharyngeal and laryngeal disorders.

It is used in digestive mixtures, liver tonics, for reducing enlarged tonsils, in prevention of postoperative adhesions, curbuncles and eschar burns. It is an allergic agent causing severe paroxysmal cough, vasomotor rhinitis and dyspnoea. It is a powerful poison when injected intravenously. In industry it is used in the manufacture of proteolytic preparations of meat, lever and casein, with dilute alcohol and lactic acid as meat tenderizer, as a substitute for rennet in cheese manufacture, in brewing industry for making chill-proof bear, for degumming natural milk, in preparation of tooth pastes and cosmetics, in tanning industry for bathing skin and hides, and as an ingredient in cleansing solutions for soft contact lenses.

Test

Papain is reacted with a gelatin solution at 80°C in the presence of an activating cysteine chloral hydrate solution for an hour. The solution is cooled to 4°C for long time. The treated solution must not regel in comparison to a blank solution under identical conditions.

Adulteration

Commercial papain is often adulterated with arrowroot starch, dried milk of cactus, gutta percha, rice flour and pepsin.

21.2. PROTEINS

A protein is a complex, high molecular weight organic compound that consists of amino acids joined by peptide bonds. The word protein is derived from Greek *'protos'* meaning *'of primary importance'*. Proteins are essential to the structure and function of all living cells. Many proteins are enzymes or subunits of enzymes. Other proteins play structural or mechanical roles, such as those that form the struts and joints of the cytoskeleton, serving as biological scaffolds for the mechanical integrity and tissue signalling functions.

They are obtained from both plant and animal sources. In plants they are stored in the form of aleurone grains.

In animals they are present in structural material in the form of collagen (connective tissue), keratin (hair, wool, hairs, feathers and horns), elastin (epithelial connective tissue), casein (milk) and plasma proteins. Casein, gelatin, heparin and haemoglobin are pharmaceutically important proteins of animal origin.

Proteins are generally large molecules, having molecular masses of up to 3,000,000 (the muscle protein titin has a single amino-acid chain 27,000 subunits long). However, protein masses are generally measured in kilodaltons

(kDa). Such long chains of amino acids are almost universally referred to as proteins, but shorter strings of amino acids are referred to as 'polypeptides', 'peptides', or rarely, 'oligopeptides'. The dividing line is undefined, though 'polypeptide' usually refers to an amino-acid chain lacking tertiary structure which may be more likely to act as a hormone (like insulin), rather than as an enzyme (which depends on its defined tertiary structure for functionality).

There are about 20 different amino acids, eight of which must be present in the diet. The eight essential amino acids required by humans are leucine, isoleucine, valine, threonine, methionine, phenylalanine, tryptophan and lysine. For children, histidine is also considered to be an essential amino acid. Unlike animal proteins, plant proteins may not contain all the essential amino acids in the necessary proportions, and so the proteins derived from plants are grouped as incomplete and from animals are grouped as complete. However, a varied vegetarian diet means a mixture of proteins are consumed, the amino acids in one protein compensating for the deficiencies of another.

The structure of protein could be differentiated into four types:

1. *Primary Structure:* The amino-acid sequence.
2. *Secondary Structure:* Highly patterned substructures—alpha helix and beta sheet—or segments of chain that assume no stable shape. Secondary structures are locally defined, meaning that there can be many different secondary motifs present in one single protein molecule.
3. *Tertiary Structure:* The overall shape of a single protein molecule; the spatial relationship of the secondary structural motifs to one another
4. *Quaternary Structure:* The shape or structure that results from the union of more than one protein molecule, usually called protein subunits in this context, which function as part of the larger assembly or protein complex.

Proteins are sensitive to their environment. They may only be active in their native state, over a small pH range and under solution conditions with a minimum quantity of electrolytes. A protein in its native state is described as folded and that is not in its native state is said to be denatured. Denatured proteins generally have no well-defined secondary structure. Many proteins denature and will not remain in solution in distilled water also they are denatured due to heat, changes in pH, treatment of organic solvents or by ultra violet radiation.

Proteins are essential for growth and repair. They play a crucial role in virtually all biological processes in the body. All enzymes are proteins and are vital for the body's metabolism. Muscle contraction, immune protection and the transmission of nerve impulses are all dependent on proteins. Proteins in skin and bone provide structural support. Many hormones are proteins. Protein can also provide a source of energy. Generally the body uses carbohydrate and fat for energy but when there is excess dietary protein or inadequate dietary fat and carbohydrate, protein is used. Excess protein may also be converted to fat and stored.

The important proteins are given hereunder.

MALT EXTRACT

Synonym

Diastase, malt extract.

Biological Source

Malt extract is the extract obtained from the dried barley grains of one or more varieties of *Hordeum vulgare* Linne, family Poaceae.

Geographical Source

Barley is widely cultivated throughout the world. The major producers are United States, Russia, Canada, India and Turkey. It is also cultivated in highlands of China and Tibet.

Cultivation, Collection and Preparation

Barley is one of the oldest cultivated cereals. It is an annual erect stout herb resembling wheat. The crop becomes ready for harvest in about four months after sowing. The grains are threshed out by beating with sticks or trampling by oxen. Dried barley grains are artificially germinated by keeping their heaps wet with water in a warm room. When the caulicle of the grains starts protruding out, the germinated grams are dried. Dry germinated barley or dry malt is subjected to extraction. The malt is infused with water at 60°C. An infusion is concentrated below 60°C under reduced pressure and then dried. Less purified malt extract contains sugars, and amylolytic enzymes. Its further purification affords diastase.

Characteristics

Malt extract contains enzymes, which are most active in neutral solution. The acidic conditions destroy the activity. It converts starch into disaccharide maltose. The enzyme is destroyed by heat. Many heat sterilized malt extracts do not contain diastase. It is completely soluble in cold water, more readily in warm water. The aqueous solution shows flocculant precipitate on standing. Limit for arsenic should not exceed one part per million.

Chemical Constituents

Malt extract contains dextrin, maltose, traces of glucose and about 8% of amylolytic enzyme diastase.

Uses

Malt extract and purified diastase, both are used as amylolytic enzymes and as an aid in digesting starch. They are used as bulk producing laxatives.

GELATIN

Synonyms

Gelfoam, puragel, gelatinum.

Biological Source

Gelatin is a protein derivative obtained by evaporating an aqueous extract made from bones, skins and tendons of various domestic animals. Some important sources are Ox, *Bos taurus* and Sheep; *Ovis aries* belonging to family Bovidae.

Preparation

The process of manufacture of gelatin vary from factory to factory. However, the general outline of the process is given below.

Raw material

Bones, skins and tendons of bovideans is collected and subjected to liming operation.

Liming Process

The raw material is first subjected to the treatment known as 'liming'. In this process, the skins and tendons are steeped for fifteen to twenty and sometimes for 40 days in a dilute milk of lime. During this, fleshy matter gets dissolved, chondroproteins of connective tissues gets removed and fatty matter is saponified. The animal skin is further thoroughly washed in running water.

Defatting

In case of bones, the material is properly ground and defatted in close iron cylinders by treatment with organic solvents such as benzene. The mineral and inorganic part of the bone is removed by treatment with hydrochloric acid.

Extraction

The treated material from bones, skins and tendons is boiled with water in open pans with perforated false bottom. This process can also be carried out under reduced pressure. The clear liquid runs of again and again and is evaporated until it reaches to above 45 per cent gelatin content.

Setting

The concentrated gelatin extract is transferred to shallow metal trays or trays with glass bottom. It is allowed to set as a semisolid jelly.

Drying

The jelly is transferred to trays with a perforated wire netting bottom and passed through series of drying compartments of 30–60°C increasing each time with 10°C. About a month is taken for complete drying.

Bleaching

In case of darker colour, finished product is subjected to bleaching by sulphur dioxide. Bleaching affords a light coloured gelatin.

Characteristics

Gelatin occurs as a colourless or slightly yellow, transparent, brittle, practically odourless, tasteless sheet, flakes or course granular powder. In water it swells and absorbs 5–10 times its weight of water to form a gel in solutions below 35–40°C. It is insoluble in cold water and organic solvents, soluble in hot water, glycerol, acetic acid; and is amphoteric. In dry condition it is stable in air, but when moist or in solution, it is attacked by bacteria. The gelatinizing property of gelatin is reduced by boiling for long time. The quality of gelatin is determined on the basis of its jelly strength (bloom strength) with the help of a bloom gelometer. Jelly strength is used in the preparation of suppositories and pessaries.

Commercially two types of gelatin, A and B, are available. Type A has an isoelectric point between pH 7 and 9. It is incompatible with anionic compounds such as acacia, agar and tragacanth. Type B has an isoelectric point between 4.7 and 5, and it is used with anionic mixtures. Gelatin is coloured with a certified colour for manufacturing capsules or for coating of tablets. It may contain various additives.

Chemical Constituents

Gelatin consists of the protein glutin which on hydrolysis gives a mixture of amino acids. The approximate amino-acid contents are glycine (25.5%), alanine (8.7%), valine (2.5%), leucine (3.2%), isoleucine (1.4%), cystine and cysteine (0.1%), methionine (1.0%), tyrosine (0.5%), aspartic acid (6.6%), glutamic acid (11.4%), arginine (8.1%), lysine (4.1%) and histidine (0.8%). Nutritionally, gelatin is an incomplete protein lacking tryptophan. The gelatinizing

compound is known as chondrin and the adhesive nature of gelatin is due to the presence of glutin.

Chemical Tests

1. *Biuret Reaction:* To alkaline solution of a protein (2 ml), a dilute solution of copper sulphate is added. A red or violet colour is formed with peptides containing at least two peptide linkages. A dipeptide does not give this test.
2. *Xanthoproteic Reaction:* Proteins usually form a yellow colour when warmed with concentrated nitric acid. This colour becomes orange when the solution is made alkaline.
3. *Millon's Reaction:* Millon's reagent (mercuric nitrate in nitric acid containing a trace of nitrous acid) usually yields a white precipitate on addition to a protein solution which turns red on heating.
4. *Ninhydrin Test:* To an aqueous solution of a protein an alcoholic solution of ninhydrin is added and then heated. Red to violet colour is formed.
5. On heating gelatin (1 g) with soda lime, smell of ammonia is produced.
6. A solution of gelatin (0.5 g) in water (10 ml) is precipitated to white buff coloured precipitate on addition of few drops of tannic acid (10%).
7. With picric acid gelatin forms yellow precipitate.

Uses

Gelatin is used to prepare pastilles, pastes, suppositories, capsules, pill-coatings, gelatin sponge; as suspending agent, tablet binder, coating agent, as stabilizer, thickener and texturizer in food; for manufacturing rubber substitutes, adhesives, cements, lithographic and printing inks, plastic compounds, artificial silk, photographic plates and films, light filters for mercury lamps, clarifying agent, in hectographic matters, sizing paper and textiles, for inhibiting crystallization in bacteriology, for preparing cultures and as a nutrient.

It forms glycerinated gelatin with glycerin which is used as vehicle and for manufacture of suppositories. Combined with zinc, it forms zinc gelatin which is employed as a topical protectant. As a nutrient, gelatin is used as commercial food products and bacteriologic culture media.

CASEIN

Biological Source

Casein is a proteolytic enzyme obtained from the stomachs of calves. It is extracted from the proteins of the milk; in the milk, casein is structured in voluminous globules. These globules are mainly responsible for the white colour of the milk. According to various species, the casein amount within the total proteins of the milk varies.

The casein content of milk represents about 80% of milk proteins. The principal casein fractions are alpha (s1) and alpha (s2)-caseins, β-casein and κ-casein. The distinguishing property of all casein is their low solubility at pH 4.6. The common compositional factor is that caseins are conjugated proteins, most with phosphate group(s) esterified to serine residues. These phosphate groups are important to the structure of the casein micelle. Calcium binding by the individual caseins is proportional to the phosphate content.

Within the group of caseins, there are several distinguishing features based on their charge distribution and sensitivity to calcium precipitation:

Alpha (s1)-Casein: (molecular weight 23,000; 199 residues, 17 proline residues).

Two hydrophobia regions, containing all the proline residues, separated by a polar region, which contains all but one of eight phosphate groups. It can be precipitated at very low levels of calcium.

Alpha (s2)-Casein: (molecular weight 25,000; 207 residues, 10 prolines).

Concentrated negative charges near N-terminus and positive charges near C-terminus. It can also be precipitated at very low levels of calcium.

β-Casein: (molecular weight 24,000; 209 residues, 35 prolines).

Highly charged N-terminal region and a hydrophobia C-terminal region. Very amphiphilic protein acts like a detergent molecule. Self association is temperature-dependent; will form a large polymer at 20°C but not at 4°C. Less sensitive to calcium precipitation.

κ-Casein: (molecular weight 19,000; 169 residues, 20 prolines).

Very resistant to calcium precipitation, stabilizing other caseins. Rennet cleavage at the Phe 105 – Met 106 bond eliminates the stabilizing ability, leaving a hydrophobia portion, para-κ-casein and a hydrophilic portion called κ-casein glycomacropeptide (GMP), or more accurately, caseinomacropeptide (CMP).

Characteristics

The isoelectric point of casein is 4.6. The purified protein is water insoluble. While it is also insoluble in neutral salt solutions, it is readily dispersible in dilute alkalis and in salt solutions such as sodium oxalate and sodium acetate. Casein does not coagulate on heating. It is precipitated by acids and by a proteolytic enzyme (rennet).

Chemical Constituents

Milk consists of 80% of milk proteins (casein). The major constituents of casein are alpha (s1) and alpha (s2)-caseins, β-casein and kappa-casein. These caseins are conjugated proteins with phosphate group(s) which are esterified into serine residues they have a low solubility at pH 4.6.

Uses

It is used in the manufacture of binders, adhesives, protective coatings, plastics (such as for knife handles and knitting needles), fabrics, food additives and many other products. It is commonly used by bodybuilders as a slow-digesting source of amino acids. There is growing evidence that casein may be addictive for some individuals, particularly those on the autism spectrum or having schizophrenia.

COLLAGEN

Synonym

Ossein.

Biological Source

It is the protein which consists of major portion of white fibres in connective tissues of the animal body specifically, from the tendons, skin, bones and teeth.

Characteristics

The molecule of collagen is similar to three strand rope, each strand consisting of polypeptide chain with molecular weight of 10,000. These three strands are left-handed helices and are wrapped together in a right-handed superhelix. The strands are held together by hydrogen bonds, which give the molecule its strength.

Collagen fibres range from 10 to 100 μm in diameter and visible by microscope as banded structure in the extra cellular matrix of connective tissues.

Chemical Constituents

Glycine and proline are the important amino acids in the central core of the triple helical molecule of collagen. It can be differentiated from other accompanying fibrous proteins like elastin and reticulin. Elastin is highly cross linked hydrophobic protein. Collagen is characterized by the presence of glycine, proline, hydroxyproline and hydroxylysine, and low tyrosine and sulphur contents, whereas elastin contains nonpolar amino acids like valine, isoleucine, and leucine. Various types of collagen exist depending upon the amino-acid sequence. Collagen is converted to gelatin by boiling with water.

Uses

It is used in the preparation of sutures, as a gel in food casings and in photographic emulsions.

FICIN

Biological Source

Ficin is found in the latex of the plants of the Genus Ficus. Commercial ficin is purified from the latex of the fig tree, *Ficus glabatra* or *Ficus carica*.

Refined ficin microgranulate is a protease, which can be used when a degradation of proteolytical stuff is required.

Characteristics

The optimum pH of ficin depends on the substrate and its concentration. Generally the optimum pH is between 5 and 8, although ficin keeps its activity over the range of pH 4–9 at 60°C. Though the optimum temperature of ficin is 45–55°C, it is effective in temperatures between 15 and 60°C. It is obtained as a white to yellow microgranular powder. The moisture content should not exceed 6%.

Uses

It is generally used in alcohol and beer industries, hydrolization of proteins, meat processing, baking industry, pet food, health food, contact lens cleaning. Cancer treatment, antiarthritis, digestive aid, etc.

Fibres, Sutures and Surgical Dressings

22.1. INTRODUCTION

Fibres may be defined as any hair-like raw material directly obtainable from an animal, vegetable or mineral source and convertible into nonwoven fabrics such as felt or paper or, after spinning into yarns, into woven cloth. A natural fibre may be further defined as an agglomeration of cells in which the diameter is negligible in comparison with the length. Although nature abounds in fibrous materials, especially cellulosic types such as cotton, wood, grains and straw, only a small number can be used for textile products or other industrial purposes. Apart from economic considerations, the usefulness of a fibre for commercial purposes is determined by such properties as length, strength, pliability, elasticity, abrasion resistance, absorbency and various surface properties. Most textile fibres are slender, flexible and relatively strong. They are elastic in that they stretch when put under tension and then partially or completely return to their original length when the tension is removed.

22.2. HISTORY

The use of natural fibres for textile materials began before recorded history. The oldest indication of fibre use is probably the discovery of flax and wool fabrics at excavation sites of the Swiss lake dwellers (seventh and sixth centuries B.C.). Several vegetable fibres were also used by prehistoric peoples. Hemp, presumably the oldest cultivated fibre plant, originated in Southeast Asia, then spread to China, where reports of cultivation date to 4500 B.C. The art of weaving and spinning linen was already well developed in Egypt by 3400 B.C., indicating that flax was cultivated sometime before that date. Reports of the spinning of cotton in India date back to 3000 B.C. The manufacture of silk and silk products originated in the highly developed Chinese culture; the invention and development of sericulture (cultivation of silkworms for raw-silk production) and of methods to spin silk date from 2640 B.C.

With improved transportation and communication, highly localized skills and arts connected with textile manufacture spread to other countries and were adapted to local needs and capabilities. New fibre plants were also discovered and their use explored. In the 18th and 19th centuries, the Industrial Revolution encouraged the further invention of machines for use in processing various natural fibres, resulting in a tremendous upsurge in fibre production. The introduction of regenerated cellulosic fibres (fibres formed of cellulose material that has been dissolved, purified and extruded), such as rayon, followed by the invention of completely synthetic fibres, such as nylon, challenged the monopoly of natural fibres for textile and industrial use. A variety of synthetic fibres having specific desirable properties began to penetrate and dominate markets previously monopolized by natural fibres. Recognition of the competitive threat from synthetic fibres resulted in intensive research directed towards the breeding of new and better strains of natural-fibre sources with higher yields, improved production and processing methods, and modification of fibre yarn or fabric properties. The considerable improvements achieved have permitted increased total production, although natural fibres' actual share of the market has decreased with the influx of the cheaper, synthetic fibres requiring fewer man hours for production.

22.3. CLASSIFICATION AND PROPERTIES

Natural fibres can be classified according to their origin.

1. The vegetable, or cellulose-base, class includes such important fibres as cotton, flax and jute.
2. The animal, or protein-base, fibres include wool, mohair and silk.
3. Regenerated and synthetic fibres include nylon, terylene, orlon, viscose, alginate fibres, etc.
4. An important fibre in the mineral class is asbestos.

The vegetable fibres can be divided into smaller groups, based on their origin within the plant. Cotton, kapok and coir are examples of fibres originating as hairs borne on the seeds or inner walls of the fruit, where each fibre consists of a single, long, narrow cell. Flax, hemp, jute and ramie are bast fibres, occurring in the inner bast tissue of certain plant stems and made up of overlapping cells. Abaca, henequen and sisal are fibres occurring as part of the fibrovascular system of the leaves.

Chemically, all vegetable fibres consist mainly of cellulose, although they also contain varying amounts of such substances as hemicellulose, lignin, pectins and waxes that must be removed or reduced by processing. The animal fibres consist exclusively of proteins and, with the exception of silk, constitute the fur or hair that serves as the protective epidermal covering of animals. Silk filaments

are extruded by the larvae of moths and are used to spin their cocoons.

With the exception of mineral fibres, all natural fibres have an affinity for water in both liquid and vapour form. This strong affinity produces swelling of the fibres connected with the uptake of water, which facilitates dyeing in watery solutions.

Unlike most synthetic fibres, all natural fibres are nonthermoplastic—that is, they do not soften when heat is applied. At temperatures below the point at which they will decompose, they show little sensitivity to dry heat, and there is no shrinkage or high extensibility upon heating, nor do they become brittle if cooled to below freezing. Natural fibres tend to yellow upon exposure to sunlight and moisture, and extended exposure results in loss of strength.

All natural fibres are particularly susceptible to microbial decomposition, including mildew and rot. Cellulosic fibres are decomposed by aerobic bacteria (those that live only in oxygen) and fungi. Cellulose mildews and decomposes rapidly at high humidity and high temperatures, especially in the absence of light. Wool and silk are also subject to microbial decomposition by bacteria and moulds. Animal fibres are also subject to damage by moths and carpet beetles; termites and silverfish attack cellulose fibres. Protection against both microbial damage and insect attacks can be obtained by chemical modification of the fibre substrate; modern developments allow treatment of natural fibres to make them essentially immune to such damage.

VEGETABLE FIBRES

COTTON

Synonyms

Raw cotton, purified cotton, absorbent cotton.

Biological Source

Epidermal trichomes of the seeds of cultivated species of the *Gossypium herbaceum* and other species of *Gossypium* (*G. hirsutum, G. barbadense*) freed from impurities, fats and sterilized, belonging to family Malvaceae.

Geographical Source

United States, Egypt, some parts of Africa and India.

History

There are about 39 species of *Gossypium* worldwide which are native to the tropics and warm temperate regions. Three species are native to South Africa, of these, *Gossypium hirsutum* from Mexico has become the predominant species in commercial cotton production worldwide. About 90% of the world commercially produces cotton from *G. hirsutum*. *G. barbadense* contributes to 8% of the market while the remaining 2% belongs to the old world cotton grown in South and South-East Asia.

Gossypium herbaceum or the African-West Asian cotton: *Gossypium herbaceum* is the indigenous species in India. It is native to semidesert conditions like in sub-Saharan Africa and in Arabia. It is a perennial shrub. It is widely cultivated in Ethiopia and also in Persia, Afghanistan. Turkey, North Africa, Spain, Ukraine, Turkestan and China (first cultivation in China reported was in about A.D. 600). It reaches a height of 2–6 feet, with palmate hairy leaves, lobes lanceolate, acute yellow petals and a purple spot in centre, capsule when ripe splits itself and exposes the loose white clump surrounding the seeds and strongly adhering to the outer coating. *G. herbaceum* requires warm weather to ripen its seeds.

Gossypium arboreum or the Pakistani-Indian cotton: It is native to Northwest India and Pakistan. The use and production of cotton dates back to 2000 B.C., by the Harappan civilization of the Indus Valley. Some of them are tall perennial while others are short annuals. People of Nubia are considered to be the first cotton weavers of Africa. This cotton variety extended into other parts of Africa (Nigeria) that became a cotton-manufacturing centre from the 9th century onwards.

Gossypium barbadense or South American cotton: G. *barbadense* gives the Sea Island, or long-stapled cotton. The oldest cotton textiles recorded from South America date to 3600 B.C. The first sign of domestication of cotton species comes from Peruvian coast where cotton balls dating to 2500 B.C. were found. Cotton became a commercial slave plantation crop in the West Indies and as a result of it Barbados in 1650s became the first British West Indian colony to export cotton. Later on around 1670, planting of *G. barbadense* also began in the British North American colonies.

Gossypium hirsutum or Mexican cotton: G. *hirsutum* are found in coastal vegetation of Central and Southern North America and also in the West Indies. There are evidences of cotton remains dating back to 3500 B.C. in the Tehuacan Caves in Mexico and even the Spanish explorers have found cotton cultivation in the 1500s.

Cultivation, Collection and Preparation

Cotton is cultivated by means of seed sowing method. The seeds are sown in rows of about 4–5 ft in distance. Proper fertilizers are provided timely. The cotton plants are shrubs or small trees that bare fruits (capsules) after flowering. The capsule consists of three to five seeds and is covered with hairs. The balls are collected when ripe, separated from the capsule, dried and subjected to the ginning press for processing. In ginning process, hairs and seeds are put before the roller with a small space, which separates the trichomes from the seeds. The short and long hair separated by delinter. Short hairs are known as 'linters', which are used in the manufacturing inferior grade cotton wool, whereas long hairs are used for preparation of cloth. The seeds remain after the removal of hair is used for the preparation of cotton seed oil and oil cake for domestic animal feed. The raw cotton so obtained is full of impurities like the colouring matter and fatty material. It is then subjected to further purification by treating it with dilute soda ash solution under pressure for about 15 hours. It is then bleached and washed properly, dried and packed. The packed cotton is then sterilized using radiations.

Description

Colour	White
Odour	Odourless
Taste	Tasteless
Shape	These are fine filaments like that of hair, which are soft and unicellular.
Size	2.2–4.6 cm in length and 20–35 μm in diameter

Chemical Constituents

It consists of 90% of cellulose, 7–8% of moisture, wax, fat and oil 0.5% and cell content about 0.5%. Purified cotton has almost cellulose and 6–7% of moisture.

Chemical Tests

1. On ignition, cotton burns with a flame, gives very little odour or fumes, does not produce a bead and leaves a small white ash; distinction from acetate rayon, alginate yarn, wool, silk and nylon.
2. Dried cotton is moistened with N/50 iodine and 80% w/w sulphuric acid is added. A blue colour is produced; distinction from acetate rayon, alginate yarn, jute, hemp, wool, silk and nylon.
3. With ammoniacal copper oxide solution, raw cotton dissolves with ballooning, leaving a few fragments of cuticle. Absorbent cotton dissolves completely with uniform swelling, distinction from acetate rayon, jute, wool and nylon.
4. In cold sulphuric acid (80% w/w) cotton dissolves; distinction from oxidized cellulose, jute, hemp and wool.
5. In cold sulphuric acid (60% w/w) cotton, is insoluble; distinction from cellulose wadding and rayons.
6. In warm (40°C) hydrochloric acid it is insoluble; distinction from acetate rayon (also silk, nylon).
7. It is insoluble in 5% potassium hydroxide solution; distinction from oxidized cellulose, wool and silk.

8. Treat it with cold Shirla stain A for 1 min and wash out. It shows shades of blue, Tilac or purple; distinction from viscose, acetate rayons, alginate yarn, wool, silk and nylon.

9. Treat it with cold Shirla stain C for 5 min and wash out; raw cotton gives a mauve to reddish-brown colour and absorbent cotton a pink one; distinction from flax, jute, hemp. The Shirla stains may be usefully applied to a small piece of the whole fabric under investigation to indicate the distribution of more than one type of yarn.

10. It does not give red stain with phloroglucinol and hydrochloric acid; distinction from jute, hemp and kapok.

Uses

Cotton is used as a filtering medium and in surgical dressings. Absorbent cotton absorbs blood, pus, mucus and prevents infections in wounds.

JUTE

Synonym

Gunny.

Biological Source

It consists of phloem fibres from the stem of various species of the *Corchorus; C. capsularis* Linn, *C. olitorius* Linn. and other species like *C. cunninghamii*, *C. junodi*, etc., belonging to family Tiliaceae.

Geographical Source

West Bengal and Assam.

History

Corchorus is a genus with 40–100 species of flowering plants. It is native to tropical and subtropical regions throughout the world. Though various species yield fibre, the chief sources of commercial jute are two Indian species the *C. capsularis* and *C. olitorius*. These species are grown in Ganges and Brahmaputra valleys.

For past many centuries, Jute has been an integral part of Bengali culture. In the late 19th and early 20th centuries, much of the raw jute fibres were exported to the United Kingdom. In '50s and '60s (when nylon and polythene were rarely used), Pakistan was the world's lead jute producer. During those periods it had earned its money through jute of East Pakistan, (now called the Bangladesh). Jute was called the 'Golden fibre' of Bangladesh because it brought the major portion of the foreign currency for the country. World's largest jute trade and jute processing economy was located in Bangladesh. Adamjee Jute Mill in Narayanganj, Bangladesh was world's largest jute mill with 1939 looms and 25,000 employees up to 2002. Presently Sonali Aansh is one of the largest jute products manufacturers in Bangladesh.

Description

They are tall, usually annual herbs, reaching to a height of 2–4 m, unbranched and if branched it has only a few side branches. The leaves are alternate, simple, lanceolate, 5–15 cm long and a finely serrated or lobed margin. The flowers are small (1.5–3 cm in diameter) and yellow, with five petals; the fruit encloses many seeds in the capsule.

Preparation

Retting is the process for the preparation of bast fibres. This process is done by three methods, that is, microbial (or water), steam and mechanical process. The microbial or water retting process is the oldest and the popular method employed for the breaking of lignin bond present between parenchyma and sclerenchyma. The breaking of this bond facilitates the easy procurement of skin from its core. Then the material is washed dried to release pectin bond which makes the hard skin to fine thread like fibres. The jute fibres are graded according to its colour, strength and fibre length. The fibres are of white to brown and 1–4 m long.

Microscopy

A thin transverse section of the strand when treated with phuloroglucinol and HCl, stains the strands deep red, indicating the presence of lignin. Each strand is a collection of polygonal cells which are surrounded by lumen with various sizes. These strands can be separated by treating it with mixture of potassium chloride and nitric acid.

Chemical Constituents

Jute fibres are composed primarily of the plant materials cellulose and lignin. Jute is composed of about 50–53% cellulose, nearly 20% of hemicellulose and 10–11% of lignin along with other constituents like moisture not more than 12–13%, fats, wax and ash contributing to 1% each.

Uses

It has a large range of use (about 1000 uses). It is listed as the second most important vegetable fibre after cotton. Jute is used chiefly to make cloth for wrapping bales of raw cotton, in the preparation of sacks and coarse cloth. They are also woven into curtains, chair coverings, carpets, Hessian cloth very fine threads of jute can be made into imitation silk and also in the making of paper. It is even used in the manufacture of tows, padding splints, filtering and straining medium. Jute is used for the preparation of coarse bags.

FLAX

Biological Source

It is the pericyclic fibres which are removed from, the stem of *Linum usitatissimum* Linn., belonging to family Linaceae.

Geographical Source

It is mainly found in United States, Russia, Ireland, Northern Europe.

History

Flax fibres are one amongst the oldest fibre crops in the world. The use of flax for the production of linen dates back to 5000 years. It was the chief source for the preparation of cloth fibre till the other fibres like jute and cotton came to market. The manufacture of cloth from flax fibre in Northern Europe dates back to the period of pre-Romans and it is also believed that the pilgrims were the ones to introduce flax to the United States.

Cultivation, Collection and Preparation

Though Eurasia is the native of flax it has been transplanted from its origin to most of the temperate zones of the world due to its favourable climatic condition (cool moist climate) for its cultivation. The most suitable soil for its growth is alluvial soil with deep friable loams, moderately fertile humus-rich soil, and it does not grow well in dry sandy and strong clays.

Linum usitatissimum is an annual plant which grows to a height of 4 ft. It bares in itself flowers with blue or white colour and these flowers mature into balls. Each ball consists of 10 seeds, which are sown by the end of March or in early April. The flowers come up in the month of June and the balls are collected after a month time before they are ripe. Flax should be pulled as soon as the lower part of the plant begins to turn yellow and soon after it is been pulled, it should be tied in bunches and put into water for retting. Standing pools are beneficial for the purpose of retting because it provides better colour and a superior quality in all aspect. The process of retting through fermentation permits bacteria to break down the woody tissues and also to dissolve the substances binding the fibre cells due to enzyme action. The branches when put in water it should be tied in small sheaves and immersed firmly with the help of a weight placed above, to facilitate equal and proper watering. In warm condition, watering process is sufficient for 10 days with proper and timely examination of the pools (after the seventh day), to check if the flax are rotten. It often happens that by the twelfth day the flax get rot irrespective of the climatic condition and it is advised to have less amount of water than excess quantity. After retting,

the stems are washed and allowed to dry on grass and beaten using a machine scutched; to separate the fibres from other material and to crush the pith. The bark remaining after the process of beating is then subjected finally for combing (hackling) for the removal of traces of nonfibrous matter like wood and parenchyma and parallel pericyclic fibres are obtained.

Description

The length of fibre cells ranges from 1.2 to 5.0 cm and the length of fibres cell bundles ranges from 30 to 90 cm. The short and broken fibres are called 'tow'. Flax is hygroscopic in nature. Flax fibre is soft, lustrous and flexible. It has more tensile strength than cotton fibre but less elasticity.

Microscopy

The flakes are a collection of 20 fibres, which are joined to each other through their pointed ends. The individual fibres when observed under the microscope show cells which are of polygonal.

Chemical Composition

The flax chiefly consists of pectocellulose.

Uses

Linen cloths can be prepared which is used as a filtering medium. The 'tow' is used in making coarse fabrics and cordage, while the long fibres are used for strong threads and fine linens. Flax fibre is also utilized as raw material for the high-quality paper industry for the purpose of printed currency notes and cigarette paper.

HEMP

Biological Source

Hemp is the pericyclic fibre obtained from *Cannabis sativa* Linn., belonging to family Cannabinaceae.

Geographical source

Hemp is grown at any altitude from Norway to the Equator. The raw materials are imported from China, Hungary, America, Germany, Switzerland, Australia, Canada, France and Norway.

History

The history of *Cannabis sativa* dates back to more than 6000 years. The history of China has in its credit of having a Hemp textile production even before 4500 B.C. which later spread to Asia in around 1000 B.C. and reaching Europe by

800 B.C. In 1175 *Cannabis sativa* was grouped under taxable goods, and in 1535 an act came into force which compelled all land owners to sow 1/4 of an acre, or otherwise they be fined was formed by Henry VIII. During this period Hemp became a major crop and till 1920s about 80% of clothing was made from Hemp textiles. Traditionally, Hemp was processed by hand, which required huge labour and was costly. In 1917 American George W. Schlichten invented and patented a new machine for separating the fibre from the internal woody core ('Hurds') reducing labour costs. By 1930, due to the tough competition by the other varieties of hemp imported by Philippines and Mexico, the hemp production by United States had fell to less than 200 acres. Later on during World War II, farmers in the United States were encouraged to cultivate both cannabis hemp and flax for the purpose of war under the banner of 'Hemp For Victory', In 1937 the production of *Cannabis sativa* was restricted except for industrial use or research purpose but in 1970 its production was categorized as illegal for all purpose. In 1992/93 the first licenses were granted for growing Hemp of the low THC varieties (THC is the narcotic substance found in the leaves) under the ruling that Hemp is grown for 'special purposes' or 'in the public interest'. At present, approximately 2500 hectares are being grown.

Chemical Constituents

Hemp mainly consist of cellulose and lignin.

Uses

Hemp is mentioned historically to have more than 25,000 diverse uses. The historically mentioned uses are printing inks, paints, varnishes, paper, bibles, bank notes, food, textiles (the original Levi's jeans were made from Hemp cloth), canvas and building materials. Due to its high tensile strength, bast fibres are ideal for such specialized paper products as: tea bags, industrial filters, currency paper, or cigarette paper.

ANIMAL FIBRES

SILK

Biological Source

Fibres obtained from the cocoons spun by the larvae *Bombyx mori* Linn., belonging to family Bombycidae/Moraceae.

Geographical Source

China, France, Iran, Italy, Japan and India.

History

It is native to northern China and Persia presently known as Iran. *Bombyx mori* is a member of a small family of about 300 moth species.

The credit for the discovery of silkworm's silk goes to an ancient empress in China, who while walking around accidentally, noticed the worms. When she touched it with her fingers, the silk came out and surrounded her finger. When the full silk had come out, she saw the small cocoon inside it; which was responsible for the formation of silk. It is even said that the Chinese princess smuggled eggs to Japan by hiding them in her hair and thus they began their love affair with silk. Due to its captivity for thousands of years, *Bombyx mori* is fully domesticated and cannot survive without the support of mankind.

The silkworm is the larva of a moth. Larvae are monophagous which takes only mulberry leaves as its diet. The cocoon is made of a single continuous thread of raw silk from 300 to 900 m long. The fibres are very fine and lustrous, about 1/2500th of an inch in diameter. One pound of silt can be made from about 2000 to 3000 cocoons, and it is estimated that almost 70 million pound of raw silk are produced each year. It requires about 1 billion pounds of mulberry leaves to produced 7 million pounds of raw silk and one pound of silk is almost equivalent to 1000 miles of filament.

Preparation

One gram of silkworm egg consists of around 15,000 eggs which are kept at 0°C to overcome the immature development. The silkworms eat mulberry leaves day and night and they grow very fast. When the colour of their heads changes darker, it indicates that the time for them to moult has come. It require almost a month time for its development into full size. During this period it takes four moulds and their body turns slightly yellow reaching a size of 4 cm long. The silkworm finally eats a meal which is about twenty to twenty five times its weight of leaves and attains a size of 9 cm length and 10 mm thick. The skin becomes tight and all these symptoms indicate that it is going to cover itself with a silky cocoon. The process of spinning cocoon continues for almost three days. After 7–8 days, the larvae changes into chrysalides, and the cocoons are collected by throwing them into boiling water, this kills the silkworms and also makes the cocoons easier to unravel. If the caterpillar is left to eat its way out of the cocoon naturally, the threads will be cut short and the silk will be useless. The cocoons are kept in hike warm water to remove the gum. Since all the eggs hatch almost the same time, the cocoons also be collected together and treated at the same period. Some amount of cocoons are retained and allowed to come out for fertilization. The females lay nearly 500 eggs and these eggs are stored till further requirement is wanted.

Description

Colour	Yellow
Size	5–25 µm in diameter and 1200 m in length
Appearance	Fine, solid, smooth to touch
Solubility	Soluble in cuoxam, in cold dilute sulphuric acid
Extra features	Hygroscopic in nature and has good elasticity and tensile strength

Chemical Constituents

Silk mainly consists of protein known as fibrion. Fibrion is soluble in warm water and on hydrolysis yields two main amino acids, glycine and alanine.

Uses

Silk is used pharmaceutically in the preparation of sutures, sieves and ligatures. The 'stiff silkworm' (dried body in the four to fifth stage of larva, which dies due to infection of the fungus *Beauveria bassiana*) is used in the traditional Chinese medicine.

WOOL

Biological Source

Wool consist of hairs from the fleece of sheep *Ovis aries* Linn., belonging to family Bovidae.

Geographical Source

The worlds leading producers of wool are Australia (25%), China and New Zealand (11%), while Turkey, Iran, India and the United States (Texas, New Mexico) contribute to 2%.

History

The use of wool for clothing and other fabrics dates back to earliest civilizations. The wool trade was a serious business during medieval times and English wool export had contributed significantly as a source of income to the crown. Smuggling of wool was considered a serious offence and was punished with cutting off the hand. Wool trade had also helped Medicis of Florence in Renaissance in building up their wealth and banking. Spain with royal permission

exported Merino lambs. By the end of 19th century German wool (from sheep of Spanish origin) overtook British wool but later by 1845 the Australian wool trade eventually overtook the German wool.

Preparation

Wool is the fibre derived from the hair of animals of the Caprinae family, mainly sheep and goats. It is produced as the outer coat of sheep. The fibre obtained from domestic sheep has two qualities which differentiate it from hair or fur. The fibres have scales which overlap like shingles on a roof and it is crimped. The amount of crimp is directly proportional with the fineness of the wool fibres and the fine wool (like merino) have up to a 100 crimps per inch, whereas coarser wools (like karakul) have one or two crimps per inch.

The hairs from sheep are removed during the shearing time. After shearing, the wool is separated into five main categories: namely fleece, pieces, bellies, crutchings and locks. It is then cleaned from dirt and high level of grease (thus 'greasy wool') which contains valuable lanolin is present on the hair. The grease is generally removed for processing by scouring with detergent and alkali. The wool is then treated with hydrogen peroxide for bleaching, it is then washed properly and spreaded on wire nettings and dried under hot air.

Description

Wool is generally a creamy white colour but some of the breeds of sheep naturally produce black, brown (also called moorit) and grey coloured wool. The wool is smooth, elastic, slippery to touch and slightly curly. Diameter of wool varies from 15 µm (superfine merino) to 30 or 40 µm. The finer the diameters the greater its value is. Wool is soluble in warm alkaline solutions, but not in dilute or strong acids.

Chemical Constituents

Wool mainly consists of a sulphur containing protein called keratin. Keratin is composed of amino acid like cystine.

Chemical Tests

1. *Solubility Test*: It is easily soluble in warm alkali.
2. Wool when treated with conc. hydrochloric acid, it does not produce any effect but dissolves silk.
3. When treated with cuoxam solution, it does not dissolve but swells the wool and produces blue colour.
4. Solution of wool treated with lead acetate produces black precipitate due to high sulphur content.

Uses

It is used as a filtering aid and straining medium and in the manufacture of clothing, carpeting, felt and it is also used to absorb odours and noise in heavy machinery and stereo speakers.

REGENERATED AND SYNTHETIC FIBRES

VISCOSE

Synonyms

Rayon, regenerated cellulose.

Source

Viscose is a viscous orange-red aqueous solution of sodium cellulose xanthogenate obtained by dissolving wood pulp cellulose in sodium hydroxide solution and treating with carbon disulphide.

Preparation

The starting material is cellulose prepared from coniferous wood (spruce), or scoured and bleached cotton linters. The wood is delignified similar to cellulose wadding. It reaches the rayon manufacturers as boards of white pulp, containing 80–90% of cellulose and some hemicellulose (mainly pentosans). The hemicellulose being alkali-soluble, are removed in the first stage of the process by steeping in sodium hydroxide solution. The excess alkaline liquor is pressed out and alkali-cellulose (sodium cellulosate) remains. This is dissolved by treatment with carbon disulphide and sodium hydroxide solution to give a viscous solution of sodium cellulose xanthate. After 'ripening' and filtering, the solution is forced through a spinneret, a jet with fine nozzles, immersed in a bath of dilute sulphuric acid and sodium sulphate, when the cellulose is regenerated as continuous filaments. These are drawn together as a yarn, which is twisted for strength, desulphurized by removing free sulphur with sodium sulphide, bleached, washed, dried and conditioned to a moisture content of 10%.

Description

The rayon is a white, highly lustrous fibre. Its tensile strength varies from two-third to one-and-a-half times that of cotton. When wetted, it loses about 60% of its tensile strength. It has a proportionately greater loss than is found with cotton. The fabric is a water repellent (e.g. cotton crepe bandage).

Chemistry

Viscose rayon is a very pure form of cellulose. Its ash contains sulphur. The cellulose molecules of the original natural material are more separated from one another in the viscose solution than in the vegetable material and in the regenerated fibres is still less closely packed. The side-to-side aggregation of the long-chain molecules is different from that in natural celluloses. The size of the molecules is also reduced. Wood cellulose has molecules of the order of 9000 glucose residue units, whereas those of viscose rayon have only about 450.

Chemical Tests

1. The fibres give the general tests for vegetable and regenerated carbohydrate fibres.
2. On ignition they behave like cotton; distinction from acetate rayon and alginate yarn, wool, silk, nylon and glass.
3. With N/50 iodine and sulphuric acid, 80%, they give a blue colour similar to that given by cotton; distinction from acetate rayon, alginate yarn, jute, hemp, wool, silk and nylon.
4. With ammoniacal copper oxide they behave like absorbent cotton; distinction from acetate rayon, jute, wool and nylon.
5. Cold sulphuric acid, 60% w/w, dissolves the fibre; distinction from cotton, oxidized cellulose, alginate yarn, flax, jute, hemp and wool.
6. Warm (40°C) hydrochloric acid does not dissolve the fibre; distinction from acetate rayon, silk and nylon.
7. It is insoluble in boiling potassium hydroxide solution (5%); distinction from oxidized cellulose, wool and silk.
8. Shirla stain A produces a bright pink; distinction from cotton, oxidized cellulose, acetate, rayon, wool, silk and nylon.
9. Phloroglucinol and hydrochloric acid produce no red stain; distinction from jute, hemp and kapok.
10. The fibres, like cotton, are insoluble in acetone, formic acid 90% or phenol 90%; distinction from acetate rayon and nylon.

Uses

Viscose rayon is used to manufacture fabrics, surgical dressings, absorbent wool, enzyme and cellophane.

ALGINATE FIBRES

Alginate fibres are composed of calcium alginate.

Preparation

An aqueous solution of sodium alginate is pumped through a spinneret which is immersed in a bath containing acidic calcium chloride solution. In the bath sodium cations are substituted with calcium cations and the insoluble calcium alginate is precipitated as continuous filaments. The filaments are collected, washed and dried for surgical purposes. The filaments are cut up to give stable form of length 1–8 inches for preparing calcium alginate wool or a fabric. Trace amounts of substances are added to the calcium alginate to inhibit mould and bacterial growth

Description

Alginate fibres are fairly lustrous and pale cream coloured. The fibres may be processed into absorbable, haemostatic dressings. They give general tests for vegetable fibres. They are soluble in ammonical copper nitrate and 5% sodium citrate solution.

Chemistry

Alginic acid is composed of polymers of both mannuronic and glucuronic acids. The properties of the two are variable and alginates of different origin have different compositions and properties. Kalostat haemostatic dressing is derived from the seaweed *Laminaria hyperborea* collected off the Norwegian coast and yields an alginate with a glucuronic-mannuronic ratio of 2:1. Other dressing is prepared from *Laminaria* and *Ascophyllum* species collected off the west coast of Scotland and gives an alginate with a glucuronic-mannuronic acid ratio of about 1:2. On a wound surface the α-linkages of the glucuronic acid polymer are not easily broken so that fibre strength is retained and a strong gel is formed on contact with the wound exudates. A high ratio of mannuronic acid polymer (β-linkages) yields a product giving a weaker gel and less retention of fibre strength. The Kalostat dressing can be removed from the wound with forceps and Sorbsan is removed by irrigation with sodium citrate solution.

Calcium alginate fibres of commerce contain substantial traces of substances used to inhibit mould and bacterial growth in the sodium alginate spinning solution. Spinning lubricants such as lauryl or cetyl pyridinium bromide (antibacterial) are also applied to the filaments. These substances must not be used in the case of bacteriological swabs.

Before use as an absorbable haemostatic dressing some calcium alginate dressing must be immersed in sodium chloride to give a fibre of the calcium alginate covered by sodium alginate. The degree of conversion is conditioned to give the desired rate of absorption when in use; the greater the proportion of sodium alginate the faster the absorption rate.

Alginate filaments are composed of salts of the long-chain molecules of alginic acid, and there is little cross-linking between the chains in the fibre.

Chemical Tests

1. The fibre burns in a flame and goes out when removed from flame.

2. With (N/50) iodine and sulphuric acid, a brownish-red colour is produced, the filaments swell and dissolve to leave a strand of insoluble alginic acid.
3. In ammoniacal copper nitrate solution they swell and dissolve.
4. The fibres are insoluble in 60% w/w sulphuric acid.
5. The fibres are insoluble in warm (40°C) hydrochloric acid.
6. The fibres are insoluble in boiling 5% KOH (swell and acquire a yellow tint).
7. The fibres are soluble in 5% sodium citrate solution.
8. Fibre, 0.1 g, boiled with 5 ml of water remains insoluble but dissolves when 1 ml 20% w/v sodium carbonate solution is added and boiled for 1 min. A white precipitate of calcium carbonate is formed, depending on the proportion of original calcium alginate present. When centrifuged and the clear supernatant acidified, a gelatinous precipitate of alginic acid is produced. The precipitate will give a purple colour after solution in NaOH and addition of an acid solution of ferric sulphate.
9. Shirla stain A gives a reddish-brown colour.
10. Alginate haemostatic fibres are invisible in polarized light with crossed Nicols.

Uses

The alginate absorbable haemostatic dressings are nontoxic and nonirritant. They have advantages over oxidized cellulose, which include selective rate of absorption, sterilization (and resterilization) by autoclaving or dry heat and compatibility with antibiotics such as penicillin. They are used internally in neurosurgery, endural and dental surgery to be subsequently absorbed. Externally, they are used (e.g. for burns or sites from which skin grafts have been taken) to arrest bleeding and form a protective dressing which may be left or later removed in a manner appropriate to the type of dressing employed. Protective films of calcium alginate may also be used by painting the injured surface with sodium alginate solution and then spraying it with calcium chloride solution.

Calcium alginate wool as a swab for pathological work or bacterial examination of such things as food processing equipment and tableware permits release of all the organisms by disintegration and solution of the swab in, for example, Ringer's solution containing sodium hexametaphosphate.

NYLON

Nylon is a synthetic thermoplastic polymer invented in 1935 by Wallace Carothers at Du Pont. It is the first commercially successful polymer and the first synthetic fibre made from inorganic ingredients like coal, water and air. It is made of repeating units linked by peptide bonds.

History

The first product was a nylon-bristled toothbrush in 1938. Nylon replaced the Asian silk in parachutes during the World War II; it was also used in making tents, ropes and other military supplies. Nylon was also used in the production of a high-grade paper for United States currency. Due to the war 80% was accounted by cotton and the rest 20% by other manufactured and wool fibres. Later in 1945, 25% of the market was taken by manufactured fibres and the hare of cotton fell down. It took Du Pont 12 years and US$27 million to refine nylon and develop the industrial processes for bulk manufacture. Nylon mania came to an abrupt stop at the end of 1941, when America entered World War II. After the war ended, Du Pont went back to selling nylon to the public, engaging in another promotional campaign in 1946 that resulted in an even bigger craze triggering off 'nylon riots'.

Chemistry

Nylons are condensation copolymers formed by reaction of equal parts of a diamine and a dicarboxylic acid, so that peptide bonds form at the both ends of each monomer in a process analogous to polypeptide biopolymers.

Uses

Nylon still remains an important plastic and not just for use in fabrics. In its bulk form, it is very wear-resistant and so is used to build gears, bearings, bushings and other mechanical parts.

TERYLENE (DACRON)

Terylene is a polyester fibre produced by condensating ethylene glycol with terephthalic acid. Its chemical formula may be represented as: $H[OCH_2CH_2OOCC_6H_4CO]_n OH$. Terylene fibres are prepared by an identical process to that for nylon. On heating the fibres with phosphoric acid (90%) for 1 minute, it retains its form. This test is negative in case of nylon. Terylene is used in the same way as nylon.

ORLON

Orlon is obtained by polymerizing acrylonitrile. It is represented as $[CH_2 CH (CH)]_n$. It is a white fibre; sticks at 235°C; ironing temperatures above 160°C may cause yellowing; sp. gr. is 1.17. Its inflammability is similar to that of rayon and cotton. Generally it has very good resistance to mineral acids; excellent resistance to common solvents, oils, greases, neutral salts, sunlight but it is degraded by strong alkalis. It resists attack by moulds, mildew and insects. The 100% polyacrylonitrile fibres are rarely used commercially due to difficulty in dyeing.

Orlon fibre is suitable for furnishing (awnings, tents and furniture), anode bags in electroplating, knitwear, rugs and dressings.

22.4. SURGICAL DRESSINGS

A material used to protect a wound and to heal is called a surgical dressing. They serve various functions for the injured site. They remove wound exudates from the site, prevent infection, and give physical protection to the healing wound and mechanical support to the supporting tissues. A good quality of dressing should be durable, easy to handle, sterilized, formed from loose threads and fibres, and it should not adhere to the granulating surface.

Surgical dressings are classified as:

Primary Wound Dressings

Primary wound dressings are applied over the wound surface to absorb pus, mucus and blood. They minimize maceration. Some dressings adhere to the wound surface and cause pain on removing them. Now nonadherent dressings are available such as petrolatum-impregnated gauge, viscose gauze impregnated with a bland, hydrophilic oil-in-water emulsion or an absorbent pad faced with a soft plastic film having openings.

Absorbents

Absorbent cotton is widely used to absorb wound secretions. Other absorbent materials are rayon wool, cotton wool, gauze pads, laparotomy sponges, sanitary napkins, disposable cleaners, eye pads, nursing pads and cotton tip applications. They are used in the shape of balls or pads.

Bandages

A bandage is a material which holds dressing at the required site, applies pressure, or supports an injured part or checks haemorrhage. The bandages may be elastic or nonelastic in nature. Common gauze roller bandage and muslin bandage rolls are employed most frequently. Elastic bandages may be woven to form elastic bandage, crepe bandage and conforming bandage.

Adhesive Tapes

Surgical adhesive tapes may be a rubber-based adhesive or an acrylate adhesive. Rubber adhesive tapes are cheap, superior and provide strength of backing. In case of operation or postoperation acrylate, adhesive tapes are used to reduce skin trauma.

Protectives

Protectives are employed to cover wet dressings, poultices and for retention of heat. They prevent the escape of moisture from the dressing. Some protectives are plastic sheeting, rubber sheeting, waxed or oil-coated papers and plastic-coated papers.

22.5. SUTURES AND LIGATURES

A surgical suture is a thread or sting used for sewing or stitching together tissues, muscles and tendons with the help of a needle. If these threads or fibres are used to tie a blood vessel to stop bleeding without the use of a needle, then they are digested in animal tissues, for example, catgut, kangaroo tendon and synthetic polyesters. If the sutures are not absorbed in the body, they are called nonabsorbable sutures, for example, silk, cotton, nylon, synthetic polyester fibres and stainless steel wire. A good quality of suture should be well-sterilized, nonirritant; having well-mechanical strength, fine gauze and with minimum time of absorption.

Absorbable Sutures

Surgical catgut

Catgut is a sterilized fibre or strand prepared from collagen of connective tissues obtained from healthy animals like sheep and cattle.

Preparation

The submucosal layer of small intestine of a freshly killed animal is used for the preparation of catgut. About 7.5 m long intestine is cleaned and split longitudinally into ribbons. The inner most mucosa and two outer layers of submucosa, muscularis and serosal layers are removed with the help of a machine leaving behind the submucosa. Up to six such ribbons are stretched, spun and dried to form a uniform strand. These fibres are polished to get smooth strings, gauzed for their diameter, cut into suitable lengths and sterilized by placing the catgut in glass tubes filled with anhydrous high-boiling liquids like toluene or xylene and then heating in an autoclave. Sterilization may be done by irradiating the suture by electron particles or by gamma rays from cobalt-60.

Kangaroo tendons, used in hernia and bone repairs, are prepared from the tails of kangaroo by the identical method adopted for the preparation of catgut. Chromicized surgical catguts are prepared by soaking the ribbons in solutions of chromium salts for tanning the tissues. These fibres are not affected by proteolytic enzymes in the body and they are not absorbed rapidly in the body.

Synthetic polyesters

The polymers obtained by condensation of cyclic derivatives of glycolic acid (glycolide) with cyclic derivatives of lactic acid (lacticide) are used to prepare synthetic absorbable sutures. These sutures have high tensile strength and are degraded by hydrolysis and absorbed in the tissue.

Nonabsorbable Sutures

Nonabsorbable sutures are not affected by the body fluid and remained unchanged for a long period. They are removed after healing of the wounds. Silk, cotton, nylon and metallic sutures are classified as nonabsorbable sutures.

Silk sutures

Silk sutures are prepared by spinning or twisting silk fibres into a single strand of varying diameters. The sutures are smooth and strong and braided by combining several twisted yarns into a compact mass. The strands are sterilized and boiled with water to soften them.

Cotton sutures

Cotton sutures have uniform size and recommended in critical parts where strength of the sutures is required for long time.

Nylon sutures

The microfilaments of nylon are braided into strands of required diameter. These sutures are strong, water resistant, and used in skin and plastic surgery.

Linen suture

A linen suture is cheap, very strong under moist condition but not uniform in diameter.

Metallic sutures

Metallic wires of silver or stainless steel are used as surgical aid. These wires are available as monofilaments, twists and braids.

CHAPTER 23

Drugs of Mineral Origin

CONTENTS

- Introduction
- Kaolin
- Asbestos
- Talc
- Bentonite
- Fuller's Earth
- Prepared Chalk
- Kieselguhr
- Calamine

23.1. INTRODUCTION

The substances of mineral origin have been used for various pharmaceutical purposes ranging from therapeutic agents to nutritional supplements to pharmaceutical excipient.

These inorganic substances are found as mineral deposits of different types such as terrestrial deposits or fossil deposition of geological origin in ocean and seabeds. The natural ores or minerals are collected by mining in open quarries, and the product is further purified for various pharmaceutical uses. Some important natural drugs of mineral origin are given in Table 23.1.

Table 23.1 Some important drugs of mineral origin

Drug	Source	Use
Kaolin	Feldspar deposits	In gastric affection
Asbestos	Hornblende	For bacterial filter
Talc	Sleatite/soap stone	Filtration
Bentonite	Mineral deposits	Emulsion, cosmetics
Fuller's Earth	Siliceous earth	Dusting powder
Prepared chalk	Calcarious remains of algae	Antacid
Kieselguhr	Fossil diatoms	Filtration aid
Calamine	Hemimorphites	Cosmetics

KAOLIN

Synonyms

China clay.

Source

Kaolin is a purified native hydrated aluminium silicate free from gritty particles. It is obtained by powdering the native kaolin, elutriating and collecting the fraction, which complies with the requirements of particle size. The native clay is derived from decomposition of the feldspar (potassium aluminosilicate) or granite rock and contains silica (47%), alumina (40%) and water (13%).

History

The word kaolin was derived from the Chinese word 'Kauling', meaning high ridge. Kaolin was first mined in colonial days in Georgia and then shipped to England. Georgia was the source of clay for famous Wedgwood Pottery and this resulted in the end of mining in Georgia for over a century. By 1876, mining here was resumed and today it continues as the major mineral production of the state by producing 72% of the total kaolin.

Collection and Preparation

Kaolin is mined from the surface layer of stones, clay and sand which are in depth up to 100 feet. The average thickness of clay varies from 12 to 15 feet. Kaolin is removed by firing a high-pressure water jet at the quarry face. The clay is then sifted and refined to remove impurities before finally being dried to reduce its moisture content. The impurities like sand are removed by washing where the impurities settle down and the slurry is then pumped into a long channel of drags. The coarse particles in the slurry settle down, whereas the lighter ones move slowly along with water and flow into a settling pits, where the clay is deposited.

Description

Kaolin is white soft plastic clay composed of well-ordered kaolinite with low iron content. In many parts of the world, it is coloured pink-orange-red by iron oxide, giving it a distinct rust hue. Lighter concentrations yield white, yellow or light orange colours also. It is made up of a loose aggregation of randomly oriented stacks of kaolinite flakes, smaller packets and sheaves and individual flakes. The median particle size of kaolin is 0.78 µm, 1.02 µm, 1.1 µm, 1.2 µm and 3.8 µm. It has loose bulk density of approximately 25 lbs/cubic feet and packed bulk density of 46 lbs/cu ft, the hardness factor is 6.0, specific gravity: 2.6 g/cc, pH: 6.0, surface area: 10–29. Odourless when dry but has clay like odour when wet. Kaolin when treated with concentrated HCl, decomposes partially but on heating it with conc. sulphuric acid, it is converted into insoluble silica and aluminium sulphates.

There are two types of kaolin: coarse (heavy) and colloidal (light). The coarser kaolin when treated with water forms a plastic and slightly sticky mass while colloidal kaolin with water forms sticky, stiff mass and if suspended in water forms a turbid solution or slurry. The standard grades of kaolin available are calcined, Sanitaryware grade, tableware grade and porcelain grade.

Chemical Constituents

Chemically kaolin is anhydrous aluminium silicate with a chemical formula: $Al_2O_3 \cdot 2SiO_2 \cdot 2H_2O$ or $H_4Al_2Si_2O_9$. The percentage composition are as follows: silicon dioxide (wt %): 56.91, iron oxide: 0.93, titanium dioxide: 0.54, aluminium oxide: 39.68, calcium oxide: 0.16, magnesium oxide: 0.16, sodium oxide: 0.60, potassium oxide: 0.60 and water: 12.6. Natural kaolinite usually contains small amounts of uranium and thorium, octahedral sheet of alumina octahedral.

Identification

Heat kaolin on charcoal black with cobalt nitrate, it forms blue mass due to alumina.

Uses

It is used as an adsorbent by oral administration, in the treatment of enteritis, dysentery and in alkaloidal and food poisoning. It is also applied externally as a dusting powder and also as clarifying agent during the filtration. Mostly, light kaolin with a particle size less than 10 µm is used in pharmaceutical preparations. Heavy kaolin with particle size up to 60 µm is only used in the preparation of kaolin poultice.

It is used as filler in paper, rubber, ceramics, cement and fertilizer industries. It is used in anticaking preparations, cosmetics, insecticides, paints and as source of alumina.

ASBESTOS

Source

Asbestos is a naturally occurring mineral which differs from other minerals in its crystal development. The crystal formation of asbestos is in the form of long thin fibres.

Geographical Source

Asbestos deposits can be found throughout the world and are still mined in Australia, Canada, South Africa and the former Soviet Union.

History

Over the years, asbestos had many uses. Its primary use is as an insulator or fire retardant, but can also be used as a binder. Due to this versatility, asbestos can be found in many types of building materials. Even though the federal government placed a moratorium on the production of most asbestos products in the early 1970s, installation of these products continued through the late 1970s and even into the early 1980s.

Description

On the basis of the crystalline structure, asbestos are divided into two mineral groups, as serpentine and amphibole. The amphiboles in their fibrous form are friable and so are the most carcinogenic. Serpentines have a sheet or layered structure, whereas amphiboles have a chain-like structure. Chrysotile (A, B) is the most common type of asbestos among serpentine group. There are five types of asbestos in amphibole group and they are amosite, crocidolite, anthophyllite, tremolite and actinolite.

Chrysotile or white asbestos is obtained from Canadian serpentine rocks. It is commonly used in industries. As it is less friable it is less likely to be inhaled. One of the formula given for chrysotile is $Na_2Fe^{2+}_3Fe^{3+}_2Si_8O_{22}(OH)_2$.

Amosite is also known as brown asbestos or grunerite is an amphibole from Africa and the formula given for amosite is $Fe_7Si_8O_{22}(OH)_2$.

Crocidolite or blue asbestos is amphibole from Africa and Australia. It is considered to be most dangerous type of asbestos and the formula given for crocidolite is $Na_2Fe^{2+}_3Fe^{3+}_2Si_8O_{22}(OH)_2$.

Anthophyllite, tremolite and actinolite have their formula $(Mg, Fe)_7Si_8O_{22}(OH)_2$, $Ca_2Mg_5Si_8O_{22}(OH)_2$, $Ca_2(Mg, Fe)_5Si_8O_{22}(OH)_2$, respectively. They are less used industrially but are found in a variety of construction materials and insulations and also in some consumer products, such as talcum powders.

Chemical Constituents

It is a double silicate of calcium–magnesium with little amount of iron which gives colour to asbestos.

Uses

It is used as filtering medium for caustic alkalies, for bacterial filters, heat resistant insulators, proof gloves, break lining and fire-proof clothing.

TALC

Synonym

French chalk, Talcum.

Source

Talc is a mineral with perfect cleavage and soapy feel, which occurs as foliated to fibrous masses and some times in coarsely granular, finely granular or cryptocrystalline masses.

Geographical Source

It is found in Austria, Canada, United States (California, Montana, Texas, etc.), France and also in Italy.

History

The origin of the name Talc came from Persian through Arabic talc. India has also been successfully exporting talc to overseas. The Indian talc industry hopes to have joint venture partnerships with international business houses with technical proficiency in the beneficiation and sterilization of talc.

Description

It is folia which is slightly flexible and is not elastic. It has perfect basal cleavage. Talc is very soft and sectile in nature, with a hardness of 1. It is the softest known solid. Talc is translucent to opaque and has specific gravity of 2.5–2.9. The colour of talc ranges from white to grey to green. The lubricating property, high luster and low conductivity to electricity and to heat determine its industrial value. Talc is chemically inert, sparingly soluble in dilute mineral acid and insoluble in water. It has no taste and odour.

Microscopy

Talc powder when observed under microscope shows colourless, irregular and sharply angular in nature.

Chemical Constituents

Talc composed of hydrated magnesium silicate with the chemical formula $H_2Mg_3(SiO_3)_4$ or $Mg_3Si_4O_{10}(OH)_2$ and usually consist of small quantities of nickel, iron and aluminium as impurities. The variation of colour of talc to greenish or greyish tint indicates the presence of iron oxide.

Chemical Tests

1. Fuse about 0.5 g talc with 0.2 g each of anhydrous sodium carbonate and potassium carbonate in a platinum crucible. Dissolve the fused mixture into 50 ml of water and to it add hydrochloric acid and until it ceases to effervescence. Add little more acid and evaporate the contents to dryness on water bath. Cool it, dissolve in 20 ml of water, boil and filter. To the filtrate, add about 2 g of ammonium chloride and 5 ml of diluted ammonia solutions. Remove the precipitate formed, if any by filtration. To the filtrate, add sodium phosphate, white crystalline precipitate of magnesium ammonium carbonate is formed.

2. Yield the reactions characteristic of silicate.

Uses

Talc is used as a cosmetic (talcum powder), as a lubricant, as a dusting powder for coating and dusting pills and as a filler in paper manufacture. It is used as astringent in baby powders for the prevention of rashes in area covered with dipper. Talc is used in making paper (as a filler), soap, lubricants, electrical insulation stoves, sinks. It is used as a filter aid for filtration and clarification of cloudy liquids.

BENTONITE

Synonyms

Whilkinite.

Source

Bentonites are clays composed of very fine particles derived usually from volcanic ash. It is chiefly composed of the hydrous magnesium–calcium–aluminium silicate called montmorillonite.

History

Bentonite, whose name derives from its type locality (San Benito County, California), is a blue plicate mineral, found in hydro thermally altered serpentinite. Bentonite fluoresces under ultraviolet light, appearing light blue in colour.

Geographical Source

It is found in Brazil, France, Britain, Germany, India, Australia, Japan, China and the United States (California, Georgia, Florida, etc.). Bentonite is the official state gem of California.

Description

Bentonite occurs slightly greenish grey or blue in colour. When observed under ultraviolet light it shows light blue colour. It is insoluble in water, HCl and H_2SO_4, it occurs as tubular dipyramidal crystals and the hardness ranges from 6 to 6.5. Bentonite has a specific gravity of 3.6, and refractive index of 1.757–1.759 and 1.802–1.804.

Microscopy

Small quantity of bentonite when mounted in glycerin and observed under microscope shows minute hexagonal crystals with 1–2.5 µm in size.

Chemical Constituents

The chemical formula of bentonite is $BaTiSi_3O_9$ (barium titanium silicate). Generally bentonite occurs along with some unique set of minerals and the frequently associated minerals are natrolite $(Na_2Al_2Si_3O_{10}2H_2O)$, albite $(NaAlSi_3O_8)$, neptunite $[KNa_2Li (Fe, Mn)_2Ti_2Si_8O_{24}]$, serpentine $[(Mg,Fe)_3Si_2O_5(OH)_4]$ and joaquinite $[NaBa_2FeCe_2(Ti, Nb)_2(SiO_3)_8(OH, F) 1H_2O]$.

Identification Test

1. Bentonite is mounted in cresol and observed on dark field polarized light, it shines brightly.
2. Bentonite acquires permanent red stain when treated with 1% solution of safranin in 70% alcohol.
3. When bentonite treated with 0.1% solution of methylene blue in absolute alcohol it takes deep blue colour.
4. Bentonite is first mounted in alcohol and then water is applied through its sides, the fragments of bentonite swells, disintegrates into small particles and forms a jelly like matrix.

Uses

The hardness of bentonite makes it suitable for its use as a gemstone. It is also used as gel in ointment, in creams as a base, in lipsticks, depilatories and rouges. Highly absorbent bentonite is used for facing the moulds and preparing the moulding sands for casting metals. The less absorbent bentonite is used chiefly in the oil industry. Bentonite is also used as suspending and emulsifying agent and base for plasters.

FULLER'S EARTH

Synonyms

Floridin, multani mitti.

History

The word Fuller's earth is derived from the ancient process of cleaning or pulling wool to remove oil and dust particles with a water slurry of earth.

Source

Fuller's earth is mined in open quarry. It is a nonplastic type of kaolin, containing aluminium magnesium silicate.

Geographical Source

It is found in Hampshire, Surrey, Somerset, Dorset and Gloucestershire.

Description

It is white to yellowish grey in colour, odourless and tasteless powder. If put into water, it swells and acquires nonplastic texture.

Chemical Constituents

Fuller's earth has the following approximate composition SiO_2, 55%; Al_2O_3, 6%; CaO, 3.5%; MgO, 2.0%; Fe_2O_3, 6%; Water, 10% representing montmorillonite 50% and silica 18%.

Uses

It is used as decolourizer for oils and other liquids, as clarifying and filtering agent and for cleansing of woollen fabrics. Due to absorbent property, it is used in the preparation of dusting powders.

PREPARED CHALK

Synonyms

Chalk, Creta, Paris-white, Whiting, English white.

Source

Chalk is a native form of calcium carbonate, freed from most of the impurities by elutriations. It contains not less than 97.0% w/w of calcium carbonate ($CaCO_3$), when dried at 100°C.

Collection and Preparation

Chalk is mined in open quarry, pulverized and then purified by elutriation. The water is removed and the insoluble chalk is settled forming flat cakes, known as 'whiting'. It is purified further for pharmaceutical use.

Description

Chalk is colourless, odourless, white earthy and soft to the touch. It is amorphous and insoluble in water. When reacted with acids, it effervesces.

Chemical Constituents

It contains calcium carbonate (96%), magnesium carbonate (0.5%), 0.5–1.0% of silica, traces of iron, manganese and aluminium oxides.

Uses

Prepared chalk is used as an antacid, a dietary supplement, a dusting powder and an antidiarrhoeal. It is used in face powders, and as an abrasive in tooth powders and toothpastes. It is also used in the manufacture of antibiotics and pharmaceuticals.

KIESELGUHR

Synonyms

Diatomaceous earth, celite supercel, industrial Earth.

Source

It is a natural diatomaceous earth consisting of siliceous skeletons of fossils, family Bacillaceae (subdivision of the algae), purified by treating with dilute hydrochloric acid, washings with water and drying.

Geographical Source

Huge quantity of this earth is available in West Germany, Denmark, Algeria, Kenya, United States. (California and Virginia), Scotland and Ireland.

Preparation

Kieselguhr is normally mined in an open quarry wherein large blocks containing moisture to the extent of 30–40% are arranged and air-dried. The blocks containing 5–10% of moisture are then pulverized to produce fine powder and subsequently graded. The powder is then subjected to acid treatment, washed thoroughly with water and finally dried.

Description

Kieselguhr is a brownish-grey to white coloured light powder. It is odourless and tasteless. Kieselguhr is very smooth, adheres to the skin after rubbing. It. is not slippery; it absorbs moisture, but does not swell when mounted in cresol. It is invisible in polarized light with crossed nicols. Diatoms vary in size from 5 to 100 to 500 μm and exhibit two shapes: elongated and circular or triangular known as discoid.

Chemical Constituents

Diatomite contains 75–90% of silica, 1–5% of aluminium oxide; calcium oxide (1.5%), magnesium oxide (1.5%) and iron oxide (5%).

Uses

It is used as a filter aid, and for clarification and decolourization of liquids. It is used for the manufacture of tooth powder, face power and nail polishes.

CALAMINE

Synonyms

Prepared calamine.

Source

Calamine is an ore and chemically it contains zinc oxide with a small amount of ferric oxide and contains after ignition not less than 98.0% of zinc oxide.

Description

It is an odourless, colourless powder, pink in colour and very fine. Calamine is insoluble in water and soluble in mineral acids.

Chemical Constituents

It contains 99% zinc oxide and 0.5% ferric oxide. The colour of calamine is due to ferric oxide only. It should not contain calcium for pharmaceutical purposes.

Chemical Tests

1. Mix 1 g of calamine in 10 ml of dilute hydrochloric acid and filter; to this solution, add ammonium sulphide a white precipitate soluble in hydrochloric acid but insoluble in acetic acid is produced.
2. Dissolve 1 g of calamine in 10 ml of diluted hydrochloric acid, boil and filter. To the filtrate, add solution of ammonium thiocyanate; red colour is produced.

Uses

It is used topically as astringent and skin protectant. It is an ingredient of lotions and cosmetics.

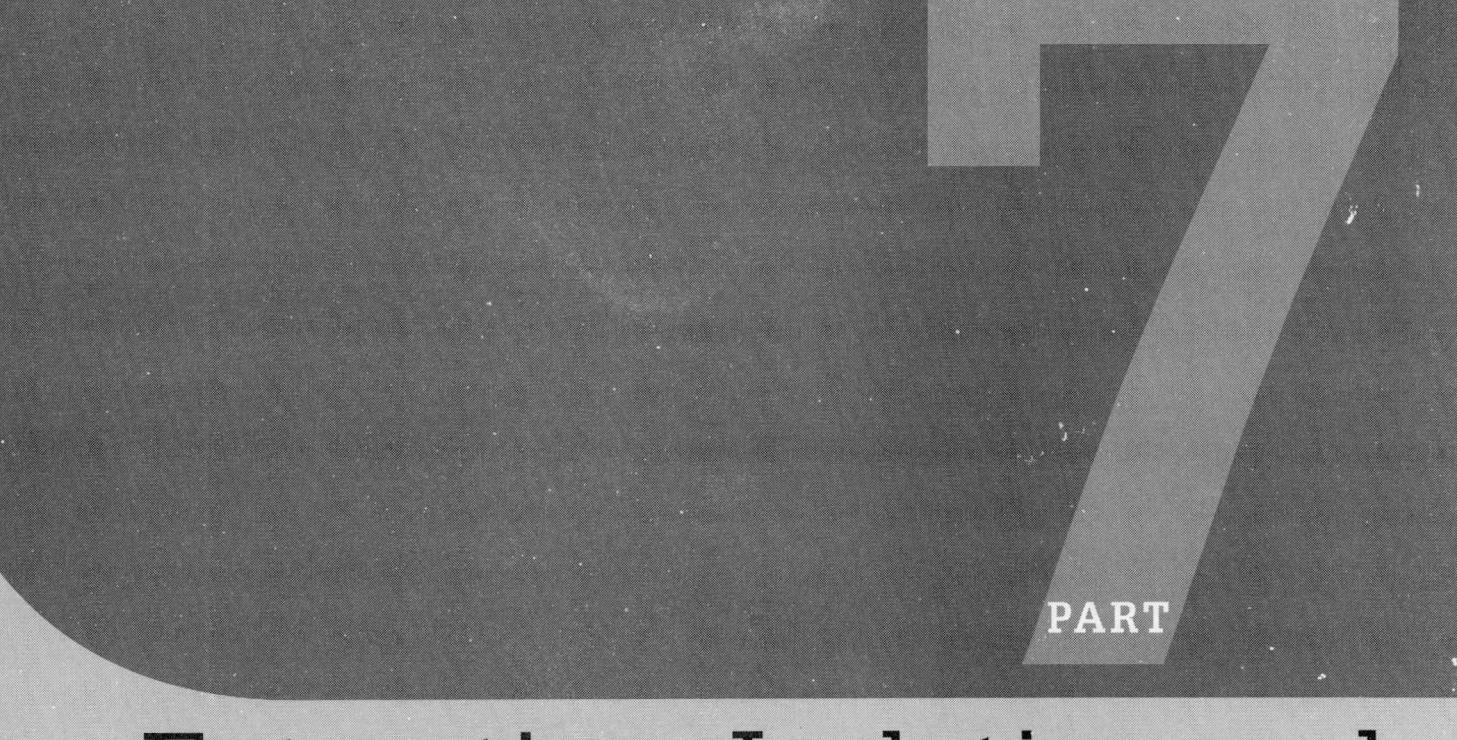

Extraction, Isolation and Purification of Herbal Drugs

Section Outline

OVERVIEW

The crude drug contains the active constituents, which can be isolated from these drugs by various methods of extraction and separation. This part provides detail information regarding various extraction and isolation techniques for crude drugs along with their identification tests. This part also provides knowledge about various recent extraction techniques adopted in the field of phytochemistry.

CHAPTER 24

General Methods for Extraction, Isolation and Identification of Herbal Drugs

CONTENTS

24.1. INTRODUCTION

The crude drug contains the active constituents, which can be isolated from these drugs by various methods of extraction and separation. Extraction is defined as the process of isolation of soluble material from an insoluble residue, which may be liquid or solid, by treatment with a solvent on the basis of the physical nature of crude drug to be extracted, i.e. liquid or solid, the extraction process may be liquid—liquid or solid—liquid extraction.

The process of extraction is controlled by mass transfer. Mass transfer is a unit operation, which involves the transfer of mass of soluble material from a solid to a fluid. If a crude drug panicle is immersed in a solvent to be used for extraction, the particle is first surrounded by a boundary layer of the solute; the solvent starts penetrating inside the particle and subsequently forms solution of the constituents within the cells. Escape of these dissolved constituents through the cell wall and through the boundary layer takes place. The process is continued till equilibrium is set up between the solution in the cells and the free solution. Few important factors, which affect the mass transfer are agitation and temperature that increase the concentration gradient to bring about an efficient extraction. Size reduction of the crude drug increases the area over which diffusion can occur. Overall extraction is also dependent on the selection of the method of extraction and the solvent selected for extraction.

24.2. EXTRACTION METHODS

Majority of the small-scale extraction processes of maceration and percolation are generally slow and time consuming and also give the inefficient extraction of the crude drugs. These processes are generally modified for more efficient and faster extraction at the laboratory scale. Large-scale industrial batch operations demand some more modifications of extraction process where the small-scale directions are inappropriate.

Maceration

Maceration process involves the separation of medicinally active portions of the crude drugs. It is based on the immersion of the crude drugs in a bulk of the solvent or menstruum. Solid drug material is taken in stoppered container as shown in Fig. 24.1, with about 750 ml of the menstruum and allowed to stand for at least three to seven days in a warm place with frequent shaking. The mixture of crude drug containing solvent is filtered until most of the liquid drains off. The filtrate and the washing are combined to produce 1000 ml of the solution.

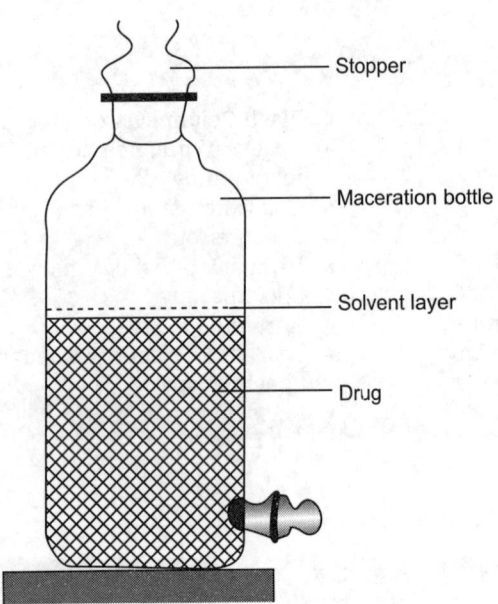

FIG. 24.1 Macerating bottle

Maceration method is modified to multiple stage extraction to increase the yield of the active ingredients in the extracts. The crude drug material is charged in the extractor, which is connected with a circulatory pump and spray distributor, along with number of connected tanks to receive the extraction solution. This is known as multiple stage extraction because the solvent added and circulated in the extractor containing drug is removed as extracted solution and is stored in the receiver tanks. This operation is repeated thrice. When the crude drug material is charged in the extractions, the stored solution is once again circulated through fresh drug and then removed as an extract. Likewise, after three extractions, the drug is removed from the extractor, again recharged with fresh drug and the whole cycle is repeated.

Percolation

As the term indicates, percolation is a continuous flow of the solvent through the bed of the crude drug material to get the extract. In this process, first the powdered drug is treated with sufficient menstruum to make it uniformly wet. Damp material is allowed to stand for about 15 min, and then transferred to a percolator winch is generally a V-shaped vessel open at both the ends. To it, sufficient menstruum is added to saturate the drug. The lid is placed on the top. When the liquid starts dripping out from the outlet of the percolator, the lower opening is closed. The drug material is allowed to macerate in the vessel for 24 h and then the percolation is continued gradually using sufficient menstruum to produce 1000 ml of solution. The percolation process is dependant on the flow of solvent through the powered drug, and it yields the products of greater concentration than the maceration process (Fig. 24.2).

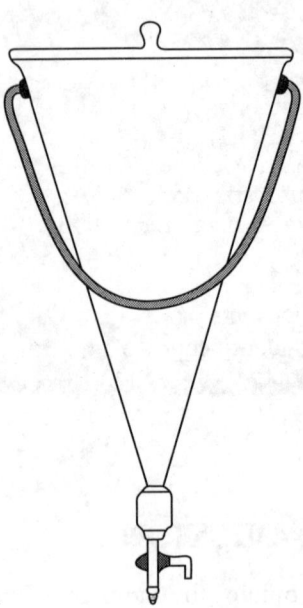

FIG. 24.2 Precolator

Modified percolation

The conventional percolation process is modified especially when the solvent is dilute alcohol. In cases when the strength of alcohol needs to be unaffected by concentration of the extract, percolation is continued and the first quantity of the percolate is collected and set aside. The subsequent quantities of the percolates are collected, concentrated and lastly, the first volume of the percolate is added in the final product. In this way it maintains the required alcohol strength and also produces the higher concentration of the products. The process is known as reserve percolate method.

In modified process of percolation techniques, continuous or semicontinuous extraction devices are used in some industries for handling the batches of varying size. The extraction batteries which consists of a number of vessels in series are interconnected through pipelines and are arranged in such a way that the solvent can be added and the product removed from any vessel. Such type of extraction battery gives maximum efficiency of extraction with minimum use of solvent. The product obtained is more concentrated and less losses of solvent take place due to evaporation.

Continuous Extraction

Soxhlet extraction

Soxhlet extraction is the process of continuous extraction in which the same solvent can be circulated through the extractor for several times. This process involves extraction followed by evaporation of the solvent. The vapours of the solvent are taken to a condenser and the condensed liquid is returned to the drug for continuous extraction.

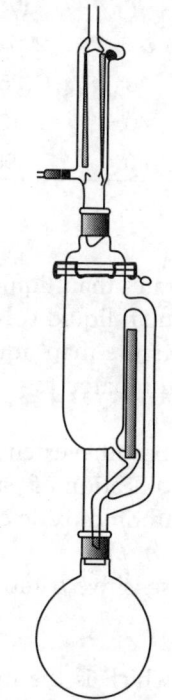

FIG. 24.3 Soxhlet extractor

Soxhlet apparatus, designed for such continuous extraction, consists of a body of extractor attached with a side tube and siphon tube as shown in Figure 24.3. The extractor from the lower side can be attached to distillation flask and the mouth of the extractor is fixed to a condenser by the standard joints. The crude drug powder is packed in the soxhlet apparatus directly or in a thimble of filter paper or fine muslin. The diameter of the thimble corresponds to the internal diameter of the soxhlet extractor. Extraction assembly is set up by fixing condenser and a distillation flask. Initially for the setting of the powder, solvent is allowed to siphon once before heating. Fresh activated porcelain pieces are added to the flask to avoid bumping of the solvent. The vapours pass through the side tube and the condensed liquid gradually increases the level of liquid in the extractor and in the siphon tube. A siphon is set up as the liquid reaches the point of return and the contents

of the extraction chamber are transferred to the flask. The cycle of solvent evaporation and siphoning back can be continued as many times as possible without changing the solvent so as to get efficient extraction. This method, although a continuous extraction process, is nothing but a series of short macerations.

Similar methodology can be adopted in large-scale production in which the operation principles may resemble the laboratory equipment. Soxhlet extraction is advantageous in a way that less solvent is needed for yielding more concentrated products. The extraction can be continued until complete exhaustion of the drug. The main disadvantage is that this process is restricted to pure boiling solvents or to azeotropes.

Large-scale extraction

As the large-scale extraction is meant for the extra large batches of drug material, the various assemblies which are generally in attachment with the body of soxhlet extractor are modified. The pilot plant extractor generally has a separate extractor and condenser unit. Separate inlet for loading the drug and an outlet for drug discharge are provided. The extractor body is divided into two parts: the upper one for drug material and the lower one as a distillation chamber. The distillation chamber is electrically heated. The vapours of the solvent are passed to condenser and the condensed liquid is sprayed on the bed of crude drug with the help of solvent distribution nozzle. Solution returns to the distillation chamber via solution return pipe. Such large-scale extractors are provided with the outlet from the lower side of the extractor, for removing the extract.

Supercritical fluid extraction

The supercritical fluid extraction (SFE) is a comparatively recent method of extraction of crude drugs. Certain gases behave like a free flowing liquids or supercritical fluids at the critical point of temperature and pressure. Such supercritical fluids have a very high penetration powers and extraction efficiency. This principle was first used in the food packing industries for the deodorization of the packed food products. The gases like carbon dioxide are held as a supercritical fluid at the critical point of 73.83 bar pressure and 31.06°C temperature. At this critical point CO_2 behaves as a liquefied gas or free-flowing liquid and assists the extraction of the phytochemical constituents from the crude drugs. The phase diagram (Fig. 24.4) of CO_2 indicates the characteristic areas for the deodorization, extraction and fractionation.

The advantages of CO_2 in SFE are that it is sterile and bacteriostatic. It is noncombustible and nonexplosive. CO_2 is harmless to environment and no waste products are generated during the process, and it is available in large amount under favourable condition.

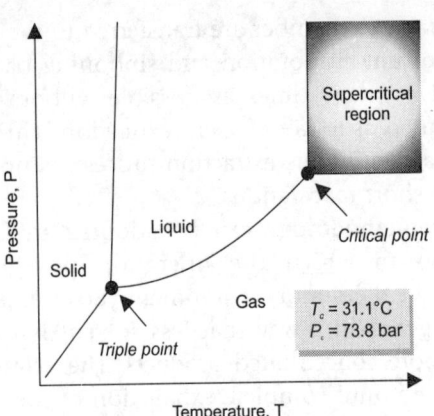

FIG. 24.4 Phase diagram of CO_2

The mixture to be fractionated is passed in the extraction column along the length of which the heater is located. CO_2 is purged through the column. Once the extraction column is pressurized, drug material gets saturated in the supercritical fluid which moves along the length of the column. The operating conditions, i.e. pressure and temperature, are selected. In the pressure controlled type of extraction, the solution is just expanded in the separation stage to precipitate the extract and then again the gas is recompressed for recycle. In temperature control type operation, the extract is precipitated by heating the solution which lowers the solvent density. The density is then increased by isobaric cooling for recycling. Operation of SFE system is controlled from a PC. PC is used to set the operating conditions like pressure, temperature and flow rate. PC is programmed to safely shut down the unit in case of overpressure or over temperature situations (Fig. 24.5).

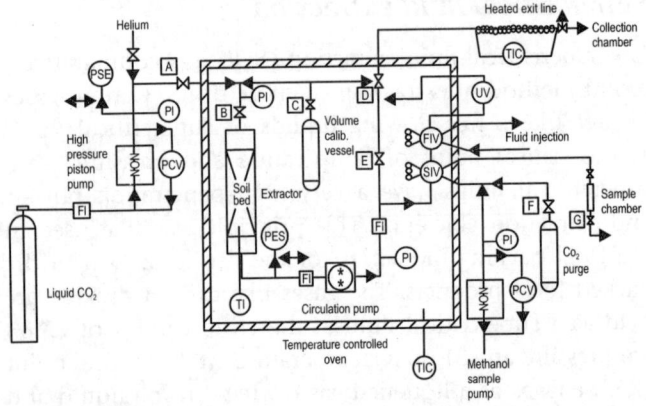

FIG. 24.5 Diagrammatic representation of supercritical extraction unit

SFE has many applications in pharmacognosy especially in the extraction and isolation of the active constituents. The process is successfully used in the decaffeination of coffee, extraction of pyrethrins and for the production of terpeneless oils. It has been successful in selectively

extracting larger proportions of active ingredients than conventional methods of hydrodistillation or extraction, i.e. in cases of acorone from *Acorus calamus*, matricin and bisabolol from chamomile flowers, heat labile sesquiterpene hydrocarbons of *Valerian* and *Nardostachys* species. It is useful for removing the off odours or 'still notes' from the freshly distilled essential oil. The temperature pressure conditions for the extraction of certain constituents from crude drugs are given in Table 24.1.

Table 24.1: Temperature and pressure conditions for SFE

Drugs	Temp (°C)	Pressure (bar)	Degree of Extraction
Caffeine from coffee	40–80°	200–300	Decaffeination
Pyrethrins	50°	250	98%
Chamomile principles	40°	160	1.4%
Acorone from calamus	40°	90	8.3%

Advantages of SFE

1. Higher diffusion rates than liquid solvents
2. Lower viscosities than liquid solvents
3. Higher vapour pressure than liquid solvents
4. Higher densities compared to gases, higher solvating power
5. Solubility and (to some extent) selectivity can be controlled by modification of parameters
6. Low polarity of carbon dioxide can be modified with cosolvents
7. Suitable for heat-sensitive compounds

Disadvantages of SFE

1. Carbon dioxide, which is the most commonly used solvent, has low polarity and hence cannot extract polar compounds
2. Presence of water may cause problems
3. Unpredictability of matrix effect
4. Need for specialized/expensive equipment

Microwave-Assisted Extraction (MAE)

Microwave assisted extraction (MAE) is also an extraction technique based on heating an organic solvent. The principle is roughly that a sample and an appropriate solvent (or solvent mixtures) are put in a vessel, which is then pressurized and heated by microwaves. After typically 5–20 minutes, the extraction is complete, and the vessels are allowed to cool down before removing the sample/solvent mixture. The solvent must be filtered to remove sample particles prior to analysis of the extracted components.

MAE is a more manual technique as it is performed in batch mode. However, many samples can be processed at the same time. Another feature of MAE is that the heating of the solvent is fast, it goes from inside the sample and outwards, and the heating capability depends on the microwave absorbing properties of the solvent. Polar solvents such as acetone will absorb microwave energy efficiently, as they have molecules with permanent dipole moment that can interact with microwaves. Nonpolar solvents such as hexane will not be heated when exposed to microwaves, but can instead be used in mixtures with polar solvents in order to obtain the desired heating properties.

Some common solvent mixtures that have been used in MAE are acetonitrile/methanol, hexane/acetone, ethylacetate/cyclohexane and isooctane/acetone.

MAE applications in the literature include, for example, extraction of capsaicinoids from capsicum fruit, PBDEs from marine biological tissues, pesticides from vegetables and pigments from paprika powder. In general, method development in MAE involves optimization of solvent composition, solvent volume, extraction temperature and extraction time. The temperature of the solvent/sample mixture is usually well above the boiling point of the solvent(s). Hence, MAE utilizes the enhanced solvent strength and faster diffusivity of a heated solvent.

There are a few different brands of equipment on the market; CEM (Matthews, NC) has the MARS-X that can process up to 14 samples simultaneously with optional sample stirring. Milestone (Shelton, CT) manufactures instruments named Ethos (6–24 vessels of volumes 100–270 ml, with sample stirring). Radient Technologies (Burlington, ON, Canada) has developed a large-scale MAE technology that they call MAP, and they design pilot plants for natural product customers. There are several MAE pilot and industrial plants around the world. For example, Archimex (Vannes, France) is doing contract research on pilot scale MAE (as well as SFE) for isolation of bioactive/high-value compounds from plant origin.

24.3. TYPES OF EXTRACTS

Numbers of different types of methods are used for the extraction of herbal drugs, and the extracts are used for different purposes ranging from internal administration, external use, for further purification of phytopharmaceuticals or for it semisynthetic conversion to some therapeutically more active compounds. The extracts are therefore prepared likewise to achieve the objectives for which it is prepared. Extracts can be in the form of aqueous, hydroalcoholic types in the form of infusion, decoction, tinctures, etc., or they can be more concentrated which may further be transformed into soft, dry or liquid extracts.

Aqueous Extracts

These are the extracts which are medicinal preparations intended to be used immediately after preparation or to be preserved for use. The following methods are generally more in utility for their preparation.

- **Decoction:** This is the ancient and more popular process of extracting water soluble and heat stable constituents from crude drugs by boiling in water for about 15 min. The boiled crude drug–water mixture is then cooled; filtered and sufficient volume of cold water is passed through the drug to produce the required volume.
- **Infusion:** An infusion is generally a dilute solution of the readily soluble constituents of crude drugs. It is nothing but a type of periodic maceration of the drug with either cold or boiling water. The infusion is filtered to remove the crude vegetable material and then produced in a required volume by addition of water.
- **Digestion:** Digestion is also a type of maceration in which moderate heating is preferred during extraction. Heating causes the digestion of drug material and increases the solvent efficiency. It is preferred for the drugs in which the use of moderately elevated temperature does not cause the degradation of constituents.
- **Tinctures:** Tinctures are the alcoholic or hydroalcoholic solutions prepared from crude drugs or from the pure organic or inorganic substances. Tinctures of crude drugs may contain 10–20 g of drug per 100 ml of tincture. The methods used for the preparation of tinctures are maceration and percolation. Iodine tincture is an example of inorganic pharmaceuticals, belladonna tincture is prepared by percolation while compound benzoin tincture, sweet orange peel tincture are prepared by maceration.
- **Liquid Extracts:** The liquid extracts are also termed as fluid extracts in some official books like USP. It is a liquid preparation of crude drugs which contain ethyl alcohol as a solvent and preservative. It may contain active constituents to the extent of 1 g of drug per ml. Pharmacopoeial liquid extracts are prepared by the percolation or modified percolation techniques.
- **Soft Extract:** The extracts which are produced as semisolid or liquids of syrupy consistency are termed as soft extracts. These extracts are used in the variety of dosage forms ranging from ointments, suppositories or can be used in the preparation of some other pharmaceuticals. Glycyrrhiza extract USP comes in the form of soft extract.
- **Dry Extract:** Dry extracts are also known as the powdered extracts or dry powders. The total extracts obtained by using suitable process of extraction, are filtered, concentrated preferably under vacuum and dried completely. The tray drying or spray drying is used for making dry extracts. Just like soft extracts, these powdered extracts can be used for the manufacture of some medicinal preparations. Powdered extracts are preferably used into a solid, dry dosage forms like capsules, powders or tablets. The Belladonna extract, Hyoscyamus extract are the official dry extracts.

24.4. ISOLATION AND IDENTIFICATION OF NATURAL PRODUCTS

The progress in the techniques for isolation and analysis has led to the identification of many unknown compounds. Various processes are involved in the isolation of the particular compound from its plant material. The isolation process possibly will depend on the nature of the active constituent present in the crude drug. For example, trapping of the components is done for the volatile chemicals while extraction of nonvolatile compounds using organic solvents is also done. The isolation of components is done for both known constituents and also for the components which are unknown and the process of the separation, purification and identification of compounds coupled with biological screening is a demanding task. After the extraction of the required crude extract from the plant, the need of the marker component to be isolated and identified is also equally important for its study with respect to chemical nature or even for the development of newer formulations. The advances in the field of chromatographic techniques have enabled the separation and purification of compounds.

Fractional Crystallization

Crystallization is an old but a very important method for the purification of the compounds from the mixture. Crystallization mostly depends upon the inherent character of the compound which forms crystals at the point of supersaturation in the solvent in which it is soluble. Many phytopharmaceuticals and natural products are crystalline compounds which tend to crystallize even in the mixtures. Compounds, such as sugars, glycosides, alkaloids, steroids, triterpenoids, flavonoids, etc., show the crystalline nature with certain exceptions. The processes, such as concentration, slow evaporation, refrigeration are used for crystallizing the products. In case of sugars, osazone formation leads to the crystallization of the derivatives in the form of various types of crystals enabling the analysis of the sugars.

Fractional Distillation

For the distillation the component should have volatile nature. Therefore, fractional distillation is mostly used for the separation of essential oil components. Most of the volatile components are steam volatile and if the process of fractional distillation is skilfully used, various low-boiling and high-boiling components can be separated from the total oil. This process is largely used for the separation of hydrocarbons from the oxygenated volatile oil components—the product referred to as terpenless essential oils. The components like citral, citronellal and eucalyptol are even now separated by fractional distillation. It is used in the separation of hydrocyanic acid from plant material.

Fractional Liberation

In the process of fractional liberation, groups of the compounds having the tendency of precipitation come out of the solution. In certain cases the nature of the compound such as alkaloids is modified by converting to their salt form or free bases. If such alkaloidal compounds are more in number with variation in basic nature, with such conversions base liberation, these may be brought about from a weaker base to relatively stronger base. The process is often used even at the industrial level for the separation of cinchona alkaloid quinine, isolation of morphine and many other alkaloids. By using the similar processes phenols, organic acids, like compounds are liberated from the solution.

Sublimation

As a matter of fact there are very few natural products which have sublimating nature. In this process the compound if subjected to heating, changes from solid state to gaseous state directly without passing through a phase of liquid. Such compounds from the gaseous state get deposited on the cooler surface in the form of crystals or cake. The process is traditionally used for the separation of camphor from the chips of wood of *Cinnamomum camphora* to obtain solid sublimate of camphor. Sublimation can also be used for the isolation of caffeine from tea or for the purification of material present in a crude extract. In the inorganic compounds, sublimation is the well-known process for the isolation and purification of sulphur.

Chromatography

Chromatography is a family of analytical chemistry techniques for the separation of mixtures. It was the Russian botanist, Mikhail Tsvet, who invented the first chromatography technique in 1901, which was based on adsorption principle. In 1952, Archer John Porter Martin and Richard Laurence Millington Synge were the two scientists who identified partition chromatography. Chromatographic techniques create a basis for analysis and separation of a wide range of physical methods used in complex mixtures. In chromatography, it has two phases: stationary phase and a mobile phase in which the components are distributed. When components pass through the system at different rates they become separated in time, like runners in a mass-start fool race. Each component has a characteristic time of passage through the system, called a retention time. Chromatographic separation is achieved when the retention time of the analyte differs from that of other components in the sample. This difference in rate of travel results in the separation of the individual component. The smaller the affinity a molecule has for the stationary phase, the shorter the time spent in the column. A chromatograph takes a chemical mixture carried by liquid or gas and separates it into its component parts as a result of differential distributions of the solutes as they flow around or over the stationary liquid or solid phase. If the right adsorbent material, mobile fluid and operating conditions are employed, any soluble or volatile component can be separated using chromatography. Even structurally very similar components can be separated with chromatography. The principle of chromatography differs according to the stationary and mobile phase used. According to this the types are following:

- **Adsorption Chromatography:** Adsorption chromatography is probably one of the oldest types of chromatography around. It utilizes a mobile liquid or gaseous phase that is adsorbed onto the surface of a stationary solid phase. The equilibration between the mobile and stationary phase accounts for the separation of different solutes.

- **Partition Chromatography:** This form of chromatography is based on a thin film formed on the surface of a solid support by a liquid stationary phase. Solute equilibrates between the mobile phase and the stationary liquid.

- **Ion Exchange Chromatography:** In this type of chromatography, the use of a resin (the stationary solid phase) is used to covalently attach anions or cations on to it. Solute ions of the opposite charge in the mobile liquid phase are attracted to the resin by electrostatic forces.

- **Molecular Exclusion Chromatography:** Also known as gel permeation or gel filtration, this type of chromatography lacks an attractive interaction between the stationary phase and solute. The liquid or gaseous phase passes through a porous gel which separates the molecules according to its size. The pores are normally small and exclude the larger solute molecules, but allow smaller molecules to enter the gel, causing them to flow through a larger volume. This causes the larger molecules to pass through the column at a faster rate than the smaller ones.

- **Affinity Chromatography:** This is the most selective type of chromatography employed. It utilizes the specific interaction between one kind of solute molecule and a second molecule that is immobilized on a stationary phase. For example, the immobilized molecule may be an antibody to some specific protein. When solute containing a mixture of proteins is passed by this molecule, only the specific protein is reacted to this antibody, binding it to the stationary phase. This protein is later extracted by changing the ionic strength or pH. There are different types of chromatographic methods like paper chromatography (PC), thin layer chromatography (TLC), column chromatography, high-performance liquid chromatography, gas chromatography and high-performance TLC. All these methods were used in the analysis, separation and isolation of the components in natural products.

Retention

The retention is nothing but a measure of the speed at which a compound moves in a chromatographic system. In continuous development systems like HPLC or GC, where the compounds are eluted with the eluent, the retention is usually measured as the *retention time R_t* the time between injection and detection. In interrupted development systems like TLC, PC the retention is measured as the *retention factor R_f*, the run length of the compound divided by the run length of the eluent front.

$$R_f = \frac{\text{Distance travelled by solute}}{\text{Distance travelled by solvent}}$$

Paper Chromatography (PC)

The main advantage of the PC is the convenience of carrying out separations simply on sheets of filter paper that serve both as the medium for separation and as support. The technique was extended to maximum all classes of natural products. The solution of components to be separated is applied as a spot near one end of a prepared filter paper strip. Usually several sample and standard spots are placed along the edge. Then the chromatogram is developed by immersing that edge of the paper in a solvent that migrates through the paper as the mobile phase. The solvent often has two, three or four components—one of which is usually water. Development is normally done in a chamber that is saturated with solvent vapour. The water from the solvent, in particular, is adsorbed and tightly held on the paper fibres, so the sample components partition between the migrating mobile phase and the tightly held water. After the separation, any strongly coloured spots are visible on the chromatogram. Colourless materials can be visualized by heating the paper in an oven so that substances (but not the paper) char and leave black spots. Sometimes the paper is first sprayed with a solution of sulphuric acid for better charring. Fluorescent materials can be visualized with ultraviolet light. Reagents specific for certain components may be sprayed on to make coloured spots. Radioactive spots can be located with a detector, or the chromatogram can be pressed against X-ray film for minutes or hours to expose the film. Sample spots can be tentatively identified if they have the same R_f values as known standard spots.

Sometimes spots, once located, are cut out so that the material in the spot can be recovered. There are also instruments that (more or less accurately) quantitative the material in the spot by measuring light absorbance.

Thin Layer Chromatography

The thin layer chromatography is a widely used, fast technique for the qualitative analysis of a mixture of compounds. The stationary phase consists of a thin layer of adsorbent like silica gel, alumina or cellulose on a flat carrier like a glass plate, a thick aluminium foil or a plastic sheet. TLC has certain advantages over PC. Fractionations can be effected more rapidly with smaller quantities of the mixture. The separated spots are usually more compact and more clearly demarcated from one another, and the nature of the film is often such that drastic reagents, such as concentrated sulphuric acid, which would destroy a paper chromatogram, can be used for the location of separated substances. TLC plates are made by mixing the adsorbent with a small amount of inert binder like calcium sulphate (gypsum) and water, spreading the thick slurry on the carrier, drying the plate and activation of the adsorbent by heating in an oven. The thickness of the adsorbent layer is typically around 0.1–0.25 mm for analytical purposes and around 1–2 mm for preparative TLC.

Several methods exist to make colourless spots visible. Often a small amount of a fluorescent dye is added to the adsorbent that allows the visualization of UV absorbing spots under a black light (UV_{254}). Even UV light without fluorescent dye could scan the compounds, both in long (365 nm) and short (254 nm) wavelength ultraviolet light. Iodine vapours are a general unspecific colour reagent.

Specific colour reagents exist into which the TLC plate is dipped or which are sprayed onto the plate. Dragendorff's reagents are used in the form of sprays for the general detection of alkaloids. Antimony trichloride in chloroform is used as a spray reagent for steroidal compounds and other terpenoids. Ammonia vapour can be used for free anthraquinone compounds and Fast Blue Salt B 'Merck' for cannabinoids and phloroglucides.

It is effective, comparatively cheap as relatively small amounts of analyte, adsorbent and solvents are required. The use of appropriate developing agents can help understand the compound properties and can be quantified by careful standardization of procedures.

High-Performance Thin Layer Chromatography

The high-performance thin layer chromatography is a sophisticated and automated form of TLC. It is useful in qualitative and quantitative analysis of natural products. The principle of separation is adsorption (same as that of TLC). In HPTLC, the precoated plates are used and the particle size of stationary phase is less than 1 μm in diameter. There is a wide choice of stationary phases like silica gel for normal phase and C18, C8, etc., for reverse phase mode. HPTLC provides a higher efficiency than TLC because adsorbents used are small and uniform in size.

A very less amount of sample is spotted on the plate so the sample prepared should be highly concentrated. The size of the sample spot should not be more than 1 mm in diameter. The samples are spotted by various techniques and commonly used method is by semiautomatic linomet V apparatus.

New types of development chambers are used in HPTLC that require less amount of solvents for developing. A linear development technique is commonly used. The plate is placed vertically in development chambers containing solvent, and chromatogram can be developed from the sides. In HPTLC, UV/VIS/fluorescence scanner is used; therefore, it scans the entire chromatogram qualitatively and quantitatively. The scanner is an advanced type of densitometer.

HPTLC is used for the standardization of herbal extracts and other formulations. By using this technique, the analytical profiles of alkaloids, cardenolides, anthracene glycosides, flavonoids, lipids, steroidal compounds, etc., have been developed.

Column Chromatography

Column chromatography utilizes a vertical glass column filled with some form of solid support with the sample to be separated placed on top of this support. The rest of the column is filled with a solvent which, under the influence of gravity, moves the sample through the column. Similarly to other forms of chromatography, differences in rates of movement through the solid medium are translated to different exit times from the bottom of the column for the various elements of the original sample.

Flash Column Chromatography

This is a fast, simple, widely used preparative separation technique, where the stationary bed is packed in a long, narrow glass lube. The flow rate of the mobile phase of the system can be accelerated either by applying pressure on the top of the column or by applying suction from the lower end of the column to decrease the time that the compounds spend in the column or to increase the flow rate of the mobile phase. Typically, silica is used as the stationary phase but other stationary beds such as reverse phase silica or cellulose are also used depending on the nature of the compounds to be separated. The particles size should be smaller than that of the column chromatography.

High-Performance Liquid Chromatography

This is a versatile natural product isolation technique which is similar to flash chromatography; however, high pressure (up to 4000–5000 psi) is applied to the system to move the mobile phase through the smaller particle sized (2–10 μm) stationary phase bed. The column is stainless steel to withstand the high pressure. It employs relatively narrow columns about 5 mm diameter for analytical work, operating at ambient temperature or up to about 200°C. The apparatus is suitable for all types of liquid chromatography columns (adsorption, partition by the use of bonded liquid phases, reversed phase, gel filtration,

ion exchange and affinity). Many stationary phases are available and the most widely used is silica based, silanol groups (SiOH).

Reversed phase packing material is produced by the bonding of octadecylsilyl groups to silica gel. In the commercial material there appears to be a considerable proportion of residual silanol OH groups, and this would lead to both adsorption and partition effects during separation. Unlike the other two methods (TLC and flash chromatography), the eluting compounds can be detected using their different physical and structural properties by connecting a detector (UV/visible UV/VIS, refractive index RI). Furthermore, the eluting compounds can be connected to a spectrophotometer (NMR, MS) to study the spectral characteristics of compounds eluting through the HPLC system. The stationary phase bed could be either silica or reverse phase C_n bonded silica, depending on the nature (polarity) of the compounds that are to be separated. The possibilities of working at ambient temperature and recovering the sample after analysis and purification associated with HPLC presents more advantages compared to gas chromatography.

Gas Chromatography

Gas chromatography is the most widely used chromatographic technique to analyse volatile compounds where those compounds are carried by an inert gas like nitrogen, helium or argon through a heated (50–350°C) stationary bed (silica supported with bonded polar or nonpolar phase). The choice of stationary phase is governed by the temperature at which the column is to operate and the nature of the material to be fractionated; it should be nonvolatile at the operating temperature and should not react with either the stationary and mobile phases or the solutes. Some commonly used, stationary phase materials are nonpolar compound like silicone oils, apiezon oils and greases, high-boiling point paraffins, such as mineral oil, squalene, moderately polar compounds high-boiling point alcohols and their esters and strongly polar compounds polypropylene glycols and their esters.

There are two general types of column, packed and capillary (also known as open tubular). Packed columns contain a finely divided, inert, solid support material (commonly based on diatomaceous earth) coated with liquid stationary phase. Most packed columns are 1.5–10 m in length and have an internal diameter of 2–4 mm.

Capillary columns have an internal diameter of a few tenths of a millimetre. They can be one of two types: wall-coated open tubular (WCOT) or support-coated open tubular (SCOT). Wall-coated columns consist of a capillary tube whose walls are coated with liquid stationary phase. In support-coated columns, the inner wall of the capillary is lined with a thin layer of support material such as diatomaceous earth, onto which the stationary phase has been adsorbed. SCOT columns are generally less efficient than WCOT columns. Both types of capillary column are more efficient than packed columns. Either a flame ionization detector (FID) or electron capture detector (BCD) detects the compounds eluting from the column producing a signal which can transform into a peak or a chromatogram. The technique is very sensitive, and low concentrations of sample (less than nanograms) can be analysed. Preparative GC also can be carried out using a thermal conductivity detector or splitting outlet to connector and FID. But the difficulties in recovering the compound after analysis are the main disadvantage over HPLC and flash chromatography. GC can be connected to a mass spectrometer to analyse the spectral characteristics of separated compounds. Once a compound is isolated, it needs to be identified to determine the chemical structure of the compound. Complete identification of a compound could be afforded using its spectral characteristics. A known compound from a new plant source can be identified using chromatographic, cochromatographic and a spectral comparison with the authentic material. With a new compound, the relationship of the chromatographic and spectral data of known compounds in the same series together with the chemical conversions, determination of the chemical formula or derivatization could help to investigate the chemical structure. The available modern advanced spectroscopic techniques and chromatography coupled spectroscopy such as gas chromatography coupled mass spectrometry (GC-MS), high-performance liquid chromatography coupled mass spectroscopy (LC-MS) and high-performance liquid chromatography coupled nuclear magnetic resonance (NMR) spectroscopy (LC-NMR) has led to the identification of new molecules more quickly than before.

Spectroscopy

The isolated and purified plant constituents should be identified and its chemical nature should be determined. The plant compounds could be identified by their spectral characteristics. Spectroscopy is the use of absorption, emission or scattering of electromagnetic radiation by atoms or molecules (or atomic or molecular ions) to qualitatively or quantitatively study the atoms or molecules or to study the physical process of a compound. The theory behind the spectroscopy is the interaction of radiation with matter. It can cause redirection of the radiation and/or transitions between energy levels of atoms or molecules. This transition could be absorption, emission or scattering. Among the number of spectroscopic methods ultraviolet visible absorption (UV-VIS), infrared (IR), NMR and mass (MS) plays a crucial role in identifying the plant compounds.

Ultraviolet–Visible Absorption Spectroscopy

Different organic molecules with certain functional groups (chromophores) that contain valence electrons of low energy can absorb ultraviolet (UV) or visible (VIS) radiation at different wavelengths. Hence the absorption spectrum of a certain molecule will show a number of absorption bands corresponding to structural groups within the molecule. Most commonly used solvent is 95% ethanol, because it solubilizes most classes of compounds. Other solvents used are water, petroleum, hexane, ether and methanol. The absorption is recorded using a detector, such as photo diode array (PDA). This phenomenon could be used to identify the functional groups of a certain molecule or when a PDA detector is connected to a HPLC system; it could be used to monitor the separation or purity of a certain mixture or a compound/s that contained different chromophores. Selection of the detection wavelength of a compound determines the nature of the chromophore within the molecule. While the compounds which possess chromophores are detected between 200–700 nm (visible), others which do not possess chromophores are detected between 200–400 nm (UV). Also, the study of the functional group or chromophore could be extended by observing the shifting (red shift or blue shift) of the maximum absorbance (λ_{max}) in the absorption spectrum of the compounds by changing the solvent in which the compound is dissolved. The value of UV and visible spectra in identifying unknown constituents is obviously related to the relative complexity of the spectrum and to the general position of the wave length maxima.

Infrared Spectroscopy

This is done by IR spectrophotometer and the plant compounds used is either in liquid, e.g. chloroform, as a mull with nujol oil or in the solid state, mixed with potassium bromide to form a thin disc. The term 'infra red' covers the range of the electromagnetic spectrum between 0.78 and 1000 µm. In the context of infra red spectroscopy, wavelength is measured in wavenumbers, which have the unit cm⁻¹.

It is useful to divide the infra red region into three sections: near, mid and far infra red.

Region	Wave length (nm)	Wave number (cm⁻¹)
Near	0.78–2.50	12,800–4000
Middle	2.5–50	4000–200
Far	50–1000	200–10

The most useful IR region lies between 4000 and 670 cm⁻¹. IR radiation does not have enough energy to induce electronic transitions seen with UV. Absorption of IR is restricted to compounds with small energy differences in the possible vibrational and rotational states.

For a molecule to absorb IR, the vibrations or rotations within a molecule must cause a net change in the dipole moment of the molecule. The alternating electrical field of the radiation interacts with fluctuations in the dipole moment of the molecule. If the frequency of the radiation matches the vibrational frequency of the molecule, then radiation will be absorbed causing a change in the amplitude of molecular vibration.

IR spectrum is the most simplest and reliable tool because many functional groups can be identified by their characteristic vibration frequencies. It has a role in structural elucidation when new compounds are identified in plants.

Nuclear Magnetic Resonance Spectroscopy

The nuclear magnetic resonance is a theoretically complex but powerful tool for providing information about the structure of a molecule in a solution. Proton NMR spectroscopy provides a means of determining the structure of an organic compound by measuring the magnetic moments of its hydrogen atom. Theoretically, subatomic particles (electrons, protons and neutrons) can be imaged as spinning on their axis. In many atoms like, ^{12}C, these spins are paired against each other. Those nuclei of atoms have no overall spin. However, in some atoms like, ^{1}H, ^{13}C, the nucleus does possess an overall spin. The sample of the substance is placed in solution, in an inert solvent between the poles of a powerful magnet and the protons undergo different chemical shifts according to their molecular environments within the molecule. It requires 5–10 mg of sample and this sample could be recovered as it is. The spin of the hydrogen atom can be promoted from the lower to higher level by interacting with and absorbing energy from electromagnetic radiation in the radio frequency region of the spectrum. The separation between the two spin energy levels is a sensitive function of the molecular environment of the hydrogen atom in the molecule. Thus, hydrogen atoms in different environments absorb photons of different energies. The NMR spectrum of the protons in a molecule is obtained by plotting the amount of energy absorbed by the spinning nuclei versus the frequency of the RF radiation applied to the molecule. This spectrum provides information about the chemical environment of the spinning proton and can be used to deduce the atomic bonding patterns in the molecule. The spin between two groups of protons result in small interactions with each other and is called spin–spin coupling where the space between each coupling is called the coupling constant. The multiplication of the coupling and the magnitude of the coupling constant in a ^{1}H NMR gives information about the number of H atoms on the nearest carbon atom of the relevant peak or proton/s and their chemical nature. But the proton NMR cannot give information on the nature of the carbon skeleton of a molecule but ^{13}C NMR could help to solve it. Even in ^{13}C NMR, the theory is the same as in ^1H NMR and both decoupled and coupled spectra are recorded. But the coupled spectrum of ^{13}C NMR is slightly different from that of ^1H NMR, and is called off-resonance proton decoupling. ^{13}C NMR helps to identify the number of unique carbon atoms in a molecule, the number of hydrogen atoms attached to that carbon atom, the environment of the carbon atom and C–C skeleton of the molecule. The modern NMR techniques like heteronuclear multiple bond correlation (HMBC), correlated spectroscopy (COSY), heteronuclear single quantum coherence (HSQC), nuclear overhauser enhancement spectroscopy (NOESY) and total correlated spectroscopy (TOCSY) have made the characterization of natural products easier.

Mass Spectroscopy

In mass spectrometry, the sample in gas or liquid or solid state is introduced to the spectrometer followed by ionization, mass analysis and ion detection/data analysis. We could get the exact molecular weights of the compounds in microgram amounts of sample. Volatilization of the sample (liquid or solid state) is done either prior to ionization or along with the ionization. The various ionization techniques commonly used are chemical ionization (CI), electron impact ionization (EI) and desorption ionization techniques. Charged molecules in the gas phase are produced by fast atom bombardment (FAB), plasma desorption (PD), and thermospray and particle beam. Then, the ion and its fragments are accelerated by electrical and magnetic fields and the ions are separated in the basis of their mass/charge (m/z) ratio and detected. The data produced by the molecular mass measurements or the fragmentation data enable us to elucidate the possible chemical structure of the molecule. The use of GC-MS, LC-MS, capillary electrophoresis–mass spectroscopy have made the identification of natural product easier.

Isolation of Phytopharmaceuticals

CONTENTS

25.1. INTRODUCTION

There is a revival of interest in the use of plants in pharmacy both from pharmaceutical industry as a source of new lead molecules find from the general public who are using plant extracts in many ways in conventional and complementary therapies. About one-quarter of all prescription drugs are of plant origin despite the fact that less than 5% of plant species have been investigated. Many of the synthetic medicine currently in clinical use have been from natural sources. It is a widely accepted fact that natural product chemistry surpasses the kind of chemistry that synthetic chemist can ever accomplish in the laboratory. Phytochemical diversity in terms of structural novelty is unprecedented in laboratory synthesis. Indeed the plant kingdom provides enormous chemical diversity. Advances in bioassay screening, isolation techniques and structural elucidation have greatly shortened and accelerated the process of drug discovery from medicinal plants. Nowadays it is a common practice among natural product chemists to use some type of bioassay to direct the progress of phytochemical investigation towards the discovery of new pure bioactive markers.

The increasing use of herbal preparations has highlighted need for adequate standards to ensure quality, safety and efficacy of such drugs and preparations. Many developing countries are becoming aware of the potential of their flora as a source of medicinally useful products. Some of the most important alkaloids, glycosides, aglycones, resin and essential oil components of commercial use have been presented here in respect to their isolation and identification.

KEY TERMS

25.2. ISOLATION OF ATROPINE

Atropine is a tropane alkaloid from the members of the Solanaceae family. It is present in *Atropa belladona* (Deadly Night shade), *Datura stramonium* (Thorn apple) and *Hyoscyamus niger* (Henbane); other important solanaceous alkaloids are hyoscyamine, hyoscine (scopolamine), apoatropine, belladonine and norhyoscyamine. Atropine is an optically inactive laevorotatory isomer of hyoscyamine.

Atropine

Isolation

Atropine is isolated from the juice or the powdered drug. *Hyoscyamus muticus* is the preferred source for the manufacture of atropine because of its high alkaloidal content, with *D. stramonium* next in order.

The powdered drug material is thoroughly moistened with an aqueous solution of sodium carbonate and then extracted with ether or benzene. The alkaloidal free bases are extracted from the solvent with water acidified with acetic acid. The acid solution is then shaken with solvent ether to remove colouring matter. The alkaloids are precipitated with sodium carbonate, filtered off, washed and dried. The dried mass is dissolved in solvent ether or acetone and dehydrated with anhydrous sodium sulphate before filtration. The filtrate after concentration and cooling yields crude crystals of hyoscyamine and atropine from the solution. The crude crystalline mass is separated from the solution. The crude crystalline mass obtained after filtration is dissolved in alcohol, and sodium hydroxide solution is added and the mixture is allowed to stand until hyoscyamine is completely racemized to atropine which is indicated by the absence of optical activity.

The crude atropine is purified by crystallization from acetone. Atropine sulphate is the most important salt of atropine. It occurs in the form of colourless crystalline powder. It is soluble in water and alcohol but insoluble in ether and chloroform.

Melting point: 115–116°C

Identification

Dilute solution of atropine, when treated with concentrated nitric acid and the mixture evaporated to dryness on the steam bath, produces a pale yellow residue. The residue gives a violet colouration when a drop of freshly prepared solution of potassium hydroxide is added. This is known as Vitali-Morin reaction.

Thin Layer Chromatography of Atropine

One percentage solution of atropine dissolved in 2 N acetic acid is spotted over silica gel-G plate and eluted in the solvent system of strong ammonia solution; methanol (1.5:100). TLC plate is spread with an acidified iodoplatinate solution. Atropine gives the R_f value 0.18. Likewise, atropine sulphate shows the R_f value 0.70 in the solvent system acetone: 0.5 M sodium chloride after spraying with Dragendorff's reagent.

25.3. ISOLATION OF ANDROGRAPHOLIDE

Andrographolide is a bitter diterpenoid lactone obtained from the dried herb of *Andrographis paniculata*; family Acanthaceae. It also consists of other bitters which includes neoandrographolide and andrographoside.

Andrographolide

Isolation

The dried herb is cleaned to remove foreign matter and then crushed to coarse powder. The powder is exhaustively extracted with 1:1 mixture of methanol and ethylene dichloride. The total extract is concentrated and subjected to treatment with activated charcoal. The solution treated with charcoal is filtered, and the filtrate is concentrated to pasty mass and then dissolved in hot methanol. The methanolic solution is again treated with charcoal or passed through mixed charcoal and Hyflo bed. The resultant clear, light yellow coloured solution is reduced to about half of its volume and subjected to crystallization in crystallizer fitted with low-speed stirrer. The crystals obtained after about 24 h are filtered off and washed with chilled methanol. The filtrate and washings are processed for second crop after concentration. The crystalline product obtained is dried in vacuum dryer at temperature not more than 50°C. This procedure yields about 1.25–1.75% of andrographolide. Melting point: 218–220°C

Thin Layer Chromatography of Andrographolide

Dissolve about 1 mg of sample in 1 ml of methanol. Apply the spots over silica gel-G plate and elute in the solvent system chloroform-methanol (7:1). Spray the eluted plate with 20% sulphuric acid in methanol and heat at 120°C for 10 min. Andrographolide appears as a visible brownish spot at R_f value 0.70, while neoandrographolide appears as a pinkish spot at R_f value 0.39.

25.4. ISOLATION OF BACOSIDES

Bacosides are the triterpenic saponins obtained from dried, whole herb, preferably leaves and stems of *Bacopa monnieri*; family Scrophulariaceae. These are the tetracyclic triterpenic saponins which consist of the crystalline mixture of several saponins including bacosides A and B.

	R	R₁
Bacoside A1	-H	-arabinosyl
Bacoside A3	-arabinosyl	-β-D-glucosyl

Isolation

The coarsely powdered drug is extracted with ethyl alcohol and the alcoholic extract is concentrated to dryness. Dry alcoholic extract is dissolved in 60% alcohol, and the solution is extracted in separating funnel with benzene to divide the constituents in benzene soluble and alcohol soluble fractions. Alcohol soluble part consists of slimy mass; it is further dissolved in alcohol and fractionally precipitated with ether and petroleum ether repeatedly leading to the separation of brown resinous material. Solution of alcohol–ether–petroleum ether mixture is concentrated and the residue is macerated with acetone

and filtered. The acetone-insoluble powder is partitioned between butanol and water. During concentration of butanol solution, a precipitate that settles down is separated and coded as A₁. The filtrate is again concentrated and precipitated with acetone and ether to afford a powder A₂. The mother liquor is concentrated to dryness to yield brownish powder A₃. Fraction A₁, A₂ and A₃ obtained consist mainly of bacoside A.

The acetone soluble fraction is left in the cold for several days when a solid settles down. It is filtered, washed with acetone, yield major amount of bacoside B.

Thin Layer Chromatography of Bacoside

The extract or the isolated glycoside dissolved in methanol and spotted over silica gel-G plates. The plates are eluted in ethyl acetate–pyridine–water (4:1:1), and the TLC plates after drying are sprayed with trichloroacetic acid (25%) in chloroform. Bacoside A of A₁, A₂ and A₃ fraction gives R_f value 0.43 while bacoside B gives R_f value 0.09.

25.5. ISOLATION OF CAFFEINE

Caffeine or 1,3,7-trimethylxanthin is a purine base present along with other related bases like theophyline and theobromine in coffee, tea, cocoa, guarana, kola and mate. Although caffeine is largely produced synthetically, it is usually isolated from tea leaves or recovered from coffee seeds during decaffeination process. Tea leaves contain 1–4% of caffeine while coffee seeds contains 1–2% of caffeine. Caffeine was first discovered by Robiquet in coffee in 1821, and mid later in 1827, Oudry found it in tea leaves.

Caffeine

Isolation

Variety of methods is in use for the isolation of caffeine from different sources. Some important processes are described below.

1. The coarse powder of tea leaves is extracted with boiling water and the aqueous extract is filtered while hot. The warm extract is treated with lead acetate to precipitate tannins and filtered. The excess of lead acetate present in the solution is precipitated as lead sulphate with dilute sulphuric acid. The filtered solution is boiled with charcoal to remove colouring

matter if any, and filtered to remove charcoal. The filtered decolourized solution is extracted with chloroform. The combined chloroform extract after evaporation affords caffeine as a white material. It is recrystallized with alcohol.

2. Finely or coarsely powdered tea leaves are extracted with ethanol in soxhlet extractor. The caffeine so extracted in ethanol is then adsorbed on magnesium oxide. Caffeine is then disorbed after treatment with 10% H_2SO_4. It is then extracted with chloroform and recrystallized.

3. Caffeine is extracted from coffee beans by the process of leaching with water. The highest yield up to about 90% was obtained when the coarse coffee powder is extracted with water at 75°C. The extraction takes about half an hour with water/coffee ratio of 9:1.

4. Decaffeination of coffee using supercritical fluid extraction. Supercritical fluid extraction has been efficiently used for the decaffeination of coffee. The process was first developed by K. Zosel using liquefied carbon dioxide. The supercritical medium in a pressure vessel is circulated through moist coffee where it becomes charged with caffeine. It is then passed through second pressurized vessel containing an adsorbing medium such as activated carbon, resin or water which retains caffeine. Adsorbed caffeine is then separated by extraction with chloroform.

Melting point: 235–237°C

Thin Layer Chromatography of Caffeine

Dissolve 1 mg of caffeine in 1 ml of chloroform or methanol. Spot the sample on TLC plate and elute it in ethyl acetate–methanol–acetic acid (80:10:10). Visualize the dried TLC plate by exposure to iodine vapour. Caffeine develops a spot at R_f value 0.41.

25.6. ISOLATION OF CAMPHOR

Camphor is a bicyclic monoterpene ketone obtained from *Cinnamomum camphora*; family Lauraceae. It is natural camphor. Camphor occurs in all parts of the camphor tree. Camphor is also produced synthetically from pinene. It is in the form of optically inactive mixture.

Camphor

Isolation

Camphor oil is obtained by steam distillation of the wood of camphor tree *C. camphor*. The main constituent of the crude oil is camphor up to about 50%, which can be separated by cooling and centrifugation. Fractionation of mother liquor gives two types of oils. The first known as white camphor oil is the first distillation fraction with cineol like odour, containing 35% of cineol. The brown camphor oil is a fraction with a higher boiling range than that of camphor. It is a pale yellow liquid containing about 80% of safrole. The production of natural camphor and camphor oils was formerly several thousands of tons per year but has declined as a result of the production of synthetic camphor.

Melting point: 179–180°C

Thin Layer Chromatography of Camphor

Dissolve 1 mg of camphor in 1 ml of methanol. Apply the spots over silica gel-G plate and elute it in benzene–ethyl acetate–glacial acetic acid (90:5:5). Spray the dried TLC plate with 1% vanillin-sulphuric acid reagent and heat at 110°C for 10 min. Camphor gives the spot with R_f value 0.33.

25.7. ISOLATION OF CAPSAICIN

Capsaicin is the pungent principle known as capsicum oleoresin obtained from the dried, ripe fruits of *Capsicum annum* var. *minimum* and small-fruited varieties of *C. frutescens*; family Solanaceae. Capsaicin is mostly present in the dissepiment of fruit. Chemically it is 8-methyl-N-vanillyl non-6-enamide. It is present to the extent of 0.02–0.14%.

Capsaicin

Isolation

Dried, ripe fruits of capsicum are coarsely powdered for the extraction of oleoresin. It is extracted with hot acetone or alcohol (90%). The extract obtained is concentrated and dried. The dried residue is further extracted with cold alcohol (90%) and the alcohol is removed by evaporation. Capsicum oleoresin thus obtained contains not less than 8% of capsaicin.

Melting point: 57–66°C

Thin Layer Chromatography of Capsaicin

The oleoresin 1 mg/ml is dissolved in alcohol and spotted on silica gel-G plate. The plate is eluted in the solvent system containing a mixture of benzene-methanol (9:1). Spray the dried plate with a 0.5% solution of 2,6-dibromoquinone-chlorimide in methanol and allow to stand in a chamber containing ammonia fumes. Blue colour and the R_f value 0.31 of the principal spot corresponds to the spots of the standard solution.

25.8. ISOLATION OF COLCHICINE

Colchicine is an alkaloid obtained from the corms or seeds of *Colchicum autumnale*; family Liliaceae and also from other species of *Colchicum*. It is a tropolone group of alkaloid. It is an active ingredient of one of the 18 plants still in use, of the approximately 700 listed in the Papyrus Ebers of ancient Egypt.

Colchicine

Isolation

Colchicum corms or seeds are exhaustively extracted with ethanol. Alcoholic extract is concentrated and dried to syrupy residue. The residue is dissolved in water to precipitate the insoluble fats and resins. The filtered aqueous extract is then repeatedly extracted with chloroform or digested with lead carbonate. It is refiltered, evaporated to a small volume and further extracted with chloroform. Colchicine is recovered as a crystalline complex with chloroform. The chloroform is distilled off and the amorphous colchicine is recovered after the evaporations of the residual solvent. Amorphous colchicine may be crystallized from ethyl acetate as pale yellow needles.

Melting point: 142–150°C

Thin Layer Chromatography of Colchicines

The dilute solution of colchicine in methanol is spotted on silica gel-G plates and eluted with chloroform-diethyl amine (9:1). Colchicine is detected by spraying with Dragendorff's reagent. It gives R_f value of 0.41.

25.9. ISOLATION OF CURCUMIN

Curcumins or curcuminoids are the diarylheptanoid compounds obtained from the dried rhizomes of turmeric, *Curcuma longa* family, Zingiberaceae. It is a major colouring principle present up to 5% in the rhizomes, which constitutes about 50–60% of the mixture of three main curcuminoids namely curcumin, desmethoxycucumin and bisdesmethoxycurcumin. The standardized extract of turmeric contains major proportion of the above curcuminoids. Commercial curcumin isolated from turmeric rhizome contains up to 97% pure product.

	R	R1
Curcumin	OCH$_3$	OCH$_3$
Desmethoxycurcumin	OCH$_3$	H
Bisdesmethoxycurcumin	H	H

Isolation

Curcumin can be obtained by different processes. Turmeric powder is extracted with alcohol in soxhlet extractor. The alcoholic extract is concentrated under reduced pressure and dried. In another procedure, turmeric powder is first extracted with hexane followed by acetone. The acetone extract is concentrated and dried to yield curcumin. The most efficient way of isolating curcumin was found to be to extract with hot ethanol, concentrate the filtrate, throw the concentrate into superior grade kerosene, when a solid mass separates. The mass is stripped off kerosene with petroleum ether and recrystallized from ethanol. The final product obtained is recrystallized from hot ethanol to yield orange–red needles.

Melting point: Curcumin 183°C, desmethoxycucumin 168°C and bisdesmethoxycurcumin 224°C.

Thin Layer Chromatography of Curcumin

Dissolve 1 mg of curcumin in 1 ml methanol. Apply the spots on silica gel-G plate and elute the plate in the solvent system chloroform–ethanol–glacial acetic acid (94:5:1). Dry the eluted plate and visualize under 366 nm light. Curcumin exhibits a bright yellow fluorescent spot at R_f value 0.79. The other spots appearing at R_f values 0.60 and 0.43 correspond to desmethoxycurcumin and bisdesmethoxycurcumin.

25.10. ISOLATION OF DIGOXIN

Digoxin or lanoxin is the most widely used cardiac glycoside obtained from the leaves of *Digitalis lanata*; family Scrophulariaceae. It is a secondary glycoside which is produced from a primary glycoside Lanatoside C. Its hydrolysis yields three molecules of digitoxose sugar and digoxigenin. It is a highly potent drug and should be handled with exceptional care.

Digoxin

Isolation

Digoxin is obtained commercially from the fresh leaves of *Digitalis lanata*. Lanatosides are the naturally occurring primary glycosides of *D. lanata* which includes Lanatoside A, lanatoside B and lanatoside C. Unstable lanatoside A is the acetyl derivative of purpurea glycoside A, and lanatoside B is the acetyl derivative of purpurea glycoside B. Lanatoside C has no counter part in *D. purpurea*. Hydrolysis of lanatosides by enzyme splits off glucose and hydrolysis by mild alkalies splits off acetyl groups leaving digitoxin, gitoxin and digoxin as the residues from Lanatoside A, B and C, respectively.

To extract lanatosides, fresh leaves are ground with neutral salt to inactivate the enzymes, and the pulp is further extracted with ethyl acetate. If the leaves are first defatted with benzene prior to extraction, better yield of the glycoside is obtained. The ethyl acetate extract is concentrated, dried and further subjected to chromatographic purification to yield lanatoside A (46%), lanatoside B (17%) and lanatoside C (37%). The fractions obtained are crystallized from alcohol. Lanatoside C after subsequent hydrolysis affords digoxin. Digoxin on acid hydrolysis yields digoxigenin as an aglycone and three moles of digitoxose.

Melting point: 230–265 °C

Thin Layer Chromatography of Digoxin

Dissolve about 1 mg of the glycoside in 1 ml of alcohol. The sample is spotted over silica gel-G plates and eluted with cyclohexane–acetone–acetic acid (49:49:2). Dried TLC plates are sprayed with 50% aqueous sulphuric acid. Digoxin appears as a blue spot under 385 nm UV light.

Identification Test

Digoxin is dissolved and diluted in hot methanol. The aliquot of the solution is evaporated to dryness. Acid ferric chloride TS is added to the residue. A green colour develops that slowly changes to a deep green blue colour.

25.11. ISOLATION OF DIOSGENIN

It is obtained from the dried tubers of *Dioscorea deltoidea* Wallich and other species of Dioscorea (Dioscoreaceae).

Diosgenin

Isolation

Alcoholic extraction method

The diosgenin tubers are cut into small pieces and dried under sun. The dried tubers are powdered, extracted with ethanol or methanol twice for 6–8 hours. It is filtered and the filtrate is concentrated to a syrupy liquid. The concentrated liquid is then hydrolysed using an acid, hydrochloric acid or sulphuric acid for 2–12 h. About 85% of the crude diosgenin is precipitated. The precipitates are filtered, washed with water and purified with alcohol.

Acid hydrolysis method

The dried tubers are powdered to a mesh size of 100–200 meshes. It is then refluxed or heated in autoclave with 2–4 N mineral acid for 2–6 h. It is filtered and the crude hydrolyte is washed with water, until neutral. Dried and extracted again for 6 h with hydrocarbon solvent. The liquid is concentrated to about 25 ml. It is allowed to stand for some time in a refrigerator for 1 h. The crystals of diosgenin are filtered out and then it's washed with acetone.

Fermentation cum acid hydrolysis method

The fresh green roots are collected and smashed in a hammer mill. The mesh is placed in the fermentation bin and allowed for fermentation for two days. The fermented mesh is dried in sun to reduce the moisture content to 7–8%. It is then subjected to hydrolysis with a mineral acid at reduced temperature. The resulting solution is extracted with heptane to obtain diosgenin.

Incubation cum acid hydrolysis method

The fresh plant material is incubated in water at 37°C for few days. It is later subjected to acid hydrolysis. The hydrolysed liquid is concentrated and extracted with hydrocarbon solvent to obtain diosgenin.

The fresh roots are homogenized with equal weight of water, concentrated acid is added until the required strength is obtained and then it is extracted with hydrocarbon solvent to obtain diosgenin.

Melting point: 204–207°C

Thin Layer Chromatography of Diosgenin

The sample dissolved in methanol is spotted in silica gel plates and developed in toluene: ethyl acetate (7:3). Dark green spot (R_f- 0.37) of diosgenin will appear when the dried plate is sprayed with anisaldehyde–sulphuric acid reagent.

25.12. ISOLATION OF EMETINE

Emetine is the major active constituent of the rhizomes and roots of *Cephaelis ipecacuanha* and *C. acuminata;* family Rubiaceae. Emetine was first isolated in a crude form by Pelletier in 1817, and recognized as an alkaloid in 1823. Ipecacuanha also consists of some other related isoquinoline alkaloids which includes cephaeline, psychotrine and emetamine.

Emetine

Isolation

The powdered ipecacuanha is extracted with about 70% ethanol or methanol. The extract obtained is concentrated and dissolved in water and the solution is made strongly basic with ammonia and extracted with di-isopropyl ether. Di-isopropyl ether extract is then treated with 10–15% aqueous potassium hydroxide to remove cephaeline. The extract is further evaporated to yield emetine. It is purified via dihydrobromide or dihydroiodide salt. These halide salts are converted to the hydrochloride by neutralizing the regenerated free base.

In another process, ipecac powder is treated with ammonia and ether. The ether extracts is subjected to dilute sulphuric acid treatment to yield alkaloids. Dilute acid extract is then nearly neutralized and washed with ether and then made strongly alkaline and treated with ether. Emetine goes into ether while cephaeline remains in the aqueous phase. The ether extract is concentrated and redissolved in methanol and converted to emetine hydrobromide with a methanolic solution of hydrobromic acid.

Melting point: 70°C

Thin Layer Chromatography of Emetine

Emetine hydrochloride is dissolved in methanol or water and spotted on silica gel-G plates. TLC is eluted in the following solvent systems and the spot is visualized under UV light or by spraying with bromocresol green or modified Dragendorff's reagent.

Solvent system	R_f
Chloroform–methanol (85:15)	0.3–0.5
Benzene–toluene–ethyl acetate–diethyl amine–methanol (35:35:10:2)	0.54
Methyl ethyl ketone–ethanol–ammonia (5:4:1)	0.70

25.13. ISOLATION OF ERGOMETRINE

Ergometrine or ergonovine is a naturally occurring indole alkaloid found in the sclerotia of *Claviceps purpurea;* family Clavicipitaceae developed on plants of rye, *Secale cereale;* family Gramineae. It is classified as one of the water-soluble, amine ergot alkaloids. It was discovered almost simultaneously in 1935 by five independent research groups. Ergot also contains ergotamine and ergotoxine groups of alkaloids which are water-insoluble groups.

Isolation

In the laboratory scale isolation technique, ergot powder is completely defatted with petroleum ether (60–80°C)

Ergometrine

Eugenol

Myrtaceae. It is also obtained from Cinnamon leaf oil obtained from *Cinnamomum zeylanicum*; family Lauraceae. Both of the oils contain 80–90% eugenol.

in soxhlet extractor. The petroleum ether extract removes about 30% fat and colouring matter. The residual marc dried below 40°C is transferred to a porcelain dish, made to semisolid mass by adding sufficient solvent ether and dilute ammonia with stirring. The material is stirred to dryness and then packed in a soxhlet and extracted with solvent ether for about 5 h. The ether extract filtered and to it little acetone added and shaken in separating funnel with three volumes of 1% of tartaric acid. The total acidic extract is combined and dried under reduced pressure to yield total ergot alkaloid.

The total alkaloid is further dissolved in dilute ammonia and extracted with four volumes of ether. The combined total ether extract is washed thoroughly with five successive quantities of water. Water-insoluble ergotamine and ergotoxine alkaloids stay with ether while the water-soluble ergometrine tartarte remains with aqueous extract. The aqueous extract is made faintly alkaline with dilute ammonia and further saturated with ether. Ergometrine free base is shifted to ethereal solution. It is again washed with water to remove impurities of other alkaloids. The ether extract is again treated with three volumes of 1% w/w tartaric acid in water. The combined acid extract is concentrated under reduced pressure to yield water soluble alkaloid. It is further purified by the column chromatographic fractionation.
Melting point: 162°C

Thin Layer Chromatography of Ergometrine

Dissolve about 1 mg/ml of alkaloid in methanol and apply on silica gel-G plates. Elute the plates in solvent system toluene–butanol NH_4Cl (saturated) (6:4) and spray the dried TLC plates with Dragendorff's reagent. Ergometrine maleate shows the R_f 0.30. The elution of the silica gel-G TLC plate in other solvent system chloroform–ethanol–acetone (6:4:4), shows the R_f value 0.23.

25.14. ISOLATION OF EUGENOL

Eugenol is a 4-allyl-2-methoxy phenol obtained from the essential oil of clove buds *Eugenia caryophyllus*; family

Isolation

Dried clove buds are hydrodistilled to yield the clove oil. Being heavier than water it makes a layer beneath water. The lower layer of clove oil is separated from water. For the separation of eugenol from clove oil, the oil is dissolved in solvent ether to make about 10% solution. It is shaken with three successive volumes of 10% potassium hydroxide solution. Eugenol being phenolic compound gets converted to phenoxide and becomes soluble in water. The total aqueous alkaline extract is combined and washed with fresh ether to remove other impurities. Eugenol is regenerated by acidifying the aqueous alkaline extract with excess of sulphuric acid. The acidified solution is extracted in separating funnel with three successive volumes of solvent ether. The combined solvent ether extract is then washed with water. Ether is removed by distillation at very low temperature to yield pure liquid eugenol.
Boiling point: 255°C

Thin Layer Chromatography of Eugenol

Dissolve about 1 mg of eugenol in 1 ml of methanol and apply the spots over silica gel-G plate. Elute the plate with pure benzene as a solvent system. Spray the dried plate with 1% anisaldehyde–sulphuric acid reagent and heat the plate at 110°C for 10 min. Eugenol shows the spot with dirty green colour at R_f 0.40 in case of normal chamber saturation at 24°C.

25.15. ISOLATION OF GINGEROLS AND SHOGAOLS

Gingerols are the oleoresin constituents of Ginger, *Zingiber officinalis*; family Zingiberaceae. These are long chain phenolic compounds responsible for the pungent taste of the drug. Ginger resin also contains their corresponding dehydration products, which are known as shogaols. Total resinous matter containing gingerols and shogaols is about 5–8% in ginger.

Gingerols (n = 0,2,3,4,5,7,9)

Shogaols (n = 4,5,7,9,10)

Isolation

Dry ginger is crushed to a coarse powder and extracted with 95% ethanol from alcoholic extract. Solvent is evaporated by distillation to obtain thick pasty mass. The thick pasty mass is suspended in water. The ginger resin precipitates in water which is removed by filtration and the residue obtained is dried under vacuum. In some cases the suspended oleoresin is extracted with solvent ether and the ether extract is evaporated to dryness at low temperature to yield total ginger oleoresin.

Identification Test

Add about 5 ml of 70% sulphuric acid and 5 mg of vanillin to the small quantity of ginger oleoresin. Allow to stand for 15 min, and then add equal volumes of water, the solution obtained turns azure blue indicating the presence of gingerol.

Thin Layer Chromatography of Gingerols

Dissolve extract or gingerol in alcohol. Apply the spots over silica gel-G plate and elute in the solvent system ether-n-hexane (7:3). Spray the dried TLC plate with 1% vanillin-sulphuric acid and heat the plate at 110°C for 10 min. Spots due to gingerols occur at R_f value 0.2.

25.16. ISOLATION OF GLYCYRRHETINIC ACID

Glycyrrhetinic acid is a pentacyclic triterpenic acid obtained from the roots and stolones of *Glycyrrhiza glabra*; family Leguminosae commonly known as liquorice. A major component of liquorice root is a sweet triterpenic saponin glycoside glycyrrhizin, which is a potassium and calcium salt of glycyrrhizic acid about 6–14%. After hydrolysis, it affords two molecules of gluconic acid and an aglycone glycyrrhetinic acid.

Glycyrrhetinic acid

Isolation

The crude drug is first extracted with chloroform. Chloroform extract is discarded. The marc is again extracted this time with 0.5 M sulphuric acid. The acid extract is cooled and shaken with chloroform. The combined chloroform extract is concentrated and dried to yield glycyrrhetinic acid. Glycyrrhizin is hydrolysed to glycyrrhetinic acid during extraction with sulphuric acid.

In another method of extraction, liquorice powder is extracted with boiling water to isolate glycyrrhizin. The aqueous extract is concentrated, dried and used as liquorice extract. The liquorice extract can be dissolved in water and acidified with hydrochloric acid to pH 3–3.4 to precipitate glycyrrhetinic acid. The precipitate is filtered, washed with water till neutral pH and then dried to yield glycyrrhetinic acid. Ammoniated glycyrrhizin, used in pharmaceutical trades is prepared by precipitating glycyrrhizic acid from liquorice extract, dissolving it in ammonia and drying the solution after spreading in a thin film on a glass plate to give shining dark brown flakes.

Melting point: 300°C

Thin Layer Chromatography of Glycyrrhetinic Acid

Dissolve 1 mg of glycyrrhetinic acid in about 1 ml of methanol–chloroform (1:1) mixture. Apply the spots over silica gel-G plates and elute in the solvent system Toluene–ethyl acetate–glacial acetic acid (12.5:7.5:0.5). Spray the dried plates with 1% vanillin–sulphuric acid or anisaldehyde–sulphuric acid and heat for 10 min at 110°C. Glycyrrhetinic acid gives purplish spot corresponding to the R_f value 0.41.

25.17. ISOLATION OF GUGGULSTERONE

Guggulsterone or gugulipid is a steroidal constituent present in the neutral fraction of the gum resin of *Commiphora mukul*; family Burseraceae known as Guggul or Indian bdellium. As guggulsterone is a major compound of the resin which comes in the lipid soluble fraction of the drug is also called as guggulipid. It is present in the form of stereoisomers, i.e. *E*-guggulsterone and *Z*-guggulsterone. The other constituent present in the neutral fraction are guggulsterol and other steroids.

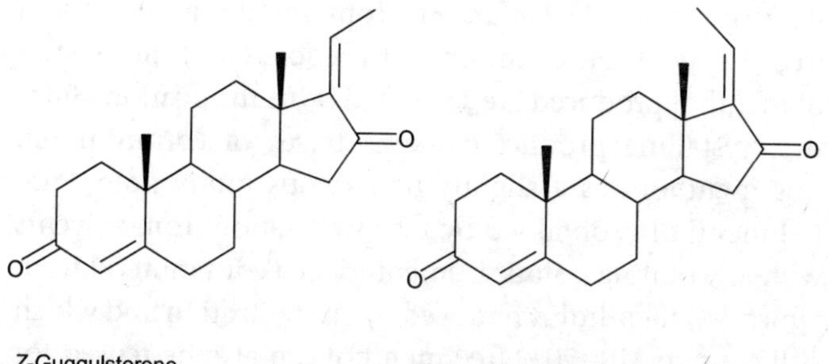

Z-Guggulsterone   E-Guggulsterone

Isolation

Gum resin of *C. mukul* coarsely powdered and extracted with ethyl acetate. The solvent is evaporated under vacuum at 50°C to yield dark brownish gummy material. It is further dissolved in ethyl acetate and extracted with 3 N HCl. The acid extract is basified to yield a basic fraction. The neutral ethyl acetate fraction obtained after treatment with acid is further divided into noncarbonyl and neutral ketonic fraction by following process. Neutral fraction is mixed with 10% semicarbazide on silica gel and toluene, stirred and heated at 60–62°C for 14 h, cooled and filtered. Silica gel is thoroughly washed with toluene to get toluene soluble noncarbonyl fraction. The above washed silica gel is mixed with aqueous 10% oxalic acid and toluene, stirred and refluxed for 2.5 h cooled and filtered. Silica gel residue is washed with ethyl acetate thrice. The combined ethyl acetate extract is further washed with water, and then concentrated and dried to yield neutral ketonic fraction.

Neutral ketonic fraction is chromatographed on silica gel and eluted with benzene–ethyl acetate to yield fractions containing mixture of *E*- and *Z*-guggulsterone. *E*- and *Z*-guggulsterone are further purified by rechromatography on silica gel.

Thin Layer Chromatography of Guggulsterone

Dissolve about 1 mg of extract or guggulsterone in 1 ml of ethyl acetate. The silica gel-G plate spotted with the sample is eluted in the solvent system toluene–ethyl acetate (80:20). The dried plate is sprayed with 1% vanillin–sulphuric acid and heated at 110°C for 10–15 min. Guggulsterone gives bluish violet spots which correspond with the R_f value 0.45 of the standard.

25.18. ISOLATION OF HESPERIDIN

Hesperidin was isolated from various citrus species like *Citrus mitis*, *Citrus aurantium*, *Citrus sinensis*, belonging to the family Rutaceae. Hesperidin decreases the fragility of blood capillaries. Hesperidin could be isolated by two methods:

Method I

Take 200 g sun-dried peel, powder and place it in a 2-litre round bottomed flask attached to a reflux condenser. One litre of petroleum ether (40–60°C) is added to the flask and heated on a water bath for 1 h. The contents of the flask are filtered while hot through a Buchner funnel, and the powder is allowed to dry at room temperature. The dried powder is taken back to the flask, and 1 litre of methanol is added to the flask. The contents are heated under reflux for 3 h and then filtered hot and the marc is washed with 200 ml hot methanol. The filtrate is concentrated under reduced pressure, leaving a syrupy residue crystallized from dilute acetic acid, yielding white needles of hesperidin.

Method II

Take 200 g of chopped orange peel in a 2-litre Erlenmeyer flask and 750 ml 10% calcium hydroxide solution is added and thoroughly mixed. The flask and its contents are left overnight at room temperature. The mixture is filtered through a large Buchner funnel containing a thin layer of celite on the filter paper. The obtained filtrate would be yellow orange colour and is acidified carefully to pH 4-5 with concentrated hydrochloric acid. Hesperidin separates as amorphous powder. It is collected on a Buchner funnel, washed with water and recrystallized from aqueous formamide.

Melting point: 252–254°C

Identification Test

1. *Ferric Chloride Test*: Addition of ferric chloride solution to hesperidin produces a wine red colour.
2. *Magnesium-Hydrochloric Acid Reduction Test*: Drop-wise addition of concentrated hydrochloric acid to an ethanolic solution of hesperidin containing magnesium develops a bright violet colour.

25.19. ISOLATION OF LEVODOPA

Levodopa or L-Dopa is a dihydroxyphenyl alanine obtained from the dried mature seeds of *Mucuna pruriens*; family Fabaceae. Two types of seeds, i.e. black or spotted variety are generally found in the market which consists of about 2.0% of L-Dopa content.

Levodopa

Isolation

Coarsely powdered Mucuna seeds are extracted with demineralized water containing 1% v/v of acetic acid at 50°C. Acetic acid extract is filtered. The filtered extract is concentrated by reverse osmosis and the liquid concentrate so obtained is kept at a low temperature (6–8°C) for about 24 h for crystallization of L-dopa. The crystals are filtered through a centrifuge, washed with cold water and dried under vacuum at 50°C. The filtrate and water washings still contain the compound of interest, i.e. L-dopa. It is mixed, concentrated and processed for second crop. The crystalline product obtained in I and II crops combiningly yield about 2.0–2.5% of L-dopa which still consists of some impurities of amino acids. It is further purified either by recrystallization or by using liquid ion exchangers.
Melting point: 283°C

Thin Layer Chromatography of Levodopa

Thin layer chromatographic study using solvent system *n*-butanol–acetic acid–water–methanol (15:7.5:7.5:1.5) and spraying the plates with Dragendorff's reagent shows the spot at R_f value 0.4.

25.20. ISOLATION OF MENTHOL

Menthol is a monoterpene alcohol obtained from diverse types of mint oils or peppermint. The sources of mint oil include black peppermint. *Mentha piperita* Var. *vulgaris*; white peppermint, *M. piperita* Var. *officinalis*; *M. arvensis*; *M. canadensis* Var. *piperascens*, etc. Peppermint contains about 1–3% of volatile oil. First two species contains not less than 45% of menthol while the later species contains menthol up to about 70–90%. Along with menthol the oil contains (+) neomenthol, (+) isomenthol, menthone, menthofuran, menthyl acetate and cineol. The menthol obtained from the natural sources is. Levorotatory (l-menthol) or racemic (dl-menthol). Menthol can be synthetically prepared by hydrogenation of thymol.

Menthol

Isolation

Mentha oil is obtained from the hydrodistillation or steam distillation of fresh above-ground parts just before flowering. For (−) menthol isolation from peppermint oil the oil is subjected to cooling. The crystals of menthol crystallize out from the oil which is separated by centrifugation.

Cornmint oil obtained from the steam distillation of the flowering herb *Mentha arvensis* contains about 70–80% of free (−) menthol. Cornmint oil is cooled and the crystals of menthol produced are separated by centrifugation. Since the crystalline product contains traces of cornmint oil, this menthol has a slightly herbaceous minty note. Pure (−) menthol is obtained by recrystallization from solvents with low boiling points. Dementholized corn mint oil from which (−) menthol is removed by crystallization and which still contains 40–50% free menthol can also be reused for producing (−) menthol.
Melting point: 41–44°C

Thin Layer Chromatography of Menthol

Dissolve about 1 mg of menthol in about 1 ml of methanol. Apply the spot on silica gel-G plate and elute it in pure chloroform. Spray the dried plates with 1% vanillin-sulphuric acid reagent and heat the plate at 110°C for 10 min. Menthol gives R_f value 0.48–0.62 in case of normal chamber saturation at 24°C.

25.21. ISOLATION OF NICOTINE

Nicotine is a pyridine alkaloid obtained from the dried leaves of tobacco plant *Nicotiana tabacum*; family Solanaceae. Tobacco leaves contains 2–8% of nicotine combined as maleate or citrate.

Nicotine

Isolation

Nicotine is generally isolated from the tobacco waste as the main tobacco crop has always to enter the normal consumption channel because it is a very high revenue earning commodity; it is extremely costly to use it as a raw material for nicotine extraction. However, tobacco waste material with less than 2% nicotine content is uneconomical for nicotine recovery.

For the isolation of nicotine, tobacco waste is thoroughly mixed with lime and extracted with water. Nicotine present in the aqueous solution is further extracted with organic solvents like chloroform or kerosene. The organic solvent extract of nicotine is then treated with dilute sulphuric acid to obtain nicotine sulphate solution. The product is separated as a heavy layer and denicotinated solvent is recovered and recycled in the procedure of extraction.

As kerosene is not an ideal solvent due to its very high distribution coefficient and undesirable odour that it leaves in the final product, ion exchange chromatography is used for recovery of nicotine from aqueous solution. Nicotine is absorbed on a cation exchanger and subsequently eluted with a suitable medium. The exchanger can also be regenerated by washing with dilute acid and reuse several times. This process yields good quality insecticide grade nicotine from tobacco waste.

Boiling point: 247°C

Thin Layer Chromatography of Nicotine

Dissolve 1 mg of sample in 1 ml of methanol. Apply the spot over silica gel-G plate, and elute the plate in chloroform–methanol–ammonium hydroxide (60:10:1). Spray the dried TLC plate with a mixture of equal volumes of 2% p-aminobenzoic acid in ethanol and 0.1 M phosphate buffer. After drying the plate for 15 min, expose it to bromine cyanide vapour for visualization. Nicotine gives the spot corresponding to the R_f value 0.77. Reaction involved in the visualization of nicotine is known as Konig reaction.

25.22. ISOLATION OF OPIUM ALKALOIDS

Morphine and codeine are the two important isoquinoline alkaloids present in the air-dried milky exudates obtained by incision of unripe capsules of *Papaver somniferum* Linn (Papaveraceae).

	R	R₁
Morphine	-H	-H
Codeine	-CH₃	-H
Thebaine	-CH₃	-CH₃

Isolation

The powdered drug is extracted with boiling water and to the aqueous phase calcium chloride is added and concentrated to get salts of morphine and codeine as crystals. It is treated with chloroform. The soluble portion consists of codeine and the insoluble portion consists of morphine.

The powered drug is shaken with calcium chloride and filtered. To the filtrate add 10% of sodium hydroxide solution. It is filtered. The marc consists of narcotine, papaverine, thebaine and the filtrate consists of morphine, codeine. The filtrate is extracted with chloroform. The chloroform layer is separated. It consists of codeine while the aqueous layer consists of morphine and narceine. The aqueous layer is first acidified and later on slightly alkalized with ammonia. Morphine is precipitated on the addition of ammonia and the aqueous layer consists of narceine. The marc consisting of narcotine, papaverine and thebaine is dissolved in alcohol and then acidified with acetic acid. To the acidified solution, add three volumes of boiling water. Precipitates of narcotine and papaverine are formed and thebaine still remains in the aqueous solution. Papaverine is separated from narcotine by the addition of 0.3% oxalic acid solution and allowed to cool. On cooling the papaverine crystals are obtained. The aqueous solution is made alkaline with ammonia for the precipitation of noscapine which is recrystallized using water.

Melting point: Morphine 254°C, Thebaine 193°C, Codeine 154–156°C

Identification Tests

1. Opium alkaloids when treated with ferric chloride solution, deep reddish purple colour is produced which persist even after the addition of few drops of hydrochloric acid.
2. Morphine when treated with concentrated sulphuric acid and formaldehyde gives dark violet colour.

Thin Layer Chromatography of Opium Alkaloids

Opium alkaloids are spotted in silica gel-G plates and developed with two different solvent systems separately, solvent system I, chloroform:acetone:diethylamine (5:4:1) and solvent system II, xylene:methyl ethyl ketone:methanol:diethylamine (20:20:3:1). The dried plates are sprayed with Dragendorff's reagent. The spots of the alkaloids will be reddish brown in colour and the R_f values of the alkaloids in both the solvent systems are:

- Solvent system I: Morphine (R_f - 0.10), codeine (R_f - 0.38), thebaine (R_f - 0.65), papaverine (R_f - 0.67) and narcotine (R_f - 0.72).
- Solvent system II: Morphine (R_f - 0.12), codeine (R_f - 0.26), thebaine (R_f - 0.45), papaverine (R_f - 0.59) and narcotine (R_f - 0.74).

25.23. ISOLATION OF PIPERINE

Piperine is isolated from unripe fruit (black pepper) and the kernel of the ripe fruit (white pepper) of *Piper nigrum*, from the fruit of ashanti *(Piper clusii)*, from long pepper *(Piper longum)*, seeds of *Cubeba censii*, *Piper fainechotti* and *Piper chaba*. The piperine content of black pepper varies from 6 to 9%.

Piperine

Isolation of Piperine

Finely powdered 20 g of black pepper is extracted with 300 ml 95% ethanol in a soxhlet extractor for 2 h. The solution is filtered and concentrated in vacuum on a water bath at 60°C. 20 ml of alcoholic potassium hydroxide is added to the filtrate residue and after it while decanted from the insoluble residue. The alcoholic solution is left overnight, whereupon yellow coloured needle shaped crystals are deposited. The yield of piperine is 0.3 g.
Melting point: 125–126°C

Thin Layer Chromatography of Piperine

The extracted piperine is spotted on TLC plate made up of silica gel-G and developed with benzene:ethyl acetate (2:1). When detected at UV$_{365}$ piperine exhibits blue fluorescence. When sprayed with anisaldehyde sulphuric acid reagent and heated at 110°C for 10 min, piperine appears as yellow spot at R_f 0.25.

Dissolve about 1 mg of piperine in 1 ml methanol. Apply the test solution on the silica gel-G plate and elute the plate with toluene–diethyl ether–dioxane (9.4:3.2:2.4). Visualize the dried plate under UV light of 254 nm. Piperine appears as a violet coloured spot at R_f value 0.48. If the TLC plate is sprayed with anisaldehyde–glacial acetic acid–methanol–conc. sulphuric acid reagent (0.5:10:85:5) and heated at 110°C for 10 min, piperine appears as a yellow spot.

25.24. ISOLATION OF PODOPHYLLOTOXIN

Indian podophyllum is the root and rhizome of *Podophyllum hexandrum* Royle (Berberidaceae).

Isolation

Commercial podophyllin is obtained by extraction of powdered rhizome/roots of *P. emodii* with methanol. Then it is reduced under vacuum. Semisolid mass is put into acidulated water (10 ml HCl in 100 ml water). The precipitates are allowed to settle. Filtrate is decanted and then washed with cold water. Resin obtained is dried,

Podophyllotoxin

and upon drying, it gives dark brown amorphous powder called podophyllin. The obtained powder is extracted with chloroform and further purification is done by repeated recrystallization from benzene alone or alcohol benzene mixture followed by washing with petroleum ether/hexane yield podophyllotoxin.

Another method of extraction to obtain pure podophyllotoxin is by dissolving the CHCl$_3$ soluble fraction in alcohol. Then it is refluxed with neutral aluminium oxide so that solution becomes light yellow. To alcoholic solution benzene is added which yielded podophyllotoxin of 95–98%.

Another method of isolating podophyllotoxin from crude (*P. emodii* roots/rhizome) podophyllin/crude podophyllotoxin involves extraction over a bed of neutral alumina with solvents like benzene, toluene, xylene, etc., for about 1.5–4 h. Recrystallization from organic solvents such as hot benzene, toluene and xylene yields pure podophyllotoxin (95–97%). Podophyllotoxin is a tetrahydronapthalin derivative with OH and lactone groups. The attachment at cis-position is responsible for the purgative property and the attachment at *trans*-position corresponds for anticancer property of the drug.
Melting point: 114–118°C

Thin Layer Chromatography of Podophyllotoxin

Podophyllotoxin is dissolved in methanol and is spotted on the TLC plate; the solvent used is toluene:ethyl acetate (5:7) and detecting agent is sulphuric acid. Spot of podophyllotoxin under day light has violet colour (R_f 0.39).

25.25. ISOLATION OF QUININE AND QUINIDINE

Cinchona is the dried bark of the stem or of the root of *Cinchona calisaya* Wedd, *Cinchona ledgeriana* Moens, *Cinchona officinalis* Linn and *Cinchona sucirubra* Pavon or hybrids of any of the first two species with any of the last two species (Rubiaceae). Quinine is laevorotatory while quinidine is dextrorotatory stereoisomer.

Quinine   Quinidine

Isolation

The powdered cinchona bark is mixed with about 30% of its weight of calcium hydroxide or calcium oxide and sufficient quantity of 5% sodium hydroxide solution. Make it into a paste and allow it to stand for few hours. The moistened mass is then transferred into soxhlet and extracted with benzene. To the benzene extract, add 5% sulphuric acid and mix well. The benzene layer is separated from that of the aqueous layer, the benzene layer is discarded and to the aqueous layer sodium hydroxide is added to adjust the pH to 6.5. Cool and on cooling precipitates of quinine sulphate is formed. The precipitate is filtered and separated. The separated precipitate is then recrystallized from hot water to free the salts from cinchonine and cinchonidine. The colouring matter is removed by treating it with activated charcoal. The quinine sulphate obtained is dissolved in dilute sulphuric acid, and it is later made alkaline with ammonia. Quinine precipitates become crystalline, which are washed and dried at 45–55°C. The mother liquor consisting of quinidine, cinchonine and cinchonidine are slightly made alkaline with ammonia, and the precipitate formed is again subjected to extraction with ether. Two portions are obtained: the first is ether insoluble fraction consisting of cinchonine crystals and the other is the ether extract with quinidine and cinchonidine. The ether soluble fraction consisting of quinine and cinchonidine is first stirred with dilute hydrochloric acid followed by the addition of 25% of solution of sodium potassium tartarate. The resulting solution is allowed to stand for some time, and on standing, precipitates of cinchonidine tartarate is formed. The cinchonidine is recrystallized from alcohol. To the liquor obtained after the separation of cinchonidine tartarate add potassium iodide solution. Addition of potassium iodide results in the precipitation of quinidine hydroiodide. This on treatment with an alkali (ammonia) liberates a base, which is dissolved in acetic acid. The colouring matter is removed by the treatment with activated charcoal. The quinidine obtained is finally recrystallized from alcohol.

Melting point: Quinine 177°C, Quinidine 174–175°C

Identification Tests

Thalleioquin Test: To the sample add one drop of dilute sulphuric acid and 1 ml of water. Add bromine water drop-wise till the solution acquires permanent yellow colour and add 1 ml of dilute ammonia solution, emerald green colour is produced.

Thin Layer Chromatography of Quinine and Quinidine

Alkaloids are dissolved in methanol and spotted in silica gel-G plate. The solvent system used are chloroform:diethyl amine (9:1) and chloroform:acetone:diethyl amine (5:4:1). Dried plates are sprayed with dragendorff's reagent, the R_f value of quinine and quinidine in the first solvent system are 0.17 and 0.28, respectively, and in solvent system second, 0.17 and 0.26.

25.26. ISOLATION OF RESERPINE

Reserpine is an indole alkaloid obtained from the roots of *Rauwolfia serpentina*, family Apocynaceae and also from other different species of *Rauwolfia*, such as *R. micrantha*, *R. vomiforia* and *R. tetraphylla*. The material obtained from natural sources may contain closely related alkaloids, which includes ajmaline, ajmalicine, ajmalinine, rescinnamine, reserpinine, serpentine and yohimbine. In *R. serpentina*, reserpine and rescinnamine both respond to the extraction procedures and extracted as a mixture of both while in *R. tetraphylla*, reserpine and deserpidine are extracted together.

Reserpine

Isolation

Rauwolfia root powder is exhaustively extracted with 90% alcohol by suitable method of extraction such as percolation. The alcoholic extract is concentrated and dried under reduced pressure below 60°C to yield rauwolfia dry extract containing about 4% of total alkaloids. Rauwolfia dry extract is extracted further with proportions of ether–chloroform–90% alcohol (20:8:2.5). To the extract obtained, add little dilute ammonia with intermittent shaking. Alkaloid is converted to water-insoluble base. Add water and allow the drug to settle after few vigorous shakings. Fitter off the solution and extract the residue with 4 volumes of 0.5 N H_2SO_4 in separating funnel. Combine the total acid extract which contains the alkaloidal salt. The extract is filtered, made alkaline with dilute ammonia to liberate alkaloid. Finally, it is extracted with chloroform. The total chloroform extract is filtered; chloroform is removed by distillation and the total alkaloidal extract is dried under vacuum to yield total rauwolfia alkaloids. Total rauwolfia alkaloid consists of the mixture of over 30 different components. It is subjected to column chromatographic fractionation for the separation of reserpine.

Melting point: 270°C

Chromatographic Study

Paper Chromatography: Dissolve about 1 mg of the sample of rauwolfia extract/standard reserpine in methanol. Immerse a 20 × 20 sheet of Whatman No. 1 filter paper in the immobile solvent formamide–acetone (3:10). Blot the paper between filter paper toweling and allow the acetone to dry. Apply the spots of the sample solution and standard on the filter paper and dry the spots. Immerse the spotted paper in the chromatographic chamber containing the mobile solvent isooctane–carbon tetrachloride–piperidine–ter. butyl alcohol (90:60:4:2) and elute the paper by ascending chromatography. Remove the chromatogram when the mobile solvent has raised approximately 7/8th of the height of the paper. Dry the chromatogram at 90°C in a current of air, spray the paper evenly with 25% trichloroacetic acid in methanol and again dry at 90°C for 10 min. Samples yield spots corresponding in position and colour to those of the standard solution.

Thin Layer Chromatography: Dissolve 1 mg of rauwolfia alkaloidal extract or pure reserpine in methanol. Apply the spots over the TIC plate. In case of silica gel-G plates elute the plate in solvent system chloroform–acetone–diethylamine (50:40:30). In case of alumina-G plate, elute in the solvent system cyclohexane–chloroform (30:70). Dry the eluted plates and spray with Dragendorff's reagent. In both the cases orange spot is given by the alkaloidal components of rauwolfia and by reference standard. In cases of silica gel-G plate, reserpine gives R_f value 0.72 while in case of alumina G plate, it gives R_f value 0.35.

25.27. ISOLATION OF SENNOSIDES

Sennosides are isolated from Tinnevelly senna, consists of dried compound leaflets of *Cassia angustifolia* Vahl (Leguminosae).

Method I

The leaves are dried and powdered. The powdered drug is shaken with benzene for 2 h on an electronic shaker.

Sennoside A (trans)
Sennoside B (meso)

Filter and distill off the solvent and marc is dried at room temperature and extracted with 70% methanol for 4–6 hours. The extract is filtered under vacuum and it is re-extracted with 70% of methanol for 2 h, and filtered. The methanolic extract is combined and concentrated to 1/8th portion of its original volume. The concentrated solution is acidified with hydrochloric acid to a pH of 3.2. The acidified solution is kept aside for 2 h at a temperature of 5°C. The solution is filtered and to the filtrate add anhydrous calcium chloride dissolved in 25 ml of denatured spirit with constant and vigorous stirring. The pH is again adjusted to 8 by ammonia and it is set aside for 2 h. The solution is filtered; the precipitate obtained is dried over P_2O_5 in a dessicator.

Method II

Powdered drug is extracted by shaking with ethanolic chloroform (93 parts of chloroform and 7 parts of ethanol) for 30 min. Filtered and the leaves are again extracted with acidic methanol (1.2 g of oxalic acid per litre of methanol). Both the extracts are combined and concentrated. It was kept for whole night in room temperature. Sennoside A precipitates out, Sennoside B remains in solution. Sennoside A is recrystallized using triethylamine. Sennoside B solutions is precipitated by 10% methanolic solution of $CaCl_2$. Further separated by methanolic ammonia solution (40 ml ammonia + 60 ml methanol). Dried washed with water and kept for one day. It is then recrystallized using glycolmonoethylether.

Melting point: Sennoside A 200–240°C, Sennoside B 180–186°C

Identification tests: To the crude extract, organic solvent like benzene, ether or chloroform is added and shaken. The organic layer is separated and to it ammonia solution is added, the ammoniacal layer produces pink to red colour indicating the presence of anthraquinone glycoside.

Thin Layer Chromatography of Sennosides

Sennosides are spotted in silica gel-G plates and developed using ethyl acetate:methanol:water (100:16.5:13.5) as solvent system. Red coloured spots will appear when the spots are sprayed with 25% nitric acid and turns to yellow when sprayed after drying with alcoholic potassium hydroxide solution.

25.28. ISOLATION OF SOLASODINE

Solasodine is an aglycone of steroidal glycoalkaloid found in many species of Solanaceae family. The various sources commonly used for the preparation of solasodine include the berries of *Solanum incanum* (1.8–2%), *S. khasianum* (1–1.75%) and *S. xanthocarpum*. Solasonine is a steroidal glycoalkaloid which yields an aglycone solasodine and the sugar such as mannose, glucose and galactose on hydrolysis.

Solasodine

Isolation

The dried berries are first powdered and subjected to defecting with petroleum ether to yield greenish yellow oil which is rejected as it is devoid of the glycoalkaloid. The defatted material is extracted thrice with ethyl alcohol; the extracts are combined and concentrated to 1/10th of its volume. Concentrated hydrochloric acid is then added to it until the final concentration reaches 5–6%. The whole mass is refluxed for about 6 h to attain complete hydrolysis of glycoalkaloid. The reaction mixture is then basified with ammonia and again refluxed for 1 h. The cooled reaction mixture is filtered and the residue obtained is thoroughly washed with water till neutral pH and dried. The dried material is then dissolved in chloroform. Solasodine goes into chloroform. The solution is filtered and the solvent is evaporated to yield the residue containing solasodine. It is further purified by crystallizing it from methanol or by sublimation in high vacuum.
Melting point: 200–202°C

Thin Layer Chromatography of Solasodine

Dissolve 1 mg of sample and standard in 1 ml of methanol separately. Apply the test solution and standard on the silica gel-G plate and develop the plate in solvent system toluene–ethyl acetate-diethyl amine (7:2:1). Spray the dried plates with modified Dragendorff's reagent. Allow the plate to dry and again spray with 10% sulphuric acid in methanol. An orange to red spot of R_f value 0.60, corresponding to solasodine is visible on both test and standard solution track.

25.29. ISOLATION OF STRYCHNINE AND BRUCINE

Strychnine and brucine are isolated from the seeds of *Strychnos nuxvomica*. Strychnine and brucine are virulent poison and is used medicinally as a tonic and stimulant. Nuxvomica seeds contain about 3% alkaloids.

Strychnine

Brucine

Isolation of Strychnine

100 g of powdered nux vomica seeds are mixed thoroughly with 100 ml of 10% calcium hydroxide in water and left overnight at room temperature. The air dried slurry is extracted with chloroform in a soxhlet extractor for 3 h. The chloroform solution is then extracted several times with 5% sulphuric acid solution and subsequently basified with 10% aqueous sodium hydroxide solution. Cooled and the crystals are filtered. Required amount of 50% ethanol is added, and the mixture is refluxed until most of the solid has dissolved. The solution is filtered after adding charcoal. The filtered crystals of strychnine are washed with a little 50% ethanol. The mother liquor and washings are used for the isolation of brucine.

The crude strychnine is dissolved in 9 volumes of boiling water, and 15% sulphuric acid solution is added slowly with stirring, until the reaction is slightly acid to Congo red. Activated charcoal is added to the solution and the solution is refluxed for 1 h and filtered hot. On cooling strychnine sulphate crystallizes out, filtered and washed with cold water. The obtained crystals are dissolved in 15 volumes of water,

heated at 80°C and neutralized with 10% aqueous sodium carbonate: after addition of charcoal, the solution is filtered hot. Strychnine precipitates on addition of aqueous sodium carbonate and cooling. The precipitate is filtered and washed with cold water. It is recrystallized using ethanol.
Melting point: 286–288°C

Isolation of Brucine

The mother liquor remaining after separation of strychnine is concentrated *in vacuo* on a water bath until most of the alcohol is removed. The residue is acidified to pH 6 with dilute sulphuric acid and then concentrated to a volume of 3–4 ml overnight. It is kept in a refrigerator and the product is filtered and washed with cold water. Adding 4.5 volumes of hot distilled water and boiling with a little charcoal for 1 h purify brucine sulphate. It is filtered while hot and kept in a refrigerator for several days. Brucine is recovered from the sulphate using the similar procedure used for strychnine. It is recrystallized using aqueous acetone.
Melting point: 178°C

Identification Tests

1. Strychnine when treated with sulphovanadic acid gives purple red colour.
2. Strychnine when treated with sulphuric acid and crystals of potassium dichromate gives purple colour, which slowly changes to red, while brucine gives immediate red colour.
3. Brucine when treated with nitric acid gives blood red colour, which is discharged by the addition of stannous chloride solution.

Thin Layer Chromatography of Strychnine and Brucine

Both the alkaloids are dissolved in methanol and spotted in silica gel-G plate. The solvent system used is benzene:chloroform:diethylamine (9:4:1). After the development the plate is sprayed with Dragendorff's reagent, R_f values of both the alkaloids corresponds respectively.

25.30. ISOLATION OF VASICINE

Vasicine is a pyrrolazoquinazoline alkaloid obtained from the leaves of *Adhatoda vasica*; family Acanthaceae. *A. vasica* known as vasaka is a highly reputed ayurvedic medicinal plant used for the treatment of respiratory ailments, particularly for the treatment of cough, bronchitis, asthma and tuberculosis. Vasicine is present in vasaka up to about 1.3%. The other alkaloids present include vasicinone, vasicinol, vasicinolone, vasicol and adhatonine.

Vasicine

Isolation

Vasaka leaves are dried, coarsely powdered and basified to pH 9 with ammonia solution. It is further extracted with chloroform. The total chloroform extract is combined and washed with water and dried over anhydrous sodium sulphate. The solvent evaporated to get the total alkaloid extract containing vasicine as a major alkaloid. Vasicine can be further purified from the dry extract by crystallization.
Melting point: 210°C

Thin Layer Chromatography of Vasicine

Dissolve 1 mg of vasicine in 1 ml of methanol with little warming. Apply the spots of test solution on the silica gel-G plate and elute with toluene–methanol–dioxane–ammonia (1:1:2.5:0.5). Spray the dried TLC plate with Dragendorff's reagent. Vasicine gives orange coloured spot.

25.31. ISOLATION OF VINCA ALKALOIDS

Vinblastine is isolated from the dried entire plant of *Catharanthus roseus* Linn (Apocynaceae).

Extraction and Isolation

The dried leaf material is taken and is extracted with a solution of hot ethanol–water–acetic acid in a ratio of 9:1:1. The solvent is removed and to the residue hot hydrochloric acid solution of 2% is added. The pH of the acidic extract is adjusted to 4, for the precipitation of the nonalkaloidal components, which can be separated by filtration. The pH of the aqueous acidic solution is now adjusted to 7 and then extracted with benzene. The benzene layer is evaporated to obtain vinblastine and other alkaloids.

Isolation of Vinblastine and Vincristine

The phenolic materials are removed by the washing the extract with dilute alkali. The washed extract is subjected to chromatography on alumina and elution is carried out in 18 fractions starting with benzene–methylene chloride (65:35) mixture to pure methylene chloride. Vinblastine recovered in the ninth fraction. Further elution of the column results in separating the fractions of vincristine.
Melting point: Vinblastine: 284–285°C, Vincristine: 273–281°C

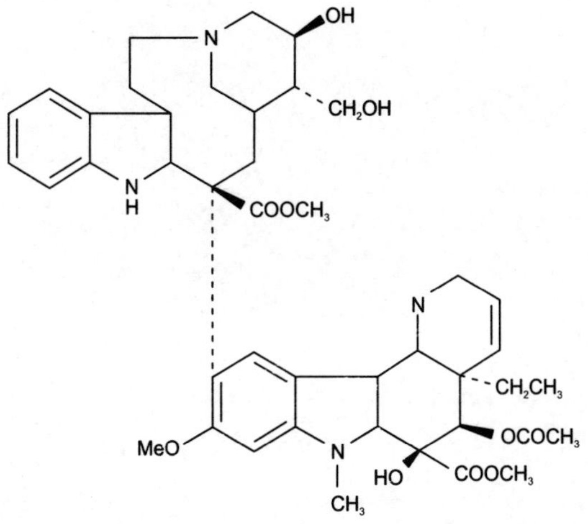

Vinblastine

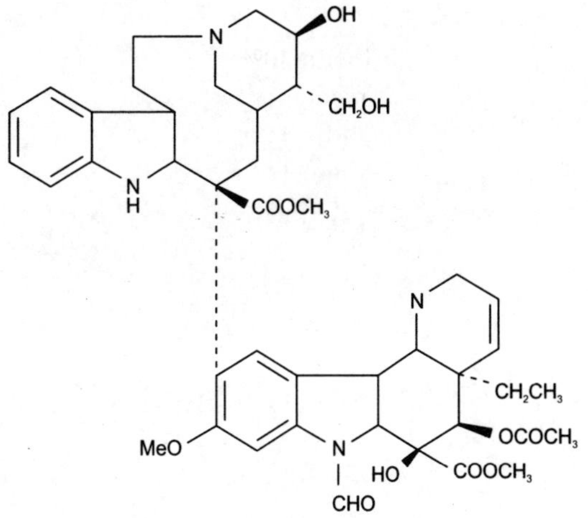

Vincristine

Thin Layer Chromatography of Vincristine

Vincristine dissolved in 25% water in methanol solution, spotted in silica gel-G plate and developed using the solvent, acetonitrile:benzene (30:70). The dried plates are sprayed with 1% solution of ceric ammonium sulphate in 85% phosphoric acid. The R_f value of the appeared spot would be 0.39.

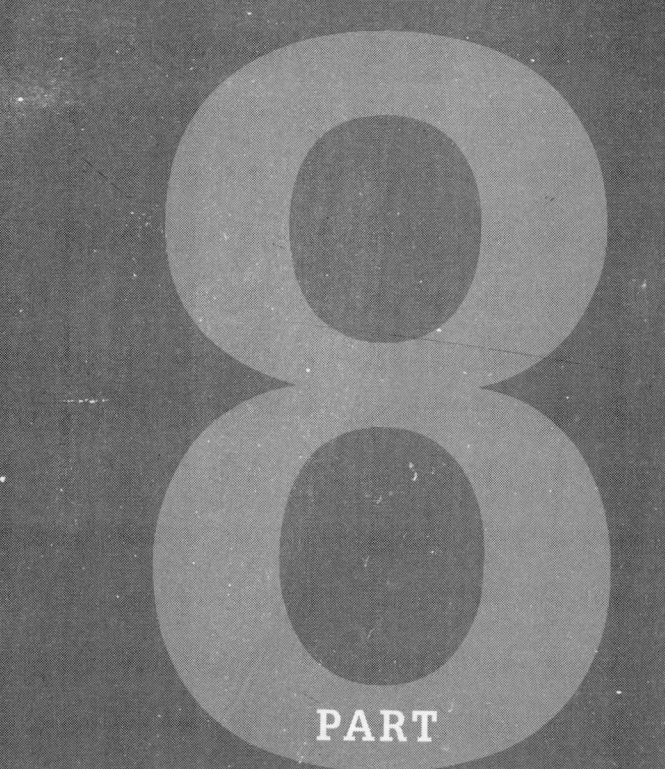

PART

Medicinal Plant Biotechnology

Section Outline

OVERVIEW

Biotechnology is the emerging voice and demand in the current scenario. This part provides basic information of plant tissue culture and various techniques used in it. This technique affords alternative solution to problems arising due to current rate of extinction and decimation of flora and ecosystem.

Plant Tissue Culture

CONTENTS

26.1. INTRODUCTION

Tissue culture is *in vitro* cultivation of plant cell or tissue under aseptic and controlled environmental conditions, in liquid or on semisolid well-defined nutrient medium for the production of primary and secondary metabolites or to regenerate plant. This technique affords alternative solution to problems arising due to current rate of extinction and decimation of flora and ecosystem.

The whole process requires a well-equipped culture laboratory and nutrient medium. This process involves various steps, viz. preparation of nutrient medium containing inorganic and organic salts, supplemented with vitamins, plant growth hormone(s) and amino acids as well as sterilization of explant (source of plant tissue), glassware and other accessories inoculation and incubation.

Advantages of Tissue Culture Technique Over the Conventional Cultivation Techniques

Availability of raw material

Some plants are difficult to cultivate and are also not available in abundance. In such a case, the biochemicals/bioproducts from these plants cannot be obtained economically in sufficient quantity. Unlimited cutting of plants also leads to deforestation, natural imbalance and sometimes may lead to extinction of a particular species. Hence, tissue culture is considered a better source for regular and uniform supply of raw material, manageable under regulated and reproducible conditions in the medicinal plants industry for the production of phytopharmaceuticals.

Fluctuation in supplies and quality

The production of crude drugs is subject to variation in quality due to changes in climate, crop diseases and seasons. The method of collection, drying and storing also influence the quality of crude drug. All these problems can be overcome by tissue culture techniques.

Patent rights

Naturally occurring plants or their metabolites cannot be patented as such. Only a novel method of isolation can be patented. For R and D purpose, the industry has to spend a lot of money and time to launch a new natural product but can't have patent right. Hence, industries prefer tissue culture for production of biochemical compounds. By this method, it is possible to obtain a constant supply and new methods can be developed for isolation and improvement of yield, which can be patented.

Political reasons

If a natural drug is successfully marketed in a particular country of its origin, the government may prohibit its export to up-value its own exports by supplying its phytochemical product, e.g. *Rauwolfia serpentina* and *Dioscorea* spp. from India. Similarly the production of opium in the world is governed as such by political consideration, in such case, if work is going on the same drug; it will be either hindered or stopped. Here also, plant tissue culture is the solution.

Easy purification of the compound

The natural products from plant tissue culture may be easily purified because of the absence of significant amounts of pigments and other unwanted impurities. With the advancement of modern technology in plant tissue culture, it is also possible to biosynthesize those chemical compounds which are difficult or impossible to synthesize.

Modifications in chemical structure

Some specific compounds can be achieved more easily in cultured plant cells rather than by chemical synthesis or by microorganism.

Disease-free and desired propagule

Plant tissue culture is advantageous over conventional method of propagation in large-scale production of disease-free and desired propagules in limited space and also the germplasm could be stored and maintained without any damage during transportation for subsequent plantation.

Crop improvement

Plant tissue culture is advantageous over the conventional cultivation technique in crop improvement by somatic hybridization or by production of hybrids.

Biosynthetic pathway

Tissue culture can be used for tracing the biosynthetic pathways of secondary metabolites using labelled precursor in the culture medium.

Immobilization of cells

Tissue culture can also be used for plants preservation by immobilization of cell further facilitating transportation and biotransformation.

26.2. HISTORY

Although the feasibility of aseptic culture of cells, tissues and organs on defined nutrient medium had been recognized at the beginning of the century, but it is only some few decades ago that modern developments in the cultivation of plants cell as a callus or as a suspension liquid culture actually came into existence. It is only in the last two decades that its implication has been realized and in particular pharmaceutical importance of this modern technique was appreciated. The principles of tissue culture were involved as early as 1838–1839 in cell theory advanced by Schleiden and Schwaiin. But according to noted biologist Gautheret (1985), the discovery of tissue culture could be considered with the Henri-Louis Dubamel du Monceau's (1756) pioneering experiment on wound healing in plants, demonstrated spontaneous callus formation on the decorticated region of the Elm plant. Further contribution to plant tissue culture could be attributed with the Haberblandt's hypothesis (1902) that a cell is capable of autonomy and have potential for totipotency (the potential of cell to develop into an organism by regeneration is termed as totipotency by Morgan); hence, the isolated plant cell should be capable of cultivation on artificial medium.

The development of multicellular or multiorganed body of a higher organism from a single cell (zygote) supports the totipotent behaviour of a cell. But Haberblandt and coworker have tried to demonstrate the hypothesis but could not succeed. In 1904, another physiologist Hannig started research work, by taking embryogenic tissue instead of single cells for *in vitro* cultivation in an artificial medium consisting of mineral salts and sugar solution. He excised nearly matured embryos of some crucifers (*Raphanus sativus, R. landra, R. caudatus* and *Cochlearia donica*) and successfully cultivated them up to maturity. Thus, it became an important area of investigation, using an *in vitro* technique.

Simon (1908) obtained more promising results as he achieved success in the regeneration of bulky callus, buds and roots from popular stem segments, and thus he succeeded in establishing the basis for callus culture and to some extent also micropropagation.

In vitro technique of culture was carried out further by many biologists. In 1922, Kotte (Germany) and Robbin (United States) simultaneously conceived a new approach to tissue culture, and reported that true *in vitro* culture could be made easier by using meristematic cells (root tips or buds). Kotte carried out number of experiments and successfully cultivated small excised root tips of pea, and grew the culture for two weeks by using a variety of nutrients containing salts of Knop's solution, glucose and several nitrogenous compounds (such as asparagine, alanine and yeast extract). Robbin working independently maintained maize root tip culture for longer period by sub-culturing, but growth gradually diminished and ultimately culture was lost.

White (1934–39) carried out the *in vitro* technique of tissue culture by changing the nature of media. He replaced the yeast extract in a medium containing inorganic salts and sucrose, with three vitamins (pyridoxine, thiamine and nicotinic acid) and was able to maintain the root tip culture; hence, White's synthetic media later proved to be one of the basic media for cell and tissue culture.

Gautheret (1934) successfully cultured cambium cells of some tree species (*Acer pseudoplatanus, Ulmus campestre, Robinia pseudoacacia* and *Salix caprea*) on the surface of the media (Knop's solution containing glucose and cysteine hydrochloride) solidified with agar and observed that after six month, proliferation of callus was ceased but on addition of auxin enhanced the proliferation of cambial culture and making it possible to prepare subculture.

Van Overbeek et al. (1941) used coconut milk (embryo sac fluid) for embryo development and callus formation in *Datura*, which proved to be turning point in the development of embryo culture, which latter on proved to be helpful in the development of several hybrids.

Loo (1945) got success in developing whole plant from stem tip culture. He obtained excellent cultures from stem tips of Dodder and Asparagus. Subsequently, Ball (1946) was able to identify the exact part of the shoot meristem, which gave rise to whole plant. This method is now being used in plant propagation at industrial scale throughout the world.

Muir (1953) demonstrated that on transferring the callus tissues of these two plants into liquid medium and on subsequent agitating on a shaking machine, it is possible to break down the callus tissue into single cell and small cell aggregates, which on subculturing into fresh liquid medium can multiply while remaining in the medium under constant shaking. Muir and associates (1954) reported that the pieces of callus of *Tagetes erecta*

and *Nicotiana tabacum* can be cultured in the form of cell suspension.

Van Overbeek et al. (1941) had suggested earlier that liquid endosperm (coconut milk) is a good medium for embryo culture. Later in 1955, Skoog and coworker finally isolated adenine derivative from the embryo sac known as kinetin which helps in the proliferation of embryo.

Skoog and Miller (1957) proposed the concept of hormonal control of organ formation. They demonstrated that root and bud initiation were conditioned by balance between auxin and kinetin addition to other ingredients of the define medium. High proportions of auxin promoted rooting, whereas proportionately more kinetin initiated bud or shoot formation.

Bergmann (1960) developed plating technique for cloning a large number of isolated single cells. He demonstrated the technique by using callus culture of *Nicotiana tabacum* and *Phaseolus vulgaris* and reported population of nearly 90% of free cells. In the same year, i.e. 1960, Jones et al. used hanging drops of free cells for the microculture propagation. This technique proved useful to have continuous observation of cell growth in the culture.

In 1960, Cocking introduced protoplasmic plant tissue culture. He succeeded in isolating the protoplasts of plant tissue by using cell wall enzymes like cellulase, hemicellulase, pectinase and protease. The enzyme was extracted from fungus *Trichoderma viride*. Earlier, Michel (1939) had demonstrated the role of sodium nitrate fusion of protoplasts. In the same year, Steward and coworker had successfully raised a large number of plantlets from carrot root suspension culture. In year 1960, Moral initiated micro-propagation technique and produced virus-free orchid, *Cymbidium*.

Steward and coworker in 1966 raised large number of plantlets from carrot root suspension culture via somatic embryogenesis. Actually Rienert (1968) introduced somatic embryogenesis callus, cultured on a semisolid medium. This phenomenon of somatic embryogenesis for the production of plantlets was later reported in many species. All these discoveries contributed to the establishment of totipotency power of the cells under suitable environment thereby accomplishing theory introduced by Haberblandt.

In 1970, Power et al. demonstrated the intra and interspecific fusion between the protoplasts of different plant roots; subsequently, in 1972, Carlson et al., succeeded in obtaining the first interspecific somatic hybrid by protoplasts fusion of *Nicotiana* species (*N. glauca* and *N. longsdorfi*). In 1981, Vilnken brought new approach of electrical fusion of protoplasts. Later Gamborg and Neabors (1987) described a number of variations in protoplasts fusion.

During last two decades, procedures for culture of somatic cells, pollens and protoplasts have been refined and many new developments in regenerating plants from such cultured cells have been made. Protoplast fusion has been used to obtain novel somatic hybrid plants among several sexually incompatible species and to produce hybrids, difficult to obtain through conventional methods. Defined tissue culture procedures have made it possible to introduce foreign DNA and cloned genes into cultured cells, protoplasts and plant organs from diverse biological systems and to regenerate transgenic plants.

26.3. BASIC REQUIREMENTS FOR A TISSUE CULTURE LABORATORY

For the successful achievement of any type of tissue culture technique, a tissue culture laboratory should have the following general basic facilities:

- Equipment and apparatus
- Washing and storage facilities
- Media preparation room
- Sterilization room
- Aseptic chamber for culture
- Culture rooms or incubators fully equipped with temperature, light and humidity control devices
- Observation or recording area well equipped with computer for data processing

Equipment and Apparatus

Culture vessels and glassware

Many different kinds of vessels may be used for wing cultures. Callus culture can be grown successfully in large test tubes (25 × 150 mm) or wide mouth conical flasks (Erlenmeyer flask). In addition to the culture vessels, glassware such as graduated pipettes, measuring cylinders, beakers, filters, funnel and petri dishes are also required for making preparations. All the glasswares should be of pyrex or corning.

Equipment

Scissors, scalpels and forceps for explant preparation from excised plant parts and for their transfer.

- A spirit burner or gas microburner for flame sterilization of instruments
- An autoclave to sterilize the media
- Hot air oven for the sterilization of glassware, etc.
- A pH meter for adjusting the pH of the medium
- A shaker to maintain cell suspension culture
- A balance to weigh various nutrients for the preparation of the medium
- Incubating chamber or laminar airflow with UV light fitting for aseptic transfer of explants to the medium and for subculturing

- A BOD incubator for maintaining constant temperature to facilitate the culture of callus and its subsequent maintenance

Washing and storage facilities

First and foremost requirement of the tissue culture laboratory is provision for fresh water supply and disposal of the waste water, and space for distillation unit for the supply of distilled and double distilled water and deionized water. Acid and alkali resistant sink or wash basin for apparatus/equipment washing and the working table should also be acid- and alkali-resistant.

Sufficient space is required for placing hot air oven, washing machine, pipette washers and the plastic bucket or steel tray for soaking or drainage of the detergent bath or extra water. For the storage of dried glassware separate dust proof cupboards or cabinet should be provided. It is mandatory to maintain cleanliness in the area of washing, drying and storage.

Media preparation room

Media preparation room should have sufficient space to accommodate chemicals, lab ware, culture vessels and equipments required for weighing and mixing, hot plate, pH meter, water baths, Bunsen burners with gas supply, microwave oven, autoclave or domestic pressure cooker, refrigerator and freezer for storage of prepared media and stock solutions.

Sterilization Room

For the sterilization of culture media, a good quality ISI mark autoclave is required and for small amount domestic pressure cookers, can also serve the purpose. For the sterilization of glassware and metallic equipments hot air oven with adjustable tray is required.

Aseptic chamber/area for transfer of culture

For the transfer of culture into sterilized media, contaminant-free environment is mandatory. The simplest type of transfer area requires an ordinary type of small wooden hood, having a glass or plastic door either sliding or hinged fitted with UV tube. This aseptic hood can be conveniently placed in a quiet corner of the laboratory.

These days, modern laboratory have laminar airflow cabinet having vertical or horizontal airflow, arrange over the working surface to make it free from dust particles/microcontaminants.

The air coming out of the fine filter (a 0.3-μm HEPA filter) is ultraclean (free from fungal or bacterial contaminant) and having adequate velocity (27±3 m/min) to prevent microcontamination of the working area by worker sitting in front of the cabinet.

Inside the cabinet, there is arrangement for Bunsen burner and a UV tube fitted on the ceiling of the cabinet (to make area free from any live contamination). The advantage of working in the laminar airflow cabinet is that the flow of air does not hamper the use of Bunsen burner and moreover, the cabinet occupies relatively small space within the laboratory (Fig. 26.1).

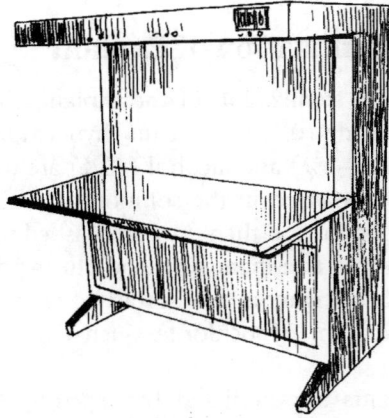

FIG. 26.1 Laminar air flow

Incubation room or incubator

Environmental factors have great effect on the growth and differentiation of cultured tissues. Therefore, it is very much essential to incubate all types of cultures in well-controlled environmental conditions, like temperature, humidity, illumination and air circulation. A typical incubation chamber or area should have both light and temperature controlled devices managed for 24 h period. Air conditioners or room heaters are required to maintain the temperature at 25±2°C. Light is adjusted in the terms of photo period duration (specified period for total darkness as well as for higher intensity light). Further the requirement for humidity range of 20–90% controllable to ±3% and uniform forced air circulation can be achieved.

The incubation chamber or room should have the provision for storing the culture vessels (flask, jars and petri dishes). Shelves should be designed in such a way so that the culture vessels can be placed in the shelf or trays in such a way that there should not be any hindrance in the light, temperature and humidity maintenance. A label having full detail about date of inoculation, name of the explant, medium and any other special information should stuck on each tray and rack to ensure identity and for maintaining the data of experiment. In the case of suspension culture arrangement for shaker should also be made.

These days BOD incubators (Fig. 26.2) with all the requisite environmental condition maintenance are available in the market, they occupy less space and manageable with small generator or automatic invertor in the case of electricity failure to maintain the necessary light and temperature conditions.

Failure of electricity may spoil important experiment and in the case of suspension culture the whole culture may get damaged due to stoppage of the shaker.

BOD incubators required to maintain the culture conditions should have the following characteristics:

- Temperature range, 2–40°C
- Temperature control ±0.5°C
- Automatic digital temperature recorder
- 24-h temperature and light programming
- Adjustable fluorescent lighting up to 10,000 lux
- Relative humidity range 20–98%
- Relative humidity control ±3%
- Uniform forced air circulation
- Shaker
- Capacity up to 0.7 m³ of 0.5 m² shelf space

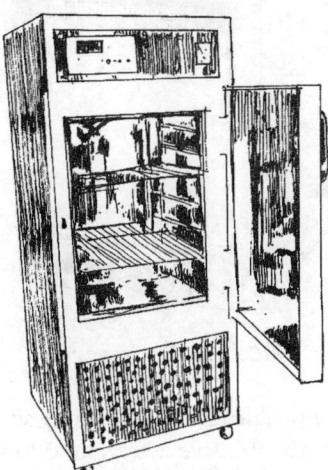

FIG. 26.2 BOD incubator

Data collection and recording the observation

The growth and maintenance of the tissue culture in the incubator should be observed and recorded at regular intervals. All the observations should be done in aseptic environment, i.e. in the laminar airflow. Whereas for microscopic examination, separate dust-free space should be marked for microscopic work. All the recorded data should be fed into the computer.

26.4. GENERAL PROCEDURES INVOLVED IN PLANT TISSUE CULTURE

In vitro culturing of plant tissue involves the following steps:

- Sterilization of glassware tools/vessels
- Preparation and sterilization of explant
- Production of callus from explant
- Proliferation of cultured callus
- Subculturing of callus
- Suspension culture

Sterilization of Glassware Tools/Vessels

Cleaning of glassware

All the glassware to be used in tissue culture laboratory should be of pyrex or corning. To make them free from any dirt, waxy material or bacteria, all the glassware should be kept overnight dipped in sodium dichromate-sulphuric acid solution. Next morning, glassware should be washed with fresh running tap water, followed by distilled water and placed in inverted position in plastic bucket or trays to remove the extra water. For drying the glassware, it is placed in hot air oven at high temperature about 120°C for 1/2–1 h (Fig. 26.3).

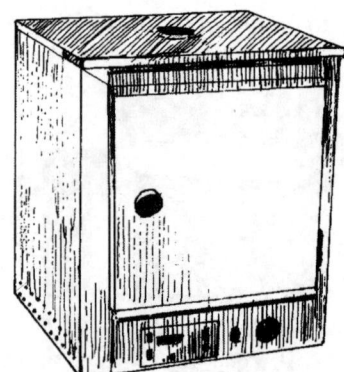

FIG. 26.3 Hot air oven

In the case of plastic labware, washing should be carried out with a mild nonabrasive detergent followed by washing under tap water or the plasticware after general washing with dilute sodium bicarbonate and water followed by drainage of extra water, rinsed with an organic solvent such as alcohol, acetone and chloroform. Washed and dried glassware or plasticware should be stored in dust proof cupboards.

To prevent reinfection following sterilization, empty containers are wrapped with aluminium foil. Stainless steel, metal tools (knives, scalpels, forceps, etc.) are also wrapped with the aluminium foil and pads of cotton wool are stuffed into the opening of the pipettes, which are either also wrapped in aluminium or placed in an aluminium or stainless steel box. The period of sterilization usually ranges between 1 and 4 h.

Preparation of Explant

Explant can be defined as a portion of plant body, which has been taken from the plant to establish a culture. Explant can be obtained from plants, which are grown in controlled environmental conditions. Such plants will be usually free from pathogens and are homozygous in nature. Explant may be taken from any part of the plant like root, stem, leaf or meristematic tissue like cambium, floral parts like anthers, stamens, etc.

Age of the explant is also an important factor in callus production. Young tissues are more suitable than mature tissues. A suitable portion from the plant is removed with the help of sharp knife, and the dried and mature portions are separated from young tissue. When seeds and grains are used for explant preparation, they are directly sterilized and put in nutrient medium. After germination, the obtained seedlings are to be used for explant preparation.

Surface Sterilization of Explant

For the surface sterilization of the explant, chromic acid, mercuric chloride (0.11%), calcium hypochlorite, sodium hypochlorite (1–2%) and alcohol (70%) are used. Usually the tissue is immersed in the solution of sterilizing agent for 10 s to 15 min, and then they are washed with distilled water. Repeat the treatment with sodium hypochlorite for 20 min, and the tissue is finally washed with sterile water to remove sodium hypochlorite. Such tissue is used for inoculation.

The explants are sterilized by exposing to aqueous sterilized solution of different concentration as shown in Table 26.1. In the case of leaf or green fresh stem the explant needs pretreatment with wetting agent (70–90% ethyl alcohol, Tween 20), 5–20 drops in 100 ml of purified water or some other mild detergent to be added directly into the sterilization solution to reduce the water repulsion (due to waxy secretion).

Table 26.1 Surface sterilizing agent

Name of Chemical	Concentration (%)	Exposure (min)
Bromine water	1–2	2–10
Benzalkonium chloride	0.01–0.1	5–20
Sodium hypochlorite	0.5–51	5–30
Calcium hypochlorite	9–10	5–30
Mercuric chloride	1–2	2–10
Hydrogen peroxide	3–10	5–15
Silver nitrate	1–2	5–20

Procedure to be followed for respective explant is as follows:

Seeds

- *1st Step:* Dip the seeds into absolute ethyl alcohol for 10 s and rinse with purified water.
- *2nd Step:* Expose seeds for 20–30 min to 10% w/v aqueous calcium hypochlorite or for 5 min in a 1% solution of bromine water.
- *3rd Step:* Wash the treated seeds with sterile water (three to five times) followed by germination on damp sterile filter paper.

Fruits

- *1st Step:* Rinse the fruit with absolute alcohol.
- *2nd Step:* Submerge into 2% (w/v) solution sodium hypochlorite for 10 min.
- *3rd Step:* Washing repeated with sterile water and remove seeds of interior tissue.

Stem

- *1st Step:* Clean the explant with running tap water followed by rinsing with pure alcohol.
- *2nd Step:* Submerge in 2% (w/v) sodium hypochlorite solution for 15–30 min.
- *3rd Step:* Wash three times with sterile water.

Leaves

Clean the leaf explant with purified water to make it free from dirt and rub the surface with absolute ethyl alcohol. Dip the explant in 0.1% (w/v) mercuric chloride solution, wash with sterile water to make it free from chloride and then dry the surface with sterile tissue paper.

Production of Callus from Explant

The sterilized explant is transferred aseptically onto defined medium contained in flasks. The flasks are transferred to BOD incubator for maintenance of culture. Temperature is adjusted to 25 ± 2°C. Some amount of light is necessary for callus (undifferentiated amorphous cell mass) production. Usually sufficient amount of callus is produced within three to eight days of incubation.

Proliferation of Callus

If callus is well developed, it should be cut into small pieces and transferred to another fresh medium containing an altered composition of hormones, which supports growth. The medium used for production of more amount of callus is called proliferation medium.

Subculturing of Callus

After sufficient growth of callus, it should be periodically transferred to fresh medium to maintain the viability of cells. This subculturing will be done at an interval of 4–6 weeks.

Suspension Culture

Suspension culture contains a uniform suspension of separate cells in liquid medium. For the preparation of suspension culture, callus is transferred to liquid medium, which is agitated continuously to keep the cells separate. Agitation can be achieved by rotary shaker system attached within the incubator at a rate of 50–150 rpm. After the production of sufficient number of cells subculturing can be done.

26.5. CULTURE MEDIA

Nutritional requirements for optimal growth of a tissue culture may vary with the species. Even tissues from different parts of a plant may have different requirements for proper satisfactory growth. As such no single medium can be suggested as being entirely sufficient for the satisfactory growth of all types of plant tissues and organs; hence, with every new system it is essential to work out a medium by hit and trial that would fulfil the specific requirements of that particular tissue. List of several culture media developed by scientists to culture diverse tissues and organs are Gautheret (1942), White (1943), Haberblandt et al. (1946), Haller (1953), Nitsch and Nitsch (1956), Murashige and Skoog (1962), Eriksson (1965) and B5 (Gamberg et al., 1968) (Table 26.2).

Media Composition

To maintain the vital functions of a culture, the basic medium consisting of inorganic nutrients (macronutrients and micronutrients) adapted to the requirements of the object in question, must be supplemented with organic components (amino acids, vitamins), growth regulators (phytohormones) and utilizable carbon (sugar) source and a gelling agent (agar/phytogel).

Inorganic nutrients

Mineral elements play very important role in the growth of a plant. For example, magnesium is a part of chlorophyll molecule, calcium is a component of cell wall and nitrogen is an important element of amino acids, vitamins, proteins and nucleic acids. Iron, zinc and molybdenum are parts of certain enzymes. Essentially about 15 elements found important for whole plant growth have also been proved necessary for the growth of tissue(s) in culture.

Macronutrients: The macronutrients include six major elements: nitrogen (N), phosphorus (P), potassium (K), calcium (Ca), magnesium (Mg) and sulphur (S) present as salts that constitute the various above mentioned defined media. The concentration of the major elements like calcium, phosphorus, sulphur and magnesium should be in the range of 1–3 mmol l^{-1} where as the nitrogen in the media (contributed by both nitrate and ammonia) should be 2–20 mmol l^{-1}.

Micronutrients: The inorganic elements required in small quantities but essential for proper growth of plant cells or tissues are boron (B), copper (Cu), iron (Fe), manganese (Mn), zinc (Zn) and molybdenum (Mo). Out of these, iron seems more critical as it is used in chelated forms of iron and zinc in preparing the culture media, as iron tartrate and citrate are difficult to dissolve. The concentration generally prescribed for all these elements are in traces.

These are added to culture media depending upon the requirement of the objective. In addition to these elements, certain media are also enriched with cobalt (Co), iodine

Table 26.2 Composition of some plant tissue culture media

Constituents	Media (in mg l⁻¹)						
	White	Heller's	MS	ER	B	Nitsch	NT
Micronutrients							
$MnSO_4 \cdot 4H_2O$	5	0.1	22.3	2.23	–	25.0	22.3
$MnSO_4 \cdot H_2O$	–	–	–	–	10.0	–	–
$ZnSO_4 \cdot 7H_2O$	3	1	8.6	–	2.0	10.0	–
$ZnSO_4 \cdot 4H_2O$	–	–	–	–	–	–	8.6
$CuSO_4 \cdot 5H_2O$	0.01	0.03	0.00025	–	0.025	0.025	0.025
$CoSO_4 \cdot 7H_2O$	–	–	–	–	–	–	0.03
$Fe_2(SO_4)_3$	2.5	–	–	–	–	–	–
$FeSO_4 \cdot 7H_2O$	–	–	27.8	27.8	–	27.8	27.8
KCl	65	750	–	–	–	–	–
KI	0.75	0.01	0.83	–	0.75	–	0.83
H_3BO_3	1.5	1	6.2	0.63	3.0	10.0	6.2
$Na_2MoO_4 \cdot 2H_2O$	–	–	0.25	0.025	0.25	0.25	0.25
MoO_3	0.001	–	–	–	–	–	–
$CoCl_2 \cdot 6H_2O$	–	–	0.025	0.0025	0.025	–	–
$AlCl_3$	–	0.03	–	–	–	–	–
$NiCl_2 \cdot 6H_2O$	–	0.03	–	–	–	–	–
$FeCl_3\, 6H_2O$	–	1.00	–	–	–	–	–
EDTA							
$Zn \cdot Na_2EDTA$	–	–	–	15.0	–	–	–
$Na_2EDTA \cdot 2H_2O$	–	–	37.3	37.3	–	37.3	37.3
Vitamins							
Nicotinic acid	0.05	–	0.5	0.5	1.0	5.0	–
Pyridoxine HCl	0.01	–	0.5	0.5	1.0	0.5	1.0
Thiamine HCl	0.01	–	0.10	0.5	10.0	0.5	1.0
Glycine	3.0	–	2.0	2.0	–	2.0	–
Folic acid	–	–	–	–	–	0.5	–
Macronutrients							
NH_4NO_3	–	–	1650	1200	–	720	825
HNO_3	80	–	1900	1900	2527.5	950	950
$NaNO_3$	–	600	–	–	–	–	–
$Ca(NO_3)4H_2O$	300	–	–	–	–	–	–
$CaCl_2 \cdot 2H_2O$	–	75	440	440	150	–	220
$CaCl_2$	–	–	–	–	–	166	–
$MgSO_4 \cdot 6H_2O$	750	250	370	370	246.5	185	1233
$(NH_4)_2SO_4$	–	–	–	–	–	–	–
KH_2PO_4	–	–	170	340	–	68.0	68.0
$NaH_2PO_3 \cdot H_2O$	19	125	–	–	150	–	–
Growth regulators							
Inositol	–	–	100	–	100	100	100
2,4-D	–	–	0.1	1.0	–	–	–
IAA	–	–	1.0	30.0	–	–	–
Kinetin	–	–	0.04	10.0	0.02	0.1	–
NAA	–	–	–	1.0	–	–	–
Myo-inositol	–	–	100.0	–	100	–	–
pH	–	–	5.7	5.8	5.5	–	–
Sucrose	2%	–	3%	4%	2%	2%	1%

MS = Murashige and Skoog; ER = Eriksson; B = Gamberg et al.; NT = Nagata and Takebe

(I) and sodium (Na) but exact cell growth requirement is not well established.

The composition of some plant tissue culture media reveal that the chief difference in the composition of various commonly used tissue culture media lies in the quantity of various salts and ions. Qualitatively, the inorganic nutrients required for various culture media appear to be fairly constant. The active factor in the medium is the ions of different types rather than the salt (mineral salts on dissolving in water undergo dissociation and ionization). A single ion may be contributed by more than one salt. For example, in Murashige and Skoog's medium, NO_3^- ions are contributed by NH_4NO_3 as well as KNO_3 and K^+ ions are contributed by KNO_3 and KH_2PO_4.

White's medium, one of the earliest plant tissue culture media, includes all the necessary nutrients and was widely used for root culture. The experience of various investigators has however revealed that quantitatively the inorganic nutrients are inadequate for good callus growth (Murashige and Skoog's, 1962); hence, most plant tissue culture media that are now being widely used are richer in mineral salts (ions) as compared to White's medium. Aluminium and nickel used by Heller's (1953) could not be proved to be essential and, therefore, were dropped by subsequent workers, but sodium, chloride and iodide are indispensable.

In Heller medium, special emphasis was given to iron and nitrogen. In the original White's medium iron was used in the form of $Fe_2(SO_4)$, but Street and coworkers replaced it by $FeCl_3$ for root culture because of the impurities due to Mn and some other metallic ions. However, $FeCl_3$ also did not prove to be an entirely satisfactory source of iron. In this form iron is available to the tissue culture at or around pH 5.2 and within a week of inoculation the pH of the medium drift from 4.9–5.0 to 5.8–6.0, and the root culture started showing the iron deficiency symptoms. To overcome this difficulty, in most medium, iron is now used as FeEDTA; in this form, iron remains available up to a pH of 7.6–8.0. However, unlike root, callus cultures can utilize $FeCl_3$ to pH 6.0 by secreting natural chelates. FeEDTA may be prepared by using $Fe_2(SO_4)_3 7H_2O$ and $Na_2EDTA\, 2H_2O$.

Organic nutrients

Nitrogenous Substances: Most cultured plant cells are capable of synthesizing essential vitamins but not in sufficient amount. To achieve best growth it is essential to supplement the tissue culture medium with one or more vitamins and amino acid. Among the essential vitamins thiamine (vitamin B_1) has been proved to be essential ingredient. Other vitamins, especially pyridoxine (vitamin B_6), nicotinic acid (vitamin B_3) and calcium pentothenate (vitamin B_5) and inositol are also known to improve growth of the tissue culture material. As shown in Table 26.2, there is variation in the quantities of essential vitamins used by various standard media.

Numerous complex nutritive mixtures of undefined composition, like casein hydrolysate, coconut milk, corn milk, malt extract, tomato juice and yeast extract have also been used to promote growth of the tissue culture, but these substances specifically fruit extracts may affect the reproducibility of results because of variation in the quality and quantity of growth promoting constituent in these extracts.

Carbon Source: It is essential to supplement the tissue culture media with an utilizable source of carbon to the culture media. Haberblandt (1902) attempted to culture green mesophyll cells, probably with the idea that green cells would have simple nutritive requirement, but this did not prove to be true. In fact even fully organized green shoot in cultures, and it also did not show proper growth and proliferation without the addition of suitable carbon source in the medium.

The most commonly used carbon source is sucrose at a concentration of 2–5%. Glucose and fructose are also known to be used for good growth of some tissues. Ball (1953, 1955) demonstrated that autoclaved sucrose was better than filtered sterilized sucrose. Autoclaving may do the hydrolysis of the sucrose thereby converting it into more efficiently utilizable sugar such as fructose. In general, excised dicotyledonous roots grow better with sucrose where as monocots do best with dextrose (glucose). Some other forms of carbon that plant tissues are known to utilize include maltose, galactose, mannose, lactose and sorbitol. It has been reported that some tissues can even metabolize starch as the sole carbon source, e.g. tissue cultures of sequoia and maize endosperm.

Plant growth regulators

Plant growth regulators are the critical media components in determining the developmental pathway of the plant cells. The plant growth regulators used most commonly are plant hormones or their synthetic analogues.

Classes of plant growth regulators: There are five main classes of plant growth regulator used in plant cell culture, namely:

(1) auxins, (2) cytokinins, (3) gibberellins, (4) abscisic acid and (5) ethylene.

Auxins: Auxins promote both cell division and cell growth. The most important naturally occurring auxin is IAA (indole-3-acetic acid), but its use in plant cell culture media is limited because it is unstable to both heat and light. Occasionally, amino acid conjugates of IAA (such as indole–acetyl–L-alanine and indole–acetyl–L-glycine), which are more stable, are used to partially alleviate the problems associated with the use of IAA. It is more common, though, to use stable chemical analogues of IAA as a source of auxin in plant cell culture media. 2,4-Dichlorophenoxyacetic acid (2,4-D) is the most commonly used auxin, and is extremely effective in most circumstances. Other auxins are available (Table 26.3), and some may be more effective or 'potent' than 2,4-D in some instances.

Cytokinins: Cytokinins promote cell division. Naturally occurring cytokinins are a large group of structurally related

Table 26.3 Commonly used auxins

Abbreviation/Name	Chemical Name
2,4-D	2,4-Dichlorophenoxyacetic acid
2,4,5-T	2,4,5-Trichlorophenoxyacetic acid
Dicamba	2-Methoxy-3,6-dichlorobenzoic acid
IAA	Indole-3-acetic acid
IBA	Indole-3-butyric acid
MCPA	2-Methyl-4-chlorophenoxyacetic acid
NAA	1-Naphthylacetic acid
NOA	2-Naphthyloxyacetic acid
Picloram	4-Amino-2,5,6-trichloropicolinic acid

Table 26.4 Commonly used cytokinins

Abbreviation/name	Chemical Name
BAP[a]	6-Benzylaminopurine
2iP (IPA)[b]	[N6-(2-isopentyl)adenine]
Kinetin[a]	6-Furfurylaminopurine
Thidiazuron[c]	1-Phenyl-3-(1,2,3-thiadiazol-5-yl)urea
Zeatin[b]	4-Hydroxy-3-methyl-*trans*-2-butenylaminopurine

[a] Synthetic analogues.
[b] Naturally occurring cytokinins.
[c] A substituted phenylurea-type cytokinin.

(they are purine derivatives) compounds. Of the naturally occurring cytokinins, two have some use in plant tissue culture media (Table 26.4). These are zeatin and 2iP (2-isopentyl adenine). Their use is not widespread as they are expensive (particularly zeatin) and relatively unstable. The synthetic analogues, kinetin and BAP (benzylaminopurine), are therefore used more frequently. Nonpurine based chemicals, such as substituted phenylureas, are also used as cytokinins in plant cell culture media. These substituted phenylureas can also substitute for auxin in some culture systems.

Gibberellins: There are numerous, naturally occurring, structurally related compounds termed gibberellins. They are involved in regulating cell elongation, and are agronomically important in determining plant height and fruit set. Only a few of the gibberellins are used in plant tissue culture media, GA_3 being the most common.

Abscisic acid: Abscisic acid (ABA) inhibits cell division. It is most commonly used in plant tissue culture to promote distinct developmental pathways such as somatic embryogenesis.

Ethylene: Ethylene is a gaseous, naturally occurring, plant growth regulator most commonly associated with controlling fruit ripening in climacteric fruits, and its use in plant tissue culture is not widespread. It does, though, present a particular problem for plant tissue culture. Some plant cell cultures produce ethylene, which, if it builds up sufficiently, can inhibit the growth and development of the culture. The type of culture vessel used and its means of closure affect the gaseous exchange between the culture vessel and the outside atmosphere and thus the levels of ethylene present in the culture.

Solidifying agents for solidification of the media

Due to improved oxygen supply and support to the culture growth, solid media are often preferred to liquid cultures. For this purpose, substance with strong gelling capacity is added into the liquid media. These reversibly bind water and thus ensure the humidity of the medium desired for culturing depending on the concentration.

Gelling agent used to solidify liquid media

The most commonly used substance for this purpose is the phycocolloid agar–agar obtained from red algae (*Gelidium gracilaria*). It is generally used at a concentration of 0.8–1.0%, with higher concentration medium becoming hard and does not allow the diffusion of nutrients into the tissues medium. However, agar is not an essential component of the nutrient medium. Single cell and cell aggregates can be grown as suspension cultures in liquid medium containing inorganic, organic nutrients and other growth factors. Such culture should however be regularly aerated either by bubbling sterile air or gentle agitation. In nutritional studies, the use of agar should be avoided because of the impurities present in all the commercially available agar–agar especially of Ca, Mg, K, Na and trace elements.

Agar (Agarose) is extraordinary resistant to enzymatic hydrolysis at incubation temperature, and only a few bacteria exist which are capable of producing degrading enzyme—agarase. This resistance to hydrolysis is the fundamental importance to the use of agar–agar in cell culture medium. It is also neutral to media constituents and thus do not react with them.

pH of the medium is generally adjusted between 5.0 and 6.0 before sterilization. In general pH higher than 6.0 gives fairly hard medium and pH below 5.0 does not allow satisfactory gelling of the Agar.

Media Preparation

For media preparation, there are two possible methods, i.e.:

1. To weigh the required quantity of nutrient, dissolve them separately and mix at the time of medium preparation.
2. To prepare the stock solution separately for macro-nutrients, micro-nutrients, iron solution and organic components are stored in the refrigerator till not used, e.g. Murashige and Skoog's media stock solution is prepared as is shown in the table.

Procedure

All the ingredients may be grouped into following four groups:

Stock Solution Ingredients	Amount (mg/l)
Group I	
NH_4NO_3	1650
KNO_3	1900
$CaCl_2 \cdot 2H_2O$	440
$MgSO_4 \cdot 7H_2O$	370
KH_2PO_4	170
Group II	
KI	0.83
H_3BO_3	6.2
$MnSO_4 \cdot 4H_2O$	22.3
$ZnSO_4 \cdot 7H_2O$	8.6
$Na_2MoO_4 \cdot 2H_2O$	0.25
$CuSO_4 \cdot 5H_2O$	0.025
$CoCl_2 \cdot 6H_2O$	0.025
Group III	
$FeSO_4 \cdot 7H_2O$	27.8
$Na_2EDTA \cdot 2H_2O$	37.3
Group IV	
Inositol	100
Nicotinic acid	0.5
Pyridoxine HCl	0.5
Thiamine HCl	0.1
Glycine	2

Concentration of the ingredients

For the preparation of stock solution, the Group I ingredient are prepared at 20x concentrated solution, Group II at 200x, Group III Iron salts at 200x and Group IV organic ingredient except sucrose at 200x.

Solution preparation

For the preparation of stock solution, each component (analar grade) should be weighed and dissolved separately in glass distilled or demineralized water and then mixed together. Stock solution may be prepared at the strength of 1 mmol l^{-1} or 10 mmol l^{-1}. All the stock solutions are stored in refrigerator till used.

For iron solution, dissolve $FeSO_4 \cdot 7H_2O$ and Na_2EDTA $2H_2O$ separately in about 450 ml distilled water by heating and constant stirring. Mix the two solutions, adjust pH of the medium to 5.5 and final volume adjusted to 1 l with distilled water.

Semisolid media preparation

Required quantities of agar and sucrose are weighed and dissolved in wafer by 3/4th volume of medium, by heating them on water bath. Adequate quantities of stock solution (for 1 l medium 50 ml of stock solution of Group 1, 5 ml of stock solution II, III and IV group) and other special supplements are added and final volume is made up with double distilled water. After mixing well, pH of the medium is adjusted to 5.8 using 0.1 N NaOH and 0.1 N HCl.

Sterilization of Culture Media

Culture media packed in glass containers or vessels are sealed with cotton plugs and covered with aluminium foils and are autoclaved at pressure of 2–2.2 atm at 121°C for 15–40 min (time to be fixed from the time when temperature reaches the required temperature). The exposure time depends on the volume of the liquid to be sterilized as given below (Table 26.5).

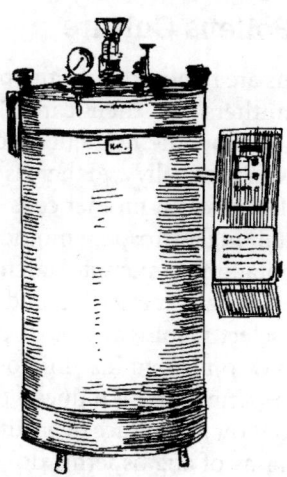

FIG. 26.4 Autoclave

Table 26.5 Minimum autoclaving time for plant tissue culture media

Volume of the Media Per Vessel (ml)	Minimum Autoclaving Time (min)
25	20
50	25
100	28
250	31
500	35
1000	40
2000	48
4000	63

Minimum autoclaving time includes the time required for the liquid volume to reach the sterilizing temperature (121°C) and 15 min at this temperature. Time may vary due to difference in autoclaves. Moreover, the actual success of sterilization can be tested using a bio-indicator, commonly spores of the bacterium *Bacillus stearothermophilus* are used as such as a test organism. Together with culture medium and a pH indicator in ampoules sealed by melting, both autoclaved material and nonautoclaved controls are incubated for 24–48 h at 60°C. If the spores are dead, the colour of the pH indicator in the solution remains unchanged indicating no change in pH (Fig. 26.4).

26.6. TYPES OF PLANT TISSUE CULTURES

Plant tissue culture is a general term to culture the isolated plant organs (particularly of isolated roots but, to a lesser extent of stem tips, immature embryo, leaf primordia, flower structures and even the cells and the protoplasts) under aseptic environment.

Root Tip Culture

Tips of the lateral roots are sterilized, excised and transferred to fresh medium. The lateral roots continue to grow and provide several roots, which after seven days, are used to initiate stock or experimental cultures. Thus, the root material derived from a single radicle could be multiplied and maintained in continuous culture; such genetically uniform root cultures are referred to as a clone of isolated roots.

Leaves or Leaf Primordia Culture

Leaves (800 µm) may be detached from shoots, surface sterilized and placed on a solidified medium where they will remain in a healthy condition for a long period. Growth rate in culture depends on their stage of maturity at excision. Young leaves have more growth potential than the nearly mature ones.

Shoot Tip Culture

The excised shoot tips (100–1000 µm long) of many plant species can be cultured on relatively simple nutrient media containing growth hormones and will often form roots and develop into whole plants.

Complete Flower Culture

Nitsch in 1951 reported the successful culture of the flowers of several dicotyledonous species; the flowers remain healthy and develop normally to produce mature fruits. Flowers (2 days after pollination) are excised, sterilized by immersion in 5% calcium hypochlorite, washed with sterilized water and transferred to culture tubes containing an agar medium. Often fruits that develop are smaller than their natural counterpart, but the size can be increased by supplementing the medium with an appropriate combination of growth hormones.

Anther and Pollens Culture

Young flower buds are removed from the plant and surface sterilized. The anthers are then carefully excised and transferred to an appropriate nutrient medium. Immature stage usually grows abnormally and there is no development of pollen grains from pollen mother cells. Anther at a very young stage (containing microspore mother cells or tetrads) and late stage (containing binucleate starch-filled pollen) of development are generally ineffective, and hence, for better response always select mature anther or pollen.

Mature anther or pollen grains (microspora) of several species of gymnosperms can be induced to form callus by spreading them out on the surface of a suitable agar media. Mature pollen grains of angiosperms do not usually form callus, although there are one or two exceptions.

Ovule and Embryo Culture

Embryo is dissected from the ovule and put into culture media. Very small globular embryos require a delicate balance of the hormones. Hence, mature embryos are excised from ripened seeds and cultured mainly to avoid inhibition in the seed for germination. This type of culture is relatively easy as the embryos require a simple nutrient medium containing mineral salts, sugar and agar for growth and development.

The seeds are treated with 70% alcohol for about 2 min, washed with sterile distilled water, treated with surface sterilizing agent for specific period, once again rinsed with sterilized distilled water and kept for germination by placing them on double layers of presterilized filter paper placed in petri dish moistened with sterilized distilled water or placed on moistened cotton swab in petri dish. The seeds are germinated in dark at 25–28°C and small part of the seedling is utilized for the initiation of callus.

Apart from abovementioned cultures, there are two more methods for culturing of plant tissues/cells:

- Protoplast culture and
- Hairy roots culture.

Protoplast Culture

Protoplasts are the naked cells of varied origin without cell walls, which are cultivated in liquid as well as on solid media. Protoplasts can be isolated by mechanical or enzymatic method from almost all parts of the plant: roots, tubers, root nodules, leaves, fruits, endosperms, crown gall tissues, pollen mother cells and the cells of the callus tissue but the most appropriate is the leaves of the plant.

Fully expanded young leaves from the healthy plant are collected, washed with running tap water and sterilized by dipping in 70% ethanol for about a minute and then treated with 2% solution of sodium hypochlorite for 20–30 min, and washed with sterile distilled water to make it free from the trace of sodium hypochlorite.

The lower surface of the sterilized leaf is peeled off and stripped leaves are cut into pieces (midrib). The peeled leaf segments are treated with enzymes (macerozyme and then treated with cellulase) to isolate the protoplasts.

The protoplasts so obtained are cleaned by centrifugation and decantation method. Finally, the protoplast solution of known density (1×10^5 protoplasts/ml) is poured on sterile and cooled down molten nutrient medium in petri dishes. Mix the two gently but quickly by rotating each petri dish. Allow the medium to set and seal petri dishes with paraffin film. Incubate the petri dishes in inverted position in BOD incubator. The protoplasts, which are capable of dividing undergo cell divisions and form callus within 2–3 weeks. The callus is then subcultured on fresh medium. Embryogenesis begins from callus when it is transferred to a medium containing proper proportion of auxin and cytokinin, where the embryos develop into plantlets which may be transferred to pots (Fig. 26.5).

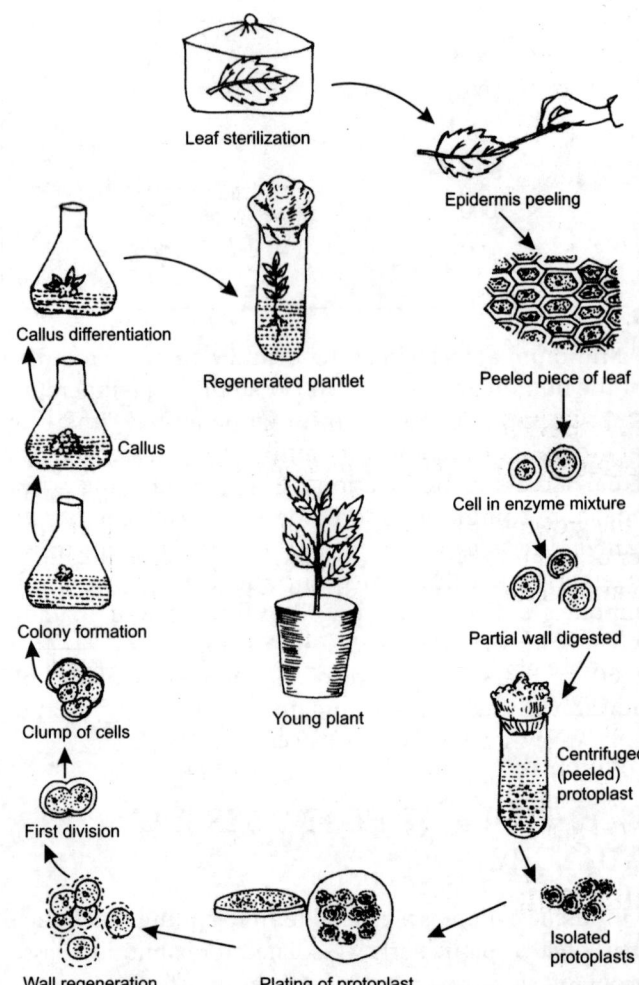

FIG. 26.5 Schematic diagram showing the isolation, culture and regeneration of young plant from leaf protoplast

Hairy Root Culture

The name 'hairy root' was mentioned in the literature by Steward et al. (1900). A large number of small fine hairy roots covered with root, hairs originate directly from the explant in response to *Agrobacterium rhizogenes* infection are termed hairy roots. These are fast-growing, highly branched adventitious roots at the site of infection and can grow even on a hormone-free culture medium. Many plant cell culture systems, which did not produce adequate amount of desired compounds, are being reinvestigated using hairy root culture methods. A diversified range of plant species has been transformed using various bacterial strains. One of the most important characteristics of the transformed roots is their capability to synthesize secondary metabolites specific to that plant species from which they have been developed. Growth kinetics and secondary metabolite production by hairy roots is highly stable and are of equal level and even they are higher to those of field grown plants (Fig. 26.6).

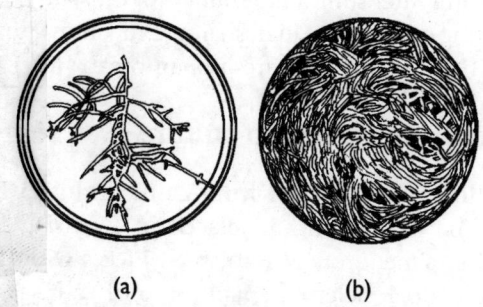

(a)   (b)

FIG. 26.6 Hairy root culture of Vinca in (a) solid media and (b) liquid media

26.7. ESTABLISHMENT AND MAINTE-NANCE OF VARIOUS CULTURES

For the growth establishment and maintenance of various types of plant tissue cultures, there are three main culture systems, selected on the basis of the objective.

1. Growth of callus masses on solidified media (callus culture also known as static culture).
2. Growth in liquid media (suspension culture) consists of mixture of single cells or cell aggregates.
3. Protoplast culture:
   (a) Callus culture (static tissue culture) or
   (b) Suspension culture.

Callus Culture

Callus is an amorphous aggregate of loosely arranged parenchyma cells, which proliferate from mother cells. Cultivation of callus usually on a solidified nutrient medium under aseptic conditions is known as callus culture; unlike tumour tissue, the cell division takes place periclinally.

Initiation of callus culture

1. Selection and preparation of explant

Selection: For the preparation of callus culture, organ or culture is selected such as segments of root or stem, leaf primordia, flower structure or fruit, etc.

Preparation:

(a) Excised parts of the plant organ are first washed with tap water, and then sterilized with 0.1% of mercuric chloride ($HgCl_2$) or 2% w/v, sodium hypochlorite (NaOCl) solution for 15 min. In the case of plant organ containing waxy layer, the material is either pretreated with wetting agents [ethanol 70–90%; tween 20 (polyoxyethylene sorbitan monolaurate): 1–20 drops into 100 ml distilled water]; or other detergents are added to the sterilization solution to reduce the water repulsion.

(b) Wash the sterilized explants with sterile glass distilled water and cut aseptically into small segments (2–5 mm).

2. Selection of culture medium

The organ is to be cultured in well-defined nutrient medium containing inorganic and organic nutrients and vitamins. The culture of the medium depends on the species of the plant and the objective of the experiment. The MS medium is quite suitable for dicot tissues because of relatively high concentration of nitrate, potassium and ammonium ions in comparison to other media (Table 26.2).

Growth hormones (auxin, cytokinin) are adjusted in the medium according to the objective of the culture. For example, auxins, 1BA and NAA are widely used in medium for rooting and in combination with cytokinin for shoot proliferation. 2,4-D and 2,4,5-T are effective for good growth of the callus culture. This is also quite favourable for monocot tissues or explant.

The selected semisolid nutrient is prepared. The pH of the medium is adjusted (5.0–6.0) and poured into culture vessels (15 ml for 25 × 150 mm culture tubes or 50 for 150 ml flasks) plugged and sterilized by autoclaving.

3. Transfer of explant

Surface sterilized organs (explant) from stem, root or tuber or leaf, etc., are transferred aseptically into the vessel containing semisolid culture medium.

4. Incubation of culture

The inoculated vessels are transferred into BOD incubator with autocontrolled device. Incubate at 25–28°C using light and dark cycles for 12-h duration. Nutrient medium is supplemented with auxin to induce cell division. After three to four weeks, callus should be about five times the size of the explant. Many tissue explants possess some degree of polarity with the result that the callus is formed most early at one surface. In stem segment, callus is formed particularly from that surface which *in vivo* is directed towards the root.

The unique feature of callus is its ability to develop normal root and shoot, ultimately forming a plant. Commercially important secondary metabolites can also be obtained from static culture by manipulating the composition of media and growth regulators (physiological and biochemical conditions), but on the whole it is a good source for the establishment of suspension culture.

Callus is formed through three stages of development, such as:

- Induction
- Cell division
- Cell differentiation

Induction

During this stage, metabolic activities of the cell will increase; with the result, the cell accumulates organic contents and finally divides into a number of cells. The length of this phase depends upon the functional potential of the explant and the environmental conditions of the cell division stage.

Cell division

This is the phase of active cell division as the explant cells revert to meristematic state.

Cell differentiation

This is the phase of cellular differentiation, i.e. morphological and physiological differentiation occur leading to the formation of secondary metabolites.

Maintenance

After sufficient time of callus growth on the same medium following change will occur, i.e.

- Depletion of nutrients in the medium
- Gradual loss of water
- Accumulation of metabolic toxins

Hence for the maintenance of growth in callus culture it becomes necessary to subculture the callus into a fresh medium. Healthy callus tissue of sufficient size (5–10 mm in diameter and weight 20–100 mg) is transferred under aseptic conditions to fresh medium; subculturing should be repeated after even four to five weeks.

Many callus cultures however remain healthy and continue to grow at slow rate for much longer period without subculturing, if the incubation is to be carried out at low temperature, 5–10°C below the normal temperature (16–18°C). Normally, total depletion takes about 28 days.

Callus tissue may appear in the following different colours:

- *White:* If grown in dark due to the absence of chlorophyll

- *Green:* If grown in light
- *Yellow:* Due to development of carotenoid pigments in greater amounts
- *Purple:* Due to the accumulation of anthocyanins in vacuole
- *Brown:* Due to excretion of phenolic substance and formation of quinones

Callus culture may vary widely in texture appearance and rate of growth. Some callus growth is heavily lignified and hard in texture while others are fragile. The cells in callus tissue vary in shape from spherical to elongated.

Suspension Culture

Suspension culture contains a uniform suspension of separate cells in liquid medium. For the preparation of suspension culture, callus fragments is transferred to liquid medium (without agar), which is agitated continuously to keep the cells separate. Agitation can be achieved by rotary shaker system attached within the BOD incubator at a rate of 50–150 rpm. After sufficient numbers of cells are produced, subculturing can be done in fresh liquid medium. Single cells can also be obtained from fresh plant organ (leaf).

Initiation of suspension culture

1. Isolation of single cell from callus culture: Healthy callus tissue is selected and placed in a petri dish on a sterile filter paper and cut into small pieces with the help of sterile scalpel. Selected small piece of callus fragment about 300–500 mg and transferred into flask containing about 60 ml of liquid nutrient media (i.e. defined nutrient medium without gelling agent), the flasks is agitated at 50–150 rpm to make the separation of the cells in the medium. Decant the medium and resuspend residue by gently rotating the flask, and finally transfer 1/4th of the entire residue to fresh medium, followed by sieving the medium to obtain the degree of uniformity of cells.

2. Isolation of single cell from plant organ: From the plant organ (leaf tissue) single cell can be isolated by any of the following methods:

(a) Mechanical method
(b) Enzymatic method

Mechanical method: The surface sterilized fresh leaves are grinded in (1:4) grinding medium (20 µmol sucrose, 10 µmol $MgCl_2$, 20 µmol tris-HCl buffer, pH 7.8) in glass pestle mortar. The homogenate is passed through muslins (two layers) cloth, washed with sterile distilled water, centrifuged with culture medium, sieved and placed on culture dish for inoculation.

Enzymatic method: Leaves are taken from 60- to 80-day-old plant and sterilized by immersing them in 70% ethanol solution followed by hypochlorite solution treatment, washed with sterile double distilled water, placed on sterile tile and peeled off the lower surface with sterile forceps. Cut the peeled surface area of the leaves into small pieces (4 cm²). Transfer them (2 g leaves) into an Erlenmeyer flask (100 ml) containing about 20 ml of filtered sterilized enzyme solution (macerozyme 0.5% solution, 0.8% mannitol and 1% potassium dextran sulphate). Incubate the flask at 25°C for 2 h. During incubation, change the enzyme solution with the fresh one at every 30 min, wash the cell twice with culture medium and place them in culture dish.

Growth pattern of suspension culture

Cell suspension culture is generally initiated by transferring an established (undifferentiated) callus tissue to a liquid nutrient medium, in flask culture vessel, which is agitated continuously during culture period. Agitation serves both, to aerate the cultures and to disperse the eel in medium. The composition of the medium for the establishment of suspension culture could be the same as for the callus culture except for the addition of agar. After transferring the cells into a suitable liquid medium they divide after lag phase and linearly increase their population. The soft callus generally forms a suspension culture without much difficulty. The release of cells and tissue fragments from less friable callus masses and the maintenance of good degree of cell separation may often be promoted by the presence of liquid medium of a high auxin concentration—an appropriate balance between yeast extract and auxin or between auxin and kinetin. After sometime depending upon the nutrient level and the rate of cell division, it comes to stationary phase (Fig. 26.7).

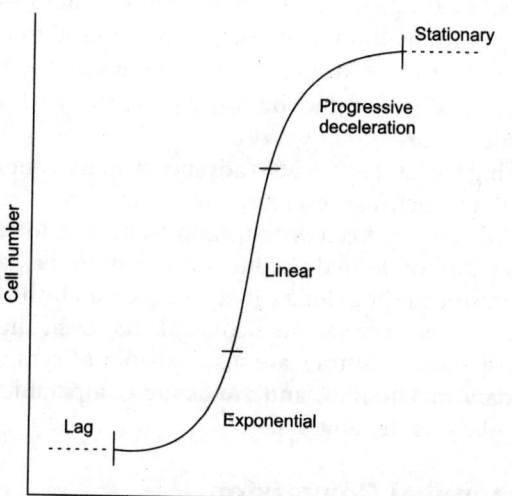

FIG. 26.7 Curve showing the growth pattern in the suspension culture

Stationary phase: The suspension culture is usually incubated at 25°C in darkness or low intensity fluorescent light at this stage, cell cultures are subcultured by dilution of stock culture 5–10 times (v/v) depending upon the growth of cells. The growth of suspension culture is higher than callus culture, and therefore it requires rapid subculture (7–21 days) as compared to callus culture (4–8 weeks).

The incubation period from culture initiation to the stationary phase is determined primarily by:

1. Initial cell density
2. Duration of lag phase and
3. Growth rate of cell type

The cell density used to subculture is critical and depend largely on the type of suspension culture to be maintained. The low initial cell density will prolong the lag phase and exponential phase of growth. At an initial cell density of 9–15 × 10³ ml, the cell will generally undergo eightfold increases in cell number before entering the stationary phase. Normal incubation time of stock culture is 21–28 days, while for subculture it is 14–21 days.

There are several parameters for measuring growth of cultured cells such as measurement of fresh and dry weights, cell mass, cell number, mitotic index or indirectly by the conductivity of the medium (King et al., 1973).

1. *Fresh weight:* The value of callus cultures, frequently determined as total weight of callus medium layer and petri dish. However, in this method, there are variations due to evaporation via the medium's surface. Hence, more exact values are obtained by determining the weight after complete separation from the culture medium. This is possible when the material is cultured on separate layers of cellulose or nylon.

2. *Dry weight:* It requires repeated drying usually at 60°C to the point of constant weight, up to fresh weight of 500 mg, a linear relationship between fresh and dry weight is assumed. This method excludes error due to varying endogenous water contents.

3. *Cell mass:* It may be determined by densification by centrifugation (Ca 2000 g, 5 min) of a particular percentage of the volume (4–7 ml) in graduated conical centrifuge tubes. In order to avoid error, due to water absorption by the cells, the so-called packed cell volume (PCV) must be recorded immediately following the separation process.

4. *Cell number:* To determine the number of cell per unit volume, existing cell clumps or aggregates must be separated into isolated cell (callus culture and in most suspension cultures). This is commonly done using chrome-trioxide alone or in combination with hypochlorous acid. Possible alternative are EDTA and pectinase.

5. *Conductivity:* The inverse relationship between the conductivity and fresh or dry weight of the medium allows the determination of growth without taking samples (which would affect the sterility of the culture); in fully synthetic media, conductivity is determined almost exclusively by salt concentration. As long as the pH of the medium remains above 3, the concentration of hydrogen ions does not affect conductivity.

6. *Cellulose concentration:* Calcofluor-white ST (0.1% aqueous) allows monitoring of changes in the concentration of cell wall polymers from β-glucoside

bond glucose molecule such as cellulose or callose. The textile brightener specifically bonds to β-1,4 glucans and intensely fluoresces following stimulation with short wave blue light. In this way even traces of these compounds may be identified.

Maintenance of suspension culture

Maintenance of suspension culture can be done by following three ways (Fig. 26.8):

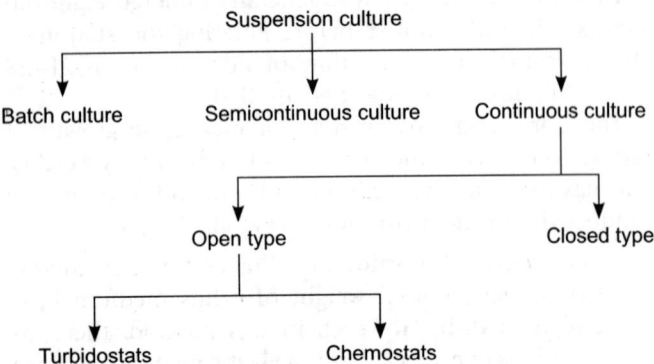

FIG. 26.8 Maintenance of suspension culture

1. Batch suspension culture: In this technique, the cells are allowed to multiply in liquid medium, which is continuously agitated to break up cell aggregates. The system is closed with respect to additions or removal of culture, except for circulation of air. In this technique to commence the growth again on the stationary phase, more amount of nutrient medium is added to the original culture or the cells are to be transferred into fresh medium. Each fresh medium containing culture (suspension) constitutes a batch. Such cultures are grown again and again for the purpose of experiment to achieve certain specific objectives. In batch culture there is no steady state of growth; hence, it is not ideal for commercial production of secondary metabolites.

2. Semicontinuous suspension culture: In this type, the system is open. It is designed for periodic removal of culture and addition of fresh medium. Hence, the growth is continuously maintained.

3. Continuous suspension culture: Here, the volume of culture remains constant and fresh medium and culture are continuously added and withdrawn respectively. The important feature of the continuous culture is the proliferation of cell occurs under constant conditions. In this very suspension culture technique, a steady state is achieved by adding medium in which single nutrient has been adjusted so as to be growth limiting. Continuous culture is closed and open type.

In the closed type, addition of fresh medium is balanced by the outflow of spent medium. The cell passing through the outgoing medium are separated mechanically and reintroduced into the culture for the continuous growth of the cell biomass.

Open continuous system involves regulated new medium and balancing harvest of equal volume of culture. The open system is further of two types depending upon regulation technique: chemostat and turbidostat.

In chemostat, the desired rate of growth is maintained by adjusting the level of concentration of nutrient by constant inflow of fresh medium.

In turbidostat, on the contrary, the input of medium is intermittent, and it is mainly required to maintain the cell density in the culture.

26.8. APPLICATIONS OF PLANT TISSUE CULTURE

Plant tissue culture technology has been used in almost all the field of biosciences. The desirable products produced by plant tissue cultures are as diversified as is industry itself. Its applications include:

- Production of phytopharmaceuticals
- Biochemical conversions
- Clonal propagation (micropropagation)
- Production of immobilized plant cells

Production of Phytopharmaceuticals

The use of plant tissue culture for the production of phytopharmaceuticals was started in 1959 when Wenstein et al., studied Agave, for the production of steroids using tissue culture method. Dioscorea was reported to contain industrially useful steroids by 1966, but it was 1969, when Kaul reported the production of 1.2% dry weight diosgenin by tissue culture of *D. sylvatica*.

During the last two decades advancement in tissue culture technology such as development of hairy root cultures, immobilized plant cell systems and technique to enhance the excretion of desired product into medium has resulted in promising findings for a variety of medicinally important substance from several medicinal plants. Even the callus and suspension cultures are also capable of synthesizing secondary metabolites, and yields are comparable to the intact plant as in Table 26.6.

Biochemical Conversion (Biotransformation)

The conversion of small part of a chemical molecule by means of biological systems is termed biotransformation. It is a process in which the substrate can be modified. For example, *Digitalis lanata* cell cultures have ability to effect hydroxylation, acetylation, glycosylation, etc. It is reported that *D. lanata* strain 291 can convert β-methyl

Table 26.6 Production of phytopharmaceuticals

Compound	Plant Species	Culture Type
Ajmalicine	Catharanthus roseus	S
Atropine	Atropa belladonna	Hairy root
Berberine	Coptis japonica	C and S
Caffeine	Coffea arabica	C
Cardenolides	Digitalis purpurea	S and C
	Digitalis lanata	S (biotransformation)
Codeine	Papaver somniferum	S
Glycyrrhizin	Glycyrrhiza glabra	S
Morphine	Papaver somniferum	S
Nicotine	Nicotiana tobacum	S
Papain	Carcia papaya	C
Psoralen	Ruta graveolens	S

S = Suspension and C = Callus culture

digitoxin into β-methyl digoxin. Cell suspension culture of *Strophanthus gratus* affects various biochemical conversions of digitoxigenin. Monoterpene bioconversions are reported with *mentha* cell culture. It can convert (–)menthone to (+)neomenthol and pulegone to isomenthone.

Podophyllum peltatum in semicontinuous culture can produce anticancer drugs by biotransformation of synthetic dibenzyl butanolides to lignans—suitable for conversion to etoposide.

In some tissue culture stereospecific biotransformation is also reported, which is important for the isolation of optically active compound from racemic mixture. Example of cell culture of *Nicotiana tabacum* selectively hydrolyses R-configurational form of monoterpenes like bornyl acetate and isobornyl acetate.

Apart from the abovementioned biochemical conversions, many other, like saponifications, esterification, epoxidation, oxidation, methylation and isomerization are also reported.

Clonal Propagation (Micropropagation)

Clonal propagation (micropropagation) is the technique to produce entire plant from single individual by asexual reproduction. This fact can be commercially utilized to produce high-yielding crops of the desirable characters in a short period of time, which otherwise show variation when grown using seeds. For example, *Foeniculum vulgare* (fennel) shows wide variations in the yield and composition of the volatile oil, and by this technique, it has been reported to have uniform clones of fennel with narrow variation in the volatile oil composition, in comparison to the normal cultivation.

Somaclonal Variation

In clonal propagation, clones are produced from tissue culture with uniform characters but few clones may show variations among the population of clones, which were not present in the parent cells. This formation of variant clones from cultured tissue is called as somaclonal variations. Variants are of two types: (1) desirable variants and (2) undesirable variants.

Desirable variants can be used for the improvement of crops. The clone showing high productivity can be used for commercial purposes.

Immobilization of Plant Cells

The immobilization of plant cell or enzymes has increased the utility of plant cell biotechnology for production of pharmaceuticals. The plant cells can be immobilized by using matrices, such as alginates, polyacrylamides, agarose and polyurethane fibres. The immobilized plant cells can be utilized in the same way as immobilized enzymes to effect different reactions.

Immobilized cell systems may be used for bioconversions, such as (–)codeinone to (–)codeinine and digitoxin to digoxin or for synthesis from added precursors, e.g. production of ajmalicine from tryptamine and secologanin. The suspension cultures of *Anisodus tanguticus* have been reported to convert hyoscyamine to anisodamine in good quantity. Subsequently, the cultures convert anisodamine into scopolamine. The biotransformation reactions, such as glycosylations, hydroxylation, acetylation, demethylation, etc., have been successfully attempted in immobilized cell systems. The hydroxylation or glycosylation of cardiac glycosides in cultures of *Digitalis lanata* and *Daucus carota* have also been reported.

Immobilized plant cells can be used for tracing the biosynthetic pathways of secondary metabolites and also can be used for carrying out biotransformation or biochemical reactions.

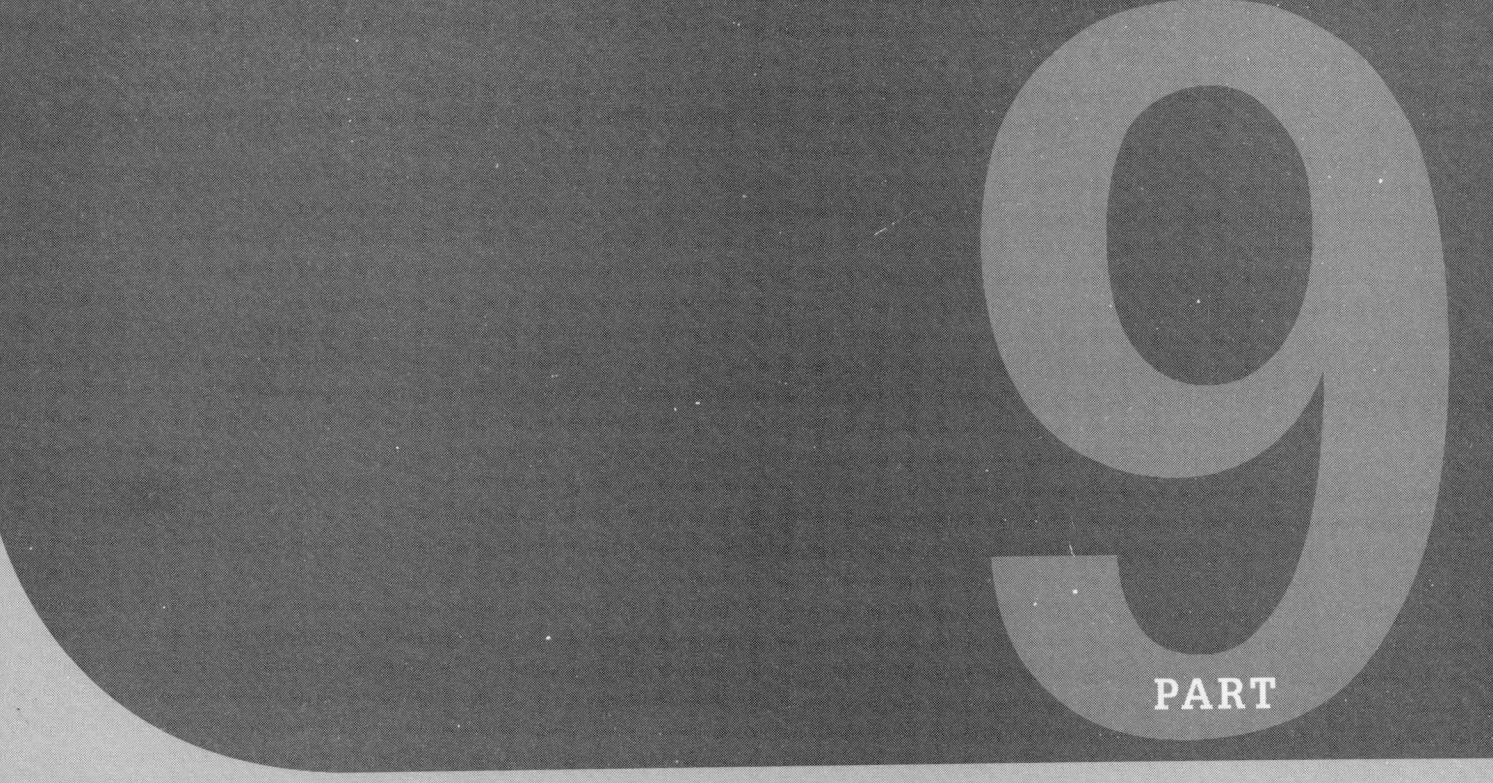

PART

9

Miscellaneous

Section Outline

OVERVIEW

This part provides information regarding various topics, which include development and standardization of ayurvedic formulations, marine pharmacognosy, natural colours and dyes, natural pesticides, nutraceuticals, poisonous plants and natural allergents.

Ayurvedic Pharmacy

CONTENTS

27.1. INTRODUCTION

Ayurveda means the science of life. Since ancient times a variety of pharmaceutical have been used in Ayurvedic system of medicine and some of them are in practice even today, obtaining maximum therapeutic benefit and making recipe palatable. Different pharmaceutical processes are prescribed in ayurveda, called *Aushadhana kalpna* (medicinal formulations), which are prepared for the convenience of administration through various routes in different forms for different disease condition. These processes not only help in the isolation of the therapeutically active parts of the drugs, but also easily administrable, palatable, digestible, therapeutically more tolerable and more preservable.

Ayurvedic dosage forms (formulations) can be grouped into four types depending upon their physical nature:

1. Solid dosage forms, e.g. *vatika, gutika, guggulu*
2. Semisolid dosage forms, e.g. *kalka, avaleha*
3. Liquid dosage forms, e.g. *asava, arishta, swarasa, taila*
4. Powder dosage forms, e.g. *churna*

All the ayurvedic preparations consist of two words. The first word may indicate either the disease for which the preparation is used (*Jwarantaka vati*), or the property of the preparation (*Kameshwara modaka*), or the drug contained (*Arjuna arishta*), or the name of some god or saint (*Narayana taila*) and the second word always indicates the type of preparation (*Jwarantaka vati, Kameshwara modaka, Arjuna arishta, Narayana taila*).

27.2. MARKET POTENTIAL

There is more recognition for nonallopathic system of medicines in the country now than in the past few decades. The concept of alternative system of treatment notably herbal and Ayurvedic medicines therapy is gaining ground and attracting attention worldwide. There is more and more scientific research being conducted in our country for treatment of various diseases by ayurvedic and herbal therapy. A large number of diseases have ayurvedic treatment much superior to the other system of medicines, and this has been recognized world over.

Thus, ayurvedic medicines/drugs are becoming popular day-by-day, and demand for its usage is increasing not only in the country but also worldwide for the inherent quality of having negligible side/after effects, which has made great potential for its production. A large number of medicinal plants, herbs, shrubs, etc., are available in our country in the hilly/forest regions. In order to boost the production of ayurvedic/herbal drugs, Govt of India has also set up a board namely Indian System of Medicine and Homoeopathy to encourage production of ayurvedic medicines especially in the regions, where basic raw materials are available in plenty. Thus, there is a great potential for ayurvedic medicines not only in the country but for export purpose also.

27.3. ASAVA AND ARISHTA

Definition

Asavas and *Arishtas* are medicinal preparations made by soaking the drugs, either in powder form or in the form of decoction (*kasaya*) in a solution of sugar or jaggery, as the case may be for a specified period of time, during which it undergoes a process of fermentation generating alcohol, thus facilitating the extraction of the active principles contained in the drugs. The alcohol, so generated, also serves as a preservative.

Method of Preparation for *Arishta*

The drugs are coarsely powdered and *kasaya* is prepared. The *kasaya* is strained and kept in the fermentation pot, vessel or barrel. Sugar, jaggery or honey, according to the formula, is dissolved, boiled, filtered and added. Drugs mentioned as *praksepa dravyas* are finely powdered and added. At the end, *dhataki puspa*, if included in the formula, should be properly cleaned and added. The mouth of the pot, vessel or barrel is covered with an earthen lid and the edges sealed with clay-smeared cloth wound in seven consecutive layers. The container is kept either in a special room, in an underground cellar or in a heap of paddy to ensure a constant temperature is maintained during fermentation, since varying temperatures may impede or accelerate the fermentation.

After the specified period, the lid is removed, and the contents examined to ascertain whether the process of fermentation (*sandhana*) has been completed. The fluid is first decanted and then strained after two or three days. When the fine suspended particles settle down, it is strained again and bottled.

Method of Preparation for *Asava*

The required quantity of water, to which jaggery or sugar as prescribed in the formula, is added, boiled and cooled. This is poured into the fermentation pot, vessel or barrel. Fine powder of the drugs mentioned in the formula is added. The container is covered with a lid and the edges are sealed with clay-smeared cloth wound in seven consecutive layers. The rest of the process is as in the case of *Arishta*.

General Precautions

If the fermentation is to be carried in an earthen vessel, it should not be new. Water should be boiled first in the vessel. Absolute cleanliness is required during the process. Each time, the inner surface of the fermentation vessel should be fumigated with *pippali churna* and smeared with ghee before the liquids poured into it. In large-scale manufacture, wooden vats, porcelain-jars or metal vessels are used in place of earthen vessels.

Characteristics

The filtered *Asava* or *Arishta* should be clear without froth at the top. It should not become sour (*cukra*). The preparation has the characteristics of aromatic alcoholic odour.

Preservation

Asavas and *Arishtas* can be kept indefinitely. They should be kept in well stoppered bottles or jars.

Examples: *Asavas*—Arvindasava, kumaryasava, vasakasava.

Arishtas—Dasmularishta, asvagandhadyarishta, ashokarishta.

27.4. ARKA

Definition

Arka is a liquid preparation obtained by distillation of certain liquids or of drugs soaked in water using the *Arkayantra* or any convenient modern distillation apparatus.

Method of Preparation

The drugs are cleaned and coarsely powdered. Some quantity of water is added to the drugs for soaking and kept overnight. This makes the drugs soft and when boiled releases the essential volatile principles easily. The following morning it is poured into the *Arkayantra* and the remaining water is added and boiled. The vapour is condensed and collected in a receiver. In the beginning, the vapour consists of only steam and may not contain the essential principles of the drugs. It should therefore be discarded. The last portion also may not contain therapeutically essential substance and should be discarded. The aliquots collected in between contain the active ingredients and may be mixed together to ensure uniformity of the *arka*.

Characteristics

Arka is a suspension of the distillate in water having slight turbidity and colour according to the nature of the drugs used and smell of the predominant drugs.

Examples: *Ajamodarka, jatamamsyarka, satapusparka*.

27.5. AVALEHA OR LEHYA

Definition

Avaleha or *lehya* is a semisolid preparation of drugs, prepared with addition of jaggery, sugar or sugar candy and boiled with prescribed drug juice or decoction. They are also known as *modaka, guda, khanda, rasayana, lehya*, etc.

Method of Preparation

These preparations are made up of *kasaya* or other liquids, jaggery or sugar or sugar candy, powders or pulps of certain drugs, ghee or oil and honey. Jaggery, sugar or sugar candy is dissolved in the liquid, strained to remove the foreign particles and boiled over a moderate fire. After the *paka* is ready or in other words, when it sinks in water without getting easily dissolved, it is removed from the fire. With continuous and vigorous stirring, fine powders of drugs are added in small quantities to form a homogeneous mixture. Required amount of ghee or oil is added while the preparation is hot and mixed well. Honey is added at last when the mass is cool and mixed uniformly.

Characteristics

The *lehya* should neither be hard nor be a thick fluid. When pulp of the drugs is added and ghee or oil is present in the preparation, this can be rolled between the fingers. Growth of fungus over it or fermentation is, among others, signs of deterioration. When metals are mentioned, the *bhasmas* of the metals are used. In the case of drugs like *bhallataka*, purified drugs alone are included in the preparation. The colour and smell depend on the drugs used.

Preservation and Storage

The *lehya* should be kept in glass or porcelain jars. It can also be kept in a metal container which does not react with it. Normally, *lehyas* should be used within one year.

Examples: *Asvagandhadi lehya, kantakaryavaleha, kalyanaka guda*.

27.6. TAILA

Definition

Tailas are preparations in which *tail* (fixed oil) is boiled with prescribed *kasayas* (decoction) and *kalkas* (pastes) of drugs according to the formula. The process of manufacturing of *taila* ensures the absorption of therapeutically active constituents of the ingredients used in the formula.

Method of Preparation

The *kalkas* (fine paste of drug(s)), the *drava* (liquid juice or decoction) and *sneha* (oil) are added and mixed together. It is boiled and stirred continuously to prevent the adherence of *kalka* to the vessel. When the *taila* is cooked properly, foam appears on the surface of the oil. The cooked material is strained properly and packed in well-closed bottles. Salts can be added only after the preparation is strained and mixed properly.

Characteristics

Taila will generally have the colour, odour and taste of the drugs used and have the consistency of the oil. When considerable quantity of milk is used in the preparation, the oil becomes thick due to *ghrta* and in cold season may condense further.

Preservation

Tailas are preserved in glass, polythene or aluminium containers. Preparations for internal use keep their potency for about 16 months.

Examples: *Narayana taila, bhringaraja taila*, etc.

27.7. CHURNA

Definition

Churna is a fine powder of drug or drugs.

Method of Preparation

Drugs mentioned in the yoga are cleaned and dried properly. They are finely powdered and sieved. Where there are a number of drugs in yoga, the drugs are separately powdered and sieved. Each one of them (powder) is weighed separately, and well mixed together. As some of the drugs contain more fibrous matter than others, this method of powdering and weighing them separately, according to the yoga, and then mixing them together, is preferred.

In industry, however, all the drugs are cleaned, dried and powdered together by disintegrators. Mechanical sifters are also used. Salt, sugar, camphor, etc., when mentioned are separately powdered and mixed with the rest at the end. Asafoetida (*hingu*) and salt may also be roasted, powdered and then added. Drugs like *satavari, guduci*, etc., which are to be taken fresh, is made into a paste, dried and then added.

Characteristics and Preservation

The powder is fine of at least 80 mesh sieve. It should not adhere together or become moist. The finer the powder, the better its therapeutic value. They retain potency for one year and should be kept in airtight containers.

Examples: *Triphla churna, sitopaladi churna*, etc.

27.8. LEPA

Definition

Medicinal preparations in the form of a paste used for external application are called *lepas*.

Method of Preparation

The drugs are made into a fine powder and it is mixed with some liquid or other medium, according to the requirement of the preparations and made into a soft paste. The commonly used media for mixing are water, cow's urine, oil and ghee.

Characteristics and Preservation

They are stored in airtight containers. The *lepas* prepared from vegetable powders will retain their potency for 30 days, and those prepared using mineral and metallic preparations last indefinitely.

Examples: *Sinduradi lepa, dasanga lepa*, etc.

27.9. VATI AND GUTIKA

Definition

Medicines prepared in the form of tablet or pills are known as *Vati* and *Gutika*. These are made of one or more drugs of plant, animal or mineral origin.

Method of Preparation

The drugs of plant origin are dried and made into fine powders separately. The minerals are made into *bhasma* or *sindura*, unless otherwise mentioned. In cases where *parada* and *gandhaka* are mentioned, *kajjali* is made first and other drugs are added, one by one according to the formula. These are put into a *khalva* and ground to a soft paste with the prescribed fluids. When more than one liquid is mentioned for grinding, they are used in succession. When the mass is properly ground and is in a condition to be made into pills, *sugandha dravyas*, like *kasturi, karpura*, which are included in the formula, are added and ground again. The criterion to determine the final stage of the formulation before making pills is that it should not stick to the fingers when rolled. Pills may be dried in shade or in sun as specified in the texts. In cases where sugar or jaggery (*guda*) is mentioned, *paka* of these should be made on mild fire and removed from the oven. The powders of the ingredients are added to the paka and briskly mixed. When still warm, *vatakas* should be rolled and dried in shade.

Characteristics and Preservation

Pills and *vatis* should not lose their original colour, smell, taste and form. When sugar, salt or *ksara* is an ingredient, the pills should be kept away from moisture.

Pills made of plant drugs when kept in airtight containers can be used for two years. Pills containing minerals can be used for an indefinite period.

Examples: *Gandhaka vati, khadiradi gutika*, etc.

27.10. VARTTI, NETRABINDU AND ANJANA

Definition

Medicines used externally for the eye come under category of *Vartti, netrabindu* and *anjana*.

Method of Preparation

Vartties are made by grinding the fine powders of the drugs with the fluids in the formula to form a soft paste. This is then made into thin sticks of about 2 cm in length and dried in shade.

Netrabindu is prepared by dissolving the specified drugs in water or *kasaya* and used as eye drop.

Anjanas are very fine semisolids of drugs to be applied with *netra salaka*.

Characteristics and Preservation

Colour and smell depend on the drugs used. These can be preserved for one year if kept in airtight container. In case of formulations in which minerals are used, the drugs are preserved indefinitely.

Examples: *Danta vartti, nalikeranjana*, etc.

27.11. BHASMA

Definition

Bhasmas are the powdered forms of a substance obtained by calcination. It is applied to the metals, mineral and animal products which are prepared by two special processes, *Shodhana* and *Marana* in closed crucibles in pits and with cow dung cakes (*puta*).

Method of Preparation

Shodhana: The process of purification is called *shodhana* in ayurveda. The process of purification is of different types, which depends upon the type of drugs used. The first one is *Samanya shodhana* and the second is *Visesa shodhana*, the first is applicable to a large number of metals or minerals by heating the thin sheets of the metals and immersing them in *gomutra, taila, takra*, etc., for removing toxicity—the latter is applicable only to certain drugs and in certain preparations.

Marana: This stage is regarding the preparation of *bhasma*. The drug that is purified by *shodhana* process is ground with juices of the specified plants or decoction of drugs mentioned for a particular mineral or metal in a *khalva* (mortar and pestle). After the specified period of time, small cakes (*cakrikas*) are made and dried well under sunlight. The dried cakes are kept on a shallow earthen plate in single and closed with another plate. The edge of the plates are wound with clay-smeared cloth in seven consecutive layers and dried. The closed earthen container is kept in a pit half filled with cow dung. After keeping inside the pit the remaining portion of the pit is filled with cow dung cakes, and fire is put on all the sides. Once the burning is over, it is allowed to cool and the earthen container is removed. The contents of the earthen container is taken out and ground into a fine powder in a *khalva*. The process of *marana* is repeated as many times as prescribed in the procedure. The fine powders are packed in airtight glass or earthen containers.

Bhasmas are yellowish, black, white, grey, reddish black and red coloured powders and do not have any characteristic taste. They are stable preparations and maintain their potency for indefinite period.

Examples: *Svarna bhasma, tamra bhasma*, etc.

27.12. SATTVA

Definition

Sattva is water extractable solid substance collected from a drug.

Method of Preparation

The drug is cut into small pieces, macerated in water and kept overnight. Then it is strained through cloth, and the solid matter is allowed to settle. The supernatant liquid is decanted and the *sattva* is washed by repeating the process by adding water and decanted.

Preservation and Characteristics

This can be preserved in a closed container. The colour varies from drug to drug.

Example: *Guduchi sattva*.

27.13. GUGGULU

Definition

Guggulu is an exudate (*niryasa*) obtained from the plant *Commiphora mukul*. Preparations having the exudates as main effective ingredient are known as *guggulu*. There are five different varieties of *guggulu* described in the texts. However, two of the varieties, namely *mahisaksa* and *kanaka guggulu* are usually preferred for medicinal preparations. *Mahisaksa guggulu* is dark greenish brown and *kanaka guggulu* is yellowish brown in colour.

Process of *Shodhana*

1. Sand stone, glass, etc., are first removed
2. Then broken into small pieces
3. Thereafter it is bundled in a piece of the cloth and boiled in *dola yantra* containing any one of the following fluids:

    (a) *Gomutra*
    (b) *Triphalakasaya*
    (c) *Vasapatra kasaya*
    (d) *Vasapatra svarasa*
    (e) *Nirgundi patra svarasa* with *haridra churna*
    (f) *Dugdha*

The boiling is continued till the *guggulu* becomes a soft mass. It is then taken out of the cloth and spread over a smooth wooden board smeared with ghee or oil.

By pressing with fingers the sand and other remaining foreign impurities are removed. It is taken out and again fried with ghee and ground in a stone mortar (*khalva*). This is called *sodhita guggulu*.

The other method is to suspend the bundle of *guggulu* in *dola yantra* so as to remain immersed in the specified fluid as it is boiled. The boiling of *guggulu* in *dola yantra* is carried until all the *guggulu* passes into the fluid through the cloth. The residue in the bundle is discarded. The fluid is filtered and again boiled till it forms a mass. This mass is dried in sunlight and then pounded with a pestle in a stone mortar, adding ghee in small quantities till it becomes waxy.

Characteristics

Sodhita guggulu is soft, waxy and brown in colour. Characteristics of preparations of *guggulu* vary depending on the other ingredients added to the preparations.

Preservation and Storage

It should be kept in glass or porcelain jars free from moisture and stored in a cool place. The potency is maintained for two years when prepared with ingredients of plant origin, and indefinitely when prepared with metals and minerals.

Examples: *Triphala guggulu, yogaraja guggulu, laksa guggulu,* etc.

27.14. KVATHA CHURNA

Definition

Certain drugs or combination of drugs are made into coarse powder (*javkut*) and kept for preparation of *kasaya*. Such powders are called *kvatha churna*.

Method of Preparation

Drugs are cleaned and dried. They are coarsely powdered (*javkut*), weighed as per formula and then mixed well.

Characteristics and Preservation

Kvatha churnas retain potency for one year and should be kept in an airtight container. They are also called *srta, niryuha* and *kasaya. Kvatha churna* can be used for preparing *kasaya, hima, phanta,* etc.

Examples: *Amrtottara kvatha churna, ardhabilva kvatha churna,* etc.

27.15. STANDARDIZATION OF AYURVEDIC PREPARATIONS

Ayurvedic medicines are manufactured under different pharmaceutical process to result in various dosage forms, such as extracts, tinctures, decoctions, pills, powders, tablets, capsules and semisolid pastes, jellies, syrups, etc. The general standardization protocols to determine the percentage of active medicaments could not be followed for ayurvedic herbal preparations. The procedures have to be modified in order to make the preparation safe. This is because of few reasons like:

1. Ayurvedic preparations are polyherbal or herbomineral preparations.
2. Even a single herb used in the preparation contains multiple constituents.
3. Bioactive chemical constituents are not known in the herbal preparations, and even if it is known and compared with a marker, it does not necessarily reflect its connection with biological effects.
4. The principle of holistic approach does not permit assaying a single marker.

So the approach has to be made from raw materials to finished products for the successful out come.

Raw Material Standardization

- *Collection:* Plants should be collected when their active principles are maximum.
- *Botanical identity:* Plants should be identified by botanist/taxonomist to distinguish from its related species.
- *Identification of adulterants and substitutes:* Quantitative microscopy, macroscopic and microscopic characters.
- *Analytical data:* (1) Ash values, (2) Solubility profiles, (3) Extractives values, (4) Loss on drying, (5) Acid values, (6) Saponification values and (7) Foreign matter.
- *Chemical identity tests:* Tests for chemical constituents like alkaloids, glycosides, saponins, tannins, etc.
- *Instrumental analysis:* Main active constituents are quantified using chromatographic techniques and spectrophotometric methods.
- *Pesticide/herbicide residues:* Check whether these remedies are well within the limits.
- *Absence of mycotoxins or aflatoxins:* These toxins should be absent.
- Efficacy and toxicity testing.

Standardization of Manufacturing Process

Next to the raw material standardization the manufacturing process should be taken into considerations. Various process evaluation parameters in general are as follows:

For liquid/extractive formulations

1. Solvent blend composition
2. Ratio of crude drug to solvent
3. Temperature
4. Length of time of extraction
5. Method of collection of extractives
6. Method of concentration
7. Light sensitivity during processing
8. Storage conditions, precautions during processing

For solid dosage formulation (powders, pills, capsules, tablets, etc.)

1. Particle size distribution of drugs
2. Blending order and time of blending
3. Granulating fluid, binder concentration, granulating time
4. Drying temperature and time
5. Moisture content
6. Tablet hardness
7. Tablet characters, such as disintegration, friability, etc.
8. Tablet weight and thickness control
9. Spray rate of film coating solution

Semisolid formulations

1. Solvent blend composition

2. Extraction process parameters, such as amount of solvent, temperature, length of time, method of collection of extractives, etc.
3. Method of concentration
4. Semisolid blending time
5. Blend homogeneity
6. Viscosity/rheological characters
7. Light sensitivity, storage and other precautions during processing

Finished products standardization

1. *Organoleptic properties:* Colour, odour, taste and touch
2. *Physical characteristics:* Viscosity, particle size, specific gravity, refractive index, etc.
3. *Chemical characteristics:* pH, chemical tests/chemical identity/assay
4. *Biological characteristics:* Efficacy and toxicity tests
5. *Microbiological parameters:* Total viable count, yeast and mould counts, tests for the absence of pathogenic microorganisms
6. *Stability testing:* To define shelf life of the product
7. Storage condition
8. Packaging systems/unit

Marine Pharmacognosy

CONTENTS

28.1. INTRODUCTION

Marine pharmacognosy is a subbranch of pharmacognosy, which is mainly concerned with the naturally occurring substances of medicinal value from marine source. It is not a new area for pharmacognosy; even the early civilizations of Greece, Japan, China and India have explored marine life as a source of drugs. In the western medicine agar, alginic acid, carrageenan, protamine sulphate, spermaceti, and cod and halibut liver oils are the established marine medicinal products.

The oceans cover more than 70% of the earth's surface and contain over 200,000 invertebrates and algal species.

Macroalgae or seaweeds have been used as crude drugs in the treatment of iodine deficiency states such as goitre, etc. Some seaweed have also been utilized as sources of additional vitamins and in the treatment of anaemia during pregnancy. Marine products have also been used for the treatment of various intestinal disorders as vermifuges, hypochloesterolaemic and hypoglycemic agent, e.g. *Cystoseria barbata*, *Sargassum confusam* and *Jania rubens*.

Seaweeds have also been employed as dressing materials, ointments and in gynaecology. For example, *Porphyra atropurpurea* have been used in Hawaii to dress wounds and burns; *Durvillaea antarctica* to treat scabies in New Zealand. Prepared, sterilized stripes of *Laminaria digitala* in conjunction with prostaglandins have been used to dilate the cervix, as the strips swell up to several times to their original diameter when moistened.

During the last 30–40 years numerous novel compounds have been isolated from marine organisms having biological activities such as antibacterial, antiviral, antitumour, antiparasitic, anticoagulants, antimicrobial, anti-inflammatory and cardiovascular active products.

Marine flora and fauna play a significant role as a source of new molecular entity. The oceans of the world contain over five million species in about 30 phyla. Because of the diversities of marine organism and habitats, marine natural products enclose a wide variety of chemical classes, including terpenes, shikimates, polyketides, acetogenins, peptides, alkaloids of varying structures and a multitude of compounds of mixed biosynthesis.

While terrestrial sources have yielded numerous drugs, marine natural products represent a relatively untapped resource for new drug development. The marine environment may contain over 80% of the world's plant and animal species. During the past 30–40 years, numerous novel compounds have been isolated from marine organisms and many of these have been reported to have biological activities, some of which are of interest from the point of view of potential drug development. On the other hand, some of the compounds pose potential risk to human health. In this latter category are the paralytic or diarrhoetic and amnesic shellfish toxins. The former can be fatal, but the latter, although producing very unpleasant effects, are not fatal. Both paralytic and diarrhoetic shellfish toxins are produced by dinoflagellates, while amnesic shellfish, poisoning result from the ingestion of shellfish contaminated with diatoms. The ingestion of other marine organisms, which can also lead to serious poisoning, include the potent neurotoxin, tetrodotoxin, resulting from eating pufferfish and ciguatoxin, associated with ingestion of tropical fish which have fed on the dinoflagellate, *Gambierdiscus toxicus*.

28.2. MARINE ORGANISMS AS POTENTIAL SOURCE OF DRUGS

Knowledge of biological activities and/or chemical constituents of marine organisms is important not only for the discovery of new therapeutic agents but such information may also be of immense value in exploring, new sources of economic materials, precursors for the synthesis of complex chemical substances and compounds of novel chemical structure, thereby prompting the chemist for the synthesis of a series of modified compounds of therapeutically importance. Thus, in recent years, considerable importance is attached to the discovery of new biodynamic agents from marine source to search new source of drugs from sea.

A survey of literature indicated that extracts from marine organisms had been evaluated for various biological activities. This has led to the isolation of substances possessing antimicrobial, antibiotic, antiviral, anticancer, cardioactive, anti-inflammatory, anthelmintic, anticoagulant neurophysiological and insecticidal activities.

Although numerous compounds have been isolated from marine organisms and the biological activities attributed to too many of them, still very few of them have been marketed or are under development. There are number of reasons that are why more number of compounds originating from marine plants and animals has not been developed. There is no doubt that much of the work undertaken in the 1960s, 1970s and probably the early 1980s was driven by an interest in the chemistry of new compounds rather than in their biological activities. The earlier studies on chemistry of marine natural products were limited to the isolation, structure elucidation and phylogenetic relationship of specific substances, such as quinonoid pigments and sterols. Now this field attracted the attention of not only the natural product chemists but also those of marine biologist, biochemist, pharmacologist, etc. The invention of the aqualung and the advent of new technology in the past few decades led to the awareness that the oceans may be a new frontier of biomedical research, as it has vast resources for the discovery of marine-derived medicine. Increasing sophistication of the tools available to explore the deep sea has expanded the habitats, which can be sampled and has greatly improved the opportunities for discovery of novel metabolites.

Much of the earlier work limited the biological testing to antimicrobial activity, but this was often extended later to testing for cytotoxic properties, which may provide useful leads for anticancer drugs. This latter area is one that most of the compounds in various stages of clinical trials are located. Screening for other activities has, of course, also been undertaken, for example, for antiviral, anti-inflammatory, anticoagulant, antiparasitic and prostaglandins.

Many of the marine compounds have shown promising biological properties but have complicated chemical structures, the synthesis of which would be hard and expensive. These organisms are valuable as source of new biologically active chemical structures, but unless either the compounds or a derivative of them can be readily synthesized, they are of little commercial interest to the pharmaceutical industry.

28.3. ANTIVIRAL AGENTS

Ara-A

Ara-A is a semisynthetic antiviral agent based on the arabinosyl nucleoside isolated from the marine sponge *Tethya crypta*. The compound shows a prominent therapeutic activity.

Eudistomins

Eudistomins are the β-caboline derivatives which are isolated from sponges and gorgonians *Eudistoma olivaceum*, family Polycitoridae. These compounds are also found in tunicates. Eudistomin compounds can be classified into four groups, i.e. pyrrolyl substituted, pyrrolinyl-substituted, unsubstituted and tetrahydro-β-carboline derivatives with a 1,3,7-oxathiazepine ring.

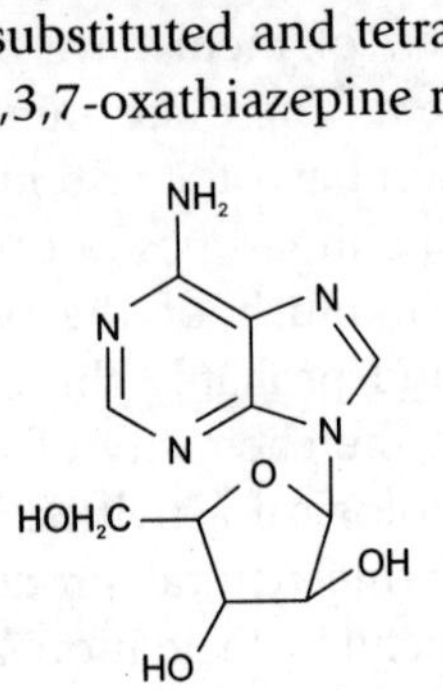

Ara-A

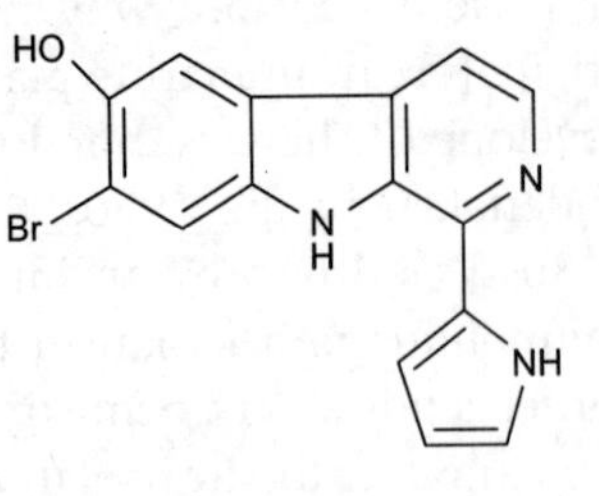

Eudistomin A

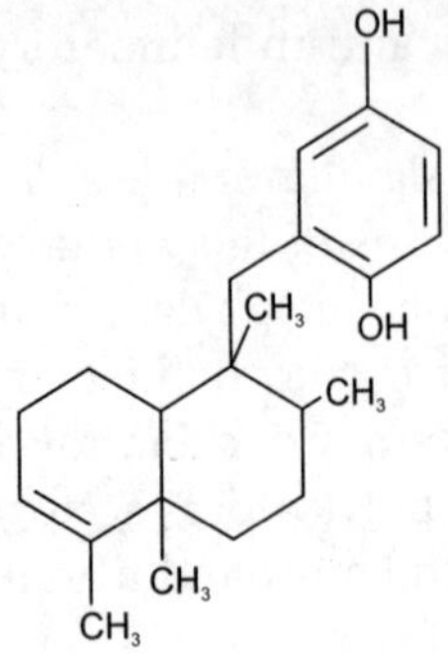

Avarol

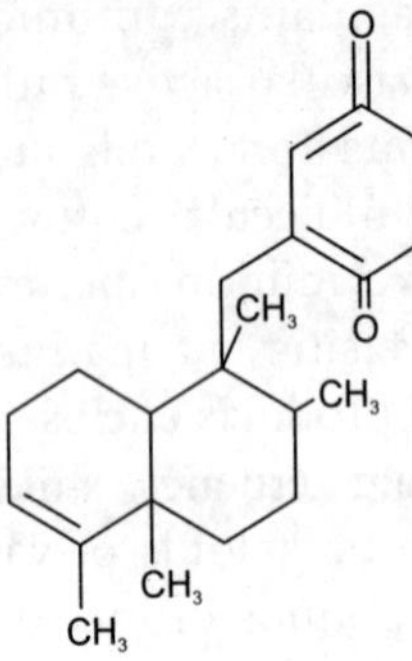

Avarone

Didemnins

Didemnin compounds are the promising antiviral and antitumour agents isolated from *Trididemnum* spp. family Didemnidae. A compound Didemnin B is found to be a potential antitumour agent during its clinical trials.

Avarol and Avarones

These two sesquiterpene benzenoids are derived from the sponge *Disidea avara*. It has exhibited strong anti-HIV activity against the human immunodeficiency virus (HIV). It shows the greater promises in the treatment of AIDS.

Patellazole B

Patellazole B is a complex derivative isolated from the ascidian *Lissoclinum patella*. It has shown the potent activity against *Herpes simplex* virus.

Fucoidan

Fucoidan, a sulphated polysaccharide compound extracted from brown algae *Laminaria* has shown the activity against HIV and *Herpes simplex* viruses.

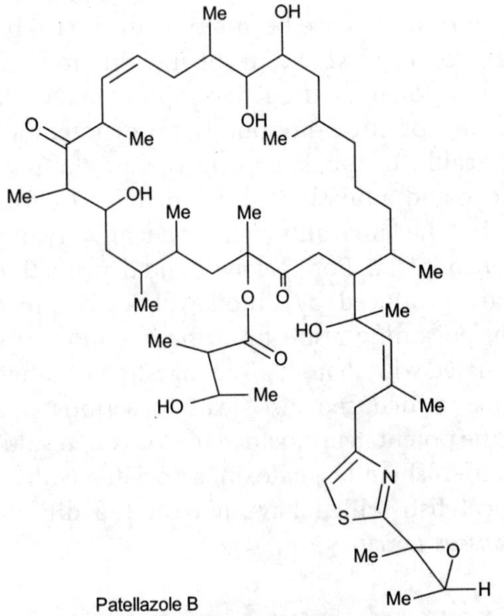

Patellazole B

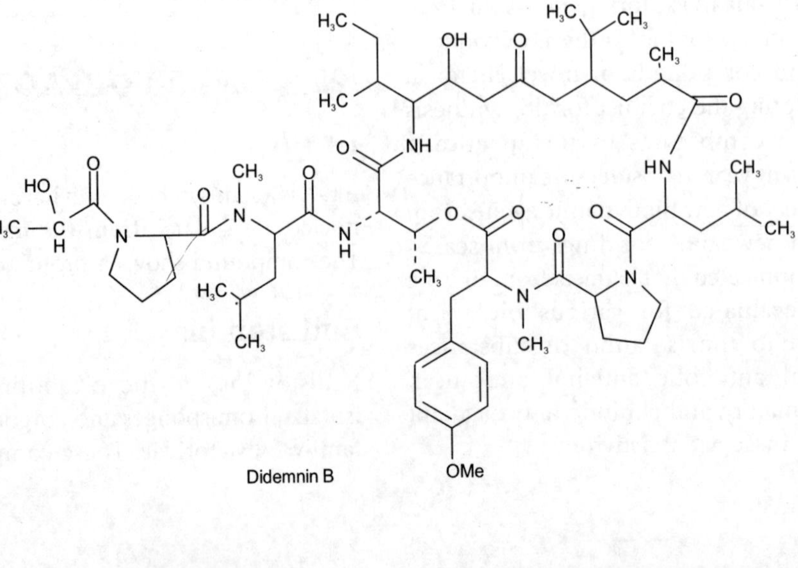

Didemnin B

Antimicrobial Agents

Verongia fistularis
V. cauliformis
V. thiona
(Marine sponges)

3,5-Dibromo-1-hydroxy-4-oxo-2,5-cyclohexadiene-1-acetamide

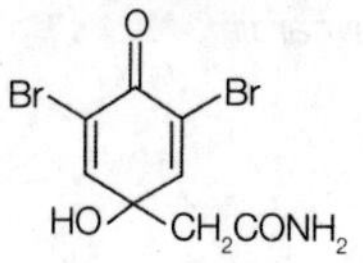

V. aerophoba
(Marine sponge)

(-) Aeroplysinin-1

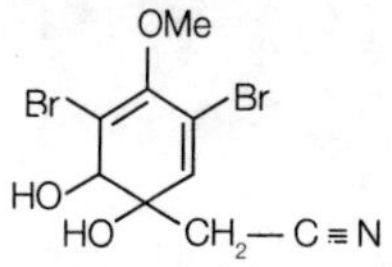

V. archeri
(Marine sponge)

2,4-Dibromo-3,6-dehydrobenzen-1-acetamide

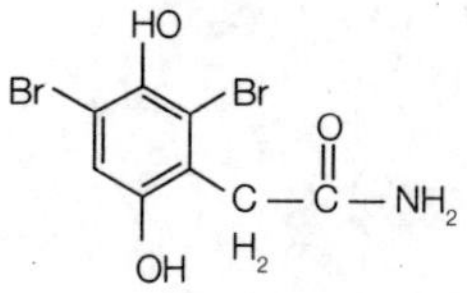

Agelas oroids
(Marine sponge)

2-Cyano-4,5-dibromopyrrole

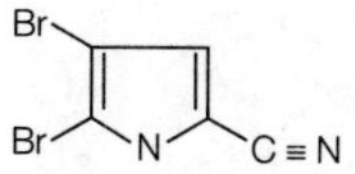

Phakellia flabellate
(Marine sponge)

Bromophakellin

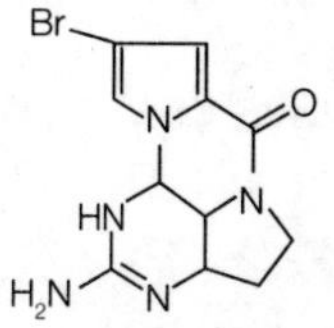

Laurencia johnstonii
(Red algae)

Laurinterol

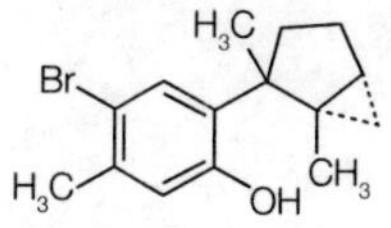

Ptilonia australasica
(Red algae)

Bromopyrones

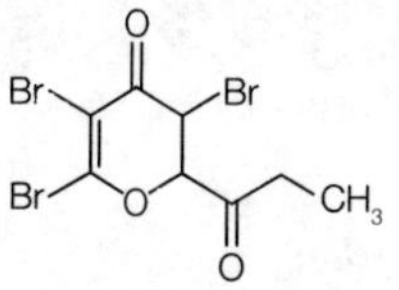

Delisea fimbriata
(Red algae)

Fimbrolide

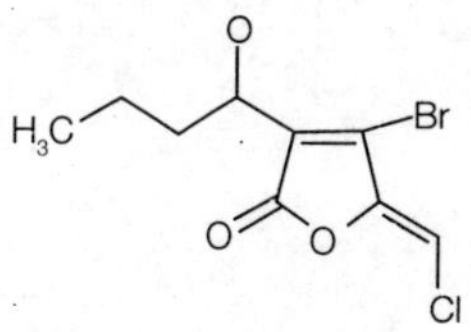

Condria californica
(Red algae)

1,2,3,5,6-Pentathiepane

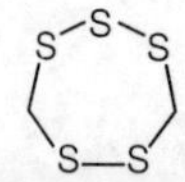

Antibacterial Agents

Acanthella acuta
(Marine sponge)

Acanthellin-1

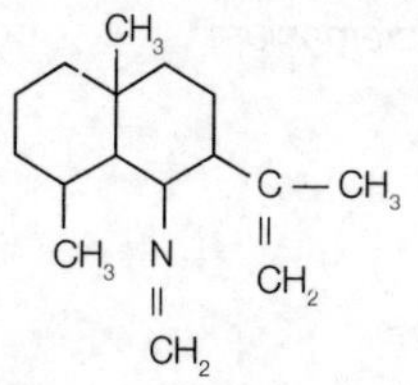

Ircinia strobilina
(Marine sponge)

Ircinin-1

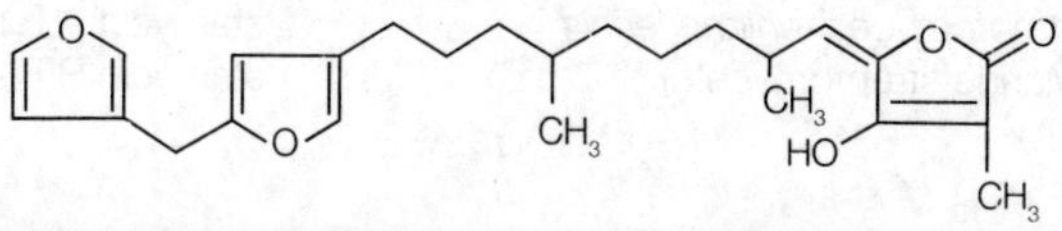

Polyfibrospongia maynardii
(Marine sponge)

5,6-Dibromo-1-H-Indole-3-ethanamine

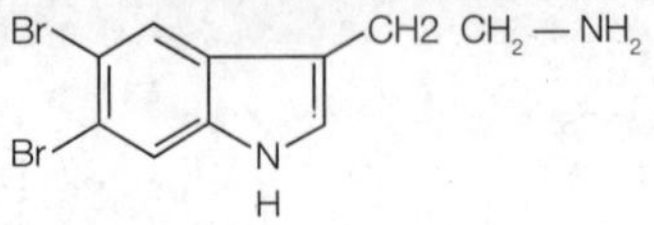

Spongia officinalis
(Marine sponge)

Furospongin

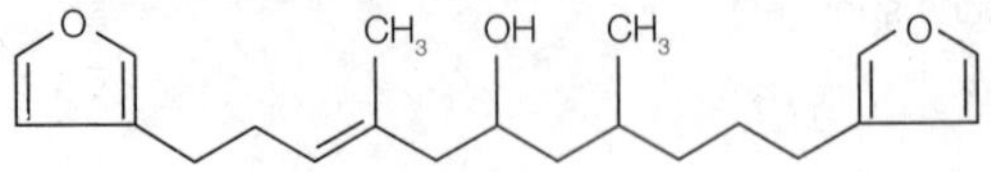

L. filiformis
(Red algae)

Chondriol

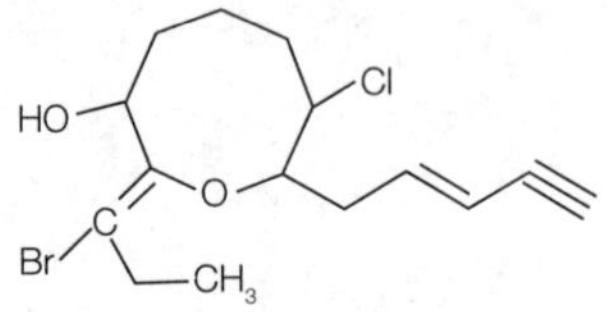

Laurencia johnstonii
(Red algae)

Prepacifenol

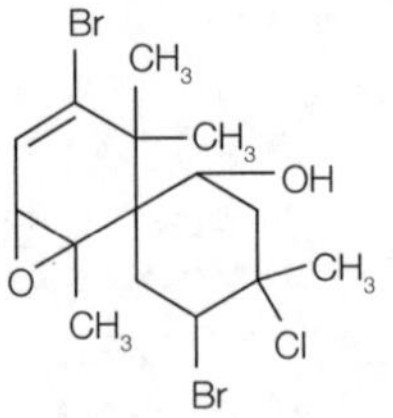

Antiprotozoal Agents

Eunicea mammosa

Eunicin

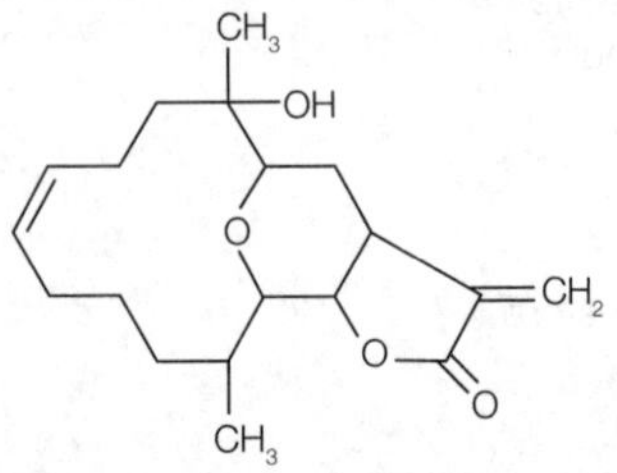

Antifungal Agents

Dictyopteris zonoroid
(Brown algae)

Zonorol, isozonorol

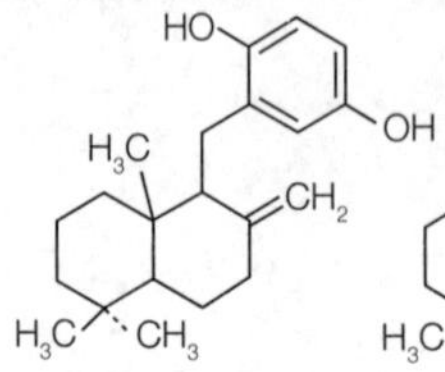

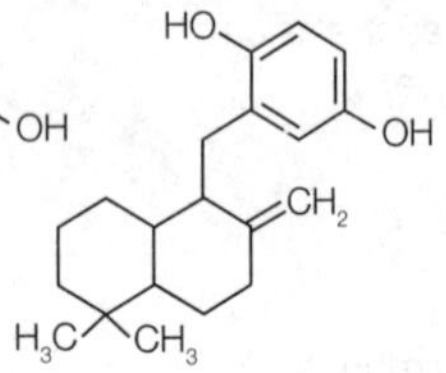

Thelepus setosus
(Annelida)

Thelpin

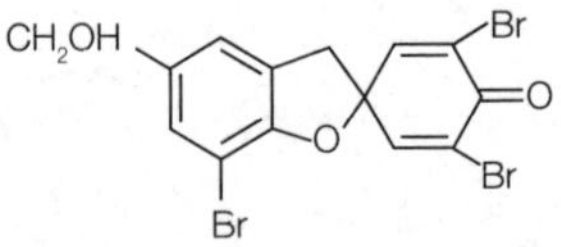

Antibiotics

Cephalosporium acremonium
(Marine fungus)

Cephalosporin-C

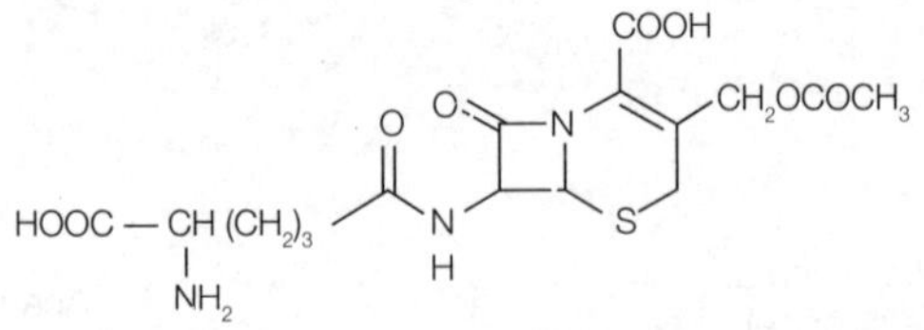

Streptomyces tenjimariensis
(Marine streptomycets)

Istamycin A R1 = H, R2 = NH₂
Istamycin B R1 = NH₂, R2 = H

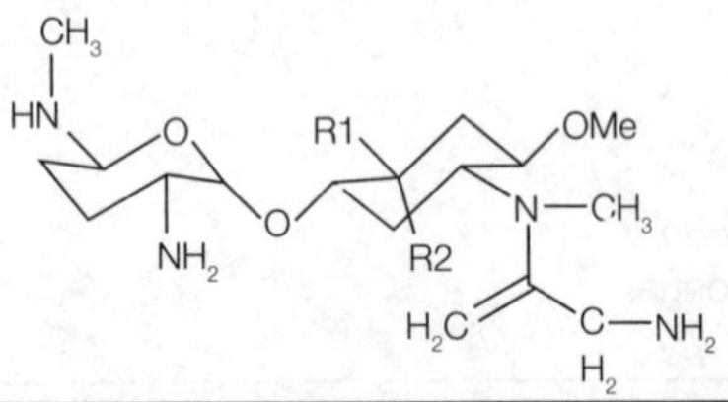

| Chondria oppositicladia (Red algae) | Cycloeudesmol | 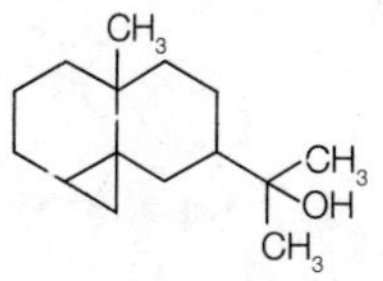 |
| Acanthella spp. (Porifera) | Kalihinol A | 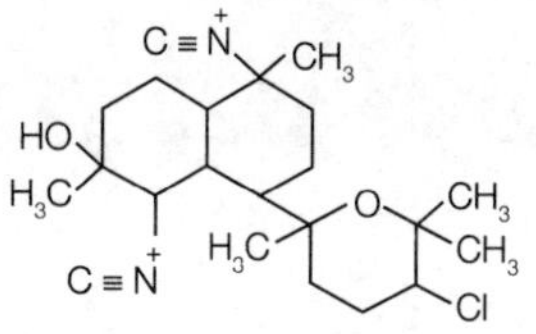 |

28.4. ANTIMICROBIAL AGENTS

A large variety of antimicrobial agents are produced by number of marine organisms, such as sponges, algae, gorgonian corals, annelids, etc., and many of them are active against gram +ve and gram –ve microorganisms, protozoal and fungal strains. Various antimicrobial, antibacterial, antifungal and antiprotozoal agents from marine sources are given below. A list of antibiotics agents derived from marine organisms have also been enumerated.

28.5. ANTIPARASITIC AGENTS

Various compounds isolated from the marine organisms have demonstrated remarkable antiparasitic activities. Some of the important agents have been listed below.

α-Kainic Acid

α-Kainic acid isolated from the red algae, *Digenea simplex* shows the broad spectrum anthelmintic activity against the parasitic round worms, tape worms and whip worms. Dried powder of *D. simplex* has been widely used for the treatment of ascariasis. A Japanese pharmaceutical company, Takeda Pharmaceuticals, produces various preparations of this drug.

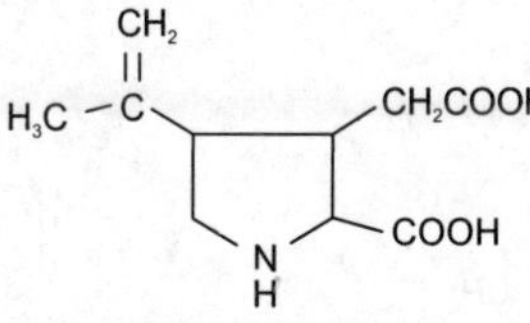

α-Kainic acid

Domoic Acid

Domoic acid is a compound chemically related to kainic acid. It has been isolated from red algae *Chondria armata* and *Alsidium corallinum*. It has shown prominent anthelmintic activities.

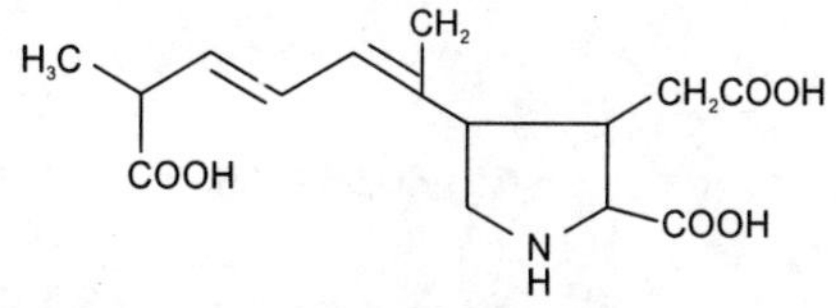

Domoic acid

Laminine

Laminine is a methylated lysine derivative found in the marine red algae of the order Laminariales as well as in brown algae. Laminarine also shows the hypotensive and smooth muscle relaxant activities, along with its potential antiparasitic activity.

$$CH_3 - N^+ - CH_2 - CH_2 - CH_2 - CH_2 - C - COO^-$$

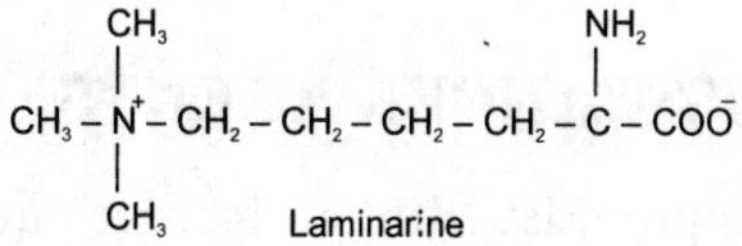

Laminarine

Bengamide F

Bengamide F is the recently isolated and characterized compound from marine sponge. It has demonstrated a remarkable antiparasitic activity during *in vitro* studies.

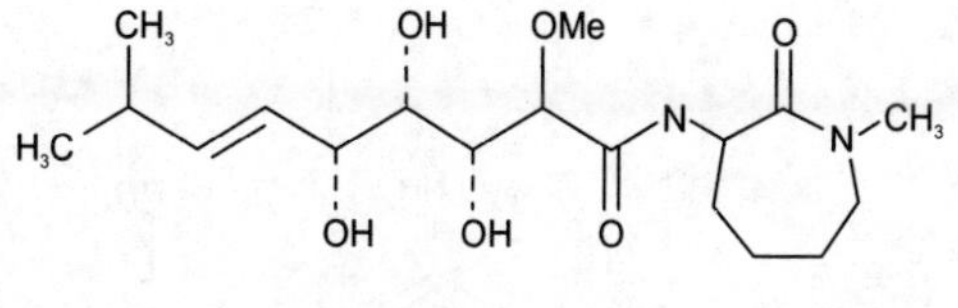

Bengamide F

Cucumechinoside F

Cucumechinoside F is a complex tetracyclic triterpenic glycoside obtained from sea cucumber. It has been reported to have a prominent antiprotozoal activity.

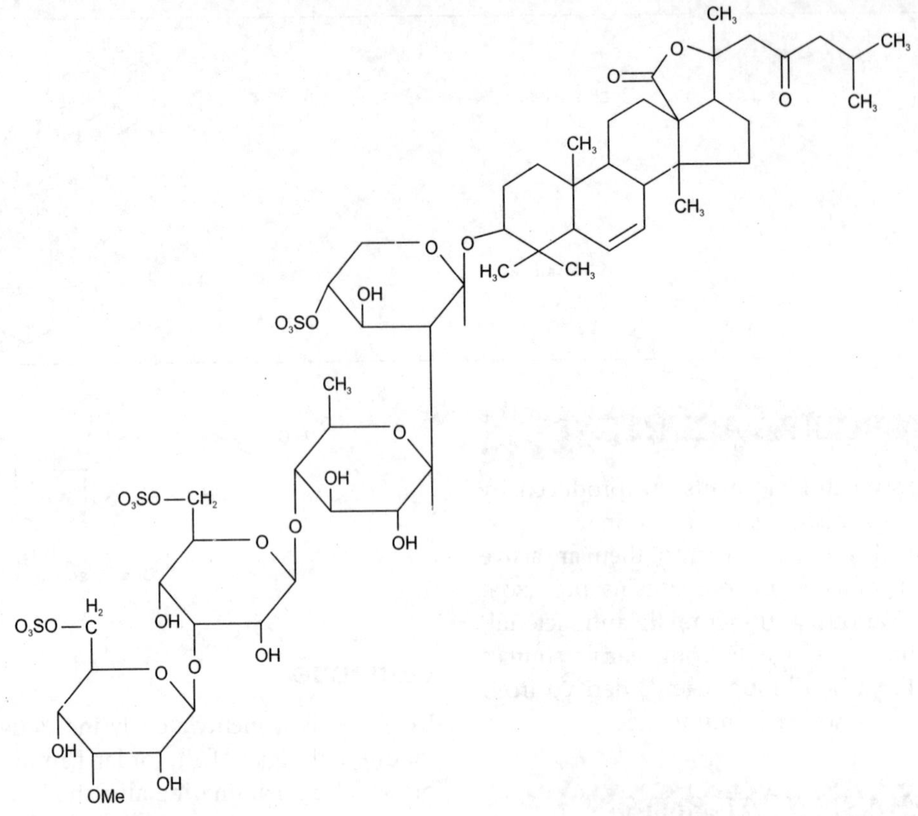

Cucumechinoside F

28.6. ANTICANCER AGENTS

Several compounds with anticancer and cytotoxic activities have been isolated and characterized from various marine organisms, such as marine sponges, gorgonian corals, sea algae, sea hares and sea cucumbers. One of the most prominent synthetic anticancer agents is cytosine arabinoside, also known as Ara-C. It originates from the natural marine substance spongothymidine isolated from Caribbean sponge (*Cryptotethya crypta*). It is marketed under the trade name Cytosar by Upjohn pharmaceutical company for the treatment of acute myelogenous leukaemia and human acute leukaemia. Ara-C is a potent inhibitor of the tumours in cases of sarcoma-180, Erlich carcinoma and L-1210 leukaemia in mice. Ara-A adenine arabinoside, another synthetic analog developed on the prototype of spongothymidine is effective for the treatment of herpes encephalitis. The other compounds isolated from the above Caribbean sponge are spongosine and spongouridine.

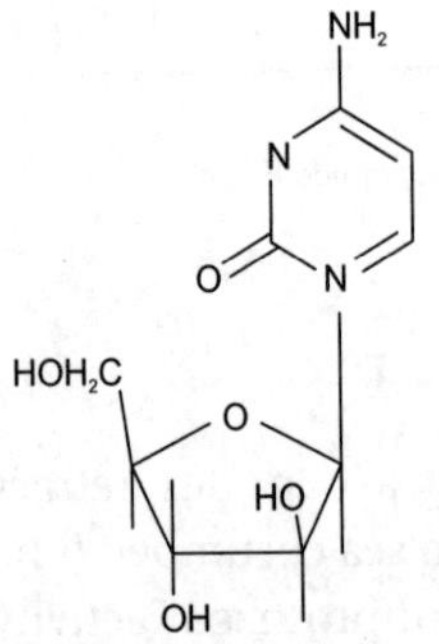

Ara-C

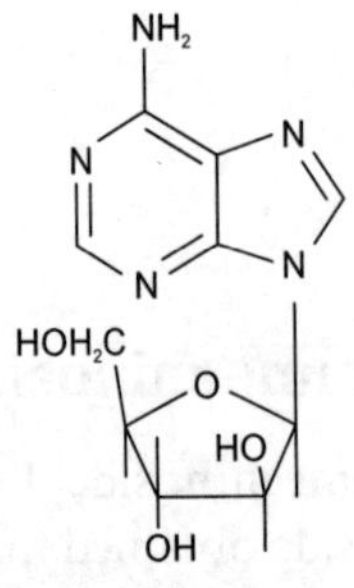

Ara-A

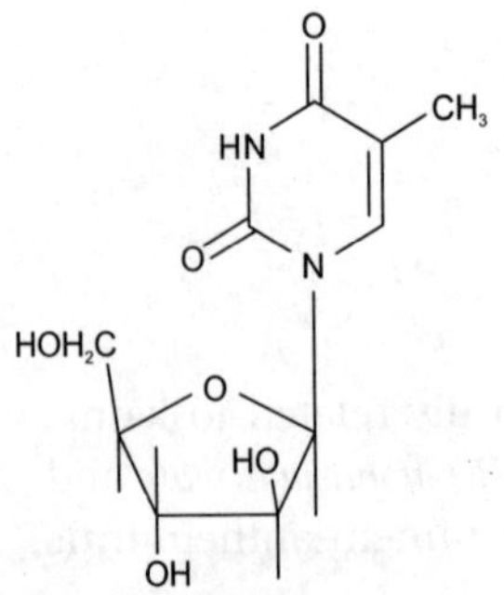

Spongothymidine

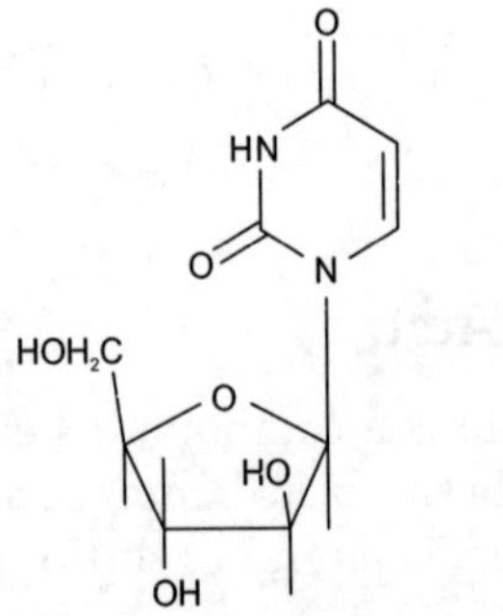

Spongouridine

Bryostatin I

Isolated from *Bugula neritina* a bryozoal marine organism showed highly potent antineoplastic activity in an extremely low dose level.

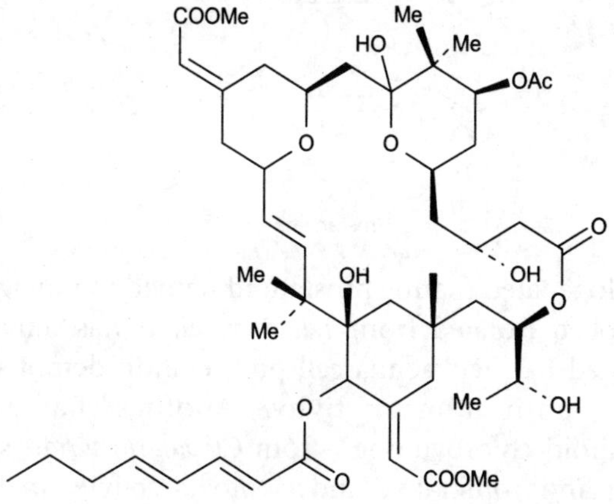

Bryostatin-I

28.7. ANTISPASMODIC AGENTS

Agelasidine A

A sesquiterpene derivative isolated from Okinawa sea sponge *Agelas* spp. has demonstrated very good antispasmodic activity in animal models. Agelasidine A is the first marine natural products containing guanine and sulfone units.

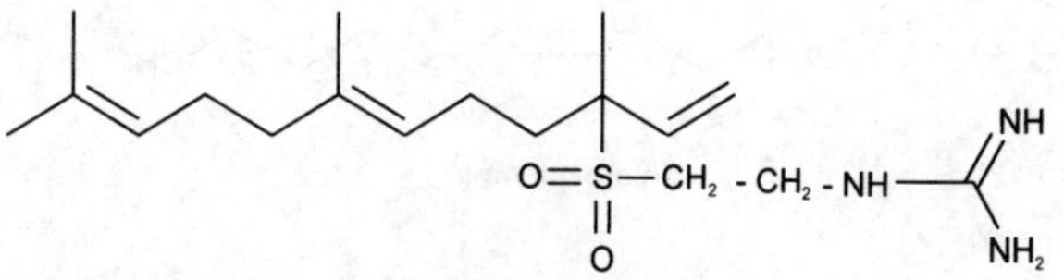

Agelasidine A

28.8. CARDIOVASCULAR AGENTS

Several cardiovascular agents have been isolated and characterized from marine organisms. Their chemical nature ranging from steroidal compounds to polypeptide of 49 amino acids residues have been isolated from the sea anemone *Anthopleura xanthogrammica*. It is a highly potent heart stimulant with about 5000 times more activity than cardiac glycosides.

Eledoisin

Eledoisin, a peptide compound has been isolated from posterior salivary glands of Cephalopod *Eledone moschata* and other related species. It has shown potent hypotensive and vasodilatory activity. It is found to be about 50 times more potent than acetyl choline, histamine or bradikinin in provoking hypotension.

OH
|
H - Pyr - Pro - Ser - Lys - Asp - Ala - Phe - Ile - Gly - Leu - Met - NH$_2$
Eledoisin

Octopamine

D(−)-Octopamine a simple phenolic derivative isolated from salivary glands of *Octopus vulgaris*, *O. macropus* and *Eledone moschata* has shown remarkable cardiotonic activity.

A toxic compound tetramine isolated from the salivary glands of *Neptunea antiqua* showed curare like effect in mammals. A basic amino acid laminine isolated from red algae *Laminaria angustata* has also shown hypotensive activity similar to that of choline.

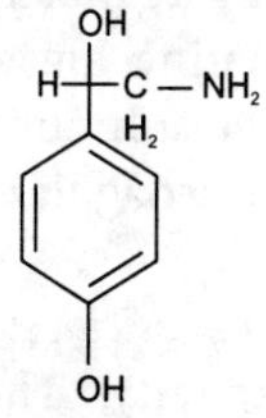

Octopamine 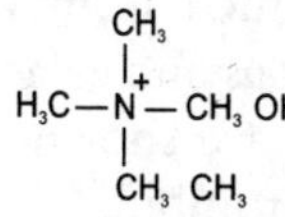   Tetramine 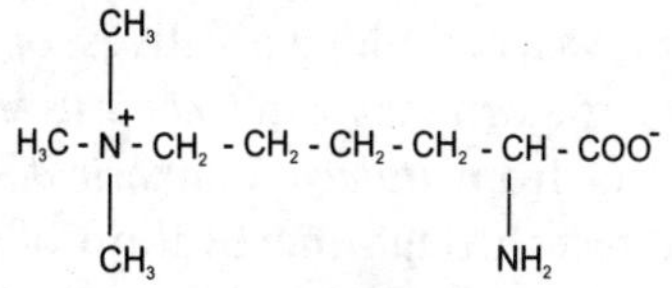   Laminine

28.9. ANTI-INFLAMMATORY AGENTS

Marine organisms have shown the presence of novel anti-inflammatory agents. A series of bio-indole derivatives isolated from marine cyanobacterium *Rivularia firma* has shown potential anti-inflammatory activity in the models of carrageenan-induced rat paw oedema. In another study, the butanolide derivatives obtained from *Euplexaura flava* have demonstrated a significant anti-inflammatory effect in a low dose of 100 µg/ml. The sulphated polysaccharide carrageenan isolated from Irish moss, *Chondrus crispus*, a red algae is used as a phlogistic agent for inducing inflammation in the rat paw oedema model for the study of anti-inflammatory activity.

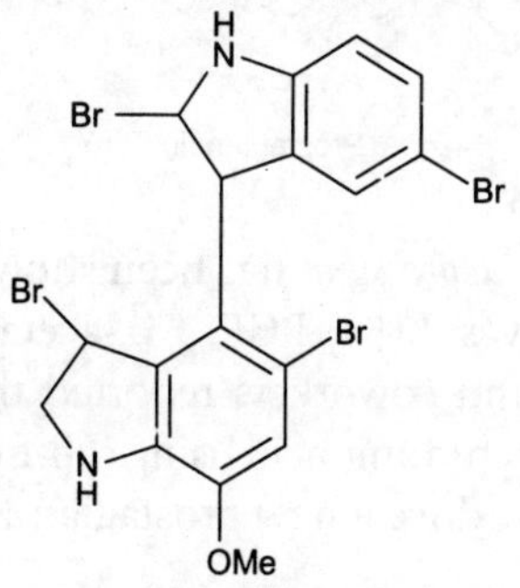

Bio-indole

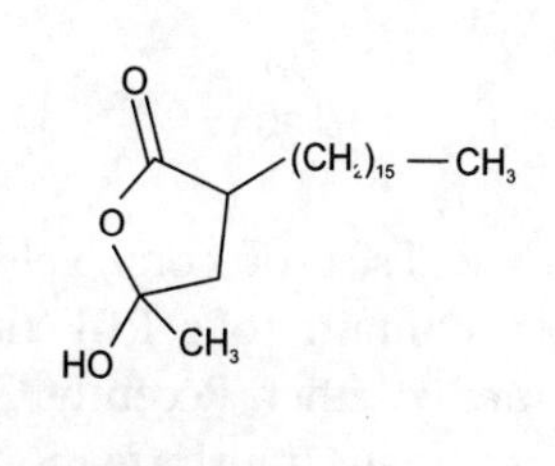

Butanolide derivative

28.10. INSECTICIDES

Nereistoxin an insecticidal compound has been isolated from the marine annelid *Lumbriconereis heteropoda*. Many semisynthetic and synthetic analogs have been produced on the structural model of nereistoxin. One of the derivative named as cartap is used as an insecticide in Japan.

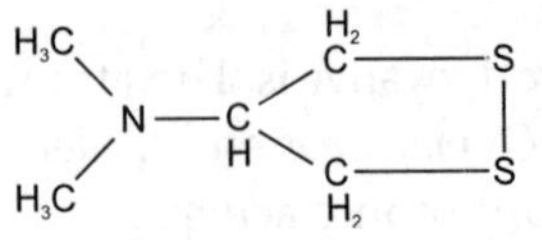

Nereistoxin 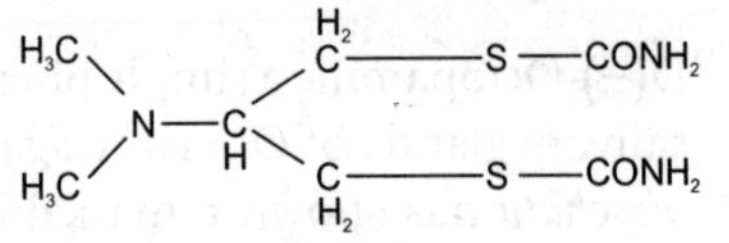   Cartap

28.11. ANTICOAGULANTS

Anticoagulants reported from the marine sources are mostly polysaccharide derivatives obtained from marine algae. Carrageenans from *Chondrus crispus* and galactan sulphuric acid from *Iridaea laminarioides* have shown anticoagulant effect through inactivation of thrombin.

Fucoidin isolated from the brown algae *Fucus vesiculosus* has shown a very good anticoagulant activity. The antithrombin effect of fucoidin is mediated through heparin cofactor II.

28.12. PROSTAGLANDINS

Prostaglandins constitute a class of natural products with variety of therapeutic activities. Varieties of these substances are found in marine algae and corals. Soft coral, *Plexaura homomalla*, is regarded as a rich source of these compounds, 15 epi-PGA$_2$ found in the form of its acetate and methyl ester derivative.

PGE$_2$ and PGF$_{2a}$ types of prostaglandins have been isolated from the red algae *Gracilaria lichenoides*. PGE$_2$ have also been derived from *G. verrucosa*.

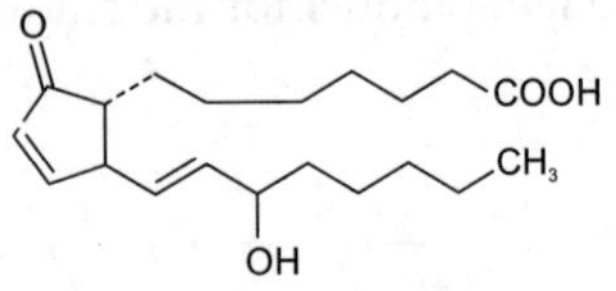

15 epi-PGA$_2$ 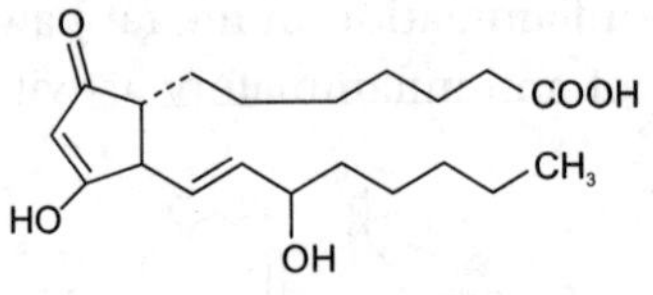   Prostaglandin E$_2$

Red sea soft coral, *Lobiphyton depressum*, has been shown to contain four PGF derivatives (15s)-PGF$_{2a}$ 11-acetate methyl ether. Recently Corey and coworkers reported the enzymatic transformation of arachidonic acid using cell-free extract of *Clavularia viridis* to produce a new prostaglandin derivative I (Prostanoide).

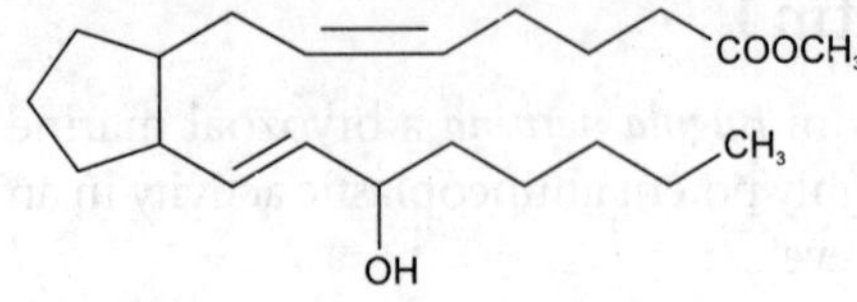

15s-PGF$_2$ 11-acetate methyl ether

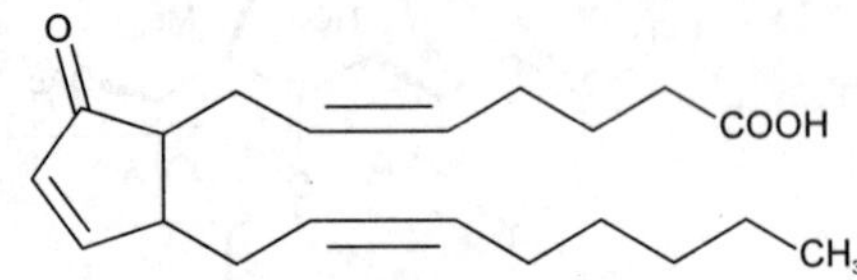

Prostanoide

Halogenated marine prostanoid named as punaglandin have been isolated from *Telesto riisei*. It has remarkably inhibited L$_{1210}$ leukaemia cell proliferation demonstrating strong antitumour activity. Another halogenated prostanoid chlorovulone I from *Clavularia viridis* showed strong antiproliferative and cytotoxic activity in human promyelocytic leukaemia (HL-60) cells.

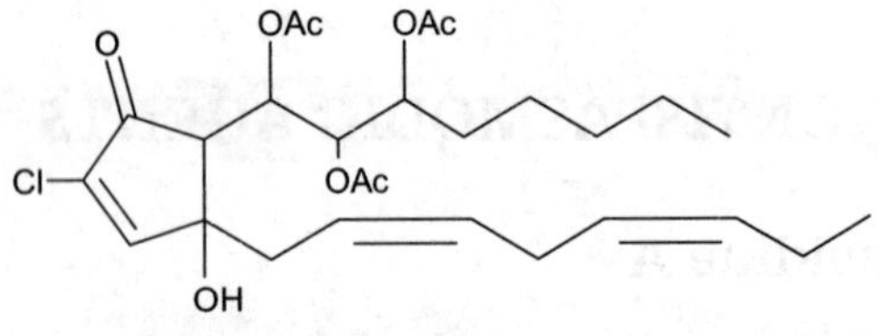

Punaglandin

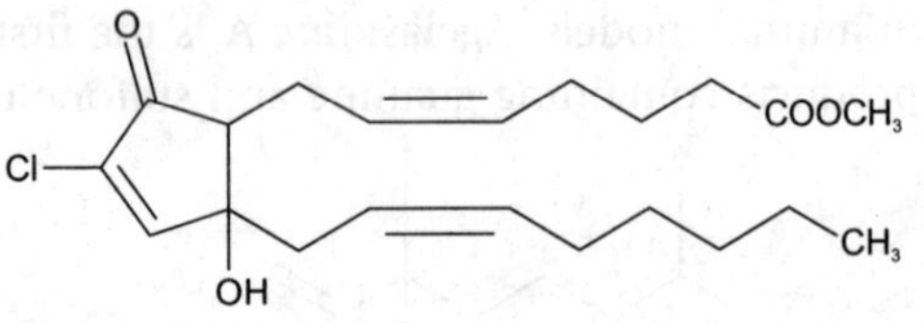

Chlorovulone-I

28.13. MARINE TOXINS

Many marine organisms produce potentially toxic compounds which may work for their safety and protect them from predators. These toxins may pose potential hazards to human health. Many of these toxins had also shown remarkable biological activities in comparatively lower doses. Some of these marine toxins are discussed below:

Tetrodotoxin

Tetrodotoxins is a potent neurotoxin produced by the pufferfish of family Tetraodontidae. It is present in other animals including *Gobius criniger*, *Taricha torosa*, *Atelopus chiriquensic* marine crabs and also produced by marine bacteria. This dangerous toxin shows the cardiovascular and neurophysiological activity in experimental animals. Tetrodotoxin containing puffer fish is considered as a delicacy in Japan, but great care is exercised to avoid the toxin during its preparation for culinary purpose.

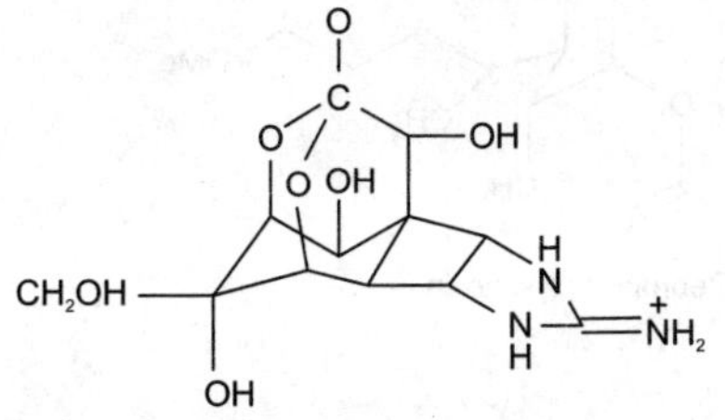

Tetrodotoxin

Saxitoxin

Saxitoxin is a purine skeleton containing toxic compound produced by the butter clam *Saxidomus giganteus* and California mussel *Mytilus californianus*. It is also found in two toxic species of mollusc, *Zolimus aeneus* and *Platypodia granulosa*. Saxitoxin is identical with toxin isolated from the dinoflagellate *Gonyaulax catenella* upon which the butter clam feeds. In lower doses this toxin produces a marked hypotensive effect.

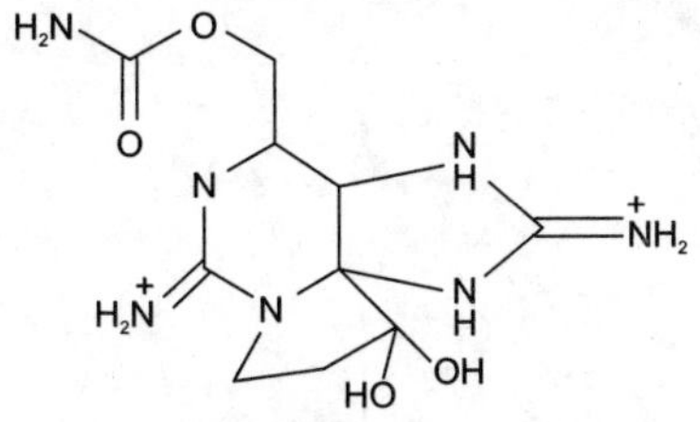

Saxitoxin

Ciguatoxin

Ciguatoxin is the poisonous compound found in the dinoflagellate *Gambierdiscus toxicus*. In many cases it is responsible for ciguatera fish poisoning associated with the utilization of tropical fish resources. Ciguatoxin shows the cardiovascular and neurophysiological properties. Another toxin, Maitotoxin, present in *G. toxicus* is found to be powerful calcium channel activator in a very low dose of pico- to nanomolar range.

Holothurin A

Holothurin A is a toxic saponin isolated from the sea cucumber of Holothurian group *Helix pomatia*. It is recognized as a mixture of triterpenic aglycones which are linked to four sugar molecules and a molecule of sulphuric acid as a sodium salt. It has shown haemolytic and neurotoxic properties.

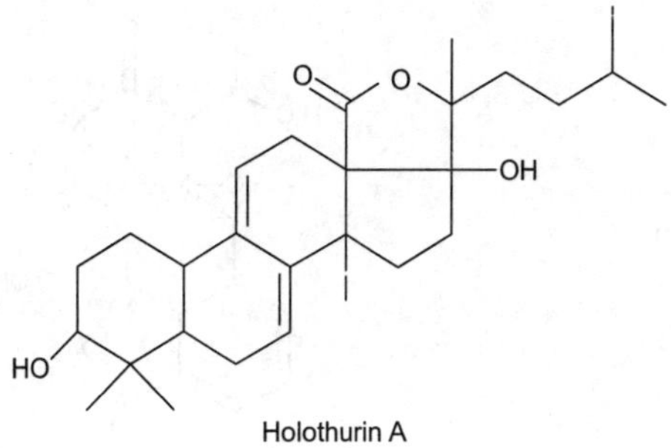

Holothurin A

Aplysins

Aplysins is a group of toxic compounds isolated from Mediterranean Sea hares *Aplysia depilans*. Aplysins contains an unpleasant, colourless fluid secreted by the skin. These are the white viscous liquid by opaline gland and purple secretion from another gland present in sea hares. Aplysins causes paralysis when injected into cold-blooded animals.

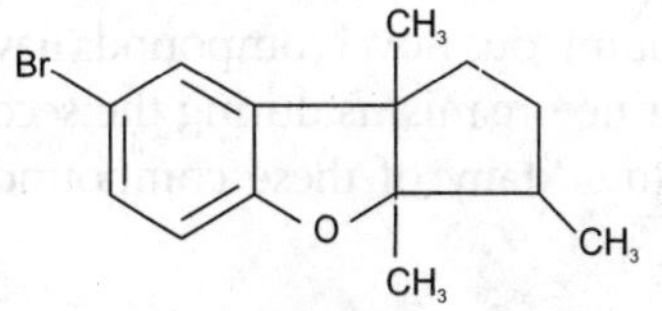

Aplysin

Lophotoxin

Lophotoxin is a diterpene lactone present in the gorgonian corals of the genus *Lophogorgia*. It produces an irreversible postsynaptic blockage at neuromuscular junction.

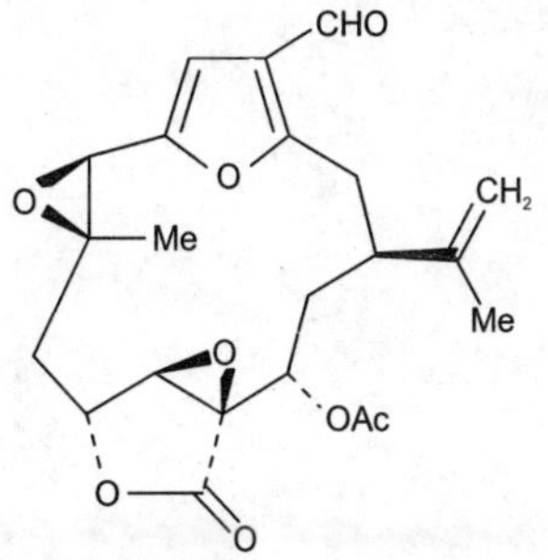

Lophotoxin

Lyngbyatoxin

Lyngbyatoxin is an indole group of alkaloid produced by the marine cyanobacterium *Lyngbya majuscula*. It is responsible for the contact dermatitis known as 'swimmer's itch' in the humans. Some other organisms of the same species *L. majuscula* have been found to produce totally unrelated skin irritant; debromoaplysiatoxin winch also demonstrates antineoplastic activity.

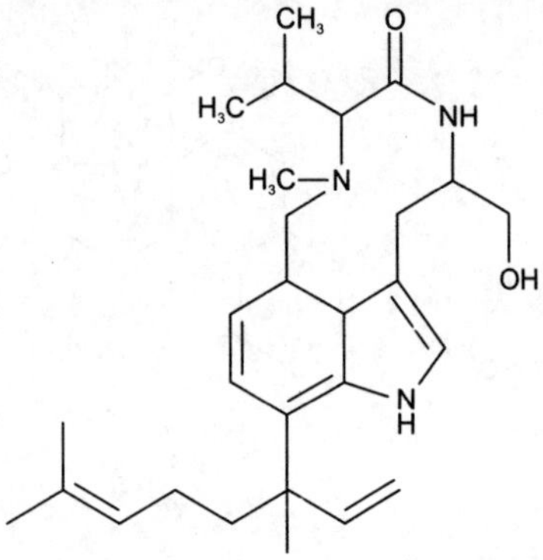

Lyngbyatoxin

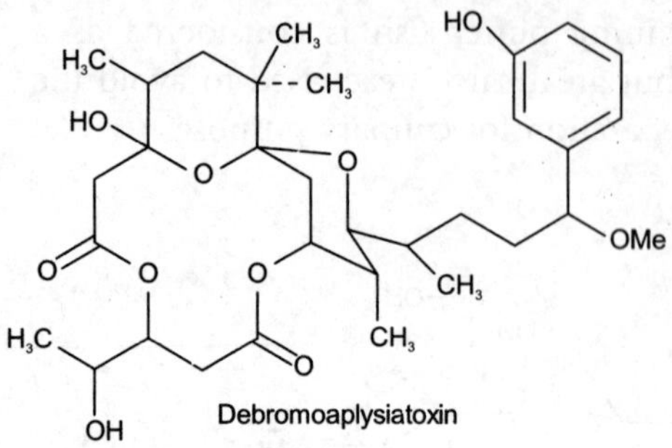

Debromoaplysiatoxin

28.14. CONCLUSION

The greater part of the earth surface is covered by seas and ocean, which contains about 500,000 species of marine organisms. Since the natural products chemists diverted their attention to exploit the vast resources of marine flora and animal world, numerous novel compounds have been isolated from these marine organisms during the second half of the twentieth century. Many of these compounds have shown pronounced biological activity. However, the compounds which have failed to show the activities for which those were assayed cannot be regarded as not having other biological activities. Many of these compounds might show some other activities if studied extensively during the course of time. Although the impact of marine natural products is presently lesser on the pharmaceutical industry, it may come forward in a big way to provide new lead compounds for the development of potential therapeutically active compounds.

Nutraceuticals and Cosmeceuticals

29.1. NUTRACEUTICALS

Food and drugs from nature plays quite a significant role in public healthcare system throughout the world. Human inquisitiveness and search for specific constituents of plant, animals, minerals and microbial origin which are beneficial to our overall health have caused coining of terminologies such as functional foods or nutraceuticals. The idea of nutraceuticals has evolved from the recognition of the link between diet and health. Nutraceuticals have caused heated debate because they blurred the traditional dividing lines between food and medicine. Dr Stephen L. Defelice defines nutraceuticals as any substance that may be considered as food or part of food which in addition to its normal nutritive value provides health benefits including prevention of disease. The American Association of Nutritional Chemists mentions nutraceuticals as the products that has been isolated or purified from food and generally sold in medicinal forms not usually associated with food. When nutraceuticals are referred to as functional foods, most of the researchers of concerned field agree that they are foods marketed as having specific health effects. Functional foods are ordinary foods that have components or ingredients incorporated in them to give them a specific medical or physiological benefit other than a purely nutritional effect.

All foods are functional in the sense that we eat it, and it provides the energy and nutrients we needed to live. As we approach towards the 21st century, nutritional science has come into its own with manufacturers and consumers, placing for more emphasis on the benefits to be derived from food. Nutraceuticals or functional foods have been found to be associated with the prevention and/or treatment of many chronic diseases and ailments, such as cancer, diabetes, heart diseases, hypertension, arthritis, osteoporosis, etc. Statistical data indicates that 35% of all cancers are related to the food that we eat and certain dietary habits have long been associated with cancer risk. It certainly makes the old saying 'you are what you eat', more relevant in the context of the health benefits of the food. As the importance of dietary changes to optimize health is gaining recognition and acceptance, the food industry is responding to consumer demand for more healthful, nutrients-rich food products. The figure of 1997 statistical data shows that the European market for functional foods was estimated at £830 million.

Classification

Nutraceuticals or functional foods can be classified on the basis of their natural sources, pharmacological conditions or as per chemical constitution of the products. On the basis of natural source, these are the products obtained from plants, animals, minerals or microbial sources.

The classification of nutraceuticals based upon its therapeutical implications for the treatment or prevention of specific condition may produce a big list. Some of the important conditions in which the nutraceuticals are specially directed for its treatment, prevention or support are given in Table 29.1.

A systematic classification on the basis of therapeutically important compounds of the nutraceuticals products responsible for the specific health benefit can be done as given in Table 29.2.

However, in many cases the health benefit is not mainly due to a single group of compounds but the overall effect of variety of proteins, lipids, carbohydrates, vitamins and mineral constitution of the product.

Inorganic mineral supplements

Large number of elements control variety of physiological and biochemical functions of human body. Most of these minerals are provided through the diet but their deficiently in diet may develop variety of health-related problems and diseases.

Calcium: Calcium is an important element in the treatment of bone loss and prevention. Calcium deficiency is found in 25% of women, even though much higher percentage has osteopenia or osteoporosis. Prepuberty is the best time to begin supplementing the diet with calcium-rich minerals along with exercise regimen. Sufficient intake of calcium and vitamin D postmenopausally can significantly reduce the risk for fracture.

Magnesium: Magnesium is an essential element involved in well over 300 enzymatic processes and critical in the proper use and maintenance of calcium. Many individuals with calcium deficiency are actually magnesium deficient which prevent proper use of calcium.

Manganese: Manganese is required in several enzymatic reactions and necessary for proper bone and cartilage formation.

Boron: Boron is reported to be helpful in supporting the calcium and oestrogen levels in postmenopausal women.

Copper: Copper is an essential element needed by all tissues in the body; copper and zinc must be in proper proportion. Copper is best absorbed when bound to an amino acid.

Zinc: Zinc is one of the most important trace mineral. Zinc supports the body's overall antioxidant system by

Table 29.1 Nutraceuticals used in various disease conditions

Conditions	Nutraceuticals
Allergy relief	*Ginkgo biloba*
Arthritis support	Glucosamine
Cancer prevention	Flax seeds, Green tea
Cardiac diseases	Garlic
Cholesterol lowering	Garlic
Digestive support	Digestive enzymes
Diabetic support	Garlic, Momordica
Female hormone support	Black Cohosh, False Unicorn
Immunomodulators	Ginseng
Prostate support	Tomato lycopenes

Table 29.2 Classification of nutraceuticals as per chemical groupings

S. No.	Class	Examples
1.	Inorganic mineral supplements	Minerals
2.	Vitamin supplements	Vitamins
3.	Digestive enzymes	Enzymes
4.	Probiotics	Helpful bacteria
5.	Prebiotics	Digestive enzymes
6.	Dietary fibres	Fibres
7.	Cereals and grains	—
8.	Health drinks	—
9.	Antioxidants	Natural antioxidants
10.	Phytochemicals	
	Polysaccharides	Arabinogalactans
	Isoprenoids	Carotenoids
	Flavanoids	Bioflavanoids
	Phenolics	Tea polyphenols
	Fatty acids	Omega-3-fatty acids
	Lipids	Sphingolipids
	Proteins	Soya proteins
11.	Herbs as a functional foods	—

scavenging free radicals. It also performs many other vital functions.

Phosphorous: Phosphorous is important in maintaining bone structure and modulating plasma and bone formation.

Silicon: Silicon is concentrated in the active growth areas of the bone. It influences bone formation and calcification.

Vitamin supplement

Vitamins are the complex substances of organic origin which in small quantities are necessary for the maintenance of human and animal life. Some of the important water-soluble and water-insoluble vitamins are discussed below.

Vitamins B complex: Specific B vitamins are recommended as the daily requirement to combat high levels of homocysteine, a known risk factor for heart diseases. Homocysteine accumulates in the blood secondary to protein intake, especially from meat. Vitamins B extra is generally recommended to those who use caffeine, alcohol, excessive sugar or oral birth pills in their diet, since B vitamins are water soluble and easily excreted. Vitamins B_1 or thiamine deficiency is mostly observed in white rice eaters. Riboflavin-5-phosphate is a cofactor for vitamin B_2 which is beneficial in people who lack the enzyme to convert vitamin B_2 because of nutritional factors or disease condition. Niacinamide deficiency may cause neurological and skin problems. The body can also synthesize niacin from tryptophan. Pantothenic acid-A deficiency affect adrenal gland, immune and cardiovascular system. Vitamin B_6 is crucial for glucose production, hormone modulation and neurotransmitter synthesis. Pyridoxal 5-phosphate is considered as an active form of vitamin B_6. Vitamin B_{12} deficiency may be observed in vegetarian people as plants have no appreciable vitamins B_{12}. Folic acid is a B complex vitamin which contributes to healthy bone formation.

Among the other vitamins, vitamin C is the body's main water-soluble antioxidant. It is necessary for proper maintenance of bones. Inositol helps move fatty material from the liver into intestine. Biotin produced by several species of intestinal flora prevents yeast from converting to a more pathogenic fungal form. Choline bitartrate is helpful in moving fat out of liver into the bile.

Digestive enzymes

Much of the reflux is not caused by too much acid in the stomach but from poor digestion because of too little acid. As we ages, stomach cells responsible for acid production slow down, this in turn slows the transit time of food in the stomach causing reflux of food from the oesophagus. Taking antacids often worsen the problem. Variety of digestive enzymes can be used as digestive aid to help absorb and digest the food material. Pepsin, principal digestive enzymes in gastric juices is a digestive aid for proteins. Pancreatin, an enzyme from pancreas is often found in enzymatic formulation.

Pancrelipase helps the body to break down fat in small intestine while amylase helps in improve digestion of carbohydrates and sugars. Betaine HCl is used as a phase I digestive aid for proper digestion. The plant proteolytic enzyme, papain obtained from *Carica papaya* fruits and bromelain derived from stem and fruit of pineapple are used as an aid in digestion and are commonly found in digestive products.

Probiotics

Probiotics (for life) can be described as a live microorganism which when ingested with or without food improves the intestinal microbial balance and consequently the health and functioning of large intestine. Probiotics or friendly bacteria present in the dairy food are another area of functional foods. Approximately 95% of all bacteria found in human body are located in colon; some of which are desirable and helpful while others harmful. The natural balance between these two groups of microbes plays an important role in the health and functioning of the large intestine. Probiotics bacteria promote gut health. Bioyoghurts containing *Lactobacillus acidophilus* and *Bifidobacteria* lead the probiotics. *Lactobacillus acidophilus* can reduce the incidence of vaginal infections including thrush and bacterial vaginosis. Specially fermented products such as yakult containing *L. Casei*, *L johnsonii* and *Lactobacillus GG* are also used as probiotics to restore the imbalance; *Biofidobacteria* may help fight wide range of harmful food poisoning bacteria including potentially harmful *E.coli-0157*. *Bifidobacteria* and *Streptococcus thermophilus* both found in yoghurt can prevent young children suffering from diarrhoea. *Lactobacillus* GG may also be helpful in treating antibiotics associated diarrhoea. It has also been reported to be effective at treating causes of travellers' diarrhoea and rotavirus infection—the most common cause of diarrhoea in children throughout the world. Probiotics may also help reduce certain food allergies. Probiotics only have a transient effect and regular daily intake is needed to bring about health benefits.

Prebiotics

Prebiotics are the food components that escape digestion by normal human digestive enzymes and safely in intact form reach the colon after passage through the stomach and small intestine, where they selectively promote the growth of probiotics. Probiotics alone can hardly survive the rigours of digestive enzymes and acids in the upper gut before reaching the colon. Such difficulties have emphasized the alternative ways of boosting the levels of probiotics in the large intestine by supply of probiotics. Insulin as fructosan obtained commercially from Jerusalem artichoke tubers, *Helianthus tuberosus*, family Compositae or raw chicory is the best known prebiotics. Fructo-oligosaccharides (FOS) are increasingly used in food supplements and can have more long-lasting effect as they encourage the growth of *Bifidobacteria* already present in the gut. At least, 10 g FOS is needed daily.

Unlike probiotics, prebiotics are easier to formulate into regular foods and therefore offer a better chance of success in restoring natural balance of the colonic microflora and enriching the health of the large intestine.

Dietary fibres

Dietary fibres play critical role in keeping good health in human individuals and animals. Fibres are those parts of the plant, leaves, stem, fruits and seeds which cannot be digested or absorbed in the body. These fibres are necessary for our body to function properly. Dietary fibres can be divided into two broad categories such as water-insoluble and water-soluble fibres. Water-insoluble fibres absorb water to a certain extent and mainly contribute to bulking of stool, and allow quick passage of wastes through the elementary canal. Soluble fibres get dissolved in water and form a gel that binds the stool. It slows down the absorption of glucose and reduces blood cholesterol levels.

It has been recommended that about 30–40 g of dietary fibre should be consumed daily in order to obtain significant health benefits. The major sources of water insoluble fibres include whole grain cereals, whole wheat products, brown rice, fruits and vegetables with the peels. The sources of water soluble fibres are oats, dried beans, legumes, lentils, fruits and vegetables. Processed food can also be formulated to contain significant properties of both soluble and insoluble dietary fibres. The examples of such marketed processed products include breads, breakfast cereals and high-fibre beverages.

Cereals and grain

Cereals and grain are largely used throughout the world as the major food material in the form of entire cereals and grains, sprouted cereals and grains and their milled flours. These products of cereals and grains are rich with normal food nutrients, vitamins, minerals and specific phytochemicals. Breads of soya flour and linseed provide phyto-oestrogenic natural substances that mimic the structure of the hormone oestrogen. Phytoestrogens have been documented to enhance oestrogen levels when hormonal levels are low to weaken the effects of oestrogen when levels are high. This action may protect against both hot flushes and breast cancer. Cereals and grains helps in calcium fortification, maintaining healthy heart and a healthy immune system.

Health drinks

Drinks are the fast-developing area of functional foods. Some of these health drinks are fortified with the antioxidants, vitamins A, C, E and others with herbal extracts. The fruits and vegetable juices have also been shown to produce the health benefits. A new range of herb and vitamin-enhanced drinks claims to help overcome problems ranging from PMS to lack of energy. A Tropicana fruit juice fortified with calcium provides about 365 mg calcium per 250 ml glass. Drinks containing caffeine can also be described as functional foods as it vitalizes body and mind, increases physical endurance, improves and increases concentration and reaction speed.

Antioxidants

Antioxidants are the nutraceuticals whose deficiency states are associated with variety of dreaded disease conditions, viz. cardiovascular diseases, diabetes, cataracts, rheumatoid arthritis, Alzheimer disease and many others.

Phytochemicals might exert antioxidant action *in vivo* or in food by inhibiting generation of reactive oxygen species (ROS) or by directly scavenging free radicals. Certain compound may act *in vivo* as antioxidants by raising the levels of endogenous antioxidants defenses by up-regulating expression of the genes encoding superoxide dismutase (SOD), catalase or glutathione peroxidase.

Antioxidants can be broadly divided into three categories: (a) true antioxidants, (b) reducing agents and (c) antioxidant synergists. True antioxidants react with the free radicals and block the chain reaction of free radical. Reducing agents have a lower redox potential and readily get oxidized and are found effective against oxidizing agents while antioxidant synergists are the substance which on their own have little antioxidant effect but may enhance the effect of true antioxidants by reacting with heavy metals ions which catalyse auto-oxidation.

Natural antioxidant compounds can be classified as vitamins, carotenoids, hydroxycinnamates and flavonoids. Among the all above, flavonoid is a largest group of antioxidant which are almost ubiquitous in nature in most of the fruits, vegetables and plants. The various types of natural antioxidants and their dietary sources are given in Table 29.3.

Vitamins C or ascorbic acid is often claimed to be an important antioxidant *in vivo*. Its antioxidant property is regarded to be due to free radical scavenging by ascorbate and dehydroascorbate radical. Vitamin E or α-tocopherol delays lipid peroxidation by reacting with chain-propagating peroxy radicals faster than these radical can react with proteins or fatty acid side chains; β-carotene has remarkable antioxidant properties by interacting with a free radical to form β-carotene-derived radical which in the presence of oxygen forms a peroxyl radical. Antioxidants act at different levels in the oxidative sequence involving lipids and the extent to which oxidation of fatty acids and their esters occurs depends on the chemical nature of the fatty acid.

Polyunsaturated fatty acids

Human body is capable of synthesizing most of the fatty acids it needs except the two major polyunsaturated fatty

Table 29.3 Naturally occurring antioxidants

Antioxidants	Sources
Vitamins	
Vitamin C	Citrus fruits, vegetables
Vitamin E	Grains, nuts, oils
Carotenoids	
Carotenes	
Lycopene	Tomatoes
β-Carotene	Carrots, sweet potato, green vegetables
Xanthophylls	
β-Cryptoxanthin	Mango, papaya, oranges
Lutein	Banana, egg yolk, green vegetables
Zeaxanthin	Paprika
Hydroxycinnamates	
Ferulic acid	Cabbage, spinach, grains
Caffeic acid	White grapes, olive, spinach
Flavonoids	
Flavone	
Rutin	Buckwheat, tobacco, *Eucalyptus* spp.
Luteolin	Lemon, red pepper, olive
Flavonols	
Quercetin	Onion, apple skin, black grapes
Kaempferol	Grape fruit, tea
Flavanone	
Naringin	Citrus peel
Taxifolin	Citrus fruits
Chalcones	
Liquiritin	Liquorice
Anthocyanidins	
Cyanidin	Grapes, strawberry
Delphinidin	Aubergin skin
Catechins	
Epicatechin gallate	Green tea polyphenols
Epigallocatechin gallate	Green tea polyphenols

acids (PUFA), i.e. omega-3-fatty acid and omega-6-fatty acids. These fatty acids are required to be supplemented from the diet. The PUFA are the known precursors for arachidonic acid (AA), eicosapentaenoic acid (EPA) and docosahexanoic acid (DHA). These fatty acids have been found to regulate blood pressure, heart rate, blood clotting and immune response. Omega-3-fatty acids have been reported to be important fatty acids in the prevention of heart diseases and also in the treatment of arthritis. Omega-3 fatty acids are mostly found in cold water fishes, such as tuna, salmon and mackerel. It is also present in dark green leafy vegetables, flaxseed oil and in certain vegetable oils. The fatty acids such as AA and DMA are essential for the development of the foetus and also during the first six months after birth. The deficiency of these fatty acids may result in poor development of foetus and may also cause a variety of problems such as premature birth to underweight babies. Breast milk is a very rich source of DHA. Most of the infant formulas which are used as a substitute of breast milk should be supplemented with DHA, as per the recommendation by WHO.

Herbs as functional foods

A great attention has nowadays been given to discover the link between dietary nutrients and disease prevention. Large numbers of herbs which had been in use since unknown time have been shown to play a crucial role in the prevention of disease. In addition to the macro- and micronutrients such as proteins, fats, carbohydrates, vitamins or minerals necessary for normal metabolism—a plant based diet contains numerous nonnutritive phyto-constituents which may also play an important role in health enhancement. A brief overview of the role of various herbs in disease prevention, with a focus on bioactive components from flaxseeds, spirulina, ginseng, garlic, green tea, citrus fruits, soya bean, tomato, *Ginkgo biloba*, turmeric, black cohosh and fenugreek has been given in this part of the nutraceuticals.

Flaxseeds

Flaxseeds are the dried ripe seeds of *Linum usitatissimum*, family Linaceae. Canada is the largest producer and exporter of flaxseeds which is about 40% of the world supply. It is also cultivated in the Mediterranean countries, the Middle East, United States, Russia and India. Generally flaxseed is cultivated for the oil but many medicinal properties are found to be associated with flaxseeds and its constituents. It is an abundant source of gamma-linolenic acid (GLA), viscous fibre components and phytochemicals such as lignans and proteins. The components are of great interest as functional food. Flaxseed incorporations into the diet are particularly attractive from the perspective of specific health benefit. Flaxseed has been recorded as one of the six plant materials as cancer-preventive foods. Alpha-linolenic acid (ALA) has a broad spectrum of health advantages. It inhibits the production of ecosanoids, alters the production of several prostanoids, reduces blood pressure in hypertensive patients and lowers triglycerides and cholesterol. Dietary ALA may retard tumour growth and plays an important role in metastasis. It has been suggested that ALA is dietary essential for optimal neurological development of humans especially during fetal and early postnatal life. GLA and its metabolites are effective in suppression of inflammation, in the treatment of diabetic neuropathy, atopic eczema and certain cancers like malignant human brain glioma.

Dietary fibres of flaxseeds contain about 6% mucilage which has nutritional value. It appears to play a role in reducing diabetes and coronary heart disease risk, preventing colon and rectal cancer and reduces the incidence of obesity. Flaxseed mucilage has hypolipidaemic, cholesterolaemic and atherogenic effects in animals and humans.

The lignan compounds of flaxseeds such as secoisolariciresinol diglycoside (SDG) have been reported to be the precursors for enterodiol and enterolactone. It has also been reported to be a protective agent against mammary and colon cancer. Flaxseed extract and purified lignans exhibit antioxidant effect and inhibits the activation of promutagens and procarcinogens.

Ginkgo biloba

Ginkgo biloba, family Ginkgoaceae, known as fossil tree is an important drug used in traditional Chinese medicine since more than 2800 years. Mainly leaves and edible seeds are used as drugs. The leaves contain dimeric flavones such as bilobelin, ginkgetin, isoginkgetin and flavonols along with their glycosides. The diterpenoids ginkgolides A, B, C and bilobalide are also the therapeutically active constituents. Leaf contains 6-hydroxykynurenic acid, a metabolite of tryptophan.

Ginkgolide

The leaves are recommended as being beneficial to the heart and lungs. Ginkgolides present in the leaves are able to alleviate the adverse effects of platelet-activating factor in a number of tissues and organs both in animals and in humans. It is also effective in the treatment of arterial insufficiency in the limbs and in the brain. Inhalation of the decoction of leaves is used for the treatment of asthma. Ginkgo preparations are beneficial in the treatment of geriatric illness, including impairment of memory. Standardized concentrated extracts of *G. biloba* leaves are marketed throughout the world.

Spirulina

Spirulina is a blue green algae obtained from *Spindina platensis* or *S. maxima*, family Oscillatoriaceae. It is a simplest photosynthetic algae which grows in fresh water in planktonic form. The major producers of the algae are United States, China, Thailand, Mexico and India.

Spirulina is a potential source of food containing nutraceuticals. It contains about 50–70% of proteins and 5–6% of lipids. Lipids mostly contain essential fatty acids, such as γ-linoleic, linoleic and oleic acid. It also contains glycolipids and sulpholipids. Spirulina is rich in vitamins B contents and also possesses β-carotenes. Its mineral content, which is about 3–6%, contains the appreciable proportion of iron which is shown to be better absorbed as compared to other natural irons.

Spirulina has been reported to have immunostimulant activities and shows promises for the treatment and management of HIV and other viral infection, such as herpes, cytomegalovirus, influenza, mumps and measles virus. The glycolipid part of the spirulina is reported to be responsible for its anti-HIV potential. It stimulates the activity of spleen, thymus and bone marrow stem cells. Spirulina also acts as an antioxidant due to the presence of enzyme superoxide dismutase and thereby found helpful in the treatment of atherosclerosis, arthritis, cataract, diabetes and aging process.

Ginseng

Ginseng roots obtained from *Panax ginseng* or from various other *Panax* spp., family Araliaceae have been extensively studied for its wide range of pharmacological activities. White ginseng represents the peeled and sun-dried roots whilst red ginseng is unpeeled steamed and dried. Ginseng contains variety of tetracyclic dammarane-type sapogenins such as protopanaxadiol and their glycosides. It also contains other constituents which include traces of volatile oil, polyacetylenes, sterols, polysaccharides, starch, β-amylase, free sugars, choline, fats and minerals along with vitamins B_1, B_2, B_{12}, pantothenic acid and biotin.

Ginseng is widely renowned for its adoptogenic properties as it is used to help the body cope with stress and fatigue and to promote recovery from diseases like hypertension or hypoglycaemia. In many countries it is self administered and taken in the form of tablets or capsules containing dried extracts of the roots. Ginseng preparations with multivitamins and trace elements have been shown to modify metabolic and liver function in elderly patients. It has been shown to reduce blood sugar concentrations in diabetics and nondiabetics and has been reported to successfully treat cases of diabetics polyneuropathy, reactive depression, psychogenic impotence and various child psychiatric disorders. When used appropriately, ginseng appears to be relatively nontoxic. Ginseng products are available in most of the developed countries as food supplements in combination with vitamins and minerals.

Garlic organosulphur compounds

Garlic consists of the fresh or dried bulbs of *Allium sativum*, family Liliaceae. It is a perennial, erect bulbous herb indigenous to Asia but commercially cultivated in most countries. The bulb shows a number of concentric bulblets which has a characteristics strong alliaceous odour and very persistently pungent and acid taste.

Garlic is used as an adjunct to dietic management in the treatment of hyperlipidaemia and in the prevention of athrosclerotic (age-dependent) vascular changes. Fresh garlic juice, aged garlic extract or the volatile oil, all lowers cholesterol and plasma lipids, lipid metabolism, and atherogenesis both *in vitro* and *in vivo*. The mechanism of garlic's antihypercholesterolaemic and antihyperlipidaemic activity appears to involve the inhibition of hepatic HMG-CoA reductase and remodelling of the plasma lipoprotein and cell membrane. The overall activity of garlic is mainly due to the presence of sulphur compound, such as alliin, allicin, ajoene and others.

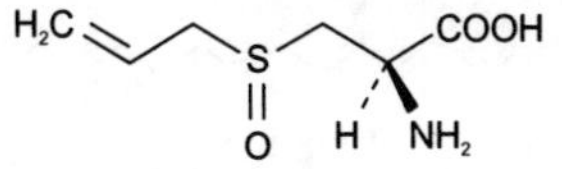

Alliin

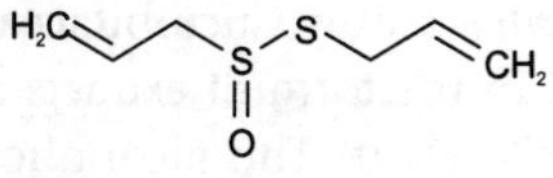

Allicin

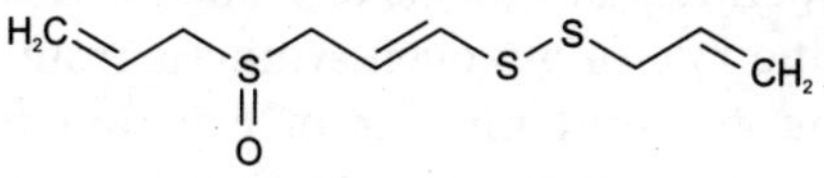

Ajoene

Cancer-preventive effect of garlic has been observed in a number of epidemiologic studies with stomach cancers appearing to be the type of neoplasia whose risk is clearly reduced by garlic consumption. Garlic has been reported to reduce the risk of colon cancer and lung carcinoma. Consumption of one or more servings of fresh or powdered garlic per week resulted in a 50% lower risk of cancer of the distal colon and a 35% lower risk of cancers anywhere in the colon. Garlic also shows antihypertensive, hypoglycaemic and antispasmodic activities.

Tea catechins

Tea is second only to water as the most widely consumed beverage in the world. About two to five million ton of dried tea is annually manufactured out of which about 78% is black tea, the reminder 20% is green tea while a smaller 2% is of oolong tea. Approximately 30% of the total dry weight of fresh is due to the presence of polyphenols, referred to as catechins. The four major green tea catechins are (−)-epicatechin (EC), (−)-epicatechin-3-gallate (ECG), (−)-epigallocatechin (EGC) and (−)-epigallocatechin-3-gallate (EGCG). Green tea polyphenols have been shown to

afford protection against cancers of skin, lung, forestomach, oesophagus, duodenum, pancreas, liver breast and colon. Tea consumption is likely to have preventive effect in reducing cancer risk.

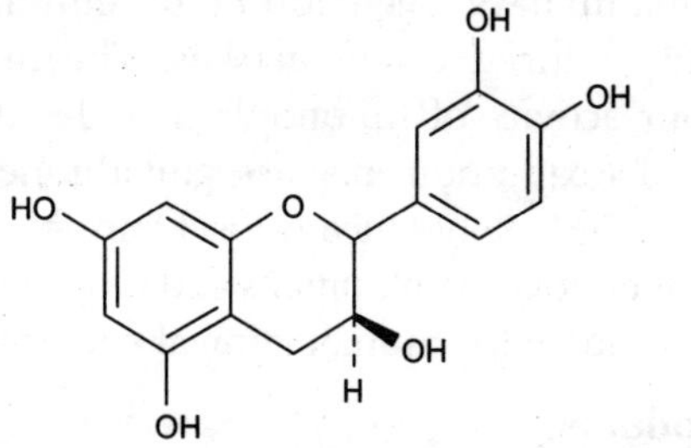

Catechin

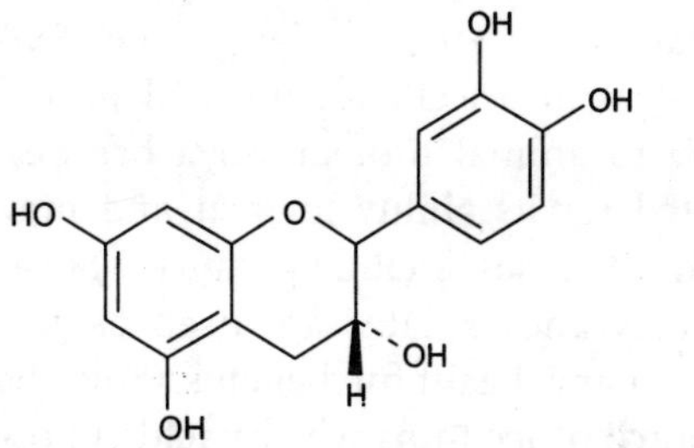

Epicatechin

Citrus limonoids

Citrus fruit consumption has been shown to protect against a variety of human cancers. The citrus fruits such as oranges, lemons, limes and grapefruits are the principal source of important nutrients like vitamins C, folate, fibres and vitamins E, but the other monoterpene compounds known as limonoids are reported to be responsible for the anticancer activity, D-limonene—a predominant monocyclic monoterpene found in essential oil of citrus fruits has

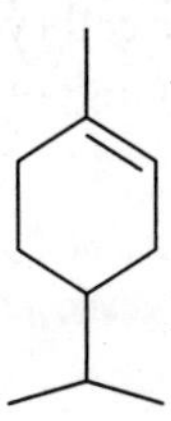

Limonene

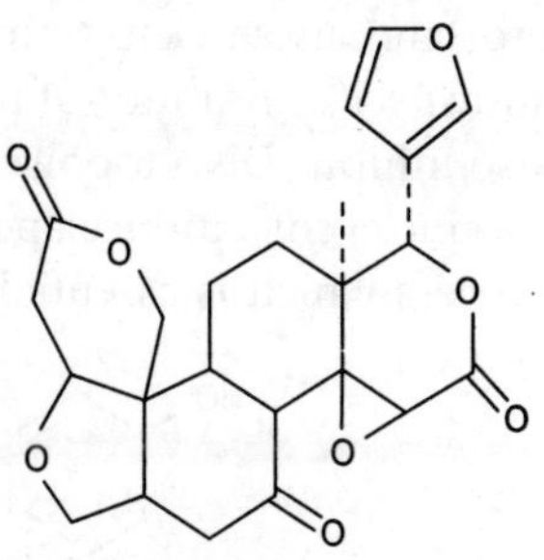

Limonin

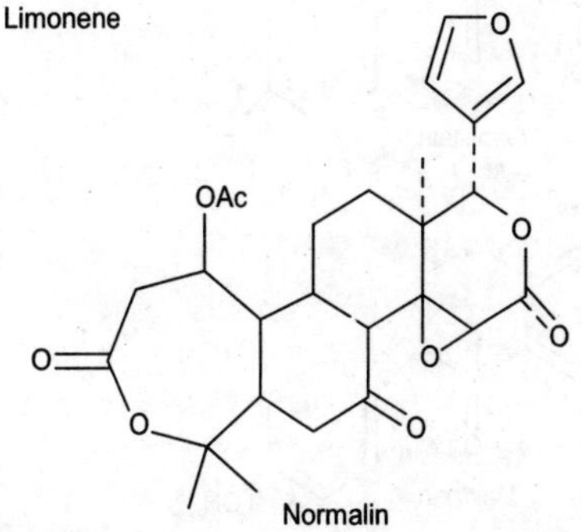

Normalin

been reported to be a cancer-chemopreventive agent. This compound has been shown to be effective against both spontaneous and chemically induced rodent mammary tumours. Two most abundant limonoids of citrus, limonin and normalin have been found to inhibit or prevent chemically induced carcinogenesis. The mechanism of antitumour activity of limonoids includes the induction of hepatic detoxification enzymes, glutathione S-transferase and uridine diphosphoglucoronosyl transferase. Limonene has little or no toxicity in humans and has been suggested as a good candidate for human clinical chemoprevention.

Soya products

Soya bean, *Glycin max*, family Leguminosae has clearly been a plant food in the spotlight in the 1990s. It has been recognized as an excellent source of protein, equivalent to quality to animal protein. Soya has been extensively investigated for its ability to treat and prevent a variety of chronic diseases including cancer. Soya bean meals, concentrates and isolates are used as meat substitute and have many healthful benefits. Soya bean is also a major source of lecithins which yields liposomes used to formulate stable emulsions and finds major use in food technology.

The primary isoflavones in soya, genistein and daidzein are structurally similar to the oestrogenic steroids and have been reported to have oestrogenic and antioestrogenic activities. Due to their weaker activity, isoflavones may act as antioestrogens by competing with the more potent, naturally occurring oestrogens for binding to the oestrogen receptor. Due to this, soya consumption may reduce the risk for oestrogen-dependent cancers. South East Asian populations who consume 20–80 mg of genistein per day are found to have significantly lower incidence of breast and prostate cancer. Genistein has been reported to be a potent and specific inhibitor of protein tyrosine kinase. Genistein also inhibits DNA topoisomerase II activity, alters cell cycle specific events, induce apoptosis and inhibits angiogenetic process which is essential for tumour growth.

Tomato lycopenes

Lycopene is a carotenoid principle present in lycopersicon family Solanaceae known throughout the world as tomato. Clinical studies have indicated that lycopene significantly lowered the risk of prostate cancer. The candidates that consumed processed tomato products about 10 times per week had less than one-half the risk of developing prostate cancer. Lycopene activity is likely to be related to its antioxidant function because lycopene has been reported to be the most efficient quencher of singlet oxygen in biological system. Lycopene has also been shown to reduce risk of other types of cancers of digestive tract, pancreas, cervix, bladder and skin. Recently, it has been proved that low-plasma lycopene levels may be an independent risk factor for lung cancers especially in smokers.

Lycopene

Momordica charantia

Momordica charantia, family Cucurbitaceae, known in India as karela is used in the form of extracts and health drinks as an antidiabetic agent. The alcoholic extract of karela pulp demonstrates a significant hypoglycemic activity in various experimental models of diabetes. The extract also increases the rate of glycogen synthesis from 14c-glucose by four- to five-fold in liver of experimental animals. Momordica antidiabetics activity could be partly attributed to increased glucose utilization in the liver rather than an insulin secretion effect.

Turmeric curcuminoids

The tuber of *Curcuma longa*, family Zingiberaceae known as turmeric is used as a spice in the culinary all over the world. It contains diaryl heptanoid compounds consisting mainly curcumin, desmethoxycurcumin and bisdesmethoxycurcumin. Curcumin has been shown to

Genistein

Daidzein

Curcumin

Desmethoxycurcumin

Bisdesmethoxycurcumin

protect the experimental animals against decrease in heartbeat rate, blood pressure and biochemical changes It also demonstrates significant hepatoprotective activity. It is used as condiment, colouring agent and as a drug in various condition in various traditional systems of medicine. Recent findings indicate the potential of turmeric as an inhibitors of integrase enzyme of HIV virus.

Black cohosh

Black cohosh consists of roots and rhizomes of *Cimicifuge racemosa*, family Rananculaceae is also known as Black snakeroot and is listed by the Food and Drug Administration (FDA) as a herb of unlimited safety. Black cohosh roots and rhizomes contain quinolizidine alkaloid *N*-methylcytisine, terpenoids like actein, 12-acetylactein and cimigoside, tannins and 15–20% of cimicifugin.

Black cohosh is stated to possess antirheumatic, antitussive, sedative and emmenagogue properties. It has been used for intercostal myalgia, sciatica, whooping cough, dysmenorrhoea and specially for rheumatism and rheumatoid arthritis. It has shown promises in reducing luteinizing hormone levels which are thought to be responsible for postmenopausal symptoms.

Fenugreek

Fenugreek seeds obtained from *Trigonella foenum-graecum*, family Leguminosae is an important food material as well as drug. Fenugreek is listed by the Council of Europe as a natural source of food flavouring. In United States, fenugreek extracts are permitted in food. Fenugreek seeds contain variety of constituents, such as alkaloids, flavonoids, coumarins, proteins and amino acids, steroidal saponins, vitamins and lipids.

Gentianine and trigonelline are the major alkaloids. Steroidal sapogenins, such as diosgenin and yamogenin are the major saponins. Fenugreek is stated to possess mucilaginous demulcent, laxative, nutritive, expectorant and orexigenic properties. Traditionally, it has been used in the treatment of anorexia, dyspepsia, gastritis and convalescence. Fenugreek has found to be a potential hypoglycaemic agent. Fenugreek seeds contain a high proportion of mucilaginous fibre which works as the dietary fibres. In addition, hypocholesterolaemic action has been documented for fenugreek.

Market Scenario of Nutraceuticals

In a wider context, there is a growing demand for plant-based medicines, health products, pharmaceuticals, food supplements, cosmetics, etc., in the national and international markets. Global demand for nutraceuticals ingredients will grow 5.8% annually through 2010. Best prospects include probiotics, soy additives, lycopene, lutein, sterol-based additives, green tea, glucosamine, chondroitin and coenzyme Q10. China and India will be the fastest growing markets, while the US will remain the largest. This study analyses the 11.7 billion dollars world nutraceutical industry. Nutraceuticals is one huge business opportunity awaiting the Indian pharmaceutical industry in the coming years. At least a dozen large companies currently produce and market nutraceuticals today. Many of these are just food supplements with no specific curative values. South based Parry Nutraceuticals, a leading player, has a well-known product, Spirulina. Some of the other major players are Wockhardt, Lupin, Morepen, Laboratories, Dabur and Himalaya. The largest Indian pharmaceutical company Ranbaxy is also planning to enter into this segment in a big way. According to an industry estimate, the current nutraceuticals market in India is about Rs. 1600 crore with an annual growth rate of 25%. The explosive growth, research and developments, lack of standards, marketing zeal, quality assurance and regulation will play a vital role in its success or failure. Nutrients, herbals and dietary supplements are major constituents of nutraceuticals which make them instrumental in maintaining health, act against various disease conditions and thus promote the quality of life. Nutraceuticals are found in a mosaic of products emerging from (a) the food industry, (b) the herbal and dietary supplement market, (c) pharmaceutical industry and (d) the newly merged pharmaceutical/agribusiness/nutrition conglomerates.

Regulatory Obstacles

In connection with the regulatory aspect, the main hurdle appears to be at the level of quality and claim parameters. It is essential to govern the disorganized sector with rational attitude. Ayurvedic and Unani medicines are herbomineral based. Modern medicine has certain parameters related to drug discovery but these parameters are unreasonable to validate nutraceuticals. Moreover, marketability of medicinal plants and their products in the country is today unorganized due to several problems. Current practices of harvesting are unsustainable and many studies have highlighted depletion of resource base. The guidelines should, therefore, be similar to regulatory requirements for ayurveda, siddha, unani or homoeopathy.

Standards and Quality Control

The regulatory body should classify the products as purely herbal, which should be endorsed through the PFA act and formulations containing minerals and vitamins through the drug authorities. All the GMP parameters applicable to ayurvedic manufacturing units should be applicable to herbomineral formulations. The magic remedy act applied to

Ayurvedic manufacturers should be stringently followed by nutraceutical manufacturers. They should be allowed to insert printed material with information to empower the user.

Emerging Scenario

Export opportunities of natural products are tremendous, as the world market is looking towards natural sources for the purposes of therapeutic use as well as nutritional dietary supplements. The present accumulated knowledge about nutraceuticals represents undoubtedly a great challenge for nutritionists, physicians, food technologists and food chemists. Public health authorities consider prevention and treatment with nutraceuticals as a powerful instrument in maintaining health and to act against nutritionally induced acute and chronic diseases, thereby promoting optimal health, longevity and quality of life.

Conclusions

Evidences are rapidly emerging that nonnutrient components in plants foods may play a critical role in the prevention of chronic diseases. New products and ingredients developed as nutraceuticals or functional foods offer large growth potential for both the food and pharmaceuticals industry. Herbal and nonherbal extract would provide the strongest growth opportunities in healthcare products. *Ginkgo biloba* for enhanced cognitive properties, ginseng for energy boosting and saw palmetto for benign prostatic hyperplasia would become the fastest selling products among herbal extracts. In most of the cases, nutraceuticals or functional foods would be much more expensive and it would be beneficial to get the same beneficial ingredients more chiefly and more naturally from a healthy balanced diet. For example, a calcium-fortified fruit drink is much more expensive than a glass of milk which contains the minerals naturally. A stimulation drink costs about twice the price of a can of cola and yet is perhaps no more effective. Nevertheless the functional foods will continue to appeal because they are convenient for today's lifestyle. Some are also genuinely researched products and offer novel ingredients that can bring about health benefits quicker than would normally be the case through eating conventionally healthy food alone. But real danger would arise if people begin to rely on these foods as a healthy diet.

29.2. COSMECEUTICALS

Today a new hot topic in the cosmetic industry is 'cosmeceuticals', which is the fastest growing segment of the natural personal care industry. Cosmeceuticals (or alternatively, cosmaceuticals) are topical cosmetic-pharmaceutical hybrids intended to enhance the beauty through ingredients that provide additional health-related function or benefit. They are applied topically as cosmetics, but contain ingredients that influence the skin's biological function. The Drug and Cosmetic Act defines cosmetics by their intended use, as 'articles intended to be rubbed, poured, sprinkled or sprayed on, introduced into, or otherwise applied to the human body for cleansing, beautifying, promoting attractiveness or altering the appearance.' Among the products included in this definition are skin moisturizers, perfumes, lipsticks, fingernail polishes, eye and facial makeup preparations, shampoos, permanent waves, hair colours, toothpastes and deodorants, as well as any material intended for use as a component of a cosmetic product. These cosmeceuticals, serving as a bridge between personal care products and pharmaceuticals, have been developed specifically for their medicinal and cosmetic benefits. Tracing the origin of cosmetics, the first recorded use of cosmetics is attributed to Egyptians, circa 4000 B.C. The ancient Sumerians, Babylonians and Hebrews also applied cosmetics. In other cases, such as European cosmetic known as Ceruse was used from the second century to the 19th century. Cosmeceutically active ingredients are constantly being developed by big and small corporations engaged in pharmaceuticals, biotechnology, natural products and cosmetics, while advances in the field and knowledge of skin biology and pharmacology have facilitated the cosmetic industry's development of novel active compounds more rapidly. Desirable features of cosmeceutical agents are efficacy, safety, formulation stability, novelty and patent protection, metabolism within skin and inexpensive manufacture.

Skin Cosmeceuticals

Cosmetics and skin care products are the part of everyday grooming. Protecting and preserving the skin is essential to good health. Our skin, the largest organ in the body, separates and protects the internal environment from the external one. Environmental elements, air pollution, exposure to solar radiation as well as normal aging process cause cumulative damage to building blocks of skin, i.e. DNA, collagen and cell membranes. Use of cosmetics or beauty products will not cause the skin to change or heal; these products are just meant to cover and beautify. Cosmeceuticals being cosmetic products having medicinal or drug-like benefits are able to affect the biological functioning of skin owing to type of functional ingredients they contain. There are skin care products that go beyond colouring and adorning the skin. These products improve the functioning/texture of the skin by encouraging collagen growth by combating harmful effects of free radicals, thus maintaining keratin structure in good condition and making the skin healthier. Some of the common cosmeceutical contents are given in Table 29.4.

Table 29.4 Common cosmeceutical contents

Ingredient	Purported Action	Source
Vitamins	Antioxidant	Vitamins A, C and E
α-Hydroxy acids (AHAs)	Exfoliates and improves circulation	Fruit acids (glycolic acid, lactic acid, citric acid, tartaric acid, pyruvic acid, maleic acid, etc.)
β-Hydroxy acids (BHAs)	Antibacterial	Salicylic acid
Essential fatty acids	Smoothens, moisturizes and protects	Linoleic, linolenic and arachidonic acids
Coenzyme Q10 (Ubiquinone)	Cellular antioxidant	Naturally occurring in skin
Allantoin	Soothes	Comfrey
Aloe vera	Softens skin	Aloe vera
Arnica	Astringent and soothes	Arnica montana
Calendula	Soothes, softens and promotes skin-cell formation	Calendula officinalis
β-Bisabolol	Anti-inflammatory, antibacterial and calms irritated skin	Chamomile flower
Cucumber	Cools, refreshes and tightens pores	Cucumber
Lupeol	Antioxidant and skin conditioning agent	Crataeva nurvala
Ginkgo	Antioxidant that smoothes, rejuvenates and promotes youthful appearance	Ginkgo biloba
Ivy	Stimulates circulation and helps other ingredients penetrate skin	Hedera spp. (ivy family)
Panthenol	Builds moisture and soothes irritation	Provitamin B
Witch hazel	Tones	Hamamelis virginiana
Green tea extract	Antioxidant	Green teas
Neem oil limonoids	Antimicrobial	Azadirachta indica
Pycnogenol	Antiaging effect	Grape seed extract
α-Lipoic acids, resveratrol, polydatins	Potent free-radical scavengers and antioxidant	Fruits and vegetables
Furfuryladenine	Improves hydration and texture of skin	Plant growth hormone
Kinetin	Free-radical scavenger and antioxidant	Plants and yeast
Sodium hyaluronate	Lubricant between skin tissues and maintains natural moisture	Natural protein
β-Carotene	Minimizes lipid peroxidation and cellular antioxidant	Carrots and tomatoes
Retinoic acid	Smoothes skin, promotes cell renewal and improves circulation to skin	Vitamin A
Tetrahydrocurcuminoides	Antioxidant and antiaging	Curcuma longa
Centella	Skin conditioning agent, increases collagen production, improves texture and integrity of skin and reduces appearance of stretch marks	Centella asiatica
Boswellia	Anti-inflammatory and antiaging	Boswellia serrata
Coriander seed oil	Anti-inflammatory and anti-irritant, skin-lightening properties	Coriandrum sativa
Turmeric oil	Antibacterial and anti-inflammatory	Curcuma longa
Coleus forskoflii oil	Antimicrobial, aromatherapy/perfumer	Coleus forskoflii
Arjunolic extract	Antioxidant and anti-inflammatory	Terminalia arjuna
Ursolic acid	Anti-inflammatory, collagen build-up	Rosmarinus officinalis
Oleanolic extract	Antioxidant, antifungal, improves texture and integrity of skin	Olive leaf
Rosemary extract	Antioxidant, antimicrobial and anti-inflammatory	Rosmarinus officinalis
Dry extract from yarrow	Treatment of oily hair	Achillea millefolium
Licorice extract	Skin whitening properties, antioxidant, antimicrobial and anti-inflammatory	Glycyrrhiza glabra
Horse chestnut extract	Supports blood circulation, wound healing effect and anti-inflammatory	Aesculus hippocastanum

OLAY vitamin line, which includes vitamins A, C, D, E, selenium and lycopene, pycnogenol plus zinc and copper, is a well-known skin care line. The treatment of aging skin with a cream containing a hormone such as oestrogen results in a fresh appearance with a rejuvenating effect. Kuno and Matsumoto had patented an external agent for the skin comprising an extract prepared from olive plants as a skin-beautifying component, in particular, as an antiaging component for the skin and/or a whitening component. Dry emollient preparation containing monounsaturated Jojoba esters was used for cosmeceutical purpose. Martin utilized plant extract of genus Chrysanthemum in a cosmetic composition for stimulating skin and/or hair pigmentation. Novel cosmetic creams or gels with active ingredients and water-soluble barrier disruption agents such as vitamin A palmitate have been developed to improve the deteriorated or aged skin.

Sunscreens

Regular use of an effective sunscreen is the single most important step to maintain healthy, youthful-looking skin. Mainly, it is the effect of ultraviolet light from the sun that causes most of the visible effects of 'aging' skin. Traditional chemical sunscreens act primarily by binding to skin protein and absorbing ultraviolet B (UVB) photons (280–320 nm) and most are based on *p*-aminobenzoic acid (or its derivatives), cinnamates, various salicylates and benzophenones, dibenzoylmethanes, anthralin derivatives, octocrylene and homosalate. Avobenzone (Parsol-1789) is a benzophenone with excellent ultraviolet A (UVA) protection. Physical agents, or sun blocks, act as barriers, which reflect or scatter radiation. Direct physical blockers include metal-containing compounds such as iron, zinc, titanium and bismuth. Zinc oxide and titanium dioxide are highly reflective white powders, but submicron zinc oxide or titanium dioxide powder particles transmit visible light while retaining their UV blocking properties, thus rendering the sun block invisible on the skin. Some commercially available sunscreens are Benzophenone-8, Neo Heliopan MA and BB, Parsol MCX and HS, Escalol 557, 587 and 597. Govier *et al.* patented sunscreen composition comprising activated platelet factor as an ingredient in a cosmeceutically acceptable carrier. Such a composition in the form of a shaving cream or foam, after shave lotion, moisturizing cream, suntan lotion, lipstick, etc., assist in restoring the skin to its natural condition when the skin is damaged by cuts, abrasions, sun, wind and the like.

Moisturizers

Moisturizers function to smooth out the age lines, help brighten and tone the delicate skin. Moisturizers usually incorporate emollients to smoothen the skin surface by working their way into the nonliving outer layers of the skin, filling spaces between the layers and lubricating and humectants to help skin cells absorb and retain moisture in these layers. Healthy Remedies Balancing Lotion has been created for menopausal women containing ingredients, which diminish the appearance of fine lines and wrinkles, uplift the neck area and moisturize the dry, sagging skin. Some of those ingredients include black cohosh, soy extract and vitamins A and E. Augmenting the skin's natural moisture balance are a nourishing complex containing hyaluronic acid and a revival complex containing green tea leaf extract, and glutathione.

Bleaching agents

Bleaching agents are used for bleaching/fading the various marks and act to block the formation of the skin pigment melanin. Hydroquinone is the most commonly used agent for 'bleaching' brown marks, liver spots, melasma, etc. Kojic acid, extracted from mushrooms, is a slightly less-effective agent, either may be compounded with tretinoin or topical steroids α-and β-hydroxy acids. As with any bleaching agent, aggressive exfoliation and sun protection are necessary for good results. A synthetic detergent bar was developed containing hydroquinone as a skin-bleaching agent. The bar is maintained at about a pH of between 4 and 7 and includes a compressed mixture of a synthetic anionic detergent, hydroquinone, a stabilizer for hydroquinone, water, a buffer which maintains the pH of the bar and excipients such as waxes, paraffin, dextrin and starch. Similarly, a skin-bleaching preparation comprising hydroquinone, tertiary butyl hydroquinone and optionally an additional stabilizer can additionally contain a buffer to maintain the pH between about 3.5 and 7.5. Because of the maintenance of low pH and the presence of a stabilizer, hydroquinone is not oxidized and thus the product is characterized by an extended shelf life.

Hair Cosmeceuticals

The appearance of the hair is a feature of the body over which humans, unlike all other land mammals, has direct control. One can modify the length, colour and style of hair according to how one wish to appear. Hair care, colour and style play an important role in people's physical appearance and self-perception. Among the earliest forms of hair cosmetic procedures in ancient Egypt were hair setting by the use of mud and hair colouring with henna. In ancient Greece and Rome, countless ointments and tonics were recommended for the beautification of the hair, as well as remedies for the treatment of scalp diseases. Henry de Mondeville was the first to make a distinction between medicinal therapies intended to treat diseases and cosmetic agents for the purpose of beautification. But today's delineation of cosmetics from pharmaceuticals has become more complex through the development of cosmetics with physiologically active ingredients, i.e. cosmeceuticals. Shampooing is by far the most frequent form of cosmetic hair treatment. While shampoos have primarily been products aimed at cleaning the hair and scalp, current formulations are adapted to the variations associated with hair quality, hair care habit and specific problems such as treatment of oily hairs, dandruff and for androgenic alopecia related to the superficial condition of the scalp.

Cosmetics for the treatment of hair are applied topically to the scalp and hair. While they can never be used for therapeutic purposes, they must be harmless to the skin and scalp, to the hair and to the mucous membranes and should not have any toxic effect, general or local, in normal conditions of their use. Mausner has patented a shampoo composition, which cleans the hair and scalp without doing any damage to the fragile biological equilibrium of the scalp and hair. A haircare cosmetic compositions comprising iodopropynyl butylcarbamate and/or a solution of zinc pyrithione in *N*-acyl ethylenediamine triacetate has been patented, which includes an appropriate carrier and a nonallergenic dry extract of yarrow (*Achillea millefolium* L.), obtained by oxidation of a water-alcohol solution extract of flower tops of yarrow. The extract contains less than 0.5% by weight of polyphenolic derivatives, is used for the treatment of hair, in particular oily hair, based on extract of yarrow. Buck has patented a method for treatment for androgenic alopecia wherein Liquor Carbonic Detergents are topically administered. It is generally accepted that genetic hair loss arises from the activation of an inherited predisposition to circulating androgenic hormones.

A hair cosmeceutical product includes conditioning agents, special care ingredients and hair growth stimulants. Conditioning agents are intended to impart softness and gloss to reduce flyaway and to enhance disentangling facility. A number of ingredients may be used, mostly fatty ingredients, hydrolysed proteins, quaternized cationic derivatives, cationic polymers and silicons. Special care ingredients are aimed at modifying specific problems relating to the superficial scalp. These shampoos are formulated around one or more specific ingredients selected for their clinical effectiveness in these conditions. Accordingly, current antidandruff ingredients are virtually all-effective antifungal agents—zinc pyrithione, octopirox and ketoconazole. Hair growth stimulants cannot be expected to have any impact on hair growth due to short contact time and water dilution. A minoxidil-related compound (2,4-diamino-pyrimidine-3-oxide) is a cosmetic agent with claim of acting as a topical hair growth stimulant. Its target of action has been proposed to be the prevention of inflammation and perifollicular fibrosis. Some degree of efficacy of 2,4-diamino-pyrimidine-3-oxide has been claimed in the prevention of seasonal alopecia. Recent approval in the United States of two new products, Propecia and Rogaine Extra Strength (Minoxidil) 5%, indicated in men to promote scalp hair growth have added a new dimension to treatment options offered by physicians in treating androgenetic alopecia.

Other Cosmeceuticals

The skin beneath the eye lacks subcutaneous fat and has virtually no oil glands. This delicate skin needs protection and plenty of moisture to replenish and repair, which helps to reduce the signs of premature aging. As the skin ages, it becomes thinner, drier and rougher. Overexposure to the elements and to environmental pollution aggravates this condition. Many topical skin-soothing products intervene in this process, but products for this area need to be particularly gentle and specially formulated with ingredients that work from the inside out by interacting with the cells under the skin's surface without irritating the eyes. There are numerous cosmeceutical eye creams that nourish the skin with natural emollients and beneficial nutrients. The other functional ingredients include butcher's broom, chamomile and vitamin E, antioxidants—vitamins A, C and E, green tea and tiare flower, *Ginkgo biloba* and also cucumber, calendula and α-bisabolol, an active constituent of chamomile, to calm irritated skin. A key ingredient in the eye lifting moisture cream that treats puffiness, irritation and also protects against future skin damage is yeast which helps to plump up the wrinkles. The eye wrinkle cream helps forestall the signs of aging and generally contains wheat germ and corn oil, squalene and carrot extract. Eye-firming fluid has aosaine—an algae extract from seaweed that helps the skin to maintain elasticity. Lawlor had developed dental care compositions, which are useful for providing a substantive composition on the surfaces of oral cavity, which can provide prophylactic, therapeutic and cosmetic benefits.

Regulatory Aspects

The claims made about drugs are subject to high scrutiny by the FDA review and approval process, but cosmetics are not subject to mandatory FDA review. Much confusion exists regarding the status of 'cosmeceuticals.' Although there is no legal class called cosmeceuticals, this term has found application and recognition to designate the products at the borderline between cosmetics and pharmaceuticals. Cosmeceuticals are not subject to FDA review and the Federal Food, Drug and Cosmetic Act do not recognize the term itself. It is also often difficult for consumers to determine whether 'claims' about the actions or efficacies of cosmeceuticals are in fact valid unless the product has been approved by the FDA or equivalent agency. Some experts are calling for increased regulation of cosmeceuticals that would require only proof of safety, which is not mandatory for cosmetics. Some countries have the classes of products that fall between the two categories of cosmetics and drugs, for example, Japan has 'Quasi-drugs', Thailand has 'controlled cosmetics' and Hong Kong has 'cosmetic-type drugs'. The regulations of cosmeceuticals have not been harmonized between the United States, European, Asian and other countries.

Conclusions

The global trend in the cosmetic industry towards developing 'medicinally' active cosmetics and in the pharmaceutical industry towards 'cosmetically' oriented medicinal products is part of a current 'lifestyle' ideology. The future promises increasingly sophisticated formulations for cosmetics and skin care products. Cosmetic companies are finding ways to deliver small-dose ingredients that do not require medical regulations and to introduce steroids and hormones into lip balms, which would result in production of cosmeceuticals that could help to improve body mass, nail and hair growth. New challenges will also be presented to government regulatory agencies as more chemicals with true biological activity are invented and tested. Claim substantiation and premarketing testing must also evolve to accurately assess efficacy and safety issues with important implications for total body health. The new vehicles and delivery systems combined with established ingredients will alter percutaneous absorption, requiring re-evaluation of substances with an assumed good safety profile. Biotechnology will also compete directly with the pharmaceuticals and cosmetic businesses. The most influential angle over the coming five years will be the links between internal health, beauty and antiaging. The next big beauty trend will include skingestibles that will promote beauty from inside out, borrowing of pharmaceutical terms for cosmetic applications, amino peptides to make the skin more elastic, neuromediators which are chemicals to tell the brain to be happy and the blurring of boundaries between surgery and cosmetics. The trend towards therapeutic cosmetics is sure to result in the need to obtain a better understanding of modern ingredients and assessment techniques.

Natural Pesticides

CONTENTS

30.1. INTRODUCTION

Pest is any animal, plant or microorganism that causes trouble, injuries or destruction; therefore, pesticide may be defined simply as chemical agents used to control or eliminate pest. Many kinds of insects transmit serious diseases, such as malaria and typhus. Some insects destroy or cause heavy damage to valuable crops, such as corn, cotton, wheat and rice. Other common pests include bacteria, fungi, rats and such weeds as ragweed and poison ivy. An understanding of genesis of pest status is important in the design and execution of pest control strategies incorporating the substance of natural origin. Worldwide, the traditional pesticide represents the big business in which the majority of the synthetic pesticides are utilized for agriculture or other purposes.

30.2. METHODS OF PEST CONTROL

The methods used for the control of pest can be of natural or artificial controls, which are discussed below.

Natural Controls

Nature is full of the example of prey–predator relationships. Every pest is more or less hindered in its increase by other predacious organisms. Parasitic pests, predators and the diseases caused by the pest are usually the most important factors in natural methods insect controls. As the use of specific pesticides against a major pest on a crop might lead to a serious outbreak of a secondary pest due to the destruction of natural enemies, this may lead to an upset in the balance between destructive and useful insects.

Topographical influence of the season changes, changing temperatures, rainfall, soil, atmospheric humidity and other natural factors also shows their effect on insects and their hosts. However, in tropical, temperate and frigid climates, the pest control methods are generally adapted to the topographic conditions.

Artificial Control

Artificial controls of pest have been developed by man. These methods can be categorized as agriculture, chemical and biological controls as discussed below.

Mechanical control: It employs manual labour as well as mechanical devices for collection or destruction of pest. Techniques, such as handpicking, pruning, trapping and burning are employed for the destruction of eggs, larvae, pupae and adult insects.

Agricultural control: Agriculture control is the oldest in its approach. Deep plugging for the eradication of weeds and early stages of insects, alternate crop rotation or changing environmental conditions are some methods that leads to obstruction of the life cycle of pests. Nowadays advanced plant breeding techniques like hybridization, mutation, polyploidy and biotechnological manipulations are greatly used for the production of pest resistant species.

Chemical controls: Chemical agents are the major pesticides agents used for the control of pest throughout the world. These are the materials used for the purpose of killing pests or for protecting crops, animals or other properties against the attack of the pest. Insect repellents, attractants, fumigants like insecticides, parasiticides are used for killing mites, ticks and sterilizing agents which employ radioisotopes or chemicals to interfere with reproductive capabilities are nowadays widely used.

New groups of compounds called as insect growth regulators (IGR) pesticides or bioinsecticides consists of the natural chemicals presents in the insects that control their developments. For example, methoprene prevent the pupate stage which develops the reproductive adults. In such cases, larvae grow larger, molt repeatedly and eventually die. Biopesticide of this type is very specific for their toxicity and safety.

Biological controls: Biological approach is of a natural approach, as the nature in which predators, parasites and weed-feeding invertebrates and living organisms are used for controlling the pest or their biological activities. All these are referred to as 'biorational pesticides'. Microorganisms may be used to kill by causing fatal disease in insects. For example, *Bacillus thuringiensis* selectively kills only larvae of butterflies and moths and *B. papillae* kill the grubs of Japanese beteles. *B. thuringiensis* Var. *israelensis* is a new strain which specifically attack only mosquito larvae. Microbial controls are safer for most of the nontargeted organisms and also human and pets. Biologically derived pest control agents, such as pheromones, allomones and kairomones combinely known as 'semiochemicals' and

hormones also attract, retard, destroy or otherwise exert a pesticide activity.

30.3. CLASSIFICATION

Pesticides are classified according to the pest they control. The four most widely used types of pesticide are briefly discussed below.

Insecticides

Farmers use insecticides to protect their crops from insect damage. In urban localities, public health officials use these chemicals to fight mosquitoes and other insects. Insecticides are widely utilized in homes and other outdoor conditions to control such pests as ants, moths, cockroaches and termites.

Herbicides

Three groups of pesticide agents control weeds or eliminate plants that grow where they are not wanted. Farmers use herbicides to reduce weeds among their crops. Herbicides are also used to control weeds in such public and recreational areas as parks, lakes and ponds. It is also used as garden pesticide or in yards to get rid of crab grass and dandelions.

Fungicides

Many of the fungi are pathogenic and many infect both plants and animals including human beings. Fungicides are used to control fungal diseases of plants and food crops. Most disinfectants used in homes, hospitals and restaurants contain fungicides.

Rodenticides

These agents are used especially in urban areas where rats and other rodents are a major health problem. Rats carry many of the pathogenic bacteria that cause disease, such as rabies, rat-bite, fever, tularemia and typhus fever. Rats also destroy large amounts of food and grain, so rodenticides help protect areas where these products are stored. Other pesticides that help to control variety of organisms are given below.

Class	Protection from
Acaricide	Controls ticks and mites
Algicides	Algae and other aquatic vegetation
Antiseptics	Microorganisms
Arbericides	Defoliate and destroy trees and shrubs
Bactericides	Bacterial infection
Molluscicides	Control mollusks including gastropods
Nematicides	Nematodes

It is difficult to classify all pesticide chemically or biologically. Some of the important natural pesticides have been categorized in Table 30.1 enlisting few important examples of each class.

Pesticides are often classified according to the type of action that results in destruction of the pest. Three broad categories, namely stomach poisons, contact insecticides and fumigants are recognized. Stomach poisons kill by being taken into the stomach, absorbed in the blood and leads to the death of the pest due to the toxic action. Contact insecticides kill by direct or indirect contact with the insect or sometimes it penetrate inside the body and causes oxidation and suffocate the insect. Fumigants can be applied only in enclosed areas where it surrounds the insect, enters their breathing pores and kills. Most of the pesticides are used in the form of dust preparations, spray preparations, suspensions or bait preparations. Sometimes they are dispensed in the form of aerosol or liquefied gas propellants. Equipments used for the application of pesticides might vary from small hand sprayers, paint brushes for use in home to large power sprayers for treating livestock and field crops. For the dispersal in vast areas of forms, airplanes and helicopters are also used.

30.4. ESSENTIALS OF A GOOD PESTICIDE

For an agent to be a good and ideal pesticide, it should bear certain important characteristics as given below.

1. A pesticide should have a high margin of safety for plants and animal causing very little or no damage to the foliage or livestock, respectively.
2. It should be safer.
3. It should be easier to handle and easy for application.
4. It should not show toxicity in case of warm blooded animals.
5. It should not have flammable or explosive character.
6. It should have safety and palatability of the food products exposed to insecticides and should not show the residual effects of pesticides.
7. It should be available easily at affordable cost.

PYRETHRUM FLOWERS

Synonym

Insect flowers, pyrethrum flowers.

Biological Source

Pyrethrum consists of the dried flower heads of *Chrysanthemum cinerariaefolium* (Trev.) Vis., family Composite.

Table 30.1 Pesticides of natural origin

Class and chemical groups	Sources	Pest
Insecticides		
Pyrethroids	*Pyrethrum cinerariaefolium*	Insects
Rotenoids	*Derris elliptica*	Lice, fleas and larvae
Nicotinoids	*Nicotiana tabacum*	Soft bodies insects
Veratrine	*Schoenocaulon officinale*	Insects
Ryanodine	*Ryania speciosa*	Lepidopterous larvae
Neem products	*Azadirachta indica*	Larvae
Rodenticides		
Scillirosides	*Urginea maritima*	Rats, mice
Strychnine	*Strychnous nuxvomica*	Rats, mice
Fungicides		
Neem products	*A. indica*	Tinea, Trychophyton
Copper sulphate	—	Fungi
Molluscicides		
Bidesmodic saponins	*Phytolacca dodecandra*	Fresh water snails
Swartzia saponin	*Swartzia madagascariensis*	Mollusc, fish
Saponins	*Tetrapleura tetraptera*	Mollusc, fish
Antifeedants		
Neem products	*A. indica*	Grain insects
Attractants		
Masculare	*Musca domestica*	Common flus
Bollweevil sex attractants	—	Boll weevil
Repellants		
Citronellal	*Cymbopogon* Spp.	Insects
Neem products	*A. indica*	Insects
Pesticide synergist		
Piperonyl butoxide	*Brazilian sassafras*	Pesticide additive

Geographical Source

Pyrethrum is indigenous to Balkan areas of Dalmatia, Herzegovina and Montenegro. The flowers were known as Dalmatian insect flowers as they were formally exported from Dalmatia. Nowadays it is principally cultivated and produced in Kenya, Tanzania, Rwanda, Ecuador and Belgium Congo. On similar scales, it is grown in Japan, Brazil,

Yugoslavia, Switzerland, Spain and India. Before World War II, Japan produced almost 80% of the world's production, but presently Kenya is the largest exporter of pyrethrum.

Cultivation and Collection

Pyrethrum is a perennial plant propagated by seeds and pieces of stems bearing roots known as splits. The best and favourable condition for pyrethrum cultivation is at an attitude of 1900–2700 m and an annual rainfall of 76–180 cm. Seeds are raised in nurseries. About 4-month old seedlings are planted out in the fields in rows about 1 m apart during sunny days. Low night temperature about 5–15°C favours the maximum bud formation. First collection of flower heads is made after about 4 months, but the best time for collection is when two-third of the disc florets are open. Collection is generally done by hand pickers at roughly 3-week intervals. The flowers are dried immediately after collection in the sun or in drying chambers at a temperature not exceeding 50°C. In Kenya, after gradation, the flowers are compressed into bales and exported. Kenyan pyrethrum production is controlled by pyrethrum marketing board at Nakuru. The flowers are directly exported or made into powder or standard liquid extract.

Characteristics

The closed pyrethrum flower heads are about 6–9 mm in diameter while the open flowers are about 9–12 mm diameter. The flowers bear a short, longitudinally striated peduncle. The involucre consists of two or three rows of yellowish or greenish yellow lanceolate hairy bract. The flat receptacle bears a single row of 15–23 cream or straw-coloured ligulate ray florets. Lignite corollas are 10–20 mm length with about 17 veins and three-rounded apical teeth of which the central one is suppressed. Disc florets are about 200–300 with tubular corolla. Pyrethrum flowers have a slight aromatic odour and a bitter acrid taste. It is interesting to note that before drying the flower heads are not toxic to insect.

The powder of pyrethrum flowers shows the presence of parenchymatous tissues, with aggregate crystals, sclerenchymatous tissues, t-shaped hairs, spherical pollen grains and tracheas. Dried flowers or powder should be stored in well-closed container, protected from air and light and should not be kept for more than two years. Pyrethrum extract is comparatively more stable than pyrethrum flowers.

Chemical Constituents

Pyrethrum flowers owe its insecticide properties to two groups of esters: the first group consists of pyrethrin I, jasmolin I and cinerin I, which have chrysenthemic acid (chrysanthemum monocarboxylic acid) as their acid

component and the second group of esters that consists of pyrethrin II, jasmolin II and cinerin II, which have pyrethric acid (monomethyl ester of chrysanthemum dicarboxylic acid) as their acid component. The alcohol component of the pyrethrin present in the form of keto-alcohol pyrethrolone and that of cinerine as cinerolone. The flowers of pyrethrum also consist of a triterpene alcohol pyrethrol and sesquiterpene lactones, pyrethrocin. Other constituents includes pyretol, pyrethroloxic acid, chrysenthemine and chrysathemumic acid.

Pyrethrocin

Allethrin

Component	R	R'
Pyrethrin I	-CH$_3$	-CH = CH$_2$
Cinerin I	-CH$_3$	-CH$_3$
Jasmolin I	-CH$_3$	-CH$_2$-CH$_3$
Pyrethrin II	-COOCH$_3$	-CH = CH$_2$
Cinerin II	-COOCH$_3$	-CH$_3$
Jasmolin II	-COOCH$_3$	-CH$_2$CH$_3$

Various pyrethrins are called as pyrethroids. These components occur in the oleoresin secretion of certain floral parts, known as achenes. Pyrethrum extract contains up to about 50% active constituents. Pyrethrum extract (BP) consists of about 25% of pyrethrins. These commercial extracts are generally obtained by supercritical fluid extraction techniques at 100–250 bar pressure and 50°C temperature conditions. The concentrated extracts are usually diluted with kerosene to a pyrethrin strength of about 0.2%. Pyrethrin assays are based on the total chrysanthemum acid and the total pyrethrin acid; therefore, the content of pyrethrums is in effect the content of pyrethrins, cinerins and jasmolins.

Uses

Pyrethrum flowers are mainly used for the preparation of pyrethrum extract which is the form of pyrethrin usually employed in the compounding of pyrethrum preparation. Pyrethrum brings about its pesticide activity by an instantaneous knock down action on insects within few seconds. It has no appreciable effect on insects as a stomach poison but acts by contact, producing a characteristic effect on the nervous system that results in muscular excitation, convulsion and paralysis. However, it is less persistent and less stable. The compounds like piperonyl butoxide, bucarpolate, sesamin and DDT act synergistically and potentiate the insecticidal properties of pyrethrin.

The synthetic pyrethrin-like compound, allethrin, also shows the potential insecticidal activity but its activity is not synergistic when combined with synergists available at present.

Pyrethrum is widely used in domestic and agricultural insecticidal sprays, dusting powders and aerosol preparations for controlling a variety of garden pests and fleas, lice and ticks on pets. A noninflammable preparation is used as a spray in aircraft to kill insect vectors and so prevent the transmission of insect borne diseases.

The toxic effects of pyrethrum include irritation to the eyes and mucosa. Maximum permissible atmospheric concentration is up to 5 mg per m³.

DERRIS ROOTS

Synonym

Derris roots, tuba roots, Tauba.

Biological Source

Derris root consists of the dried rhizomes and roots of *Derris elliptica* (Roxb.) Benth. and *D. malaccensis* Prain, family Leguminosae.

Geographical Source

Derris is indigenous to Malaya. It is cultivated in Burma, Thailand, East Indies and tropical African countries. It is also produced in Singapore, Borneo and in Sumatra.

Characteristics

Derris roots are slender pieces of about 2 m long with a diameter of about 8–10 mm. Externally the root bark is dark reddish brown in case of *D. elliptica* and greyish brown in cash of *D. malaccensis*, while the inner wood is yellowish and porous in both the cases. It shows the fine longitudinal furrows on the outer surface of roots. It is flexible, tough and hard and breaks in the fibrous fracture. It shows slightly aromatic odour and bitter and numbing taste. Derris rhizomes constitute a very small proportion of the commercial drug. It consists of short but thick brown coloured pieces with numerous longitudinal wrinkles, transverse cracks and circular lenticels. The transversely cut surface of roots shows thick cork followed by rings of sclerenchyma containing strands of phloem.

Microscopy

The transverse section of the derris root consists of the layers of cork cells followed by phelloderm and pericyclic parenchyma with numerous groups of lignified sclereids and starch grains. The phloem is stratified by the altering bands of phloem fibres and sieve tissue. Phloem parenchyma contains longitudinal small cells and prismatic crystals of calcium oxalate. Two types of xylem vessels of larger and smaller size are present in groups of two to six. Groups of xylem fibres and vessels are usually embedded in cellulosic parenchyma. The fibres of both phloem and xylem are unlignified except the middle lamella. One to six cell thick medullary rays are radially arranged.

Chemical Constituents

Derris roots contains about 3–10% of a flavone derivative rotenone. It is colourless to brownish crystalline compound or a white to brownish white odourless tasteless crystalline powder. It is insoluble in water but soluble in alcohol, acetone and other organic solvents. Rotenone is incompatible in the alkalies and oxidizing agents. Derris in powder should be protected from light. The overall evaluation of drug depends both on rotenone content and on the amount of chloroform extractive that the root yields. Rotenone is rapidly degraded by sunlight, lasting a week or less.

Uses

Derris is a widely used agricultural and horticultural insecticide and larvicide. It is a contact and stomach poison.

Rotenone

Its action is more persistent but less rapid than pyrethrum. The insecticidal preparations of rotenoids at concentrations ranging from 0.75 to 1.0% are effective against a wide range of insects, such as Mexican bean beetle, cabbage worms, leaf hoppers and other insects attacking a variety of vegetable. It is especially useful for application to vegetable near the time of harvest when certain other insecticides cannot be used because of potentially excessive residues. Derris and rotenoids are also useful in controlling insect parasites of animals such as cattle, grubs, lice, fleas and ticks on pets and live stocks.

In general rotenone insecticides are considered low in hazard. It is irritant to eyes and mucosa and may cause convulsions and stupor if inhaled. Rotenoids are generally harmless to mammals but are extremely toxic to fish and used to kill unwanted fish in a pond to restocking.

LONCHOCARPUS ROOTS

Synonym

Lonchocarpus roots, cube roots, timbo, barbasco.

Biological Source

Lonchocarpus consists of the dried roots of *Lonchocarpus utilis*, *L. urucu* and other species of *Lonchocarpus*, family Leguminosae.

Geographical Source

Lonchocarpus is indigenous to Peru and Brazil. It is also produced in British and Dutch Guiana.

Characteristics

Lonchocarpus roots usually occur in pieces to 30 cm long and 12–25 mm in diameter. Outer surface is brownish-grey with longitudinal reticulated wrinkles. Microscopically it resembles Derris but may be distinguished by the abundant starch grains, comparatively larger and lignified xylem. The freshly cut transverse surface of lonchocarpus roots appears greyish-green under UV light, and its ethereal extract shows bright blue fluorescence.

Chemical Constituents

Lonchocarpus roots contain about 3–10 % rotenone.

Uses

Lonchocarpus roots owe its action to the presence of constituents similar to those of Derris and are used for the same purpose.

TOBACCO

Synonym

Tobacco.

Biological Source

Tobacco consists of the dried leaves of *Nicotiana tabacum*, family Solanaceae, known as Virginian tobacco and *N. rustica* referred to as Turkish tobacco.

Geographical Source

Tobacco is indigenous to tropical America. It is cultivated on large scale in China, United States and India. It is also produced in Brazil, Turkey, Russia and Italy. In India tobacco is mainly cultivated in Andhra Pradesh, Karnataka, Tamil Nadu, Orissa, Gujarat, Bihar, West Bengal and Assam.

Cultivation, Collection and Preparation

Although tobacco is tropical in origin and thrives best in the warm climate, it is grown under wide range of conditions. Tobacco is an annual crop attaining 1–3 m height. It tears about 20 large leaves. Tobacco is generally propagated by seeds. Seedlings are developed in the seedbeds during early spring and the seedlings of about 12 weeks are transplanted in the field. Cutting of the flowering tops encourages the growth of the foliage. The crop is harvested after about three to three-and-a-half months. Tobacco is subjected to curing by any of the three procedures, namely flue curing, fire curing and air curing, which modifies the aroma and flavour characteristics of tobacco. Loss of nicotine during flue-curing is negligible but sun-curing causes considerable loss of nicotine content.

Characteristics

Tobacco is a crop which is mostly used for the preparation of cigarettes, bidi, cigar, cheroot, hookah, snuff and chewing tobacco. Nicotine is the characteristic alkaloid prepared commercially from waste material of tobacco industry. Nicotine is a colourless to pale yellow, very hygroscopic, oily liquid with an unpleasant pungent odour and a sharp burning persistent taste. It gradually becomes brown on exposure to air or light. It is soluble in water, alcohol, chloroform, kerosene and fixed oils. It should be stored in airtight containers.

Chemical Constituents

Levels of nicotine content in various tobacco types vary drastically, but it is in the range of about 1–10%. Nicotine is a pyridine–pyrrolidine group of alkaloid mainly responsible for its pesticidal activity. Along with nicotine, tobacco leaf has several other alkaloids especially narcotine and anabasine which may have some insecticidal properties in association with nicotine.

| Nicotine | Nornicotine | Anabasine |

Most of the tobacco waste materials obtained from the tobacco industry are used as the potential source of raw material for production of commercial grade insecticidal nicotine. Nicotine is isolated by mixing tobacco waste with lime and extracting with water. Aqueous extract is further extracted with kerosene and the subsequent kerosene extract is treated with sulphuric acid to obtain nicotine sulphate solution from which it is separated.

Uses

Insecticidal use of nicotine dates back to the 17th century. During 18th century, aqueous tobacco extract or dust was employed as an insecticide in the vegetable gardens of Europe, and the commercial preparation of nicotine sulphate was put into market by 1910 as a potential insecticidal agent. Nicotine acts by its triple action insecticidal property, acting as stomach, contact and fumigant poison. Its free base is more toxic than the sulphate or hydrochloride salt. It is mostly effective against minute soft bodied insects, such as aphides and also against white flies, red spidermites, leaf rollers, moths, fruit tree borers, termites, cabbage butterfly larvae, etc. Nicotinoids are active as a spray solution containing 0.04–0.05% active ingredients.

One of the advantages of the insecticidal use of nicotine is its high margin of safety for plants. Nicotine preparations are safer, easier to handle and much less toxic to warm-blooded animals. Due to the volatile nature of nicotine, it disappears quickly leaving no residue on treated plants. The above properties make nicotine preparation a very ideal insecticide.

NEEM

Synonym

Neem, Margosa, Azadirachta.

Biological Source

Neem consists of almost all parts of the plants which are used as drug. Some important morphological parts are the dried stem bark, root bark, leaves and fruits of *Azadirachta indica* also, known as *Melia azadirachta*, family Meliaceae.

Geographical Source

Neem is native of the arid region of India and Pakistan. Neem is found abundantly in India, Pakistan, Bangladesh, Sri Lanka, Thailand, Malaysia and Mauritius, countries of East and South Africa and in tropical Australia.

Characteristics

Neem is large subtropical shade tree. It is known for centuries as being free of insects, disease and nematodes. All the parts of the tree, such as bark, leaves, fruits and especially the seeds are resistant. The bark is grey to reddish brown with numerous furrows. Leaves are imparipinnate, alternate or opposite and bluntly serrate. Flowers are white to pale yellow which gives green drupaceous fruits turning yellow on ripening. Fruit contains single exalburainous seed.

Neem oil or margosa oil is a fixed oil expressed from seed kernels. It gives about 10% of the oil which is yellow in colour with garlic-like odour and bitter taste. It is soluble in organic solvents and practically insoluble in alcohol and water.

The cake left after the expression of oil is used as such. It may be subjected to alcoholic extraction to yield neem cake extract.

Chemical Constituents

Neem has been found to possess several types of chemicals that could be exploited for pest management. Neem seeds mostly contain the complex tetranorterpenoid lactones azadirachtin, nimbin, nimbidin, salanin and nimbolin B out of which azadirachtin is the most active component responsible for the antifeedant activity of neem. Other antifeedent components identified are meliantrol a triterpenoid alcohol and salanin. Neem oil obtained from seeds also shows the presence of these constituents along with other compounds such as nimbolides, olichinolide B and azadiradione. The leaves also contain azadirachtin, meliantrol, salanin, β-sitosterol, stigmasterol and flavonoids such as nimatone, quercetin, myrecetin and kaempferol.

The bark shows the presence of nimbin, nimbidin and nimbinin like antiviral agents and margolone and margolonone like antibacterial principles.

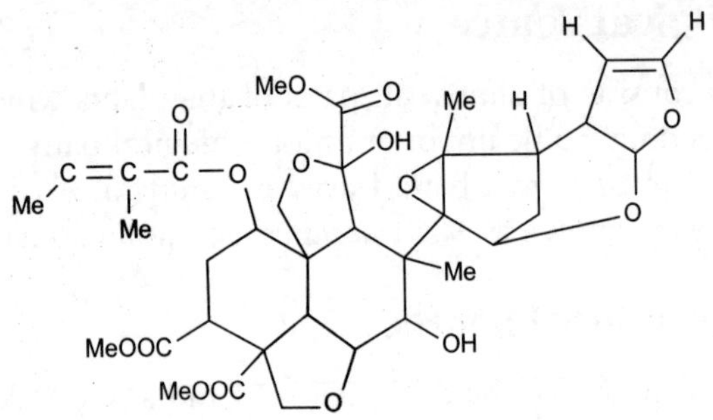

Azadirachtin

Uses

The pest control usage of neem and neem products can be properly exploited depending upon the nature of the pest. The various reported pest control activities are given in Table 30.2 along with the neem and neem products used on specific pests.

Neem seeds can be directly extracted to yield neem seed extracts. The oil expressed from the seed is known as neem oil, while the residual marc is called as neem cake which may be extracted using alcohol to obtain neem cake extractives. Neem oil extractive is a resinous dark byproduct of neem oil refining. It is well known that neem possesses low- to medium-contact toxicity which is restricted to soft body insects, and its use as an insecticide alone does not carry much conviction with the user.

Table 30.2 Neem products and their pest control usages

Activity	Neem Products	Pests
Antifeedant	Neem seed extract	Locust, grain insects
	Neem oil	Brown plant hoppers
Attractants	Neem leaves and twigs	White grub
Repellant	Neem cake	Termites
	Neem oil	Potato tuber moth
Insecticide	Seed kernel	Aphicidal
	Neem cake extract	Aphicidal
	Neem oil extractive (0.04%)	Mosquito larvicide
Nematicide	Neem cake	Reduces root galls of tomato and okra
Growth disruptor	Neem oil extractive (0.01%)	Diamond back moth, cabbage caterpillar, army worm, etc.
Antimicrobial	Neem cake extractive (3%)	Soil microorganisms (inhibitor of pesticide degradation)

CEVADILLA

Synonym

Cevadilla, Sabadilla, Caustic Barley.

Biological Source

Cevadilla consists of the dried ripe seeds of *Schoenocaulon officinale*, family Liliaceae.

Geographical Source

Cevadilla is a tall, herbaceous plant found in Mexico to Venezuela. It also grows in Guatemala.

Collection and Preparation

Sabadilla plant is 3–4 feet high. The seeds and fruits are collected from the plant after maturity. It is not quite certain whether the seeds are obtained from *Veratrum sabadilla* or from *Veratrum officinale* which differs slightly in appearance and morphological characteristics.

Characteristics

Dried mature seeds of cevadilla are dark brown to blackish about 6-mm long but narrow and sharply pointed at the ends. The seeds are bitter and acrid in taste. The seed powder is sternutatory and causes violent sneezing.

Chemical Constituents

Cevadilla seeds contain about 2–4% of mixed alkaloids known combinely as 'Veratrine'. The major alkaloids cevadine (crystalline veratrine), sabadine, sabadilline and veratridine shows the close relationship to the ester alkaloids of veratrum. Sabadilla is less toxic to mammals than rotenone or pyrethrin. The acute oral LD_{50} is greater than 4000 mg/kg.

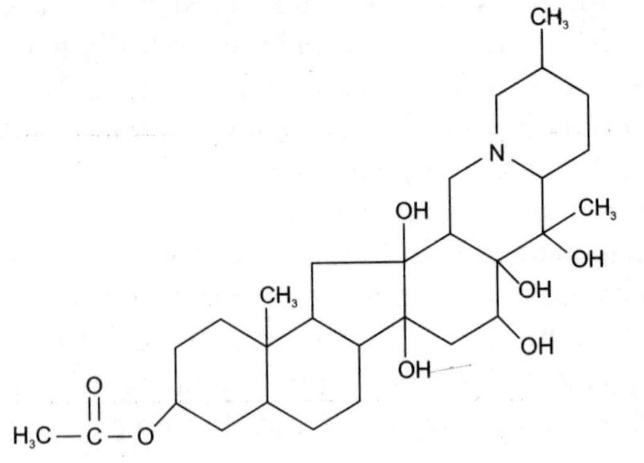

Sabadine

Uses

Cevadilla was formerly used as pesticide especially for pediculosis coptis in the form of ointment. Powdered cevadilla is used for killing house flies, thrips and vegetable attacking bugs in the form of sprays or dust in overdoses capable of producing fatal results. It is also used as a taenicide.

RYANIA

Synonym

Ryania.

Biological Source

Ryania consists of the roots and stems of *Ryania speciosa*, family Flacourtiaceae.

Geographical Source

Ryania is indigenous to South America. It is mostly found in Trinidad.

Collection

The roots and stem of Ryania are collected after flowering and fruiting. It is the most expensive material and is not as readily available as rotenone or pyrethrin.

Chemical Constituents

Ryania contains about 0.16–0.2 % of alkaloids. Ryanodine is the major pyrrole alkaloid that is esterified with a complex polyhydroxy diterpenoid.

Ryanodine

Uses

Ryania extracts containing the alkaloid ryanodine are used as insecticide for various lepidopterous larvae which attacks fruits. It is also used for controlling moths and corn borer. Ryanodine is formulated as a wettable powder and is labelled to be used against the codling moth in apples. It is more persistent than rotenone or pyrethrin and more selective. It is generally not very harmful to pest predators and parasites. It may also be used up to 24 h before harvest. It is toxic to fish.

RED SQUILL

Red squill and white squill are the two important varieties of *Urginia maritima*, family Liliaceae. Red squill either the whole bulb or dried scales and powder is distinguished from that of white variety on the basis of its reddish colour.

Red variety of *U. maritima* contains in addition to cardiac glycosides, an active principle, scilliroside, which is very toxic to rats. It acts on the central nervous system (CNS). Unlike other mammals rodents do not regurgitate the red squill and death follows convulsions and respiratory failure. Red squill was not considered acceptable to animals other than rodents but poisoning has been reported in catties, sheep, chicken and dogs. It is incorporated as a pesticide in rat pastes. Since it is extremely irritating to the skin it should be handled with rubber gloves. Its use as a poison for animals is prohibited in England and is considered as a cruel poison. WHO expert committee on insecticides had endorsed its use from the standpoint of safety.

STRYCHNINE

Strychnine is an alkaloid obtained from the dried seeds of *Strychnous nuxvomica*, family Loganiaceae. It occurs as odourless translucent, colourless crystalline powder with a very bitter metallic taste. The symptoms of poisoning by strychnine are mainly those arising from stimulation of CNS. The first signs are tremors and slight twitching of limbs followed by sudden convulsions quickly involving all muscles. The jaw is rigidly cramped. Respiration is arrested and death occurs from asphyxia or medullary paralysis. Strychnine was used as rodenticide in olden days, and it was recommended that strychnine should only be used by trained pest control operators in areas to which access by unauthorized persons and useful animals could be completely prevented. In England use of strychnine for killing of animals is prohibited under the Animal (Cruel poisons) regulations 1963. Strychnine is traditionally used for the extermination of moles. Its toxicity and painful poisonous action do not make it a rodenticide of choice.

MOLLUSCICIDES

A number of organisms from the Mollusca class cause a variety of diseases in human beings and animals. The pharmaceutical interest in molluscicides is concerned primarily to kill such parasitic organisms. The blood flukes, *Schistosoma haematobium* and its other species causes intestinal and bladder damage in South America and Africa. Fresh water snails act as an intermediate host to produce numerous cercaria which emerge into fresh water and causes infection to humans by penetrating through the skin into the blood. The berries of *Phytolacca dodecandra*, family Phytolaccaceae is an Ethiopian plant which have shown molluscicidal activity against fresh water snails which works as a host for Schistosoma. The berries contain a triterpenoid saponin glycoside oleanolic acid which is responsible for its poisonous effect on snails.

The pods of *Swartzia madagascariensis* and *S. simplex,* family Leguminosae, contain oleanolic acid glycosides and certain other saponins. Locally these are used as insecticidal and piscicidal agents. Another leguminous plant *Tetrapleura tetraptera* which consists of saponins is used as a potential piscicidal and molluscicidal agents in Nigeria.

CITRONELLA OIL

Citronella oil is a pale to deep yellow oil with a pleasant characteristic odour. It is obtained by distillation from *Cymbopogon nardus* and *C. wintcrianus,* family Gramineae and also from other varieties and hybrids of these species. The commercial oil is found in two types which are known as Ceylon oil and Jawa oil. Both the oils contain a monoterpene aldehyde citronellal as a major component of essential oil. Both citronella and citronellal oil have been used as a constituent of insect repellant products. However, it shows lesser effectivity than diethyltoluamide or dimethyl phthalate. It is used as an outdoor insect repellant.

Some of the other Indian medicinal plants which have shown the promising results in several pesticidal studies are mentioned in Table 30.3.

Table 30.3 Indian medicinal plants having pesticidal activity

Warm wood	*Artemisia vulgaris* (Herb)	Insect repellant
	Cassia galuca (Leaves)	Antifeedant
Clove	*Eugenia caryophyllus* (buds)	Moth repellant
Walnut	*Juglan regia* (leaves)	Antitermite
Indian olean-der	*Nerium indicum* (bark)	Insecticide
Nirgundi	*Vitex negundo* (leaf oil)	Mosquito repellant

30.5. FACTORS INFLUENCING DEVELOPMENT OF NATURAL PESTICIDES

Discovery

The secondary compounds of plants are a vast repository of compounds with a wide range of biological activities. This diversity is largely the result of coevolution of hundreds of thousands of plant species with each other and with an even greater number of species of microorganisms and animals. Thus, unlike compounds synthesized in the laboratory, secondary compounds from plants are virtually guaranteed to have biological activity and that activity is highly likely to function in protecting the producing plant from a pathogen, herbivore or competitor. Thus, knowledge of the pests to which the producing plant is resistant may provide

useful leads in predicting what pests may be controlled by compounds from a particular species. This approach has led to the discovery of several commercial pesticides such as the pyrethroid insecticides. Isolation and chemical characterization of the active compounds from plants with strong biological activities can be a major effort compared to synthesizing a new synthetic compound. However, the assurance of biological activity and improvement in methods of purification and structural identification is shifting the odds in favour of natural compounds.

Considering the probability of plant secondary products being involved in plant–pest interactions, the strategy of randomly isolating, identifying and bioassaying these compounds may also be an effective method of pesticide discovery. Biologically active compounds from plants will often have activity against organisms with which the producing plant does not have to cope. Many secondary compounds described in the natural product, pharmacological and chemical ecology literature have not been screened for pesticidal activity. This is due, in part, to the very small amounts of these compounds that have been available for screening.

The discovery process for natural pesticides is more complicated than that for synthetic pesticides (Fig. 30.1). Traditionally, new pesticides have been discovered by synthesis, bioassay and evaluation if the compound is sufficiently promising, quantitative structure–activity relationship-based synthesis of analogues is used to optimize desirable pesticidal properties. The discovery process with natural compounds is complicated by several factors.

First, the amount of purification initially conducted is a variable for which there is no general rule. Furthermore, secondary compounds are generally isolated in relatively small amounts compared to the amounts of synthesized chemicals available for screening for pesticide activity. Therefore, bioassays requiring very small amounts of material will be helpful in screening natural products from plants. A number of published methods for assaying small amounts of compounds for pesticidal and biological activities are available in the allelochemical and natural product literature. At some point in the discovery process, structural identification is a requirement. This step can be quite difficult for some natural products. Finally, synthesis of the compound and analogues must be considered. This is generally much more difficult than identification. Despite these difficulties, modern instrumental analysis and improved methods are reducing the difficulty, cost and time involved in each of the above steps.

Development

Few pesticides that are found to be highly efficacious in testing are ever brought to market. Many factors must be

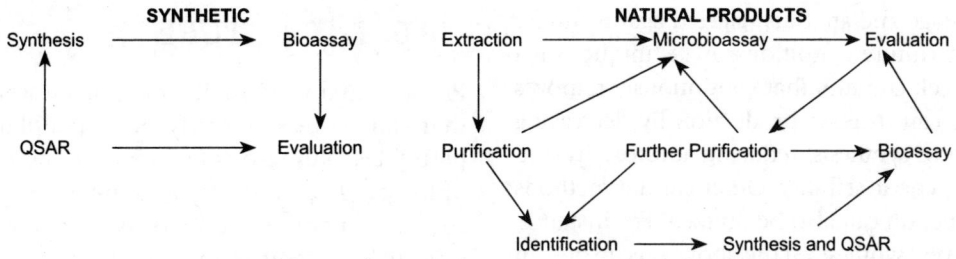

FIG. 30.1 Pesticide discovery strategies for synthetic versus natural products

considered in the decision to develop and market a pesticide. An early consideration is the patentability of the compound. A patent search must be done for natural compounds as with any synthetic compound. Prior publication of the pesticidal properties of a compound could cause patent problems. Compared to synthetic compounds, there is a plethora of published information on the biological activity of natural products. For this reason, patenting synthetic analogues with no mention of the natural source of the chemical family might be safer than patenting the natural product in some situations.

The toxicological and environmental properties of the compound must be considered. Simply because a compound is a natural product does not ensure that it is safe. The most toxic mammalian poisons known are natural products and many of these are plant products. Introduction of levels of toxic natural compounds into the environment that would never be found in nature could cause adverse effects. However, evidence is strong that natural products generally have a much shorter half-life in the environment than synthetic pesticides. In fact, the relatively short environmental persistence of natural products may be a problem, because most pesticides must have some residual activity in order to be effective. As with pyrethroids, chemical modification can increase persistence.

After promising biological activity is discovered, extraction of larger amounts of the compound for more extensive bioassays can be considered. Also, analogues of the compound should be made by chemical alteration of the compound and/or chemical synthesis. Structural manipulation could lead to improvement of activity, toxicological properties, altered environmental effects, or discovery of an active compound that can be economically synthesized. This has been the case with several natural compounds that have been used as a template for commercial pesticides (e.g. pyrethroids).

Before a decision is made to produce a natural pesticide for commercial use, the most cost-effective means of production must be found. Although this is a crucial question in considering the development of

any pesticide, it is even more complex and critical with natural products. Historically, preparations of crude natural product mixtures have been used as pesticides. However, the potential problems in clearing a complex mixture of many biologically active compounds for use by the public may be prohibitive in today's regulatory climate. Thus, the question that will most probably be considered is whether the pure compound will be produced by biosynthesis and purification or by traditional chemical synthesis.

Before considering any other factors, there are two advantages to the pesticide industry to industrial synthesis. They have invested heavily in personnel and facilities for this approach. Changing this approach may be difficult for personnel trained in disciplines geared to use it. Secondly, in addition to the patent for use, patents for chemical synthesis often further protect the investment that a company makes in development of a pesticide.

However, many natural products are so complex that the cost of chemical synthesis would be prohibitive. Even so, more economically synthesized analogues with adequate or even superior biological activity may tip the balance towards industrial synthesis. If not biosynthesis must be considered. There are a growing number of biosynthetic options.

The simplest method is to extract the compound from field-grown plants. To optimize production, the species and the variety of that species that produce the highest levels of the compound must be selected and grown under conditions that will optimize their biosynthetic capacity to produce the compound. Genetically manipulating the producing plants by classical or biotechnological methods could also increase production of some secondary products. For instance, low doses of diphenyl ether herbicides can cause massive increases in phytoalexins in a variety of crop species.

Another alternative is to produce the compound in tissue or cell culture. With these methods, cell lines that produce higher levels of the compound can be rapidly selected. However, genetic stability of such traits has been a problem in cell culture production of secondary products. Cells that produce and accumulate massive amounts of possibly autotoxic secondary compounds are obviously at a metabolic disadvantage and are thus selected against under many cell or tissue culture conditions. A technique, such as an immobilized cell column, that continuously removes secondary products can increase production by decreasing feedback inhibition of synthesis, reducing autotoxicity and possibly increasing generic stability. Other culture methods that optimize production can also be utilized. For instance, supplying inexpensively synthesized metabolic precursors can greatly enhance biosynthesis of many secondary products. Also, plant growth regulators, elicitors and metabolic blockers can be used to increase production.

Genetic engineering and biotechnology may allow for the production of plant-derived secondary products by gene transfer to microorganisms and production by fermentation. This concept is attractive because of the existing fermentation technology for production of secondary products. However, it may be prohibitively difficult for complex secondary products in which several genes control the conversion of several complex intermediates to the desired product.

Genetic engineering might also be used to insert the genetic information for production of plant-produced pesticides from one plant species to another species to be protected from pests. However, such transgenic manipulation of the complex metabolism of a higher plant might be extremely difficult. A simpler alternative might be to infect plant-colonizing microbes with the desired genetic machinery to produce the natural pesticide, as has been done with bacterial-produced insecticides.

30.6. THE FUTURE

Plants contain a virtually untapped reservoir of pesticides that can be used directly or as templates for synthetic pesticides. Numerous factors have increased the interest of the pesticide industry and the pesticide market in this source of natural products as pesticides. These include diminishing returns with traditional pesticide discovery methods, increased environmental and toxicological concerns with synthetic pesticides, and the high level of reliance of modern agriculture on pesticides. Despite the relatively small amount of previous effort in development of plant-derived compounds as pesticides, they have made a large impact in the area of insecticides. Minor successes can be found as herbicides, nematicides, rodenticides, fungicides and molluscicides. The number of options that must be considered in discovery and development of a natural product as a pesticide is larger than for a synthetic pesticide. Furthermore, the molecular complexity limited environmental stability, and low activity of many biocides from plants, compared to synthetic pesticides, is discouraging. However, advances in chemical and biotechnology are increasing the speed and ease with which man can discover and develop secondary compounds of plants as pesticides. These advances, combined with increasing need and environmental pressure, are greatly increasing the interest in plant products as pesticides.

Poisonous Plants

CONTENTS

31.1. INTRODUCTION

Spread over 1,575,107 square miles and endowed by nature with a wide variety of physical and climatological conditions, India possesses what is perhaps the richest and certainly the most varied flora of all other areas of similar size on globe. India has an area of culturable land of about 450 million acres, excluding a forest area of 83 million acres of which the total gross cropped area sown each year is approximately 285 million acres.

Plants are of great importance to us. India abounds in all kinds of food plants, spices, perfumes, timber, fibres, gums, etc., which have been known all over the world from ancient times. There are about 700 species of food and fodder plants including 260 species of valuable fodder grasses. Nearly 2000 species of medicinally active plants have been found in India.

Many other plants are also present which contain certain constituents which, if introduced in the body in relatively small quantity, act deleteriously and may cause serious impairment of body functions or even death. They primarily injure the basic living principle the protoplasm. These plants are known as poisonous plants.

Recent studies have revealed that in India there are about 700 poisonous species belonging to over 90 families of flowering plants. Some of these are Ranunculaceae, Euphorbiaceae, Leguminosae, Solanaceae, Compositae, Apocyanaceae, Asclepiadaceae, Liliaceae, Gramineae, Araceae, etc.

31.2. DEFINITION OF POISONOUS PLANTS

A poisonous plant is one which, as a whole or a part thereof, under all or certain conditions and in a manner and in amount to be taken or brought into contact with an organism will exert or cause death either immediately or by reason of cumulative action of the toxic property due to the presence of known or unknown chemical substance in it, and not by mechanical method.

The points which should be borne in mind before terming a plant as poisonous are:

1. The seeds of certain plants like aristida may pierce the skin giving rise to subcutaneous or intramuscular abscesses. These seed have bored into the salivary ducts of the cattle and caused injury. This action is purely mechanical, so it cannot be termed as poisonous plants.

2. All parts of the plant may not be poisonous. Seed of family Rosaceae contain dangerous amount of prussic acid but the outer fleshy portion of the fruit is eaten.

3. Certain plants are poisonous to one species and the same quantity may not affect the other species. Example; Belladonna is poisonous to most species but rodents like rabbit can have it in large quantities.

4. Some plants if eaten affect only a particular organ of the body. It does not cause serious body harm but render the organ unable to carry on their normal functions, e.g. *Senecio* of sunflower family causes hepatic cirrhosis in man and animals and prevent the liver from carrying out its normal functioning.

5. Certain plants loose their toxicity on being dried or cooked, e.g. species of Ranunculaceae is toxic in green state but can be used as food when dried.

6. Certain plants provide food but under certain conditions produce varying amount of poisonous substance, e.g. potato is a vegetable but at time of sprouting produces dangerous amount of solanine.

7. Certain plants like khesari (*Lathyrus sativus*) give rise to pathological conditions when fed in large doses for prolonged use.

31.3. TOXIC CONSTITUENTS OF THE PLANTS

By the metabolic activity the plants not only produce food material but also certain other substances such as alkaloids, glycosides, toxic proteins, bitter principles, etc. Many of these constituents are harmful to animal life, at least under certain conditions and the plants containing these principles which are capable of producing harmful effect are known as poisonous plants. These constituents can be divided into different groups:

1. *Vegetable Base:* It constitutes nitrogenous vegetable bases like amines, purines and alkaloids.

   (a) *Amines:* Derived from amino acid and are building materials for proteins. Gives poisonous character to certain mushrooms.

   (b) *Purines:* Form active principle of certain tropical plants such as tea, coffee, guaraila.

   (c) *Alkaloids:* Alkaloids form the most important group of vegetable base. These are complex heterocyclic nitrogenous compounds having a basic nature and are mostly tertiary amines. These have profound physiological action and in many cases are of intense poisonous nature. These plants contain bitter taste and sufficient protection from being eaten by cattle. Some of the poisonous alkaloids are—aconitine from aconite root, morphine from poppy capsules, emetine from ipecacuanha root, strychnine from nux vomica seeds, nicotine from tobacco leaves, curarine from curare, etc.

2. *Glycosides:* These are compounds which when split up with help of acids or enzymes yield a sugar and a carbohydrate known as aglycone. Among the glycosides, one of the important classes is cyanogenetic glycosides. These glycosides are harmless but give rise to toxic acids, e.g. amygdalin found in bitter almonds, phaseolunatin found in flax, prunasin found in wild cherry, etc. Some other glycosides which produce harmful components on hydrolysis are sinigrin in black mustard seeds, sinalbin in white mustard seed. Certain glycosides have direct toxic action such as digitoxin in Digitalis, cerberin in cerebra, thevetin in Thevetia, antiarin in Antiaris.

3. *Saponin:* Occurs in about 400 species belonging to 50 families. They are particularly toxic to cold blooded animals, such as fishes, frogs, insects, etc. Poisonous saponins are known as 'sapotoxins'.

4. *Bitter Principles:* These possess a bitter taste and are found in a number of plants. Bitter principle include the different aloe bitter, which are found in inspissate juice of several species of aloe. These possess a characteristic nauseous and bitter taste and have purgative action, e.g. Santonin—a lactone found in sonic species of Artemmisia, Picrotoxin from *Anamirta cocculus*.

5. *Toxic Proteins:* These are also known as toxalbumin and have been observed in Leguminosae and in Euphorbiaceae, e.g. Abrin from *Abrus precatorius*, ricinin from *Ricinus communis*, crotin from *Croton tiglium*. These toxalbumins are essentially blood poisons and are characterized by their property of agglutinating and precipitating the RBC's.

6. *Fixed Oils:* These are compounds of glycerol with different kind of fatty acids containing sterols and other substances dissolved in them when heated they decompose giving of acrid acrolein vapours. These are insoluble in water and sparingly soluble in alcohol, freely soluble in ether, chloroform, benzene, etc. These generally have laxative property. The croton oil expressed from the seeds of *Croton tiglium* produces irritation to the skin; the vesicating action of croton oil is due to resin dissolved in it.

7. *Essential Oils:* These are odourous principles which are generally responsible for the odour of plants.

They are generally found in combination with glycosides. They are volatile in steam. They sometime possess sharp burning taste, and locally have an irritating action. Large doses causes irritation to the GIT with diarrhoea, vomiting, pain, etc. They may cause haemorrhage and abortion, e.g. oils of juniper, savin, rue, parsley and pennyroyal. Some plants containing oils with toxic constituents are Artemisia, Ruta, Mentha, Petroselinum, Anemone, ranunculus, Piper, Ferula, etc.

8. *Organic Acids*: Organic acids significant in poisonous point of view is oxalic acid, protoplasmic poison occurring in large number of plants in form of oxalates. Formic acid an irritant is also found in some plants especially in family utricaceae.

31.4. FACTORS DETERMINING THE TOXICITY OF PLANTS

It is surprising that some plants are fairly harmless to humans and animals under certain conditions, while in certain circumstances, they may prove to be poisonous. Some species of plants when grown in different environment produce different amount of active principles. Variability in the poisonous content of the plant depends on various factors. Some of these are:

1. *Correct Identification*: Proper identification of the plants is very important and if there are several varieties of some species present each should be carefully examined in order to determine which contain highest amount of active principles, e.g. there are two forms of *Artemisia maritima* present; in early stages of growth one has deep reddish stem and other greyish. Both form brownish stems at maturity but it is only the form with deep reddish stem at early stages contains santonin.

2. *Stages of Growth*: The stages of growth of plants are perhaps the most important factor in determining the toxicity, e.g. sorghum when young and wild or stunted contain fatal quantity of hydrocyanic acid. The green berries of *Solanum nigrum* are harmful while the ripe one is edible. The unopened flower heads of *Artemisia maritima* yield greater amount of santonin than the opened ones.

3. *Condition of Plant*: Certain plants like potato and grasses which normally provide valuable food to man and animal may acquire toxic properties during sprouting; yams and certain aroids are poisonous when fresh, but lose their toxicity on drying or boiling.

4. *Soil and Cultivation*: Structure of soil, moisture present and temperature influence the metabolic activity of a plant. The difference in soil modifies the production of poison in plants, e.g. cinchona and oleander cultivation can enhance the active principles of the plants.

5. *Climatic Conditions*: Climatic conditions such as temperature, light, humidity may influence the metabolic properties of the plants. Ephedra contains large amount of active principles in areas of low rainfall. Alkaloid contents in these plants are less in rainy areas than in dry areas.

6. *Toxic Part of the Plant*: Different part of plant varies considerably in the amount of toxic principals contained in them. Thus the toxicity of the root, stem, leaves, flowers, fruits vary considerably even at same stage of growth. One part of the plant may he poisonous while other may not be, e.g. peach, plum kernels contain dangerous amount of hydrocyanic acid but outer portions of fruit are edible.

31.5. CLASSIFICATION OF POISONOUS PLANTS

Poisonous plants have been classified in a number of ways. The commonly acceptable classification is as follows.

Poisoning by Plants with Anticholinergic (Antimuscarinic) Poisons

Examples of plant genera associated with this syndrome:

Atropa	Brugmansia	Datura
Hyoscyamus	Solandra	Solanum

Toxic Mechanism: Competitive antagonism of acetylcholine at the muscarinic subtype of the acetylcholine receptor, which is primarily located in the parasympathetic nervous system and the brain.

ATROPA BELLADONNA L. (Fig. 31.1)

Family

Solanaceae.

Common Names

Belladonna, black nightshade, deadly nightshade, nightshade, sleeping nightshade.

Description

These perennial plants are about 3-feet high and are often cultivated in flower gardens. The stems are very branched with 6-inch ovate leaves. Solitary flowers, which emerge from the leaf axils, are blue-purple to dull red and about 1-inch long. The fruit is nearly globular, about 0.5 inch in diameter, and is purple to shiny black when mature. The root is a thick rhizome. The sap is reddish.

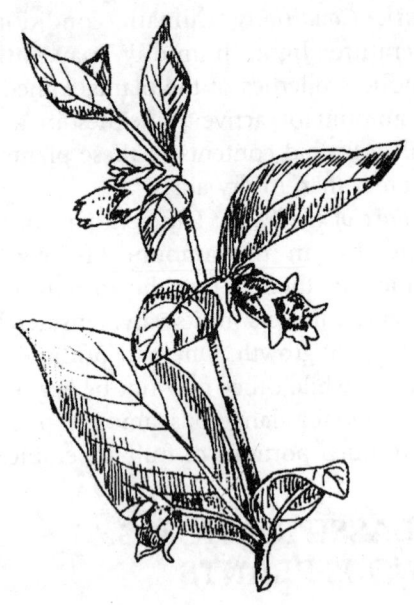

FIG. 31.1 *Atropa belladonna*

Toxic Part

The whole plant is toxic.

Toxins

Atropine, scopolamine and other anticholinergic alkaloids.

Clinical Findings

Intoxication results in dry mouth with dysphagia and dysphonia, tachycardia and urinary retention. Elevation of body temperature may be accompanied by flushed, dry skin. Mydriasis, blurred vision, excitement and delirium, headache and confusion may be observed.

Management

Initially, symptomatic and supportive care should be given. If the severity of the intoxication warrants intervention (hyperthermia, delirium), an antidote, physostigmine, is available. Consultation with a Poison Control Centre should be considered.

Poisoning by Plants with Calcium Oxalate Crystals

Examples of plant genera associated with this syndrome:

Alocasia	Arisaema	Brassaia
Caladium	Caryota	Colocasia
Dieffenbachia	Epipremnum	Monstera
Philodendron	Spathiphyllum	

Toxic Mechanism: Upon mechanical stimulation, as occurs with chewing, crystalline calcium oxalate needles, bundled in needle-like raphides, release from their intracellular packaging (idioblasts) in a projectile fashion. These needles penetrate the mucous membranes and induce the release of histamine and other inflammatory mediators.

ALOCASIA SPECIES (Fig. 31.2a and b)

Family

Araceae.

Common Names

Ahe Poi, Ape, Cabeza de Burro, Chine Ape, Elephant's Ear, Malanga Cara de Chivo, Malanga de Jardín, Papao-Apaka, Papao-Atolong, Taro.

Description

These erect perennials have single, long-stemmed, spearhead-shaped leaves that are prominently veined and often varicoloured. Flowers appear on a spadix subtended by a greenish spathe similar to *Colocasia*. Individual plants may develop from runners (rhizomes).

Toxic Part

The leaves, stems and tubers may be injurious.

Toxins

Raphides of water-insoluble calcium oxalate and unverified proteinaceous toxins.

Clinical Findings

A painful burning sensation of the lips and mouth result from ingestion. There is an inflammatory reaction, often with oedema and blistering. Hoarseness, dysphonia and dysphagia may result.

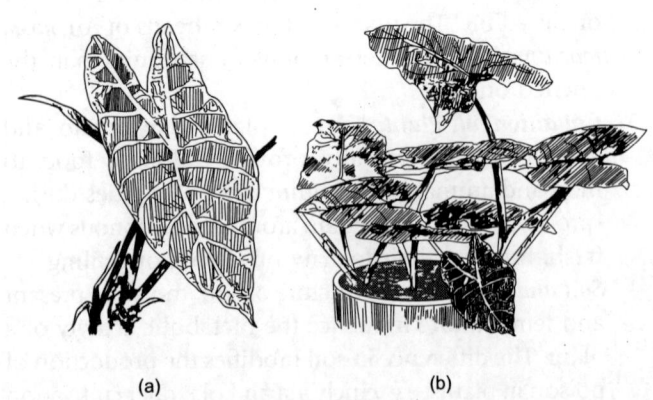

(a) (b)

FIG. 31.2 (a) *Alocasia watsoniana* and (b) *Alocasia macrorrhiza*

Management

The pain and oedema recede slowly without therapy. Cool liquids or demulcents held in the mouth may bring some relief. Analgesics may be indicated. The insoluble oxalate in these plants does not cause systemic oxalate poisoning. Consultation with a Poison Control Centre should be considered.

Poisoning by Plants with Cardioactive Steroids/Cardiac Glycosides

Examples of plant genera associated with this syndrome:

Acokanthera	Adenium	Adonis
Calotropis	Cryptostegia	Digitalis
Helleborus	Ornithogalum	Convallaria
Nerium	Pentalinon	Thevetia
Urginea	Strophanthus	Scilla

Toxic Mechanism: Cardioactive steroids, termed cardiac glycosides when sugar moieties are attached, inhibit the cellular Na^+/K^+-ATPase. The effect is to indirectly increase intracellular Ca^{2+} concentrations in certain cells, particularly myocardial cells. Therapeutically, this both enhances cardiac ionotropy (contractility) and slows the heart rate. However, excessive elevation of the intracellular Ca^{2+} also increases myocardial excitability, predisposing to the development of ventricular dysrhythmias. Enhanced vagal tone, mediated by the neurotransmitter acetylcholine, is common with poisoning by these agents, and produces bradycardia and heart block.

CALOTROPIS SPECIES

Family

Asclepiadaceae.
   Calotropis gigantea (L.) W. T. Aiton.
   Calotropis procera (Aiton) W. T. Aiton.

Common Names

Calotropis gigantea (Fig. 31.3a): Bowstring Hemp, crown flower, giant milkweed, mudar, mudar crown plant, pua kalaunu.
   Calotropis procera (Fig. 31.3b): Algodón de Seda, French jasmine, giant milkweed, mudar, mudar small crown flower, small crown flower, tula.

Description

These treelike shrubs have ovate or elliptical thick, glaucous, rubbery, opposite leaves. The flowers appear in clusters along the branches; they have a prominent crown with recurved petals and a sweet, pleasant odour. Colours vary from creamy white to lilac, mauve and purple. The seeds have silky attachments (like other types of milkweed seeds), which emerge from pods as they split on drying. The two species differ in size: *Calotropis gigantea* grows to 15 feet; *C. procera* generally grows to under 6 feet and has correspondingly more diminutive plant parts.

Toxic Part

The latex has a direct irritant action on mucous membranes, particularly in the eye. Skin reactions to this plant may be caused by allergy rather than to a direct irritant action. All parts of the plant contain a cardioactive steroid and calcium oxalate crystals.

Toxins

An unidentified vesicant allergen in the latex, calcium oxalate crystals and cardioactive steroids resembling digitalis.

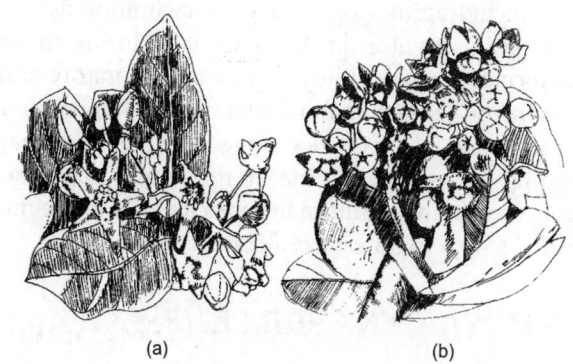

FIG. 31.3 (a) *Calotropis gigantea* (b) *Calotropis procera*

Clinical Findings

Human intoxications from this plant have not been reported in modern times. Ingestion of calcium oxalates causes a painful burning sensation of the lips and mouth. There is an inflammatory reaction, often with oedema and blistering. Hoarseness, dysphonia and dysphagia may result. Poisoning would be expected to produce clinical findings typical of cardioactive steroids. Toxicity has a variable latent period that depends on the quantity ingested. Dysrhythmias include sinus bradycardia, premature ventricular contractions, atrioventricular conduction defects or ventricular tachydysrhythmias. Hyperkalaemia, if present, may be an indicator of toxicity.

Management

Calcium oxalate toxicity: The pain and oedema recede slowly without therapy. Cool liquids or demulcents held in the mouth may bring some relief. Analgesics may be indicated. The insoluble oxalate in these plants does not cause systemic oxalate poisoning.

Poisoning by Plants with Convulsant Poisons (Seizure)

Examples of plant genera associated with this syndrome:

Aethusa	Anemone	Blighia
Caltha	Caulophyllum	Cicuta
Clematis	Conium	Coriaria
Gymnocladus	Hippobroma	Laburnum
Lobelia	Menispermum	Myoporum
Nicotiana	Pulsatilla	Ranunculus
Sophora	Spigelia	Strychnos

Toxic Mechanism: A convulsion is the rhythmic, forceful contraction of the muscles—one cause of which is seizures. Seizures are disorganized discharges of the central nervous system that generally, but not always, result in a convulsion. There are various toxicological mechanisms that result in seizures including antagonism of gamma-aminobutyric acid (GABA) at its receptor on the neuronal chloride channel, imbalance of acetylcholine homeostasis, excitatory amino acid mimicry, sodium channel alteration or hypoglycemia. Strychnine and its analogues antagonize the postsynaptic inhibiting activity of glycine at the spinal cord motor neuron. Strychnine results in hyperexcitability of the motor neurons, which manifests as a convulsion.

AETHUSA CYNAPIUM L. (Fig. 31.4)

Family

Umbelliferae (Apiaceae).

Common Names

Dog parsley, dog poison, false parsley, fool's cicely, fool's parsley, lesser hemlock, small hemlock.

Description

This carrot-like plant is 8–24 inch high. The leaves resemble parsley but have a glossy shine on both sides and an unpleasant garlic-like odour. The white flowers and seedpods are inconspicuous and are formed on the stem tips. As the common name suggests, this plant may be consumed if mistaken for parsley.

Toxic Part

The whole plant is poisonous.

Toxin

Unsaturated aliphatic alcohols (e.g. aethusanol A) closely related to cicutoxin (from *Cicuta* species) and traces of coniine.

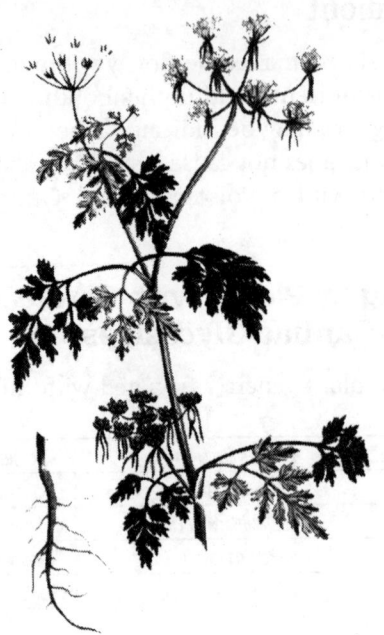

FIG. 31.4 *Aethusa cynapium*

Clinical Findings

Ingestion can cause nausea, vomiting, diaphoresis and headache. Toxicity resembles poisoning from cicutoxin. However, the concentration of toxin is insufficient to cause serious effects in most cases. If poisoning occurs, onset of effect is rapid, usually within 1 h of ingestion. Symptoms include nausea, vomiting, salivation and trismus. Generalized seizures also may occur. Death may occur if seizures do not terminate.

Management

If toxicity develops, supportive care—including airway management and protection against rhabdomyolysis and associated complications (e.g. electrolyte abnormalities and renal insufficiency)—is the mainstay of therapy. Rapidly acting anticonvulsants, (i.e. diazepam or lorazepam) for persistent seizures may be needed. Consultation with a Poison Control Centre should be considered.

Poisoning by Plants with Cyanogenic Compounds

Examples of plant genera associated with this syndrome:

Eriobotrya	Hydrangea	Malus
Prunus	Sambucus	

Toxic Mechanism: Cyanogenic compounds, most commonly glycosides, must be metabolized to release cyanide. Cyanide inhibits the final step of the mitochondrial electron transport chain, resulting rapidly in cellular energy failure.

MALUS SPECIES (Fig. 31.5)

Family

Rosaceae.

Common Names

Apple, Crabapple, Manzana, Pommier.

Description

The apple is a deciduous tree with flowers that form in simple clusters. The fruit is a pome with seeds.

Toxic Part

Seeds are poisonous.

Toxin

Amygdalin, a cyanogenic glycoside.

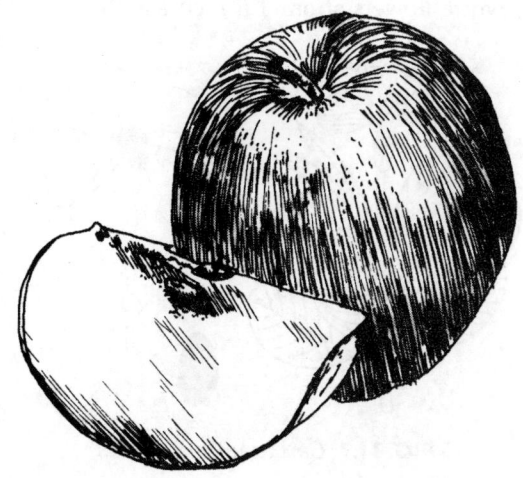

FIG. 31.5 Malus spp., fruit

Clinical Findings

Apple seeds that are swallowed whole or chewed and eaten in small quantities are harmless. A single case of fatal cyanide poisoning has been reported in an adult who chewed and swallowed a cup of apple seeds. Because the cyanogenic glycosides must be hydrolysed in the gastrointestinal tract before cyanide ion is released, several hours may elapse before poisoning occurs. Abdominal pain, vomiting, lethargy and sweating typically occur first. Cyanosis does not occur. In severe poisonings, coma develops and may be accompanied by convulsions and cardiovascular collapse.

Management

Symptomatic and supportive care should be given. Antidotal therapy is available. Consultation with a Poison Control Centre is strongly suggested.

Poisoning by Plants with Gastrointestinal Toxins

Many and various plant genera are associated with this syndrome.

Pachyrhizus	Phytolacca	Ranunculus
Pedilanthus	Physalis	Sapindus

Toxic Mechanism: Several different mechanisms are utilized by plant toxin to produce gastrointestinal effects, generally described as either mechanical irritation or a pharmacologic effect. Irritant toxins indirectly stimulate contraction of the gastrointestinal smooth muscle. The pharmacologically active agents most commonly work by stimulation of cholinergic receptors in the gastrointestinal tract to induce smooth muscle contraction, e.g. cholinergic, including nicotine-like alkaloids. Some plant toxins, e.g. mitotic inhibitors, toxalbumins alter the normal development and turnover of gastrointestinal lining cells and induce sloughing of this cellular layer. Hepatotoxins may directly injure the liver cells, commonly through the production of oxidant metabolites. Indirect hepatotoxicity may occur, as with the pyrrolizidine alkaloids.

SAPINDUS SPECIES

Family

Sapindaceae.
Sapindus saponaria L.
Sapindus drummondii.

Common Names

Sapindus saponaria (Fig. 31.6): A'e, Bois Savonnette, False Dogwood, Indian Soap Plant, Jaboncillo, Manele, Savonnier, Soapberry, Wild China Tree, Wingleaf.
Sapindus drummondii: Western Soapberry, Soapberry.

Description

Sapindus drummondii: A deciduous tree growing to 50-feet tall with pinnate leaves containing eight to ten leaflets, each about 3-inch long. Flowers are small, yellowish-white, in panicles. Fruits are yellow, turning black, up to 0.5 inch long.

Sapindus saponaria: A tropical evergreen tree growing to 30 feet, leaves with seven to nine leaflets, each 4-inch long. Flowers are white and fruits are shiny orange-brown, about 0.75 inch in diameter. The fruit of these species has been employed as soap.

Toxic Part

The fruit is poisonous.

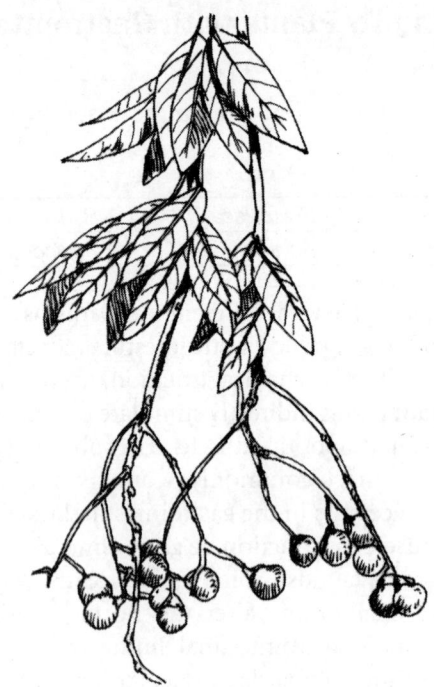

FIG. 31.6 *Sapindus saponaria*

Toxin

Saponin, a gastrointestinal irritant, and a dermal irritant/sensitizer.

Clinical Findings

Most ingestions result in little or no toxicity. The saponins are poorly absorbed, but with large exposures gastrointestinal effects of nausea, vomiting, abdominal cramping and diarrhoea may occur. Allergic sensitization to this plant is common and can cause severe dermatitis.

Management

If severe gastrointestinal effects occur, intravenous hydration, antiemetics and electrolyte replacement may be necessary, particularly in children. Consultation with a Poison Control Centre should be considered.

Poisoning by Plants with Mitotic Inhibitors

Examples of plant genera associated with this syndrome:

Bulbocodium	Catharanthus	Colchicum
Gloriosa	Podophyllum	

Toxic Mechanism: These agents interfere with the polymerization of microtubules, which must polymerize for mitosis to occur, leading to metaphase arrest. Rapidly dividing cells, e.g. gastrointestinal or bone marrow cells typically are affected earlier and to a greater extent than those cells that divide slowly. In addition, microtubules are important in the maintenance of proper neuronal function.

CATHARANTHUS ROSEUS (Fig. 31.7)

Family

Apocynaceae.

Common Names

Madagascar periwinkle, Bigleaf Periwinkle, Large Periwinkle, Periwinkle, Vinca (formerly known as *Vinca rosea*).

Description

The Madagascar periwinkle is a perennial herb with milky sap that is often cultivated on an annual basis. It has erect stems that bear dark glossy green, opposite, oblong-lanceolate leaves, 1–2 inch long, and bear solitary rose pink to white flowers about 1.5 inch across.

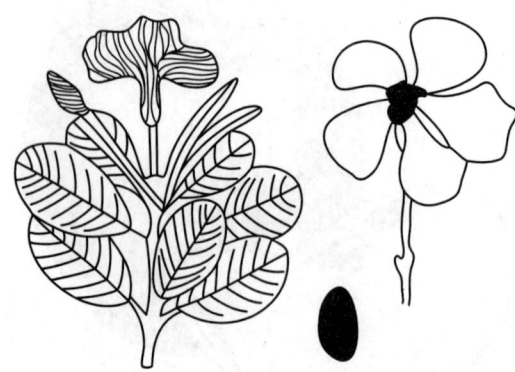

FIG. 31.7 *Catharanthus roseus*

Toxic Part

The whole plant is poisonous. A tea made from the leaves and stems is used in folk medicine in the Caribbean and elsewhere.

Toxins

Vinca alkaloids, e.g. vincristine, clinically similar to colchicine—a cytotoxic alkaloid capable of inhibiting microtubule formation.

Clinical Findings

Ingestion may cause initial oropharyngeal pain followed in several hours by intense gastrointestinal symptoms. Abdominal pain and severe, profuse and persistent diarrhoea may develop causing extensive fluid depletion and its sequelae. Vinca alkaloids may subsequently produce peripheral neuropathy, bone marrow suppression and cardiovascular collapse.

Management

Aggressive symptomatic and supportive care is critical, with prolonged observation of symptomatic patients. Consultation with a Poison Control Centre should be strongly considered.

Poisoning by Plants with Nicotine-Like Alkaloids

Examples of plant genera associated with this syndrome:

Nicotiana	Caulophyllum	Conium
Gymnocladus	Hippobroma	Laburnum
Lobelia	Baptisia	Sophora

Toxic Mechanism: These agents are direct acting agonists at the nicotinic subtype of the acetylcholine receptor in the ganglia of both the parasympathetic and sympathetic limbs of the autonomic nervous system (NN receptors), the neuromuscular junction (NM receptors) and the brain.

NICOTIANA SPECIES (Fig. 31.8)

Family

Solanaceae.
Nicotiana attenuata Torr. ex S. Watson.
Nicotiana glauca Graham.
Nicotiana longiflora Cav.
Nicotiana rustica L.
Nicotiana tabacum L.

Common Names

Paka, Tabac, Tabaco, Tobacco.

Description

Nicotiana species may be annual or perennial; the latter generally are large shrubs or small trees. The five-lobed flowers, in large terminal panicles, are distinctively tubular, flare at the mouth, and may be white, yellow, greenish-yellow or red. The fruit is a capsule with many minute seeds. The leaves are simple and alternate, usually have smooth edges and often are broad, hairy and sticky.

Toxic Part

The whole plant is poisonous.

Toxin

The specific toxin depends on the species but involves chemically related alkaloids, for example, nicotine in *Nicotiana tabacum* and anabasine in *N. glauca*.

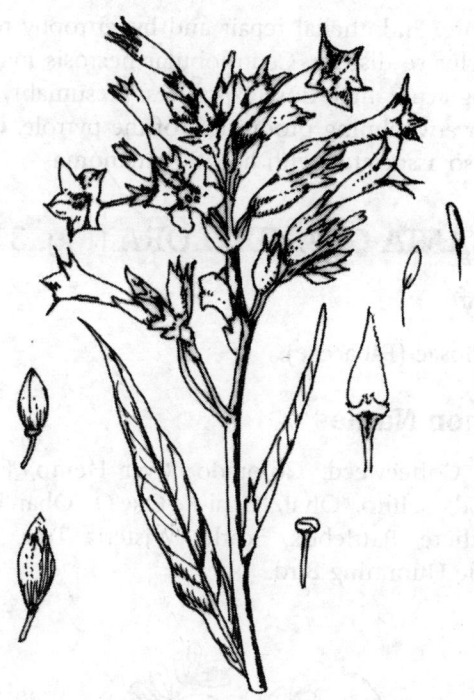

FIG. 31.8 *Nicotiana tabacum*

Clinical Findings

Acute intoxications result from ingestion of the leaves as a salad (particularly *Nicotiana glauca*) from the use of *N. tabacum* infusions in enemas as a home remedy, from the cutaneous absorption of the alkaloid during commercial tobacco harvesting, or from the ingestion of cigarettes or purified nicotine. Initial gastrointestinal symptoms may be followed by those typical of nicotine poisoning; these include hypertension, large pupils, sweating and perhaps seizures. Severe poisoning produces coma, weakness and paralysis that may result in death from respiratory failure.

Management

Symptomatic and supportive care should be given, with attention to adequacy of ventilation and vital signs. Atropine may reverse some of the toxic effects. Consultation with a Poison Control Centre should be strongly considered.

Poisoning by Plants with Pyrrolizidine Alkaloids

Examples of plant genera associated with this syndrome:

Crotalaria	Echium	Heliotropium
Senecio	Sesbania	

Toxic Mechanism: Pyrrolizidine alkaloids are metabolized to pyrroles, which are alkylating agents that injure the endothelium of the hepatic sinusoids or pulmonary vasculature. Endothelial repair and hypertrophy result in veno-occlusive disease. Centrilobular necrosis may occur following acute, high-dose exposures, presumably caused by the overwhelming production of the pyrrole. Chronic use is also associated with hepatic carcinoma.

SESBANIA GRANDIFLORA (Fig. 31.9)

Family

Leguminosae (Fabaceae).

Common Names

Báculo, Coffeeweed, Colorado River Hemp, Egyptian Rattlepod, Gallito, 'Ohai, 'Ohai-Ke'Oke'O, 'Ohai-'Ula'Ula, Pois Valière, Rattlebox, Scarlet Wisteria Tree, Sesban, Vegetable Humming Bird.

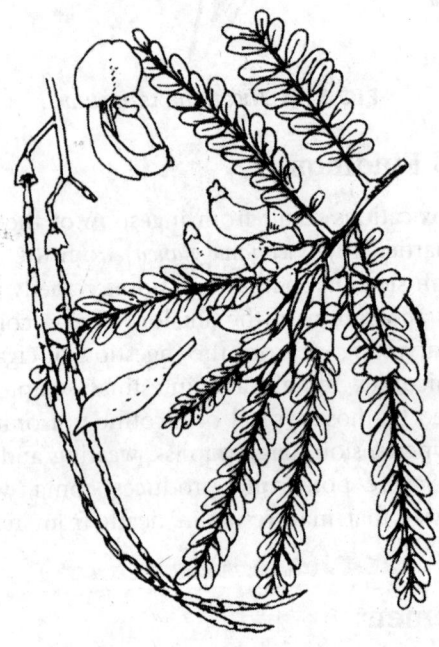

FIG. 31.9 *Sesbania grandiflora*

Description

These annuals have green stems 3–8 feet tall that become woody; the entire plant can be shrublike. The compound leaves have numerous linear leaflets. The small, sweetpea-shaped flowers are yellow dotted with purple. The fruits are curved seed pods.

Toxic Part

All parts of this plant are poisonous.

Toxin

Pyrrolizidine alkaloids.

Clinical Findings

There are no adequately documented human poisonings, and clinical descriptions are based on the nature of the toxin. Substantial short-term exposure may cause acute hepatitis, and chronic exposure to lower levels may cause hepatic veno-occlusive disease (Budd–Chiari syndrome), and in some cases pulmonary hypertension.

Management

There is no known antidote. Supportive care is the mainstay of therapy. Consultation with a Poison Control Centre should be considered.

Poisoning by Plants with Sodium Channel Activators

Examples of plant genera associated with this syndrome:

Aconitum	Kalmia	Leucothoe
Lyonia	Pernettya	Pieris
Rhododendron	Schoenocaulon	Veratrum

Toxic Mechanism: These agents stabilize the open form of the voltage-dependent sodium channel in excitable membranes, such as neurons and the cardiac conducting system. This causes persistent sodium influx (i.e. persistent depolarization) and prevents adequate repolarization leading to seizures and dysrhythmias, respectively. In the heart, the excess sodium influx activates calcium exchange, and the intracellular hypercalcemia increases both ionotropy and the potential for dysrhythmias.

ACONITUM SPECIES (Fig. 31.10)

Family

Ranunculaceae.
   Aconitum columbianum Nutt.
   Aconitum napellus L.
   Aconitum reclinatum Gray.
   Aconitum uncinatum L.

Common Names

Aconite, Friar's Cap, Helmet Flower, Monkshood, Soldier's Cap, Trailing Monkshood, Wild Monkshood, Wolfsbane.

Description

These perennial plants are usually erect, sometimes branched, 2–6 feet in height and have tuberous roots. They resemble delphiniums. The char acteristic helmet-shaped flowers grow in a raceme at the top of the stalk and appear in summer or autumn. The flowers are usually blue but may be white, pink or flesh toned. The dried seedpods contain numerous tiny seeds. *Aconitum napellus* is the commonly cultivated monkshood.

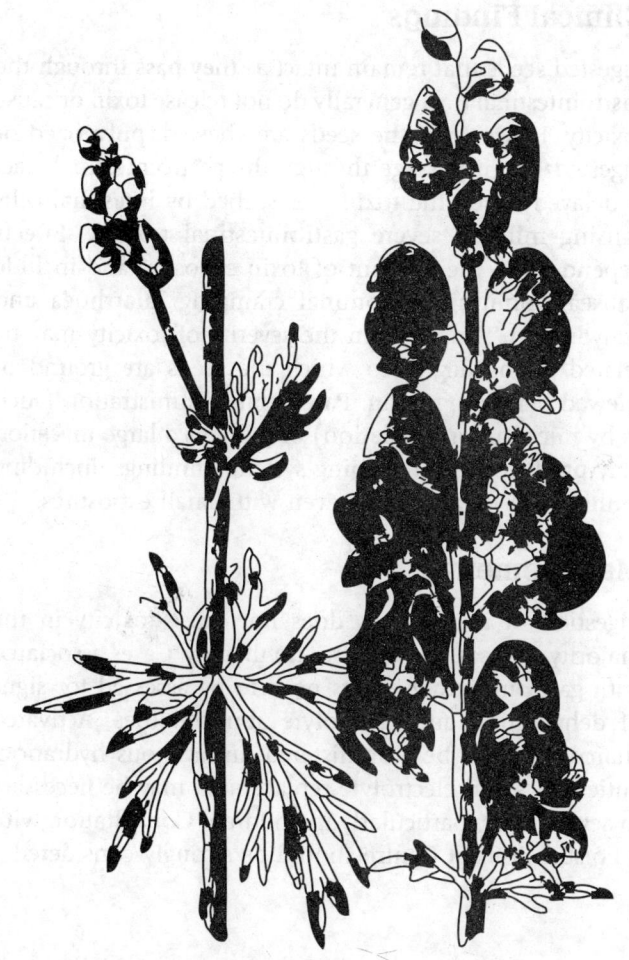

FIG. 31.10 *Aconitum napellus*

Toxic Part

The whole plant is poisonous, especially the leaves and roots.

Toxin

Aconitine and related alkaloids, sodium channel activators.

Clinical Findings

Exposures are relatively uncommon. However, these plants are utilized in some herbal products (e.g. chuanwu, caowu, fuzi). Symptoms are predominantly neurological and cardiac. There is transient burning in the mouth after ingestion, followed after several hours by increased salivation, vomiting, diarrhoea and a tingling sensation in the skin (paresthesia). The patient may complain of headache, muscular weakness and dimness of vision. Bradycardia and other cardiac dysrhythmias can be associated with severe blood pressure abnormalities. Coma may develop, and convulsions may be a terminal event.

Management

Fluid replacement should be instituted with respiratory support if indicated. Heart rhythm and blood pressure should be monitored and treated with appropriate medications and supportive care. Recovery is generally complete within 24 h. Consultation with a Poison Control Centre should be strongly considered.

Poisoning by Plants with Toxalbumins

Examples of plant genera associated with this syndrome:

Momordica	Ricinus	Abrus
Jatropha	Phoradendron	Robinia

Toxic Mechanism: The protein toxins derived from these plants work specifically by inhibiting the function of ribosomes—the subcellular organelle responsible for protein synthesis. The toxins typically have two linked polypeptide chains. One of the chains binds to cell surface glycoproteins to allow endocytosis into the cell. The other chain upon cell entry binds the 60S ribosomal subunit and impairs its ability to synthesize protein.

RICINUS COMMUNIS L. (Fig. 31.11)

Family

Euphorbiaceae.

Common Names

African Coffee Tree, Castor Bean, Castor Oil Plant, Higuereta, Higuerilla, Koli, La'Au-'Aila, Man's Motherwort, Mexico Weed, Pa'Aila, Palma Christi, Ricin, Ricino, Steadfast, Wonder Tree.

Description

The annual growth is up to 15 feet or higher in the tropics. The large, lobed leaves are up to 3 feet across. It is also grown as a summer ornamental in temperate areas, where, depending on the cultivar, the leaves can be green to red-purple. Spiny fruits form in clusters along spikes. The fruits contain plump seeds resembling fat ticks in shape, usually mottled black or brown on white. The highly toxic seeds have a pleasant taste.

Toxic Part

The toxin is contained within the hard, water-impermeable coat of the seeds. The toxin is not released unless the

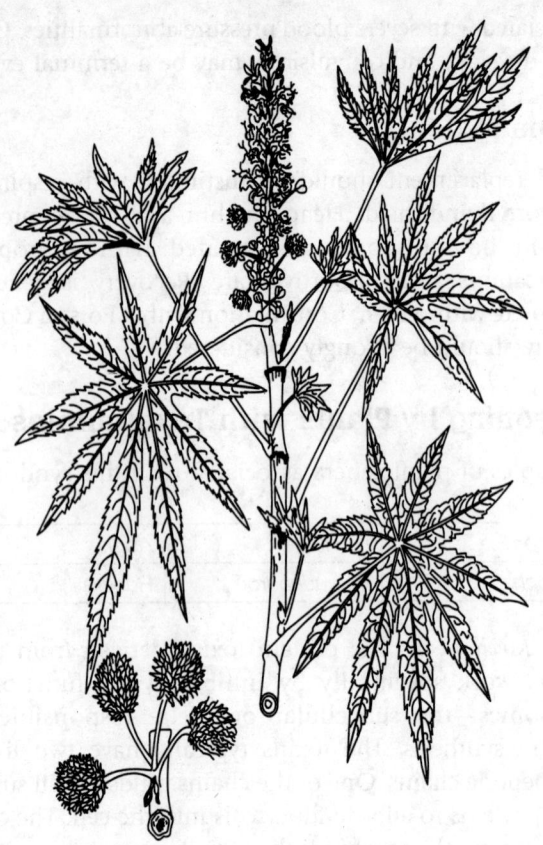

FIG. 31.11 *Ricinus communis*

seed coats are broken (e.g. chewed) and the contents digested.

Toxin

Ricin.

Clinical Findings

Ingested seeds that remain intact as they pass through the gastrointestinal tract generally do not release toxin or cause toxicity. However, if the seeds are chewed, pulverized or digested (i.e. if passage through the gastrointestinal tract is delayed), then the toxin is absorbed by intestinal cells causing mild to severe gastrointestinal toxicity. Effects depend upon the amount of toxin exposure and include nausea, vomiting, abdominal cramping, diarrhoea and dehydration. Variations in the severity of toxicity may be related to the degree to which the seeds are ground or chewed before ingestion. Parenteral administration (such as by injection or inhalation) or perhaps a large ingestion may produce life-threatening systemic findings, including multisystem organ failure, even with small exposures.

Management

Ingestion of intact seeds does not cause toxicity in the majority of cases and requires no therapy. Cases associated with gastrointestinal effects need to be assessed for signs of dehydration and electrolyte abnormalities. Activated charcoal should be administered. Intravenous hydration, antiemetics and electrolyte replacement may be necessary in severe cases, particularly in children. Consultation with a Poison Control Centre should be strongly considered.

Natural Allergens

CONTENTS

32.1. ALLERGENS

Allergens are inciting agents of allergy, i.e. the substances capable of sensitizing the body in such a way that an unusual response occurs in hypersensitive person. Allergen may be biologic, chemical or of synthetic origin. It is common to speak about the substances, such as pollens, danders, dust, etc., as natural allergens. Although the chemical identity of allergen is unknown, but most known allergens are protein or glycoprotein and do not have much difference from other immunogens except perhaps being somewhat smaller in size (mol. wt. 10,000–70,000). Most allergenic substances are mixture in composition. Allergens from related sources often are similar chemically and cross allergenic.

A number of low molecular weight chemicals (allergenic haptens) are partial immunogens and induce allergy after combining covalently with a suitable protein carrier, viz. drug allergy.

32.2. WHAT IS ALLERGY

The allergy (hypersensitivity) may be defined as a specific immunologic reaction to an immunogen—a normally harmless substance (allergen). It was first defined in 1906 by von Pirquet who described allergy as changed or altered reaction in the body of an individual, in response to a substance or condition that is harmless to others.

Sneezing is always considered to be a symptom of a cold but sometimes it is an allergic reaction to some thing in the air. According to reports available approximately 30% population suffers from some sort of allergic syndrome. However, few persons develop symptoms that are sufficiently severe to require the services of allergist or physician. The occurrence of allergic disease is determined by the characteristic of the individual as well as those of the allergen and even the condition of exposure.

Following are predisposing factors which make the person hypersensitive to allergens:

1. Hereditary tendency to allergic response
2. Dysfunction of the endocrine glands
3. Increased excitability of sympathetic and parasympathetic nervous systems
4. Absorption of metabolic and catabolic substances
5. Hepatic dysfunction
6. Psychic influences

32.3. TYPES OF ALLERGENS

The allergens can be classified on the basis of types of symptoms, which depend on the shock organs affected by the particular allergens and its route of entry into the body:

1. Inhalant allergens
2. Ingestant allergens
3. Injectant allergens
4. Contactant allergens
5. Infectant allergens

Inhalant Allergens

Inhalant allergens are airborne substances as chemicals, causing respiratory disease, inflammation in the nose and lungs. Inflammation in the nose is manifested by sneezing, lacrimation, itching and swelling of nose and eyes. The condition is known as sinusitis or hay fever. The odour emanating from new-mown hay is often responsible for the fever or stuffiness of the nasal passages. Inflammation of lungs is often expressed as asthma. Air pollution, both indoor and outdoor, plays a significant role in the aggravation of airway disease in the asthmatics and may contribute to the overall increase in asthma morbidity.

Symptoms of allergies to airborne substances are following:

1. Sneezing often accompanied by a runny or clogged nose
2. Coughing and postnasal drip
3. Itching eyes, nose and throat
4. Allergic shiner (dark circles under the eyes caused by increased blood flow near the sinuses)
5. The 'allergic salute' (in a child, persistent upward rubbing of the nose that causes mark on the nose)
6. Watering eyes, conjunctivitis (an inflammation of the membrane that lines the eye lids causing red-rimmed, swollen eyes and crusting the eyelids)

As soon as the allergens land on mucous membrane, an inside lining of the nose, a chain reaction occurs that leads the mast cells in these tissue to release histamine and other chemicals. These powerful chemical contract certain cells of some small blood vessels in the nose, which allow fluid to escape causing the nasal passage to swell resulting in nasal congestions.

The allergens that can cause airborne allergies (inhalant allergens) include pollens, dust, mites, mould spores and animal allergy (epidermis or dander).

Pollen allergens

Pollens are the tiny, egg-shaped, round, angular, square, rectangular or otherwise shaped male cells (organ) of flowering plants. These microscopic, powdery granules are necessary for plant fertilization. The average pollen particle size is less than the width of an average human hair.

Most pollen grains are single entities but some may be two-compound, three-compound, tetrad or so forth. They may either have no germinal apertures as such (a colpate) or have many pores (multicolpate) or range in between (dicolpate, tricolpate, tetracolpate). The surface appearance of outer wall (exine) is characteristic; it may range from smooth (psilate) to spiny (echinate) with various intervening gradations (reticulate granulate, cophate).

These pollens can be further classified into two types:

1. Anemophilous (wind pollinated)
2. Entomophilous (insect pollinated)

Anemophilous: Anemophilous pollens are usually small 15–45 μm in diameter, light, nonadhesive and relatively smooth and are produced by plain looking plants, e.g. trees (oak and walnut), grasses (bermuda grass and timothy) and weeds (ragweed and plantain).

Entomophilous: Entomophilous pollens are usually larger in size (up to 200 μm in diameter), heavier, adhesive and may be somewhat spiny. Plants are scented, with coloured flowers such as clover, hollyhock, honey suckle and rose.

Most common allergic reactions are produced by wind-pollinated (anemophilous) pollens, because of their light weight and the dry nature; these pollen grains are carried for long distances.

List of plant or tree producing pollens (allergens):

Alfalfa, almond, apple, acacia, barley, blue grass, canary grass, cherry, eucalyptus, gladiolus, hazelnut, juniper, mulberry, mustard, lemon and related species of citrus.

Ingestant Allergens

Allergens which are present in food stuff and swallowed are termed ingestant (food allergy). A food allergy is an immune system response to a food. Once the immune system decides that a particular food is harmful, it creates specific antibody to it.

The gastrointestinal symptoms are mainly affected by the food allergens, but they also cause skin rash, puffed lips and tongue, migraine, rhinitis or other symptoms like severe eczema of hand and feet. The effects of food allergens are not localized to one organ or area of the body, but it may transfer to other organs by the blood. Thus, an atopic dermatitis, such as tomato rash, strawberry rash, or that caused by eating oranges, chocolate or shellfish, is developed by patients.

Some most common food allergens ingested by patients are milk, egg, peanut, tree nut (walnut, cashew nut, etc.), fish, shellfish, soy, wheat, orange juice, cod liver oil or other vitamins containing fish liver oils. In addition to the above-mentioned normal food, there are food additive, which also could be allergic to any individual, viz. mannitol, sorbitol, polysorbates, malt-dextrins, citrus, bioflavonoids, artificial preservatives, artificial colours, citrus pectin, talc, soy lecithin, gluten, soy flour, rice flour, alfalfa, potato starch and gum acacia.

Most satisfactory method of combating food allergens is elimination of the offending substance from the diet. Dairy milk allergy is a specific immunologic antibody–antigen reaction due to a lactoalbumin, because heating and boiling alter this protein. Milk allergy may result in severe dermatitis, recurrent rhinorrhoea, bronchitis and asthma. Its antigenicity can be avoided by the use of commercial milk substitutes that are prepared from soya bean isolates.

Injectant Allergens

Injectant allergens cause symptoms similar to those of the antibiotics, e.g. penicillin, cephalosporin and semisynthetic penicillin, etc. Itching of the palms of the hands and the soles of the feet, erythema and peeling of the skin are characteristic. In severe cases anaphylactic shock may occur.

The natural sources of injectable allergens are produced by the sting of bees, hornets and wasps. The allergens injected by the stings of such insects can induce severe local and constitutional reactions sometimes causing death.

In addition to penicillin products, other injectable that may cause allergies are liver extract, antitoxins and the glandular products.

Contactant Allergens

A number of plants and their products have been identified as the causes of contact allergies. The plant most responsible for contact dermatitis in North America belongs to the Ancardiaceae family, primarily the genus Toxicodendron (Rhus) and includes poison ivy, oak and sumac. The allergen component of these plants, called urushiols (a phenolic compound) are found in the oleoresin fraction and are derivatives of pentadecylcatechol or heptadecylcatechol. Many plants of compositae family, which include the ragweeds, also cause contact dermatitis and the allergens responsible had been identified as Sesquiterpenoids lactone.

Other plants species, which can give rise to contact allergic reactions are *Ruta graveolens*, asparagus, ornamental 'dumb cane' *(Dieffenbachia seguine)*, buck wheat, butter cups, catalpa leaves, chrysanthemums, ginkgo leaves, lobelia, marigolds, may-apple, osage orange, flowering spurge, snow on the mountains and smart weeds.

Infectant Allergens

Allergy caused by the metabolic product of living microorganism in the human body, such as the continual presence of certain types of bacteria, protozoas, moulds, helminthes and other parasites in the body of human being that are responsible for chronic infection for which patients are not aware. Often the metabolic product of their growth causes some patient sensitized and the patient may exhibit allergic symptoms, which does not response positively to routine skin test for inhalant allergens. In such patients, bacterial metabolic wastes are considered to be infectant allergens.

The continuous presence of growth products and metabolic waste of parasitic organism such as hookworms, tape worms, pinworms, threadworms and dermatophytes are referred as infectant allergens.

Natural Colours and Dyes

CONTENTS

33.1. INTRODUCTION

To understand the concepts of natural dyes and dye-yielding plants, there are three basic questions to be addressed: Why only certain plants are able to yield dyes? How does the plant benefit by producing dyes? What is the evolutionary explanation for production of dyes? Answers to the first two questions can be substantiated with two further questions, i.e. 'Why do plants have so many different colours?' and 'What purpose might they serve for the plant?' Green in most leaves is surely the most ubiquitous plant colour. The green pigment chlorophyll in leaves helps capture the sun's energy and converts it to chemical energy, which is then stored and used as food for the plant. Colours in flowers are adaptations that attract insects and other animals that in turn pollinate and help the plants reproduce. Some plants have colourful fruits that attract animals to eat them, thus inadvertently spreading the plant's seeds as they do so. Scientists believe that other pigments may help protect plants from diseases. Despite what we know about the role of a few of the thousands of plant pigments, the role of most colours in plants remains a mystery to us till date.

Although plants exhibit a wide range of colours, not all of these pigments can be used as dyes. Some do not dissolve in water, some cannot be adsorbed on to fibres, whereas others fade when washed or exposed to air or sunlight. It remains a mystery: Why plants reward us with vibrant dyes? India has a rich biodiversity and it is not only one of the world's 12 mega-diversity countries, but also one of the eight major centres of origin and diversification of domesticated taxa. It has approximately 490,000 plant species of which about 17,500 are angiosperms; more than 400 are domesticated crop species and almost an equal number their wild relatives.

Thus, India harbours a wealth of useful germ plasm resources and there is no doubt that the plant kingdom is a treasure house of diverse natural products. One such product from nature is the dye. Natural dyes are environment friendly, for example, turmeric—the brightest of naturally occurring yellow dyes—is a powerful antiseptic which revitalizes the skin, while indigo gives a cooling sensation.

Natural Colours and Dyes

After the accidental synthesis of mauveine by Perkin in Germany in 1856, and its subsequent commercialization, coal tar dyes began to compete with natural dyes. The advent of synthetic dyes caused rapid decline in the use of natural dyes, which were completely replaced by the former within a century.

However, research has shown that synthetic dyes are suspected to release harmful chemicals that are allergic, carcinogenic and detrimental to human health. Ironically, in 1996, Germany became the first country to ban certain azo dyes.

In this chapter, we review the origin of natural dyes, plants and animals yielding dyes, chemical nature of these dyes, their advantages with limitation, technology involved with natural dyes production and present status of these dyes.

33.2. HISTORY

Natural dyes, dyestuff and dyeing are as old as textiles themselves. Man has always been interested in colours; the art of dyeing has a long past and many of the dyes go back into prehistory. It was practised during the Bronze Age in Europe. The earliest written record of the use of natural dyes was found in China dated 2600 B.C. Dyeing was known as early as in the Indus Valley period (2500 B.C.); this knowledge has been substantiated by findings of coloured garments of cloth and traces of madder dye in the ruins of the Indus Valley Civilization at Mohenjo-daro and Harappa (3500 B.C.). Natural matter was used to stain hides, decorate shells and feathers, and in cave paintings. Scientists have been able to date the black, white, yellow and reddish pigments made from ochre used by primitive man in cave paintings. In Egypt, mummies have been found wrapped in dyed cloth. Chemical tests of red fabrics found in the tomb of King Tutankhamen in Egypt show the presence of alizarin—a pigment extracted from madder. In more modern times, Alexander the Great mentioned having found purple robes dating to 541 B.C. in the royal treasury when he conquered Susa, the Persian capital. Kermes (from the Kermes insect) is identified in the *Book of Exodus* in the *Bible*, where references are made to scarlet coloured linen. By the 4th century A.D., dyes such as woad, madder, weld, Brazilwood, indigo and a dark reddish-purple were known. Brazil was named after the woad found there.

Henna was used even before 2500 B.C., while saffron is mentioned in the *Bible*. The first use of the blue dye, woad, by the ancient Britons may have originated in Palestine, where it was found growing wild. The most famous and highly prized colour through the ages was Tyrian purple (noted in the *Bible*)—a dye obtained from the spiny dyemurex shellfish. The Phoenicians prepared it until the seventh century, when Arab conquerors destroyed their dyeing installations in the Levant. In the prehistoric times man used to crush berries to colour mud for his cave paintings. Primitive men used plant dyestuff for colouring animal skin and to their own skin during religious festivals as well as during wars. They believed that the colour would give them magical powers, protect them from evil spirits and help them to achieve victory in war.

Dyes might have been discovered accidentally, but their use has become so much a part of man's customs that it is difficult to imagine a modern world without dyes. The art of dyeing spread widely as civilization advanced.

Primitive dyeing techniques included sticking plants to fabric or rubbing crushed pigments into cloth. The methods became more sophisticated with time and techniques using natural dyes from crushed fruits, berries and other plants, which were boiled into the fabric and which gave light and water fastness (resistance), were developed. Some of the well-known ancient dyes include madder, a red dye made from the roots of the *Rubia tinctorum L.*, blue indigo from the leaves of *Indigofera tinctoria L.*, yellow from the stigmas of the saffron plant (*Crocus sativus L.*) and from turmeric (*Curcuma longa L.*). Today, dyeing is a complex and specialized science. Nearly all dyestuffs are now produced from synthetic compounds. This means that costs have been greatly reduced and certain application and wear characteristics have been greatly enhanced. However, practitioners of the craft of natural dying (i.e. using naturally occurring sources of dye) maintain that natural dyes have a far superior aesthetic quality, which is much more pleasing to the eye. On the other hand, many commercial practitioners feel that natural dyes are non-viable on grounds of both quality and economics. In the West, natural dyeing is now practised only as a handcraft, while synthetic dyes are being used in all commercial applications. Some craft spinners, weavers and knitters use natural dyes as a particular feature of their work.

33.3. TYPES OF NATURAL DYES AND MORDANTS

Natural dyes can be sorted into three categories: natural dyes obtained from plants, animals and minerals. Although some fabrics such as silk and wool can be coloured simply by being dipped in the dye, others such as cotton require a mordant.

Mordant

Dyes do not interact directly with the materials they are intended to colour. Natural dyes are substantive and require a mordant to fix to the fabric, and prevent the colour from either fading with exposure to light or washing out. These compounds bind the natural dyes to the fabrics. A mordant is an element which aids the chemical reaction that takes place between the dye and the fibre so that the dye is absorbed. Containers used for dying must be non-reactive (enamel, stainless steel). Brass, copper or iron pots will do their own mordanting.

Not all dyes need mordants to help them adhere to fabric. If they need no mordants, such as lichens and walnut hulls, they are called substantive dyes. If they need a mordant, they are called adjective dyes. Common mordants are alum (usually used with cream of tartar, which helps evenness and brightens slightly); iron (or copper) (which saddens or darken colours, bringing out green shades); tin (usually used with cream of tartar, which blooms or brightens colours, especially reds, oranges and yellows); and blue vitriol (which saddens colours and brings out greens shades).

There are three types of mordant:

1. *Metallic mordants*: Metal salts of aluminium, chromium, iron, copper and tin are used.
2. *Tannins*: Myrobalan and sumach are commonly used in the textile industry.
3. *Oil mordants*: These are mainly used in dyeing turkey red colour from madder. The main function of the oil mordant is to form a complex with alum used as the main mordent.

33.4. NATURAL DYES OBTAINED FROM PLANTS

Many natural dyestuff and stains were obtained mainly from plants and dominated as sources of natural dyes, producing different colours like red, yellow, blue, black, brown and a combination of these (Table 33.1). Almost all parts of the plants like root, bark, leaf, fruit, wood, seed, flower, etc., produce dyes. It is interesting to note that over 2000 pigments are synthesized by various parts of plants, of which only about 150 have been commercially exploited. Nearly 450 taxa are known to yield dyes in India alone, of which 50 are considered to be the most important; 10 of these are from roots, four from barks, five from leaves, seven from flowers, seven from fruits, three from seeds, eight from wood, and three from gums and resins.

Some important dye-yielding plant habitats, their distribution and colouring pigments are given in Table 33.2. The increasing market demand for dyes and the dwindling number of dye-yielding plants forced the emergence of synthetic dyes like aniline and coal tar, which threatened total replacement of natural dyes. Even today, some dyes continue to be derived from natural sources, for example, dyes for lipstick are still obtained from *Bixa orellena* L. and *Lithospermum erythrorhizon* Sieb and Zucc., and those for eye shadow from indigo. The content or amount of dye present in the plants varies greatly depending on the season as well as age of the plants.

There are also several factors which influence the content of the dye in each dye-yielding plant. In some cases, the dye content has not been thoroughly studied so far.

Table 33.1 Sources of different coloured dyes and mordants

Colour	Botanical Name	Parts Used	Mordants
Red Dye			
Safflower	Carthamus tinctorius L.	Flower	—
Caesalpinia	Caesalpinia sappan L.	Wood	Alum
Madder	Rubia tinctorum L.	Wood	Alum
Log wood	Haematoxylon campechianum L.	Wood	—
Khat palak	Rumex dentatus L.	Wood	Alum
Indian mulberry	Morinda tinctoria L.	Wood	Alum
Kamala	Mallotus philippinensis Muell.	Flower	Alum
Lac	Coccus lacca Kerr.	Insect	Stannic chloride
Yellow Dye			
Golden rod	Solidago grandis DC.	Flower	Alum
Teak	Tectona grandis L.f.	Leaf	Alum
Marigold	Tagetes sp.	Flower	Chrome
Saffron	Crocus sativus L.	Flower	Alum
Flame of the forest	Butea monosperma (Lam) Taubert.	Flower	Alum
Blue Dye			
Indigo	Indigofera tinctoria L.	Leaf	Alum
Woad	Isatis tinctoria L.	Leaf	—
Sunt berry	Acacia nilotica (L.) Del.	Seed pod	—
Pivet	Ligustrum vulgare L.	Fruit	Alum and iron
Water lily	Nymphaea alba L.	Rhizome	Iron and acid
Black Dye			
Alder	Alnus glutinosa (L.) Gaertn.	Bark	Ferrous sulphate
Rofblamala	Loranthus pentapetalus Roxb.	Leaf	Ferrous sulphate
Custard apple	Anona reticulata L.	Fruit	—
Harda	Terminalia chebula Retz.	Fruit	Ferrous sulphate
Orange Dye			
Annota	Bixa orellena L.	Seed	Alum
Dhalia	Dhalia sp.	Flower	Alum
Lily	Convallaria majalis L.	Leaf	Ferrous sulphate
Nettles	Urtica dioica L.	Leaf	Alum

Table 33.2 Important dye-yielding plants with pigments

Plant	Colour Obtained	Pigment
Acacia catechu (L.f.) Willd.	Brown, black	Catechin, catechutanic acid
Adhatoda vasica Nees.	Yellow	Adhatodic acid, carotein, luteolin, quercetin
Bixa orellena L.	Orange, red	Bixin, norbixin
Butea monosperma (Lam) Taubert.	Yellow or orange	Butrin
Carthamus tinctorius L.	Yellow, red	Carthamin
Curcuma longa L.	Yellow	Curcumin
Indigofera tinctoria L.	Blue	Indigotin, Indican
Lawsonia inermis L.	Orange	Lawsone
Mallotus philippensis Muell.	Red	Rottlerin
Morinda citrifolia L.	Yellow, red	Morindone
Oldenlandia umbeliata L.	Red	Alizarin, rubicholric acid
Pterocarpus santalinus L.	Red	Santalin
Punica granatum L.	Yellow	Pelargonidon-3,5-diglucoside
Rubia cordifolia L.	Red	Purpurin
Semecarpus anacardium L.f.	Black	Bhilawanol
Toddalia asiatica (L.) Lam.	Yellow	Toddaline
Wrightia tinctoria R. Br.	Blue	β-Amyrine

Medicinal Properties of Natural Dyes

Many of the plants used for dye extraction are classified as medicinal, and some of these have recently been shown to possess antimicrobial activity. *Punica granatum* L. and many other common natural dyes are reported as potent antimicrobial agents owing to the presence of a large amount of tannins. Several other sources of plant dyes rich in naphthoquinones such as lawsone from *Lawsonia inermis* L. (henna), juglone from walnut and lapachol from alkannet are reported to exhibit antibacterial and antifungal activity.

Singh *et al.* studied the antimicrobial activity of some natural dyes. Optimized natural dye powders of *Acacia catechu* (L.f.) Willd., *Kerria lacca*, *Rubia cordifolia* L. and *Rumex maritimus* were obtained from commercial industries, and they showed antimicrobial activities. This is clear evidence that some natural dyes by themselves have medicinal properties. Another example is lycopene—a carotenoid pigment responsible for red colour in tomato, watermelon, carrot and other fruits—also used as a colour ingredient in many food formulations. It has received considerable attention in recent years because of its possible role in the prevention of chronic diseases such as prostate cancer.

Epidemiological studies have also shown that increased consumption of lycopene-rich food such as tomatoes is associated with a low risk of cancer. Also it is interesting to note that lycopene is the precursor to bixin and norbixin, pigments from *Bixa orellena*, commonly used for colouring foodstuff. Apart from dye-yielding property, some plants are also used traditionally for medicinal purposes.

33.5. NATURAL DYES OBTAINED FROM MINERALS

Ocher is a dye obtained from an impure earthy ore of iron or ferruginous clay, usually red (hematite) or yellow (limonite). In addition to being the principal ore of iron, hematite is a constituent of a number of abrasives and pigments.

33.6. NATURAL DYES OBTAINED FROM ANIMALS

Cochineal is a brilliant red dye produced from insects living on cactus plants. The properties of the cochineal bug were discovered by pre-Columbian Indians, who dried the female insects under the sun, and then ground the dried bodies to produce a rich red powder. When mixed with water, the powder produced a deep, vibrant red colour. Cochineal is still harvested today on the Canary Islands. In fact, most cherries today have a bright red appearance through the artificial colour 'carmine', which is obtained from the cochineal insect.

33.7. CHARACTERIZATION OF DYES

A dye can be defined as a highly coloured substance used to impart colour to an infinite variety of materials like textiles, paper, wood, varnishes, leather, ink, fur, foodstuff, cosmetics, medicine, toothpaste, etc. As far as the chemistry of dyes is concerned, a dye molecule has two principal chemical groups, viz. chromophores and auxochromes. The chromophore, usually an aromatic ring, is associated with the colouring property. It has unsaturated bonds such as $-C=C$, $=C=O$, $-C-S$, $=C-NH$, $-CH=N-$, $-N=N-$ and $-N=O$, whose number decides the intensity of the colour. The auxochrome helps the dye molecule to combine with the substrate, thus imparting colour to the latter

33.8. CHEMISTRY OF NATURAL DYES

Dyes are classified based on their chemical structure (Table 33.1), method of application, colour, etc. As a model study here the author explains chemistry as described by Vankar.

They are classified into the following groups based on chemical structure:

1. *Indigo dyes*: This is considered to be the most important dye obtained from the plant *I. tinctoria* L.
2. *Anthroquinone dyes*: Some of the most important red dyes are based on the anthroquinone structure. These are obtained from both plants and insects. These dyes have good fastness to light. They form complexes with metal salts and the resultant metal complex dyes have good fastness.
3. *Alpha-hydroxy naphthoquinones*: The most prominent member of this class of dye is henna or lawsone (*L. inermis* L.).
4. *Flavones*: Most of the natural yellow colours are hydroxy and methoxy derivatives of flavones and isoflavones.
5. *Dihydropyrans*: Closely related to flavones in chemical structure are substituted dihydropyrans.
6. *Anthocyananidins*: Carajurin obtained from *Bignonia chica* Bonpl.
7. *Carotenoids*: In these the colour is due to the presence of long conjugated double bonds. Typical examples for this group are annato (*B. orellena*) and saffron.

33.9. PREPARATION OF DYES

The dye is generally prepared by boiling the crushed powder with water, but sometimes it is left to steep in cold water. The solution then obtained is used generally to dye coarse cotton fabrics. Alum is generally used as a mordant. Flowers of *Butea monosperma* (Lam) Taubert yield an orange-coloured dye, which is not fast and is easily washed away. For the purpose of colouring, the material is steeped in a hot or cold decoction of the flowers. A more permanent colour is produced either by first preparing the cloth with alum and wood ash, or by adding these substances to the dye bath. The dye indigo is produced by steeping the plant in water and allowing it to ferment. This is followed by oxidation of the solution with air in a separate vessel. *Mallotus philippinensis* Muell. yields an orange colour, used for dyeing silk and wool. To prepare the annatto dye from *B. orellena* L., the fruits are collected when nearly ripe. The seeds and pulp are removed from the mature fruit and macerated with water. Thereafter, they are either ground up into an 'annatto paste' or dried and marketed as annatto seeds. Sometimes when the seeds and pulp are macerated with water, the product is stained through a sieve and the colouring matter which settles out is collected and partially evaporated by heat and finally dried in the sun.

33.10. ADVANTAGES AND LIMITATIONS OF NATURAL DYES

Natural dyes are less toxic, less polluting, less health hazardous, noncarcinogenic and nonpoisonous. Added to this, they are harmonizing colours, gentle, soft and subtle, and create a restful effect. Above all, they are environment-

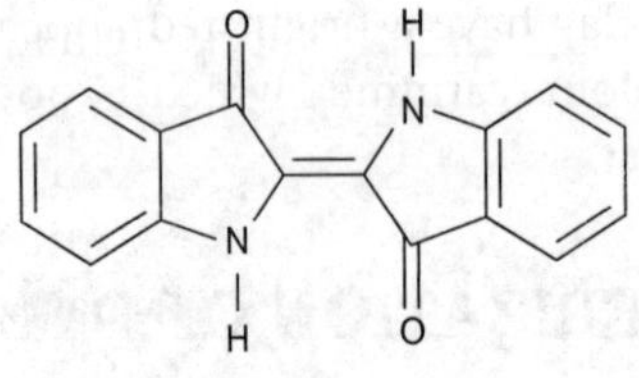

Indigo

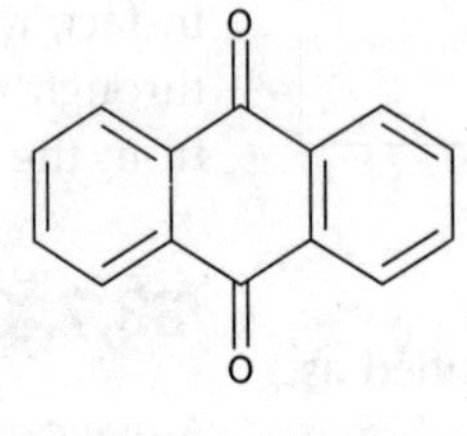

Anthraquinone

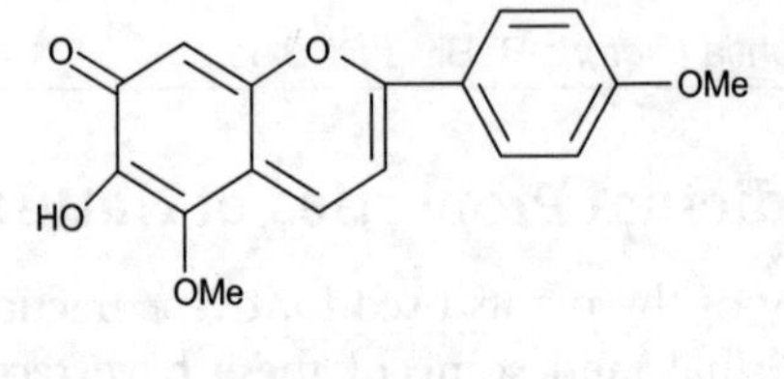

Anthocyananidin

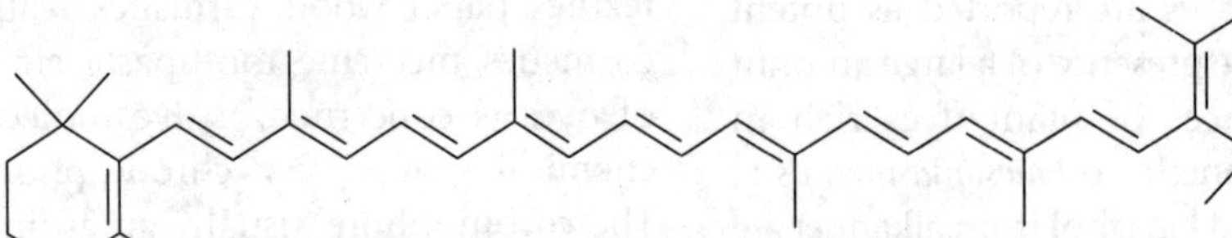

Beta-carotene

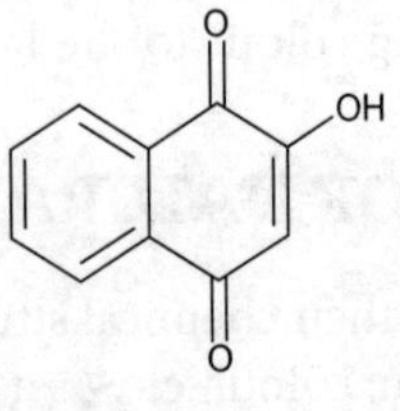

α-Hydroxynaphthoquinone

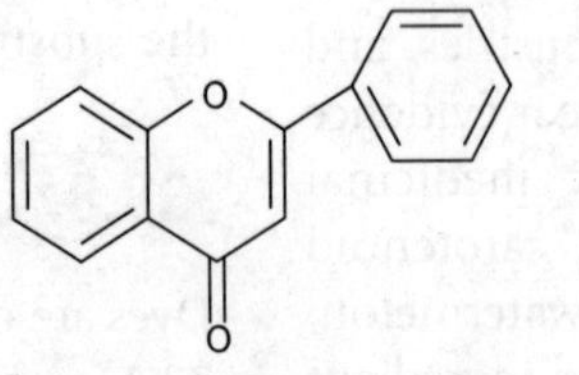

Flavone

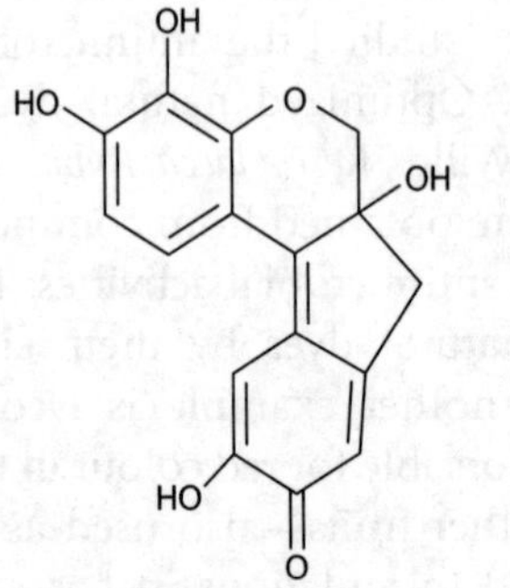

Dihydropyrans

friendly and can be recycled after use. Although natural dyes have several advantages, there are some limitations as well. Tedious extraction of colouring component from the raw material, low colour value and longer time makes the cost of dyeing with natural dyes considerably higher than with synthetic dyes. Some of the natural dyes are fugitive and need a mordant for enhancement of their fastness properties. Some of the metallic mordants are hazardous. Also there are problems like difficulty in the collection of plants, lack of standardization, lack of availability of precise technical knowledge of extracting and dyeing technique and species availability. Tyrian purple is obtained from the rare Mediterranean molluse *Murex brandavis*. In order to obtain 14 g of the dye, about 1200 molluses are needed.

33.11. TECHNOLOGY FOR PRODUCTION OF NATURAL DYES

Technology for production of natural dyes could vary from simple aqueous to complicated solvent systems to sophisticated supercritical fluid extraction techniques depending on the product and purity required. Purification may entail filtration or reverse osmosis or preparatory HPLC, and drying of the product may be by spray or under vacuum or using a freeze-drying technique. Use of biotechnological methods to increase the yield of colourants in plants is also being attempted in several laboratories in India.

33.12. GENETIC VARIATION AND DYE CONTENT

Siva and Krishnamurthy studied an important dye-yielding plant, *B. orellena*, for understanding the relationship between degree of genetic diversity (using isozymes) of various populations and their pigment content. Bixin ($C_{25}H_{30}O_4$) and norbixin ($C_{24}H_{28}O$) are carotenoid pigments that form the main components of *B. orellena*. The total amount of these two pigments in seed materials collected from 10 different geographical localities was estimated using HPLC. It was interesting to learn that the lowest band frequency shows the least total pigment and bixin content. Similarly, greater band frequency (i.e. genetic diversity) shows greatest dye content. In other words, it is likely that individuals with greater genetic diversity may have high dye content. Further critical study is needed to establish the relationship between the geographical localities with the dye content.

33.13. CONCLUSIONS

Nowadays, fortunately, there is increasing awareness among people towards natural products. Due to their nontoxic properties, low pollution and less side effects, natural dyes are used in day-to-day food products. Although the Indian subcontinent possesses large plant resources, only little has been exploited so far. More detailed studies and scientific investigations are needed to assess the real potential and availability of natural dye-yielding resources and for propagation of species in great demand on commercial scale. Biotechnological and other modern techniques are required to improve the quality and quantity of dye production. Due to lack of availability of precise technical knowledge on the extraction and dyeing technique, it has not commercially succeeded like synthetic dyes. Also, low colour value and longer time make the cost of dyeing with natural dyes considerably higher than with synthetic dyes.

Mahanta and Tiwari identified a few rare, endangered and endemic dye-yielding plant species during their study in Arunachal Pradesh. They reported that species of *Ilex embelioides*, *Phaius tankervilliae* and *Entada purseatha* are rare treasures amidst the rich floral diversity of Arunachal Pradesh. Numerous plant species are found to have an important role in the day-to-day life of the ethnic and local people. However, it is a matter of concern that the indigenous knowledge of extraction, processing and practice of using of natural dyes has diminished to a great extent among the new generation of ethnic people due to easy availability of cheap synthetic dyes. It has been observed that the traditional knowledge of dye-making is now confined only among the surviving older people and few practitioners in the tribal communities of Arunachal Pradesh. Unfortunately, no serious attempts have been made to document and preserve this immense treasure of traditional knowledge of natural dye-making associated with the indigenous people. Lack of a focused conservation strategy could also cause a depletion of this valuable resource. It is time that steps are taken towards documenting these treasures of indigenous knowledge systems. Otherwise, we are bound to lose vital information on the utilization of natural resources around us. To conclude, there is an urgent need for proper collection, documentation, assessment and characterization of dye-yielding plants and their dyes, as well as research to overcome the limitation of natural dyes.

Hallucinogenic Plants

CONTENTS

34.1. INTRODUCTION

Hallucinogens are natural and synthetic (synthesized) substances that, when ingested (taken into the body), significantly alter one's state of consciousness. Hallucinogenic compounds often cause people to see (or think they see) random colours, patterns, events and objects that do not exist. People sometimes have a different perception of time and space, hold imaginary conversations, believe they hear music and experience smells, tastes and other sensations that are not real. The other names of hallucinogens are Cartoon acid, Microdot, California sunshine, Psilocybin and Magic mushrooms.

Many types of substances are classified as hallucinogens, solely because of their capacity to produce such hallucinations. These substances are sometimes called psychedelic, or mind-expanding drugs. They are generally illegal to use in the United States, but are sometimes sold on the street by drug dealers. A few hallucinogens have been used in medicine to treat certain disorders, but they must be given under controlled circumstances. Hallucinogens found in plants and mushrooms were used by humans for many centuries in spiritual practice worldwide. Unlike such drugs as barbiturates and amphetamines (which depress or speed up the central nervous system (CNS), respectively), hallucinogens are not physically addictive (habit forming). The real danger of hallucinogens is not their toxicity (poison level), but their unpredictability. The actual causes of such hallucinations are chemical substances in the plants. These substances are true narcotics. Contrary to popular opinion, not all narcotics are dangerous and addictive. A narcotic is any substance that has a depressive effect, whether slight or great, on the CNS. People have had such varied reactions to these substances, especially to lysergic acid diethylamide (LSD) that it is virtually impossible to predict the effect of a hallucinogen that will have on any given individual. Effects depend upon the person's mood, surroundings, personality and expectations while taking the drug.

Natural hallucinogens are formed in dozens of psychoactive plants, including the peyote cactus, various species of mushrooms and the bark and seeds of several trees and plants.

KEY TERMS

Marijuana and hashish—two substances derived from the hemp plant (*Cannabis sativa*)—are also considered natural hallucinogens although their potency (power) is very low when compared to others. Marijuana—a green herb from the flower of the hemp plant—is considered a mild hallucinogen. Hashish is marijuana in a more potent, concentrated form. Both drugs are usually smoked. Their effects include a feeling of relaxation, faster heart rate—the sensation that time is passing more slowly, and a greater sense of hearing, taste, touch and smell.

A form of LSD was first produced in 1938, when Albert Hoffman, a Swiss research chemist at Sandoz Laboratories, synthesized many important ergot alkaloids (organic plant bases), including Hydergine, LSD-25 and psilocybin. The physical effects of hallucinogens are considered small compared to their effects on the mind. Death from an overdose of hallucinogens is highly unlikely, but deaths have resulted from accidents or suicides involving people under the influence of LSD. LSD is so powerful that a tiny amount can have a hallucinogenic effect.

34.2. MEDICAL USES OF HALLUCINOGENS

Hallucinogens have been studied for possible medical uses, including the treatment of some forms of mental illness, alcoholism and addiction to the drug opium. They have also been given to dying patients. Most of these uses have been abandoned, however. A synthetic form of the active chemical in marijuana, tetrahydrocannabinol (THC) has been approved for prescription use by cancer patients, who suffer from severe nausea after receiving chemotherapy (treating cancer with drugs). THC is also used to reduce eye pressure in treating severe cases of glaucoma. Phencyclidine (PCP) is occasionally used by veterinarians as an anaesthetic and sedative for animals.

Hallucinogenic plants have played an important role in many developing cultures of the world, including our own. They have been used in healing, as entheogens, and as religious sacraments, as well as having recreational utility. It is only a recent development that use of all hallucinogens has been frowned upon. A vast amount of resources has been put into controlling common psychoactive substances (Marijuana, LSD, PCP, etc.), which may be turning curious experimenters back towards the use of plants and other unregulated substances as a means of getting 'high'. There are many different species of hallucinogenic plants. Much information is available on many of them; yet, some are less studied than others.

Some of the important plant hallucinogens are as follows: Belladonna (*Atropa belladonna*), Betel Nut (*Areca catechu*), the Brooms (misc. sp.), Cabeza de Angel (*Calliandra anomala*), Calamus (*Acorus calamus*),

California Poppy (*Eschscholzia californica*), Catnip (*Nepeta cataria*), Chicalote, Prickly Poppy (*Argemone mexicana*), Coleus (*Coleus* sp.), Colorines (*Erythrina flabelliformis*), Damiana (*Turnera diffusa*), Daturas (*Datura* sp.), Donana (*Coryphantha macromeris*), Fennel (*Foeniculum vulgare*), Hawaiian Baby Woodrose (*Argyreia nervosa*), Hawaiian Woodrose (*Merremia tuberosa*), Heliotrope (*Valeriana officinalis*), Henbane (*Hyoscyamus niger*), Hops (*Humulus lupulus*), Hydrangea (*Hydrangea paniculata*), Iochroma (*Iochroma* sp.), Kava Kava (*Piper methysticum*), Khat (*Catha edulis*), Lion's Tail (*Leonotis leonurus*), Lobelia (*Lobelia inflata*), Madagascar Periwinkle (*Catharanthus rosea*), Mandrake (*Mandragora officinarum*), Maraba (*Kaempferia galanga*), Maté (*Ilex paraguayensis*), Mescal Beans (*Sophora secundiflora*), Mormon Tea (*Ephedra nevadensis*), Morning Glory (*Ipomoea* sp.), Nutmeg (*Myristica fragrans*), Ololiuqui (*Rivea corymbosa*), Passionflower (*Passiflora incarnata*), Pipiltzintzintli (*Salvia divinorum*), Psilocybe Mushrooms (misc. sp.), Rhynchosia (*Rhynchosia phaseoloides*), San Pedro (*Trichocereus pachanoi*), Sassafras (*Sassafras albidum*), Shansi (*Coriaria thymifolia*), Silvervine (*Actinidia polygama*), Sinicuichi (*Heimia* sp.), So'ksi (*Mirabilis multiflora*), Syrian Rue (*Peganum harmala*), Tobacco (*Nicotiana tabacum*), Wild Lettuce (*Lactuca virosa*), Wormwood (*Artemisia absinthium*).

BELLADONNA

Atropa belladonna L.; Nightshade family (Solanaceae).

A perennial branching herb growing to 5-feet tall, with 8-inch-long ovate leaves. The leaves in first-year plants are larger than those of older plants. The flowers are bell-shaped, blue-purple or dull red, followed by a shiny, black or purple 0.5 inch berry. The plant is native of Europe and Asia.

Constituents

Atropine, hyoscyamine, belladonnine and hyoscine.

Medicinal Uses

Belladonna can be fatal to most carnivorous animals and humans, but the same doses have very little effect upon most birds and plant-eating animals. Children are often poisoned by the berries, mistaking them for cherries or other sweet fruit. In large doses, belladonna acts upon the cerebrospinal system, as showing such symptoms as dilatation of the pupils (mydriasis), presbyopia, obscurity of vision, blindness (amaurosis), visual illusions (phantasms), suffused eyes, occasionally disturbance of hearing (as ringing in the ears, etc.), numbness of the face, confusion of head, giddiness and delirium. Belladonna has been and is being used as a recreational drug, diuretic, sedative, antispasmodic and mydriatic. It is used very successfully to treat eye diseases, because of its effect of dilating the pupil. Atropine, an extract of belladonna, is what an eye doctor uses when they put liquid in your eye before testing you for glasses. Atropine has also been used as an antidote to opium, Calabar bean and chloroform poisoning.

BETEL NUT

Areca catechu L.; Palm family (Palmaceae).

A very slender, graceful palm that grows up to 100-feet tall with a 6-inch diameter trunk. This is topped by a crown of three 6-foot-long leaves that are divided into many leaflets. The fruits are the size and shape of a hen's egg and are yellowish to scarlet with a fibrous covering. It is native to Malaysia.

Constituents

Betel nut contains arecaine and arecoline alkaloids which are comparable to nicotine in its stimulating, mildly intoxicating and appetite-suppressing effects on the mind. It also contains the alkaloids arecaidine, arecolidine, guracine (guacine) and guvacoline.

Medicinal Uses

Stimulant, stroke recovery, schizophrenia, anaemia, dental cavities, ulcerative colitis and saliva stimulant. It is also used as alcohol, aphrodisiac, appetite stimulant, asthma, cough, digestive aid, diphtheria and as diuretic. The findings of a prior study indicating a therapeutic relationship between consumption of betel nut and symptoms of schizophrenia were tested. These findings have clinical significance in betel-chewing regions and broader implications for theory of muscarinic neurophysiology in schizophrenia.

CABEZA DE ANGEL

Calliandra anomala (*Kunth*) Macbride; Bean family (Leguminosae).

This plant is tall and evergreen shrub. Leaves are bipinnate, rachis covered with dense brown hairs. Pinnae 15 pairs or more; leaflets 30–60 pairs, densely crowded and oblong. Pods are 7.5–10 cm long and 1.2–1.8 cm wide, densely villous with red hairs.

Constituents

Mainly contains triterpenoidal saponins. Three triterpenoidal saponins were identified by FAB-MS spectrum, viz. Calliandra saponin M, N and O. Six triterpenoids like Calliandra saponins: G(1), H(2), I (3), J(4), K(5) and L(6) were isolated from the branches of *Calliandra anomala*.

Medicinal Uses

Formerly it was used by Aztecs. Cut the bark and collect resin for several days; dry, pulverize, mix with ash and used as snuff. It acts as hypnotic, often induces sleep.

CALAMUS

Acorus calamus L.; Arum family (Araceae).

A vigorous perennial herb growing up to 6-feet tall, composed of much long, slender, grass-like leaves up to 0.75 inch wide rising from a horizontal rootstock. The flowers are minute and greenish-yellow in colour, occurring on a 4-inch-long spike resembling a finger. The fruit is berrylike. It is native to eastern North America, Europe and Asia.

Constituents

Both triploid and tetraploid calamus contain asarone. Monoterpene hydrocarbons, sequestrene, ketones, (*trans-* or alpha) asarone (2,4,5-trimethoxy-1-propenylbenzene) and beta-asarone (*cis-* isomer) contained in the roots essential oils.

Medicinal Uses

It is use as an analgesic for the relief of toothache or headache, for oral hygiene to cleanse and disinfect the teeth, to fight the effects of exhaustion or fatigue and to help cure/prevent a hangover. Also used to treat a cough, made a decoction as a carminative and as an infusion for cholic. The ethyl acetate fraction of the *Acorus calamus* extract (ACE) was found to enhance adipocyte differentiation as did rosiglitazone. The results of further fractionation of ACE indicated that the active fraction does not consist of beta-asarone, which is a toxic component of this plant. This finding suggests that ACE has potential insulin-sensitizing activity like rosiglitazone, and may improve type 2 diabetes. The *in vitro* acetylcholinesterase (AChE) inhibitory potential of the hydroalcoholic extract and of the essential oil from *Acorus calamus* (AC) rhizomes and that of its major constituents were evaluated based on the Ellman's method.

CATNIP

Nepeta cataria L.; Mint family (Labiatae).

A hardy, upright, perennial herb with sturdy stems bearing hairy, heart-shaped, greyish-green leaves. The flowers are white or lilac, 0.25 inch long and occur in several clusters towards the tips of the branches. Native of Eurasia, naturalized in North America.

Constituents

Daucosterol (beta-sitosterol 3-O-beta-D-glucoside) was isolated from the plant, in addition to small amounts of beta-sitosterol, campesterol, alpha-amyrin and beta-amyrin was also isolated.

Medicinal Uses

It is used as a household herbal remedy, being employed especially in treating disorders of the digestive system and, as it stimulates sweating, it is useful in reducing fevers. The herb's pleasant taste and gentle action makes it suitable for treating cold, flu and fever in children. It is more effective when used in conjunction with elder flower (*Sambucus nigra*). The leaves and flowering tops are strongly antispasmodic, antitussive, astringent, carminative, diaphoretic, slightly emmenagogue, refrigerant, sedative, slightly stimulant, stomachic and tonic.

CHICALOTE, PRICKLY POPPY

Argemone mexicana L.; Poppy family (Papaveraceae).

It is an annual herb, 1–3 feet high with prickly stems, leaves and capsules. The flowers are yellow or orange, up to 2.5 inches across and followed by an oblong seed capsule. The leaves are white-veined and 4–6 inch long. It is native to tropical America.

Constituents

The plant contains alkaloids as berberine, protopine, sanguinarine, optisine, chelerythrine, etc. The seed oil contains myristic, palmitic, oleic, linoleic acids, etc.

Medicinal Uses

The whole plant is analgesic, antispasmodic, possibly hallucinogenic and sedative. The fresh yellow, milky, acrid sap contains protein-dissolving substances and has been used in the treatment of warts, cold sores, cutaneous affections, skin diseases, itches, etc. It has also been used to treat cataracts. The sensitivity of two Gram positive (*Staphylococcus aureus* and *Bacillus subtilis*) and two Gram negative (*Escherichia coli* and *Pseudomonas aeruginosa*) pathogenic multidrug resistant bacteria was tested against the crude extracts (cold aqueous, hot aqueous and methanol extracts) of leaves and seeds of *Argemone mexicana* L. (Papaveraceae) by agar well diffusion method. Though all the extracts were found effective, yet the methanol extract showed maximum inhibition against the test microorganisms followed by hot aqueous extract and cold aqueous extract.

COLORINES

Erythrina flabelliformis Kearney; Bean family (Leguminosae).

A shrub or small tree growing up to 10-feet high with spiny branches and leaves composed of fan-shaped leaflets. The flowers are bright scarlet, in short crowded racemes. The pods are up to 1-foot long, containing bright scarlet oval seeds. It is native to southern Arizona, New Mexico and Mexico.

Constituents

The first compounds isolated from *Erythrina* were alkaloids, i.e. β–Erythroidine. Homoerythrina alkaloids were also isolated.

Medicinal Uses

Erythrina has been used in folk medicine for treatment of insomnia, malaria fever, venereal disease, asthma and toothache. South American Indians used *Erythrina* as a fish poison. In addition, there are reports of its use as a narcotic and antihelmintic, anticancer and relaxant in Mesoamerica.

DAMIANA

Turnera diffusa; Turnera family (Turneraceae).

A small shrub with smooth inch long, pale green leaves which have dense hairs on the underside. The flowers are yellow, rising from the leaf axils, followed by a one-celled capsule, which splits into three pieces. This plant is native to the Southwest and Mexico.

Constituents

It contains Arbutin, volatile oil, tetraphyllin B, resins, gums, starch and tannins.

Medicinal Uses

It is used as stimulant, mild diuretic, mild laxative, testosteromimetic action, nervous restorative, antidepressant, urinary antiseptic anxiety and depression. It also is used as sexual inadequacies with a strong psychological or emotional element and to establish normal menstruation at puberty. A phytochemical investigation of *Turnera diffusa* afforded 35 compounds, comprised flavonoids, terpenoids, saccharides, phenolics and cyanogenic derivatives, including five new compounds (1–5) and a new natural product (6).

DATURAS

Nightshade family (Solanaceae).

This genus has 15–20 species ranging from annual and perennial herbs to shrubs and trees, with trumpet-shaped flowers. All of these are hallucinogenic.

Datura fastuosa L., formerly known as *D. metel*: It is an annual herb, 4–5 feet tall, with ovate 7- to 8-inch leaves. The flower is 7-inch long, white inside, violet and yellowish outside, with a purple calyx. The fruit is a 1.25 inch diameter spiny capsule. There are also double-flowered and blue-, red- and yellow-flowered varieties. It is native to India and naturalized in the tropics of both hemispheres.

D. inoxia Mill: It is a low-growing, spreading perennial with hairy 2- to 4-inch leaves. The flowers are white, 6–7 inch long, 10-lobed. The fruit is spiny, 2-inch or more in diameter. It is native to Mexico and the Southwest.

D. meteloides DC: It is an erect perennial herb with 2–5 inch leaves. The flowers are white, 8-inch long, often tinged with rose or violet, fragrant. The capsule is intensely spiny, 2 inches in diameter. It is native to the Southwest and Mexico.

D. stramonium L. 'Jimson weed': It is a green-stemmed, hairless annual, 2–4 feet tall, with few branches and two 8-inch-long ovate leaves. The flowers are white, 4-inch long. The capsule is egg-shaped, 2-inch long, filled with many black seeds. In *D. Stramonium* var. *tatula*, the flower is violet-purple or lavender; the stems are purple. They are easily grown from seeds, which sprout quickly even without bottom heat. It does well in rich soil in a dry, sunny location. Thin out all but the healthiest plant after sprouting.

D. chlorantha Hook: It is a hairless, perennial shrub, occasionally reaching 10-feet tall, with almost triangular, wavy-margined leaves. The flowers are yellow, drooping, followed by a prickly capsule. This is not a true tree datura although it occasionally reaches similar heights.

Constituents

One steroidal constituent, daturasterol and a tricyclic diterpene, daturabietariene, have been isolated for the first time from the stem bark of Datura metel Linn. along with beta-sitosterol and atropine. The structures of the new compounds have been elucidated as 24-beta-methylcholest-4-ene-22-one-3alfa-ol and 15-,18-dihydroxyabietatriene, respectively, on the basis of the spectral data analyses and chemical reactions.

Medicinal Uses

The whole plant, but especially the leaves and seed, is anaesthetic, anodyne, antiasthmatic, antispasmodic, antitussive, bronchodilator, hallucinogenic, hypnotic and mydriatic.

DONANA

Coryphantha macromeris (Engl.) Lem.; Cactus family (Cactaceae).

A low, cylindrical cactus to 8-inch-tall branching at the base, covered with several inch long, soft, spine-tipped tubercles. The flowers are purple, 5 inches across. It is native to Mexico and West Texas.

Constituents

Mainly it contains macromerine, normacromerine. It also contains phenethylamines, normacromerine (*N*-methyl-3,4-dimethoxy-beta-hydroxyphenethylamine) abundantly.

Medicinal Uses

It is a strong narcotic or hallucinogenic drug.

FENNEL

Foeniculum vulgare Mill.; Carrot family (Umbelliferae).

It is a perennial herb growing to 5-feet high, with blue-green stems and leaves. The leaves are finely divided into threadlike leaflets. The flower cluster is a large umbel, composed of 15–20 yellow flowers. This plant is native of southern Europe; naturalized in the Western United States.

Constituents

The major biologically active constituent of Foeniculum fruit oil was characterized as (+)-fenchone and (*E*)-9-octadecenoic acid. It also contains anethole, methyl chavicol, D-apenine, camphene, etc.

Medicinal Uses

The plant is analgesic, anti-inflammatory, antispasmodic, aromatic, carminative, diuretic, emmenagogue, expectorant, galactagogue, hallucinogenic, laxative, stimulant and stomachic. The essential oil is bactericidal, carminative and stimulant. Pectin's from *Foeniculum vulgare* were extracted under acidic conditions. The obtained pectins were mainly composed of uronic acid but also contained traces of rhamnose, galactose and arabinose. Extracted pectin's were used as a carbohydrate source to prepare biopolymer films in the absence and in the presence of phaseolin protein. The antiulcerogenic and antioxidant effects of aqueous *Foeniculum vulgare* (FVE) extract was studied on ethanol-induced gastric lesions in rats. It was found that pretreatment with FVE significantly reduced ethanol-induced gastric damage.

HAWAIIAN BABY WOODROSE

Argyreia nervosa Bojer.; family (Convolvulaceae).

A large, perennial climbing vine with heart-shaped leaves up to 1 foot across backed with silvery hairs. The flowers are 2–3 inch long, rose-coloured, on 6-inch stalks. Pods dry to a smooth, dark brown, filbert-sized capsule containing one to four furry brown seeds. The capsule is surrounded by a dry calyx divided into five petal-like sections. It is native to Asia.

Constituents

It contains argyroside, a new steroidal glycoside, (24R)-ergost-5-en-11-oxo-3beta-ol-alpha-D-glucopyranoside. It also contains ergoline alkaloids and D-lysergic acid amide.

Medicinal Uses

Used as psychotropic agent; in India, it is an Ayurvedic medicinal plant.

HELIOTROPE

Valeriana officinalis L.; Valerian family (Valerianaceae).

It is a perennial herb, 2–5 feet high with pinnately divided leaves and clusters of small, whitish, pinkish or lavender flowers. This plant is native of Europe and N. Asia.

Constituents

It is of complex composition, containing valerianic, formic and acetic acids. The alcohol is known as borneol and pinene. The root also contains two alkaloids—Chatarine and Valerianine.

Medicinal Uses

Valerian is a powerful nervine, stimulant, carminative and antispasmodic. It has a remarkable influence on the cerebro-spinal system, and is used as a sedative to the higher nerve centres in conditions of nervous unrest. The effect of valerian extract preparation (BIM) containing valerian extract, golden root (*Rhodiola rosea* L.) extract and L-theanine (gamma-glutamylethylamide) on the sleep-wake cycle using sleep-disturbed model rats in comparison with that of valerian extract. A significant shortening in sleep latency was observed with valerian extract and the BIM at a dose of 1000 mg/kg.

HENBANE

Hyoscyamus niger L.; Nightshade family (Solanaceae).

An annual or biennial herb, to 2.5-feet high, with hairy, 3- to 8-inch-long leaves. The flowers are 1 inch across, greenish-yellow with purple veins; they grow in spikes from June to September. The seed capsule is filled with many pitted seeds.

Constituents

The main constituents are hyoscyamine, hyoscine, scopolamine and hyoscipicrin.

Medicinal Uses

It causes deranged vision, headache, giddiness, dilated pupils, dry throat, hoarseness, weakness of the lower limbs, spasms, cramps, paralysis, loss of speech or loquacious delirium with hallucinations, followed by a dreamy sleep, according to the dosage. The cDNA from *Nicotiana tabacum* encoding Putrescine *N*-methyltransferase (PMT), which catalyses the first committed step in the biosynthesis of tropane alkaloids, has been introduced into the genome of a scopolamine-producing *Hyoscyamus niger* mediated by the disarmed *Agrobacterium tumefaciens* strain C58C1, which also carries *Agrobacterium rhizogenes* Ri plasmid pRiA4, and expressed under the control of the CaMV 35S promoter.

HOPS

Humulus lupulus L.; Hemp family (Cannabinaceae).

A perennial twining vine growing from 15- to 30-feet long with oval three- to five-lobed leaves having coarsely toothed edges. Male and female flowers occur on separate plants. It is native to Eurasia.

Constituents

It contains up to 1% volatile oil (humulene, myrcene, caryophylline, farnesene); 15–25% resinous bitter principles and phloroglucinol derivatives known as alpha acids (humulone, cohumulone, adhumulone, valerianic acid) and beta acids (lupulone, colupulone, adlupulone); condensed tannins and phenolic acids, flavonoid glycosides (astragalin, quercetin, rutin), fats, amino acids, unidentified oestrogenic substances, choline, asparagine. The oil and bitter resins together are known as lupulin.

Medicinal Uses

Hops are an aromatic bitter and hence may be useful in atonic dyspepsia. By many they are believed to have a sedative effect on the nervous system and are used in hysteria, restlessness, insomnia. It also used as sedative, soporific, visceral spasmolytic, aromatic bitter, digestive tonic, hypnotic, astringent, diuretic. The *in vivo* and *in vitro* effect of hop beta-acids on CNS function was investigated. Oral administration of beta-acids (5–10 mg/kg) in rats produced an increased exploratory activity in the open field, a reduction in the pentobarbital hypnotic activity and a worsening of picrotoxin-induced seizures.

Xanthohumol (XN) is a prenylated chalcone with antimutagenic and anticancer activity from hops. A nonaqueous reverse polarity capillary electrophoretic method for the determination of XN in hop extract was developed and validated.

HYDRANGEA

Hydrangea paniculata Sieb. var. *grandiflora*; family (Saxifragaceae).

This is the commonest hardy hydrangea in cultivation. It is a treelike shrub 8–30 feet high, with 3- to 5-inch-long oval leaves. The flowers are whitish, in dense clusters 8–15 inch long. The flowers sometimes change to pink and purple with age. It is native to China and Japan.

Constituents

It contains flavonoids, a cyanogenic glycoside (hydrangein), saponins and a volatile oil.

Medicinal Uses

It is helpful in the treatment of kidney and bladder stones. It is also used in genitourinary system, including cystitis, urethritis, enlarged prostate and prostatitis.

KAVA KAVA

Piper methysticum Forst.; Pepper family (Piperaceae).

It is a perennial, soft-wooded shrub growing 8–10 feet tall, with 8-inch ovate to heart-shaped leaves. The flower spikes are opposite to the leaves; male and female flowers occur on separate plants. This plant is native to the Pacific Islands.

Constituents

Kava pyrones (including kavalactones, kawahin, yangonin, methysticin) and Mucilage. It also contains pipermethystine, a kava alkaloids obtained from leaves.

Medicinal Uses

It is used as diuretic, urinary antiseptic, circulatory stimulant antispasmodic, analgesic, anaesthetic (topically), anaesthetic effect in the gastric mucosa and bladder mucosa, mental stimulant in small doses depressant in large, rubefacient (topically) and as antifungal. Serial plasma concentration-time profiles of the P-gp substrate, digoxin, were used to determine whether supplementation with goldenseal or kava kava modified P-gp activity *in vivo*. The current study compared short-term toxic effects of pipermethystine in F-344 rats to acetone-water extracts of kava rhizome (KRE).

Traditional Drugs of India

Section Outline

OVERVIEW

A large number of natural plant species, specifically those used extensively in various Indian traditional herbal drugs, have been and are still being investigated for ascertaining their specific inherent vital pharmacological and microbiological activities. In the recent past, stretched over to almost two decades, the spectacular thrust generated enough interest, inquisitiveness and incredible latest scientific approach to search for new drugs of tremendous potential value and worth in comparison to the modern allopathic system of medicine. This part focuses on such traditionally used herbal medicines and gives detail information on their pharmacological and phytochemical prospects.

CHAPTER 35

Detail Study of Traditional Drugs of India

CONTENTS

35.1. INTRODUCTION

A large number of natural plant species, specifically those used extensively in various Indian traditional herbal drugs, have been, and are still being investigated for ascertaining their specific inherent vital pharmacological and microbiological activities.

In the recent past, stretched over to almost two decades the spectacular thrust generated enough interest, inquisitiveness and incredible latest scientific approach to search for new drugs of tremendous potential value and worth in comparison to the modern allopathic system of medicine.

Based upon the high quality, proper standardization procedures, ultramodern packaging concepts and ideas, exhaustively informative drug-usage literatures, and above all the broad-spectrum methodical promotions both in India and abroad, the Indian traditional herbal drugs have undoubtedly made their presence felt amongst the valued consumers. An overwhelmingly plausible and sound confidence amongst the consumers to make use of such available drugs as: OTC products, prescribed medications, long-term usage in chronic ailments, have really turned them into a widely accepted alternative saga of safer and effective medications not only in India but also across the entire globe.

The importance of 'medicinal plants' right from the very dawn of civilization up to the last couple of decades have witnessed a tremendous cumulative, informative and educative volume of researches carried out in the ever-expanding field of pharmaceutically significant naturally occurring plant products. Interestingly, the better understanding of the plants as a whole vis-a-vis their important chemical constituents have undoubtedly broadened and strengthened one's acceptability and overall confidence in their usages amongst the consumers. Hence, the prevailing biodynamism of the 'active principles' strategically located in the plant kingdom would certainly provide the mankind with an eternal storehouse of clinically beneficial herbal drugs.

Indian plant drug caught the attention of west since the beginning of colonial days. Garcia da Orta, the personal physician of the then Portuguese governor in India was the first to publish his treatise on Indian drugs in 1563. During the period of 1678–1703, Henrich Van Reed, the Dutch governor of Cochin, published his work in twelve volumes on the medicinal plants of Kerala. In the later period, most of the systematic work on Indian medicinal plants has been published by Indian authors such as Nadkarni (1908), Kirtikar and Basu (1918), Chopra (1956), Aiyer and Kolammal (1960–66), Moose (1976–79) and Nambiar (1986). The aspects of cultivation and utilization of medicinal and aromatic plants were edited in details by Atal and Kapoor (1982) and as we see in recent days Handa (1998) published *Indian Herbal Pharmacopoeia* with an emphasis on the standardization and quality control of traditional drugs of India.

Some of the commonly used traditional drugs have been discussed in this chapter.

ADUSA

Synonym

Vasaka.

Regional Names

Sansk: atarusa, Vasaka; Guj: aduso, ardusi; Hindi: adusa, arusa; Kan: atarusha, adsole, adasale; Mar: adulsa.

Biological Source

Vasaka consists of the fresh or dried leaves of *Adhatoda vasica* Nees (Fig. 35.1).

Family

Acanthaceae.

Habitat

The plant is distributed all over the plains of India and in the lower Himalayan ranges, ascending to a height of 1500 m.

Macroscopy

Leaves are entire when fresh and crumpled or broken when dried. Shape is lanceolate-ovate lanceolate, crenate to entire margin, acuminate apex, base tapering; petiole 2- to 8-cm long. The leaves are 10- to 30-cm long and 3- to 10-cm broad, pinnate venation, glabrous or slightly pubescent green when fresh, on drying the colour changes from brown to grey. Odour is characteristic and bitter in taste.

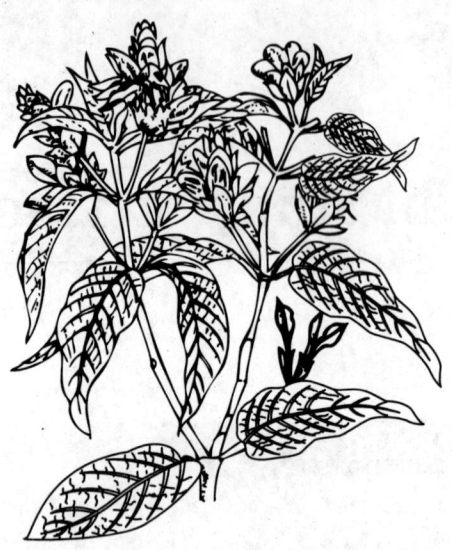

FIG. 35.1 *Adhatoda vasica*

Microscopy

Leaf shows dorsiventral structure with two layers of palisade cells below upper epidermis, epidermal cells sinuous walls with anomocytic stomata on both surfaces; one to three, rarely up to five-celled uniseriate covering trichomes few, and glandular trichomes with unicellular stalk and four-celled head are seen; acicular and prismatic forms of calcium oxalate crystals are also present in mesophyll.

Standards

Foreign matter	Not more than 2%
Total ash	Not more than 21%
Acid-insoluble ash	Not more than 1%
Alcohol-soluble extractive	Not less than 3%
Water-soluble extractive	Not less than 22%

Chemical Constituents

Vasaka contains several alkaloids but the major ones include pyrroloquinazoline alkaloids vasicine about 1.3% accompanied by vasicinol, vasicinone and adhatonine. Aliphatic hydroketones such as 37-hydroxy hexateracont-1-en-5-one and 37-hydroxy hentetracontan 19-one have also been reported from vasaka.

Uses

The leaf extract has been used for treatment of bronchitis and asthma for many centuries. It relieves cough and breathlessness. It is also prescribed commonly in ayurveda for bleeding due to idiopathic thrombocytopenic purpura, local bleeding due to peptic ulcer, piles, menorrhagia, etc. Large doses of fresh juice of leaves have been used in

Vasicine

Vasicinone

Adhatonine

tuberculosis. Its local use gives relief in pyorrhoea and in bleeding gums.

Marketed Formulations

It is one of the ingredients of the preparations known as Vasavaleha (Dabur), Kasamrit Herbal (Baidyanath) and Vasaka capsule (Himalaya Drug Company).

AMLA

Synonyms

Indian gooseberry, Emblic myrobalan.

Regional Names

Sansk: amalaka, dhatriphala; Guj: ambala, amala; Hindi: amla; Kan: nellikayi; Mar: anvala, avalkathi.

Biological Source

Amla consists of the fresh or dried fruit of *Emblica officinalis* Gaertn. (syn. *Phyllanthus emblica* Linn.) (Fig. 35.2).

Family

Euphorbiaceae.

Habitat

A deciduous tree, small to medium in size, the average height being 5.5 metres, commonly found in India, Sri Lanka, China and Malaya ascending to 1500 m on the hills.

Macroscopy

Fruits, fleshy, almost depressed to globose, 1.5- to 2.5-cm in diameter. It is distinctly marked in six lobes. The fruit is

green when tender but the colour changes to light yellow or brick red on maturity. Taste is sour and astringent initially and sweet afterwards.

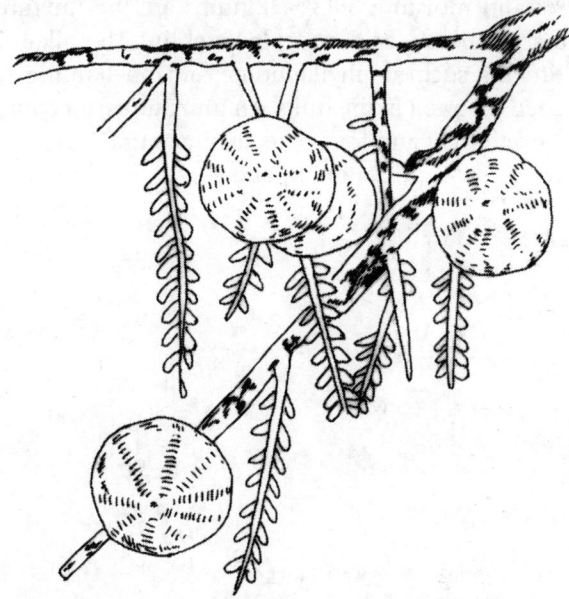

FIG. 35.2 *Emblica officinalis*

Microscopy

Fruit shows an epicarp consisting of epidermis with a thick cuticle and two to four layers of hypodermis; the cells in hypodermis is tangentially elongated, thick-walled, smaller in dimension than epidermal cells; mesocarp consists of thin-walled isodiametric parenchymatous cells; several collateral fibrovascular bundles scattered throughout mesocarp; xylem composed of tracheal elements, fibre tracheids and xylem fibres; tracheal elements, show reticulate, scalariform and spiral thickenings; mesocarp also contains large aggregates of numerous irregular silica crystals.

Standards

Foreign matter	Not more than 3%
Total ash	Not more than 7%
Acid-insoluble ash	Not more than 2%
Alcohol-soluble extractive	Not less than 40%
Water-soluble extractive	Not less than 50%

Chemical Constituents

It is highly nutritious and is an important dietary source of Vitamin C, minerals and amino acids. The edible fruit tissue contains protein concentration 3-fold and ascorbic acid concentration 160-fold compared to that of the apple. The fruit also contains considerably higher concentration of most minerals and amino acids than apples. The pulpy portion of fruit, dried and freed from the nuts contains: gallic acid 1.32%; tannin, sugar 36.10%; gum 13.75%; albumin 13.08%; crude cellulose 17.08%; mineral matter 4.12%; and moisture 3.83%. Tannins are the mixture of gallic acid, ellagic acid and phyllemblin. The alkaloidal constituents such as phyllantidine and phyllantine have also been reported in the fruits. An immature fruit contains indoleacetic acid and four other auxins: a1, a3, a4 and a5, and two growth inhibitors R_1 and R_2.

Vitamin C

Gallic acid

Ellagic acid

Uses

The fruits are diuretic, acrid, cooling, refrigerant and laxative. Dried fruit is useful in haemorrhage, diarrhoea, diabetes and dysentery. They are useful in the disorders associated with the digestive system and are also prescribed in the treatment of jaundice and coughs. It has antioxidant, antibacterial, antifungal and antiviral activities. Amla is one of the three ingredients of the famous ayurvedic preparation, triphala, which is given to treat chronic dysentery, biliousness and other disorders, and also it is an ingredient in Chyawanprash.

Marketed Formulations

It is one of the ingredients of the preparations known as Jeevani malt (Chirayu Pharmaceuticals), Triphala churna (Zandu) and Chyawanprash (Dabur).

APAMARGA

Synonym

Prickly Chaff flower.

Regional Names

Sansk: apamarga; Hindi: chirchira; Mar: aghada.

Biological Source

The drug consists of dried whole plant of *Achyranthes aspera* Linn. Syn. *A. canescens* (Fig. 35.3).

Family

Amaranthaceae.

Habitat

It is found commonly as a weed through out India up to an altitude of 900 m.

Macroscopy

Root

Tap root are cylindrical in shape that are slightly ribbed. They are 0.1- to 1.0-cm thick and the outer surface is rough due to presence of some root scars, secondary and tertiary roots are present. It is yellowish brown in colour and devoid of odour.

Stem

The stems are cylindrical, erect, branched, hollow, 0.3- to 0.5-cm in cut pieces with yellowish brown in colour.

Leaf

Simple, obovate, opposite, subsessile, exstipulated with wavy margin; slightly acuminate apex and pubescent.

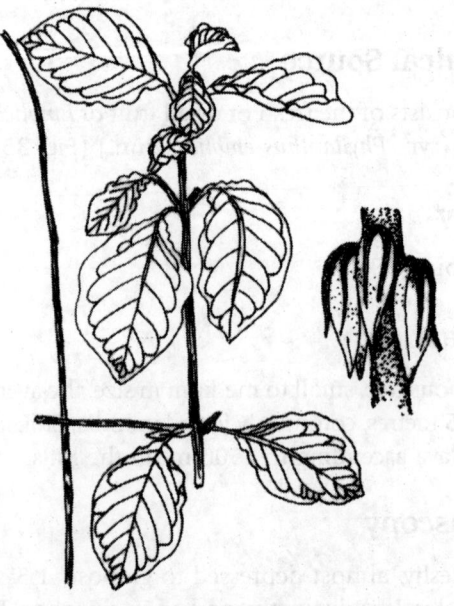

FIG. 35.3 *Achyranthes aspera*

Saponin C = L-Rhamnopyranosyl

Saponin D = L-Rhamnopyranosyl-(1-4)-D-glycopyranosyl

Structure formula of Saponin C and D

Flower

They are greenish white arranged as inflorescence on a long spikes, bisexual, actinomorphic, hypogynous, gynoecuim bicarpellary, syncarpous with superior ovary.

Seed

Subcylindrical, truncate at the apex, rounded at the base, endospermic, black and shiny.

Microscopy

Root

The outer most layers are the cork cells which are three- to eight-layered, rectangular, tangentially elongated and thin walled. The cortex consist of six to nine layers; the cells are thin-walled, oval to rectangular shape, parenchymatous cells with hardly any scattered stone cells either single or in groups. Below this it has four to six discontinuous rings of secondary thickening with vascular tissues; sieve tubes are distinct in phloem parenchyma and xylem rings are also present. The xylem is composed of pitted vessels. Medullary rays are one- to three-cells wide with small prismatic crystals of calcium oxalate.

Stem

Stem shows six to ten outstanding ridges. Epidermis is single layered and covered by thick cuticle having uniseriate covering trichomes and glandular trichomes which are two to five celled. The cortex has parenchymatous cells, six to ten layered, with rosette crystals of calcium oxalate. Cortex has collenchymatous cells with vascular bundles capped by pericyclic fibres. The mature stem shows thin-walled lignified cork cells. Vascular tissues show anomalous secondary growth with four to six incomplete rings of xylem and phloem.

Leaf

Epidermis is the outer layer which is covered with cuticle and consists of both covering and glandular trichomes. The stomata present are anomocytic stomata in the epidermis; the lower epidermis has numerous stomata. The ground tissues consisting of thin-walled parenchymatous cells containing of rosette type of calcium oxalate crystals. In the midrib it has four- to five-layered collenchyma just below the upper epidermis and two- to three-layered above the lower. Vascular bundle is present in the middle of the midrib, and the remaining is filled with parenchyma cells with calcium oxalate crystals.

Chemical Constituents

A. apsera contains triterpenoid saponins as the major constituents of the whole drug. The triterpenoid saponins yield oleanolic acid as an aglycone. It also shows the presence of an insect moulting hormone Ecdysterone, long-chain alcohols such as 17-pentatriacontanol, 27-cyclohexyIheptacosan-7-ol, long-chain ketones and a water-soluble base betaine. Two new saponins C and D have been isolated from the fruits.

Uses

A. aspera is much valued in the indigenous medicine. It is reported to be an astringent and diuretic. A decoction of the plant is useful in pneumonia and renal dropsy, while the juice is useful in ophthalmia and dysentery. The leaves are used to cure gonorrhoea, whereas the flowers are used in the treatment of menorrhagia. The roots are astringent and their paste is applied to clear opacity of cornea. It is also reported to be useful in cancer. The plant shows significant abortifacient activity in mice and rabbit. The plant also shows hypoglycaemic activity in the normal and diabetic rabbits.

Marketed Formulations

It is one of the ingredients of the preparation known as Cystone tablet (Himalaya Drug Company).

ARJUNA

Synonym

Arjuna Myrobalan.

Regional Names

Sansk: kakubha, svetavaha; Guj: arjuna, sajada; Hindi: arjuna; Kan: matti, neermatti, mathichakke; Mar: adurta, sadada.

Biological Source

It is the dried bark of *Terminalia arjuna* W. and A. (Fig. 35.4).

Family

Combretaceae.

Habitat

This herb has been known from as early as the Vedic period. It is grown in flowerpots in most Hindu homes. Its leaves are used in the worship of gods and goddesses and partaken as prasad. It is native to India. It reached Western Europe only in the 16th century. It is widely grown throughout the world.

Macroscopy

Bark is available in pieces, flat, curved, recurved, channelled to half quilled 0.2- to 1.5-cm thick, 10 cm in length and up to 7 cm in width; inner surface fibrous and pinkish, short fracture; taste is bitter and astringent.

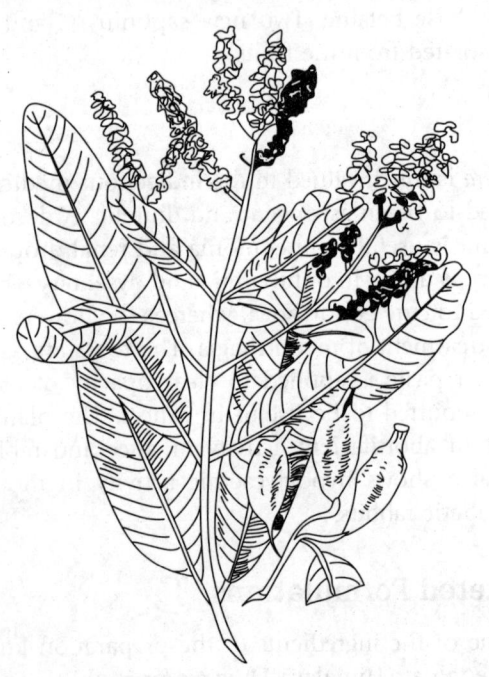

FIG. 35.4 *Terminalia arjuna*

Microscopy

Outer cork consists of 9–10 layers of tangentially elongated cells; cork cambium and secondary cortex are not distinct. Medullary rays are seen traversing almost up to outer bark secondary phloem occupies a wide zone, consisting of sieve tubes, companion cells, phloem parenchyma and phloem fibres; phloem fibres are distributed in rows and present in groups of 2–10; rosette type of calcium oxalate crystals and starch grains are also present.

Standards

Foreign matter	Not more than 2%
Total ash	Not more than 25%
Acid-insoluble ash	Not more than 1%
Alcohol-soluble extractive	Not less than 20%
Water-soluble extractive	Not less than 20%

Chemical Constituents

The dry bark from the stem contains about 20–24% of tannin, whereas that of the bark obtained from the lower branches is up to 15–18%. The tannins present in arjuna bark are of mixed type consisting of both hydrolysable and condensed tannins. The tannins are reported to be present are (+) catechol, (+) gallocatechol, epicatechol, epigallocatechol and ellagic acid. The flavonoids such as arjunolone, arjunone and baicalein have been reported from the stem bark. The triterpenoid compounds arjunetin, arjungenin, arjunglucoside I and II, and terminoic acid have also been reported from the bark. The root contains number of triterpenoids such as arjunoside I and II, terminic acid, oleanolic acid, arjunic acid, arjunolic acid, etc. The fruits also contain 7–20% of tannins. A pentacyclic triterpenic glycoside arjunoglucoside III has been reported from the fruits along with hentriacontane, myristyl oleate and arachidic stearate.

Uses

Arjuna bark is used as a diuretic and astringent. The diuretic properties can be attributed to the triterpenoids present in fruits. It causes decrease in blood pressure and heart rate. It is used in the treatment of various heart diseases in indigenous systems of medicines. The bark was extensively used in the past by the local tanneries for tanning animal hides. It yields a very firm leather of a colour which is similar babool tanned leather.

Marketed Formulations

It is one of the ingredients of the preparations known as Abana, Geriforte, Liv 52, Mentat (Himalaya Drug Company); Arjun Ghrita, Arjun Churna (Baidyanath Company); and Madhudoshantak (Jamuna Pharma).

Arjunolone

Arjunone

Arjuglucoside III

Terminoic acid

ASHOKA

Synonym

Ashok.

Regional Names

Hindi and Bengali: asok; Mar: ashoka.

Biological Source

The drug consists of the dried bark of *Saraca indica* auct. non Linn., syn. *S. asoca* (roxb). De Wilde (Fig. 35.5).

Family

Leguminosae.

Habitat

Ashoka tree is evergreen tree, grown all over India, in Burma and Ceylon. In India, it is cultivated in states like Madhya Pradesh, Rajasthan, Punjab, Haryana, Uttar Pradesh, Tamil Nadu, Kerala, Karnataka, Maharashtra and Andhra Pardesh.

Macroscopy

S. indica is a small evergreen tree of 6–9 m height distributed throughout India up to an altitude of 750 m in the central and the eastern Himalayas, and the Khasi, Garo and Lusai hills. It is found wild along streams or in the shade of evergreen forests. The bark of the plant is bark brown to grey or almost black with warty surfaces. Leaves are paripinnate, oblong-lanceolate and rigidly subcoriaceous. Flowers are orange to orange-yellow eventually turning vermillion in dense axillary corymbs. Fruits consist of the flat leathery pods with four to eight ellipsoid-oblong seeds.

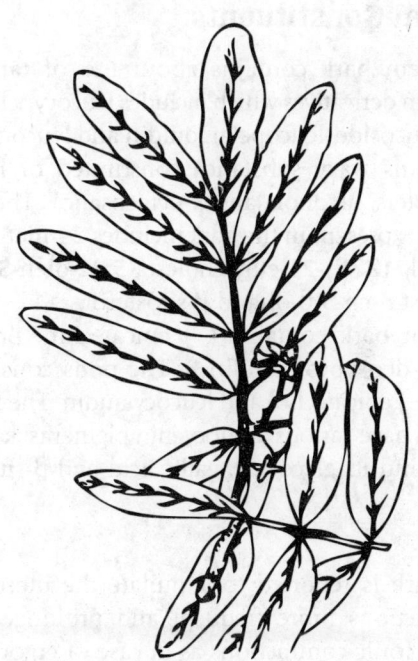

FIG. 35.5 *Saraca indica*

Microscopy

The outer most layers consist of few layers of phellem and phelloderm. Phelloderm contains stone cells in large numbers in the form of distinct rings and also large strands. The transverse section also reveals the presence of phloem fibres in small groups, crystal fibres and funnel-shaped, uniseriate medullary rays in the inner bark. Starch is also present to small extent.

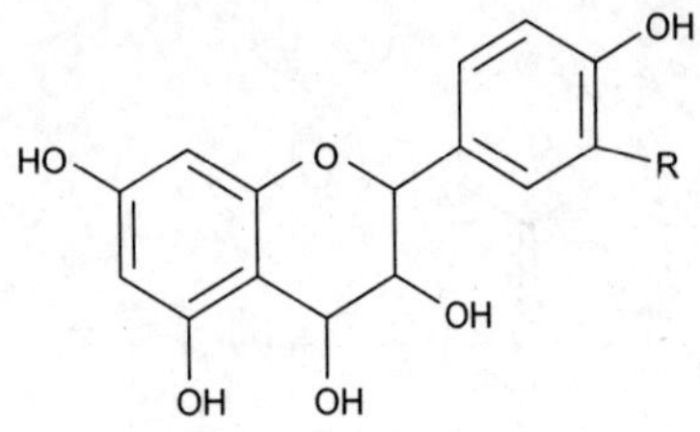

Leucocyanidin R = OH

Leucopelargonidin R = H

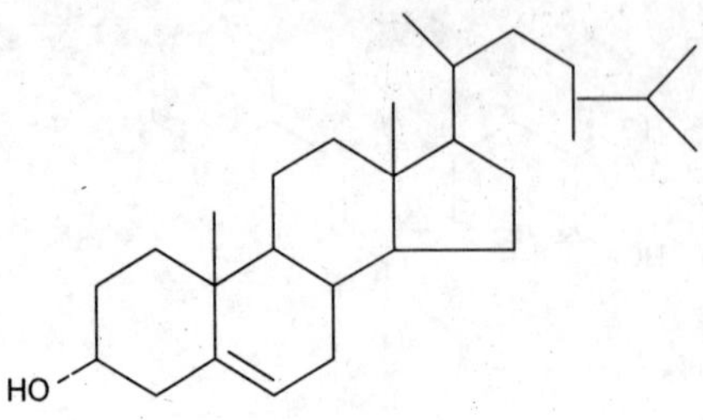

24-Methylcholest-5-en-3β-ol

Standards

Foreign matter	Not more than 2%
Total ash	Not more than 11%
Acid-insoluble ash	Not more than 1%
Alcohol (90%)-soluble extractive	Not less than 15%
Water-soluble extractive	Not less than 11%

Chemical Constituents

Ashoka stem bark contains about 6% of tannins and anthocyanin derivatives which includes leucocypelargonidin-3-O-β-D-glucoside. leucopelargonidin and leucocyanidin. It also contains waxy substance constituted of long-chain alkanes, esters, alcohols and *n*-octacosanol. The steroidal components present in the bark includes 24-methylcholest-5-en-3-β-ol, (ZZE)-24-ethylcholesta-5,22-dien-3-β-ol, 24-ethylcholest-5-en-3-β-ol and β-sitosterol.

The root bark contains (–) epicatechin, procyanidin B$_2$ and 11'-deoxyprocyanidin B. The pods consists of (+) catechol, (–) epicatechol and leucocyanidin. The flowers are reported to have various anthocyanin pigments, kaempferol, quercetin and its glycoside, gallic acid and β-sitosterol.

Uses

Ashoka bark is reported to stimulate the uterus making the contractions more frequent and prolonged without producing tonic contractions as in case of ergot alkaloids. The phenolic glycoside is reported to be responsible for the specific oxytocic activity in vitro and in vivo on uterus and isolated myometrial strips and fallopian tube. The bark is reported to have a stimulating effect on the endometrium and ovarian tissue and is used in the treatment of menorrhagia due to uterine fibroids. It is also used in leucorrhoea and in internal bleeding, haemorrhoids and haemorrhagic dysentery. Alcoholic extract of the bark shows significant antimicrobial activity against a wide range of bacteria and aqueous extract has been found to enhance the life span of mice infected with Ehrlich ascites carcinoma.

Marketed Formulations

It is one of the ingredients of the preparations known as Pmensa (Lupin Herbal Lab.), Femiplex (Charak Pharma) and Ashokarishta (Baidyanath Company).

BAHERA

Synonym

Belleric Myrobalan.

Regional Names

Sansk: aksa, aksaka; Guj: bahedan; Hindi: bahera; Kan: tare kai, shanti kayi; Mar: baheda.

Biological Source

Bahera is the dried ripe fruits of *Terminalia belerica* Roxb. (Fig. 35.6).

Family

Combretaceae.

Habitat

It is a large deciduous tree found through out India, Burma and Sri Lanka, common in plains and forests of about 1000 m. Except in dry and arid regions.

Macroscopy

Globular 1.3- to 2.5-cm in diameter, ovoid, suddenly narrowing into a short stalk. Outer surface is velvet in nature, irregularly wrinkled containing five longitudinal ridges. The upper end is depressed and a prominent, sound scar of pedicel is present at one end of the fruit. It is very hard and when broken surface will be yellow in colour. It is devoid of odour and taste is astringent.

Microscopy

T.S. shows an outer epicarp consisting of a layer of epidermis, most of the epidermal cells elongate to form hair-like protuberance with swollen base; next to epidermis it contains a zone of parenchymatous cells, slightly tangentially elongated and irregularly arranged. Stone cells of varying shape and size are present in between these parenchymatous cells. Mesocarp traversed in various directions by numerous vascular bundles collateral, endarch; simple starch grains and rosettes of calcium oxalate crystals are present in parenchymatous cells.

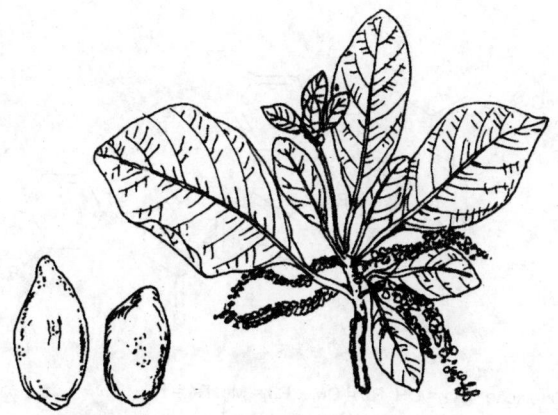

FIG. 35.6 Fruit and flowering branch of *Terminalia belerica*

Standards

Foreign matter	Not more than 2%
Total ash	Not more than 7%
Acid-insoluble ash	Not more than 1%
Alcohol-soluble extractive	Not less than 8%
Water-soluble extractive	Not less than 35%

Chemical Constituents

Bahera contains tannins (20–25%) like gallic acid, ellagic acid, ethyl gallate, galloyl glucose and chebulagic acid. Minor contents phyllemblin, β-sitosterol, mannitol, glucose, fructose and rhamnose. The fixed oil in the fruit contains the esters of palmitic, stearic, oleic and linoleic acids. A new cardiac glucoside bellericanin has also been reported from the fruits.

Uses

The fruit has bitter, astringent, tonic, laxative, demulcent, mild diuretic, hypolipidaemic, hepatoprotective, antipyretic activities, and is also used in piles and dropsy. It is a

Gallic acid

Ellagic acid

constituent of Triphala and is prescribed in disease of liver and gastrointestinal tracts.

Marketed Formulations

It is one of the ingredients of the preparation known as Sage Triphala syrup (Sage Herbals).

BHILAMA

Synonyms

Marking nut tree, oriental cashew.

Biological Source

It is the tree of *Semecarpus anacardium* Linn. f. (Fig. 35.7).

Family

Anacardiaceae.

Habitat

It is a moderate-sized deciduous tree, 12–15 m high, found in the outer Himalayas from Sutlej to Sikkim, Assam and in hotter parts of India.

Macroscopy

The bark is dark brown, rough, leaves large, simple, obovate-oblong; flowers small, greenish-yellow, in terminal panicles, drupes ovoid, smooth, shining, black when ripe. The pericarp is abundant in a black, oily, bitter and highly vesicant juice used for marking linen, in varnish, paints and plastics. The juice, known in the trade as Bhilwan shell liquid, is a rich source of phenols. It is obtained from the nuts by extraction with petroleum ether or other solvent, by hot expression in a hydraulic press, or by roasting in a specially designed retort, or by subjecting the nuts to superheated steam at 180–230°C in a close retort with an inlet for steam and an outlet for the expelled liquid.

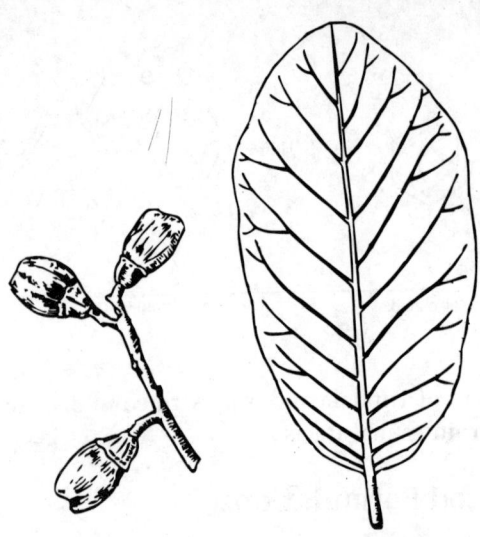

FIG. 35.7 *Semecarpus anacardium*

Galluflavanone	R1 = H, R2, R3 = OH
Jeediflavanone	R1 = OH, R2,R3 = H
Semecarpuflavanone	R1,R2 = H, R3 = OH

Nallaflavanone	R1 = OH, R2 = OMe, R3 = Me, R4 = H
Semecarpetin	R1, R2, R3 = H, R4 = Me

Chemical Constituents

The juice is a dark brown oily liquid or a semisolid depending on the method of extraction. The major constituent is bhilawanol, (46%). It is an O-dihydroxy compound with a catechol nucleus and an unsaturated C_{15}-side chain. It is a mixture of *cis*- and *trans*- isomers of urushenol [3-(pentadecenyl-8')-catechol]. A small quantity of a monohydroxy phenol, semicarpol, is also present. The dark tarry residue left after distillation contains high boiling phenols and hydrocarbons. Thermal degradation of the shell liquid at 400°C gives catechol and a mixture of phenols and hydrocarbons.

The fruits contain nicotinic acid, riboflavin, thiamine and essential amino acids. The nuts yield anacardic acid, aromatic amines, bhilawanol, 1-pentadeca-7,10-dienyl-2,3-dihydroxy benzene, biflavanoids A, B and C, (3',8-binaringenin and 3',8-biliquiritigenin), tetrahydrobustaflavone, tetrahydroamentoflavone and nallaflavone. The nutshell contains galluflavanone and jeediflavanone. The seed oil is composed of glycerides of linoleic, myristic, oleic, palmitic and stearic acids. Anacarduflavanone is present in nutshells. Amentoflavone is present in the leaves. The plant also contains biflavanones A_1 and A_2.

Uses

The tree is a host plant of the lac insect. The bark is astringent. The tree exudes a gum or gum-resin, which is used in leprous affections and nervous debility, also in scrofulous and venereal affections. The fruits are used in asthma, ascites, epilepsy, neuralgia, tumours, warts, psoriasis and rheumatism; as abortifacient, anthelmintic and vermifuge. A decoction of the fruits mixed with milk and butter fat is useful in asthma, gout, hemiplegia, neuritis, piles, rheumatism and syphilitic complaints. The kernel is anthelmintic, cardiotonic, carminative and digestive. The seed oil is used externally in gout, leprosy and leucoderma. The root cooked in sour rice water causes sterility in women when eaten. The juice of the pericarp and tree trunk is a powerful counter-irritant and vesicant. It causes painful blisters. The juice is used for tattooing and for chobing elephant feet. The pericarp juice has antibacterial properties.

Marketed Formulations

It is one of the ingredients of the preparations known as Prasarini Tail, Patrangasava and Sanjivani vati (Dabur).

BRAHMI

Synonyms

Indian Pennywort, Mangosteen.

Regional Names

Sansk: manduki, darduracchada; Guj: khodabrahmi, khadbhrammi; Hindi: brahma manduki, brahmi; Kan: ondelaga, brahmi soppu; Mar: karivana.

Biological Source

Brahmi is the fresh or dried herb of *Centella asiatica* (L.) (syn. *Hydrocotyl asiatica* Linn.) (Fig. 35.8).

Family

Umbelliferae.

Habitat

The plant is found in swampy areas of India, commonly found as a weed in crop fields and other waste places throughout India up to an altitude of 600 m and also in Pakistan, Sri Lanka and Madagascar.

Macroscopy

It is a slender, herbaceous creeper. Stems are long, prostate, filiform, often reddish and with long internodes, rooting at nodes. Leaves are long-petioled, 1.3–6.3 cm in diameter, several from rootstock and 1–3 cm from each node of stem. They are orbicular, reniform, rather broader than long, glabrous on both sides and with numerous slender nerves from a deeply cordate base. Fruit 8 mm long, ovoid, hard with a thick pericarp.

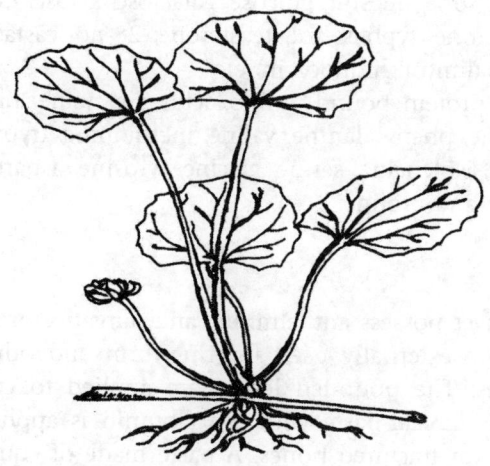

FIG. 35.8 *Centella asiatica*

Microscopy

Root

Outer cork consisting of three- to five-layered, exfoliated rectangular cells, followed by cortex region consisting three or four layers of parenchyma cells containing oval to round, simple, starch grains and microsphenoidal crystals of calcium oxalate; secondary cortex composed of thin-walled, oval to polygonal parenchymatous cells. Secretory cells are also present.

Stem

Single-layered epidermis composed of round to cubical cells covered by striated cuticle. Two or three layers of collenchymatous cells are found below the epidermis, collenchymatous cells are followed by six to eight layers of thin-walled, isodiametric, parenchymatous cells with intercellular space present; vascular bundles collateral, open, arranged in a ring, capped, by patches of sclerenchyma and traversed by wide medullary rays. Resin ducts are also present in parenchymatous cells of cortex; pith consists of isodiametric parenchyma cells with intercellular spaces.

Leaf

Single-layered epidermis covered by a thick cuticle, two- or three-layered collenchyma in the midrib region on both surfaces, central zone occupied by vascular bundles, mesophyll consists of two or three layer of palisade cells, five to seven layers of loosely arranged, more or less isodiametric spongy parenchyma cells. Rosette type crystals of calcium oxalate and anisocytic stomata are also present. Few anomocytic stomata are also seen.

Standards

Foreign matter	Not more than 2%
Total ash	Not more than 17%
Acid-insoluble ash	Not more than 5%
Alcohol-soluble extractive	Not less than 9%
Water-soluble extractive	Not less than 20%

Chemical Constituents

The drug contains triterpenoid saponin glycosides, indocentelloside, brahmoside, brahminoside, asiaticosides, thankuniside and isothankuniside. The corresponding triterpene acids obtained on hydrolysis of the glycosides are indocentoic, brahmic, asiatic, thankunic and isothankunic acids. These acids, except the last two, are also present in free form in the plant from isobrahmic and betulic acids. The presence of mesoinositol, a new oligosaccharide, centellose, kaempferol, quercetin and stigmasterol, have also been reported.

	R1	R2
Asiatic acid	-H	-OH
Madecassic acid	-OH	-OH
Asiaticoside	-H	-O-glu-glu-rha
Madecassoside	-OH	-O-glu-glu-rha

Uses

The plant is used as tonic, in diseases of skin, nerves, blood, and also to improve memory. It also strengthens our immune system. Asiaticosides stimulate the reticuloendothelial system where new blood cells are formed and old ones destroyed, fatty materials are stored, iron is metabolized, and immune responses and inflammation occur or begin. The primary mode of action of centella appears to be on the various phases of connective tissue development, which are part of the healing process. Centella also increases keratinization, the process of building more skin in areas of infection such as sores and ulcers. Asiaticosides also stimulate the synthesis of lipids and proteins necessary for healthy skin. Finally centella strengthens veins by repairing the connective tissues surrounding veins and decreasing capillary fragility.

Marketed Formulations

It is one of the ingredients of the preparations known as Iqmen (Lupin Herbal Lab.) and Abana, Geriforte, Menosan, Mentat (Himalaya Drug Company).

CASSIA TORA

Synonyms

Chakunda, Panevar, Wild Senna, Foetid Senna.

Biological Source

It consists of the leaves and seeds of *Cassia tora* Linn.; syn. *C. obtusifolia* L. (Fig. 35.9).

Family

Caesalpiniaceae.

Habitat

It is distributed throughout the tropical parts of India as a weed up to an altitude of 1550 m in the Himalayas.

Macroscopy

A foetid, annual herb or undershrub; up to 1–2 m in height, leaves paripinnate; leaflets three pairs, membranous, ovate-oblong, with glands in the last two pairs; flowers small, yellow, in pairs, on short axillary peduncles; pods stout, slender, sub-4-angled; seeds green, many, flat.

Chemical Constituents

The seeds contain fatty acids, physcion, rubrofusarin, its 6β-gentiobioside, aloe-emodin, chrysophanol, norrubrofusarin, 8-hydroxy-3-methyl anthraquinone-1β-gentiobioside, emodin, rhein, β-sitosterol, amino acids, chrysophanic acid, its 9-anthrone, obtusin, aurantio-obtusin, toralactone,

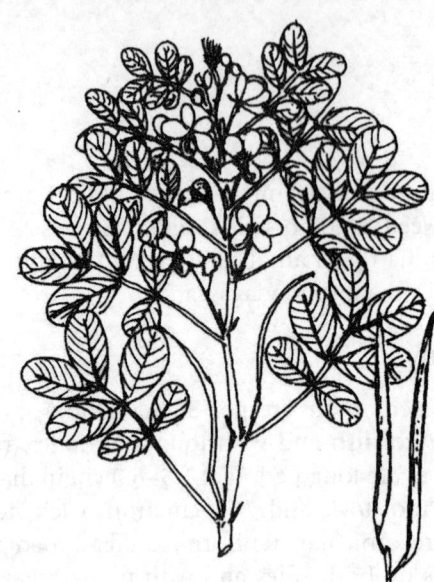

FIG. 35.9 *Cassia tora*

torachrysone, questin, glucose, galactose, xylose, raffinose, castasterone, typhasterol, teasterone, 28-nor-castasterone, monopalmitin, monoolein, etc.

The protein bound amino acids are lysine, histidine, theonine, phenylalanine, valine, methionine, tryptophan, leucine, isoleucine, serine, glycine, tyrosine, aspartic acid, alanine and proline.

Uses

The leaves possess anthelmintic and purgative properties. They are externally used for ringworm and other skin diseases. The pounded leaves are applied to cuts and wounds. A leaf-paste with egg albumin is applied as a plaster for fractured bones. A paste made of equal parts of the leaves and seeds are given in jaundice. A leaf extract showed antifungal activity against *Curvularia verruculosa* and *Microsporon nanum*. The seeds are official in Japanese Pharmacopoeia. They are used as a stomachic and tonic. A paste of the seeds with lime juice is used for ringworm and other skin diseases. The seeds are used in eye diseases, liver complaints and earache. A decoction of the seeds is taken as a blood purifier and for the inflammation of the skin.

Marketed Formulations

It is one of the ingredients of the preparation known as Mahamarichadi Tail (Dabur).

CHIRATA

Synonyms

Indian Gentian, Indian Balmony, Chirayta, *Ophelia chirata*, *Swertia chirayita*.

Biological Source

Chirata consists of the entire herb of *Swertia chirata* Buch-Ham (Fig. 35.10). It contains not less than 1.3% bitter constituent.

Family

Gentianaceae.

Habitat

India, Nepal and Bhutan.

Macroscopy

It is an annual, about 3 feet high; branching stem, upper part of the stem is yellow to brown, thinner and 2 mm broad. The lower part is purplish or brown to dark brown; 6-mm broad cylindrical and exfoliated at some places showing dull wood. Leaves are smooth entire, opposite, very acute, lanceolate dark brown up to 8-cm long, 1.5- to 2-cm broad. Flowers numerous; peduncles yellow; one-celled capsule. Rhizome is angular to 5-cm long, pale yellow to brown in colour and covered with dense scale leaves. Root is primary, 5- to 10-cm long, light brown, oblique somewhat twisted, tapering, longitudinally wrinkled and with transverse ridges. Drug has no odour but taste is very bitter.

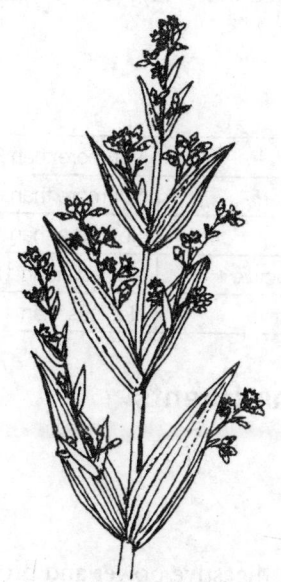

FIG. 35.10 *Swertia chirata*

Microscopy

Root

The microscopy presents 2–4 layers of cork; cortex region consists of 4–12 layers of thick-walled, parenchymatous cells with sinuous walls; secondary phloem composed of thin-walled sieve tubes, companion cells and phloem parenchyma; secondary xylem composed of lignified and thick-walled vessels, parenchyma, tracheids and xylem fibres; minute acicular crystals present in abundance in secondary cortex and phloem region; resin are also present as dark brown mass in secondary cortex cells.

Leaf

Single-layered epidermis covered with a thick, striated cuticle and anisocytic stomata; single-layered palisade tissue below the upper epidermis, four to seven layers of loosely arranged spongy parenchyma cells in mesophyll, mucilage and minute acicular crystal are present in mesophyll cells; parenchyma cells contain oil droplets also.

Stem

Single-layered epidermis, externally covered with a thick striated cuticle present in young stem, in older epidermis remains intact but cells flattened and tangentially elongated; endodermis distinct, showing anticlinal or periclinal walls, followed by single-layered pericycle consisting of thin-walled cells; cambium, between external phloem and xylem composed of a thin strip of tangentially elongated cells, internal phloem, similar in structure as that of external phloem excepting that sieve tube strand is more widely separated; xylem is continuous and composed mostly of tracheids, a few xylem vessels present; vessels and fibre tracheids have mostly simple and bordered pits and fibres with simple pits on the walls; medullary rays are absent; pith is present in the central part consisting of rounded and isodiametric cells with prominent intercellular spaces; acicular crystals, oil droplets and brown pigments are also present.

Standards

Foreign matter	Not more than 2%
Total ash	Not more than 8%
Acid-insoluble ash	Not more than 2%
Alcohol-soluble extractive	Not less than 13%
Water-soluble extractive	Not less than 11%

Chemical Constituents

Chirata contains chiritin, gentiopicrin and amarogentin. Amarogentin is phenol carboxylic acid ester of sweroside a substance related to gentiopicrin. Ophelic acid a noncrystalline bitter substance is present. It also contains gentianine and gentiocrucine.

Uses

It is an important ingredient in the well-known ayurvedic preparations Mahasudarshan churna and Sudarshan churna used successfully in chronic fever. The whole plant is an

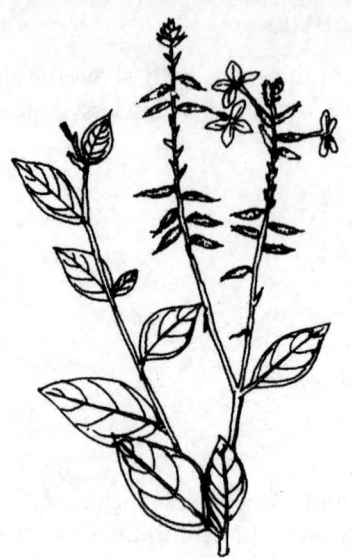

Amarogentin

extremely bitter tonic digestive herb that lowers fevers and is stimulant. The herb has a beneficial effect on the liver, promoting the flow of bile. It also cures constipation and is useful for treating dyspepsia.

Marketed Formulations

It is one of the ingredients of the preparations known as Diabecon (Himalaya Drug Company), Mehmudgar bati (Baidyanath), Sabaigo (Aimil Company), J.P. Liver syrup (Jaumana Pharma), Fever end syrup (Chirayu), Sage Chirata (Sage Herbals) and Safi (Hamdard Laboratories).

CHITRAK

Synonym

White Leadwort.

Regional Names

Sansk: agni, vahni, hutasa, dahana, hutribhuk, sikhi; Guj: chitrakmula; Hindi: chira, chitrak; Kan: chitramula, vahni, bilichitramoola; Mar: chitraka.

Biological Source

Chitraka consists of dried mature root of *Plumbago zeylanica* Linn. (Fig. 35.11).

Family

Plumbaginaceae.

Habitat

This herb is found throughout India. It grows wild as a garden plant in all part of India and Ceylon.

Macroscopy

Roots are above 30 cm in diameter, reddish to deep brown in colour, scars of rootlets are present. It has disagreeable odour and acrid in taste.

FIG. 35.11 *Plumbago zeylanica*

Microscopy

Outer cork consists of five to seven rows of cubical to rectangular dark brown cells; cortex consists of two to three rows of thin-walled rectangular. The parenchymatous cells below the cortex region contain starch grains. Phloem fibres are in groups lignified with pointed ends and narrow lumen. Straight medullary rays one to six seriate. Stone cells are absent.

Standards

Foreign matter	Not more than 3%
Total ash	Not more than 3%
Acid-insoluble ash	Not more than 1%
Alcohol-soluble extractive	Not less than 12%
Water-soluble extractive	Not less than 1.2%

Chemical Constituents

Plumbagin.

Uses

Root increases the digestive power and promotes appetite. It is hypoglycaemic, hypolipidaemic, CNS stimulant, and also used in dyspepsia, piles, anasarca, diarrhoea, skin diseases, etc.

Marketed Formulations

It is one of the ingredients of the preparations known as J.P. Liver syrup (Jaumana Pharma), Piles care and Mansulate (Chitrayu Company), and Chitrakadi bati Avaleha (Baidyanath).

LODH

Biological Source

It consists of the stem bark of *Symplocos racemosa* Roxb. (Fig. 35.12).

Family

Symplocaceae.

Macroscopy

It is an evergreen tree or shrub, 6- to 9-m height, abundant in the plains, and lower hills throughout northern and eastern India, in Himalayas up to 1400 m and southwards up to Chota Nagpur. The leaves are dark green above, orbicular, oblong. The flowers are white or yellow, aromatic. The fruits are drupes, purple-black, subcylindrical, smooth; seeds 1–3.

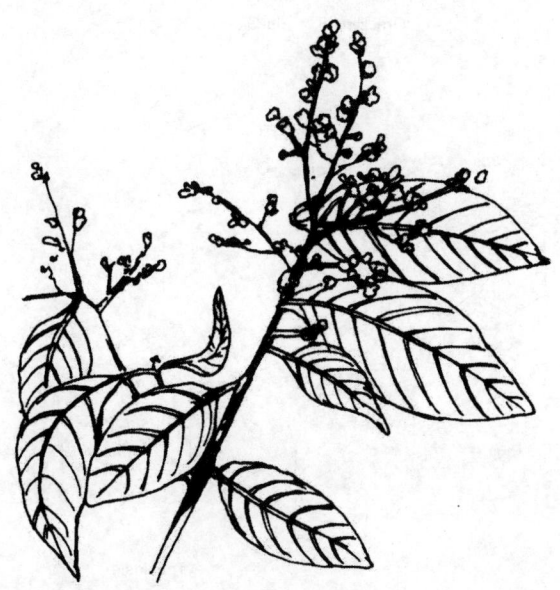

FIG. 35.12 *Symplocos racemosa*

Chemical Constituents

The bark contains oxalic acid, 3-monoglucoside of 7-O-methyl leucopelargonidin, pelargonidin-3-O-glucoside, betulinic, acetyloleanolic, oleanolic and ellagic acids; flavan glycoside symposide; β-sitosterol, 28-hydroxy-20α-urs-12,18(19)-dien-3β-yl-acetate, 3-oxo-20α-urs-12,18(19)-dien-28-oic, 24-hydroxyolean-12-en-3-one and butelin.

Uses

A yellow dye is extracted from the leaves and bark. Mainly the bark is used as a mordant with other drugs. For dyeing silk yellow, it is used combination with turmeric and *Plecospermum spinosum*. It is one of the ingredients of *abir*, a red powder used during the festival of Holi.

Marketed Formulations

It is one of the ingredients of the preparations known as Evecare, Styplon (Himalaya Drug Company).

GOKHRU

Synonym

Caltrops fruit.

Regional Names

Sansk: goksuraka, trikanta, svadamstra; Guj: bethagokharu, nazagokharu, mithagokhru; Hindi: gokhru; Kan: sannaneggilu, neggilmullu; Mar: sarate, gokharu.

Biological Source

In ayurveda two types of gokhru are used. The smaller or chota gokhru is the dried ripe seeds of *Tribulus terrestris* Linn. (Fig. 35.13).

Family

Zygophyllaceae.

Habitat

The plant is an annual, prostrate herb growing throughout India up to 3500 m in Kashmir.

Macroscopy

The fruits are yellowish in colour, globose, 1.2 cm in diameter containing five woody, densely hairy, spiny cocci. Large pointed spines are present in each coccus. Two smaller and shorter spines are directed downwards. Several seeds are present in each coccus.

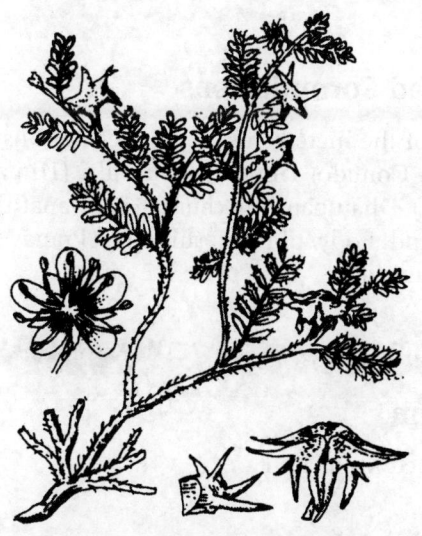

FIG. 35.13 *Tribulus terrestris*

Microscopy

Fruit section shows small rectangular epidermal cells of each coccus. Unicellular trichomes are found on the surface; 6–10 layers of large parenchymatous cells forms mesocarp, next to mesocarp 3–4 compact layers of small cells are present which contains rosette of calcium oxalate crystals.

Standards

Foreign matter	Not more than 2%
Total ash	Not more than 15%
Acid-insoluble ash	Not more than 2%
Alcohol-soluble extractive	Not less than 6%
Water-soluble extractive	Not less than 10%

Chemical Constituents

The dried fruits of *T. terrestris* consist of steroidal saponins as the major constituents. It includes terestrosins A, B, C, D and E; desgalactotigonin, F-gitonin, desglucolanatigonin and gitonin. The hydrolysed extract consists of sapogenins such as diosgenin, chlorogenin, hecogenin and neotigogenin. Certain other steroidal such as terestroside F, tribulosin, trillin, gracillin, dioscin have also been isolated from the aerial parts of the herb. The flavonoid derivatives reported from the fruits includes tribuloside and number of other glycosides of quercetin, kaempferol and isorhamnetin. It also consists of common phytosterols, such as β-sitosterol and stigmasterol, and cinnamic amide derivative, terestiamide.

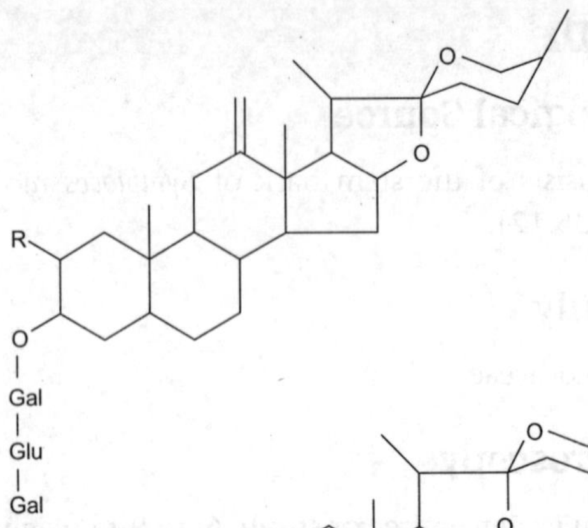

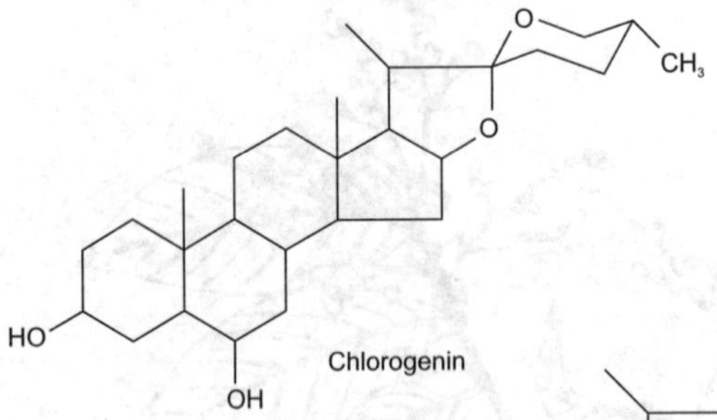

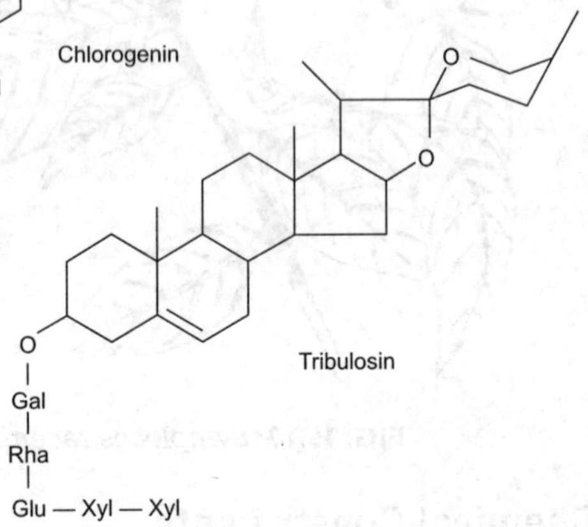

Uses

The fruit has cooling, anti-inflammatory, antiarthritic, diuretic, tonic, aphrodisiac properties. It is used in building immune system, in painful micturition, calculus affections and impotency. It improves and prolongs the duration of erection and also exerts a stimulating effect on reproductary organs.

Marketed Formulations

It is one of the ingredients of the preparations known as Bonnisan, Confido, Himplasia, Renalka (Himalaya Drug Company), Dhatupaushtik churna (Baidyanath), Semento (Aimil) and Body plus capsule (Jay Pranav Ayurvedic Pharmaceuticals).

GUDUCHI

Synonym

Heart-leaved Moonseed.

Teresterosin A R = H
Teresterosin E R = OH

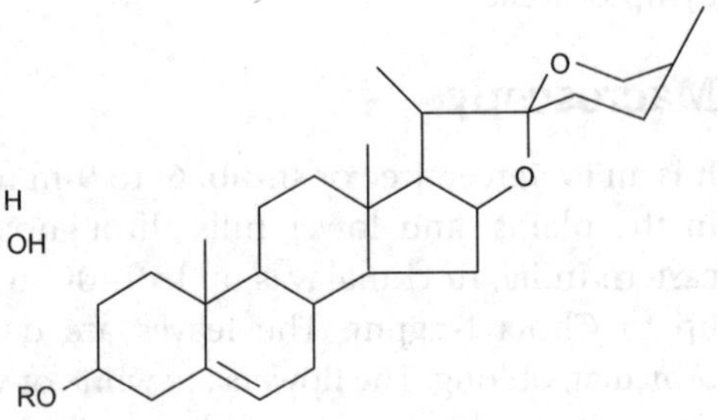

Trillin   R = Glu
Gracillin R = Glu-Glu-Rha

Chlorogenin

Tribulosin

Regional Names

Sansk: anirtavallf, amrta, madlitiparni, guducika, criinnodbhavd; Guj: galac, garo; Hindi: giloe, gurcha; Kan: amrutaballi.

Biological Source

It consists of dried, matured pieces of stem of *Tinospora cordifolia* (Willd.) Miers. (Fig. 35.14).

Family

Menispermaceae.

Habitat

This herb is a perennial climber found in the Himalayas and in many parts of the South India and Sri Lanka.

Macroscopy

Stem rather succulent with long filiform flesh aerial roots from the branches. It occurs in pieces of varying thickness in market ranging from 0.6 to 5 cm in diameter; young stems are green in colour with smooth surfaces and older ones are light brown in colour, circular lenticels are present on the surface, and is bitter in taste.

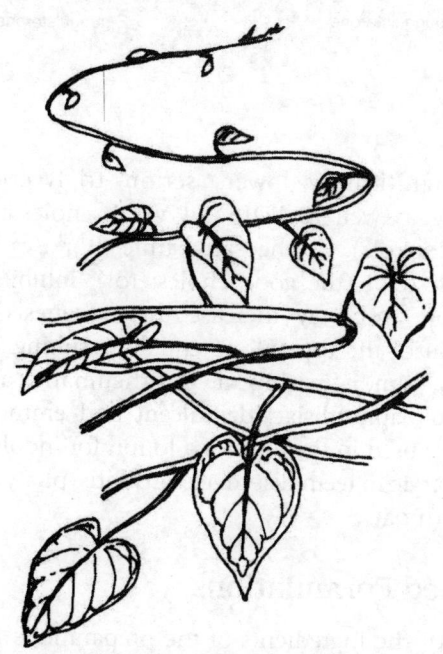

FIG. 35.14 *Tinospora cordifolia*

Microscopy

The outer cork is differentiated in to two layers, outer layer consists of thick-walled brownish and compressed cells, inner layer by thin-walled colourless, tangentially arranged three to four rows of cells; cortex consists of five or more rows of cells, and groups of sclereids are also found in cortex. Cortex cells are filled with plenty of starch grains, simple ovoid or irregularly ovoid-elliptical, several secretory cells; pericyclic fibres are lignified with wide lumen and pointed ends, associated with a large number of crystal fibres containing a single prism in each chamber; vascular bundles with 15–20 or more cells wide medullary rays are in middle; cambium composed of one to two layers of tangentially elongated cells; central pith composed of large, thin-walled cells mostly containing starch grains.

Standards

Foreign, matter	Not more than 2%
Total ash	Not more than 16%
Acid-insoluble ash	Not more than 3%
Alcohol-soluble extractive	Not less than 3%
Water-soluble extractive	Not less than 11%

Chemical Constituents

It contains clerodane furanoditerpenes like columbin, tinosporaside, a lignan, 3,4-bis-(-4-hydroxy-3-methoxy benzyl) tetrahydrofuran and alkaloids like, jactrorhizine, palmatine, berberine, tembeterine. The drug also contains a sesquiterpene glucoside, tinocordifolisoide; phenylpropene disaccharides like cordifolioside A and B; others include choline, tinosporic acid, tinosporal, tinosporone.

Uses

The drug is used as rejuvinator, hypoglycaemic, immunomodulatory, astringent, antipyretic, blood purifier, antineoplastic, cardiotonic and antiasthmatic. It is also used in general debility, pyrexia, skin diseases, gout and rheumatic arthritis.

Tinosporoside

Columbin

Tinosporaside

Marketed Formulations

It is one of the ingredients of the preparations known as Guduchi tablet, Abana, Bonnisan and Rumalaya (Himalaya Drug Company).

GUGGAL

Synonyms

Gumgugul, Salai-gogil.

Regional Names

Sansk: purd, kaugika, palahkas; Guj: gugal, gugar; Hindi: gugal, guggui; Kan: kanthagana, guggala; Mar: guggul, mahishaksh.

Biological Source

Guggal is a gumresin obtained by incision of the bark of *Commiphora mukul* (H. and S.) Engl.

Family

Burseraceae.

Habitat

The mukul myrrh (*Commiphora mukul*) tree is a small, thorny plant distributed throughout India.

Collection

Guggal tree is a small thorny tree, 4–6 feet tall, branches slightly ascending. It is sometimes planted in hedges. The tree remains without any foliage for most of the year. It has ash-coloured bark, and comes off in rough flakes, exposing the inner bark, which also peels off. The tree exudes a yellowish resin called gum guggul or guggulu that has a balsamic odour. Each plant yields about 1 kg of the product, which is collected in cold season.

Macroscopy

Guggal occurs as viscid, brown tears; or in fragment pieces, mixed with stem, piece of bark; golden yellow to brown in colour. With water it forms a milk emulsion. It has a balsamic odour and taste is bitter, aromatic.

Standards

Foreign matter	Not more than 4%
Total ash	Not more then 5%
Acid-insclube ash	Not more than 1%
Alcohol-soluble extractive	Not less than 27%
Water-soluble extractive	Not less than 53%

Chemical Constituents

Guggal conthins gum (32%), essential oil (1.45%), sterols (guggulsterols I to VI, β-sitosterol, cholesterol, Z- and E-guggulsterone), sugars (sucrose, fructose), amino acids, α-camphorene, cembrene, allylcembrol, flavonoids (quercetin and its glycosides), ellagic acid, myricyl alcohol, aliphatic tetrols, etc.

Z-guggulsterone   E-guggulsterone

Uses

Guggal significantly lowers serum triglycerides and cholesterol as well as LDL and VLDL cholesterols (the bad cholesterols). At the same time, it raises levels of HDL cholesterol (the good cholesterol), inhibits platelet aggregation and may increase thermogenesis through stimulation of the thyroid, potentially resulting in weight loss. Also gum is astringent, aritirheumatic, antiseptic, expectorant, aphrodisiac, demulcent and emmenagogue. The resin is used in the form of a lotion for indolent ulcers and as a gargle in teeth disorders, tonsillitis, pharyngitis and ulcerated throat.

Marketed Formulations

It is one of the ingredients of the preparations known as Arogyavardhini Gutika (Dabur) and Abana, Diabecon, Diakof (Himalaya Drug Company).

KALEJIRE

Synonyms

Small Fennel, Nigella Seed, Black Cumin, Fitch (Biblical), Love in the Mist, Fitches.

Regional Names

Sansk: sthfilajiraka, upakufici, susavi; Guj: kalonji jeeru; Hindi: kalounji, kalaunii, mangaraila; Kan: karijirige; Mar: kalaunji jire, kalejire.

Biological Source

It consists of seeds of *Nigella sativa* Linn. (Fig. 35.15).

Family

Ranunculaceae.

Habitat

Nigella sativa is an annual flowering plant, native to southwest Asia, Africa and India.

Macroscopy

Seeds are flattened, oblong, angular, funnel shaped, size 0.2 cm long and 0.1 cm wide, black in colour, slight aromatic odour and bitter in taste.

Microscopy

T.S. of seed shows single layer of thick-walled epidermis covered by cuticle containing reddish-brown content. Epidermis is followed by two to four layers of tangentially elongated, parenchymatous cells. Under this parenchyma cell, few layer of cells with reddish brown pigments are seen; endosperm is composed of thick-walled, rectangular to polygonal cells, with oil globules; embryo is embedded in endosperm.

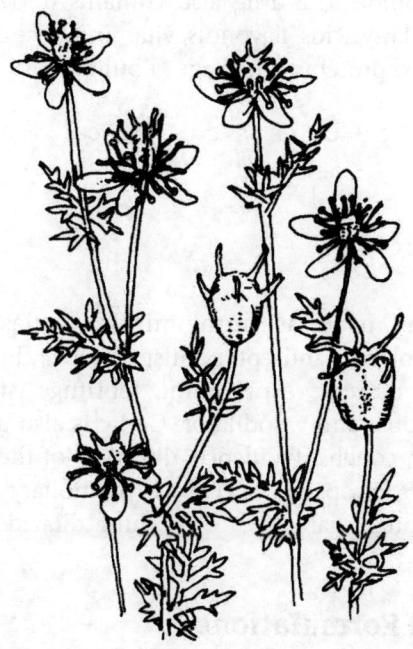

FIG. 35.15 *Nigella sativa*

Standards

Foreign matter	Not more than 2%
Total ash	Not more than 6%
Acid-insoluble ash	Not more than 0.2%
Alcohol-soluble extractive	Not less than 20%
Water-soluble extractive	Not less than 15%

Chemical Constituents

The seeds contain numerous esters of structurally unusual unsaturated fatty acids with terpene alcohols; furthermore, traces of alkaloids are found which belong to two different types: isochinoline alkaloids are represented by nigellimin and nigellimin-*N*-oxide, and pyrazol alkaloids include nigellidin and nigellicin. The essential oil contains thymoquinone (50%) besides *p*-cymene (40%), α-pinene (up to 15%), dithymoquinone and thymohydroquinone. Other terpene derivatives are found only in trace amounts: carvacrol, carvone, limonene, 4-terpineol and citronellol. The drug also contains resin, saponin and tannin.

Uses

It is mainly used in upper respiratory conditions, allergies, coughs, colds, bronchitis, fevers, flu, asthma and emphysema. It also possesses anti-inflammatory, antihypertensive, anti-diarrhoeal and hypolipidemic activities.

Marketed Formulations

It is one of the ingredients of the preparations known as Antidandruff shampoo (Himalaya Drug Company) and Kankayan Gutika (Dabur).

KANTAKARI

Synonyms

Kateli, yellow-berried nightshade.

Biological Source

It consists of the whole plant of *Solanum surattense* Burm. f. (syn. *S. xanthocarpum* Schrad and Wendl.).

Family

Solanaceae.

Habitat

It is very spiny diffuse herb, up to 1.2-m high, found all over India. The leaves are ovate or elliptic, flowers blue and berries globose, glabrous green.

Chemical Constituents

The berries contain caffeic, chlorogenic, isochlorogenic and neochlorogenic acids; esculin, esculetin, cycloartanol, cycloartenol, cholesterol, diosgenin, campesterol, cholesterol derivatives, solasodine, solamargine, β-solamargine, solasonine, solasurine, β-sitosterol and stigmasterol glucoside. The fruit oil is composed of glycerides of arachidic, linoleic, oleic, palmitic and stearic acids, and solanocarpine. The flowers yield diosgenin, apigenin and quercetin glycoside.

Uses

The root is reputed as antiasthmatic, antiemetic, diuretic and expectorant, used to prepare an ayurvedic medicine, *Dasamula*. It is given in asthma, cough and pain in the chest. A decoction of the root in combination with *Tinospora cordifolia* is useful in cough and fever. The leaves are anodyne. Leaf juice is given with black pepper in rheumatism. The stem, flowers and fruits are bitter and carminative; useful in burning sensation of the feet accompanied by vesicular watery eruptions. The leaves are applied to relieve pain and leaf juice with black peppers is given in rheumatism. The juice of berries is used in sore throat. The seeds are given as an expectorant in asthma and cough and to relieve toothache. A powder of the berries is mixed with honey and given to children in cough. The plant has alternative, antiasthmatic, aperient, diuretic, digestive and febrifuge properties, and is used to cure bronchitis, cough, constipation and dropsy. The plant is a part of an ayurvedic formulation *Arkadhi*, which is prescribed in bronchitis, dengue fever and chest affections. A decoction of the plant is used in gonorrhoea and to promote conception.

Marketed Formulations

It is one of the ingredients of the preparations known as Diakof, Koflet, Chyawanprash (Himalaya Drug Company) and Khadiradi Gutika (Dabur).

LAHSUN

Synonyms

Garlic.

Regional Names

Sansk: rasona, yavanesta; Guj: lasan, lassun; Hindi: lahasun; Kan: balluci; Mar: lasun.

Biological Source

It consists of bulb of *Allium sativum* Linn.

Family

Liliaceae.

Habitat

Europe, Central Asia, United States and India.

Macroscopy

It is a small plant. The leaves are green, slender, flat and elongated. The stem is smooth and solid. The bulbs are composed of several bulbils (cloves), enclosed in white skin of the parent bulb. The inflorescence is an umbel initially enclosed in a spathe. Drug occurs either as entire bulb or isolated cloves; bulb is subglobular, 4–6 cm in diameter and consists of 8–20 cloves. The bulb is surrounded by 3–5 whitish papery membranous scales, cloves are irregular, ovoid, tapering at upper end with dorsal convex surface, 2- to 3-cm long, 0.5- to 0.8-cm wide, each cloves surrounded by two very thin papery whitish and brittle scales. Odour is characteristic and aromatic. Aromatic and pungent in taste.

Standards

Foreign matter	Not more than 2%
Total ash	Not more than 4%
Acid-insoluble ash	Not more than 1%
Alcohol-soluble extractive	Not less than 2.5%
Loss on drying	Not less than 60%

Chemical Constituents

The chief active constituent of garlic is volatile oil containing allyl disulphide, alliin, allicin, allyl propyl disulphide and diallyl disulphide. The drug also contains thioglycoside, amino acids, fatty acids, flavonols, vitamins, trace elements, carbohydrates, proteins, mucilage, albumin, etc.

$$CH_2 = CH - CH_2 - S - S - CH_2 - CH = CH_2$$

$$\underset{\underset{\text{Allicin}}{O}}{\|}$$

Uses

The bulb is used as anthelmintic, antiasthmatic, anticholesterolemic, antiseptic, antispasmodic, cholagogue, diaphoretic, diuretic, expectorant, febrifuge, stimulant, stomachic, tonic and vasodilator. Garlic is also useful for colon cancer, coughs, flatulence, disorders of the nervous system, agues, dropsical affections, pulmonary phthisis, whooping cough, gangrene of the lung dilated bronchi, etc.

Marketed Formulations

It is one of the ingredients of the preparations known as Lasuna tablet (Himalaya Drug Company) and Lashunadi bati (Baidyanath).

MALKANGNI

Synonyms

Black-Oil tree, intellect tree, climbing-staff plant.

Regional Names

Sansk: jyotishmati, kanguni, sphutabandhani, svarnalota; Guj: malkangana, velo; Hindi: malkakni, malkamni, malkangni; Mar: kangani, malkangoni.

Biological Source

It consists of seeds and leaves of plant *Celastrus paniculatus* Wild. (Fig. 35.16).

Family

Celastraceae.

Habitat

Celastrus paniculata belonging to the genus of woody, climbing shrubs is distributed almost all over the India.

Macroscopy

Leaves simple, alternate, very variable, elliptic, ovate, broadly obovate, glabrous, sometimes pubescent beneath along the venation, up to 6 × 11 cm; base, cuneate, obtuse or rounded, apex acute, acuminate or obtuse; panicles large, terminal, pubescent; male flowers minute, pale green; calyx lobes suborbicular, toothed; petals oblong or obovate-oblong, entire; disk copular; female flowers having sepals, petals and disk similar to those of male flowers; capsule subglobose, bright yellow, trivalved, three to six seeded; seeds ellipsoid, yellowish brown, enclosed in a red fleshy aril. The seeds are bitter in nature.

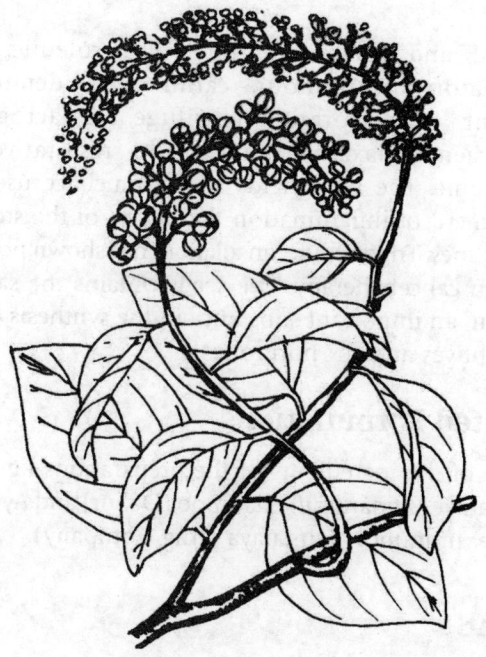

FIG. 35.16 *Celastrus paniculatus*

Chemical Constituents

C. paniculatus seeds contain a number of sesquiterpene polyesters namely malkangunins I to VIII and sesquiterpene alkaloids such as celapanine, celapagine and celapanigine. It also contains about 42–45% of fixed oil. The major fatty acids presents are palmitic, oleic, linoleic and linolenic. The oil also contain α,α'-dipalmitoylglycerol the unsaponifiable matter (6%) contains phytosterol and celastrol.

Malkangunin

Malkanguninol

Uses

Celastrus paniculata is used in treating mental depression. It is used as an aphrodisiac, as a powerful brain tonic to stimulate intellect, as a stimulant, to increase cognitive recognition (helps with dreams), sharpen memory. It also showed tranquillizing effect. Leaves are emmenagogue.

In folk medicine the seeds are boiled and taken for purification of body and mind through the cleansing of blood. The seeds constitute the drug; they are slightly bitter and hence used almost always with a natural sweetener like Liquorice root (which enhances its effects) or stevia leaves.

Marketed Formulations

It is one of the ingredients of the preparations known as Iqmen (Lupin Herbal Lab.), Abana, Geriforte, Himcolin, Mentat (Himalaya Drug Company), J.P. Massaj oil, J.P. Painkill oil (Jamuna Pharma) and Syrup Learnol Plus (Dalmia Industries).

METHI

Synonyms

Fenugreek, Greek hay.

Regional Names

Sansk: methini; Guj: methi; Hindi: methi; Kan: menthe, mente.

Biological Source

It consists of dried seeds of *Trigonella foenum-graecum* Linn. (Fig. 35.17).

Family

Fabaceae.

Habitat

It is 30- to 60-cm tall; annual herb; grown in India, Europe, Africa and the United States.

Macroscopy

Seeds are oblong or rhomboidalin in shape, 0.2- to 0.5-cm long, 0.15- to 0.35-cm broad, dull yellow in colour, surface smooth, very hard; it has a pleasant odour and bitter in taste.

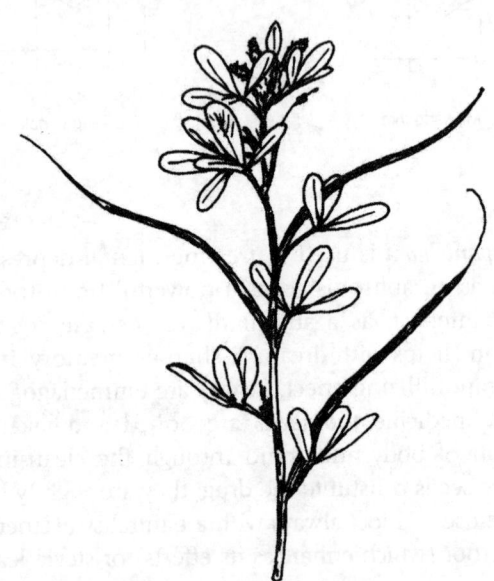

FIG. 35.17 *Trigonella foenum-graecum*

Microscopy

Epidermis covered with thick cuticle followed by four to five layers of tangentially elongated, thin-walled, parenchymatous cells; endosperm consists of a layer of thick-walled cells containing aleurone grains, cotyledons consists of three to four layers of palisade cells varying in size with long axis containing aleurone grains and oil globules. The cells in endosperm contain mucilage.

Standards

Foreign matter	Not more than 2%
Total ash	Not more than 4%
Acid-insoluble ash	Not more than 0.5%
Alcohol-soluble extractive	Not less than 5%

Chemical Constituents

Fenugreek seed contains steroidal saponins as their main chemical constituents. These saponins includes trigofoenoside A, B, C, D, E, F and G. The other saponins includes trigonelloside C, yamogenin tetroside B and C, tenugrin B, trigogenin, neotigogenin, yemogenin, diosgenin and gitogenin. The seeds contain glycosides of diosgenin, that is graecunins A, B, C, H, I, J, K, L, M and N. The seed also consists of number of flavonoid compounds such as quercetin, luteolin, vitexin, isovitexin, saponaretin, homoorientin, vicenin-1 and vicenin-2. Fenugreek seed is a rich source of 4-hydroxyisoleucine. Coumarin derivatives, such as trigocoumarin, trigoforin, 4-methyl-7-acetoxycoumarin and *p*-coumaric acid, have also been reported from seeds.

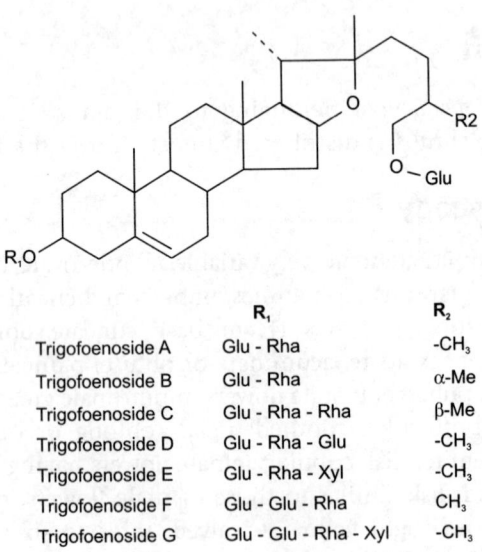

	R₁	R₂
Trigofoenoside A	Glu - Rha	-CH₃
Trigofoenoside B	Glu - Rha	α-Me
Trigofoenoside C	Glu - Rha - Rha	β-Me
Trigofoenoside D	Glu - Rha - Glu	-CH₃
Trigofoenoside E	Glu - Rha - Xyl	-CH₃
Trigofoenoside F	Glu - Glu - Rha	CH₃
Trigofoenoside G	Glu - Glu - Rha - Xyl	-CH₃

Uses

The seed and leaves are anticholesterolemic, anti-inflammatory, antitumour, carminative, demulcent, emollient, expectorant, febrifuge, galactogogue, hypoglycaemic, laxative, parasiticide, restorative and uterine tonic. The seed yields strong mucilage useful in the treatment of inflammation and ulcers of the stomach and intestines. Trigonelline, an alkaloid has shown potential for use in cancer therapy. The seed contains the saponin diosgenin, an important substance in the synthesis of oral contraceptives and sex hormones.

Marketed Formulations

It is one of the ingredients of the preparations known as Dabur Vatika Antidandruff Shampoo (Dabur) and Ayurslim, Geriforte, Immunol (Himalaya Drug Company).

PALAS

Synonyms

Dhak, bastard teak, Bengal kino tree, flame of the forest.

Biological Source

It is the whole plant of *Butea monosperma* (Lam.) Tomb; syn. *B. frondosa* Koenig ex Roxb. (Fig. 35.18).

Family

Papilionaceae.

Habitat

It is commonly found throughout India, except in the arid regions; in Burma, outer Himalayas up to 1008 m and Sri Lanka.

Macroscopy

The plant is a deciduous tree with crooked trunk, up to 15 m in height; bark bluish grey or light brown; branches irregular; leaves long-petioled, three-foliolate, leaflets coriaceous, obovate, from a cuneate base, glabrescent above, densely finely silky below; flower buds dark brown, flowers bright orange-red, sometimes yellow, in 15 cm long racemes on bare branches; pods pendulous, silky tomentose, containing one seed at the apex, reticulately veined; seeds flat, reniform.

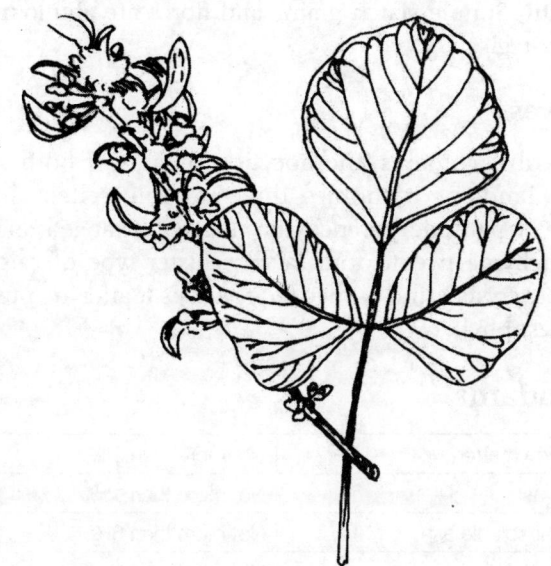

FIG. 35.18 *Butea monosperma*

Chemical Constituents

Butea gum contains leucocyanidin, its tetramer, procyanidin, gallic acid, riboflavin and thiamine. The flowers contain flavonoid glycosides, butin, butein, butrin, isobutrin, palasitrin, coreopsin, isocoreopsin (butin-7-glucoside), isomonospermoside, sulfurein, palasitrin, chalcone, aurones, β-sitosterol, 4-carbomethoxy-3,6-dioxo-5-hydro-

1,2,4-triazine, fructose and amino acids. The aqueous extract of the flowers contains mainly chalcone and isobutrin. The unsaponifiable matter consists mainly of myricyl alcohol and β-sitosterol. The fatty acids isolated from the wax are palmitic, stearic, arachidic, behenic, lignoceric and cerotic acids. Palasimide is present in pods.

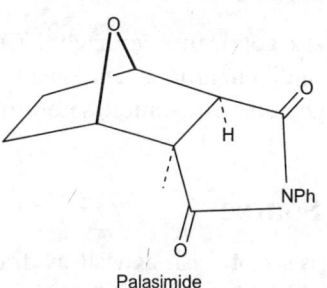

Palasimide

Uses

The hot alcoholic extract of the seeds showed significant anti-implantation and antiovulatory activity in rats and rabbits, respectively. The alcoholic extract of the seeds inhibits the growth of *Escherichia coli* and *Micrococcus pyogenes* var. *aureus*. A crude, saline extract (0.9%) of the seeds agglutinates the erythrocytes in experimental animals. The glycosides palasitrin and butrin reduced the number of implants in the mated rats. The seed oil showed a marked and prolonged fall in the blood pressure in animals. The seeds given orally are effective in roundworm and threadworm infections but ineffective in case of tapeworm. The side effects observed are nausea, vomiting, dizziness, general weakness and pain in the abdomen. The extracts of the seeds and seed coat administered daily from day one postcoitum for 10 days prevented pregnancy in female rats. The fruits possess anthelmintic property. They are used in abdominal problems, eye diseases, inflammation, piles, skin diseases, tumours and urinary discharges. The ether, alcoholic and aqueous extracts of flowers showed antioestrogenic activity in mice. A fraction containing sodium salt of phenolic constituents, isolated from the bark, is a potent antiasthmatic agent. They are active against the fungus *Helminthosporium sativum*. An alcoholic solution of the petals showed antioestrogenic activity in mice. A decoction of the flowers is given in diarrhoea and to puerperal women. The aqueous extract of the flowers shows significant anti-implantation activity in rats. Flower extract exhibited antihepatotoxic activity.

Marketed Formulations

It is one of the ingredients of the preparations known as Lukol (Himalaya Drug Company) and J.P. Nikhar oil (Jamuna Pharma).

PUNARNAVA

Synonym

Hogweed.

Regional Names

Sansk: punarnava, gophaghni, gothaghni; Guj: dholisaturdi, motosatodo; Hindi: punarnava; Kan: sanadika, kommeberu, komma; Mar: ghetuli, vasuchimuli, satodirnula, punarnava, khaparkhuti.

Biological Source

Punarnava consists of fresh as well as dried whole plant of *Boerhaavia diffusa* Linn. (Fig. 35.19).

Family

Nyctaginaceae.

Habitat

The plant is a weed found throughout India and Sri Lanka during rainy season.

Macroscopy

Stem is greenish purple in colour, slender, stiff, cylindrical, swollen at nodes, minutely pubescent or nearly glabrous. Roots are long, cylindrical, 0.2–1.5 cm in diameter; yellowish brown to brown in colour, longitudinal striations and root scars on surface; short fracture, odourless and bitter in taste. Leaves are opposite, larger ones 2.5- to 3.5-cm long and smaller ones are 1.2- to 1.8-cm long, ovate-oblong, apex rounded or slightly pointed, base subcordate, glabrous on upper, entire margin. Flowers are very small and white or pink in colour. Two chief varieties are described based on the flower colour, one with white flowers is 'Sweta Punarnava' while the other with red flowers is referred to as 'Rakta Punarnava'. Fruits are 6-mm long, rounded with one seed.

Microscopy

Stem

T.S. shows epidermal layer containing multicellular uniseriate glandular trichomes consisting of 9–12 cells, cortex consists of 1–2 layers of parenchyma; endodermis indistinct; 1–2 layered pericycle, isolated fibres; small vascular bundles joined together in a ring and many big vascular bundles scattered in the ground tissue, cambium is also present.

Roots

Cork is composed of thin-walled elongated cells with brown walls in the outer few layers. Cork cambium consists of

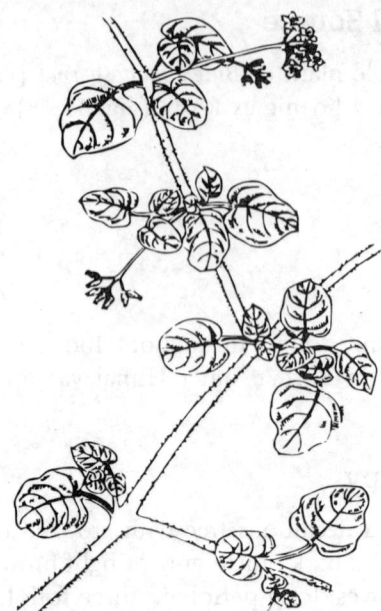

FIG. 35.19 *Boerhaavia diffusa*

1–2 layers of thin-walled cells. Cortex is composed of 5–12 layers of thin-walled polygonal cells; central regions of root are occupied by primary vascular bundles; moreover, numerous raphides of calcium oxalate crystals are also present. Simple starch grains and fibres are abundant in cortex region.

Leaves

Epidermis contains anomocytic stomata on both sides and glandular trichomes three- to four-celled, single layer of palisade parenchyma; loosely arranged spongy parenchyma two to four layers; cluster type of calcium oxalate crystals and orange red resinous matter are present in mesophyll.

Standards

Foreign matter	Not more than 2%
Total ash	Not more than 15%
Acid-insoluble ash	Not more than 6%
Alcohol-soluble extractive	Not less than 1%
Water-soluble extractive	Not less than 4%

Chemical Constituents

Punarnava contains a phenolic glycoside punarnavoside up to 0.03–0.05%. It also shows the presence of rotenoids, such as, boeravinones A, B, C, D and E. Lignan derivatives such as liridodendrin and syringaresinol mono-β-D-glucosides have been reported. The root contains purine nucleoside-hypoxanthine-9-arabinofuranoside and boeravine, ursolic acid and β-sitosterol. The root also contains an insect moulding hormone, β-ecdysone.

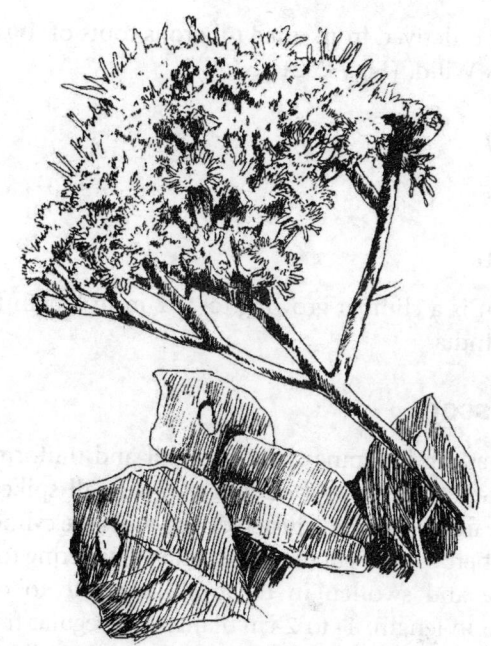

Punarnavoside

Boeravinone A

Liridodendrin

Uses

Punarnava possess potent antifibrinolytic, anti-inflammatory and diuretic properties. Punarnavoside has been found to be responsible for antifibrinolytic activity. Punarnava is a very useful drug for the treatment of inflammatory renal diseases and nephritic syndrome. It is also recommended for the treatment of IUD menorrhagia. Plant extract also shows hepatoprotective activity and is effective in cases of oedema and ascites resulting from early cirrhosis of liver and chronic peritonitis. Liridodendrin and hypoxanthine-9-arabinofuranoside exhibits, antihypertensive activity, the former being a Ca^{2+} channel antagonist. Root extract on oral administration was found to stop intrauterine contraceptive device-induced bleeding in experimental animals. The whole herb in the form of juice is given internally as a blood purifier. It is eaten as a vegetable in curries and soups.

Marketed Formulations

It is one of the ingredients of the preparations known as Deepact (Lupin Herbal Lab.), Abana, Immunol, Diabecon (Himalaya Drug Company), Punarnawadi, Guggulin, Punarnavarista (Baidyanath), Sobigol (Aimil) and Painkill oil, J.P. Liver syrup (Jamuna Pharma).

RASANA

Biological Source

It consists of the whole plant of *Pluchea lanceolata* (DC) Clarke (Fig. 35.20).

Family

Asteraceae.

Habitat

It is found in the saline or sandy soil of Punjab, Rajasthan and Gangetic plain, and in Delhi as a weed.

Macroscopy

It is an erect undershrub, 30- to 60-cm tall; stem and branches terete, grey-pubescent. Leaves sessile, coriaceous, oblanceolate, obtuse, narrowed at the base, entire. Flower heads in compound corymbs, white, yellow lilac or purple.

FIG. 35.20 *Pluchea lanceolata*

Chemical Constituents

The leaves of *P. lanceolata* contain quercetin, moretenol, its acetate, neolupenol, isorhamnetin and quercitrin. The flowers yield pluchine, sorghumol acetate, moretenol, its acetate, stigmasterol, neolupenol, cycloart-23-en-3β,25-diol, β-sitosterol-D-glucoside, nonacosane, heptacosane, hentriacontane and octacosane.

Uses

The herb possesses analgesic, antipyretic, laxative and nervine tonic properties. A decoction of the plant is used in bronchitis and inflammation. In Tibet, the drug is used to treat asthma, cough, hiccough, poisoning and diseases caused by *vayu*. The leaves are substituted for senna leaves.

Marketed Formulations

It is one of the ingredients of the preparations known as Ashwagandharishta, Rheumatil tablet (Dabur).

SHATAVARI

Synonym

Asparagus.

Regional Names

Sansk: narayani, vari, abhiru, atirasa; Guj: satavari; Hindi: satavar, satamul; Kan: ashadi poeru, halavu bau, narayani, makkala; Mar: shatavari.

Biological Source

The drug is derived from dried tuberous roots of *Asparagus racemosus* Willd. (Fig. 35.21).

Family

Liliaceae.

Habitat

The plant is a climber growing to 1–2 m in length found all over India.

Macroscopy

The leaves are like pine-needles, small and uniform. The inflorescence has tiny white flowers, in small spikes. The roots are finger-like and clustered. The roots are cylindrical, fleshy raberous, straight or slightly curved, tapering towards the base and swollen in the middle; white to colour, 5–15 cm in length, 1- to 2-cm diameter, irregular fracture, longitudinal furrows and minute transverse wrinkles on upper surface, and bitter in taste.

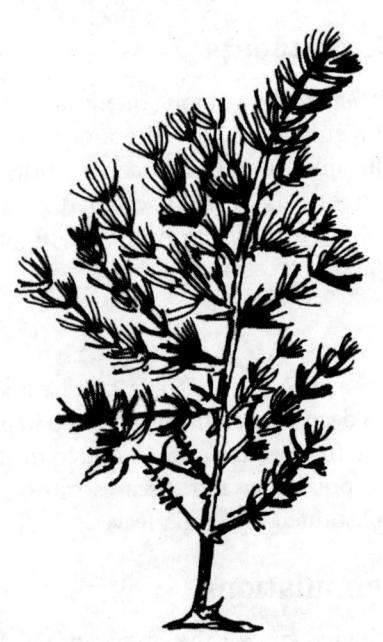

FIG. 35.21 *Asparagus racemosus*

Standards

Foreign matter	Not more than 1%
Total ash	Not more than 5%
Acid-insoluble ash	Not more than 5%
Alcohol-soluble extractive	Not less than 10%
Water-soluble extractive	Not less than 45%

Chemical Constituents

The active constituents are steroidal saponins, such as shatavarin I-IV (0.1—0.2%). The aglycone unit is sarsapogenin. In shatavarin I three glucose and one rhamnose molecules are attached whereas shatavarin IV possesses two glucose and one rhamnose molecules. The other compounds isolated from *A. racemosus* are β-sitosterol, stigmasterol, their glycosides, sarsasepogenin, spirostanolic acid, furostanolic saponins, 4,6-dihydroxy-2-O-(2'-hydroxy-isobutyl) benzaldehyde, undecanyl cetanoate and polycyclic alkaloid asparagamine A.

Shatavarin

Uses

The root is alterative, antispasmodic, aphrodisiac, demulcent, diuretic, galactogogue and refrigerant. It is taken internally in the treatment of infertility, loss of libido, threatened miscarriage, menopausal problems, hyperacidity, stomach ulcers and bronchial infections. Externally it is used to treat stiffness in the joints. The root is used fresh in the treatment of dysentery.

Marketed Formulations

It is one of the ingredients of the preparations known as K.G. Tone (Aimil), Menosan, Diabecon, Galactin, Abana (Himalaya Drug Company), Dhatupaushtik churna, Rhuma oil, Brahmi Rasayan, Mahanarayan tel (Baidyanath), J.P. Massaj oil, Painkill oil (Jamuna Pharma), Memoplus, Jeevani malt (Chirayu), and Satavari kalp and Satavarex granules (Zandu).

SHANKHPUSHPI

Synonym

Sankhapushpi.

Regional Names

Sansk: sankhapushpi; Guj: shankhavali; Hindi: sankhapushpl; Kan: bilikantlsoppu, shankhapushpl; Mar: shankhavela, sanklmhull, sankhapuspi.

Biological Source

Shankhpushpi consists of the whole aerial parts of *Convolvulus pluricaulis* Choisy (Fig. 35.22).

Family

Convolvulaceae.

Habitat

The plant grows wildly in plains of India.

Macroscopy

Root

1- to 5-cm long, 0.1- to 0.4-cm thick, yellowish-brown to light brown in colour.

Stem

Slender, light green, cylindrical in shape, about 0.1 cm or less in thickness with clear hair nodes and internodes.

Leaf

Shortly petiolate, linear-lanceolate, acute apex, hairy on both surfaces; 0.5- to 2-cm long and 0.1- to 0.5-cm broad, light green in colour.

Flowers

White or pinkish in colour.

Fruit

Oblong globose with caraceous, pale brown pericarp.

Seed

Brown in colour, minutely puberulous.

Microscopy

Root

Outer cork composed of 10–15 layers of tangentially elongated thick-walled cells, cortex composed of 6–10

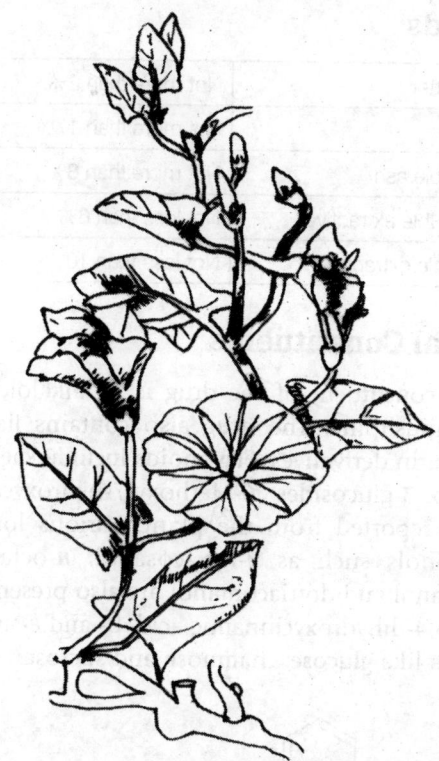

FIG. 35.22 *Convolvulus pluricaulis*

layers of oval to elongated, elliptical, parenchymatous cells. Yellowish-brown tanniniferous, secretory cells are present in cortex region; phloem is composed of sieve elements, phloem parenchyma and phloem rays; xylem consisting of usual elements; medullary rays are 1–3 cells wide and multicellular in length; starch grains are also present.

Stem

Single-layered epidermis, covered with thick cuticle and contains unicellular hairs. Cortex is divided in two zones, two to three upper collenchymatous and one to two lower parenchymatous layers; pericycle present in the form of single strand of fibres in endodermis; phloem mostly composed, of sieve element and parenchyma; xylem consists of vessels fibres and parenchyma; medullary rays and tacheids are not distinct and in centre slightly lignified pith is seen.

Leaf

Single-layered epidermis is covered with thick cuticle, unicellular covering trichomes. Epidermis followed by two to three layers of chlorenchymatous cells; two-layered palisade cells below epidermis in mesophyll region, spongy parenchyma four to five layered, vascular bundles bicollateral composed of usual elements of phloem and xylem, rest of tissue between chlorenchyma and vascular bundles composed of four to five layers of parenchymatous cells.

Standards

Foreign matter	Not more than 2%
Total ash	Not more than 17%
Acid-insoluble ash	Not more than 8%
Alcohol-soluble extractive	Not less than 6%
Water-soluble extractive	Not less than 10%

Chemical Constituents

The chief constituent of the drug is an alkaloid known as shankhpushpine. The drug also contains flavonoids and coumarin derivatives. Flavonoids include kaempferol, kaempferol-3-glucosides. 6-Methoxy-7-hydroxycoumarin has been reported from the plant. Various long-chain fatty alcohols such as *n*-hexacosanol, *n*-octacosanol, *n*-triacontanol and dotriacontanol are also present. It also contains 3,4-dihydroxycinnamic acid, β- and ε-sitosterols, and sugars like glucose, rhamnose and sucrose.

Kaempferol-3-O-glucoside

6-Methoxy-7-hydroxycoumarin

Uses

The drug is used as a brain tonic, antihypertensive and tranquilliser. The plant is used as a vegetable in northern India. The fresh juice is used as a nervine tonic in case of epilepsy, insanity and nervous debility. It has been reported to improve memory. The possible potentiation of cognitive process by *C. pluricaulis* is reported to be due to the increased supply of proteins to hippocampus, thus enhancing the learning process. It also reduces spontaneous motor activity and reduces fighting response.

The aerial parts of *Canscora decussata* family Gentianaceae is used as a substitute for shunkhpushpi in Karnataka and Konkan region in India. It consists of xanthone derivatives, triterpenoids and bitter substances. *Chitoria ternate* family Papilionaceae is a plant with blue colours which is used in Kerala as shunkhpushpi.

Marketed Formulations

It is one of the ingredients of the preparations known as Mentat, Anxocare (Himalaya Drug Company), Shankhapushpi syrup (Baidyanath) and Shankhpushpi churna (Shantikunj Pharmacy).

TULSI

Synonyms

Holi basil, Sacred basil.

Regional Names

Sansk: surasa, suresam sahumaniari, bhutaghni; Guj: tulsi, tulsi; Hindi: tulasi; Kan: tulasi, sritulasi; Mar: tulasi.

Biological Source

It consists of the dried leaves of *Ocimum sanctum* Linn. (Fig. 35.23).

Family

Labiatae.

Habitat

This herb has been known from as early as the Vedic period. The plant is cultivated throughout India especially in Hindu houses and temples for worship of gods and goddesses. It has widely grown throughout the world.

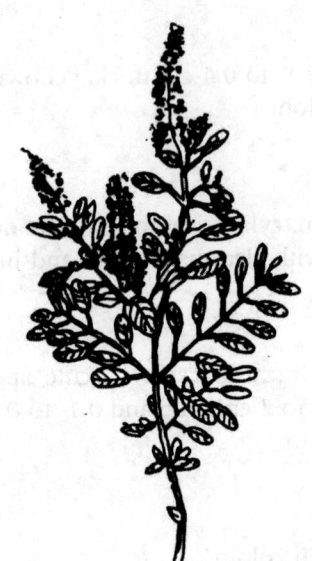

FIG. 35.23 Ocimum sanctum

Macroscopy

Tulsi is an annual herb, grows 30- to 75-cm height. The stems are branched, generally purplish in colour, and covered with soft hairs. Leaves are oblong, obtuse or acute, margin entire or serrate, 2- to 5-cm long, 1.5- to 14-cm wide, petiole slender 1.3- to 2.5-cm long, pubescent on both sides. Seeds sub globose, brown or red in colour with mucilaginous outer covering slightly notched at the tip and broadly rounded at the base; odourless; taste, slightly pungent and mucilaginous.

Standards

Foreign matter	Not more than 2%
Total ash	Not more than 8%
Acid-insoluble ash	Not more than 2%
Alcohol-soluble extractive	Not less than 4%

Chemical Constituents

Leaves contain volatile oil 0.4–0.8% containing chiefly eugenol 21% and β-caryophyllene 37% (eugenol content reaches maximum in spring and minimum in autumn), sesquiterpenes and monoterpenes like bornyl acetate, β-elemene, methyleugenol, neral, β-pinene, camphene, α-pinene, etc. It also contains ursolic acid, campesterol, cholesterol, stigmasterol, β-sitosterol and methyl esters of common fatty acids.

Eugenol

Bornyl acetate

Caryophylline

Ursolic acid

Uses

The leaves are used as aromatic, carminative, stimulant and flavouring agent. Leaves have hypoglycaemic, immunomodulatory, antistress, analgesic, antipyretic, anti-inflammatory, antiulcerogenic, antihypertensive, CNS depressant, radioprotective, antitumour, antibacterial, expectorant, diaphoretic, antiperiodic, anticatarrhal, antiseptic and spasmolytic properties, and are used in bronchitis, cold, cough, fever and gastric disorders. Seeds are demulcent and used in genitourinary disorders. It is also used in scorpion sting and snakebite.

Marketed Formulations

It is one of the ingredients of the preparations known as Respinova (Lupin Herbal Lab.), Abana, Diabecon, Diakof, Koflet, Tulsi Pure Herb (Himalaya Drug Company), Amylcure (Aimil), Nomarks cream (Nyle Herbals), Sualin (Hamdard) and Kofol syrup (Charak Pharma).

TYLOPHORA

Synonyms

Anantmul, *Tylophora asthmatica* W. and A.

Biological Source

The drug consists of dried leaves and roots of *Tylophora indica* Burm f. (Fig. 35.24).

Family

Asclepiadaceae.

Habitat

Tylophora is a perennial climbing plant native to the plains, forests, and hills of southern and eastern India.

Macroscopy

Leaves, ovate or elliptic-oblong shape, acute or acuminate apex, cordate base, 5- to 10-cm long, 2.5- to 5.3-cm wide, glabrous, pubescent beneath. The whole part of the plant is pale yellow-brown in colour and devoid of odour but has a sweetish and subsequent acrid taste.

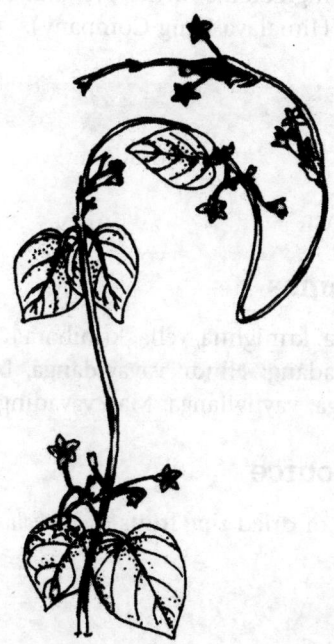

FIG. 35.24 *Tylophora indica*

Chemical Constituents

The active constituents are phenanthroindolizidine alkaloids like tylophorine, tylophorinine, tylophorinidine, and septicine. The plant also contains a phytosterol (cetyl alcohol, wax, resin, pigments, tannin, glucose, calcium salts, potassium chloride, α-amyrin and flavonoids like quercetin, kaempferol and tyloindane.

Tylophorine

Uses

The dried leaves are used in the treatment of bronchial asthma, bronchitis, rheumatism and dermatitis. It is also used as emetic, diaphoretic, anti-inflammatory, antibacterial and expectorant. The roots have stimulant, emetic, cathartic, expectorant, stomachic, antidysentery, antidiarrhoeal and diaphoretic properties.

Marketed Formulations

It is one of the ingredients of the preparation known as Geriforte Aqua (Himalaya Drug Company).

VIDANG

Synonym

False black pepper.

Regional Names

Sansk: jantughna, krmighna, vella, krmihara; Guj: vavding, vavading, vayavadang; Hindi: vayavidanga, bhabhiranga; Kan: vayuvidanga, vayuvilanga; Mar. vavading, vavding.

Biological Source

Vidang consists of dried ripe fruits of *Embelia ribes* Burm. (Fig. 35.25).

Family

Myrisinaceae.

Habitat

These climbing herbs are found in India, central and lower Himalayas, Sri Lanka, Burma, South China and Singapore.

Macroscopy

Fruits are globular to subglobular, brownish black, 24 mm in diameter, style at apex, often short, thin pedicel and persistent calyx with usually three or five sepals present; pericarp brittle enclosing a single seed covered by a thin membrane; seed, reddish in colour and covered with yellowish spots, aromatic odour, astringent in taste.

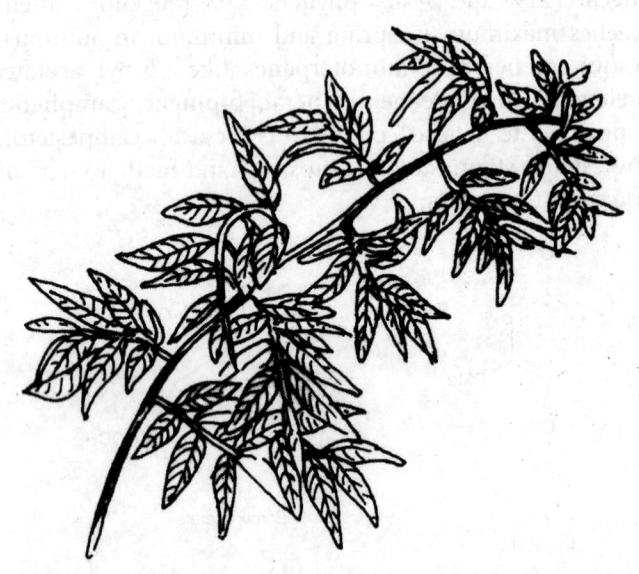

FIG. 35.25 *Embelia ribes*

Microscopy

Fruit T.S. shows epicarp consisting of single row of tabular cells of epidermis with wrinkled cuticle; mesocarp consists of a number of layers of reddish brown-coloured cells and numerous fibre vascular bundles. Mesocarp and endodermis composed of stone cells; endodermis consisting of single-layered, thick-walled large, palisade like stone cells; seed coat is composed of two- to three-layered reddish brown-coloured cells; the cells in endosperm are irregular in shape and thick walled, containing fixed oil and proteinous masses; mesocarp contains few prismatic crystals of calcium oxalate and a small embryo is seen.

Standards

Foreign matter	Not more than 2%
Total ash	Not more than 6%
Acid-insoluble ash	Not more than 1.5%
Alcohol-soluble extractive	Not less than 10%
Water-soluble extractive	Not less than 9%

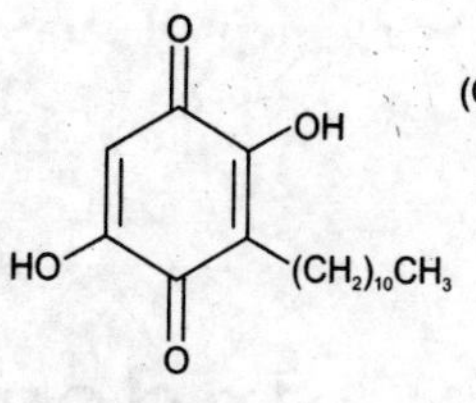

Embelin

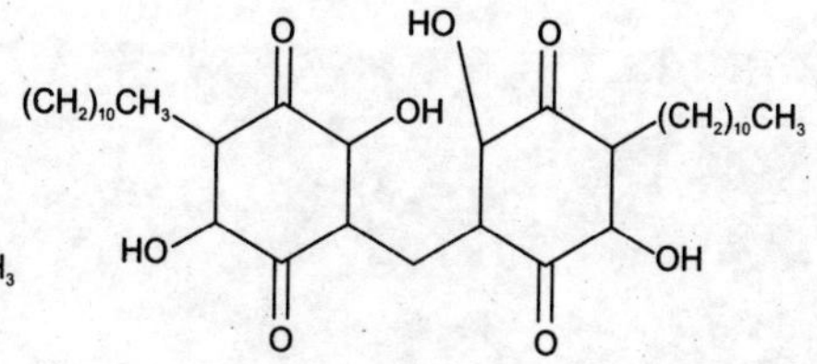

Vilangin

Chemical Constituents

Vidang contains hydroquinone derivative embelin, embellic acid, a dimer of embelin known as vilangin, an alkaloid christembine, tannins and quercitol. It also contains volatile oil and fats. In fruit embelin occurs in golden yellow needles and is insoluble in water but soluble in alcohol, chloroform and benzene.

Uses

It is anthelmintic, carminative and stimulant. It is also used in abdominal disorders, lung diseases, insanity, constipation, fungus, gas, indigestion, headache, heart disease, toothache, haemorrhoids, mouth ulcers, obesity, pneumonia, sore throat, worms, etc.

Marketed Formulations

It is one of the ingredients of the preparations known as Gasex, Diakof, Herbolax and Koflet (Himalaya Drug Company).